W9-BMB-687

A DICTIONARY OF PRACTICAL MATERIA MEDICA

The amount of matter dealt with in this volume having been found to require much more space than was anticipated (upwards of 1,600 pages), it has been deemed advisable to bind it in two parts. It is paged throughout as one.

A DICTIONARY OF PRACTICAL MATERIA MEDICA

By

JOHN HENRY CLARKE, M.D.

IN THREE VOLUMES

VOL-III

B. JAIN PUBLISHERS (P) LTD

NEW DELHI

Note

Any information given in this book is not intended to be taken as a replacement for medical advice. Any person with a condition requiring medical attention should consult a qualified practitioner or therapist.

Export Quality

Reprint edition: 1999

Price: [illegible]*0* **3 vols**

Published by :

Kuldeep Jain

For

B. Jain publishers (P.) Ltd.

1921, Street No. 10, Chuna Mandi,
Paharganj, New Delhi 110 055 (INDIA)
Phones: 7770430; 7770572; 7536418
FAX 011-7510471 & 7536420
Email: kjain@nda.vsnl.net.in

Printed in India by:

J.J. Offset Printers

7, Wazirpur, Delhi - 110 052

ISBN : 81-7021-013 - 5
ISBN : 81-7021-021 - 6

BOOK CODE : BC-2159

Penthorum Sedoides.

Penthorum sedoides. Virginia Stone-crop. *N. O.* Crassulaceæ.
Tincture of fresh plant.

Clinical.—Coryza. Diarrhœa. Hæmorrhoids. Headache. Post-nasal catarrh. Sacrum, pain in. Varicocele.

Characteristics.—*Penth.* was proved by Dr. D. B. Morrow (twice), Dr. Scudder, and a young man, who all took substantial doses. The majority of the symptoms are Morrow's, including the catarrhal symptoms, which have been verified in practice : "A peculiar wet feeling in nares as though a violent coryza would set in," but it did not ; the secretion became thickened and pus-like but not increased. The same "wet feeling" was experienced at the same time in trachea and bronchi, which passed from above down as if coryza would set in, followed by a slight feeling of constriction in the chest, which also passed from above down. The next day the nose felt stuffed. The third day the first symptoms were repeated, and the discharge became thick, pus-like, and streaked with blood, and there was an odour in the nose as if from an open sore. Scudder had "fulness in nose and ears." Morrow experienced itching at anus, hæmorrhoids, and pains and sensations in rectum, sacrum, and sacro-iliac joints ; his first proving cured "heat and soreness in sacrum with a dull, heavy headache." Hale says *Penth.* is reputed to be curative in catarrh and in diarrhœa. A scalded sensation in the tongue is one of the symptoms. A sense of levitation was also produced. The symptoms proceed from above downward. Morrow (*Med. Adv.*, xviii. 540) reports these cures : (1) Miss P., 17, blonde, had severe cough of several weeks' duration. < Talking or singing. Frothy, greenish sputa. *Pul.* and *Pho.* failed ; *Penth. s.* soon cured. (2) Decrepit old lady, 75, sufferer from eczema for twelve years. Previous winter cured of asthma (probably from suppressed eczema) with *Sul.* c.m. Now paretic right side, for which *Pho.* was given. But *Pho.* did not relieve a loose, continual, rattling cough, caused by tickling at bifurcation of bronchi, with raising much thick, frothy, greenish sputa. *Penth.* ϕ pellets quickly cured.

Relations.—*Compare :* Sedum., Hydrangea. In scalded sensation on tongue, and in catarrh, Sang. Catarrh, Puls. Levitation, Can. i., Coccul., Phos. ac., Sticta, Sul., Thu. Jerking of limbs, Meny., Pso.

SYMPTOMS.

1. **Mind.**—Dull ; discouraged ; desponding.—Mind is dull, study impossible.

2. **Head.**—On closing eyes, felt like floating ; vertigo.—Dull, heavy headache, with heat and soreness in sacrum (cured during proving).—Catarrhal aching in forehead.—Weight in sinciput.—Itching of hairy scalp.

3. **Eyes.**—Inner, upper tarsal borders itched and burned.—Full sensation in supra-orbital region.

4. **Ears.**—Ringing and singing in both ears.

5. **Nose.**—Discharge from nares thick, pus-like, streaked with blood, and an odour as if from an open sore.—A peculiar wet feeling in nares, as though a violent coryza would set in, which did not; the secretion from the nose became thickened and pus-like, but not increased.—Nose: stuffed as if swollen; fulness of nose and ears.—Contractile feeling of muscles of side of nose affected with catarrh (a secondary symptom).—Itching in nares.

8. **Mouth.**—Prickling, burning sensation on tongue as though scalded. —Increased flow of saliva (bloody).

9. **Throat.**—Posterior nares feel raw as if denuded of epithelium.

11. **Stomach.**—Appetite increased.—Forcible eructation and dejections of small quantities of odourless flatus.—Disgust and nausea.

12. **Abdomen.**—Borborygmus.—Parieties of abdomen felt thickened.—A clawing, uneasy sensation about umbilicus, which gradually passed to lower bowel.—Twitching in muscles of abdomen.

13. **Stool and Anus.**—Crawling in lower rectum as though a worm tried to escape.—Burning in rectum at stool, continuing after.—Itching of anus; hæmorrhoids with aching in sacrum and sacro-iliac joint.—After being constipated, semi-fluid evacuation next morning.—Constipation; an atonic condition of bowels and rectum.

14. **Urinary Organs.**—Dull aching in kidneys.—Bladder sore to pressure.—Urine increased; burning along urethra when micturating.—Urine alkaline.

15. **Male Sexual Organs.**—Sexual orgasm.—Erethism, almost satyriasis; followed by long-continued depression, approaching impotence.—Varicocele (cured).

17. **Respiratory Organs.**—(Connected with wet feeling in nose) wet feeling in trachea and bronchi; passing from above down, as if a coryza would set in, followed by a slight feeling of constriction, which passed from above down through chest.—In morning a cough (dry, "as though he would cough his insides out") from deep in chest, with soreness throughout chest.

20. **Neck and Back.**—Aching through basilar region from back to front.—Aching in sacrum and sacro-iliac joint.—Heat in sacrum with headache (cured).

22. **Upper Limbs.**—Arm numb.—Hand felt swollen.

23. **Lower Limbs.**—Trembling feeling of legs for several days, with soreness of knees.—While on lounge muscles of l. leg suddenly contracted, jerking foot up as in stepping; in a moment r. leg performed same manœuvre.

24. **Generalities.**—General malaise, headache, weakness of limbs, inability to attend to business.

25. **Skin.**—A long-cured impetiginous eczema reappeared on both legs. —A few hot prickings in skin.—Itching on face and forehead.

26. **Sleep.**—Dreams: fantastic; voluptuous and increased desire sympathetic with urinary excitement.

27. **Fever.**—A very few cold chills rushed in succession up spinal column.

Pepsinum.

A proteolytic ferment found in the gastric juice. The Pepsin in general use is extracted from the stomach of the pig. [Alcohol, tannin, and the alkaline carbonates destroy its power. It is prepared in granular form or in glycerinated extract for general use. Homœopathic attenuations may be made by triturating the secretory layer of a fresh pig's-stomach; by triturating the granular Pepsin with sugar of milk; or by making the lower attenuations of the liquid extracts with distilled water.]

Clinical.—Dyspepsia.

Characteristics.—*Pepsin.* has been supposed to act purely as a *digestive*, but recent discoveries in regard to the action of the sarcodes makes this now scarcely tenable. *Pepsin.* may digest the contents of the stomach; but, like the secretions of other glands, it will in all probability act also, by its specific affinity, on the secretory tissues of the stomach itself.

Persica.

Amygdalus persica. Peach. *N. O.* Rosaceæ. Tincture of the flowers. Infusion of the bark. Infusion of the leaves.

Clinical.—Eyes, irritation of. Gastric irritation. Genital weakness. Smell, loss of. Sprains. Taste, loss of. Toe-nails, affections of. Vision, disordered. Wrists, affections of.

Characteristics.—The symptoms were obtained by Demeures whilst pounding the flowers for the purpose of making a tincture, and from later provings with the tincture on himself. The sense of vision was disordered and the eyes irritated. The senses of smell and taste were abolished. Pains in vertical lines in abdomen, heart, limbs; weak wrists; pains under great toenails and persistent itching were the chief effects observed. O. S. Haynes (*H. R.*, v. 214) relates a case *apropos* of remarks by C. C. Edson on the value of an infusion of Peach *bark* in the gastric irritability of children. An infant in its second summer had acute dyspeptic diarrhœa, with persistent vomiting of all food. No remedy helped, and the child was sent to the mountains; but the change made it worse, and death was hourly expected, when an old local practitioner was called in and prescribed: Two or three fresh Peach *leaves* to be put into a cup of boiling water; the infant to have a drink of the infusion at frequent intervals. The effect was rapid; food was soon retained and the child got well.

Relations.—*Compare:* Amyg. (the peach is hardly distinguishable from the almond, *A. communis*, botanically; almonds have been known to have fleshy drupes), Pru. spi., Pru. virg.

SYMPTOMS.

3. **Eyes.**—Pressure and itching in eyes from reading, evening; sensation of foreign body in eyes.—Lachrymation from reading.—Dazzling before eyes; objects wave in zigzags; reading impossible; < candle-light.

4. **Ears.**—Tumour size of nut on lobe of r. ear, very painful to touch.

5. **Nose.**—Nasal cartilage and upper jaw painful as if bruised (only when touched); nasal cartilage feels thinner than usual.—Persistent loss of smell.

6. **Face.**—Raw pain middle of lower lip.—Swelling on l. lower jaw.

8. **Mouth.**—Persistent loss of taste.

12. **Abdomen.**—Vertical internal pain in line from tip of l. tenth rib cartilage to anterior superior spine of l. ilium.

15. **Male Sexual Organs.**—During stool ejaculation of semen, without erection, followed by empty feeling in hypogastrium and pain in genitals as after excess; painful lassitude in legs, then pain above hips, < in sacral region.

18. **Chest.**—During dinner stinging pain under false ribs, as from a sharp point, also under scapulæ.—Severe deep-seated prickings above l. nipple.

19. **Heart.**—Sharp vertical pains in heart region.

22. **Upper Limbs.**—Wrists sprain easily.—Fatiguing pains in both wrists, and at same time in feet.

23. **Lower Limbs.**—Vertical lancinations in r. thigh.—Pain in both knees and r. ankle.—Pricking and lancinations, numbness, stiffness of legs.—Itching and sharp pains under great toenails.

24. **Generalities.**—A single glass of wine is sufficient to intoxicate him.

25. **Skin.**—Obstinate, intolerable itching on different parts of body, pimples appear.—Sudden local itching.

Persicaria Urens, *see* Polygonum.

Pestinum.

Plaguinum. Nosode of Plague. Trituration of the virus.

Clinical.– Bubo. Plague. Typhus.

Characteristics.—The prophylaxis and treatment of plague with injections of more or less modified virus of plague by old-school practioners affords evidence that the nosode of plague is available, like other nosodes, for the treatment of cases of the disease from which it is derived.

Petiveria.

Petiveria tetrandra (Gom.). Erva de Pipi. *N. O.* Phytolaccaceæ. Trituration of fresh root.

Clinical.—Conjunctivitis. Paralysis. Paraplegia.

Characteristics.—Mure proved *Petiv.*, and I have given his terminology. Allen says in a note that it is probably identical with the

Mexican and West Indian species, *P. alliacea.* Mure's figure corresponds to this, and he says the roots, which are branching and fibrous, "smell strongly of garlic." *P. alliac.* (according to *Treas. oj Bot.*) is called "Guinea-hen Weed" in West Indies," and "Raiz de Guine" in Brazil, in which country "it is put into warm baths to restore motion to paralysed limbs." Mure does not mention these names or this fact; but his proving brings out some strongly confirmative symptoms in numbness and paralytic sensations; weariness and weight of eyelids. Cold saliva; internal coldness; coldness inside bones were experienced. The symptoms in general were < by movement; in the morning on waking and on rising; after breakfast and during and after dinner; bending backward.

Relations.—*Compare:* Botan., Phytolacc. In paralysis, Rhus. Cold saliva, Cist.

SYMPTOMS.

1. **Mind.**—Excessive gaiety; inclination to sing, laugh, jest; followed by sadness and tears.—Vanishing of thought.

2. **Head.**—Head heavy.—Compressed feeling as if head bound with a warm cloth.—Head feels as if it would split.—Headache > by motion.—Sensation of hot water on scalp penetrating to brain.—Weight at vertex pressing into brain.

3. **Eyes.**—Eyes half-closed, swollen, surrounded by blue rings, esp. next to nose.—Rapid inflammation of l. eye while at dinner, lasts three days.—Weight on lids compelling to close eyes; on doing so sees a variety of figures.—Pain in eyes as if the balls were pushed out of their sockets.—Painful burning at margin of lids, < on closing them.—Lachrymation.—Conjunctivitis.—Dim sight.

4. **Ears.**—R. ear deaf, as if stopped.

5. **Nose.**—Coryza.—Veins of nose swollen, bluish.—Redness of l. wing of nose and cheek.—Dull pain over root of nose, evening.—Nose slightly inflamed and shining.—Intense and sudden itching of bridge of nose.

6. **Face.**—Redness of l. cheek.—Bruised pain in zygomatic process.—Sensation as if needle stuck in upper lip from within out.

8. **Mouth.**—Burning tongue as if scalded, morning, on rising.—Dry mouth.—Flow of watery cold saliva, depositing ashy sediment and whitish granules.—Offensive breath.

9. **Throat.**—Sensation in throat as after eating something astringent.—Pain in throat with difficulty of swallowing saliva.

11. **Stomach.**—Sharp lancinations in epigastrium from within out; evening; after dinner; on rising.—Stomachache with sensation of internal coldness.

12. **Abdomen.**—Long blue horizontal spots on r. hypochondrium.—Lancinations: in hypochondria; through spleen from below up.—Borborygmi, on moving in bed.—Dull pain in hypogastrium.—Circumscribed acute pains in groins.—Colic of descending colon.

13. **Stool.**—Diarrhœa of dark mucus, mixed with fecal matter in separate hard pieces.—Constipation.

14. Urinary Organs.—Micturition every five minutes from 11 a.m. till evening, with heat in urethra.—Urine : pale, copious.

17. Respiratory Organs.—Voice seems to come from afar.—Voice hoarse from coughing.—Suffocation, with cold feet.

18. Chest.—Deep-seated, dull pain beneath sternum, < moving neck or bending head forward.—Violent lancinations under r. breast at each inspiration.

19. Heart.—Contraction and throbbing in region of heart, evening.

20. Back.—Strained feeling in spine, < sitting upright and bending back, > bending forward.

21. Limbs.—Paralytic numbness, heaviness, and weariness in all limbs ; after rising from bed.—Bruised pains in arms and legs.

22. Upper Limbs.—Twitching sensation in shoulder-joint on stooping. —Pricking, burning, crampy pains in arms ; with inflammatory redness.—Numbness ; at r. arm ; at wrist ; at fingers (r.) ; at finger-tips.—Lancinating and heat as from whitlow at tip of r. thumb.—Itching in l. palm.

23. Lower Limbs.—Weakness of lower limbs.—Sudden numbness of knees with dull pain in tibia.—Numbness, itching and weakness of legs ; from knees to soles.

24. Generalities.—General rigor when lying down.—Prostration as from drowsiness but without inclination to sleep.—When walking seems as if she does not touch the ground and would fall.—On lying down body numb.

25. Skin.—Itching, pricking, and formication of skin.

26. Sleep.—Drowsy : all day ; with frequent yawning ; after dinner.—Sleep deep and prolonged.—Dreams : of corpses and starts up in cold sweat ; sad ; unpleasant ; of quarrels.

27. Fever.—Excessive coldness of hands and feet piercing to bones.—Cold feeling in interior of bones.—Febrile heat with pale face and cold hands. —Dry heat all over, esp. of palms.—Profuse cold sweat all over, with shuddering, after first sleep.—Sweat in palms.

Petroleum.

Oleum petræ. Rock-oil. Coal Oil. Trituration and tincture of the rectified oil. (Preparations of the non-rectified oil should also be made.)

Clinical.—Addison's disease. Albuminuria. *Anæmia.* Angina pectoris. Anus, fissure of. Bed-sores. *Breath, offensive.* Burns. *Chilblains.* Chlorosis. Constipation. *Cracks in skin.* Deafness. *Diarrhœa.* Dysmenia. Dyspepsia. *Ear, affections of. Eczema. Face, rough.* Facial paralysis. *Feet, soles painful. Fester, tendency to.* Fistulæ. Frost-bite. Gastric ulcer. Gonorrhœa. Hæmorrhoids. *Hands, chapped.* Headache ; occipital. Herpes. Herpes preputialis. *Irritation. Jaw, easily dislocated.* Myopia. *Nose, sore.* Otorrhœa. *Perspiration, offensive. Pregnancy, sickness of.* Presbyopia. Prostatitis. *Psoriasis.* Rheumatism. *Sea-sickness. Skin, affections of.* Sprains. Syphilis. Tabes mesenterica. Toothache. Urethra, stricture of ; chronic inflammation of. Varices. *Vomiting.* Warts.

Characteristics.—The *Petrol.* proved by Hahnemann is made by agitating the liquid commercial Petroleum with Sulphuric Acid and then rectifying the portion which this acid does not act upon. It is "a light oily fluid, colourless or of a pale straw colour, and strong characteristic naphthalic smell. Dropped on white paper it evaporates completely, leaving no greasy stain." Under PARAFFIN I have described the relation between *Petrol.*, *Naph.*, and *Paraff.* Commercial "Petroleum" and commercial "Paraffin oil" are one and the same. The *Petrol.* of homœopathy is this substance purified and rectified. But in the pathogenesis are included effects observed on those engaged in petroleum works, and those who use "Paraffin oil" in various trades; it would therefore be well to have also a preparation of the crude, non-rectified liquid. *Petrolatum* (Vaseline) consists of hydrocarbons of the Paraffin series, obtained from residues after distillation of lighter oils from crude petroleum; or deposited from crude petroleum on standing. The affections met with in petroleum extractors and refiners are—(1) Diseases of the skin and subcutaneous tissue; depressed nutrition, anæmia, dyspepsia, nerve troubles, irritability, insomnia, respiratory affections. In addition to these is a species of intoxication. A man, a patient of mine who suffered from inveterate eczema, and who had formerly been employed in a factory where much petroleum was used, noticed that his eczema was much better whilst working with petroleum. He told me that the vapour had the singular effect of making some of the workmen insane, causing: Desire to kill; hallucinations, they will see things not actually visible; for instance, "they will see the rails in a station when a train is on them." Boys (who are much affected) will jump at a straight wall and try to scramble up it. A rickety boy, æt. 2½, who had an unconquerable desire to drink anything liquid within his reach, took one day a good draught of paraffin oil. An Ipecacuanha emetic and a Castor Oil purge got rid of a good deal of it, and a month after he was brought to me with these symptoms: Appetite bad. Pale, dark rings round eyes. Every now and then seems to collapse; goes into a corner and will not play; after tea quite bright. Cold sweat in bed; complains of burning heat; then goes cold and clammy. I prescribed *Phos.* 2. In three weeks he was brought back much better. He had lost the pallor and dark rings round the eyes, and had ceased to mope; but he had come out all over small boils which discharged, the discharge having the odour of paraffin. There was a slight recurrence of the old symptoms a fortnight later, and after that I did not see the boy again till a year later, when he was brought to me for diphtheritic paralysis. Two years after this he was brought to me again. He was now well grown and had no sign of rickets, but some of the old symptoms came back: Languid; inclined to be quiet; averse to play. At times clammy all over body. This time *Petrol.* 30 soon put him right. In the case of a woman who drank paraffin oil when intoxicated, there was epigastric pain so severe that she thought she would go out of her mind, > lying with knees drawn up; tenderness of ileo-cæcal region and of epigastrium; swollen feeling of abdomen, without actual swelling; blood and albumen in urine; pain in back and slight return of menses, which had ceased a week before. These cases show the profound action of *Petrol.* on the organism. It is one of Hahnemann's leading antipsorics, and is especially closely related to *Graph.* It is *suited to* long-lasting, deep-seated, wasting diseases ; lingering gastric and intestinal troubles with or without ulceration. In my experience no remedy corresponds to more cases of chlorosis in young girls, with or without ulceration of the stomach. *Petrol.* (says Kent) corresponds to low conditions in which there is inability to throw out eruptions on the skin ; or conditions in which an eruption has disappeared without improvement in health : to reflexions of disease on mucous membranes setting up catarrh. Ozæna ; intestinal catarrh. Soreness and cracks about muco-cutaneous orifices. Irritability of skin and irritability of mind are both found in *Petrol.*, as in many other remedies : Excitable ; angry at trifles. Anxiety with fear. Mental weakness and forgetfulness are also very characteristic, and are generally met with in connection with deep-seated disease. An illusion that there is another person, or another baby in bed, is very characteristic of the remedy, and has led to cures with *Petrol.* of cases of typhoid and puerperal fever. "Falling out of the hair" is a characteristic symptom of *Petrol.*, and accounts for the popularity of Petroleum hair-restorers. [*Petrol.* "probably acts on the sebaceous rather than the sudoriferous secretions of the skin, and its local action is on parts where the sebum is abundant."—R. T. C.]. The use of these hair-restorers has caused many violent headaches. So has the use of "Coal Oil" (a tablespoonful to a bucketful of water) by washer-women to improve the colour of linen. M. T. Bleim (quoted *H. W.*, xxvi. 318) thus describes the result in one case : Severe occipital headache, loss of strength, emaciation, diarrhœa, dyspepsia with fulness on eating very little ; accumulation of gas ; very severe attacks of suffocation, > by eructations of gas. The headaches of *Petrol.* may be in any part, but they are most marked in occiput. Heaviness like lead ; pressure, sticking ; pulsating ; < on shaking head or any jar. Pain travels from occiput to eyes, and is associated with temporary loss of sight and fainting. The vertigo and heaviness of *Petrol.* are often associated with nausea and bilious vomiting. This (nausea with or without vomiting) is one of the grand characteristics of the remedy. It is < by motion in a carriage or on the sea ; hence *Petrol.* is one of the first remedies in train-sickness or sea-sickness. The other side of this nausea is another grand characteristic : Awful ravenous hunger, the "sinking" of the chief antipsorics. It is particularly noticed immediately after a stool, in diarrhœa, nervous affections, spinal disease, &c. (Kent). In pulmonary affections *Petrol.* has gained much repute of late in the form of an emulsion. A leading indication for it is "Oppression of the chest ; < in cold air." *Petrol.* has a peculiar cough, not infrequently met with in young girls and boys, coming from deep down in the chest, and frequently waking the patient up at night. A student who had a deep, hollow-sounding, hacking cough, excited by laughing, waking him up in the middle of the night, I cured with *Petrol.* 30 after *Arg. n.* and *Arg. met.* had failed to do anything. The cough had persisted some time and caused his family no little anxiety. The discharges of *Petrol.* are thick, purulent, and yellowish green. For the cracked nostrils accompanying and following cold in the head I find the application of vaseline more often useful than other forms of unguent. The *localities* of *Petrol.* are very like those of *Graph.*: Scalp, behind ears, scrotum, genitals. The modality "< in winter" has given Nash the key to several cases of eczema, chapped hands, chilblains, and one case of chronic diarrhœa, as soon as he discovered that the patient had eczema of the hands in winter. *Petrol.* 200 was given. The skin is extremely sensitive; all clothing is painful; slight injuries suppurate. Allen's *Appendix* quotes an important case reported by O. Lassar in Virchow's *Archiv.* A man used for four days extensive inunctions with *Petrol.* to relieve himself from scabies. A week later his feet began to swell, and the dropsy, increasing rapidly, spread over abdomen and thorax. In a fortnight it disappeared, but eight days later returned and persisted till death, four months after the inunction. The urine was highly albuminous, and contained hyaline and granular cylinders; but the necropsy revealed no lesion of any organ to account for the dropsy. The body was extremely œdematous; there was œdema of the lungs and dropsy of the cavities, and whilst in hospital the wrist pulse was small, empty, and of low tension; the blood corpuscles were few, but their relative proportions were normal. Temperature normal, and the skin showed localised areas of inflammation. Along the veins and lymphatics a small-celled growth existed, and in all the layers of the cutis there was a widely distributed nuclear proliferation. *Peculiar symptoms* are: Brain as if wrapped in a fog. As if everything in head were alive. As if head made of wood, or as if bruised. As if a cold breeze were blowing on head. As if head would burst. Veil before eyes. Sand in eyes. As if skin over bridge of nose drawn stiff and tight. As if something were tearing off from pit of stomach. As if a cold stone at heart. Splinter in heel. Upper and lower limbs as if stiff without joints. Jaw as if distended. There is great weakness; fainting; tremor; twitching of limbs; catalepsy; tonic spasms; left-sided paralysis. The notes of the skin affections are: Itching; burning; rawness; bleeding. Burning sensations are very marked; and as *Petrol.* is accountable for so many burning accidents it is fitting that it should make a very good application for burns in the form of vaseline, cosmoline, or *Petrol.* mixed with equal parts of olive oil. *Petrol.* is *suited to*: Persons with light hair and skin. Especially for lean, slender persons. The symptoms are < by touch; by contact of clothing; by scratching; by riding in carriage or ship. Pinching the parts > hæmorrhoids. < From mental exertion. Headache < on shaking head; > by epistaxis; < from light and noise. After stool: hunger immediately. Ravenous hunger; frequently awakened by it at night; easily satisfied, with aversion to meat, fats, cooked or hot food; desire only for dainties, which are eaten with avidity. Eating > gastralgia. Gastralgia comes on whenever the stomach is empty. Empty, weak sensation in stomach. < After eating or drinking. After eating: giddiness; heat in face; cutting in abdomen; eructations; drowsiness; uneasiness. Cabbages, saurkraut = diarrhœa. Colic > by bending double. Exertion, motion, riding, sitting <. Lying down < cough, and distension of abdomen. Vertigo when head lies low. < Cold air. < Winter. < Open air. < Before and during thunderstorm. < Bathing. > Warmth and warm air. < Warmth of bed (itching). Cough is < at night and 2, 4, and 6 a.m. Smoking befogs him ; = cough. < After coitus (nervous irritability). Cough < by laughing (cured). < During day (diarrhœa and dysentery). Throat affections go right to left. Headache back to front.

Relations.—*Antidoted by:* Coccul., Nux, Phos. (in my case), *Antidote to:* Lead poisoning (one of the best remedies), Nit. ac. *Complementary:* Before Sep. *Compatible:* Bry., Calc., Lyc., Nit. ac., Nux, Puls., Sep., Sil., Sul. *Compare:* Graph., Naph., Paraf., Eupn., Kreas., and other Carbons. In sea-sickness, Arn., Coccul., Tab. Nausea of pregnancy, Coccul., Sep. Cracking of joints, Caust. Gastralgia > by eating, Chel., Anac., Graph., Lach. Imagines he has a limb double ; illusions of shape, Bap., Stram. Epistaxis > headache (Borax <). Aversion to hot food, Pho. (opp. Lyc.). < From thunderstorms, Pho., Merc., Sil., Rho., Pso. Head as if made of wood ; eruptions behind ears and on genitals, Graph. Cold feeling about heart, Nat. m. (< when exerting mind), K. chlo., Graph., K. nit., Ruta. Diarrhœa in early morning, Sul. (Petro. also during day). Loses his way in well-known streets, Glo. (from heat or sun). Moist eruptions about genitals, Thuj. Hot, burning eructations, K. ca., Sep. Faintness during or connected with evacuations, Crot. t., Dulc., Ox. ac., Sul. (these have it with scanty stools ; the rest with copious stools :) Apis, Nux m., Pul., Spi., Ver. Sinking immediately after meals, Ars., Cina, Lyc., Sil., Stp., Urt. ur., Calc., Iod. Brownish scattered spots on dark-haired people, Nit. ac. Loquacity, Lach. (Petrol. on one subject). Hunger after stool (Alo. during stool). Symptoms appear and disappear rapidly, Bell., Mag. p., Lyc.—opp. Plat., Stan. Imagines two babies in bed, Val. Vertigo on rising, Bry. Skin sensitive to clothing ; every injury suppurates, Hep. Tender feet, which are bathed in foul-smelling sweat, Graph., Sanic., Sil. Heat and burning of soles and palms, Sang., Sul. Skin < in winter, > in summer, Alm.

Causation.—Vexation. Riding in carriage or ship. Nitric acid (deafness from). Cabbage. Suppressed eruptions. Sprains.

SYMPTOMS.

1. Mind.—Anxious and timorous disposition.—Sadness and mental dejection.—Great irresolution.—Uneasiness respecting the future.—Hypochondriacal humour.—Inclination to anger and to scold.—Violent, irascible, insolent temper.—Frequent tears ; on slightest provocation.—Loss of memory.—Does not know where she is in the street.—Unfitness for reflection.—Weakness of apprehension.—Delirium ; thinks another person is lying with him in bed (or that he is double, or one limb is double) ; or always and continuously delirious talk of the same distressing subject.—Imagines he has a third leg which will not keep quiet.—Desire to kill.—Hallucinations of vision.

2. Head.—Head bewildered.—Feeling as if brain wrapped in fog.—Frequent vertigo, esp. on raising eyes.—Vertigo, like that produced by a swinging motion.—Vertigo on stooping, or on rising from bed, or from a seat.—Headache after a fit of anger, or when fasting in morning, as also after a walk in evening.—Attacks of semi-lateral headache, which compel patient to lie down.—Heaviness and fulness in head in morning, and when stooping.—Pressive or lancinating pressive pains in head, esp. in occiput.—Headache < by all kinds of intellectual labour, to the extent of complete stupefaction.—Tension in head, as if dura mater were tightened.—Cramp-like, drawing, pinching pains in head.—Neuralgic headache, beginning in occiput and extending forward.—Occipital headache, extending to vertex, with vertigo.—Occipital headache, with nausea, esp. in sea-sickness.—Pulsative headache, esp. in occiput (cerebellum).—Pressing stinging in the cerebellum.—Sensation as if all were alive in head.—Scalp painful to touch, as if bruised or ulcerated (followed by numbness and very sore on scratching, < in morning and on becoming heated).—Headache in forehead ; every mental exertion causes him to become quite stupid.—Drawing pains in head, forehead, and temples, extending into teeth.—Seborrhœa of scalp.—Eruption on head and nape of neck.—Œdematous swelling and scabs on scalp.—Hair falls off.

3. **Eyes.**—Itching in eyes.—Itching of lids ; obliged to rub them.—(Lids everted.)—Aching, smarting, shooting, and burning pain in eyes.—Conjunctivitis and blepharadenitis.—Inflammation of eyes (with itching and stitches in eyes).—Lachrymal fistula (with dryness of r. side of nose).—Lachrymation.—Jerking and quivering of eyes and lids.—Convulsion of eyes.—Myopia or presbyopia.—Diplopia.—Scintillation and appearance as of a veil before sight ; or sparks and black spots.

4. **Ears.**—Inflammation and painful swelling of meatus auditorius.—Otalgia, with cramp-like and jerking pain.—Dryness, and distressing sensation of dryness, in interior of ear.—Discharge of blood and pus from ears.—Eruption of ears.—Redness, excoriation, and oozing behind ears.—Deafness.—Tinkling, rolling, roaring, ringing, rumbling, cracking, and buzzing in ears.—Excessive secretion of cerumen.

5. **Nose.**—Epistaxis.—Slight epistaxis > headache.—Purulent blisters on nose.—Ulcerated nostrils (and stopped catarrh).—Ozæna, scabs, purulent mucus, cracked nostrils.—Swelling of nose, with discharge of pus, and pain above root of nose.—Stoppage of nose.—Dryness, and distressing sensation of dryness, in nose.—Much mucus in nose.—Itching on tip of nose.—Coryza with hoarseness.

6. **Face.**—Heat in face, sometimes after a meal, and with thirst.—Dryness and constriction of skin of face and eyelids as though covered with a thin layer of albumen ; cheeks look glazed and contracted.—Pale, yellowish complexion.—Facial paralysis (from inflammatory products in Fallopian canal).—Eruption of pimples on face.—Scurfs around mouth.—Scabby pimples, with shooting pain on lips, and commissures.—Furuncles on lower lip.—Swelling of sub-maxillary glands.—Easy dislocation of maxillary joint in bed in morning with sharp pains.

7. **Teeth.**—Toothache from contact with open air, < at night, with swelling of cheek.—Numbness of teeth, with pain on clenching them.—Pustule above a hollow tooth like a fistula.—Fistulous vesicles in gums.—Swelling of gums, with shooting pain on being touched.

8. **Mouth.**—Fetid breath, sometimes like garlic.—Ulcers on inner surface of cheeks (painful when closing teeth).—Much mucus in mouth and throat.—Tongue coated white.—Painful soreness on chewing.—Great dryness of mouth (and throat in morning) with violent thirst (for beer).

9. **Throat.**—Sore throat, with shooting pain during deglutition.—Swelling and great dryness of throat.—Swelling of the submaxillary glands.—Rawness (stitching and burning) in pharynx, < on swallowing.—Tickling on swallowing, extending to ear.—Dryness and burning in pharynx.—When swallowing the aliment rises towards nasal fossæ.—Hawking up of mucus in morning.

10. **Appetite.**—Putrid, mawkish, mucous, or else bitter or acid taste.—Excessive thirst for beer.—Bulimy.—Hunger with speedy satiety.—Voracity.—Daintiness.—Anorexia.—Repugnance to meat and fat, also to hot and cooked aliments; < by eating cabbage.—Uneasiness during digestion, after almost every kind of food, however little may have been eaten.—After a meal: obscuration and vertigo; nausea; heaviness and pressure at stomach; sleep; or colic, with eructations; or sour risings, congestion in head, cramp in chest, &c.

11. **Stomach.**—Noisy eructations.—Sour (or bitter eructations or) risings and regurgitations.—Pyrosis.—Frequent nausea, esp. in morning, often with accumulation of water in mouth, obstructed respiration, sour risings, tongue dry and white, stitches in hepatic region, heat in face, vertigo, &c.—After eating, vertigo and giddiness.—Nausea from motion of a carriage.—Nausea and vomiting of pregnant women.—Water-brash.—Heartburn toward evening.—Inclination to vomit.—Greenish, bitter vomiting.—Aching of stomach.—Cramps in stomach.—Pressure on the stomach; colic (at night).—Sensation of emptiness and weakness in stomach.—Weak digestion.—Diarrhœa from suppressed eruptions.—Pain in epigastrium, as if something were being torn away.—Swelling of epigastrium, with pain when touched.—Sensation of fulness in epigastrium.

12. **Abdomen.**—Pain (cutting) in abdomen, shortly after a meal.—Sensation of great emptiness in abdomen.—Distension and tension in abdomen, with cramp.—Pinchings and cuttings in abdomen, sometimes with pressing want to evacuate.—Colic, with diarrhœa, at night, towards morning.—Colic > from bending double.—Borborygmi in abdomen, with sensation as if abdomen were entirely empty.—Inguinal hernia.—Fetid flatus.—Sensation of coldness in abdomen.

13. **Stool and Anus.**—Difficult, hard, knotty, and insufficient evacuations.—Frequent diurnal stools, sometimes with evacuation of serous, yellowish matter.—Diarrhœa, often preceded by cuttings (colic only during the day).—Mucous stools, often mixed with blood.—Burning pain in rectum after evacuation.—Itching tetters in perineum.—Diarrhœa < from riding in carriage.—In anus burning itching; pressure.—Weakness of rectum.—Piles with great itching, < at night from heat of bed; < from rubbing or scratching.—Fissure with great rawness.

14. **Urinary Organs.**—Constant dribbling of urine after micturition.—Discharge of mucus with the urine.—Frequent emission of urine, with scanty stream of a red or brown and fetid urine.—Urine bloody and turbid; it deposits a red, slimy sand, that adheres tightly to vessel; urine contains albumen, hyalin, and granulated casts; covered with a glistening film and with a red sediment.—Involuntary discharge of urine.—Emission of urine at night.—Wetting the bed.—Burning in urethra.—Stricture of urethra.—(Chronic urethritis.)

15. **Male Sexual Organs.**—Burning pain, itching, redness, excoriation, and oozing, or itching pimples and tetters, on scrotum and between scrotum and thigh.—Diminished sexual desire.—Frequent pollutions.—Discharge of prostatic fluid.—(Prostatitis.)—Weakness and nervous irritability after coition. —Reddish eruption on glans, with itching.

16. **Female Sexual Organs.**—Itching, soreness, and moisture on external parts.—Repugnance to coition.—Catamenia too early, with a menstrual flux which excites itching.—Leucorrhœa like white of egg.—Leucorrhœa with lascivious dreams.—During pregnancy diarrhœa and vomiting.—Itching and furfur on the mammæ ; the nipples itch, and have a mealy coating.

17. **Respiratory Organs.**—Hoarseness, with or without coryza.—Cough, with dryness in throat.—Vexatious cough that takes away the breath ; cannot cough it out.—Suffocating cough at night.—Dry cough at night, or in evening, after lying down.—At night dry cough, coming deep from chest, caused by a scratching in throat.—Cough from low down in chest.—Hollow, hacking cough, coming on when laughing, waking him in middle of night (cured).—Dry cough, with shootings under sternum.

18. **Chest.**—Respiration obstructed in cold air.—Rattling and snoring in trachea.—Sensation of heaviness, anxiety, and uneasiness in chest.—Oppression of chest at night.—Shootings in sides of chest.—Herpes on chest.

19. **Heart.**—Palpitation of heart.—Feeling of coldness about heart ; as if there was a cold stone in heart.—Fainting, with ebullitions, heat, pressing on heart, palpitation.

20. **Neck and Back.**—Herpes on nape of neck.—Heaviness and pain in nape of neck.—Painful drawing extending from nape to occiput.—Swelling of glands and eruption on nape of neck.—Sacral pains, which do not permit standing upright.—Coccyx painful on sitting.—Stiffness in coccyx.—Pain in back, which obstructs every movement.—Weakness and stiffness in back and loins.—Suppuration of the axillary glands.

21. **Limbs.**—Cracking of the joints.—Inflexibility of the joints.—Sprains ; chronic sprains.

22. **Upper Limbs.**—Fetid sweat of axillæ.—Drawing pains in arms and fingers.—Great weakness of arms.—Stiffness of arms and fingers.—Erysipelatous inflammation in arms.—Brown or yellow spots on arms.—Furunculi on forearm.—Tearings in hands.—Burning sensation in palms of hands.—Sweating of hands.—Pain in wrist-joint as if sprained.—Brown spots on wrist.—Bleeding fissures in hands and fingers, esp. in winter.—Salt-rheum, red, raw, burning ; moist or covered with thick crusts.—Chilblains and warts on fingers. —Pricking and pain in warts on fingers, evening in bed.—Arthritic stiffness in joints of fingers.—Finger-nails painful when touched as if bruised.—Finger-tips rough, cracked, fissured, with sticking, cutting pain.

23. **Lower Limbs.**—Cracking in joints of legs.—Cramps in thighs, calves, and feet (all day ; in soles at night).—Furunculi in thighs and calves. —Tension in the ham.—Lancinations in knee.—Weakness of knee.—Herpes on knee.—Tuberous, itching eruption on calves of legs.—Herpes on ankle bones.—Burning sensation in soles.—Profuse perspiration on feet.—Fœtid perspiration of feet with tenderness.—Coldness of feet.—Swelling of feet.—Hot swelling of soles.—Swelling and redness of heel with burning pain and shootings, < by walking.—Heels blistered.—Sensation of splinter in heel.—

Chilblains on toes, esp. when they itch and are moist; itch and burn; inflamed in cold weather.—Ulcers on the toes, originating in blisters on the toes.—Corns on feet.—Burning and stitching in corns.—Obstinate superficial ulcers on toes, with elevated margins and red bases, with oozings.—Eruption between toes.

24. **Generalities.**—Affections in general of any kind, appearing on the r. eye; internal or external occiput; behind ears; inner surface of thighs; ball or under part of toes; knee-joint.—Drawing pains in limbs.—Stiffness and tendency to numbness of limbs.—Cracking of joints, with arthritic rigidity and drawing, tearing pains.—Swelling and induration of glands, also after a contusion.—Jerking of limbs by day and during sleep.—Catalepsy; tonic spasms.—Epileptic fits.—Fainting fits, with ebullition of blood, heat, palpitation, and pressure at heart.—Great weakness after least exertion, sometimes with confused sight, trembling of body, buzzing in ears, and nausea.—Weakness, nausea, and other sufferings, from motion of a carriage.—Weakness in morning in bed.—Many of the symptoms appear, or are <, during stormy weather.—Transient heat, ebullition of blood, and perspiration after a walk, or after a fit of anger.—Emaciation; also in children.—Sensation of insupportable and general uneasiness, with trembling and dejection.—Heaviness and lassitude in all limbs.—Great lassitude morning and evening.—Great tendency to take cold.—Repugnance to open air, with shivering when exposed to it.—Several symptoms manifest themselves in morning.

25. **Skin.**—Swelling and induration of the glands; also after contusions.—Great sensibility of the surface of skin.—Miliary urticaria.—Itching tetters.—Itching, excoriated, and running spots on skin.—Brown and yellow spots on skin.—Eruption of itching and burning pustules.—Pruritus of the aged.—Dreadful irritation all over body, very intense in vagina, anus and perineum, preventing sleep (cured—R. T. C.).—Papular eruptions, esp. on face and lips.—Skin sore, crawling sensations.—Rhagades.—The skin is hard to heal.—Skin unhealthy; every injury tends to ulceration.—Furunculi.—Ulcers with shooting pains; often deep ulcers, with raised edges.—Proud flesh in ulcers.—When a person complains of eruption or itching at night (affecting scrotum particularly), the eruption being either dry or moist.—Chilblains particularly where they itch a good deal and are moist.—Exanthema corroding and spreading; very difficult to heal.—Sensibility of the skin in general.—Sores produced by lying in bed.—Warts.—Corns on feet.—Chilblains, sometimes painful.

26. **Sleep.**—Disposition to sleep by day and in evening when sitting quietly (yawning).—Broken and agitated sleep at night, with many vivid, anxious, and frightful dreams (as if somebody were lying alongside of him in bed), frequent awakening with a start, and heat with anxiety.—Sensation in morning as of having slept too short a time.

27. **Fever.**—Shivering with headache, and coldness in hands and face.—Chilliness in open air.—Frequent shivering over whole body, and, on becoming warm, excessive itching of skin.—Shivering or coldness, generally in evening (with heat at the same time), and sometimes with blueness of nails.—Sweat immediately after shivering.—Intermittent fever: Violent chilliness and coldness of hands and face at 10 a.m.; half an hour later heat in the face, esp. in the eyes, with thirst.—Shaking fits, 7 p.m., followed by perspiration, first in

face, later all over, except in legs, which are quite cold.—Fever in evening, with hot face and cold feet, after shivering.—Frequent flushes of heat.—Heat after midnight and in morning in bed.—Fever, with full pulse and burning sensation in skin.—Pulse accelerated from every exertion ; as soon as reposing, pulse becomes again slow.—Nocturnal heat.—Nocturnal sweat.

Petroselinum.

Carum petroselinum. Petroselinum sativum. Apium petroselinum: *N. O.* Umbelliferæ. Tincture of whole fresh plant when coming into bloom.

Clinical.—Catheter fever. Cystitis. Dysuria. Gleet. Gonorrhœa. Gravel. Intermittent fever. Night-blindness. Priapism.

Characteristics.—*Petrosel.* is referred to by Hahnemann as a gonorrhœal remedy when frequent desire to urinate exists. It was proved by Bethmann. He obtained only thirty-six symptoms, all in the genito-urinary sphere, but these were very characteristic, and have given the remedy a definite place in homœopathic medicine, especially in gonorrhœa and gleet. The leading indication is : *Sudden urging* to urinate ; and drawing, tingling, crawling, or itching in navicular fossa. During micturition, burning and tingling from perineum through whole urethra. After micturition cutting biting in fossa navicularis. Milky or yellow discharge. Parsley tea is a recognised remedy for gonorrhœa in domestic country practice. Parsley eaten after meals, with or without salad oil, is reputed to act as a solvent on uric acid if there is a tendency to its formation in the urine. I have seen a case in which this effect was apparently produced. In gonorrhœa and gleet I have confirmed its efficiency, given in ten-drop doses of the tincture. In a case of dysuria from prostatic enlargement (quoted in *Critique*, vii. 84) there was frequent urging to urinate every half to three-quarters of an hour, with burning pains in bladder and urethra. *Petrosel.* 4x, three drops every hour, took away all the pains and relieved the tenesmus in a few days. The prostate gland itself was not influenced. Hering has collected symptoms from other observers. Farrington says *Petrosel.* is a great "baby medicine" in urinary difficulties. It has cured numbers of cases of intermittent fever ; and traumatic or other urethral fevers. [Parsley is said to be poisonous to ferrets. Fresh butter and parsley applied warm is an old remedy for bruises. An infusion is given to all children recovering from scarlatina by the matron of a suburban infectious hospital. An old gleet has been known to disappear from parsley infusion ; and an old Edinburgh surgeon used to give it in all nephritic and vesical diseases that were chronic.—R. T. C.]

Relations.—*Compare :* In gonorrhœa with sudden and frequent urging, Cann. s., Canth., Merc. Screams before urinating from irritation of mucous membrane, Aco., Caust., Borax (Sars., Lyc., and Benz. ac. have screaming before urinating when due to gravel). Gonorrhœa, strangury, frequent urging to urinate ; white stools, Dig. (Dig. has slow pulse ; often puffed prepuce ; Sul. indurated prepuce). Cystitis, Con. (Con. has *intermittent* urination ; Petrosel. has inflammation that has travelled back, *sudden*, irresistible desire). Bubbling in back ; urinary disorders, Berb. Uric acid tendency, intermittent fevers, Urt. ur.

SYMPTOMS.

3. **Eyes.**—Blind at night, with swelling of eyes.

4. **Ears.**—Shrill singing in ears, like a bell ringing out of tune, which affects the whole organism.

11. **Stomach.**—Thirsty and hungry, yet as soon as they begin to eat or drink they lose all desire.—Twitching, jerking pains in epigastrium, flatulent eructations, colic, nausea, and vomiting.

13. **Stool and Anus.**—Whitish evacuations, like clay ; chronic diarrhœa.—Burning at anus.

14. **Urinary Organs.**—Sudden urging to urinate.—Child suddenly seized with desire to urinate ; if not gratified immediately, jumps up and down with pain.—So much pain when he passes urine as to cause him to shiver and dance round room in agony.—Discharge of a milky fluid from urethra.—Albuminous yellow discharge from urethra ; gonorrhœa.—Orifice of urethra agglutinated with mucus.—Creeping and crawling throughout whole length of urethra.—Frequent and almost fruitless want to urinate, every half-hour.—Tingling, lancinating, pressure and drawing, in urethra.—Crawling and pressure in region of Cowper's glands in morning in bed, > while standing and sitting.—During micturition, burning and tingling from perineum through the whole urethra.—Drawing, afterwards itching in fossa navicularis ; burning in navicular fossa while urinating.—Frequent desire to urinate, caused by crawling stitch behind navicular fossa.—Frequent voluptuous tickling in navicular fossa.

15. **Male Sexual Organs.**—Priapismus, without curvature of penis.—Pollutions ; profuse emission toward morning.

20. **Back.**—Jerking (or bubbling sensation) in muscles of back and arms.

25. **Skin.**—Urticaria.

26. **Sleep.**—Sleep late, with many anxious dreams.

27. **Fever.**—Ague, esp. quotidian ; marked periodicity ; stages regular ; acute fevers from defective assimilation or perverted innervation, accompanied by flatulent dyspepsia.—Intermittents, complicated with abdominal affections.—Intermittent fevers ; complicating traumatic or chronic inflammation of urethra, or even stricture.

Phallus Impudicus.

Stinkhorn. *N. O.* Fungi. Tincture or infusion of whole fungus.

Clinical.—Gastro-enteralgia. Sweat, viscid. Vertigo. Vomiting.

Characteristics.—Kalieniczensko took five or six teaspoonfuls of an infusion of *Phallus* in twenty-four hours, and the symptoms of the

Schema are the effects observed. There is a general resemblance to the effect of the *Agarici*—vertigo, disordered vision, gastro-enteric disturbance and viscid sweat.

SYMPTOMS.

2. **Head.**—Vertigo.

3. **Eyes.**—Vision: difficult; obscured.—Objects seem coloured grey, as in smoke.

8. **Mouth.**—Profuse salivation.

9. **Throat.**—Great dryness of throat, with irritation as from black pepper.

11. **Stomach.**—Loss of appetite.—Devouring thirst.—Violent vomiting with profuse salivation.—Gastro-enteralgia.

12. **Abdomen.**—Painful sensitiveness of whole abdomen.

13. **Stool.**—Watery diarrhœa.

14. **Urinary Organs.**—Urine deep red, depositing a sediment of urates of lime and soda.

17. **Respiratory Organs.**—Dry, oppressive cough.

24. **Generalities.**—Great feebleness of whole body.

26. **Sleep.**—Sleepiness.

27. **Fever.**—After four days all the pores became opened, profuse, viscid perspiration.

Phaseolus.

'PHASEOLUS NANUS. Dwarf-bean. N.O. Trituration of the dried bean. Decoction of dried beans and pods.

PHASEOLUS VULGARIS. Kidney-bean. Leguminosæ. Trituration of the dried bean. Decoction of dried beans and pods.

Clinical.—Albuminuria. Breast, tumour of. Diabetes. Dropsy. Hæmaturia. Headache. Heart, affections of; failure of; palpitation of. Hernia. Hydrothorax. Impotence. Pericarditis. Pleurisy. Prostate, diseases of; hæmorrhage from. Wounds, punctured.

Characteristics.—I have included under the heading *Phaseolus* both *P. nanus* and *P. vulgaris*, as I cannot discern any difference in their action. The proving of *P. vulg.* is by Demeures. Some effects of eating mildewed beans in a child recorded by W. Dale are distinguished in the Schema by (D). A. M. Cushing proved *P. nanus*, but has only published the symptoms observed on the heart. These are distinguished by (C). Cured symptoms are bracketed. Some symptoms observed in patients taking the remedy are included in the Schema. The *New Eng. Med. Gaz.* (quoted by Lambert, *H. W.*, xxxi. 125) published a translation of a pamphlet by Dr. Heinrich Ramm on the uses of "Bean tea." A lady whom Ramm had treated in vain for mitral disease with liver and kidney complications and dropsy, presented herself one day apparently cured by drinking Bean tea. This led Ramm to try it in other cases, and he found that renal and cardiac dropsies were speedily relieved; urine largely increased in quantity, and in cases of albuminuria, the albumen quickly disappeared. Dropsical effusion into pleura, pericardium, and peritoneum, according to Ramm, also yield to it; and all chronic disorders of the urinary tract from kidneys to urethra; pyelitis, vesical catarrh, gravel, calculi, uric acid, he says, quickly disappear; Ramm considers *Phas.* a most important remedy in gout and in diabetes. Ramm used a decoction of the whole dried ripe pod "of the taller variety." He names it *P. vulgaris.* [The inside of the pod rubbed on warts is said to cure them. —R. T. C.] We owe to A. M. Cushing (*New Eng. Med. Gaz.*, January, 1897) the best definition of the power and sphere of action of this remedy. He names it from Gray *P. nanus*, "the common white bean." His paper was read in Boston, and he refers to the "bean-eating city" and to its reputation "for sudden deaths from brain or heart trouble," and for premature ageing of young men. I am not quite sure whether this was jest or earnest, but it points the action of the remedy which in Cushing's proving caused disturbance of the nervous system, genital organs (impotence), stomach, bowels, and kidneys, and this symptom, which brought the proving to an abrupt close: "I suddenly felt a curious sensation in the region of the heart. It was so sudden and strange I immediately felt my pulse, and found it very irregular and feeble, so much so I think I was frightened; at least, I did not take any more of the medicine." "Irregular, weak pulse," "Heart failure," are the chief keynotes of the remedy in heart cases, and correspond with the one heart symptom recorded by Allen. Demeures in his proving experienced severe headache from *fulness* in the brain. Cushing relates two experiences bearing on this. (1) He gave a decoction of the dried pods in a hopeless case of uterine cancer with severe general dropsy with apparent relief. Calling one day and expecting to find the patient comfortable, he found her dead. "She suddenly screamed, 'Oh, my head!' grasped it with both hands and was dead." (2) A lady doctor, 30, married, no children, never ill except with children's diseases, had had much mental trouble two years before, and had done much cycling. Since then her heart had given trouble. About five times in a minute the heart would give one hard, unpleasant throb, then omit one beat. During the night it was much worse and prevented sleep. *Phas.* 10 was given. Thirty-six hours later the heart would beat a hundred beats without varying, and improvement continued; but the patient had to give up the remedy on account of the headache it caused, "as if something were pressing hard against each temple, much worse after each dose of the medicine. The patient was never subject to headaches. Other cases of Cushing's were: (3) Man, 45, dropsy, heart, and other complications. Bean pod decoction enabled him to lie down on a couch, and markedly diminished the dropsy. (4) Clergyman, 69, many years invalided on account of heart disease, after unusual exertion was greatly exhausted, and became entirely pulseless, and so remained four days in spite of treatment till *Phas.* 9x was given. In a few hours pulse returned. In thirty-six hours it was regular and strong, and so remained till his death, which occurred two weeks later. (5) Lady, 50, weak, tired, badly acting heart for some years. *Phas.* 9x was given, and in forty-eight hours "her heart wheeled into line all right and remains so." (6) Lady, 87, heart acted badly, every third beat omitted. After taking *Phas.* two days pulse quite right. (7) Confinement case, primapara, urine loaded with albumen, frightful convulsions, forceps delivery. Two hours later the heart failed and no stimulants would start it. *Phas.* 9x was given, and in ten minutes the heart was all right. Twice in the night the dose had to be repeated, but that was all. The albumen rapidly disappeared and a quick recovery was made. (8) Man, 92, had been passing bloody urine (apparently as much blood as urine) for a week. Had previously had urinary troubles, urinating several times in the night, and passing catheter twice in twenty-four hours; but for a little time past had not had to use the catheter. Cushing diagnosed prostatic trouble and gave *Phas.* 4x, No. 25 globules in water, a teaspoonful every two hours. (9) Another case of prostatic hæmorrhage in a man, 70, was cured by *Phas.* 4x globules dry on the tongue. Well in four days. (10) Cushing gives an interesting account (*Med. Vis.*, xiii. 375) of *Phas.* as a vulnerary. Fifty years ago he accidentally ran one tine of a hay fork into the top of his foot. A backwoods doctor promised to have him all right next day. He split a medium-sized white bean, bound one half, the flat, split side, on the wound. The pain was so severe Cushing became delirious, went to sleep, and woke well. In forty-one years of practice he has tried it in punctured wounds by rivets, nails, &c., and with perfect success every time. (11) A lady, 30, took a tablet containing gr. 12½ of Morphine placed in the middle of a baked bean with suicidal intent. It was in the evening, having fasted since noon. She went to sleep and woke at 7 a.m. next morning, surprised to find herself in this world. She slept again till 11 a.m., when she had to get up, but could not walk. A doctor was sent for. She vomited a little mucus, some dark specks like blood, and a small piece of lettuce, eaten the previous noon. Query: Did *Phas.* antidote *Morph.*? (12) Robust man, 50, had grippe, which developed rheumatism, worse in arms, occasionally below elbows. Pain so severe he could not lie in bed at nights. Drank much water. Passed much urine, which Cushing found to contain 3·5 per cent. of sugar. *Phas.* 5x every four hours removed all but a trace of sugar in eight days, and the patient was in other respects well. S. R. Stone (*Amer. Hom.*, xxiv. 123) reports the case of Mr. T., 69, whom he found semi-conscious, yet suffering severely, having been seized with distress in heart region; respiration laboured; pulse 51. Had had attacks previously, but lighter, and the pulse in them had always been slow. *Phas.* 6x was given, at first every half-hour, then every hour. Next day patient was nearly well, and said he "could feel every dose working." In a case reported by Cushing, a nurse, 50, "had fearful time with her heart palpitating and feeling as if she should die;" *Phas.* 15x cured. Patient "never took anything in her life that did her so much good" (*H. R.*, xii. 237). Remarkable symptoms of the proving were: *Soreness to touch*—eyeballs, right rib, epigastrium, right humerus. The headache was < by movement of the head or any mental exertion, reading, writing, &c. Pressure <. Breathing slow; pulse slow or extinct.

Relations.—*Compare :* The Leguminosæ. In heart, Dig., Cratæg. Spig., Lach., Thyr. Punctured wounds, Hyper., Led. Diabetes Syzyg., Thyr., Nat. sul., Uran. nit.

SYMPTOMS.

1. **Mind.**—Could only be roused by speaking loudly (D).—Frightened by irregular action of heart (C).—(Feeling that she would die, with palpitation.)

2. **Head.**—Headache, chiefly in forehead and orbits, from fulness of brain ; < every movement of head ; from 12 noon to bedtime ; > in bed, < again 10 a.m. next day.—Pain r. side forehead while writing.—Severe headache, as if something pressing hard against each temple, much < after each dose of *Phas.* (in patient cured of heart symptoms, not a subject of headaches).—Suddenly screamed, "Oh, my head !" grasped it with both hands and was dead (in cancer case taking a decoction of *Phas.*, including dried pod, C).

3. **Eyes.**—Eyeballs (esp. r.) painful to touch as from a blow.—Scalding pain in r. orbit.—Pain in r. orbit when wrinkling skin of forehead.—Very smart itching in inner canthi.—Pain over r. orbit < by any mental exertion.—Pupils widely dilated and insensible (D).

6. **Face.**—Features expressed suffering (D).

11. **Stomach.**—Pain in epigastrium when touched, esp. in region of pylorus.—(*Severe,* dull pain in epigastrium, vomiting, &c., *Phas.* 4x cured.)

12. **Abdomen.**—Pressure on abdomen apparently gave pain, child shrank from it and drew up legs (D).—Pain like hernia in r. inguinal ring, lasting all day.

14. **Urinary Organs.**—Bloody urine.—Diabetes.—Uric acid gravel.

15. **Male Sexual Organs.**—Complete impotence (C).—Prostate, enlargement of.

17. **Respiratory Organs.**—Breathing slow and sighing (D).—(Respirations eight a minute.)

18. **Chest.**—Cartilage of last true r. rib painful as if bruised.—A hard, rounded, projecting, movable tumour, painful to touch, appears suddenly, above r. nipple, in full state of development (15th day).—(Hydrothorax.)

19. **Heart.**—Pulse at wrists rapid and almost imperceptible (D).—Sudden curious sensation in region of heart ; so sudden and strange he immediately felt his pulse and found it very weak and irregular ; was frightened and discontinued the proving (C).—(Sick feeling about heart with weak pulse.)—(Last stage of heart disease, pulseless.—*Phas.* 9x restored pulse, and it remained good till death, three weeks later.)—(For two years, about five times each minute heart would give one hard throb, then omit one beat ; < night. *Phas.* 10 cured this and caused headache.)—(Restored heart action in case of puerperal convulsions and albuminuria when heart failed.)—(Unconscious, pulseless, respirations eight a minute.)—(Distress in region of heart, pulse very slow.—Stone.)—Dropsy of pericardium.)—(Fearful palpitation and feeling that she should die.)

22. **Upper Limbs.**—Pain to touch in extremity of head of r. humerus.

27. **Fever.**—Bedewed with cold perspiration (D).

Phellandrium.

Œnanthe phellandrium. Phellandrium aquaticum. Water dropwort. Fine-leaved water-hemlock. Horse-bane. *N. O.* Umbelliferæ. Tincture of fresh ripe fruit.

Clinical.—Abdomen, coldness in. Asthma. Breasts, affections of. Bronchitis. Catarrh. Ciliary neuralgia. Coryza. Cough. *Headache*, Influenza. Intermittent fever. *Nipples, painful.* Phthisis. Sleeplessness, excessive. Tongue, soreness of.

Characteristics.—*Phelland.* which, like *Œnanthe croc.*, grows in moist places, and even in the water itself, has not shown the poisonous properties of the latter. The provings were made by Nenning and Richter with tincture of the seeds. The symptoms show a general resemblance to those of the poisonous Umbelliferæ—vertigo, headache, nausea, vomiting, diarrhœa, drowsiness and weakness, but *Phelland.* is easily distinguished from the rest in its particular features. The provings developed many symptoms in both mammæ, especially the right, stitches shooting inward being most marked. Clinical experience in nursing women has further brought out its characteristics. The keynote is "Intolerable pain in lactiferous tubes between the acts of nursing." It has also "Pain in nipples on each application of child." Either breast may be affected, but the right breast and nipple were more affected than the left. The breast and chest symptoms have led to the use of *Phelland.* in phthisis and other chest affections, and it is in right-side affections that *Phelland.* has done its best work. The cough is continuous and suffocating; the sputa purulent and horribly offensive. There are also offensive eructations, smelling of bed-bugs. There is burning as from vesicles on the tongue, and again the right border is most affected. Nausea; sick, empty, faint feeling at epigastrium. Burning and stitches. "Desire for acids" is a leading symptom. The headaches and eye-pains are a leading feature of *Phelland.* Headaches involving the eyes; with inflammation of the eyes. Heavy headaches; as if a crushing weight were on vertex; as if the head would be drawn back by a weight in the nape. Ciliary neuralgia. Obscured vision. *Phelland.* has the sense of enlargement of the head with fulness. Abnormal sleepiness following confinement has been cured by it. Goullon, junr., calls attention to the value of *Phelland.* as a cough remedy (*H. R.*, iii. 151). He regards it as a "universal cough remedy," but particularly useful in phthisicy coughs. He gives this case: Mrs. E., of spare build, has almost always a slight cough, and has had repeated attacks of influenza of weeks' and even months' duration. Of late she suffers early in the morning with continuous cough for an hour or more accompanied by dyspnœa and prostration. *Phelland.* 2x in water, thrice daily, effected a rapid cure. *Phelland.* 2x also cured a young teacher who was harassed by a chronic persistent cough. A. J. T. (*H. R.*, i. 170) with *Phelland.* 200 removed in an inveterate coffee-drinker this symptom: "In the evening turns purplish-red in the face, with staring eyes and extreme difficulty in breathing." He found in an old repertory under

Phelland. : "Livid redness of face 7 to 8 p.m." Ussher (*H. W.*, xxiv. 20) had a patient who suffered from excessive sleepiness after the birth of her last child. She would even go to sleep standing over her washtub. *Phelland.* φ, and later 200, repeated thrice daily, quickly relieved her. *Peculiar sensations* are : As if head were moving to and fro. Sound in brain as if striking a piece of silver. As if a stone or lump of lead on vertex. As if a red-hot iron were moved close to left side of neck. As if blood-vessels in whole body were in vibrating motion. Though there were many symptoms of heat and burning, symptoms of coldness are also pronounced. Coldness of head with headache (also sweat with headache) ; coldness in abdomen, with movements ; icy coldness after stool. *Phelland.* is *suited to* : Persons of a feeble, irritable, lymphatic temperament, with weak and deficient nutrition. The symptoms are < in open air ; after dinner ; during and after eating ; on appearance of menses ; sitting ; standing ; lying down ; after spirituous drinks ; after drinking water ; while swallowing ; after stool (coldness in abdomen). > In open air (vertigo and head symptoms) ; during dinner (headache) ; eating bread (sore throat) ; motion, in open air ; lying on left side ; scratching ; rubbing. Chilliness predominates, and the catarrh and asthma of *Phelland.* are > in warm and < in cold seasons. Open air = sense of intoxication ; < vertigo. < During increasing moon.

Relations.—*Antidoted by* : Rheum (diarrhœa). *Compare* : Breast symptoms, Con., Phyt., Bry., Ol. an. (Ol. an. has stitches shooting *out* ; Phelland. stitches shooting *in*). Painful nursing, Crot. t. (pains in breast go through to back when nursing), Bov. (empty feeling). Stitches, K. ca. Headache involving eyes, Onos. Pains in right chest, Zn. (right apex, Calc., Ars. ; r. middle, Sep. ; right base, Chel., Lachn., K. ca., Sep. ; left apex, Ars. ; left base, Ox. ac., Sul.). Last stage of phthisis, sputa terribly offensive, Sil. Offensive breath with cough, Caps. Sleepiness, Op., Nux m.

SYMPTOMS.

1. **Mind.**—Character sad, anxious, profoundly meditative, sometimes given to extravagant merriment.—Peevish arrogance.

2. **Head.**—Confusion in head, as from intoxication.—Heaviness of head, as if too large and too full ; as if it would be drawn back by a weight in nape.—Vertigo, which almost occasions falling backward, forward, or sideways, esp. to side to which one turns in room ; < (sometimes >) in open air, > by lying down.—Sound in brain as if one were beating on a metal that was freely swinging, which woke him, after which the sound died away (5 a.m.).—Headache, which disappears in open air, and during dinner.—Headache with perspiration on top of head, fifteen minutes after dinner, soon followed by coldness of the head.—Dizzy headache in (l.) forehead with increased warmth of head and hands without perspiration.—Headache involving nerves going to eyes, crushing feeling on vertex with burning of eyes and lachrymation.—Painful heaviness of vertex as if a hard body were lying on it.—Pain like weight on vertex with aching, burning, shooting pains in temples.—Compressive pain in sides of head.—Digging pain in head.—Ebullition of blood, with

heat and throbbing in head.—In occiput: intermitting pressure; burning, constrictive sensation; tearing; burrowing; stitches.—Itching, biting like flea-bites in scalp.

3. **Eyes.**—Itching in eyes.—Burning sensation in lids, morning and evening.—Frequent twitching of l. lids.—Twitching of lids, which close easily from a sensation of heaviness and sleepiness.—Dryness of eyes, with shooting and burning pain.—Frequent tearing in upper r. orbital margin in the bone.—Ciliary neuralgia, $<$ attempting to read or sew; fearful intolerance of light; lids swollen and half-closed.—Lachrymation, esp. in open air.—Sight cloudy, as if directed through a fog, $<$ when looking intently at any object.

4. **Ears.**—Tearings and boring in ears.—Singing and noises in r. ear.

5. **Nose.**—Nostrils red, burning, and (with upper lip) swollen.—Itching, confluent vesicles in nostrils.—Loss of smell.—Coryza, with obstruction of nose, can only breathe through mouth.

6. **Face.**—Heat in face.—Livid redness of face from 7 to 8 p.m.—Tension in skin of face.—Violent, and almost tearing, quivering in cheek.

8. **Mouth.**—Toothache with tearing or shooting pain.—Gums red, swollen, and painful.—Dryness of mouth and throat at night.—Increase of frothy saliva in mouth, which it is necessary to expectorate.—Burning pain and burning vesicles on tongue (r. margin towards lip).—Clammy or cheese-like taste.—Sweetish taste after drinking water.—Beer has a bitter taste.

9. **Throat.**—Sore throat, with pressive and shooting pain when not swallowing, and during empty deglutition, but not when swallowing food.

11. **Stomach.**—Thirst for milk and for beer, with repugnance to and dread of water.—Desire for acid drinks with thirst.—Disgust and nausea with inclination to vomit and to eructate.—Offensive risings, which have the smell of bugs, or with taste of food.—Pain in stomach, as if it were empty.—Sensation as if stomach were full of water, that would run up, followed by a sensation as if a large round body were twisting about in stomach, that afterwards fell downward, followed by rumbling in stomach.—Burning pain in stomach.

12. **Abdomen.**—Pinchings in the abdomen.—Sensation of coldness in the abdomen, with movements in intestines.—Icy coldness in intestines; after stool; after spirituous drinks.—Burning extending from abdomen up into stomach, following eructations of the drug.—Pinching and cutting pains as if diarrhœa would come on.—Cutting and pinching in hypogastrium.—Dull stitch in r. flank; on bending to that side violent shock in r. inguinal region, after dinner.—Incarcerated flatus in hypochondria and lumbar region.

13. **Stool and Anus.**—Hard fæces, with clawing and pressure at anus.—Liquid evacuation, with tenesmus, followed by pain as of excoriation in anus.—Abundant expulsion of flatus during and after the evacuation.—Burning in anus.—Itching in anus that becomes a burning after rubbing.

14. **Urinary Organs.**—Pale and scanty urine.—Desire to urinate, but only very little passed, with violent burning in evening.—Urine pale, almost greenish.

15. **Male Sexual Organs.**—Itching on prepuce, $>$ by scratching.

16. **Female Sexual Organs.**—Menses too early.—At commencement of menses, lassitude, yawning, and bruised pain in thighs.—She could neither sit, stand, nor lie for the pain.—Menses flowed only morning and evening,

and rather more profusely than usual.—Menses that had just begun ceased.—Menses twelve days early, lasting only a day and a half, very scanty, though without any difficulties, quite unusual.—Pain in nipples on each application of child.—Always after nursing intolerable pain in r. breast along course of lactiferous tubes; physical and mental distress; hysterical weeping; this occurred some time after micturition, the nipples were sore with purulent discharge, the pain appearing after nipples were healed.—Intolerable pains in lactiferous tubes between the acts of nursing.

17. **Respiratory Organs.**—Hoarseness and roughness in throat and fluent coryza.—Suffocating, dry cough, with shortness of breath.—Nocturnal cough from accumulation of mucus in throat.—Frequent expectoration of mucus, without cough, in morning.—Shortness of breath, esp. when walking.

18. **Chest.**—Oppression of chest when standing and taking a deep inspiration.—Stitches in chest.—(Phthisis, esp. of r. lung; cavity; burning on breathing; continuous cough; profuse sweat; diarrhœa; vomiting of food; copious purulent sputa, terribly offensive; emaciation.)—Pressure on side of chest in bed in morning, which disappears when lying on the side affected.—Sharp stitches, extending inward beneath l. mamma, not affected by breathing.—Painful tearing stitches extend through whole l. mamma.—Violent stitch through r. mamma, near sternum, extending to back between shoulders, then down into r. side of sacrum, that was very painful on breathing, immediately after dinner.—Biting sticking in r. nipple, evening before lying down.

20. **Neck and Back.**—Sensation on l. side of neck below jaw as if red-hot iron were moved along close to the part.—Tearing in l. side of neck to jaw.—Stitches: between shoulders; in lower end of l. scapula; in sacrum.—Pain as from a bruise in loins when seated.

22. **Upper Limbs.**—Tearing in shoulders and arms.

23. **Lower Limbs.**—Tearing along anterior surface of r. thigh.—Vibration in calves.—Sensation as of congested blood in knees.

24. **Generalities.**—Tearing pains in limbs.—Sensation of trembling in all the vessels of the body.—The majority of symptoms appear when patient is quietly seated, standing, or lying down; they are > by movement and in open air.—Great dejection and lassitude.

25. **Skin.**—Itching, sometimes burning or smarting, disappearing quickly when the parts are scratched.—Small blue spots, like petechiæ.

26. **Sleep.**—Sleepiness during day, with frequent yawning.—So sleepy would fall asleep standing at work, lasting an hour.—Retarded sleep.—Frequent and early waking, or prolonged sleep in morning.—Dreams: of lightning with fright; of a robbery in which he received many blows.

27. **Fever.**—Predominance of shivering, sometimes with shaking chills, generally neither accompanied nor followed by heat or thirst.—Shuddering, generally in evening, sometimes as if cold water had been poured over body.—Inability to urinate the day after ague attack.—Accelerated pulse.

Phenacetinum.

Para-acetphenatidine. $C_6H_4OC_2H_5NHC_2H_3O$.

Clinical.—Cyanosis. Face, eruption on. Fevers. Headache. Perspiration, excessive. Typhoid fever. Uræmia.

Characteristics.—*Phenacet.* belongs to the Aniline group, and was introduced into old-school practice as a remedy in febrile states and neuralgias, free from the dangers of *Antfeb.*, *Antipyr.*, *Exalg.*, &c. Though not so dangerous as these, it is not free from ill effects. These have been well summed up by F. G. Oehme (*H. R.*, xv. 506), and I have put them in Schema form, and added a symptom observed by myself on a young lady who had taken *Phenacet.* for headaches: A circumscribed rash on both cheeks which came out red, lasted four days and then peeled, and as soon as it was clear the process was repeated. I tried many remedies with varying success, but it finally disappeared under *Alm.* 30, one powder at bedtime.

SYMPTOMS.

1. **Mind.**—Anxiety.

2. **Head.**—Vertigo, faintness.—Headache and flushed face.

3. **Eyes.**—Œdema of lower lids and fingers.

4. **Ears.**—Permanent deafness.

6. **Face.**—Circumscribed, erythematous, exfoliating eruption on both cheeks; fading away and recurring for several weeks (finally cured with *Alm.* 30).

11. **Stomach.**—Nausea; epigastric pains.

14. **Urinary Organs.**—Large doses may cause uræmia.—Frequent urination at night (cured in two cases).

17. **Respiratory Organs.**—Dyspnœa.

19. **Heart.**—Decrease of cardiac vigour; pulse slow, almost imperceptible.

24. **Generalities.**—Severe cyanosis, esp. of limbs, chilliness, nausea, epigastric pains, faintness, vertigo.—Trembling from nervous excitement.—Weakness and numbness of whole body, cold perspiration, collapse.

25. **Skin.**—Febrile exanthema; patches profusely scattered on limbs, scanty on trunk; disappearing on pressure, headache, flushed face (from five grains daily).

26. **Sleep.**—Incessant yawning; drowsiness.

27. **Fever.**—Chilliness.—Sweating; frequently profuse in low states of the system.

Phlorizinum.

Phlorizin. (A substance discovered in the fresh bark of the Apple, Pear, Cherry, and Plum.) $C_{21}H_{24}O_{10}$. Solution. Trituration.

Clinical.—Diabetes. Herpes preputialis. Intermittent fever.

Characteristics.—*Phloriz.* exists in fine, silky, four-sided, colourless needles, soluble in water. It has a bitter and slightly astringent taste, and has been used in old-school practice as a remedy for intermittent fever, and whilst being administered for this it has produced glycosuria. This observation has led to its successful use by homœopaths in cases of diabetes. Successes with the 3x and 6 have been reported. A patient to whom it was given by Burnett accused him of having given him *a preparation of apples*. The man discovered it because it produced herpes along the dorsum of the penis, an effect which invariably occurred whenever he ventured to eat apples. V. Mering. (*H. W.*, xxiv. 535) produced glycosuria in dogs with *Phlor.*; but if *Syzyg.* was given simultaneously with *Phlor.*, no glycosuria appeared.

Phosphoricum Acidum.

Phosphoric acid. H_3PO_4. Dilution. (The dilute acid of B.P. forms the homœopathic 1 x. In U.S. the first solution is made of glacial Phosphoric Acid.)

Clinical.—*Amblyopia.* Asthma. Boils. *Brain-fag.* Bronchitis; capillary. Chancre. Chilblains. Cholera. Climacteric flushes and vertigo. Coccygodynia. Condylomata. Corns. Cough. Coxalgia. *Debility. Diabetes. Diarrhœa.* Dyspepsia. *Emissions. Enteric fever.* Enuresis. *Feet, sore.* Flatulence. Ganglion. Gout. *Gravel. Hair, falling off. Headache*; of school children. Hectic. Herpes. *Hip-joint disease. Home-sickness. Impotence. Joints, scrofulous.* Lactation defective. Levitation. Lienteria. Locomotor ataxy. Love, disappointed. Masturbation. *Mental weakness.* Mercurial syphilis. Navel, pains in. Neurasthenia. Nymphomania. Osteo-myelitis. *Perspiration, profuse.* Phosphaturia. *Physometra.* Pimples. *Pregnancy, diarrhœa of*; nausea of. Prepuce, warts on. Psoas abscess. Puerperal eclampsia. *Purpura.* Rheumatism. Sciatica. Scurvy. *Self-abuse. Spermatorrhœa.* Spinal caries. Sycosis Hahnemanni. Syphilis. Tetters. Typhus fever. Ulcers. *Urine, phosphatic.* Uterus, prolapse of. Varices. Vertigo. Warts. Wens. Worms.

Characteristics.—*Phos. ac.* is less poisonous than *Phos.* Our chief knowledge of it is derived from Hahnemann's provings in *M. M. P.* These show a marked action on the emotional and sensorial faculties, a drowsy, depressed, apathetic state being produced, such as is not unfrequently met with in typhoid fevers. The keynote of the *Phos. ac.* stupor is that the patient is easily aroused and then is fully conscious. Indifference; prostrated and stupefied with grief; effects of disappointed love. Home-sick. The mind is confused; thoughts cannot be connected; thinking makes him dizzy. The legs tremble in walking and the limbs are as difficult to control as the thoughts. Many symptoms of vertigo are produced, and one is peculiar. *Phos.* has a sensation as if the chair he was sitting on was rising; *Phos. ac.* has this: Sensation as if the feet were rising until he stood on his head. This very symptom occurred in a patient of Skinner's suffering from small-pox. The disease had been cut short by *Variol.*, when the patient, a lady, complained that her feet were rising to the ceiling, and begged her nurses to keep them down. *Phos. ac.* speedily put her straight. *Phos. ac.* causes illusions of the senses as well as of the sensorium, bells are heard, ciphers, sparks, &c., are seen. At the same time there is exalted sensitiveness to light, sound, and odours; "odours take away his breath." A remarkable effect was noted by Becher, one of Hahnemann's provers (the same who experienced the topsy-turvy symptom just mentioned), namely, that the right pupil became widely dilate while the left remained normal: the more he strained the eye the wider the pupil became until the iris almost disappeared. Franz had this symptom: "Sees things lying near him (outside the sphere of vision) moving." Meyer had a somewhat analogous mental symptom: "When reading a thousand other thoughts came into his head, and he could not rightly comprehend anything; what he read became as if dark in his head, and he immediately forgot all; what he had long known he could only recall with difficulty." Such states of mind and the senses are frequently observed in those under the influence of grief and other depressing emotions; from over-study; and in the subjects of venereal excesses and seminal loss. But whilst these losses produce extreme weakness of mind and body, and an abashed, sad state of mind with despair of cure, there is one drain which does *not* debilitate—a diarrhœa. "Persistent, painless, watery diarrhœa, often containing undigested particles of food, and which does not debilitate," is a keynote of *Phos. ac.* Another characteristic in connection with the debility of *Phos. ac.* is that though the weakness is very great the patient is *rested by a short sleep.* (*Phos.* also has > by sleep, but not so markedly by a *short* sleep.) The copious discharges of *Phos. ac.* appear in the sweat and urine. The keynote of the enuresis of *Phos. ac.* is that the child passes a *great quantity* of urine. The polyuria and dry mouth and throat give leading correspondences for *Phos. ac.* in diabetes; and when there is in addition a history of sexual excess, or of severe mental or emotional over-strain, the indications will be very clear. White, milky urine; and also white stools, are very characteristic of *Phos. ac.* The urine may be passed clear but turns milky at once, and is very offensive. If flatulence is to be regarded as an excretion that is another instance of the excess of *Phos. ac.* There is meteoristic distension and passing of flatus in large quantities; sometimes with odour of garlic. "Meteoristic distension; rumbling or gurgling and noise as if there were water in abdomen, < when touched and when the body is bent backward and forward." A case quoted from *H. Maandblad.* illustrates the action of *Phos. ac.* in gastric affections. A married woman, 36, mother of eight children, had for some time been so melancholy and depressed as to be unable to fulfil her household duties. There was no discoverable mental cause, though her condition had been made < by a sudden death in the family. The beginning of the illness was apparently a weakness of the stomach: small appetite; always pain and distension after eating; the food seemed to lie long in the stomach undigested. *Phos. ac.* 6x, ten drops three times a day, soon restored the patient. In connection with the flatulence of *Phos. ac.* there is even bloating of the uterus with gas. The menses are excessive and premature; and there are many symptoms connected with the pregnant and puerperal state, including debility from lactation. *Phos. ac.* has many respiratory symptoms, and this is a keynote: "Weak feeling in chest from talking, coughing, or sitting too long; > by walking." Hoarseness and nasal voice; dyspnœa; capillary bronchitis. The cough seems to be caused by tickling of a feather from middle of chest to larynx, low down in chest, about ensiform cartilage, pit of stomach; is < evening after lying down; expectoration muco-purulent; salty; bloody; offensive. Every draught of air = fresh cold. Cough = headache; nausea and vomiting of food; spurting of urine. A very prominent sensation running through the proving is that of *pressure;* pressure as from a crushing weight in vertex, forehead, sternum. Pressure in eyes; in navel; in left breast. Squeezing above the knee; in the soie. The hæmorrhages of *Phos. ac.* are dark, profuse, with passive hæmorrhages. A case of land scurvy (quoted *Amer. Hom.*, xxii. 421) contracted in mining camps presented the usual condition of the gums, and also purpureal spots covering the whole body. Patient was able to be about, and had little pain, but was despondent. Pulse weak, very slow. Had been months ill under old-school treatment. *Merc. sol.* was given but did not relieve. *Phos. ac.* given strong enough to taste acid speedily cured. A peculiar symptom of *Phos. ac.* is involuntary biting of tongue in sleep. The sphincters are weakened, and there is involuntary escape of fæces and urine, the latter especially on coughing or movement. *Peculiar sensations* are: As if intoxicated. As if head would burst. As if feet going up. As if weight in head. As if brain crushed. Bones as if scraped with a knife. As if eyeballs too large. As if white of egg had dried on face. As if lower jaw were going to break. Nausea as if in soft palate; in throat. As if stomach being balanced up and down. Heavy load in stomach. Ants crawling over body. Uterus as if filled with wind. Tickling in chest as with a feather; as with down in larynx. Red-hot coal on arm and shoulder. *Phos. ac.* is *suited to:* (1) Persons of originally strong constitution weakened by loss of fluids; excesses; violent, acute diseases; chagrin or a long succession of moral emotions. (2) Persons of mild disposition. (3) Children and young people who have grown too rapidly, tall, slender, and slim; with pains in back and limbs as if beaten; growing pains. Lutze (*Hahn. Adv.*, 1900, 664) cured with *Phos. ac.* a German woman, 66, of chronic, early morning, painless diarrhœa after the failure of *Pod.* and partial success of *Gels.* The patient had been ill two years, dating from the time she came to Brooklyn from Germany to be near her daughters. One of the latter gave Lutze the keynote of the case by telling him that her mother was *home-sick, and wanted to return to Germany, though she had not a single relative there.*—The symptoms are: < By music (every note = stitch in ears; violent pains in head). Slight shock or noise = pressure in head to be extremely violent. Odours = vomiting. Bad news; depressing emotions = cough, diarrhœa, &c. Touch <. Movement of child = escape of stool. Many symptoms are < evening and night. > After short sleep. Many symptoms are > walking. Sitting <. Standing <. < Lying on left side. < Side on which he lies. < Talking. < From mental affections; suppressed eruptions; loss of fluids, especially seminal; masturbation; perspiration; urination. There is desire for warm food; which > pressive pain in stomach. Warm room <. Warmth of bed > pains in bowels. Aversion to uncover in heat. < By draught; wind; snowy air. Cannot bear draught on chest. Every draught = fresh cold. Catching cold in summer = diarrhœa. Least cold = arthritic pains. Coldness of part < pains. Fresh air = invigoration.

Relations.—*Antidoted by:* Camph., Coff., Staph. *Compatible:* Chi., before or after, in colliquative sweats, diarrhœa, and debility; after Nux in fainting after a meal; after Rhus in typhoid. *Followed well by:* Ars., Bell., Caust., Lyc., Nux, Puls., Sep., Sul., Calc. p., Fer. p., K. ph., Nat. p. *Compare:* Effects of grief, &c., Ign. (Phos. ac. deeper, more settled despair, hair turns grey, crushing weight on vertex). Growing too fast, Calc. (Calc. fast and fat; Phos. ac. fast and tall). School headaches, Nat. m., Calc. ph. Typhoid and typhus, Rhus (both have nose-bleed at beginning of typhus, with Rhus it >; with Phos. ac. not: Phos. ac. follows Rhus; both have > by movement). Cina (bores fingers in nose). Pho. (Pho. has more dryness of tongue, more sensorial excitement and intolerance of noises or odours; if diarrhœa is present it is blood-streaked and looks like flesh water). Nit. s. d. (sensorial apathy); Arn. (more developed stupor); Op. (stertor; countenance deeper red, almost brownish red; Phos. ac. sunken hippocratic). Home-sickness, Caps. (Caps. has red cheeks). Lienteric diarrhœa, Chi. (Chi. exhausts rapidly; Phos. ac. not). Loss of seminal fluids, Chi. (Chi. acute; Phos. ac. chronic effects). Tuberculosis, Pho. (Phos. ac. better than Pho. when there is cough from tickling at ensiform cartilage, < evening and lying down at night; weakness causing dyspnœa; < from draught on chest). Diabetes, Lact. ac. Growing pains, Guaiac. Bad news, effects of, Coloc., Gels. As if white of egg had dried on face, Alm., Bar. acet. Affections of palate, Mang. Aversion to bread; effects of masturbation, Nat. m. Effects of music, Ambra, Pho. Over-lifting, Calc. Nausea at sight of food, especially during pregnancy, Eu. perf.; at sight of food, Colch., Lyc., Mosch., Phos. ac., Saba., Spi.; at smell of food, Colch., Eu. perf. Inquietude about health and life, Calc., Pho. Apathy, K. ca. (Phos. ac. sensorial; K. ca. from exhaustion—puerperal mania, puerperal fever). Cerebro-spinal exhaustion from overwork, Pic. ac. Apathy with indifference (Mur. ac. taciturnity with indifference; Sul. listless; Hell. n. not easily roused). Mild, yielding disposition, Puls. Headache > by lying down, Bry., Gels., Sil. Neurosis in stump after amputation, Cepa. Masturbation when patient distressed by culpability of act, Dros., Staph. Sycosis, Thuj., Sabi. Escape of urine during cough, Caust., Nat. m., Puls. Nausea in throat, Cupr., Cycl., Pul., Stan. Feet as if in air, Passif.

Causation.—Bad news. Grief. Chagrin. Disappointed love.

Separation from home. Loss of fluids. Sexual excesses. Injuries. Operations. Over-lifting. Over-study. Shock.

SYMPTOMS.

1. **Mind.**—Disposition to weep, as from nostalgia.—Bad effects from grief, sorrow, unfortunate love, with great emaciation, sleepiness, and morning sweat.—Sadness and uneasiness respecting the future.—Anxious inquiries respecting the disease under treatment.—Restlessness and precipitation.—Silent (sadness) peevishness and aversion to conversation.—Great indifference.—A complete indifference to everything; not a soporous, delirious, or irritable condition, but simply an indifferent state of mind to all things; patient does not want anything, nor to speak, shows no interest in the outside world (may occur in any disease in fevers of very low type).—Difficulty of comprehension, patient will think a little while about a question, perhaps answers it, then forgets all about it; dizziness of the mind.—When reading, a thousand other thoughts came into his head, could not rightly comprehend anything; what he read became as if dark in his head and he immediately forgot all; what he had long known he could only recall with difficulty.—Inability to endure noise or conversation.—Dulness and indolence of mind, with want of imagination.—Weakness of memory.—Imbecility.—Cannot connect his thoughts.—Paucity of ideas and unfitness for intellectual labour.—Illusions of the senses; hears a bell pealing; sees only ciphers before his eyes.

2. **Head.**—Vertigo: head sinks forward or backward; on closing eyes; at climaxis with flushes and sweat; in typhus; when lying in bed, as if feet were going up and he was standing on his head; after reflection.—Stupefaction in forehead, with somnolency without snoring, eyes closed.—Head bewildered, as after intoxication or immoderate pollutions.—Sensation as if intoxicated, evening, in warm room, with humming in head, which feels as if it would burst when coughing.—Stunning vertigo when standing and walking, esp. in evening.—Pressure as from a weight in head, or as if vertex had been beaten.—Headache in morning.—Aching with tingling in head.—Headache usually from behind forward.—Constant headache, which compels to lie down, < to an insupportable degree by the slightest commotion or by noise.—Heaviness of head, as if full of water.—Violent pressure in forehead in morning on waking.—As if temples and sides of head were squeezed together by forceps.—Cramp-like and hard pressure in head, < by pressing on head and by turning it; also by meditation and by going up stairs, but esp. after midnight, in the part which presses pillow.—Compression in brain.—Tearing headache.—Lancinations in temples or above eyes.—Stitches over one (the r.) eye.—Jerks or shocks, blows and hammering in head.—Drawing pains in bones of occiput.—Grey, lank hair, like tow.—The hair becomes grey early or flaxen, and very greasy, falls off; also hair of beard, esp. after grief and sorrow.—Pain in bones of skull; it feels as if somebody scraped the swollen and tender periosteum with a knife, < at rest, > from motion; caries of skull with burning pain.—Itching of scalp.

3. **Eyes.**—Eyes dull, glassy (but without lustre), downcast.—Pressure in eyes, with sensation as if eyeballs too large; as if eyeballs were forcibly pressed together and into head.—Coldness in internal surface of lids.—Eyes

dazzled on looking at bright objects.—Burning pain in lids and their angles, esp. by candle-light in evening.—Inflammation in eyes, with congestion of veins in internal angles.—Agglutination, mornings.—Inflammation of lids.—Hordeolum.—Yellow spot in sclerotica.—Lachrymation.—Pupils dilated.—R. pupil much dilated, l. pupil constantly normal.—Fixed look.—Sight confused as if directed through a mist.—Myopia.—Black band before eyes ; ciphers ; sees objects lying near him (outside sphere of vision) moving.—A dull, shooting, burning pain forced r. eyeball to its outer canthus ; could then see nothing with this eye but a limitless white expanse with fiery points falling on it ; later, expanse became fiery and the falling points dazzling white.

4. **Ears.**—Shootings in ears, sometimes with drawing in cheeks, jaws, and teeth, < only by sound of music.—At every stroke of a bell or musical note stitches in ears like earache, also on singing himself ; non-musical sounds had no effect.—Cramp-like drawings in ears.—Inability to endure music, noise, and conversation.—Every sound re-echoes loudly in the ears.—Nervous deafness, shrill sounds most painful and most distressing (R. T .C.).—Deafness for distant sounds.—Squeaking in ear on blowing nose.—Roaring in ears with difficult hearing.

5. **Nose.**—Swelling on bridge of nose with red spots.—(Redness of tip of nose with dyspepsia.—R. T. C.)—Each dose (3x) goes to his nose as effervescing waters do, and < the redness (agg.—R. T. C.).—Scabs on nose.—Disposition to put fingers into nose.—Itching on point of nose ; must scratch there.—Fetid exhalation from nose.—Discharge of (bloody) pus from nose.—Epistaxis (dark blood).—Violent coryza, with redness of margins of nostrils.—Fluent coryza, with cough and burning pain in chest and throat.

6. **Face.**—Face pale, wan, with (lustreless) hollow eyes surrounded by a blue circle, and pointed nose.—Drawings in cheeks and jaws.—Irregular features.—Heat of side of face on which he is not lying.—Heat in face, with tension of skin of face, as if the white of an egg had dried upon it.—Large pimples on face.—Burning pain in cheeks.—Humid and scabious tetters on cheeks, lips, and commissures.—Lips dry, scurfy, covered with suppurating cracks, with pains as from excoriation.—Yellow-brown, crust-like eruptions, with pus on lower lip towards corner of mouth.—Pimples and scabs on red part of lips.—Violent burning pain in r. lower lip, persisting when moving it.—Pimples on chin.—Swelling of sub-maxillary glands.—Pain in lower jaw as if dislocated.

7. **Teeth.**—Toothache with tearing pain (burning in the front teeth), < by heat of bed and by cold or hot things.—Violent pains in incisors at night.—Violent aching in a hollow tooth when particles of food get into it, going off when they have been removed.—The teeth are yellow.—Gums bleeding easily, swollen, stand off from teeth.—Painful nodosities in the gums.

8. **Mouth.**—Dryness of mouth and palate without thirst.—Viscid, tenacious phlegm in mouth and on tongue.—Shootings and burning sensation on tongue.—Involuntary biting of tongue at night.—Swelling of tongue, with pain when speaking.—Red streak in middle of tongue, widens in front.—Nasal tone of voice.—Smarting in mouth during mastication of solid food.—Excoriation and ulceration of velum palati, with burning pain.

9. **Throat.**—Pain as from excoriation in throat, with smarting, scraping,

and shooting, esp. during passage of food.—Contractive pain in pit of throat. —Hawking up of tough mucous phlegm.

10. **Appetite.**—Loss of appetite.—Putrid, acid, herbaceous taste.—Prolonged after-taste of food, and esp. of bread.—Repugnance to bread, which seems bitter.—Aversion to coffee.—Violent thirst for cold milk or for beer, as well as in general for cool and juicy things; bread appears too dry.—Insatiable thirst, excited by a sensation of dryness in whole body.—Acids excite bitter risings and other inconveniences.—Ate heartily, much oppressed after with flatulence.—After a meal pressure, or a sensation of wavering in stomach, with confusion of head, uneasiness, fulness, and disposition to sleep, or dejection, as if about to faint.

11. **Stomach.**—Sour, incomplete, or burning risings.—Constant nausea in throat.—Nausea which compels lying down.—Nausea at sight of food.—Vomiting of food.—Sour vomiting.—Pressive pain in stomach, as from a weight, when fasting, and after any food whatever (with sleepiness), as also on touching pit of stomach.—Sensation of coldness or of burning in stomach. —Feeling in stomach as if everything had stuck fast and was dry.

12. **Abdomen.**—Spasmodic aching, with (pressure and) anguish in hypochondria, and esp. in liver.—Sensation as if liver were too heavy.—Shootings in regions of liver and spleen.—General tympanites with enlarged spleen.—In navel periodical aching, squeezing.—Contractions in abdomen on both sides of umbilical region.—Spasmodic pains in abdomen, esp. in umbilical region.—Shootings and cuttings in abdomen.—Sensitiveness in lower cæcal region.—Burning sensation in hypogastrium.—Meteoristic distension of and frequent grumbling and borborygmi in abdomen, as if from water in it; esp. when it is touched, and when the body is bent backwards and forwards.—Production and expulsion of much flatus, esp. after eating acid things.—Swelling of inguinal glands.

13. **Stool and Anus.**—Hard fæces in small portions, difficult to evacuate.—Frequent evacuations.—Diarrhœa, particularly painless, which may be very fetid.—Diarrhœa lasting a long time, apparently without any weakening effect.—Stools: loose, slimy, whitish-grey; undigested, greenish-white.—Yellowish and very offensive.—Escape of stool when child is moved or turned.—Involuntary stools of the consistence of pap (bright yellow), with sensation as if flatus were expelled.—Choleraic diarrhœa as if rectum remained open.—(Chronic diarrhœa, thin and greenish, almost involuntary with gastric irritability.—A. E. Small.).—In evening great discharge of garlic-smelling flatus; great yawning.—Protrusion of hæmorrhoidal tumours from rectum during stool.—Intolerable pain in hæmorrhoids when sitting.—After stool tenesmus; sickening pain about navel.—Tearing, smarting, and itching in anus and rectum.—Itching prick on outer circumference of anus.

14. **Urinary Organs.**—Urgent want to urinate, with scanty emission of urine, paleness of face, heat, and thirst.—Frequent and profuse emission of aqueous urine, which immediately deposits a thick and white cloud.—Urine like milk, with sanguineous and gelatinous coagulum.—Fetid urine.—Flow of urine with spasmodic pains in loins.—Urgent and irresistible desire to urinate.—Urine like that which passes in diabetes mellitus.—Anguish and uneasiness before urinating.—Nocturnal enuresis.—Children pass a *great deal* of water in bed at night; persons get up in the night to urinate and pass a

great deal.—Burning pain in urethra during and after emission of urine; cutting before.—Creeping in urethra when not urinating.—Spasmodic (painful) constriction of bladder (without urging).—Incisive pains in urethra when making water.

15. **Male Sexual Organs.**—Lancinating pains in glans.—Fine pricking at point of penis.—Burning cutting in glans with an out-pressing pain in both groins.—A feeling of heaviness in glans, esp. when urinating.—Tingling and oozing vesicles round frænum.—Sycotic excrescences with heat and burning.—Crop of warts on prepuce.—A crop of pedunculated warts come round corona glandis after taking *Pho. ac.* in summer drinks (agg.—R. T. C.).—Condylomata.—Eruption on penis and scrotum.—Inflammatory swelling of scrotum.—Pain in testes when touched.—Gnawing pain in testes.—Swelling of testes (l.), while spermatic cord is enlarged, hard, and tightened.—Absence of sexual desire.—Frequent erections (in morning in bed; in morning when standing), without desire for coition.—Weakness of sexual organs, with onanism, and little sexual desire.—Exhaustion after coition.—Frequent and very debilitating pollutions, esp. where the patient is much affected by the flow.—Onanism; esp. when patient is much distressed by the culpability of the act.—Discharge of semen when straining during an evacuation.

16. **Female Sexual Organs.**—Oophoritis, metritis, or prolapsus from debilitating or emotional influences; amenorrhœa.—Very irritable uterus.—Uterine ulcer, with copious, putrid, bloody discharge, itching or corroding pain, or no pain.—Hepatic pains during menses.—Menses too early and too long; too copious; too late; dark clotted; preceded by leucorrhœa, and for one or two days by griping and rumbling in abdomen.—Yellowish, itching leucorrhœa after menses.—Distension of uterus as by gas.—Itching pricking like flea-bites between mammæ, obliging her to rise at night.—Dysuria during pregnancy; cutting pains.—Vomiting at sight of food during pregnancy.—Puerperal convulsions; albuminuria; hæmorrhage.—Scanty milk with debility and great apathy.—Deterioration of health during nursing.—Constant vomiting of milk in a suckling; waxy face; blue rings round eyes; child does not cry; mother has little milk.—Sharp pressure on l. breast; and nipple.

17. **Respiratory Organs.**—Voice nasal.—Great hoarseness and roughness in throat.—Pain in pit of throat, which contracts throat.—Cough excited by a tickling and a scraping in larynx; or above epigastrium, which is dry in evening, and with a yellowish-white expectoration in morning.—The cough is < morning and evening; during rest if one sits or lies long in the same position; after sleeping; from cold air; from loss of fluids.—(Cough after food of any kind.)—Cough with (nausea) vomiting of food and headache; involuntary emission of urine.—During cough expectoration (of dark blood, or of tough white mucus, tasting acid), having an herbaceous smell and taste.—Cough with purulent (very offensive) expectoration and pains in chest.—Salty expectoration in morning.

18. **Chest.**—Shortness of breath and inability to speak long, from weakness of chest.—Capillary bronchitis, < evenings, with fever, pain under sternum, then violent sneezing, thirst and coryza, profuse, purulent secretion.—Spasmodic and contractive oppression of chest, as if tightened.—Weakness in chest after speaking.—Pressure at chest often spasmodic or incisive.—Pressive

pain in middle of chest, < when expiring; felt as if sternum would be pressed out; < by pressure with hand, stooping, coughing, &c.—Pressure behind sternum rendering inspiration difficult.—Lancinations in sides of chest.—Burning and pressure in chest.

19. **Heart and Pulse.**—Stitches through heart.—Palpitation: in young persons growing too fast; after onanism.—Pulse irregular, with irregular beating of heart; pulse intermitting.—Swollen veins.

20. **Neck and Back.**—Tension and cramp-like drawing in muscles of neck, esp. on moving head.—Miliaria on neck.—Boils under axillæ; on nates.—Boring pain between scapulæ.—Spondylitis of cervical vertebræ.—Eruption, painful to touch, on back, shoulder-blades, neck, and chest.—Burning pain in a spot above small of back.—Itching stitch in coccyx; fine stitches in coccyx and sternum.—Crawling (formication) tingling in back and loins.

21. **Limbs.**—Bruised feeling in hips, thighs, arms, nape, like growing pains; at same time repeated single tearing stitches in all these parts at once; the stitches occur on commencing to walk, esp. to go up stairs; bruised pain continues all the time.—Bruised pain in all joints in morning, and in arms and legs.—Burning, gnawing, tearing pains in bones of extremities.—Weakness of extremities after loss of fluids.

22. **Upper Limbs.**—Boring, digging, drawing pain in l. shoulder-joint, intermittent, < lying on l. side, > moving arms.—Cramp-like pressure in arms, hands, and fingers.—Drawings and jerking tearings in arms and fingers.—Eruption of pimples on arms.—Drawing, incisive pains in joints of elbows, hands, and fingers.—Sharp, shooting, boring pains under l. forearm near elbow, < at rest.—Numbness in course of r. radial nerve.—Weakness and trembling of arms.—Trembling of hands (when writing).—Ganglion on back of hand.—Skin of hands and fingers dry, shrivelled, parched.—Fingers dead, sometimes on one side only, and within well-defined limits.—Lancinations (stitches) in fingers and joints of fingers.

23. **Lower Limbs.**—Swelling and furunculi on buttocks.—Contusive pains in hips and thighs, esp. when walking or rising from a seat.—On l. hip-joint and l. thigh, a neuralgic or rheumatic pain, from gluteal muscles or hip-joint, running down leg to knee, and often to calf or ankle; gets a little > after walking, but is still very bad.—Cramp in coxo-femoral joint, with tearing throughout the limb, insupportable when seated, and during repose.—Aching, cramp-like pains in thighs, legs, feet, and toes.—Tearing throughout leg, with heaviness in joints.—Weakness of legs, so that a false step (or tripping) occasions falling.—Burning tearing in tibia at night.—Pimples on knees and legs, which become confluent, and are transformed into easily bleeding ulcers.—Itching ulcers on legs.—Burning sensation in feet and soles, with excoriation between toes.—Swelling of feet.—Feet swollen and sore on putting on walking shoes.—In evening spasmodic drawing in feet, < r. sole and ball of great toe, preventing sleep till midnight.—Sweating of feet.—Corns on feet.—Blisters on balls of toes.—Chilblains on toes.—Swelling of joint of great toe, with burning, throbbing, and incisive, dull pains on being touched.

24. **Generalities.**—Affections of any kind in inner navel; lower part of chest, buttocks, thighs, external side.—Squeezing or contracting pain; lassitude of the body; feeling very weak.—Drawings and jerking tearings in limbs.—Cramp-like, pressive pains.—Painfulness in general in bones or

periosteum.—Sensation as if the periosteum were scraped with a knife; after contusions.—Aching, burning, tearing pains at night.—Swelling (and sponginess) of the bones or periosteum; burning sphacelus.—Caries with smarting pains.—Neurosis of stump after amputation.—Ulcers with stinking pus; painless.—Burning through lower half of body from small of back and pit of stomach downwards, while extremities are cold to touch.—Weakness from loss of fluids without any other pain than burning.—Swellings of glands.—Contusive pain in limbs and joints, as from paralysis, or like growing pains, esp. morning and evening.—Numbness and weakness of limbs.—Heaviness in limbs and joints, with great indolence.—Great fatigue after walking.—Great general weakness, physical or nervous, with strong tendency to perspire, during day (esp. in morning), or with burning sensation in body.—Very pale face; nausea in throat.—Emaciation, with sickly complexion, and eyes surrounded by a livid circle.—Sensation as if body and limbs were bruised, as from growing, esp. in morning.—Formication in different parts.—Agreeable feeling of buoyancy and lightness.—Violent ebullition of blood, with great agitation.—The pains are < during repose, and > by movement, and those which manifest themselves at night are > by pressure.—Symptoms < from mental affections; after suppression of cutaneous eruptions, *i.e.*, any bad result that ensues from such suppression; from loss of fluids, particularly seminal; sunlight; masturbation; after perspiration; sexual excesses, talking, esp. when it causes a weakness in the chest; while urinating.

25. **Skin.**—Insensibility of skin.—Crawling tingling under skin.—Formication of skin.—Red and burning spots on limbs.—Eruption like scarlatina.—Erysipelatous inflammations.—Eruption of small pimples, and of miliary pimples collected in clusters and red.—Eruption of pimples with burning pain, or pain as from excoriation.—Scabious vesicles.—Humid and dry tetters, squamous; variola.—Corns with shootings and burning pain.—Chilblains.—Wens.—Warts: large, jagged, often pedunculated, exuding moisture and bleeding readily; indented.—Condylomata.—Furunculi.—Flat, indolent ulcers, with secretion of a dirty-looking pus, and having a serrated bottom.—Itching ulcers.

26. **Sleep.**—Great tendency to go to sleep during day, early in evening, and in morning, with difficulty in waking.—Coma.—Retarded sleep and sleeplessness at night, caused by agitation and dry heat.—Arithmetical figures appear before eyes on falling asleep.—Profound sleep; can scarcely be roused in morning.—Jerking and involuntary movements of hands, moaning, talking, and singing, or an aspect during sleep at one time of laughing, at another of weeping, with eyes half-opened and convulsed.—Anxious dreams of death, with fear on waking.—Lascivious dreams, with emissions.—Awakened by: canine hunger; dry heat; sensation of falling; sad thoughts.—Patient though quite weak is rested by a very short sleep.

27. **Fever.**—Pulse irregular, sometimes intermitting one or two beats, generally small, weak, or frequent, at times full and strong.—Violent ebullitions with great restlessness.—Swollen veins.—Shuddering and shivering, sometimes with shaking, or with coldness in hands and fingers, generally in evening, and without thirst (followed by heat without thirst, or by excessive heat, depriving one almost of consciousness).—Sensation of coldness on one side of the face.—Sensation of coldness, with shiverings and coldness in

abdomen.—Internal dry heat without being hot to touch; and without any complaint at any time of the day.—General heat with loss of consciousness and somnolence.—Heat in head with cold feet.—Febrile heat in evening, without thirst, with anguish, and great activity of the circulation.—Shivering alternately with heat.—Malignant (typhus) fever with great weakness (quiet delirium with dulness of head), apathy, stupidity, aversion to conversation, diarrhœa, &c.—Tertian ague with profuse perspiration, anxiety of look, thirst and vomiting.—Night-sweat.—Sweat in morning.—Perspiration mostly on back part of head and in neck, with sleepiness during the day.—Profuse perspirations during night and in morning, with anxiety.—Great inclination to perspire during day and night; clammy perspirations.

Phosphorus.

The Element. P. (A. W. 30.96). Saturated solution in absolute alcohol. Trituration of Red amorphous Phosphorus.

Clinical.—Alopecia areata. *Amaurosis. Amblyopia. Anæmia, acute pernicious.* Anus, fissure of. *Antrum, disease of. Arteries, disease of.* Asthma. *Bone, diseases of. Brain, affections of;* softening of. Brain-fag. Breast, abscess of; fistulæ of. *Bronchitis;* membranous. *Cancer; of bone. Cataract.* Catarrh; intestinal; nasal. Chilblains. Chlorosis. Chorea. Ciliary neuralgia. Coccygodynia. Cold. Constipation. *Consumption. Corpulency. Cough.* Croup. Dandruff. Diarrhœa. Dropsy. *Ecchymosis. Enteric fever.* Ephelis. Epilepsy. *Erotomania.* Exophthalmos. Exostosis. *Eyes, affections of.* Fainting. *Fatty degeneration.* Fistula. Flatulence. Fungus hæmatoides. *Gastritis.* Glaucoma. Gleet. *Gums, ulceration of. Hæmoglobinuria. Hæmorrhagic diathesis.* Headache. *Heart, degeneration of;* murmurs of. Hydrocele. *Hydrocephalus.* Hysteria. Impotence. Intussusception. *Jaundice;* malignant; of pregnancy; of anæmia. *Jaw, disease of. Joints, affections of.* Keratitis. *Lactation, disorders of. Laryngitis.* Levitation. Lightning, effects of. Lienteria. *Liver, diseases of; acute yellow atrophy of. Locomotor ataxy. Lungs, hæmorrhage from;* œdema of; paralysis of. Marasmus. Menorrhagia. *Menstruation, symptoms before. Mollities ossium. Morphœa. Muscæ volitantes. Nævus. Nails, ulcers round. Neuralgia.* Nightmare. Nipples, sore. *Nose, bleeding from. Numbness.* Nymphomania. *Odour of body, changed. Œsophagus, pain in.* Ozæna. Pancreas, disorders of. *Paralysis; pseudo-hypertrophic; general of insane.* Periostitis. *Perspiration, abnormal.* Petit mal. *Plague. Pneumonia. Polypus.* Pregnancy, vomiting of. Proctalgia. *Proctitis. Progressive muscular atrophy.* Pruritus ani. Psoriasis. Puerperal convulsions. *Purpura. Pylorus, thickening of.* Retinitis. Rheumatism; paralytic. *Rickets. Screaming.* Scurvy. *Shiverings. Sleep, disordered.* Somnambulism. *Spine, curvature of.* Spleen, enlargement of. Sprains. Stammering. Sterility. Syphilis. *Syringo-myelia. Throat, mucus in. Tobacco habit. Trachea, tickling in.* Tuberculosis. Tumours, erectile; polypoid; cancerous. *Typhus fever. Ulcers. Urethra, stricture of.* Vaccinia. Variola. Voice, loss of. *Whitlow.* Wounds. Yellow fever.

Characteristics.—*Phosphorus* (Light-bearer, Morning Star) "was discovered in 1673 by Brandt, an alchymist of Hamburgh, and shortly afterwards by Kunkel, in Saxony." Teste, from whom I quote, says that attempts were made to use *Phos.* in medicine immediately after discovery. Kunkel made it into his "luminous pills," and Kramer claimed to have cured with it diarrhœa, epilepsy, and malignant fevers. Teste gives a list of old-school cures, which include: Continuous, bilious, and intermittent fevers; general œdema; measles two cases of pneumonia of left lung, with ataxic symptoms ; chronic rheumatism of the legs ; apoplexy ; hydrocephalus ; periodic headaches (in one case with menstrual irregularity) ; catalepsy ; epilepsy ; gutta serena ; asthenia facilis ; chronic lead poisoning,—a list which shows a very good idea of the range of action of *Phos.* Hahnemann's proving brought out the fine indications, without which the generals are of little service, and to Hahnemann's symptoms have been added those of later provings and of numerous cases of poisoning, and the effects on workers in match factories, especially necrosis of the lower jaw. The vapour given off by unignited *Phos.* is *Phosphorus oxide.* The jaw affection, called " Phossy-jaw " by the workpeople themselves, is accompanied by profound adynamia, and not unfrequently ends in death. " The form of the disease differs according to whether the upper or lower jaw is attacked. In the former case it pursues generally a chronic and mild course, ending in exfoliation, cicatrisation, and cure. In the latter the necrosis may be either acute or chronic, but is always severe, and the patients usually die of " consumptive fever " (*C. D. P.*). Here is a typical case quoted in *C. D. P.* from *B. J. H.*, iv. 287 : J. D., 21, had been four years in a match factory. For two and a half years he had only laryngeal irritation from the local action of the fumes. He then began to cough very much and expectorate thick white mucus. Then most violent toothache set in, with swelling on right side of face. A molar was extracted but without relief, and one tooth after another dropped out. He became too weak to walk. A swelling as big as an egg formed below right orbit, burst in a fortnight, and discharged a large quantity of white pus. He grew worse ; all the teeth fell out ; gums of lower jaw were retracted. Examination found right cheek swollen. At right angle of lower jaw an opening discharging laudable pus, through which a probe can be passed two inches along bare bone, and two inches anterior to this another aperture leads to the same. On opening mouth the whole lower jaw as far as ascending rami and down to reflection of mucous membrane is denuded and of leaden greyish colour. On right upper jaw probe can be passed over bare bone. Pareira (*C. D. P.*) has observed in phosphorus workers " a peculiar sallow, bloated complexion, with dull expression of eye and gastric derangement," when there was no affection of the jaws. [Wagner found *Phos.* symptoms long before local disease appeared, *e.g.*, cardialgia, anorexia, eructation of gas smelling of *Phos.*; also dizziness, faintness, and cachectic appearance. The first symptoms in the jaws are tearing pains, the teeth being sound, swelling and suppuration of the gums, and loosening of the teeth follow, and the bone becomes denuded. Langenbeck objects to the term " necrosis," stating that it is a periostatics in which bony deposit occurs, enclosing the jaws more or less as in a sheath. There is no exfoliation. This osteoperiostitis may arise from rheumatism.—*Klin. Woch*, Jan. 2, 1872.] In cases of acute poisoning the most remarkable effect noted is acute fatty degeneration of the liver and engorgement of the lungs. At first there is tenderness of the liver, but as it shrinks this passes away. The right lung is more affected than the left. The symptoms of acute *Phos.* poisoning are exceedingly painful if consciousness is retained; violent tearing pains in œsophagus, chest, stomach; vomiting and diarrhœa; rectal, vesical, uterine tenesmus; bloating of abdomen; sensitiveness to touch; hæmorrhages from all orifices. Death may take place in a few hours, or it may be delayed for months. In the case of a child of 2½ who had sucked the heads of matches, two days afterwards there was some feverish excitement, later violent convulsions, lasting three hours, and ending in death. There were found after death no fewer than ten invaginations of the small intestines, which, however, were empty, and there was no sign of strangulation (*C. D. P.*). In a woman, 45, who swallowed the *Phos.* from 120 matches, Ozanam found a typhoid febrile state, profound prostration; inability to raise herself; dry tongue; much thirst; stomach sensitive; vomiting of black, sooty matter. Death took place on the second day (*C. D. P.*). A man, 48, inhaled vapour of burning *Phos.* Among his symptoms were: A sensation as if something twitched under skin or was creeping between skin and flesh. Twitching of single bundles of fibres at different times like playing on a piano. Tongue when speaking often refuses to move, so that he stammers (*C. D. P.*). A case reported by J. O. Müller and translated in *C. D. P.* brings out some very characteristic symptoms of *Phos.* A strong woman, 30, took about three grains of *Phos.* from matches. Among her symptoms were: After eight hours violent and noisy vomitings. Prostrated, cold, pallid, as if moribund and unconscious. Cold, clammy sweat, general; skin here and there waxy yellow; complexion leaden grey; dark blue rings round eyes; pulse small, hard, slow, unrhythmic, intermitting. Abdomen distended, very sensitive all over, the slightest touch causing violent pains; could not bear weight of nightdress. Senses and mind in unconscious apathy; could only be roused by loud calling into her ear. *Aco.* 1 every ten minutes revived her. She complained of very violent burning pain in lower chest (œsophagus?), stomach, and whole abdomen < by every touch or change of posture. Vomiting and diarrhœa had ceased, but she still had retching and *ineffectual straining at stool with burning like fire in large intestine and anus.* She passed with difficulty small quantities of dark yellow urine, smelling strongly of garlic, *after micturition very severe burning.* Boring, burning pains in bones, especially of skull, palate, nose, jaws, and teeth, < taking cold or warm things into mouth or chewing, only tepid liquid nutriment could be borne. At times numb pain in teeth; they felt loose as if they would fall out. Apathy alternating with angry words and actions. After menses, burning leucorrhœa that made the parts sore. Soft parts of joints swollen. Considerable rigidity of joints. The skin, which had been pale, put on a yellow tint, bloated swellings appeared in places on eyelids and face, pitting on pressure. On nape, back, and other parts the skin could be raised by the fingers in large folds, which slowly smoothed down again. Finally a peculiar exanthema appeared on the skin about the joints like eczema; vesicles in groups turned rapidly into scabs and frequently recurred. *Sulph.* was given and gradual recovery occurred. In a youth poisoned by *Phos.* there was nausea and sour taste; milk tasted burnt; every smell (tobacco, wine, beer) < the nausea. One of the provers had: Loathing of butcher's meat and bad appetite. *Phosphorus* burns are among the most painful of all burns, and the burning sensations of the poisonings are prominent also in the provings : "Glowing sensation throughout epigastrium and chest." "A flame seemed passing through me." "Warming sensation right side of heart and below left clavicle. This heat spread to apex of left scapula and to acromion, when it left the heart." "From 11 a.m. till 4 p.m. remarkable numb feeling in left leg from knee to toes, sometimes sensation as if hot blood flowed into it." Other symptoms from the provings are : "Drawing forcing towards pelvis and rectum as if menses coming on." Intense sexual excitement in men with erections, emissions ; later impotence. Dr. Sorge, 34, had this symptom : "Weight in occiput and nape, down whole spine a dull feeling as if over-filled with blood, and in sacrum a peculiar paralytic feeling like what one feels in the limbs when exposed to unavoidable danger ; heaviness of feet, which were not placed on ground with usual energy. Walk less strong, often stumbled on a smooth road. Diminished sexual appetite, and feeling as if the penis would not become erect when excitement was present. Mental indifference (quite unusual)." E. R. Heath had some decidedly "phosphorescent" symptoms : Darting, cutting pains, causing much distress, starting from different points and flashing over whole abdomen ; imagined an aurora borealis and seemed to hear distinctly voices shouting "Beautiful, oh ! was not that splendid ?" as the pains became more severe and lasting. He sprang from bed and tried to collect his thoughts ; had numbness all over with sensation of myriads of needles slightly pricking him. Throat dry and parched ; a flame seemed to pass through him. Feet seemed glued to the floor. With great difficulty he reached the vessel, and as soon as the bowels began to act the pains changed to cramps. Stools were like scrapings of intestines, almost constant, with tenesmus, for over two hours, after which he lay down in bed, weak, sore, almost helpless. The same prover had : Intolerable thirst ; drink did not quench it, but caused cold, clammy sweat to exude the moment the water entered the stomach. Later : Involuntary passages, periodic ; rectum insensible ; sphincter paralysed ; slight prolapse after each stool. Stools inodorous save for a slight mouldy smell. H. Noah Martin proved *Red amorphous Phosphorus*. The symptoms do not differ from those of transparent *Phos.*, and are included in the Schema.—Such are the materials out of which the picture of the great remedy known in homœopathy by the name *Phosphorus* has been drawn, the characteristic features being pointed up with the added light and shade of clinical experience. The types of constitution in which *Phos.* has been found particularly *suitable* are strongly marked : (1) Tall, slender persons, of sanguine temperament, fair skin, blonde or red hair, quick, lively perceptions and sensitive nature. (2) Young people who grow too rapidly and are inclined to stoop ; chlorotic ; anæmic. [In experiments on young animals *Phos.* has produced rickets. Kessel (*H. W.*, xxxi. 394) gave *Phos.* to young dogs, in whom it caused fatal disturbance of digestion and fatty liver, and "marked atrophic process where bone was being deposited."] (3) Persons of waxy, translucent skin ; half anæmic, half jaundiced. (4) Tall, slender, narrow-chested, phthisical patients ; delicate eyelashes, soft hair. (5) Tall, slim, dark-haired persons, especially women, disposed to stoop. (6) Nervous, weak persons who like to be magnetised. (7) Hæmorrhagic patients ; slight wounds bleed profusely. *Phos.* profoundly affects the nutrition and function of every tissue, notably the hardest (bone) and the softest (nerve and blood). It causes irritation, erethism, exaltation of all the senses, and later a typhoid state and fatty degeneration. In fevers of typhoid type and in pneumonia *Phos.* has an important place. It is indicated especially when the morbid action becomes localised in the right lung, particularly the lower lobe. In the year 1876, in the course of a severe attack of typhus fever during my residence in Liverpool, my state, as I am told (for I was in delirium), suddenly became very critical through pneumonic consolidation of the right lung. *Phos.* was the remedy selected by Drs. Drysdale, Hayward, and Hawkes, who attended me, and under its action I made a rapid recovery.—Hard, dry cough, rusty sputa ; < *at twilight* and *till midnight ;* < *lying on left side ;* > *lying on right side ;* abdomen *distended, sore, very sensitive to touch ;* stools offensive, bloody, involuntary ; *the anus appearing to remain open.* Each one of the symptoms I have italicised is a keynote of *Phos.* When any of them are present (with or without the pneumonia) *Phos.* is likely to be the remedy. The delirium is low, muttering, stupid ; or violent ; or there may be a state of ecstasy ; or odd ideas, that his bones are in fragments and he cannot fit the pieces together. As a leading constituent of nervous matter *Phos.* has a deep action on the organ of mind and sensation. It produces an excitable condition, exaltation of mental faculties, and the condition which follows over-exertion. The mind, like the special senses, is too excitable and impressionable. Easily angered and becomes vehement ; actually gets beside himself with anger and suffers physically in consequence. At other times anxious and restless, especially in the dark and at twilight (the restlessness of *Phos.* is universal ; patient cannot sit or stand still a moment ; it belongs to the stage of irritation, and is succeeded by apathy if the condition is not arrested). Imagines he sees faces grinning at him from the corners of the room. Such conditions are found in cases resulting from losses of fluids ; over-work of brain ; sexual excesses and abuse, and take shape in general paralysis of the insane with mania of grandeur ; and in apoplexy and its sequelæ ; in Duchenne's pseudo-hypertrophic paralysis, in locomotor ataxy and other paralyses. A very characteristic condition of *Phos.* in nervous cases is *fibrillary twitching* of individual bundles of fibres in muscles. Numbness and formication in paralysed limbs indicate it in hemiplegia and paraplegia. Spasms on paralysed side. In other cases the burning pains of *Phos.* are prominent : burning between the scapulæ ; burning in spots along the spine ; *feeling of intense heat running up the back* (no other remedy has exactly this symptom). The uncertain gait, neuralgic pain, and fuzzy feeling of the feet, give the correspondence with locomotor ataxy, when the conditions correspond. Epilepsy from masturbation. Petit mal : epilepsy with consciousness. Mau of Itzehoe (*H. R.*, xv. 268) cured this case of sciatica : An elderly lady had for eight weeks a continual burning pain running along back of left thigh and leg, compelling her to spend most of the day in bed. Entire limb so weak that she could hardly walk. < Lying on left side. > Lying on right side or on back. < By movement. < By cold air. > Being warmly covered. < In evening. *Phos.* 6x, every two hours, caused aggravation for the first three days, and after that gave relief, but did not cure. *Phos.* 30, one powder every evening, completed the cure in a week. But the action of *Phos.* is not confined to the brain and spinal cord, it also affects the cranial bones and spinal column. I cured mainly with *Phos.* 1m a case of spinal caries with paralytic symptoms in a lady aged 67. That is, I cured the caries and removed the paralysis, though the curvature remained. There was a history of a strained back thirty-five years before, and of lumbago and sciatica five years before I saw her. She had many pains in the scapula and chest, and could not walk unless supported about the waist. Incidentally *Phos.* set up a symptom of its own : Dryness of mouth, lips, and throat. *Phos.* has burning thirst for cold water ; cold water relieves, but *as soon as it becomes warm in the stomach it is vomited*. This is one of the keynotes of *Phos.*, and distinguishes it from all other remedies in cases of vomiting. Desire for cold foods and preference for cold meat is very characteristic of *Phos.*, and the cold food, like the cold drink, may be vomited as soon as it becomes warm inside. Ice cream > the gastric pains. There is nausea on putting hands into warm water ; sneezing and coryza from putting hands in water. Regurgitation of ingesta in mouthfuls. During pregnancy the sight of water = vomiting. The appetite of *Phos.* is remarkable : *Must eat often or he faints.* Hungry soon after a meal ; hungry in the night, must eat. Craving for salt (*Phos.* remedies the effects of excessive salt-eating). The sinking, faint feeling of *Phos. is felt in the whole abdominal cavity ;* also in head, chest, and stomach. The stools of *Phos.* are peculiar, whether constipated or diarrhœic : Long, tough, hard fæces (like a dog's) ; voided with great difficulty and straining. Diarrhœa as soon as anything enters the rectum ; profuse pouring away as from a hydrant ; watery with sago-like particles ; with sensation as if the anus stood open ; involuntary ; during cholera-time ; painless ; morning of old people ; bloody stool ; blood-streaked stool ; stool like shreddy membranes. With the stool there is burning in the anus and tenesmus. There are also pains of all descriptions in the anus, notably stitches shooting up rectum. A man suffering from pneumonia, to whom I gave *Phos.* 3, after a few days developed attacks of violent pain in rectum and anus, with distension of abdomen and desire for stool ; stool light, lumpy, constipated, only passed by aid of glycerine enema ; after stool, complete relief of pain ; sometimes the attack waked him from sleep. With *Phos.* 200 I cured a very severe proctalgia coming on at every menstrual period. During urination, and also when not urinating, there is burning in the urethra. Another very characteristic burning of *Phos.* is *burning palms*, cannot bear to have the hands covered. Flashes of heat beginning in hands and spreading to face. The fever is more of the yellow fever, typhus, or typhoid, nervous or hectic, type. In intermittents when there is heat at night beginning in stomach ; faint and hungry in night ; heat of hands. There is also chilliness towards evening ; icy coldness of hands, knees, and feet, even in bed. Sweat is anxious, profuse, exhausting on slightest exertion ; profuse at night ; cold and clammy, smelling of sulphur or of garlic. *Phos.* corresponds to yellow fever in many particulars ; disorganisation of the liver and blood with jaundice ; hæmorrhages. It has caused acute fatty degeneration of the liver ; and corresponds also to fatty degeneration of pancreas with gastric symptoms and oily stools, and fatty and amyloid degeneration of the kidneys. *Phos.* stands at the head of hæmorrhagics, and corresponds to the hæmorrhagic diathesis. The blood loses its coagulability. Very small wounds bleed profusely. *Blood-streaked discharges* are very characteristic when from lungs, nose, bowels, or other orifices. Hæmorrhoids. Menses are more profuse and longer-lasting than usual. There may be vicarious menstruation in the form of hæmoptysis, epistaxis, or hæmaturia. Left ovarian pain. Leucorrhœa which causes blisters. Sexual excitement is great in both sexes, going to the extent of satyriasis and nymphomania. Frequent erections in men, and sexual thoughts entirely beyond the patient's control. Erections in spite of efforts to control passion in young men. Impotence from over-indulgence or from celibacy. The female breasts are the seat of many burning, shooting, cramping pains, and *Phos.* has proved a leading remedy in mammary abscess and fistulæ. The characteristics are : Erysipelatous appearance ; red streaks starting from opening ; thin, ichorous discharge. The hæmorrhagic action of *Phos.* is seen in many forms of pulmonary hæmorrhage and congestion : blood-streaked or rusty sputa ; tasting salty ; when patients with delicate chests bring up phlegm tinged with blood whenever they take cold *Phos.* will generally clear up the case. Phthisis florida may also need *Phos.* It has also a "stomach-" or "liver-" cough ; cough comes on after eating, and starts from a tickling in pit of stomach. Cough < when strangers enter the room. Cough < from strong odours (part of the general sensitiveness of the drug). Bronchial catarrh > in all grades may require it. Cough = tearing pain under sternum as if something was being torn loose. Suffocative pains in upper part of chest with constriction of larynx and engorgement of lungs ; mucous râles ; panting and laboured breathing, even emphysema. After the cough an asthmatic attack. The *Conditions* of *Phos.* will generally decide when it should be given. T. D. Stow (*J. of Homœopathics*, August, 1890) reports the case of H. B., 52, farmer, who had for six months a sharp pain with soreness in third intercostal space, three inches to left of sternum, limiting inspirations. Dyspnœa on exercise ; dry cough during the day till 10 p.m. Thick, yellow, sweetish sputa from 6 a.m. to 10 a.m. Cough < lying on left side ; when talking ; when eating and just after eating ; on going into cold air ; by change of weather. > In fairly warm room ; lying on right side. Prefers cold food. Has become alarmed by the persistence of the attack and loss of flesh. Three doses of *Phos.* 500 (Dunham), taken on three successive days, cured. This case was translated in *Hahn. Month.*, September, 1890, from *Alg. H. Zeit.* : Whilst walking rapidly against the west wind three months before, X. felt a pain under middle of sternum with sensitiveness of the part to pressure. Pulse rapid. *Phos.* 6 removed the symptoms for two weeks, when pain and sensitiveness returned, and with the pain a sensation as though gas would rise from epigastrium. *Phos.* 3 cured. W. A. Nicholas (*H. W.*, xxv. 495) reports the case of T. B., 51, whom he saw after a four months' illness, which began with congestion of the brain on the sudden death of his wife, and was followed by bronchitis. During all this time he was heavily drugged. A rather long walk brought on a severe attack of angina pectoris. *Bell.* 1 x gave much relief. Nicholas noticed the patient at times put his hand to the back of his neck. *Phos.* 1 relieved entirely. *Phos.* corresponds to headache and other sufferings from grief. Hot vertex after grief. It has shocks in occiput; coldness in cerebellum; congestion of brain seeming to rise from spine into head. *Phos.* has "splitting headache caused by cough." Neuralgic pains of many kinds, and impending paralysis. The attacks are induced by mental exertion; worry; *washing clothes;* and are < by music; noises; strong odours. Gale, of Quebec, discovered in *Phos.* a remedy for "washerwoman's headache" (*Organon*, iii. 30). His patient had these symptoms: Whenever she washes clothes or walks fast she has—rush of blood to head, red face and eyes, heat on head, scalp sensitive to touch, sudden shooting pains, especially in vertex. *Phos.* cm cured. I cured a somewhat similar case (*H. W.*, xxiv. 455) with *Phos.* 30 every four hours; only in my case the headaches always appeared the morning after washing: violent shooting pains left side of vertex, > wrapping head in flannel. I had given several medicines previously which had improved the general health, but had done very little for the headaches. *Phos.* affects all parts of the eye—retina, choroid, vitreous and crystalline lenses, cornea, and conjunctivæ. It has arrested cataract and glaucoma, and cured retinitis albuminuria from suppressed menses. The leading symptoms are: Colours appear black before the eyes. Always sees green. Halo round candle. Letters appear red whilst reading. As if a grey veil over everything. Blindness after typhoid; sexual excess; loss of fluids; lightning. Twitching of lids. Pustule on cornea. Burning pains. The characteristic skin of *Phos.* is *waxy*, and either clear and pale or yellow. Under a "*Phosphorus* treatment" which was in vogue a generation ago, patients had a peculiarly waxy, fine, clear complexion; and in one case which came under my observation there was also very marked enlargement of the liver. In a case of rheumatism in an old lady who had *waxy pallor*, Cooper gave *Phos.* and set free all the joints. All kinds of eruptions may be set up. Exanthema with pustules (like small-pox), ulcers, psoriasis, lichen, eczema, blood boils, purpura. Hansen cured a case of purpura in a girl of ten (*H. W.*, xxxv. 105). The disease began with loss of appetite and pains in the stomach, but as soon as the purpura spots appeared the pains ceased and the appetite returned. The inner aspects of the thighs were affected. *Phos.* 2 cured. The ulcers of *Phos.* bleed easily at the slightest touch, and open cancers or fungus hæmatodes with this characteristic have been cured with *Phos.* "Large ulcers surrounded by smaller ones." Ulcers affecting the nails. Inflammation and eruptions about joints. Fistulæ with callous edges from glands. The joints most affected by *Phos.* are the hip and knee. The left side of the lower jaw is more affected than the right. Caries and exostoses of spine and other parts have been cured with *Phos.* De Noë Walker cured with *Phos.* 6 a large exostosis of the femur which had been pronounced osteo-sarcoma by old-school authorities. There are some forms of rheumatism which only *Phos.* can cure. These are characterised by great *stiffness* of the joints, more stiffness than pain. A drawing, tearing, *tight* feeling in parts. Stiffness of old people. Paralytic rheumatism from exposure to rain. The *tight* sensation appears in the girdle pain of spinal affections; *tightness* of skin of face and forehead. (Also stiffness in brain; in eyes.) Allied to the rheumatic symptoms of *Phos.* is its sensitiveness to effects of storms, especially thunderstorms. *Phos.* has cured more cases of headache always coming on when thunderstorms are about than any other remedy in my experience. It has also cured blindness from lightning stroke. The headaches from inhaling the steam of a washtub perhaps come in the same category as effects of vapour-laden air when storms are about. Mills (quoted *H. W.*, xxxi. 33) relates a typical case of thunderstorm effect: Mrs. F., tall, thin, dark, of mild and gentle disposition, was seen by the doctor during a thunderstorm. He found her sitting on the stairs, trembling and cold and bathed in cold, clammy sweat, full of nervous dread, and almost beside herself. One dose of *Phos.* cm cured. Some weeks later she witnessed a worse storm with complete unconcern. The power of *Phos.* over septic conditions is illustrated in a case of Howard Crutcher's (quoted *H. W.*, xxxiii. 405). A girl, 16, had perforating appendicitis, operation having been delayed too long in consequence of opposition of friends. Although he deemed it useless he was persuaded to operate, and found a large abscess behind the colon, freely communicating with the peritoneal cavity. Up to the fourth day the patient progressed favourably. Then there was a collapse: pulse 130, mind wandering, urine and fæces passed without restraint. The patient was rapidly sinking; *Arsen.* gave no help. The doctor sent word to the students who were nursing the patient that they might try a hot saline enema. On attempting to give it the *rectum was found to be open*, no resistance being offered by the sphincter. *Greyish-white fæcal discharges, watery and offensive, passed constantly.* "The students, recognising the indication for *Phos.*, gave a dose of that remedy, and instead of dying the girl got well." *Peculiar sensations* are: As if about to die. As if immersed in hot water. Anxiety as if below left breast. As if he had been lying at night with head too low. As if everything had stopped in head. As if chair were rising. As if eyes would be pressed out; or pressed down by weight about them. As if painful nodes under scalp. As if pulled by hair. As if head would burst. As if something exploded in head. As if skin of face too tight. As if something were pulled tight over ears. As if dust in right eye; sand in left eye; eyeballs large. As if something lay before ears; foreign body in ears. As if nose stuck together. As if nails driven into jaws. As if food did not digest properly. As if heavy weight in stomach. Stomach as if freezing. As if something cooking in stomach. Anus as if open. Larynx as if lined with fur. As if skin on larynx. As if a piece of skin hanging loose in larynx. As if something in middle of sternum torn loose. As if heart had grown fast. As if chest eviscerated. As if a narrow band encircled body and lay upon heart. As if great weight lying on middle of sternum. Back as if broken. As if quicksilver moved up and down spinal cord. Coccyx as if ulcerated. Soles as if he had walked too much. Feet as if asleep. Ankles as if sprained. *Suddenness* is a feature of *Phos.:* Sudden prostration such as may occur in diphtheria, measles, scarlatina, or any disease in which the system has sustained a profound shock. The left side is somewhat more affected than the right, the venous more than the arterial system. The symptoms of *Phos.* are < from touch (cannot bear touch of nightdress) ; from pressure (but pressure > feeling as if something before ears and pains in chest). Rubbing >. Mesmerism >. Rest < pain in arms and shoulders. Lying down = intense pains in eyes ; < colic and tearing in jaws ; > heat of scalp and incarcerated flatus. Weakness after stool and after urinating, compelling lying down. Lying on back < diarrhœa ; asthma ; > pneumonia ; pain in arm. Lying on left side < ; on right side >. Sitting <. Motion ; exertion ; walking, especially fast walking, <. Exertion physical or mental <. Laughing < (cough). Coughing = headache. Talking < pain in larynx. < From spraining parts. < Lifting arms. < Before sleep, > after. (Some symptoms are < on waking, but this is less characteristic.) < Morning ; evening (especially *twilight*) ; before midnight. Heat < boring in teeth ; back pains ; itching spots of skin. Warm food and drink < (but hot drinks > flatulent colic). Warm water, putting hands in = toothache. Warm wraps > neuralgia of head and heat of scalp. Weather changes (either way) <. Open air > pain in forehead ; hemicrania ; stuffed feeling in nose ; < vertigo ; toothache ; cough ; = tearing in labia ; = taking cold easily. Wind <. Thunderstorm <. Washing with cold water >. Washing clothes ; wet weather <. < Light ; noise ; music ; piano playing. > In the dark.

Relations.—*Antidoted by:* Nux, Coff., Tereb. ; Kali permang. well diluted and given freely (Dr. Antal). *It antidotes:* Tereb., Rhus ven., Camph., Iod., Nat. m. (excessive use of salt), Petrol. *Complementary:* Ars., Cepa (all three have alliaceous odours), Carb. v., Ipec. *Incompatible:* Caust. *Compatible:* Ars., Bapt., Bell., Bry., Calc., Carb. v., Chi., K. ca., Lyc., Nux, Pul., Rhus, Sep., Sil., Sul. *Compare:* Ars., Merc., Petr., Sul. Asthma after cough, Ars. (Ars. before and after). Fancies himself in pieces, Bapt. Stitches up vagina, Sul., Sep., Pul., Nit. ac., Alum., Berb., Am. c. Weakening night-sweats, Chi., Calc., Lyc. Sweats towards morning, Calc., Lyc. (Phos. on awaking). Tongue glazed, Lach. (Lach. red ; Phos. dry, cracked, black). Lienteria, Chi. Cough < entering cold air from warm room (Bry. opposite). Fear of darkness, Am. m., Calc., Stro., Val., Stram. Fear of ghosts, Pul. Sense of insecurity in bowels, Alo. Piles during menses, Collins., Ign., Lach., Pul. Effect of raising arms high to lift things, Rhus. Chilblains ; general paralysis, Agar. Headache with increased intellectual powers (Phyt. with increased hearing). Hunger at night, Chi. s., Pso., Pul., Ign., Lyc. (Pho. unappeasable hunger with febrile heat). Left ovarian pain, Coloc., Thuj., Lach., Bry. Somnambulism, Can. i., Sul., Luna. Sensation of anus open, Phos. ac., Apis

(Lach. as if vagina open). < Walking fast, Pul. Regurgitation of food, Sul. Nocturnal salivation, Cham., Nux, Rhus. Difficult swallowing of liquids, Bell., Caust., Can., Hyo., Ign., Lach., Lyc. Blood from bowel, Merc., Nit. ac., Sul., Caps., Merc. c. Menorrhagia, Calc. Laughs at serious things, Anac., Lyc., Nux m., Plat. Hæmorrhage, blood does not coagulate, Sanguisuga. Fatty changes in blood, kidneys, spinal cord; brain-fag; crawling and tingling sensations; sexual excitement with erethism; backache as if it would break Pic. ac. (Phos. has more irritability and over-sensitiveness to external impressions with the weakness; the senses are too acute, or if failing, accompanied by photopsies; Pic. ac. has more intense erections and less lasciviousness than Phos.). In general features; taciturn and distrustful; inclined to be angry and scold; sensation of tension; nervous weakness and restlessness, Caust. (Phos. has great soreness of larynx, fears to cough or talk; Caust. has cough > by cold drink, Hoarseness of Phos. is < evening, of Caust. < morning). Scrofula, tuberculosis, swelling of glands, indolent ulceration, difficult learning to talk and walk (Phos. has delicate, refined skin, features sharp and rather handsome; Calc. large, swollen lips). Small ulcers surrounding large ones (Hep. pimples round sore eyes). Phthisis florida, Fer. (Fer. has apparent plethora with great oppression of chest from least exertion). Weakness and goneness in stomach at 11 a.m.; softening of brain; enervation accompanied by trembling; restlessness, Zn. (Zn. has ptosis; < from wine; restlessness of feet, Phos. of entire body). Functional paralysis from fatigue or emotion, Stan., Coccul., Ign., Nat. mur., Collins. Hoarseness, < evening, weak chest, cough, copious expectoration, hectic, Stan. (Phos. has more blood-streaked sputa; tightness across chest). Bone disease, abscess, especially of breast, with fistulous openings; over-excitability of nervous system; cough excited by speaking, Sil. Phthisis; rapidly growing young people, Iod. (Phos. is nearest Iod. in phthisis). Aphonia with rawness of larynx, Carb. v. Heat at vertex; imperfect growth of tissue; morning diarrhœa, Sul. (Sul. has hunger at 11 a.m. with the heat at vertex, Phos. has not; Phos. has green painless stools, Sul. stools changing colour, and raw sore anus). Irritation of respiratory tract, sore larynx (Phos. has irritation lower down; sore larynx, < from talking or pressure, Bell. only from pressure). Capillary bronchitis, Ipec. (Phos. more inflammatory). Prostration, Chi. (Phos. *sudden*, Chi. not). Vicarious menstruation, Bry., Puls., Senec. Typhoid, Rhus; and erotic mania, Hyo. Cold; cerebral softening, Nux (Phos. follows Nux in both; if cold goes to chest in spite of Nux). Cough from reflex nervous influence, Ambra (Amb. < when strangers in room). Irritability; intolerance of mental strain, Nux. Vomiting: after drinking cold water, Ars. (Ars. immediately; Pho. as soon as warm in stomach), Bism. (immediately after eating, with burning cardalgia), Kre. (of undigested food hours after eating). Diarrhœa as soon as he eats, Ars. Weakness after stool, Con., Nux. Sensitive to storms and electricity, Rhod., Merc., Morph. Polypi. Teuc., Calc., Sang., Pso., Lemn. > From cold drinks and food (Lyc. opposite). Hysteria, Ign. Deafness, especially to human voice (Ign. opposite). Small wounds bleed much, Lach. < Putting hands in water, Lac. d.

Apathy; weakness and prostration from loss of fluids, Pho. ac. (Phos. has more dryness of tongue and sensorial excitement). Diarrhœa blood-streaked and looking like flesh water, Canth., Rhus. Shreddy, membranous diarrhœa, Ars., Caust. < Twilight, Puls. Hepatisation of lungs, Ant. t., Sul., Lyc. (these correspond to the later breaking-up stage). Can only lie right side (Merc. can only lie left). Levitation, Phos. ac., Stict. pul. Desire for acids, Phell. Affections of skin about joints, Sep. Tongue as if burnt, Sang. Deafness after typhoid, Ars., Petrol. Nymphomania, Calc. ph., Orig. Tuberculosis, Bacil., Tuberc. Explosion in head, Alo. Jerks in head during stool, Indm. Numb, stiff feeling in brain, Graph. Duchenne's paralysis, Curar. Growing ends of bones, Conch. Effects of hair-cutting, Bell. Teste puts Phos. in three of his groups, of which Puls., Ipec., and Fer. are the types.

Causation.—Anger. Fear. Grief. Worry. Mental exertion. Strong emotions. Music. Strong odours. Gas. Flowers (fainting). Thunderstorms. Lightning (blindness). Sexual excesses. Loss of fluids. Sprains. Lifting. Wounds. Exposure to drenching rains. Tobacco (amblyopia). Washing clothes. Having hair cut.

SYMPTOMS.

1. **Mind.**—Affections of the mind in general; amativeness; dizziness of the mind.—Nymphomania.—Melancholy sadness and melancholy, sometimes with violent weeping, or interrupted by fits of involuntary laughter.—Laughs at serious things.—Stupor, low, muttering delirium; loquacious.—Thinks he is several pieces, and cannot adjust the fragments.—Stupor from which he could be aroused for a moment only to lapse back into a muttering lethargy; and forgetfulness.—Great apathy; very sluggish; dislike to talk; answers slowly or not at all.—Anguish and uneasiness, esp. when alone, or in stormy weather, principally in evening, with timorousness and fright.—Anguish respecting the future; or respecting the issue of the disease.—Susceptibility to fright.—Fear: in evening; of darkness; of spectres; of things creeping out of corners.—Hypochondriacal sadness.—Disgust to life.—Apathy alternating with angry words and acts.—Becomes easily vexed and angry, which makes him exceedingly vehement, from which he suffers afterwards.—Any lively impression = heat, as if dipped in hot water.—Great irascibility, anger, passion, and violence.—Involuntary and spasmodic weeping and laughter.—Misanthropy.—Repugnance to labour.—Shamelessness, approaching insanity.—Great indifference to everything, and even to patient's own family.—Great forgetfulness, esp. in morning.—Great flow of ill-assorted ideas.—Zoomagnetic condition; state of clairvoyance.—Ecstasy.

2. **Head.**—Cloudiness and dizziness, esp. in morning.—Vertigo when rising from bed in morning; when rising from a seat, with faintness and falling to the floor; < morning and after meals.—Dulness of head > washing face with cold water.—Frequent attacks of vertigo at different times, and at different hours in the day, esp. in morning, in middle of day, and in bed in evening.—Vertigo when seated; with hypochondriasis, during which chair appears to rise.—Vertigo with nausea and pressive pains in head.—Obstinate vertigo; falls back whenever he attempts to rise from bed.—Vertigo very

pronounced; up and down vertigo; things move up and down, or else patient feels sinking through the floor (R. T. C.).—Apoplectic unchanging vertigo (R. T. C.)—Vertigo with loss of ideas.—Stupefying headache, morning, when moving, and < on stooping; ceasing for a short time after eating; > when lying down and in cold air.—Attacks of headache, with nausea and vomiting, and throbbing, jerking pains.—Nocturnal headache, preceded by nausea in evening.—Headache caused by vexation.—Headache in morning.—Headache with increased mental power.—Weakness of head, which is fatigued by music, laughter, a heavy step, a warm room, &c.—Pain in brain as if it had been bruised.—Stunning headache, sometimes with violent ebullition of blood, and paleness of face.—Congestion to head, with burning, singing, and pulsations in head, red face, puffiness under eyes, < morning when sitting and in evening in bed.—Sensation of emptiness in head with vertigo.—Headache as if too full of blood from intense study.—Headache above l. eye with floating spots before vision.—Numb, dizzy sensation in brain, inability to work.—Feeling as if everything had stopped in brain.—Jerks in head, esp. during stool.—Sensation as if brain stiffened on remaining in open air.—Sensation of heaviness, of fulness, and pressure in head.—Tearing in head, and esp. in temples, or semi-lateral.—Lancinations in different parts of head, esp. in evening.—(Incessant shooting pains through brain with sensation as if eyes being pulled out, beginning in forehead, lasting day and night, with vomiting, > by either warmth or cold.—R. T. C.)—Shocks in occiput, loud snaps; shocks in whole head, with shattered sensation as if something had exploded; brought on by over-work or worry.—Washerwoman's headache.—Burning in forehead, with pulsations, morning and afternoon, after eating < in warm room, > in open air.—Pulsation in head, with singing and burning in it, mostly in forehead, with nausea and vomiting from morning till noon; < from music, while masticating, and in warm room.—Congestion in head, with beating, buzzing, heat, and burning sensation, esp. in forehead.—Splitting headache from cough.—Sensation of coldness in head.—The headaches are > by open air.—Neuralgia of head, when it must be kept warmly wrapped up night and day.—External shootings in side of head.—Distressing sensation, as if skin of forehead were too tight, and tension in face, as if the skin were not large enough, frequently only on one side; < from change of temperature and while eating; > after eating, with anxiety.—Tendency to suffer from a chill in head, with a sensation in open air as if brain were congealed.—(Sensation of coldness in cerebellum, with sensation of stiffness in brain.)—Inflammation of brain with pulsations and singing in head; the heat enters head from the spine, and from it extends to feet; < in warm room, > when moving about in cold air.—Headache over l. eye.—Headache extending to eyes; to root of nose.—Itching in scalp, < from scratching, with dandruff.—Falling off of hair (in large bunches on forepart of head, and) esp. above ears (alopecia areata).—Dry scabs and great scaliness of scalp.—Dry, painful heat of scalp, compelling one to uncover head; temperature of body not increased; > when lying down.—Clammy perspiration on head only, and in palms of hands, with discharge of much turbid urine.—Sensation as if pulled by the hair.—Exostosis on cranium.

3. **Eyes.**—Pains in eyes, as if in orbital bones.—Pressure in eyes as from a grain of sand.—Frequent itching in eyes.—Pressure as if eyes would

be pressed out.—Shootings, smarting, heat, and burning sensation in eyes, esp. in external canthi.—(Eyeballs feel sore, with tendency to cold sweat and giddiness.—R. T. C.)—Eyes sore to touch and feel full (cured. Qy. glaucoma ? —R. T. C.).—Congestion of blood in eyes.—Redness of sclerotica and of conjunctiva.—Yellowish colour of sclerotica.—(Episcleritis shifting from one eye to the other.—R. T. C.).—Inflammation of eyes of various kinds (with pressing and burning pains).—Lachrymation, esp. in open air, and when facing the wind.—Agglutination of eyes, morning, with lachrymation in open air, < in wind.—Sees better in morning, in twilight, or by shading eyes with hand.—Small burning spots on eyeballs.—Balls seem large, difficult to get lids over them.—Stiffness in eyes.—Nocturnal agglutination of eyes.—Hordeolum.—(Styes constantly appearing ; suppurate.—R. T. C.).—Quivering of eyelids and of their angles.—Difficulty in opening eyelids.—Swelling of eyelids.—Pupils contracted.—Œdema of the lids and about the eyes.—Amblyopia.—Weakness of sight on waking in morning.—Eyes give out while reading.—Myopia.—Diurnal blindness, which is sometimes instantaneous (as from fainting) ; everything seems to be covered with a grey veil.—As if a black veil were before the eyes.—Clouded sight by candle-light.—Weak-eyed people who see a halo around the lamplight.—Shortsightedness ; momentary loss of sight.—One sees variegated colours when there may be only one colour.—Black reflections or sparks, and black spots before sight.—Sensibility of eyes to both daylight and candle-light (aversion to light).—Greenish (or red) halo round candle.—Cataracta viridis.

4. **Ears.**—Otalgia.—Acute tearings and shootings in ears and head.—Beating and pulsation in ears.—Congestion of blood in ears.—Sensation of dryness in ears.—Yellow discharge from ears, alternating with deafness.—Acuteness of hearing.—Strong echoing of sounds, esp. of human voice, in ears, with vibration in head.—Deafness, esp. to human voice.—Feeling as if something were in front of the ears.—(Deafness after typhoid, &c.)—Deafness, l. side, and throbbing headache (produced.—R. T. C.).—Deafness from cold in head.—(Deafness with decayed teeth.—R. T. C.)—Murmuring before ears.—Buzzing in ears.—Roaring, ringing in the ears.—Aching ; tickling ; itching in ears.—Frequent tinnitus sometimes changing into beautiful tunes.—(Never-ceasing tinnitus like steam ; seems to cause vertigo and feeling of falling through floor.—R. T. C.).

5. **Nose.**—Nose red, swollen, and painful to touch.—Dry and hard scabs in nose.—Polypus in nose (bleeding easily).—Excoriation at angles of nose.—Ulcerated nostrils.—Numerous freckles on nose.—Fetid exhalation from nose.—Blowing of blood from nose (every time it is blown).—Profuse nose-bleed ; slow bleeding.—Epistaxis, sometimes during a stool or in evening.—Acute sense of smelling, esp. during the headaches.—Foul imaginary smells.—Loss of smell.—Uncomfortable (painful) dryness of nose.—Constant (profuse) discharge of yellow, greenish, bloody, purulent mucus from nose ; without coryza.—Coryza ; with inflammation (soreness) of throat and dulness (confusion) of head ; fluent and dry alternating.—Frequent sneezing.—Obstruction of nose, esp. in morning.

6. **Face.**—Face pale, wan, sallow, earth-coloured, with hollow eyes, surrounded by a blue circle.—The colour of the face is very changeable.—Paleness, alternately with redness of face, and transient heat.—Redness and

burning heat of cheeks.—Circumscribed red spots on cheeks.—Ashy, anæmic; blue lips; waxy.—Bloatedness of face, esp. round eyes.—Jerking of muscles of face.—Tension of skin of face and forehead, sometimes on one side only.—Desquamation of skin of face.—Painful sensibility of one side of face on opening mouth.—Painful, drawing, and tearing shootings in bones of face, esp. in evening, or at night in bed, or after the slightest chill.—The pains in face are renewed by speaking or by slightest touch.—Eruption of pimples and of scabs on face.—Lips bluish.—Lips dry and parched, swollen, covered with brownish scabs.—Cracked lips; crack in middle of lower lip.—Tetters and pimples round the mouth.—Ulceration of corners of mouth.—Cramp in jaw.—Necrosis of lower jaw, more rarely of upper.—Necrosis of l. lower jaw; swelling of jawbones.—Engorgement of submaxillary glands.

7. **Teeth.**—Drawing or tearing (pricking, stinging) toothache, or else gnawing, boring, pulsative, jerking, and shooting, esp. in open air, or in evening and morning, sometimes at night only, esp. in heat of bed, or else from contact with hot food.—Toothache after washing clothes; from having the hands in cold water.—Toothache with salivation, after slightest chill.—Pains as of ulceration in teeth during a morning meal.—Caries in teeth.—Teeth become very loose.—Bleeding of teeth.—Grinding of teeth.—Painful sensibility, inflammation, unfixing, ulceration, swelling and ready bleeding o[f] gums.—Gums separated from teeth, and bleed easily, esp. from touch.

8. **Mouth.**—Excoriation of mouth.—Bitter taste in mouth; sour afte[r] milk; bloody erosions on inner surface of cheeks.—Accumulation of saliva which is watery, saltish, sweetish; or excessive dryness of mouth.—Sorenes[s] of mouth.—Spitting of blood.—Viscid mucus in throat.—Hæmoptysis.—Puru[-] lent vesicles in palate.—Skin of palate shrivelled, as if about to be detached —Tongue swollen, dry, loaded with a blackish brown coating.—The tongu[e] swells (agg.—R. T. C.).—Stinging in tip of tongue.—Tongue: chalky white; dr[y] and white; dry and red; dry and brown in centre; coated yellow.—Difficul[t] articulation; speech slow; tongue refuses to move so that he stammers.

9. **Throat.**—Dryness of throat day and night.—Aching in throat.—Smarting, scraping, and burning pain in throat.—Burning in œsophagus.—(Spasmodic) stricture of œsophagus.—Tonsils and uvula are much swolle[n] —Hawking up of mucus in morning.—Pain as from excoriation in throat.

10. **Appetite.**—Clammy or cheese-like taste.—Bitterness in mouth an[d] throat after eating, with roughness.—Taste saltish, sour, or sweetish in mout[h] esp. after a meal.—Loss of taste.—Want of appetite from a sensation of fu[l-] ness in gullet and violent thirst.—Excessive craving for cooling things.—Longing for acids and spicy things.—Hunger after a meal.—Bulimy, even [at] night (during an attack of gout), with great weakness, so great that he fain[ts] if the hunger is not soon allayed.—Thirst, with longing for something refres[h-] ing.—Sensation of faintness and softness in abdomen after breakfast.—Aft[er] a meal drowsiness and indolence, heat and anxiety, burning sensatio[n] in hands, acidity increased, pressure and fulness in stomach, chest, an[d] abdomen, accompanied by obstructed respiration, vomiting of food, inflatio[n] of abdomen, or headache, risings of sour ingesta, hiccough, debility, coli[c] and many other sufferings.—Throwing up of ingesta by mouthfuls.

11. **Stomach.**—Risings, with pain in stomach, as if something we[re] being torn out of it.—Tobacco smoke produces nausea and palpitation

heart.—Frequent risings, generally empty, esp. after a meal and after drinking; sometimes also abortive, or spasmodic, or else sour, or with taste of the food.—Sour regurgitation of food.—Pyrosis.—Hiccough.—Nausea of various kinds, esp. in morning or in evening, or else after a meal.—Nausea with violent hunger or thirst, which disappears on eating or drinking water.—As soon as the water (or food) becomes warm in the stomach it is thrown up.—Waterbrash, esp. after eating acid things.—Vomiting with violent pains in stomach and great weakness.—Greenish or blackish vomiting.—Vomiting of acid matter.—Vomiting of food, esp. in evening.—Vomiting of bile or of mucus at night, sometimes with coldness and numbness of hands and feet.—Vomiting of blood.—Vomiting with diarrhœa.—Pain in stomach, esp. when it is touched and when walking.—Violent pains in stomach, > by a cold drink.—Sensation of contraction in cardia; the food, scarcely digested, returns into throat.—Fulness in stomach.—Shootings and pressure in stomach, esp. after a meal, with vomiting of food.—Pain in scrobiculus when it is touched, also in morning.—Sensation of coldness, or heat and burning sensation in stomach and scrobiculus.—Inflammation of stomach.—Ulceration of stomach in anæmic girls (R. T. C.).—Spasmodic pain, sensation of clawing and contraction in stomach, sometimes with choking.—The pains in the stomach are > by cold food (ice-cream, ice).—General uneasiness, but which is felt more particularly in stomach.—The pains in stomach manifest themselves chiefly after a meal, as well as in evening and at night.—Oppression and burning in epigastrium.—Drawing pain in pit of stomach, extending to chest.

12. **Abdomen.**—A very weak, empty, or gone sensation, felt in whole abdominal cavity (this is an indicative point whether found existing among a complication of troubles or occurring alone, and esp. when accompanied by sensation of heat in the back between shoulder-blades.—H. N. G.).—Sharp pains through abdomen.—Shootings in hepatic region.—Distension of abdomen, esp. after a meal.—Abdomen hard and distended.—(Distended abdomen with bilious tendency.—R. T. C.).—Acute yellow atrophy of the liver.—Enlargement and induration of liver, with pain.—Pain in hepatic region on pressure.—Enlargement of spleen.—Sensitiveness in hepatic region, < when lying on r. side, with pain on touch.—Painful pulsation in r. hypochondrium.—Contractive pain in abdomen.—Spasmodic colic.—Pinchings, cuttings, and tearings in abdomen, esp. in morning, in bed at night, and in evening, and often with urgent want to evacuate and diarrhœa.—Shooting pains in abdomen, sometimes with pallid face, shiverings, and headache.—Sensation of coldness, with heat and burning sensation in abdomen.—Inflammation of intestines.—Intussusception.—Uneasiness in abdomen after breakfast.—Pressure outwards against sides of abdomen.—Soreness of abdomen to touch when walking.—Flaccidity of the abdomen.—Obliged to lie down from weakness across abdomen.—Inguinal hernia.—Large yellow spots in abdomen.—Swelling and suppuration of inguinal glands.—Incarcerated flatus.—Flatulent colic, deeply seated in abdomen; < when lying down, with grumbling (rumbling and rolling in bowels) and borborygmi.—Flatus in general.

13. **Stool and Anus.**—A very characteristic symptom is found in the stool, which is long, slim, hard, and dry, and is evacuated with a great deal of difficulty; it may be compared to a dog's stool in appearance and in manner

of evacuation, is often accompanied with the same straining, trembling of the limbs, &c.—Diarrhœa : in great quantity, like water from a hydrant, and is very exhausting to the patient (often accompanied with a very weak, empty, or gone feeling in abdomen) ; painless ; stools large ; involuntary ; mucous.—(Emaciating diarrhœa, skin dry and hard.—E. A. Small).—Constipation.—Fæces hard, small, slow, interrupted, difficult to evacuate, and much too dry (like a dog's).—Urgent and distressing want to evacuate.—Prolonged looseness of bowels.—Fæces of the consistence of pap.—Serous diarrhœa.—Diarrhœa with diminished strength (< in morning).—Mucous diarrhœa.—Bloody diarrhœa.—Undigested fæces.—Greenish, grey (or whitish-grey), or black fæces (with flakes of mucus).—Stools watery, with whitish-yellow and cheesy masses ; lumps of white mucus.—Stools odourless save for a slight mouldy smell.—Stools like scraping of intestines.—Involuntary evacuations.—Discharge of mucus from anus, which remains continually open.—Tenia, or ascarides from rectum, during stool.—Discharge of blood during the evacuation.—After stool : pressure, burning pain, and tenesmus in anus and rectum, with great exhaustion.—Dartings and shakings in rectum and anus (this may occur in children, causing them to cry out, is usually < in evening or night ; they appear to have worms ; they will put their hands to the seat, and show by various signs where and what the matter is).—Nettle-like stitches in rectum when not at stool.—Stitches in anus.—Biting and itching in anus.—Tearing in rectum ; and genitals, even to sinking down.—Pain in anus so violent it seemed as though the body would be torn asunder, with cutting and movements in whole abdomen, constant ineffectual desire for stool, heat in hands and anxiety ; > only by application of warm cloths.—Shaking and clawing l. side of anus.—Crawling stitches.—Pruritus ani.—After stool, frightful tenesmus for some time.—Paralysis of lower intestines ; of sphincter ani.—Anus wide open.—Sensation of rectum paralysed.—Cramps and contraction of rectum.—Protrusion and ready bleeding of hæmorrhoidal tumours in rectum and anus, with pain as from excoriation, when sitting or lying down.—Fissure of anus.

14. **Urinary Organs.**—Increased secretion of watery urine.—Frequent emission of a scanty stream of urine (only a small quantity each time).—Urine with white, serous, sandy and red, or else yellow sediment.—Turbid urine, with sediment like brick-dust.—Pale, aqueous, or whitish urine.—Variegated pellicle on surface of urine.—Hæmaturia (with acute pain in region of kidneys and liver, and jaundice).—Smarting and burning sensation when urinating.—Tension and jerking, or burning pain in urethra when not urinating (with frequent desire to urinate).

15. **Male Sexual Organs.**—Very strong sexual desire, with constant wish for coition.—Impotence after excessive excitement and onanism.—Erections which are too energetic in evening or morning.—Frequent (involuntary) pollutions.—Feeble erections or none at all.—Feeble and too speedy emission during coition.—Pains in testes and swelling of spermatic cord.—Hydrocele.

16. **Female Sexual Organs.**—Nymphomania.—Aversion to coitus.—Tearing in genital organs, and stitches upward from vagina into uterus.—(Small pustulation of vulva with great irritation.—R. T. C.).—Œdema of labia (< l.), later gangrene.—Catamenia too early and too profuse (and of too long duration), or too early and too scanty and serous.—[*Phos.* patients

generally menstruate regularly but profusely, and not uncommon symptoms are, vertigo on rising in morning, with weakness of legs, so that for a few moments after getting out of bed, they cannot stand.—H. N. Martin.]—Discharge of blood from uterus during pregnancy.—Catamenia of too long duration, with toothache and colic.—Before menses: abundant bleeding of ulcers; leucorrhœa; want to urinate; and weeping.—Frequent and profuse metrorrhagia.—On appearance of menses; incisive, griping pains in the back and vomiting.—After menses: weakness, blue circles round eyes, and anxiety.—Menses: of too short continuance; retarded.—During menses: shooting headaches; fermentation in abdomen; expectoration of blood; pains in (small of) back; soreness of limbs; great lassitude and fever; or palpitation of heart; shiverings; swelling of gums and cheeks, and many other sufferings.—Sterility on account of excessive voluptuousness, or if the menstruation comes on too late and is too profuse.—Smarting, corrosive leucorrhœa (drawing blisters).—Hard and painful nodosities in breasts.—Inflammation (erysipelatous) of breasts, even after formation of pus.—Erysipelatous inflammation of mammæ, with swelling, burning pains, and shootings.—Anxious feeling beneath l. breast, with bitter eructations.—Burning, pinching in r. breast, heat mounting to head.—Cramp pain in breast, high up, under sternum, with eructations.—At 3.30 p.m. pain from l. nipple to r. nipple, thence to r. shoulder and r. little finger.—Pain below nipple shooting like electricity.—Nipples hot and sore.—Papular eruption on breasts.—Abscess in mammæ, also with fistulous ulcers; bluish colour.

17. **Respiratory Organs.**—Hoarseness and scraping in throat, sometimes prolonged.—Aphonia, so as to be unable to speak except in a whisper.—Catarrh with cough, fever, and fear of death.—Very painful sensibility of larynx, which prevents speaking.—Stitches, soreness, roughness, and dryness in the larynx.—Croup; bronchitis.—Great sensibility of larynx with burning pain.—Dryness in trachea and chest.—Expectoration of mucus from larynx.—Cough excited by a tickling and itching in chest, or with hoarseness and sensation as if chest were raw.—Hollow, hacking, spasmodic, tickling cough, esp. if caused by tickling in chest; at night, preventing sleep.—Cough with shootings in throat, chest, and scrobiculus, sometimes only at night.—Dry cough every day, which continues several hours, with pains in stomach and abdomen.—Cough with stitches over one eye.—Cough from a change in the weather and from strong odours; from lying on l. side or on back.—Cough from going from warm into cold room (H. N. Martin). — Dry, shaking cough, with sensation as if head were going to burst, excited by cold air, by drinking, or by reading aloud.—Cough with vomiting.—Cough excited by laughing.—Dry cough, as if caused by tubercles, or chronic pneumonia.—Cough in paroxysms, brings up a viscid, muco-purulent expectoration, branched like the bronchial tubes.—Cough with purulent and saltish expectoration, esp. morning and evening.—Cough with expectoration in morning, without expectoration in evening; expectoration frothy, pale red, rust-coloured, streaked with blood; white and tough; cold mucus, tasting sour or sweet; transparent mucus in morning after rising.—Greenish expectoration from cough.—Cough with expectoration of slimy mucus or of blood, with smarting in chest.

18. **Chest.**—Noisy and panting respiration.—Difficult respiration, esp. in

evening, with anguish in chest, < by sitting down.—Respiration oppressed, quick, anxious.—Difficult inspiration ; heaviness, fulness, and tension on chest.—Obstructed respiration and oppression of chest of various kinds, esp. in morning or evening, as also during movement.—Spasmodic asthma.—Constrictive spasms in chest.—After a cough, asthma.—Fits of suffocation at night.—Pressure at chest.—Heaviness, fulness, and tension in chest.—Contractive spasms in chest.—Tearing in chest.—Lancinations in chest, and esp. in l. side, sometimes prolonged, or else when the parts are touched.—Burning pain as from excoriation in chest.—Inflammation of lungs (l. side).—Pneumonia nervosa (lungs hepatised).—Tuberculosis (phthisis mucosa).—Sensation of fatigue in chest.—Anguish in chest.—Congestion in chest, with sensation of heat which ascends to throat.—Pain under l. breast, when lying upon it.—Yellow spots on chest.

19. **Heart and Pulse.**—Anxiety about heart with nausea and a peculiar hunger, somewhat > by eating, distressing even in bed.—Sensation of warmth about r. side of heart.—Pressure ; heaviness ; aching in heart.—Rush of blood to heart and palpitation, that becomes very violent after eating.—Palpitation of heart of different kinds, esp. after a meal, morning and evening, as also when seated, and after all kinds of mental excitement.—Palpitation of heart with obstructed respiration ; palpitation from every mental emotion.—Violent palpitation with anxiety, evenings and mornings in bed ; on slight motion.—Blowing sounds in heart.—Pressure in middle of sternum and about heart.—Pulse rapid, full, and hard ; small, weak, easily compressed.

20. **Neck and Back.**—Rigidity of nape of neck.—Pressure on shoulders.—Swelling of neck.—Engorgement of axillary glands and of those of nape of neck and of neck.—Itching and shooting under axillæ.—Fetid sweat under axillæ.—Paralysed sensation in upper sacrum and lower lumbar vertebræ.—Contusive pain in loins and back (as if back were broken), esp. after having been seated a long time, hindering walking, rising up, or making the least movement.—Pain in small of the back when rising from a stooping position.—Burning in back or small of back (esp. with delayed menses).—Tabes dorsalis.—Burning pains in loins.—Sensitiveness of spinous processes of dorsal vertebræ to pressure.—Softening of spine.—Heat or burning in back, between scapulæ.—Tearings and stitches in and beneath both scapulæ.—Pain in coccyx impeding easy motion, can find no comfortable position ; followed by painful stiffness of nape.—Coccyx painful to touch as from an ulcer.—Transient pain from coccyx through spine to vertex that drew head back during the stool.—Backache and palpitations prevail (R. T. C.).

21. **Limbs.**—Weakness in all the limbs as if paralysed ; esp. in joints, trembling from every exertion.—Swelling of hands and feet.—Bruised pain in limbs.—Extremities, esp. hands and feet, heavy as lead.—Numbness and falling asleep of limbs.—Exanthema on skin about joints.—Swelling of soft tissues of joints.—Joints stiff.

22. **Upper Limbs.**—Stiffness in morning on washing, with pressure.—Rheumatic tearing (and lancinating pains) in shoulders, arms, and hands (particularly in joints), esp. at night.—Burning pain in palms of hands and arms ; clammy perspiration in palms and on head.—Burning pain in hands and arms.—Numbness of arms and hands.—Lassitude and trembling in arms

and hands, and esp. when holding anything.—Furfuraceous tetters on arms. —Congestion of blood in hands, with swelling and redness of veins, esp. when allowing arms to hang down.—Wrenching pain in joints of hands and fingers, with tension.—Swelling of hands, even at night.—Heat in hands.—Coldness of hands at night.—Contraction and jerking of fingers.—Deadness of fingers.—Paralysis of fingers.—Numbness of finger-tips.—Skin cracked at joints of fingers.—Chilblains on fingers.

23. **Lower Limbs.**—Uneasiness, weakness, < on ascending steps, with heaviness.—Pain as from ulceration (suppurative) in buttocks when seated.—Pain in r. hip-joint.—(Exostosis of femur.)—Wrenching pain in coxo-femoral joints, and those of knees and feet, with external heat.—Swelling of tibia. —Bruised pain in periosteum of tibia.—Gangrenous periosteum of tibia, with fever; the periosteum peeled off as far as knee, leaving the bone rough.—Painful fatigue and heaviness of legs.—Heaviness in hollow of knees.—Burning sensation in legs and feet.—Tension and cramps in legs, esp. in knees.—Rheumatic stiffness of the knee.—Shocks in legs before going to sleep, day and night.—Drawing and tearing (rheumatic pain) in knees, extending into feet.—Paralytic weakness in legs, and arthritic rigidity of knees.—Tetters on knee.—Spots like petechiæ on legs.—Ulcers on legs, with surrounding small pustules.—Exostosis on tibia.—Jerking, and cramp in calves.—Tearings and shootings in feet, esp. at night (in feet of a pregnant woman).—Swelling of feet, or only of the malleoli, esp. in evening or after a walk, sometimes with shooting pain.—Sprained pain in ankles on walking.—Easy dislocation of foot.—Coldness of feet, esp. at night.—Paralytic feeling in feet.—Pain (as if bruised) as from ulceration in soles when walking.—Shocks in feet day and night before going to sleep.—Numbness of tips of toes.—Inflammation and redness of ball of great toe with lancinations.—Chilblains and corns on toes.

24. **Generalities.**—Affections of inner chest; shinbones; bones of legs; of r. upper or r. lower extremity; r. upper or r. lower side.—Profuse secretion of mucus.—Affections of axillary glands; inflammation of glands in general; glands painful, particularly stitching pains; hot swelling of glands. —Glandular diseases, esp. after contusion.—Bleeding from inner parts; threatened phthisis pulmonalis.—The pains of *Phos.* are continuous, or, at least, irregular as to time.—Arthritic and rheumatic tearings and stitching pains, principally in limbs, sometimes after a slight chill, esp. in bed at night.—Burning pain in limbs.—Tension, cramp, jerking, and distortion of some of the limbs.—Sprains, easy dislocations.—Ataxia and adynamia.—Convulsions.—Rigidity of some parts.—Fits of paleness and numbness in some of the limbs, which then appear dead.—Mucous membrane pale.—Trembling of limbs from least exertion, but chiefly during labour.—Tendency to strain the back.—Ebullition and congestion of blood, sometimes with pulsation throughout body.—Sensations: of fulness; of itching or tickling; of knocking, beating, or throbbing; of darting; darting pain; of roughness—all occurring in inner parts.—Sensation of dryness or of festering in internal parts.—Bleeding from various (internal) organs.—Inflammation and stinging pain of inner parts.—Itching of inner parts.—Small wounds bleed much.—Blood fluid non-coagulable.—Bleeding from all cavities; also from soft cancer.—Weakness and soreness in joints, esp. knees.—Great weakness and para-

lytic lassitude, which sometimes come on suddenly, esp. in bed in morning, or after a very short walk.—Can only lie on the r. side.—Lying on the l. side at night causes anxiety.—Spasms of the paralysed side.—Paralysis, formication, and tearing in limbs ; anæsthesia ; increased heat.—Exostosis, esp. of skull.—Hip-joint disease, oozing a watery pus.—Epilepsy with consciousness. —Fainting fits ; from strong odours.—Excessive sensibility of all the organs. —Hysterical lassitude.—General dejection and nervous debility.—Heaviness of limbs and sluggishness.—Paralysis with tingling in the parts affected.—Emaciation and consumption.—Inability to remain in open air, esp. when cold.—Strong tendency to take cold, which is often followed by headache and toothache, coryza, with fever, shivering, &c.—Effects of hair-cutting and chill to head.—Pains in limbs on change of weather.—The majority of symptoms manifest themselves morning and evening, in bed, as well as after dinner, while several others appear at the beginning of a meal and disappear after it.—<: In morning ; evening ; before falling asleep ; on waking ; before breakfast ; after taking cold ; while coughing ; before or after eating ; from violent bleeding ; from spraining parts ; while lying on back ; lying on l. side ; from laughing (often producing cough) ; from light in general ; light of the lamp ; warm food ("very thirsty, takes water, likes it, feels better, gets warm in stomach and is vomited") ; reading aloud ; from strong smells ; after stool (exhausted, &c.) ; while swallowing drink ; in the wind ; when singing ; when the weather changes either way.—> : In the dark ; lying on r. side ; from being mesmerised ; from rubbing ; from scratching ; after sleep ; from cold things ; cold food ; cold water (till it gets warm).

25. **Skin.**—Exanthema which comes out in pustules ; is scaly.—Ulcers in general.—Summer freckles.—Hard swellings here and there on body.—Wounds which appear to have healed break out again and bleed ; wounds that continually heal and break out again.—Desquamation of skin.—Burning in the skin.—Excoriated spots on skin, with cracks and shootings.—Round, tettery spots over whole body.—Freckles (nose).—Dry, furfuraceous tetters.—Yellow or brown spots on skin (esp. chest and abdomen).—Copper-coloured or bluish spots, like petechiæ.—Red spots.—Jaundice.—Pale skin.—Ecchymosis.—Furunculi.—Lymphatic abscess with fistulous ulcers (which have callous margins, secreting a fetid and colourless pus) and hectic fever.—Large ulcers surrounded by small ones.—Ulcers bleed on appearance of menses.—Fungus hæmatodes.—Copious bleeding even from very small wounds.—Polypus.—Chilblains (fingers and toes) and corns on feet, sometimes very painful.—Tingling in skin.—Nettle-rash.

26. **Sleep.**—Falling asleep late.—Complaints preventing sleep.—Overpowering sleep coming on after dinner, if only a moderate dinner has been eaten.—Sleeplessness before midnight.—Sleepy at 7 p.m. ; wakeful at night (produced.—R. T. C.).—Strong tendency to sleep by day, as from lethargy.—Stupefying sleep.—Sleep retarded in evening, and sleeplessness at night, or frequent waking, with difficulty in going to sleep again, caused by restlessness, with anguish, tossing, heat, vertigo, and ebullition of blood.—Inability to remain lying on back or on side.—Coma vigil.—Sleep unrefreshing ; sensation in morning as after insufficient sleep.—At night vertigo with nausea, painful sensibility of limbs, pains in stomach and abdomen, suffocating and spasmodic asthma, &c.—Frequent waking from feeling

too hot, without perspiration.—Frequent waking, with starts and fright.—During sleep, jerks in limbs, cries, talking, tears, complaints, lamentations, and moans.—Dreams: anxious, distressing; lascivious; frightful and horrible; or vivid and uneasy; of animals which bite; of robbers; fire; the business of the day (which he could not finish); bloodshed; death; quarrels; creeping things, &c.—Nightmare.—Somnambulism.

27. **Fever.**—Shuddering and shivering, esp. in bed, in evening (without thirst, with aversion to being uncovered and with swollen veins on hands), sometimes with yawning, followed by heat or otherwise.—Coldness of limbs.—Internal chilliness and chill not > by heat of stove.—Chilliness in evening till midnight, with great weakness and sleep.—Chill running down back.—Shiverings, followed by heat, with thirst and sweat, esp. at night, and in afternoon.—(Chronic feverishness with recurring albuminuria.—R. T. C.).—Internal or external heat of single parts. — Flushes of heat running up back.—Burning in back, between shoulder-blades.—Burning pain of external parts or of internal parts.—Transient or anxious heat.—Nocturnal heat (disturbing sleep).—Flushes of heat over whole body, beginning in hands.—Perspiration most profuse on head, hands, and feet, with increased secretion of urine.—Perspiration on fore part of body.—Perspiration frequently smells of sulphur or of garlic.—Intermittent fever: heat and perspiration at night, with faintness and ravenous hunger, which could not be satisfied with eating; afterwards chilliness with chattering of teeth and external coldness; the chilliness was succeeded by internal heat, esp. in hands, while the external coldness continued.—Fevers with soporous condition, dry, black lips and tongue and open mouth.—Typhus fever (often with pneumonia and bronchitis, that developed into consumption).—Hectic fever, with dry heat towards the evening, esp. in palms of hands, sweat, and colliquative diarrhœa, circumscribed redness of cheeks (l. more than r.), &c.—Pulse changed; quick, full, and hard; occasionally small and weak.—Nocturnal and viscid sweat.—Sweat in morning.—Cold, clammy sweat.

Phosphorus Hydrogenatus.

Phosphoretted Hydrogen. Phosphine. PH_3. Solution.

Clinical.—Amblyopia. Diarrhœa. Hyperæsthesia. Locomotor ataxy. Stammering. Teeth, crumbling.

Characteristics.—Breunar (quoted by Allen) relates the effects of inhaling this gas, given off in the preparation of some "hypophosphites." The symptoms began to appear after three months in visional disturbances, diarrhœa, paralysis, and a complete state of locomotor ataxia, < on closing eyes. The teeth crumbled without pain. Articulation and swallowing were difficult. The diarrhœa was accompanied by weakness of the anus.

Relations.—Electricity *antidoted* the effects. *Compare:* Locomotor ataxy, Arg. n., Alm., Helod. Visional defects, Benz. din., Carb. s.

SYMPTOMS.

3. **Eyes.**—Flickering points in field of vision, rapidly enlarging and rendering it impossible to fix vision on any object, esp. in reading.—Optic nerves very irritable to reflex stimuli.

4. **Ears.**—Auditory hyperæsthesia.

8. **Mouth.**—Teeth, both healthy and carious, crumble, without pain.—Ataxia of muscles of articulation, great effort of will required to form the word.

9. **Throat.**—Swallowing somewhat difficult.

12. **Abdomen.**—Shooting pains in limbs and abdomen.

13. **Stool and Anus.**—Diarrhœa with weakness and unsteadiness of arms.

22. **Upper Limbs.**—Weakness and unsteadiness of arms, making difficult to write.

23. **Lower Limbs.**—Limbs unsteady; gait tottering; associated with undercurrent shooting pains in limbs and abdomen.

24. **Generalities.**—Complete expression of ataxia; stood with limbs separated; walking wholly impossible when eyes closed; would stagger and fall.—No anæsthesia; electric irritability of muscles greatly increased.

Phosphorus Muriaticus.

Phosphorus pentachloride. PCl_5. Solution.

Clinical.—Asthma. Coryza. Ophthalmia.

Characteristics.—J. Meredith (*H. W.*, xxxiii. 127) has recorded the effects observed on a science student from grinding up this salt and inhaling the fumes. Eye-soreness, coryza, sore throat and chest with difficult breathing, were the main symptoms. They lasted fourteen days from the exposure; and were cured by *Bell.* 3x internally and a one per cent. *Iodine* lotion locally as a compress at night.

SYMPTOMS.

3. **Eyes.**—Great soreness of mucous membranes of eyes and nose, with copious intermittent runnings; lasts all night.—Shades eyes from light reflected from tablecloth at dinner.—Whites of eyes congested.

5. **Nose.**—Irritation and copious intermittent running.—The intolerable smell of the fumes cannot be forgotten at night, and sleep is impossible.

9. **Throat.**—Throat and chest sore.

17. **Respiratory Organs.**—In morning breathing difficult; lungs wheezy; chest and throat sore.

26. **Sleep.**—Symptoms kept him awake all night.

Physalia.

Physalia pelagica. Portuguese man-of-war. *N. O.* Physophoridæ.

Clinical.—Urticaria.

Characteristics.—G. Bennett was stung by the animal on second and ring fingers. The sensation was as if stung by a nettle, succeeded in a few minutes by violent aching, affecting the finger-joints and spreading up arm, involving elbow-joint. The pain was < by application of water; < by motion; and < when joints became affected. The pain spread to the shoulder-joint and pectoral muscles causing oppression of breathing. After half an hour the symptoms began to abate, leaving numbness of the limb and a vesicle at the spot which was stung.

Relations.—*Compare:* Medusa, Urt. ur.

Physostigma.

Physostigma venenosum. Calabar Bean. Eséré. *N. O.* Leguminosæ. Trituration of the bean.

Clinical.—Astigmatism. Bathing, effects of. Blepharospasm. Chorea. Ciliary spasm. Climacteric. Constipation. Coccygodynia. Dentition. Diarrhœa. Dyspepsia. Epilepsy. *Eyes, affections of;* injuries of; strain of. General paralysis. Glaucoma. Hæmorrhoids. Headache. Heart, affections of. Hemiplegia (l.) Herpes, preputialis. Hiccough. Hysteria. Iris, prolapsed. Leucorrhœa. Levitation. Locomotor ataxy. *Myopia.* Navel, inflammation of. *Paralysis, local;* agitans; spinal. Paraplegia. Progressive muscular atrophy. Prostration; muscular. Sleeplessness. Spinal irritation. Spinal sclerosis. Stiff neck. Tetanus. Throat, sore; fish-bone sensation. Water, effects of. Wounds.

Characteristics.—"The Ordeal-bean" of Old Calabar, the Eséré of the natives, is the type of a genus of *Leguminosæ* of the tribe *Phaseoleæ*, with flowers very like *Phaseolus*, except that its bearded style is terminated by a great oblique hood, covering the blunt stigma." It is this hood which distinguishes the genus and gives it its name. *P. ven.* is a great twining climber, and has purplish flowers. Its seeds are very poisonous, and are used by the Calabari as an ordeal, suspected persons being compelled to eat them until they either vomit or die. In the latter case they are considered guilty, in the former innocent. In cases observed in Calabar convulsions have been noted, and twitchings, especially in the back, and death in thirty minutes. A number of cases of poisoning have occurred in this country, and in these the most notable feature was complete muscular prostration. According to Brunton, the tetanising properties of the bean belong to an alkaloid, *Calabarine*, and the paralysis to *Eserine* (or *Physostigmine*, as it is now called). In animals poisoned by it speedy general paralysis is set up, and death occurs from failure of respiration; though the heart may be poisoned both directly and through its nerves. The paralysis is seated in the spinal cord itself. The muscles are affected by fluttering tremors; involuntary muscles are excited to active movements and expulsive efforts. The intestines are often twisted up in knots. All the secretions are somewhat increased (*C. D. P.*). A crowd of children in Liverpool ate beans which they found among the sweepings of a ship from Africa. Forty-six were admitted to hospital with loss of muscular power, prostration, feeble, slow pulse, cold, perspiring skin, cold extremities; vomiting in nearly all cases, diarrhœa in one-third of them. At first there was colic, but later on remarkable freedom from pain. Pupils contracted in many; in one contracted during sleep, dilated when aroused. Only one (a phthisical boy) succumbed. He staggered as he walked, then fell, kicking and rolling as if in pain, but afterwards became quiet; much purged; pulse hardly perceptible; skin cold, face livid; quite conscious and able to swallow water. Directly after drinking he died without a struggle, some froth issuing from nose and mouth. After death the blood was found to be fluid; the heart distended with it, and its muscular substance very flaccid (*C. D. P.*). Many excellent provings have been made with *Physo.*, among which one made by Christison on himself is remarkable. Simpson and Douglas MacLagan were sent for to attend him in his collapsed state, which Simpson could only compare to that produced by severe flooding, though Christison's only sensation was one of "extreme but not unpleasant faintness." MacLagan thought it like *Aconite* poisoning. Christison could not get his *will* into his muscles except by a tremendous effort. Warmth to feet and a sinapism to whole abdomen gave great relief, and he was then able to turn on his left side; but only remained there a very short time on account of the tumultuous action of the heart it set up. He became drowsy and slept; but his mind was so active in sleep that on awaking he did not know that he had slept. The tumultuous action of the heart continued on waking, but strong coffee quickly restored the whole condition and made the heart regular. A symptom observed by Christison and many other provers was one of indigestion, "as if large pieces of food had been suddenly swallowed." It began under upper sternum, descending and increasing in intensity till it reached the epigastrium; eructations then occurred, and a reversal of direction followed, the sensation ending where it began. With other provers there was a sensation of weight and hardness. Christison also had very much giddiness and dimness of vision. It is for its action on the eye, especially for its power of contracting the pupil, and thereby antagonising *Atropine*, that *Physo.* and its alkaloid *Eserine* are best known in old-school practice. The effects are more definite when the drug (tincture, extract, or solution of alkaloid) is applied to the eye direct; but one myopic prover had his myopia much diminished. In glaucoma it has been used with signal success to diminish intraocular tension; and especially when glaucoma has been the result of injury. Dudgeon (*B. J. H.*, xxxviii. 60) relates the case of A. E., 26, struck by the cork of a soda-water bottle on inferior and outer part of left eyeball. Intense burning pain and effusion into the eyeball followed. Under *Arn.*, prescribed by Mr. Engall, the effusion disappeared, and later the pain and inflammation subsided under *Aco.* and *Merc. c.* The pupil was now egg-shaped, the long diameter perpendicular, smaller end downwards; vision extremely myopic. *Bell.* dilated the pupil, but had no effect on the vision. Engall sent the patient to Dudgeon, who found the pupil was sluggish, and a book had to be held within four inches of the eye to be read. *Physo.* 3x, every three hours, was given. After the first dose objects could be seen at a considerable distance, and next day sight was nearly as good as ever. Dudgeon considers that the lens was tilted by the blow, and that *Physo.* restored the over-stretched or paralysed portion of the ciliary muscle. Woodyatt (*Org.* iii. 99) states that *Physo.* has produced corneal astigmatism in a young lady, who found any attempt at close work caused redness of tarsal edges and a hot, sandy feeling in conjunctiva. *Lil. t.* 30 cured. Paralysis and tremors predominate over the cramps, twitchings, stiffnesses, and tension of *Physo.*, but these are also characteristic, and tetanus has been cured by *Physo.* Paralysis of left side is very pro-eminent, and the numbness is more apparent on left side, especially in left arm; which may be associated with heart symptoms. The apex of the left lung is also affected. A feeling of levitation was observed in one prover on stepping. Ataxic gait and shooting pains down limbs show its appropriateness in locomotor ataxy. The inability to get the *will* into the muscles is a striking feature of many paralyses. Spinal, sacral, and coccygeal pains were experienced, and associated with some of them, numbness of the womb. The association of *muscular prostration* (in any form, of which laboured respiration is one) with any affection is a keynote of *Physo.* This case was cured: Great muscular prostration with continual inclination to sigh; leucorrhœa < by exercising during the day, especially 4 p.m.; sighing < when leucorrhœa is <; dread of cold water. This *dread of cold water* is a grand keynote of *Physo.* One of the provers (a water drinker) developed a perfect disgust for cold water and cold drinks; and though used to a cold morning plunge, was obliged to omit it on account of his horror. Other provers felt uncomfortable after bathing, and had great reluctance to their bath. Weakness was felt on change of weather, and on cold, bracing days. A paralytic state of mind and body from grief has been cured with *Physo.* Sleeplessness of a peculiar kind occurs in *Physo.* Nash (*Med. Adv.*, xx. 258) cured with *Physo.* 12 and 30 persistent sleeplessness in a patient who had been in an insane asylum, and feared she would have to go again. Her symptom was: "If she chanced to get a nap she awoke suddenly as if in a fright, and felt no > from what she had slept." *Peculiar sensations* are: As if stomach were full. As if she must lose her mind. As if a ball were coming up throat. Lower limbs as if asleep. Back as if paralysed. Tongue as if burnt (left margin); as if swollen and paralysed. Sensations of contraction and tension. Wavering in brain. Weak feeling in stomach. H. L. Chase, one of the provers, had a "very severe pain in the right popliteal space," and he afterwards cured a patient who came to him with pain in the same region two years later (*H. R.*, xiii. 117). (Allen gives the symptom as in the *left* popliteal space.) The symptoms are < by pressure (of finger between vertebræ causing wincing); by falls and blows. < Motion; descending stairs (wavering in brain). < Walking; stepping; jar of misstep. > Lying supine. < Lying l. side ; > lying on r. side. < 4 p.m. < Night (headache unbearable). If pain began at any hour it always continued till 12 o'clock following, either noon or midnight. < Cold water ; perfect horror of cold drink ; cold bath. < From bathing ; from change in weather ; on bracing days. < In church. > In cool open air. < On waking. > Closing eyes. > By sleep (hiccough). > Warmth to feet ; sinapisms to abdomen.

Relations.—*Antidoted by:* Coffee ; Sinapisms ; Arn. ; (emetics are of the first importance. Injection of Atropine antagonises its effects). Lil. t. cured astigmatism of Physo. *Compare:* Eserin. In paralyses, Lathyr., Oxyt., Strych., Ciner., Con., Gels. Heart, Phaseol., Phos. Eyes, Onos., Lil. t., Rut., Jabor., Bell. Headache with drowsiness, Brucea, Gins., Herac. Spinal irritation, hungry sensation, numbness, muscles of back rigid, wavering in brain, Act. r. Headache < by music, Phos., Phos. ac. (Physo. of organ.). Levitation, Phos., Phos. ac. Headache with inability to stop thinking (Phos. with increased mental power), Globus, Ign., Asaf. < Descending stairs, Borax. Increased irritability, tetanic spasms, cramp, tenesmus recti, stiff spine and legs, Strych. and Nux (Physo. has diminished reflexes, spinal paralysis ; unsteady gait with eyes closed ; death by paralysis, Strych. has death from respiratory spasm ; dilated pupils). Tetanus, Passif. Tongue as if scalded, Sang.

Causation.—Emotions. Grief. Bathing. Injuries. Blows.

SYMPTOMS.

1. **Mind.**—Uncommon mental activity.—Foolish actions, said it made him crazy.—Exhilarated in morning, gloomy towards noon.—Nothing was right, too many things in room ; continually counting them.—Irritable.—Nervous, cannot endure pain.—Exhaustion, cannot remember anything.—Disinclined to work.—Difficult thinking ; cannot concentrate the mind.

2. **Head.**—Vertigo : on moving, with fainting and muscæ volitantes ; with nausea ; in evening, if people stepped in front of her in the doorway ; at night ; when reading ; on getting up after dinner ; when walking ; on descending stairs, with dim vision and unsteady gait ; wavering in brain ; as if drunk ; with sensation of wavering in brain.—Confusion and dizziness ; dull, heavy, oppressive headache.—Intolerable pain over both eyes.—Head drooping listlessly.—Darting pain in various parts, < motion.—Aching in morning with epistaxis l. side.—Bruised pain in brain all day, < a heavy step ; < l. temple, with general fatigue and sensitiveness to cold or change of temperature.—Pressure encircling head, with sleepiness.—Constriction as from a bandage or tight cap pressed down as far as temples.—Severe, dull, frontal headache, esp. in the morning.—Darting pain in forehead, < motion, and in temples.—Sharp pain in supra-orbital region, running off towards nose.—Pain : over r. eye, in morning on waking, by noon pain in whole cerebrum, fulness of blood-vessels of brain, and contracted feeling in forehead, which extended to eyelids, causing an effort to open or close them ; in l. side at 10 a.m., with heat in abdomen and nausea, the pain is heavy at 11, pain over whole head from 4 till 10 p.m., with nausea and general sweat, headache next day with lame, bruised feeling in region of kidneys.—Pain in temples ; show-

ing from r. temple to 2nd bicuspid.—In evening sound of the organ caused headache, < forehead and temples.—One-sided headache with fear of opening eyes lest it should < the pain.—Inability to stop thinking with headache. —Sensation of rush of blood to frontal and temporal regions.—Sharp, shooting pains in temples.—Throbbing of temporal and carotid arteries; heart beats felt in head on lying down.—Intense, painful pressure in vertex and both temples, the pressure in vertex extending over to occiput.

3. **Eyes.**—Eyes inflamed, first r., then l.; sclerotic dry, red, and swollen; eyeballs pain and smart; lids feel sore.—Eyes bloodshot all the forenoon, with burning in them.—Pain on attempting to use binocular vision, as in reading, so that one eye must be closed, > by a weak concave glass.—Pressure; with muscæ volitantes, dark and light long worms or snakes, also tremulous vision.—Bright marks when looking at an object; dark yellowish spots covering one or two letters when reading.—Sharp, shooting pains, and drawing, twisting sensation in eyes.—Eyes sore and painful when moved from side to side.—Pain deep in, over top of eyeball, running up from inner canthus to r. frontal eminence, then down obliquely outward into temple.—Sharp stitches in r. eyeball, > by motion in open air.—The muscularis internus seems not to do its work rightly, and the axis of the eyes differs in each; eyes feel weak, with lachrymation.—Eyes convulsed.—Sight blurred, hazy, or misty, film over eyes; objects mixed; after which dull pain over the eyes and between the eyes.—Aching in posterior part of orbit, extending back into the brain; < on reading, causing nausea.—Lids (esp. l.) heavy; cannot bear to raise them; twitching of lids (upper, < l.).—Contracted sensation in lids with difficulty in opening them and lachrymation when wide open, difficulty in keeping l. eye open.—Lids immovable.—Tight feeling in ciliary region as if something were creeping about in it, with sharp pain, < reading.—Contraction of pupils; in morning; by small and rapid jerks, with sensitiveness to light; then mydriasis, < morning, seeming to depend on fatigue of sphincter, which was > during day by reflex stimulus of light.—Pupils dilated.—Pupils contracted when asleep, dilated when aroused.—Disturbed accommodation; approximation of far point (myopia) and also of near point (the accommodation recovers before the pupil).—Vision abnormally acute; double; dim and indistinct; blurred, hazy, misty.—(Lens dislocated by blow.)

4. **Ears.**—Sharp, shooting pains in the ears.—Shooting in l. ear; in r.—Pain in r. ear when writing.—Hammering in r. in evening, with feeling in external ear as from a hot wind.—Painful pressure on tympani.—Discomfort in r., with inclination to bore in with finger; after removal of wax some pain; *with eructation* a sudden pain from throat along Eustachian tube to middle ear.—Crawling in l. ear.—Fulness.—Stopped feeling.—Partial deafness of r.—Sensitive to every sound.—Singing or tuning like escaping steam, at night after lying down.—Hissing, buzzing, ringing in the ears.

5. **Nose.**—Fluent coryza, sneezing; burning, smarting, itching, and tingling of nostrils; nose stuffed and hot.—Twitchings in nose and involuntary expansion of nostrils.—Small boil inside r. nostril.—Epistaxis while at supper.—Smarting at end of nose, it feels as if burnt by hot liquid.—Tension in skin of nose and forehead.

6. **Face.**—Face pale; flushings of the face; heat.—Neuralgic pain in r. side of face.—Sensation of cramps or spasms in face extending to neck;

with numbness of l. hand.—Sensation of contraction of l. side of face, with numbness.—Severe pain in r. upper jaw like toothache (though all teeth on that side had been extracted).—Numbness of lips.

7. **Teeth.**—Dentition: nervous children with vacillating pupils who have trouble when nursing or taking food; pain in stomach as soon as they begin, but going off if they continue to nurse.

8. **Mouth.**—Tongue sore on tip and rough.—Smarting of end of tongue; feels as if burnt.—Scalding sensation l. side.—Tongue coated, more heavily at root.—Numbness and tingling of tongue and lips, with constant desire to moisten them.—Bad taste in mouth.—Profuse salivation; thick, leathery saliva.—Difficult speech.—Power of speech retained long after inability to swallow.

9. **Throat.**—Sore throat, painful swallowing.—Tonsils and soft palate dark red.—Burning, scraping, raw feeling in throat.—Tonsils enlarged; swollen, elongated uvula.—Small ulcers, with yellow centres in pharynx.—Feeling as of a fish-bone in throat; swallowing saliva very painful.—Constriction of throat and dysphagia.—Pain extending from throat to l. ear when swallowing.—Feeling as if a ball were coming up in throat.—Submaxillary gland tender and tumefied.

10. **Appetite.**—Hunger but can find nothing to satisfy it; food has a flat taste.—No appetite, disgust for food, tobacco, and coffee; and esp. for cold drinks.

11. **Stomach.**—Tasteless eructations.—Burning in stomach with hot eructations.—Violent hiccough.—Nausea and vomiting.—In stomach: prickling, sharp pains; darting pains, with paralysed feeling of l. side; heaviness and weight, as if undigested food were lying there; hard pain; griping; emptiness and weakness; sensation of nervousness and trembling.—Soreness in region of stomach.—Sensation at epigastrium as when large pieces of food are suddenly swallowed.

12. **Abdomen.**—Lancinating pains in hypochondria.—Hard, sore pain in splenic region; descending to groin and across hypogastrium, < by motion.—Soreness and pain at navel, which was found much inflamed.—Severe pain in umbilical region.—Pain and soreness in umbilical region.—Stitches in l. side of abdomen.—Much rumbling and distension in abdomen, with discharge of large quantities of flatus.—Dull pain in transverse and descending colon.—Colicky pains, with feeling as if diarrhœa would occur.—Shooting pains in l. iliac region and down thigh.—Sharp, cutting pains in lower part of abdomen.—Dull pain in groins.

13. **Stool and Anus.**—Stools: copious; soft, thin; watery; yellowish; bilious; part natural, part black like tar; lumpy, mixed with watery discharge; dark and offensive.—Constipation; from atony.—Sphincter ani swollen and rigid; evacuation painful; rectum protruding, swollen and very sensitive.—Tenesmus and burning, with diarrhœa; also tenesmus of bladder.—Stool irregular and loose, anus sore and inclined to protrude; piles (absent for three years) return.—Severe piles following childbirth.

14. **Urinary Organs.**—Bruised, sore feeling in region of kidneys.—Bladder feels distended.—Frequent desire to urinate, often ineffectual.—Frequent and copious urination.—Urine: yellow; high coloured; strong-smelling; clear; muddy; pale and copious.

15. **Male Sexual Organs.**—Frequent erections with but slight desire. —Two emissions without dreams or excitement.—Strong-smelling sweat about genitals, prepuce tender and swollen, many small vesicles on glans with burning itching.

16. **Female Sexual Organs.**—Leucorrhœa ; < exercising during day, esp. about 4 p.m. ; with inclination to sigh ; sighing < when leucorrhœa is worse ; dread of cold water.—Menses irregular.—Numbness of womb with pain in back.—Condition like that produced by flooding after delivery.—Metrorrhagia.—Pain as if menses were coming on.—Menstruation, with palpitation ; congestion of the eyes, with tonic spasms, rigidity, sighing respiration, consciousness retained.

17. **Respiratory Organs.**—Cough from tickling in throat.—Slight constant inclination to cough from filling lungs.—Laboured, sighing respiration ; yawning.

18. **Chest.**—Stitches in the chest.—Cannot fill l. lung as inspiration = dull pain at l. apex, > by pressure.—Stitches under inferior angles of scapulæ during expiration.—Heavy weight at chest.—Twitches across pectoral muscles.—Stitches in l. breast, and unable to draw long breath.

19. **Heart and Pulse.**—Dull pain, uneasiness and distress about the heart.—Violent palpitation of the heart, with feeling of pulsation through whole body.—As the fresh, bracing air strikes me, a choking sensation with fluttering of heart.—Heart's action irregular and tumultuous, when lying on l. side, > when lying on the back.—Pulse : variable ; accelerated ; small, frequent, slow, feeble, intermittent.

20. **Neck and Back.**—Inclination to stretch out the neck.—Pain at base of brain as if it were cutting off body from head ; going through to back part of throat, which is stiff and sore.—Stiffness in neck.—On waking, pain in r. head and neck as if latter was stiff.—While taking morning bath suddenly stiff neck (r.).—Drawing on turning head.—Rheumatic pains in l. neck and shoulder.—Feeling of weakness passed down from occiput through back to lower limbs.—Cramp-like stitches up and down spine ; stiffness of l. neck.—Chilly, creeping sensations up back, 7 p.m.—Back very weak, unable to stand erect.—Dull pain in back.—Backache (in renal region) kept him restless all night ; no > in any position ; passed copious colourless urine.—Creeping numbness from back of head down spine.—Cramp-like stitches up and down the spine.—Pain under r. shoulder-blade.—Dull, heavy pain in lumbar region ; also over l. hip, extending to back.—Pain in back between hips, with numbness of womb.—Pain in (l.) sacral region, as if strained by lifting, < on motion.—Contractive pain of anterior surface of coccyx ; as if dysentery coming on ; (since verified).

21. **Limbs.**—Limbs feel weary, as after great fatigue.—(Pleasant) numbness in all the limbs ; and paralytic feeling.—Neuralgic pains in the limbs. —Stiffness or bruised feeling in the joints.—Staggering gait.—Cold extremities.

22. **Upper Limbs.**—Wrists feel weak ; dull aching pain in them.—Sharp, shooting pain in l. shoulder.—Itching of l. palm.—Paroxysms of burning in palms.—Hands feel cold, then hot and red.—Pain in r. deltoid > only by violent motion.—Numbness in l. arm.—Sharp pain in l., then r. arm.

23. **Lower Limbs.**—Unsteadiness from knee downward when walking,

esp. with eyes shut.—Dragging pain in l. hip towards back.—Thrusts with aching down l. thigh from iliac region.—Stiffness in hip and knee.—Cramp-like pain in l. (and r.) popliteal space.—Sensation of a drawing cord behind leg and knee, impeding walking.—Gnawing in l. tibia.—Legs feel asleep.—Numbness in l. foot.

24. Generalities.—Indescribable torpidity as from opium ; " this is not debility but volition is inoperative " (Christison's experiment).—Great sense of fatigue and weariness ; weakness.—Convulsive twitchings.—Constant fibrillary twitchings of the muscles.—Violent trembling all over the body.—Great prostration of the muscular system.—Diminished reflex action.—Omits bath on account of horror for cold water.—Sore and stiff all over, as from a cold.—Severe, sharp pains in various parts of the body.—In nerves in front of body waves like tremblings going up and down ; at back nerves paralysed and numbed with pain as when the nerve of a tooth is being killed.—Stiff all over as after taking cold.—Paralysed feeling in l. side.—On raising foot in walking, momentary feeling as if he were floating upwards, and on foot touching ground an unpleasant feeling making a shuddering sensation pass all over him.

26. Sleep.—Irresistible desire to sleep ; soporific sleep.—Restless sleep with dreams.—During sleep mind so active was unaware he had been asleep.—Falls asleep frequently, but awakes suddenly without relief ; following night scarcely closed eyes in sleep ; thoughts very active ; an idea once started kept on with unusual persistence.

27. Fever.—Creeping, chilly sensation in back ; yawning ; every movement and draught = shuddering.—Hands and feet cold.—Cold, clammy skin.—Heat in head and face ; flushed and hot.—Heat in face and down back with chilliness of legs.—Dry burning in hands.—Perspires very easily.—Cold sweat in drops over whole body.—Strong-smelling sweat around genitals.—Copious sweat all over body.

Phytolacca.

Phytolacca decandra. Virginian Poke. Poke-root. Red Ink Plant. Garget Weed. *N. O.* Phytolaccaceæ. Tincture of fresh root dug in winter. Tincture of the ripe berries. Tincture of fresh leaves. Solution of the resinous extract, Phytolaccin.

Clinical.—Abortion, threatened. Albuminuria. Angina pectoris. Anus, fissure of. Asthma. Barber's itch. *Boils. Bone, diseases of* ; tumours of. *Breasts, affections of. Cancer.* Cholera. *Cicatrix.* Ciliary neuralgia. Constipation. *Corpulence.* Cough. Dentition, difficult. Diarrhœa. *Diphtheria.* Diplopia. Dysentery. Dysmenia. Ears, affections of. Erythema nodosum. Eustachian tubes, affections of. Glands, enlarged. Gleet. Glossitis. Gonorrhœa. Gout. Granular conjunctivitis. Hæmorrhoids. Headache. Hearing, altered. Heart, affections of ; hypertrophy of ; fatty. Impotence. Influenza. Intestinal catarrh. Itch. Lactation, abnormal. Laryngismus. Leucorrhœa. Lichen. Liver, affections of. Lumbago. Lupus. Mercury, effects of. Mouth, ulcerated. Mumps. *Neuralgia.* Nipples, sore ; painful. Nursing, painful. Orchitis. Ozæna. Panophthalmitis. Paralysis, diphtheritic. Parotitis. Prostate, affections of. Rectum, cancer of. *Respiration, abnormal. Rheumatism* ; syphilitic ; gonorrhœal. Ringworm. Rodent ulcer. Salivation.

Sciatica. *Sewer-gas poisoning.* Spinal irritation. Spleen, pain in. Stiff-neck. *Syphilis.* Syphilitic eruptions. Tetanus. *Throat, sore;* diphtheritic; herpetic; granular. Toothache. Tumours. Ulcers. Uterus, affections of. Warts. *Wens.*

Characteristics.—*Phyt. dec.* is a branching herbaceous plant, with a thick perennial root, sometimes larger than a man's leg in diameter. The young shoots, though extremely acrid, are rendered harmless by boiling, and are eaten like asparagus in the United States. The berries have a popular repute as a remedy for cancer and rheumatism. The berries of *P. octandra* are used in Mexico and the West Indies as a soap. According to Raffinesque, quoted by Hale (who introduced the remedy into homœopathy), the ash of the plant (which has been used as an escharotic in cancers, ulcers, &c.) contains 45 per cent. of caustic potash; and the plant contains besides an acid, *Phytolaccic acid*, which is closely allied to *Malic acid*. The plant is common throughout North America, the Azores, North Africa, and China. It grows in damp places. Some rather severe cases of poisoning have been reported. Vomiting, diarrhœa, frontal headache, sore throat, are the most common symptoms observed. One boy who drank two or three drachms of a tincture of the root had none of these symptoms, but developed complete tetanus: Extremities stiff; hands firmly shut; feet extended; toes flexed; lower lids drawn down; teeth clenched; lips everted and firm, general opisthotonos. Respiration difficult, râles heard all over the room. For an hour muscular rigidity increased generally, with convulsive action of muscles of face and neck; chin drawn close on sternum. This condition would last five or ten minutes, to be succeeded by perfect relaxation, and return in twenty minutes more with the same violence. After cold-water affusion, cupping, and sinapisms, the boy slept about twenty-five minutes. On awaking some twitchings, especially of lower limbs; pain in back of head and stomach. Next day he was quite recovered. A boy, 8, who ate a quantity of berries, was found in great agony, complaining that his stomach was "pinched together." He had nausea, violent vomiting; throat sore and dry; fauces dark red, tonsils swollen. After vomiting ceased, purging set in; stools dark brown and thin; severe pain in stomach on pressure, extorting cries. Later he had burning griping in umbilical region; dim vision; tongue coated white; spasmodic jerkings in arms and legs. In a woman, 45, who took *Phyt.* as a "blood purifier," a general rash, in appearance not unlike the rash of secondary syphilis, was set up. In a family of four poisoned by eating the root in mistake with their food, these symptoms were observed: Dread of movement; seems stupid; falls asleep after a paroxysm of cramping pain has ceased; pain in forehead < after eating; vomiting of clotted blood and slime; copious discharge of blood and mucus which looked like scrapings of intestines; involuntary stools from straining, which occurred even in sleep. In the mother of the family, seven months pregnant, it very nearly produced miscarriage; the uterus could be felt contracting under the hand; involuntary straining and hæmorrhage from the vagina; intense griping pain in small of back and cramps in legs coming and going suddenly, coldness and withered appearance of extremities, whole body cold. In all the above cases the spasmodic action of the drug is evident in some form. From inhaling the dust of the powdered dried root, or the odour given off on slicing the fresh root, intense irritation of eyes, nose, and throat, and severe headache and diarrhœa have occurred. Given to animals, *Phyt.* has caused convulsive symptoms, vomiting, and vomiting of worms. Wild pigeons and other birds which eat the berries acquire a highly red colour and lose their fat. This last observation has led to the use of a tincture of *Phyt.* berries as an anti-fat, and many successful results have been reported. This observation may be taken as the key to one of the great spheres of the action of this remedy—the absorption of tissues, especially new growths. There are few remedies which have a wider range in the cure of tumours and indurations, particularly of the female breast. Hale tells us that among dairymen in America the root is used to regulate any abnormality in the milk of cows—scanty ; thick ; watery ; curdy ; containing blood or pus. But its chief repute is in caked udders. In breast induration and abscesses of nursing women, and even in cancers (internally and sometimes externally as well), its action has been well confirmed. But it must not be supposed that this action is purely physiological, as is the absorption of fat in birds. A patient of mine, about forty-five, took *Phyt.* 30 for sore throat. After a few doses she was compelled to desist because of its effects on her breasts ; both became full and uncomfortable, and in the left one appeared a large lump in its upper segment, which lasted five days, and was only got rid of by dint of vigorous rubbing with camphorated oil. A case of cancer of the rectum has been cured with *Phytolaccin* 3x. In the uterus and the prostate gland (the male uterus) specific symptoms were evoked in the poisonings and provings. Muscles, joints, bones, brain, and spinal cord, as well as the special senses, were all more or less disordered. The intense action of the drug on the throat has led to its being used as a routine remedy in diphtheria. It is not a specific ; but it has some very characteristic symptoms which will indicate it when present. Among these are : Great pain at root of tongue when swallowing ; pains shooting from throat into ears on swallowing ; hot feeling as if a red-hot ball in throat ; burning < by hot drinks ; dark redness of fauces. Eclectics (*H. R.*, xi. 429) give the expressed juice of the berries in "spasmodic or membranous croup, or diphtheria." There is one form of sore throat in which I have found it of the greatest service—the so-called "diphtheritic sore throat." Dark red, swollen mucous membrane and tonsils, pain on swallowing, eruption of herpetic, whitish, or grey spots on fauces, swelling and tenderness of the glands externally at the angle of the jaw. With these symptoms there are generally headache, backache, wandering rheumatic pains and fever. I have cleared up numberless cases of this kind with *Phyt.* 30. Not infrequently epidemic influenza has taken this form, and then *Phyt.* has been my most successful remedy. (Nash has relieved chronic follicular pharyngitis in public speakers when there has been much *burning*, as if a hot substance in throat.) One of the provers had "swollen and tender gland right side of neck" ; and swollen and tender glands in many other localities have been remedied with *Phyt.* The headaches of *Phyt.* are chiefly frontal, pressive, involving eyes, < right side. One headache is peculiar, being associated with *increased sense of hearing*. The irritation of the mucous membrane of the throat extends to nose, ears, and eyes, producing characteristic symptoms in each. The discharges are tough, stringy, difficult to detach, and may take the form of clinkers. Offensiveness and acridity are also common features. The nervous irritability of *Phyt.* has led to its successful use in disorders of dentition, a keynote symptom being: Irresistible inclination to bite the teeth or gums together. The *pains* of *Phyt.* come and go suddenly; move about, radiate from a centre, or change place. Pain in sore nipples of nursing women radiate all over the body when the child is put to the breast. When pain in intestines disappears pain in extremities comes on. Pain leaves heart and appears in right arm (this association is unusual, and therefore important). Pains in head and chest go from before backward. Pains run down spine from nape; from sacrum down outer aspect of thighs to toes. The *outer* aspects of the limbs are chiefly affected. The shreddy discharge of *Phyt.* mark it as a remedy in certain forms of intestinal catarrh and dysmenorrhœa. It is hæmorrhagic and hæmorrhoidal, acting strongly on rectum and anus, curing tenesmus, bloody discharges and heat. One characteristic pain (noted in a case of constipation) is: Shooting pain from anus to lower part of rectum, along perinæum to middle of penis. "Gurgling in the prostate gland, repeatedly in the afternoon," was noted by one prover, and pains in spermatic cords. Entire suspension of sexual appetite with relaxation of the genitals was caused. *Stiffness* is a characteristic effect of *Phyt.*, noted in the tetanus case, and in others in less degree. Stiff neck, especially right side. The prostration is so rapid and profound that it has led to the successful use of *Phyt.* in diphtheritic paralysis. Faint and dizzy when standing. Soreness of all the muscles. Restlessness, but he fears to move because motion < the pains. The rheumatic swellings are hard, tender, and intensely hot. *Phyt.* is *suited to* rheumatic or syphilitic subjects who are sensitive to damp weather. *Peculiar sensations* are: Brain as if bruised. Right side of head as if pressed firmly. As if sand in eyes. As if eyes too large. As if lids granulated. As if tarsal edges raw. As if lids on fire. Nostril as if tickled with a stiff feather. Nose and eyes as if a cold would come on. Tongue as if scalded. As if a ball of red-hot iron in throat. As if lump in throat. As if apple core in throat. Throat so full it felt choked. Pharynx feels like a cavern; chest as if it were a big empty cask. Body as if bruised; pounded all over. As if joint were being chopped with an axe. The right side is most affected, and many symptoms were experienced in the liver; there were also some severe ones in the spleen. The liver-pains were < lying on right (painful) side. The spleen pain was > lying on left (painful) side. Nash has removed many breast tumours by giving a single dose of *Phyt.* cm during the wane of the moon. The symptoms are < by touch (liver, &c). There is great general sensitiveness. Pressure < pain in joints and ulcers. Pressure with hand > pain in breasts. Pressure on trachea facilitates expectoration. Rubbing > pain in hip. Riding < nose and breathing. < Stepping down high step. Rising from bed = faint feeling. Sitting up = sick and giddy. Standing = faint and dizzy. Gaslight < eyes. Swallowing <. After breakfast head and throat >, gastric symptoms <. Vomiting < headache, > nausea. Hunger soon after eating. (This is like the deadly sinking so often met with in the cancerous diathesis.) < At menstrual periods. Must lie down. < Lying right side. > Lying left side. > Lying on stomach. < Standing and < motion. < Walking. < Raising arm. < Night. < Morning ; 3, 4, or 5 a.m. ; on waking. < Damp weather ; washing ; hot drinks. < Exposure to air ; open air (but it > eyes). The external use of *Phyt.* has been attended with good results in cases of ulceration, and I have found a gargle of a few drops of the ϕ to a tumbler of water useful in many throat cases. A preparation of the *leaves* has been used successfully by Hurndall (*H. W.*, xxxi. 217) as an external application for carcinomatous growths in dogs ; and an ointment prepared with a strong tincture of the leaves as well as the juice of the leaves have been used for malignant ulcers in human beings.

Relations.—*Antidoted by :* Milk, Salt, Coffee (vomiting), Nit. sp. dulc., Bell., Ign., Merc., Mez., Sul. (eyes), Op. (large doses). *Compare :* Botan., Petiver. Diphtheria, Ar. t., Lach. [Lach. has not the great pain at root of tongue when swallowing of Phyt. S. M. Pease (*Med. Adv.*, xxv. 27) found *bleeding from the buccal cavity* a keynote symptom of Phyt. in one epidemic.] Hypertrophy of heart, Rhus (Phyt. has right arm numb ; Rhus has left arm numb, also Aco., Act. r., Puls.). Breast abscess, Bry. (Phyt. follows Bry. when suppuration seems inevitable ; pain goes from nipples all over body). < Motion, Bry. Tetanic spasms, Nux (Phyt. is slower than Nux, has everted lips, alternate relaxation and spasm). Pain in breasts when suckling, Crot. t., Phell., Lac c., Borax (Borax, like Phyt., has > from pressure ; Borax alone has empty, sucked-out feeling). Sensation of apple core in throat, Hep., Nit. ac. Stringy discharges and clinkers, electric shocks, flying pains, K. bi. Desires cold water (Physt. opp.). Symptoms fly from centre outward (Abrot. opp.) Pains in breast at menstrual period, Calc., Con. Diarrhœa with shreddy membranes, Caust., Ars. < In damp weather, Rhus, Dulc. Pains in tibia, Carb. v., Lach. < After sleep, Lach. Loss of fat (Sabal ser. opp.). Loss of sense of delicacy, Hyo. Bruised, sore feeling, Arn. Hale says K. iod. is the nearest analogue (rheumatism, syphilis, wasting) ; Merc. and its antidotes are also closely related.

Causation.—Exposure to cold and damp.

SYMPTOMS.

1. **Mind.**—Delirium.—Indisposition to mental exertion ; disgust for business on waking early in morning.—Melancholy, gloom.—Indifference to life.—Great fear ; is sure she will die.—Loss of personal delicacy, complete shamelessness and indifference to exposure of her person.—Irritability ; restlessness.—Irresistible desire to bite teeth together.—Cannot be persuaded to take nourishment.—Over-sensitive ; pain intolerable.

2. **Head.**—Vertigo : staggering with danger of falling ; with dim vision ; when rising from bed feels faint.—Headache : with nausea ; dull ; heavy ;

neuralgic ; rheumatic ; syphilitic ; with backache and bearing down ; weekly ; < from wet weather.—Sore pain over head, < on r. side.—Pain in vertex ; and sensation of soreness deep in brain as if bruised ; when slipping from a high step to ground.—One-sided pain, just above eyebrows, with sick stomach ; < in forehead, or above eyebrows (glabella most affected) ; comes every week.—Dull, pressive pain in forehead, with slight nausea, cold sweat on forehead and feeling of weakness.—Shooting pain from l. eye to vertex.—Violent pain at back of l. eye and over eyebrow extending down side of head.—Heavy aching in forehead after dinner.—Slight pain in forepart of head with increase of hearing.—Heaviness of head, with feeling in back part of tongue as if burnt.—Headache commencing in frontal region and extending backward.—Nausea and headache > by eating, but returning soon with vomiting which < headache and > the nausea.—Pressive pain on forehead and upper part of both eyes ; on vertex with dryness.—Pain in back of head and neck.—Head thrown backward.—Pain in occiput ; and stomach.—Rheumatism of r. frontal region with nausea, < morning ; of scalp when it rains, with depression.—Syphilitic nodes on skull.—Tinea capitis.—Crusta lactea, moist, fearful itching, with little raw tubercles on scalp, face, and arms.

3. **Eyes.**—Eyes staring.—Blue round eyes.—Eyes sunk deep in sockets with livid circles.—Sclerotica dark yellow.—Sharp pain through ball of eye on reading or writing.—Dull aching in eyes, < from motion, light, or exercise.—Pressure around eyes in afternoon as if eyes too large.—Circum-orbital pains in syphilitic ophthalmia.—Panophthalmitis.—Aching along lower half r. orbit.—Orbital cellulitis.—Lids feel granulated ; tarsal edges feel scalded, hot, raw.—Burning and smarting sensation (feeling of sand) in eyes and lids, with profuse lachrymation and coryza, which is > in the open air.—Smarting in inner canthi (< l.), < by gaslight in evening.—Lids agglutinated and swollen, as if poisoned.—Reddish-blue swelling of lids (< l.), < morning ; cannot close eyes without pain all forenoon, > afternoon.—Fistula lachrymalis.—Lids feel on fire.—Lupus, epithelioma, &c., of lids.—Pupils : contracted (tetanus) ; much dilated.—Photophobia.—Motion of one eye independent of that of the other.—Double vision ; with giddiness and headache.—Objects quintupled.—Far-sighted.

4. **Ears.**—Shooting in r. ear.—Pains in both ears, < r. ; < swallowing.—Obstruction in l. Eustachian tube, rushing in l. ear, a feeling as if hearing were dull, while at same time sensitive to minutest sounds.—Irritation in one Eustachian tube.—Increased sense of hearing (most r.) ; with pain in forehead.—Very peculiar pressure and tension in parotids.

5. **Nose.**—Flow of mucus from one nostril while the other is stopped.—Drawing sensation at root of nose.—Feeling in nose and eyes as if a cold would come on.—Acrid, excoriating discharge.—Wakes 3 a.m. with nose stopped up, discharges clinkers from both nostrils in morning.—Sensation in nostrils as if tickled with a stiff feather.—Total obstruction of nose, when riding must breathe through mouth ; not > by blowing nose ; mucus discharged with difficulty.—Syphilitic ozæna with bloody sanious discharge and disease of bones.—Rodent ulcer.

6. **Face.**—Face : pale ; sunken, blue, suffering ; hippocratic ; distorted.—Stupid.—Cool sweat on forehead.—Heat in face (l.) after dinner ; with redness of face, coldness of feet, eruption in upper lip (l.).—Face very red,

almost purple; alternately very pale.—Pains in bones of face and head at night, keeping her awake many nights; proceeding esp. from "nodes" on frontal bone, very much like pains of periostitis.—Pains in upper jaws.—Jaws ached awfully the whole time, it seemed he could not open or shut them.—Blotches in face, < afternoon, after washing and eating.—Swelling round l. ear and side of face, like erysipelas; thence over scalp; very painful.—Ulcers and scaly eruption on face.—Chin drawn closely to sternum by convulsive action of muscles of face and neck; lips everted and firm (tetanus).—Eruption on upper lip.—Ulcers (cancerous) on lips.

7. **Teeth.**—Teeth all ache; feel elongated and are very sore.—Shooting pains in r. upper and lower molars.—Irresistible inclination to bite teeth together.—Difficult dentition; crying, moaning, restless at night; diarrhœa in hot weather; > biting something hard.

8. **Mouth.**—The mouth fills with saliva; tenacious, yellowish, ropy, with metallic taste.—Cold, sticky, stringy saliva.—No saliva.—Taste: disagreeable; metallic; burnt; nutty; bitter at first; leaving smarting and coldness towards tip of tongue.—Burnt feeling on back of tongue (with heavy head).—Tongue: coated white; furred; thick at back; dry, and lips; feels scalded; thick; protruding.—Tongue feels rough, with blisters on both sides, and very red tip; great pain in root of tongue when swallowing.—Roof of mouth sore.—Mouth dry.—Submaxillary glands swollen.

9. **Throat.**—Sensation of dryness in throat and the posterior fauces (provoking cough, with disposition to hawk and clear the throat); tonsils swollen.—Uvula large, almost translucent.—Fauces congested and of a dark red colour.—Sore throat (roughness and rawness), swelling of soft palate in morning, with a thick, white, and yellow mucus about the fauces.—Sensation of a lump in throat (when swallowing), causing a continuous desire to swallow; also when turning head to l.—Could not swallow, throat so dry and rough.—Throat feels like a cavern.—< From hot drinks.—Difficult swallowing; with every attempt excruciating shooting pains through both ears.—Sensation of apple-core in throat.—While riding in forenoon sensation of plug in throat, not > by hawking; this sensation was replaced by increased discharge of mucus from posterior nares, discharged with difficulty, constantly exciting attempts to expel it.—Sensation of rawness and scraping in throat and tonsils.—Burning heat in throat as from coal of fire, as if red-hot iron ball lodged in fauces and whole length of œsophagus; catarrh in throat; diphtheria.—Eruption on fauces and œsophagus.—Herpes pharyngalis.—Soreness of posterior fauces extending into Eustachian tube.—Fulness in throat.

11. **Stomach.**—Intense thirst.—Canine hunger; soon after eating.—Loss of appetite.—Eructations: of air; sour fluid; food in evening.—Hiccough, with great inclination to vomit but no nausea.—Nausea followed by violent vomiting of mucus, bile, ingesta, worms; of clotted blood and slime, with retching, intense pain, and desire for death to relieve.—Vomits undigested food.—Frequent vomiting; prostration, fainting, even convulsions, followed by gripes, cramps, vomiting of dark bilious substance.—In great agony; said his stomach was pinched together.—Bruised and sore feeling at pit of stomach.—Heat in stomach.—Cutting in pit of stomach, tender to touch.—Pains in cardiac portion of stomach, < full respiration and by walking.—Pain in region of pylorus.

12. **Abdomen.**—Intense vomiting and purging, with griping pains and cramps in abdomen.—Soreness and pain in r. hypochondrium (during pregnancy).—Sore spot, r. hypochondrium, size of dollar, extremely sensitive to touch.—Digging in upper and lower portions of liver.—Lying on r. side = penetrating pain in r. hypochondrium.—Violent dull pressing pain l. hypochondrium, cannot remain in sitting posture, lies on painful side all night and pain is gone in morning.—Heavy aching pain in hypochondrium which left as soon as leucorrhœa commenced.—Chronic hepatitis, with enlargement and induration.—Burning, griping pain in umbilical region.—Much rumbling, pain in umbilicus, stools of blood and mucus; gastro-enteritis.—Bearing-down pains.—Violent pains in abdomen during menstruation in a barren female.—Rheumatism extending to abdominal muscles.

13. **Stool and Anus.**—Constipation, hard stools.—Stool with mucus and straining.—Constipation habitual; patient says the bowels will not move without the aid of purgatives; feeling of fulness in abdomen before stool, which remains after stool, as if all had not passed.—Constipation from torpor of the rectum.—Constipation: of the aged; of persons with weak heart.—Diarrhœa with sickly feeling in bowels; passage only of mucus and blood, or like scrapings from intestines.—Tenesmus.—Continual inclination to stool but passes constantly fetid flatus.—Diarrhœa early in morning after lemonade.—Dysentery.—Intense vomiting or purging, with prostration and cramps, as in cholera.—Stools: thin, dark brown; of mucus and blood; of bile; from 1 or 2 a.m. till after breakfast; mushy; yellow, then greenish, then dark, bloody; dark, lumpy.—Hæmorrhoids permanent and obstinate; bleeding and mucus.—Neuralgic pains in anus and lower part of rectum, shooting along perinæum to middle of penis; in middle of night (with constipation).—Bloody discharge with heat in rectum.—Heat in rectum with burning in stomach.—Ulceration; fissure.

14. **Urinary Organs.**—Weakness, dull pain, and soreness in region of kidneys, < r., connected with heat; uneasiness down ureters; chalk-like sediment in urine.—Albuminuria: after scarlatina or diphtheria; chills at night without special fever, accompanied by a form of insanity.—Pain in bladder before and during urination.—Slight suppression of urine, with pains in loins.—Violent, painful urging to pass urine.—Copious nocturnal urination.—Thick, chalk-like sediment.—The dark-red urine leaves a mahogany stain in the chamber.—Urine: acid and albuminous; excessive or scanty; stains clothes yellow.

15. **Male Sexual Organs.**—Sharp pains (and hard, grinding pain) running up each spermatic cord; later continued soreness in place of the pains.—Gurgling sensation in prostate gland.—Complete loss of desire, absence of erections and relaxation of parts during the proving.—Impotence.—Gonorrhœa; gleet; orchitis, with suppuration and fistulous ulcer.—Syphilis: chancres; ulcerated throat; ulcers on genitals; bubo; rheumatism.

16. **Female Sexual Organs.**—Menses: too frequent and copious; mammæ painful; increase of tears, saliva, bile, urine; rheumatic subjects.—Menses: amenorrhœa complicated with ovarian irritation or disease; very painful menstruation in apparently barren women when occurring in connection with rheumatism; shreds of membrane are passed with the menstrual

flow.—Leucorrhœa: uterine, thick, tenacious, irritating.—Profuse, thick, tenacious, from swollen Nabothian glands.—Threatened miscarriage; bearing-down pains; involuntary straining and hæmorrhage per vaginum caused in woman seven months pregnant.—Sensation as though menses would appear all the time.—Dysmenorrhœa accompanying erosion or ulceration of the cervix; menses too often; too profuse, with corresponding increase of the tears, and other secretions.—Metrorrhagia.—Inflammation, swelling, and suppuration of the mammæ.—Neuralgia of breasts.—Mastitis, where the hardness is very apparent from the first, with great burning; very sensitive nipples or breasts, which are more or less painful; even after suppuration these characteristics continue.—Fulness of both breasts; lump in upper part of l. —Abscesses; fistulæ; tumours; cancer; hypertrophy.—Irritable tumour; very sensitive and painful; < at menstrual period.—Nipples cracked and excoriated; intense suffering on putting child to breast; pains radiate from nipple all over body.—Breasts hard as stones after confinement.—Breasts full of hard, painful nodosities.—Suppression of lochia.—Pain in sacrum, down to knees and ankles, then up to sacrum, jerks here and there, after confinement.

17. **Respiratory Organs.**—Hoarseness and aphonia.—Tickling in l. side larynx with hacking cough, aching r. side of breast, great dryness of throat.—Sensation of roughness in the bronchia.—Laryngismus, thumbs and toes flexed; features distorted; eye muscles act independently.—Respiration difficult and oppressed; loud mucous râles.—Faint, with sighing, slow breathing.—Panting.—Cough: hacking, dry, hawking; from tickling in larynx or dryness in pharynx: < night, on lying down; dry, bronchial.—Cough with: scraping and tickling in throat; burning pains in trachea and larynx, sensation of contraction of glottis, laboured breathing; sensation of ulcerated spot in trachea just above breast-bone, could only expectorate (pus) by pressing on this spot; pains through mid-sternum.—Hoarse, croupy, barking cough, < at night; < out of doors.—Expectoration: thick, tough; thick, starch-like mucus, profuse and exhausting with pharyngitis.—Dryness of larynx and trachea, < evening.

18. **Chest.**—Sharp pains through upper part of chest, preventing a long breath.—Stitch from r. chest to back.—Pain and suffocation in lungs, throat, and fauces.—Pains in lungs, 7 a.m.—Tenderness and lameness of muscles of chest, as if bruised.—(Chest feels as if it were a big empty cask.)—Rheumatism of lower intercostal muscles from exposure to cold and dampness.—Spots size of lentil on chest.—Hard, tender swelling midway between nipple and sternum, but nearer latter; restless nights; (in baby a few months old).

19. **Heart.**—In night awoke with lameness near cardiac region, with much nervous restlessness, < motion, esp. < expiration; kept him awake long time.—Constrictive feeling in præcordia with pressure in temples.—Great pain in præcordia, much < walking.—Occasional shocks of pain in heart region, as soon as this ceases similar pain appears in r. arm.—Heart-beats distinctly felt.—Fatty degeneration; lassitude and indisposition to move. —Pulse: small, irregular, with great excitement in chest, esp. in cardiac region; full but soft; intermittent; weak.

20. **Neck and Back.**—Hardness of gland in r. side of neck.—Stiff neck, < on r. side; in bed; after midnight; on waking.—Back very stiff every morning.—Sensation as if cold iron were pressed on painful scapula.—Both

scapulæ ache continually.—Towards evening, while riding, laming pain began l. side back below scapula ; 9.30 p.m. it had reached spine and was a pricking stitching.—Severe pain behind scapulæ when walking.—Intense griping in small of back.—Pain running down spine from nape.—Pain in loins with suppression of urine.—Constant, dull, heavy pain in lumbar and sacral regions.—Pains shooting from sacrum down both hips to feet.

21. **Limbs.**—Intense cramps, muscles gather in large knots, hard and ridged ; come and go suddenly.—Rheumatism of all joints 3 p.m.—Sudden transference of internal pains to extremities.—Pains in limbs always in outer aspects.—Patient is subject to rheumatic pains on change of weather, esp. in hips and thighs ; rheumatic muscular or chronic rheumatism.—Rheumatic pains in arms and hands.—Cold hands and feet.

22. **Upper Limbs.**—Enlarged glands in axillæ.—Shooting in r. shoulder-joint with stiffness and paralysis.—Rheumatism of (l.) shoulder (esp. in syphilitics) ; pains fly like electric shocks from one part to another ; < night and damp weather.—Pains at attachment of deltoid.—Weakness and aching in r. humerus, < motion and extension.—Dull aching and excessive tenderness, as from a bruise, in outer muscle of r. arm.—Hands tremble.—Rheumatic pains in hands ; sudden pricking.—Painful, hard, shiny swelling of joints of all fingers.—Bony growth in palmar aspect of one finger.—Whitlow.—Ends of fingers all throb and ache as if going to suppurate.—Shooting like needles in finger-joints ; in top of l. thumb.

23. **Lower Limbs.**—Neuralgic pain in outer side of both thighs (shooting from sacrum) ; sciatica.—Sharp, cutting pain in hip, drawing, cannot touch floor ; pain runs down outside of thigh, < night, and esp. < after sleep.—Rheumatic pains in lower extremities, < damp weather.—Sensation of shortening of tendons back of knee when walking.—Leg drawn up.—Legs tremble.—Pain in dorsum of r. foot, 4 a.m.—Syphilitic and mercurial rheumatism ; nightly pains in periosteum of tibia, with nodes and irritable ulcers on lower leg.—Stitches in various parts, always from without inward and near surface.—Ankles swollen.—Feet puffed, soles burn.—Ulcers on inner sides of soles.—Aching of heels, dull, wearing ; > raising feet above level of body.—Pain in great toe waking him at night.—Corn painful.

24. **Generalities.**—Extremities stiff, hands clenched, feet extended, toes flexed, teeth clenched, lips everted, firm, chin drawn on sternum, opisthotonus.—Great desire for cold water, for bathing in it.—Pains are pressing, shooting, and sore.—Great exhaustion and prostration.—Sore and stiff.—Soreness from head to foot in all muscles.—Pains and numbness followed by itching and burning.—Pains came suddenly in full force and so continued till they ceased ; followed by drowsiness, stupor, or sleep.—Bones and glands inflamed and swollen.

25. **Skin.**—Skin cool, shrivelled, dry, lead-coloured.—Syphilitic eruptions and ulcerations—secondary and tertiary.—Squamous eruptions ; tinea capitis ; lupus.—Shingles.—Itch.—Pityriasis.—Psoriasis.—Warts.—Lipoma.—Erythematous blotches, slightly raised, pinkish, slowly desquamating, ending in purple spot, as old ones died away others came.—Suppuration of painless tumours.—Drawing in cicatrices.—Itching began on hands and feet and spread over whole body ; rash followed four hours later ; itching < by scratching ; < heat of bed.—Itching and lichen-like eruption on l. leg, <

fore part of night, preventing sleep till midnight.—Boils ; esp. near ulcers ; on back ; behind ears.—Ulcers : punched-out looking ; lardaceous base ; pus watery, fetid, ichorous ; shooting, lancinating, jerking pains ; syphilitic ; cancerous.—Warts.—Corns.

26. Sleep.—Frequent yawning ; drowsiness.—Restlessness at night, pains drive him out of bed.—On awaking feels wretched.

27. Fever.—Great coldness, withered appearance of extremities.—Coldness, faintness, dyspnœa ; limbs cold, head and face hot.—Internal shiverings during the pains.—Chill : every morning ; sudden, followed by fever after confinement ; at night without special fever.—Heat : with pain in joints ; high fever ; in face after dinner ; with red face ; on l. side of face.—Sweat : cold on forehead ; esp. under toes ; night-sweat, acrid.

Pichi.

Fabiana imbricata. *N. O.* Solanaceæ. Fluid extract.

Clinical.—Cystitis. Gall-stones. Gonorrhœa. Liver, affections of. Prostate, disease of.

Characteristics.—*Pichi* is a solanaceous shrub of South America. It is unproved, but in 1 to 20 drop doses of the fluid extract it has been used with good effect in cases of chronic cystitis with enlarged prostate ; liver affections and gall-stones ; excess of uric acid. Hansen gives these indications : Excoriating urine and urinary calculi. Inflammation of whole urethral tract, must pass water frequently ; burning pains and violent vesical tenesmus after urination. Acute or chronic cystitis, caused by gravel, painful urination, much mucus and pus. Subacute or chronic gonorrhœa, painful urination, much mucus and pus.

Picricum Acidum.

Picric Acid. Carbazotic Acid. Tri-nitro-carbolic Acid. ($C_6H_2(NO_2)_3OH$). Trituration. Solution in rectified spirit.

Clinical.—Acne. *Anæmia.* Boils. Brain, base of, pain in. *Brain-fag,* Burns. Cancerous cachexia. Condylomata. Debility. Diabetes. Ears, boils in. *Emissions.* Enuresis. Epistaxis. *Erotomania.* Erythema. *Hæmoglobinuria.* Hands, perspiration of. Headache, of students. Hemiplegia. Jaundice. *Leucocythæmia.* Liver, congestion of ; fatty. *Locomotor ataxia. Lumbago.* Myelitis. Neurasthenia. Otitis. *Paralysis.* Paraplegia. Pernicious anæmia. Priapism. Pruritus vulvæ. *Self-abuse.* Spinal exhaustion. Spinal irritation. Spinal sclerosis. Styes. Sycosis. Urine, bloody. Writer's cramp.

Characteristics.—*Pic. ac.* was discovered by Hausman in 1788. It is formed by the action of *Nitric acid* on *Carbolic acid*, *Salicin*, *Silk*, and many other substances. It crystallises in bright yellow needles or scales, of very bitter taste, sparingly soluble in water. The yellow colour is imparted to the eyes and skins of patients who take it in the crude, and it not only produces a semblance of jaundice, but actually disorganises the liver if pushed. In some experiments by Parisel (*C. D. P.*) these symptoms were observed: Buzzing and whistling in ears; sparks, whirling round of objects; heaviness of head alternately with sense of emptiness. Moderately copious, *oily-looking*, yellowish stool, with > of cerebral symptoms. Pulse slow, small, very feeble. *Great weakness, compelling to lie down;* limbs hardly able to stir themselves; *no anxiety*, profound calm. *Vivid colouration of sclerotics and integuments; urine coloured blood-red.* These were effects of 0·5 grm. doses. Slow poisoning set up an intermittent fever of quotidian type, and "anorexia, thirst, often sweat, *cancerous tint about skin, tendency to cachexia.*" These observations give the chief features of the drug's action: Fatigue, mental and bodily; symptoms < by least exertion; fatigue going into actual paralysis; brain fatigue, nerve fatigue; at the same time absence of anxiety—indifference. Like so many other *yellow* substances, *Pic. ac.* acts powerfully on the liver, and produces jaundice, cachexia, and cancerous tints. "Tired-out, washed-out feeling—must give in," is the chief keynote of *Pic. ac.* and its salts. Nash cured promptly with *Pic. ac.* 6 trit. an old man who had been failing for a year, and complained of heaviness in the occiput, inability to exert the mind, talk, or think, and general "played-out" feeling. Nash had feared brain softening. Halbert (*Clinique*, September, 1898) reports a case illustrating the power of *Pic. ac.* over the effects of fatigue in professional neuroses. A stenographer and typewriter after using her right index finger continuously for six years, noticed weakness of her thumb and index, and inability to hold pen or pencil. Next there was difficulty in striking correctly the keys of the typewriter and some wrist-drop. The finger when Halbert first saw her was quite rigid and straight, showing extreme spasticity. Massage, electricity, &c., had failed to give any relief. *Pic. ac.* 3x six times daily cured the case and made great improvement in the patient's general health. Evans has found it curative in girls and young women who, under the strain of many studies, show signs of breaking down—lose appetite, sleep lightly and lie awake (*Pic. ac.* 30 *caused* a patient of mine, previously a good sleeper, to lie awake a long time at nights.—J. H. C.), exhaustion after the day's studies, fatigue even from a short walk, twitchings of muscles when asleep or awake; hysterical state, loss of will power; constant headache, irregular menses. Such patients are usually given iron, which does little or no good. *Pic. ac.* and its compounds are among the most powerful explosives known, lyddite being an example. *Pic. ac.*, like *Glon.*, has occipital headaches and *bursting* headaches. The headache, frontal or occipital, is < on any attempt to use the mind, and it may extend down the spine. There is also a headache extending from the top of the spine up over the head to the eyes. In a case of spinal irritation I relieved with *Pic. ac.* 30 a pain which shot up from the spine into the head. The pains referable to the spinal cord are strongly marked. Any attempt to study = burning along spine; with great weakness of back and legs; soreness of muscles and joints. To the spinal congestion must be attributed the remarkable disturbance in the sexual sphere : Priapism ; penis distended almost to bursting. Terrible erections, disturbing sleep. When over-excitement of sexual system is associated with spinal or cerebellar affections in either sex. Great sexual desire with emissions. Amorous fancies. On the skin *Pic. ac.* produces jaundice with itching ; small painful furuncles, particularly in the auditory meatus ; and erythema and pruritus of abdomen and feet. Théry of Paris accidentally discovered in *Pic. ac.* solution a remedy for burns. He twice dropped burning matter on his hands whilst working with a *Pic. ac.* disinfectant, and was astonished at the absence of pain or injury. From that date *Pic. ac.* became his principal remedy for burns, and though others have complained that it caused violent pains, Théry has only once in some thousands of cases had to abandon its use on that account. A. C. Blackwood (*Clinique*, October, 1898, *H. W.*, xxxiv. 133) gives the details of its use. Burns of the first and second degree only are suitable. A saturated solution (*Pic. ac.* gr. xc to alcohol ℥iii) diluted with one quart of water is used. The clothing is removed and the burnt surface cleansed with the solution and absorbent cotton. Blisters are opened but the epithelial covering is carefully preserved. If extensive, the whole surface may be bathed with the solution, and strips of sterilised gauze soaked and applied to entirely cover it, a layer of absorbent cotton held with a light bandage over all. After three or four days the dressing is removed carefully after thorough moistening, as it adheres closely. The second dressing is applied as at first, and allowed to remain a week. Blackwood finds it painless, anodyne, antiseptic, preventing inflammation and suppuration and septic poisoning. It coagulates the albuminous exudation, and healing takes place under the coagulum. The staining of the hands and linen caused by the dressing can be removed by *Boracic acid.* Gaucher (*Sem. Méd.*, May 26, 1897) has removed acute vesicular eczema by the same treatment. The skin and kidneys are intimately related, and *Pic. ac.* has a powerful action on the latter. Among other affections it has cured diabetes. Halbert (*Clinique*, quoted *H. W.*, xxxiv. 542) reports this case : Mrs, C., 49, had " nervous prostration " since the shock of the loss of a child three years before. Wasting with great appetite. Intense thirst and copious urination, especially at night. Great perspiration and some jaundice. Heart flabby, mitral bruit, dyspnœa ; emaciation, anæmia, exhaustion. Urine 1040, 7½ per cent. of sugar and some albumen. *Pic. ac.* 6x six times daily. Rapid and continuous improvement followed. Kent (*H. P.*, viii. 168) says *Pic. ac.* cures fig-warts and gonorrhœa ; he was led to infer its relation thereto by its power over pernicious anæmia, which he has often traced to a gonorrhœal base. *Pic. ac.* is *suited to* dark complexioned persons, with dirty appearance about knuckles (from bile pigments) ; anæmic and cachectic persons ; worn-out persons, overtaxed mentally and bodily. *Peculiar sensations* are : As if sand, or sticks, in eyes. As if throat would split. As if legs enclosed in elastic stockings ; as if chest encircled in a tight band. Pricking as from needles in legs. As of a lump back of thyroid cartilage. As if stairs or ground coming up to meet him. As of ants crawling over surface. Nose-bleed accompanies heat and congestion of head.

Heaviness of head alternates with emptiness. The right upper part of the body is more affected than the left, the left leg more than the right. Touch < pimples. The headache is > by binding head tightly ; > by rest ; lying down. < By motion ; walking ; raising head ; sitting up ; stooping ; ascending stairs. < By study or slightest mental exertion. The throat is > by eating ; < empty swallowing. Turning over, and turning the head < headache. < Morning ; 5 a.m. nausea. Open air and cold room > headache. Work in open air = prostration. Wet weather < pains. > From cold air and water. Chilliness predominates. Lamplight, strong light, moving eye < pain in eyes. During and after micturition, burning.

Relations.—*Compare :* Am. pic., Calc. pic., Fer. pic., Zn. pic. Spinal exhaustion, Ox. ac. (Ox. ac. more numbness, blueness, pains in small spots ; symptoms < thinking of them. Pic. ac. more heaviness ; extreme spinal softening). Tired feeling, exhaustion from sexual excess, Phos. ac. Fatty degeneration, sexual excess and priapism, brain-fag, congestive vertigo, burning in spine, Phos. (Phos. has more irritability and excessive sensitiveness, sexual excitement very strong ; Pic. ac. has more intense erections but less marked lasciviousness). Brain-fag, inability to study, gastric symptoms, sour eructations, < morning, Nux. Brain-fag, occipital headache, sexual neurasthenia, Gels. Lascivious thoughts in presence of women, Con. Headache and backache, Arg. n. Spinal pains, Alm. (Alm. pain as if hot iron had been thrust into the part). Nervous exhaustion, sensitive spine, Sil. (Pic. ac. washed out, *must* give in ; Sil. *won't* give in). Nervous exhaustion, Zn. Violent erections, Canth., Graph., Hyo., Phos., Myg., Sil. Acne, K. bro., Bels., Arct. l. Hands sweat, Sil. Burning in back, Lyc., Phos. Writer's cramp, Gels., Plat.

Causation.—Fatigue. Study. Mental exertion.

SYMPTOMS.

1. **Mind.**—Nervous feeling, which I never have except when fever is leaving me, feeling as if about to be crushed by the bed-clothes, arms, face, tongue, and forepart of brain seemed to reach the clouds when I was going to sleep.—Although enjoying the society of men, idea of marriage unendurable.—Desire to be alone.—Irritable.—Low spirits.—Indifference, lack of will power to undertake anything.—Disinclination for mental or physical work, aversion to talking or movement, with headache.—Mental prostration after reading a little ; after writing a little.—The least study = burning along spine and other symptoms.

2. **Head.**—Vertigo : at noon, < rising from a seat ; at 6 p.m. on least motion, with nausea, both repeated at 9 p.m., with pain in forehead and vertex and inability to sit up ; on stooping or bending head or lying down ; < evening.—Headache : < rising, > open air ; > pressure ; > bandaging head ; morning, probably from over-sleeping ; in forenoon, < afternoon ; in afternoon and evening, with trembling ; in evening.—Headache in evening, with thirst and heat, chiefly in temples, and burning in external ears, < stooping, = vertigo, head feels too small, scalp sore to touch, sore aching in

infra-orbital region.—Heat and congestion of head with nose-bleed.—Pressure outward as if head would fly apart, at 8 p.m., < motion and study.—Heaviness; and dulness; alternating with emptiness.—Head feels as if falling forward.—Shooting from outside to centre of forehead in evening.—Intermittent, sharp, and vibrating pain in r. supra-orbital region.—Aching in r. supra-orbital region; and in nape.—Throbbing over r. eye.—Shooting from r. to l. temple with headache.—Neuralgic pain alternately in l. and r. temples.—Pressure outward at sides of head at 9 p.m., < turning head, moving eyes or least motion, with sensation as if frontal bones would split open.—Contracted, squeezed sensation in l. hemisphere of brain at 6.30 p.m. on going into open air.—Pain in r. lower occiput, with sensation as of a hand passing along r. parietal eminence.—Pain in occiput and in nape; pain in r. lower occiput, as if r. side of cerebellum were loose, 6 till 7 p.m., < walking, > quiet, with throbbing.—Heavy pain extending down neck and spine.—Heavy throbbing and burning pains, extending from nape to supra-orbital foramen and thence into eyes, which throb and feel sore to touch.—(Pain shooting up from spine into head.)—Confusion in base of brain.

3. **Eyes.**—Eyes yellow.—Shooting in centre of eye, extending along optic nerve to occiput, with soreness of balls on touch, and photophobia.—Sensation of sand in eyes, with smarting pain and acrid tears.—Feeling as if sticks were in eyes on waking, with inflammation, afterwards feeling as if sticks were in them in evening.—Styes; with sore feeling.—Eyes < on moving them.—Lachrymation.—Pupils dilated.—Conjunctivitis; < r. eye, > washing with cold water and by cold air, < warm room, with difficulty in keeping eyes open, and sticky feeling on reading.—Shooting from r. eyeball to l. side of occiput; pain < moving eyes, > closing them and quiet, with soreness; heavy, smarting, and burning pains, > pressure; sore pains, < strong light and by turning eyes.—Throbbing pain in l. eyeball much < going upstairs.—Inability to keep eyes open when studying.—Air looks smoky.—Vision: dim and confused; dim, can read clearly at only one point, about five inches from eyes; blurred; whirling of objects.—Vision of sparks.

4. **Ears.**—Puffy and burning sensation in ears as if worms were crawling in them.—Pain behind r. ear running down side of neck.—Painful boils in meatus.—Buzzing and hissing in ears.—(Noises in ears, with vertigo and headache at the base of brain.)—(Chronic deafness, apparently caused by excessive headache, with noises in the ears when tired, membrane pale.)

5. **Nose.**—Boil in l. nostril.—Stinging on r. side of nose.—Acne along edges and sides of nose, indurated, elevated papules, rather dark red, painless but sore to touch, very small pustules on tips.—Weight or pressure on bridge.—Nose full of mucus, can breathe only through mouth, > open air.—Bleeding from r. nostril; with heat and congestion of head.

6. **Face.**—Pustular acne on face, burning and stinging when touched; on chin.—Irregular pain in lower jaw, with beating in molars.—Tingling in lips.

8. **Mouth.**—White, frothy saliva hangs in strings to the floor.—Taste: bitter; with thirst; sour, bitter; sour; bad; bad, of gas.

9. **Throat.**—Redness of throat, with raw, scraped, stiff, and hot feeling, as if burnt, and with thick white mucus on tonsils, difficulty in swallowing, with sensation as if throat would split open.—Rawness in l. side, extending

forward to submaxillary gland, < swallowing ; rawness with roughness and scraping.—Soreness back of and above soft palate, with debility.—Dry and husky.—Feeling of a plug on swallowing saliva and afterwards.— Sensation of something in lower part of œsophagus.

10. **Appetite.**—Appetite great in evening; increased, then lost; lost; lost for breakfast.—Aversion to food; at noon.—Thirst: great, with bitter taste; unquenchable, for cold water.

11. **Stomach.**—Eructations: empty; sour, of gas and ingesta; bitter after breakfast.—Waterbrash.—Nausea: on retiring; after retiring, with headache; deathlike, in stomach and abdomen on waking at 5 a.m., < rising and moving about, returned on waking a second time, repeated next morning on waking.—Vomiting.—Sharp pain in epigastric region; when eating breakfast.—Oppression of epigastric region.—Weight in pit of stomach, with ineffectual desire to eructate.—Faint feeling in epigastrium most of the time.

12. **Abdomen.**—Sticking through hepatic region, < in muscles.—Liver full of fat granules (in animals poisoned with *Pic. ac.*).—Tendency to jaundice. —Fulness of abdomen.—Rumbling: in small intestines; at 7 a.m. on waking, with colic; with crampy pain and flatus.—Emission of flatus; during the day; in evening.—Crawling stinging.—Pain in abdomen all forenoon, with slight headache.—Pain in abdomen on waking, with strong erections, and on moving emission of much flatus.—Pain in neck of bladder.—Sticking backward through l. umbilical region.—Sharp pain l. side of umbilicus.—Shooting, wandering pain in region of coccyx, bladder, rectum, and umbilicus, caused by wind.—Sharp pain in r. iliac region, above ovary at 11 p.m., with soreness on pressure.—Pain: in lower part of large intestines; in l. groin on walking, < ascending stairs.—Occasional sensation of giving way in hypogastrium all day.—Vacant and sore feeling in hypogastric region.

13. **Stool and Anus.**—Stinging in anus during and after stool, with itching.—Shooting around anus at 9 p.m.—Stool like gruel, yellow or yellowish-grey, twice before 9 a.m.—Diarrhœa: with burning and smarting at anus; frequent with prostration, light-coloured, with cutting and smarting at anus during and after stool.—Stool: soft; light-coloured, with tenesmus, then drawing up of anus; scanty, with burning and smarting at anus; in plugs, easy, shooting away, then much flatus; yellowish, copious, oily, frequent.—Stool quick, as if greased, of sweetish smell, as of boiling sap, at night and morning, then with much wind.—Difficult stool, next day ineffectual desire for stool.

14. **Urinary Organs.**—Sharp pain in region of bladder; in evening, < r. side.—Frequent micturition in morning.—Dribbling micturition.—Urethra: jerking drawing in; pain in after micturition; burning pain during micturition.—Urine: yellow; of a milky, olive hue; dark; indications of sugar; dark yellow, with strong odour; dark yellow, scanty, afterwards profuse and yellow; red; dark, in evening.—Urine copious and pale; and light coloured, sp. gr. increased; and hot when passed, with burning pain in urethra; afterwards scanty.—Urates abundant.—Urine contained much indican, numerous granular cylinders and fatty degenerated epithelium.

15. **Male Sexual Organs.**—Erections: in morning on waking; at 11 a.m., with bruised pain in l. testicle, extending up cord to external abdominal ring; firm in morning, with pain in abdomen, next morning woke with

emission and firm erection, which lasted about ten minutes after the emission ; terrible at night, with restless sleep ; violent, all night ; violent, all night, then profuse emissions.—Lascivious thoughts in presence of any woman.—Desire : at night, with emissions ; at night, with hard erections, lewd dreams and emission, priapism night and day.

16. **Female Sexual Organs.**—Occasional aching and twinges in l. ovarian region.—Menses delayed ; during the period yellowish-brown leucorrhœa.—During menses, bruised pain in abdomen with sickening sensation.—Excessive and voluptuous pruritus at night, after retiring, making her feel irritable and exasperated (night before menses ; usually had slight pruritus *after* menses, never *before*).—(Used locally in diseases of nipples, inflammation diminishes, skin becomes tougher.)

17. **Respiratory Organs.**—Dry cough, as from dust in throat, then nausea.—Can get the breath only half-way down.

18. **Chest.**—Twitching : in l. side over eighth and ninth ribs ; in l. side over tenth and eleventh ribs from 6 till 11 p.m., with throbbing in muscles.—Pain in r. side, extending across l.—Pain in l. lung in evening.—Sharp pain under r. clavicle.—A heavy throbbing in l. chest under tenth and eleventh ribs at 11 a.m., changing at noon to region of kidneys, extending at 2 p.m. into legs, < l.—Stunning pain at 9.30 a.m., with twitching in throat.—Tightness of chest, as if encircled by a band.—Numbness in lower part of sternum.

19. **Heart and Pulse.**—Pain in apex of heart in evening.—Intermittent fluttering at base of heart all day, it seemed to move.—Palpitation.—Pulse : frequent ; slow, feeble, afterwards rapid ; slow, small, and feeble ; irregular.

20. **Neck and Back.**—Terrible pains in neck and occiput, extending to supra-orbital notch and thence into eyes.—Muscles on r. side of neck felt as if they would give way in afternoon when lying ; at night when lying on r. side, with feeling as if neck would be dislocated.—Pain in back and lower limbs, with heaviness, tired aching, and weakness.—Burning along spine and very great weakness, < by study.—Heat in lower spine ; aching and digging in loins, < from motion.—Pain extending from r. scapula to r. loin when bending forward.—Sticking : under r. scapula ; in lumbar region or bending forward when sitting.—Pain in lumbar region ; and anteriorly in thighs, in muscles, < motion, with weakness in the same, < legs ; extending down legs, < motion, legs and lumbar region sensitive to pressure ; heavy at 6 p.m.—Dragging pains in region of kidneys and at nape, extending upward and downward till they meet between scapulæ, at 2 p.m.—Weakness in sacral and lumbar regions.—(Myelitis with tonic and clonic spasms, keeps legs wide apart when standing ; looks steadily at objects as if could not make them out.—Spinal exhaustion following acute disease.)—Sharp pain in region of coccyx.

21. **Limbs.**—Rheumatic pains in joints.—Weakness from a short walk, with excessive heaviness.—Heaviness, < l. ; of arms and legs on exertion, < legs, legs weak and heavy all the time.—Extremities cold.

22. **Upper Limbs.**—Lame sensation in shoulders.—Shoulders tired and sore ; r.—Twitching of lower part of l. biceps ; in forenoon.—Shooting in l. elbow, extending down arm.—Pain in r. elbow between ulna and radius.—Shooting in hands.—L. hand goes to sleep.

23. Lower Limbs.—Weakness of limbs (< l.); on ascending stairs; and heaviness.—Numbness and crawling in legs with trembling and pricking as from needles.—Twitching on back of l. hip at 9 p.m.—Pain anteriorly in l. thigh, can hardly flex and extend legs.—Hips and legs heavy all day.—Knees weak.—Twitching of flesh of r. leg.—Sticking in legs and feet.—Pain in legs anteriorly, on touch; in calves all night.—Deep-seated, sore pain in upper part of l. Scarpa's triangle, < night, > sleep, returning on waking.—Numb, sleepy sensation, extending to soles, > cold water and in the open air.—Calves lame and sore.—Weakness of legs; < l., which trembles; with soreness; with heaviness.—Heaviness of legs, < l.—Numbness of anterior muscles.—Crawling pain in l. sole and under patella.—Feet feel as if frost-bitten.—Numbness of l. foot.—Soreness in ball of l. big toe in afternoon and evening, > continued walking.

24. Generalities.—Veins sunken and small, < l. side.—Bright yellow colour of sclerotic, skin, and urine.—Cancerous cachexia.—Trembling of all muscles.—Rheumatic stitches in different parts, with muscular debility.—Darting pains in various parts, extending into bones, every hour of the day.—All pains lasted till 8 p.m.—Soreness and lameness, < l. side, in morning when rising, with heavy, throbbing pains and dilated pupils, conjunctivitis, and lachrymation.—Tired feeling: in morning on waking, with heaviness; on least exertion; > open air; with lame sensation over whole body; with no desire to talk or do anything, indifferent to anything around, sleepiness and desire to lie down.—Numbness, with pains, as when taking cold.

25. Skin.—Yellow skin.—Pimples on face and neck that he had for years were now increased in number and size.—Reddish, painful boils about mouth and face, when opened they exude a thin, clear serum, which dries into a transparent scab, then become painful and contain pus like condensed milk.—Reddish boils on face, becoming pustular, with burning stinging on touch.—Erythema of abdomen and feet.—Tight feeling in skin over epigastrium.—Itching; at night.—(Burns.)

26. Sleep.—Frequent gaping in church.—Sleepiness, slept an hour in afternoon, then felt better.—Sleepiness in evening, > walking in open air; at 9 p.m.—Sleep sound but unrefreshing.—Sleepless all night.—Late falling asleep from a crowd of ideas.—Woke earlier than usual and dozed till time to rise.—Woke at 3 a.m., then difficulty in going to sleep.—Constant dreams; dreamt that she was pregnant.

27. Fever.—Chilliness, with cold, clammy sweat.—Cold limbs; feet; hands and feet.—Fever; and chilliness, then cold, clammy sweat.—Chilliness predominates.—Heat in head; r. side; in forehead.—Burning: along coronal suture; along spine, < trying to study, > motion.—Heat in lower dorsal and lumbar regions.—Sweat.—Cold, clammy sweat: in evening; on hands; on hands and feet in daytime; on hands in forenoon; on feet in evening, next day feet cold and sweaty all day.

Picrotoxinum.

Picrotoxin. An Alkaloid obtained from the fruit of Cocculus indicus. $C_{15}H_{16}O_6H_2O$. Trituration.

Clinical.—Dysentery. Dyspepsia. Hernia. Locomotor ataxy. Night-sweats. Urine, excess of.

Characteristics.—*Coc. ind.* is used to stupefy fishes, and when *Picro.* is added to water in which fishes are swimming "they make winding and boring movements of the body, alternating with quiet swimming, open their mouths and gill caverns frequently, fall on their side and rapidly die of asphyxia" (Falk, quoted *C. D. P.*). J. H. Henry proved *Picro.* on himself. The symptoms were so severe that he was alarmed, and took *Opium* and *Camphor* to antidote them. Nausea with tendency to faint, violent intestinal pain and purging, dysenteric diarrhœa and excessive secretion of urine, cramps and paralytic sensations were experienced. The symptom which gave the most concern was the pain in the bowels and sensation as if the bowels would protrude at left inguinal ring. Brunton says the local application of *Picro.* as an ointment to the head for tinea capitis and to destroy pediculi has been followed by convulsions and death. Hansen mentions that it has been given at bedtime to relieve the night-sweats of phthisis. With *Picrotoxicum acidum* 3x Dörr cured in a few weeks a case of advanced locomotor ataxy with amaurotic amblyopia (*B. J. H.*, xxxvii. 378).

Relations.—*Compare:* Coccul. In tetaniform convulsions, Nux (with Picro. respiration is accelerated more from spasm of glottis than of respiration, and there is less susceptibility to slight touch; more choreic symptoms.—Farrington).

SYMPTOMS.

1. **Mind.**—Sad thoughts, desires sleep.

2. **Head.**—Nausea with headache.

11. **Stomach.**—Pressure on stomach, with coated tongue and eructations.—Pain in pit of stomach.

12. **Abdomen.**—Pain extending all over bowels.—Fainting, violent subacute irritation of intestinal lining membrane.—Pain in bowels as if bruised.—Soreness in l. inguinal ring as if bowels would protrude.

13. **Stool and Anus.**—Flatulence with fetid diarrhœa, followed by tenesmus, painful and continued.—Diarrhœa and dysentery.

14. **Urinary Organs.**—Large quantity of clear urine passes twelve times a day.

17. **Respiratory Organs.**—Wants more breath; respiration impeded.—(Asphyxia in fishes.)

20. **Back.**—Bruised pain in back; drawing pain (l.).

22. **Upper Limbs.**—Dragging sensation of r. arm.—Pains in l. forearm running up to shoulder.

23. Lower Limbs.—Lower limbs feel bruised and paralysed (l.); have a tendency to draw back with the back, giving great > to limbs.—Constrictive painless sensation.—Cramp pains.

Pilocarpinum.

PILOCARPINUM. Pilocarpia. Pilocarpine. $C_{11}H_{16}N_2O_2$. Solution in distilled water.

P. MURIATICUM. Hydrochlorate of Pilocarpine. $C_{11}H_{16}N_2O_2HCl$. Solution in distilled water.

P. NITRICUM. Nitrate of Pilocarpine. $C_{11}H_{16}N_2O_2HNO_3$. Solution. Trituration.

Clinical.—Albuminuria. Alopecia. Convulsions, uræmic; puerperal. Deafness. Ménière's disease. Mumps. Myopia. Perspiration, excessive. Pregnancy, nausea of; salivation of. Salivation. Vertigo, aural.

Characteristics.—*Pilocarpin.* is one of the most characteristic of several alkaloids which have been isolated from *Jaborandi* (*Pilocarpus pinnatus*). It has been used, like *Jabor.*, to produce and cure profuse sweating; and by oculists to produce contraction of the pupil, which it does whether it is injected subcutaneously or applied directly to the eye. It has also an action on the ear. G. P. Field (*Brit. Med. Jour.*, May 17, 1890, &c.) has given it with good effect in labyrinthine deafness, tinnitus, and auditory nerve vertigo. The cases least amenable to its influence were those in which the hearing was > in a noise as of a train, &c.; and those in which the hearing is < after a cold. Subjects of syphilis, hereditary or acquired, and patients who are more deaf when tired, are the most suitable. The method of administration is as follows: A solution of *Pilo. nit.*, gr. $\frac{1}{2}$ to 10 minims, is used, and the initial dose (injected into the back of the arm) is gr. $\frac{1}{12}$, gradually increased to $\frac{1}{8}$, $\frac{1}{6}$, and, if well borne, to $\frac{1}{4}$. Salivation and sweating speedily occur. After each injection a drachm of sal volatile is given in a small tumbler of water. The patient is made to lie on a sofa, well covered with rugs, the head being wrapped in a shawl. The wraps are removed very gradually as the effects wear off. If there is any faintness brandy is given. The treatment is continued for a period of six weeks. [According to Cooper the improvement is only temporary. Moreover, the injections create tendency to take cold in some patients.] James C. Wood (*Med. Cent.*, i. 301) relates two instructive cases. (1) A primipara, 22, eight months pregnant, was seized with violent convulsions the night after a long walk in the month of June, and exposure whilst perspiring. Delivery was effected with extreme difficulty, and only under chloroform and after incision of the imperfectly dilated os and craniotomy of the fetus, which was evidently already dead. A sharp hæmorrhage followed. The week previous the urine had been examined and found normal. It was now scanty and loaded with albumen. *Apis* 3x was given. This was about noon. At 5 p.m. the convulsions returned. Two ounces of urine drawn off by the catheter became almost solid on boiling. *Pilo.* gr. ⅛ was administered hypodermically. In a few moments saliva began to pour from the mouth, drops of sweat gathered on the head, and sweating soon became general; nausea and some retching; laryngeal and nasal secretions increased; blood pressure diminished; face and entire body flushed red. These symptoms lasted four hours, when a second injection kept them up. The saliva was thick, stringy, exceedingly tenacious. The urine rapidly increased in quantity, whilst the albumen disappeared. Consciousness was restored, and the patient made a perfect recovery under *Apis*, *Arsen.*, and *Merc.* Wood has seen *Pilo.* relieve uræmic convulsions in the same way, the diaphoresis, free elimination by the skin and other secretive organs, removing the pressure on the over-burdened kidneys until they have time to recover themselves. (2) From the bedside of No. 1 Wood went to see a woman three months pregnant. She was a picture of distress and despair. For eight weeks she had saturated from six to ten handkerchiefs daily with tenacious saliva. Nausea and vomiting were constant, emaciation extreme. Nausea < by slightest movement. Alternate redness and paleness of face, flushes of heat and perspiration. Urine scanty, high coloured, depositing much uric acid. Very chilly; obstinate constipation. *Pilo.*, a tablet containing gr. ⅙, was dissolved in half a glass of water: to take a teaspoonful every two hours. Next day Wood found his patient sitting up, cheerful, and free from nausea and salivation. The improvement, with some fluctuations, continued. *Merc.*, *Ipec.*, *Nit. ac.*, *K. bi.*, *Hydrast.*, *Act. r.* had all previously failed. Lambert (*H. W.*, xxxii. 460) had under treatment a severe case of rheumatic iritis of *left* eye, for which *Atropine* (gr. iv. to the ounce) was being instilled several times in the day. There developed profuse night perspiration of the *right* half of the body, and during the day the right side was much moister than the left. *Pilo. mur.* 4x gr. iv. at bedtime reduced the excessive secretion of sweat. Lambert queries whether the *Atropine* instillations into the left eye were accountable for the absence of sweat on the left side of the body.—The hair as well as the skin is affected by *Pilo.*, which is an ingredient in many "hair restorers." Schmitz, of Cologne (*H. W.*, xiv. 180) treated two bald men with injections of *Pilo. mur.* to produce absorption of inflammatory residue within the eye. In both a secondary effect occurred—the growth of young downy hairs on the bald parts of the scalp. One, æt. 60, in four months had his head covered "partly with grey and partly with black hairs" of considerable growth, so as to entirely obliterate his previous baldness. *Pilo.* has also been known to turn white hair black.—A woman who had had *Pilo.* injections complained to Cooper that thereafter she had been constantly taking cold and in fear of bronchitis. Her skin, too, became irritable. *Pilo. mur.* 3x is Burnett's chief remedy in mumps. He regards it (and *Jaborandi*) as an organ remedy of the sweat glands, parotid, and pancreas. Frohling (*H. R.*, xii. 320) relates a case showing the power of *Pilo.* (he used *Pilo. mur.*, 4th trituration) over debilitating sweats left after acute diseases. With *Merc. sol.* 12 he had cured a case of rheumatic fever so far as the articular affection was concerned, but the sweats persisted and strength declined in spite of remedies until *Pilo.* was given, when the sweating stopped after the first dose.

Relations.—*Antidoted by:* Atrop., Amm. c. (sal volatile) ; brandy. *Follows well:* Merc. (in sweating of rheumatic fever). *Compare:* Jaborandi, Myosot., Eser., Phys.

SYMPTOMS.

2. **Head.**—Throbbing in temples with acceleration of pulse.—Turns white hair black.

3. **Eyes.**—Profuse lachrymation.—Pupils contracted to pin-head.—Sight for distance improved.

4. **Ears.**—(Labyrinthine deafness; < when tired; in syphilitics.—Aural vertigo.—Deafness with tinnitus.—Tinnitus of l. ear.)—Increases the secretion of wax.

5. **Nose.**—Nasal secretion increased.

6. **Face.**—Forehead and face red, veins stand out.—Perspiration begins on face.

8. **Mouth.**—Sudden salivation; maximum reached in fifteen minutes, continues two hours, one and a half pints of thin saliva being secreted in the time.—Saliva thick, stringy, exceedingly tenacious.

11. **Stomach.**—Intense thirst following the sweating.—Nausea; only occurring when salivation is complete; does not go on to vomiting as that of *Jaborandi* does.—Nausea and retching.

13. **Stool.**—Urging to stool.

16. **Female Sexual Organs.**—Menses two days early.

17. **Respiratory Organs.**—Increased bronchial mucus; much cough and expectoration.—Constantly taking cold and in fear of bronchitis.

19. **Heart.**—Weakness of heart.—Pulse accelerated, blood pressure diminished.—After the perspiration the pulse sinks to normal.

24. **Generalities.**—Dilatation of blood-vessels; temporal artery becomes a thick, pulsating cord; veins of forehead stand out blue.—Exhaustion (after the perspiration) during which most of the patients fell asleep.—Faintness.—In a case of lead paralysis it produced profuse salivation and perspiration, with sensation of great coldness and excessive tremors of limbs.

25. **Skin.**—Irritable skin.

26. **Sleep.**—Patients fall asleep under its influence.

27. **Fever.**—Sensation of coldness and shaking chill without fall of temperature.—Increase of temperature with feeling of intense cold.—Redness of face with sensation of warmth; perspiration at first over forehead along margin of hair, invading successively neck, chest, trunk, arms, and, finally lower limbs.—Sweat profuse; may lose from two to four pounds in the sweating.—Sweat begins about five minutes later than salivation, often accompanied by feeling of intense cold, chattering of teeth and desire for wraps.—After sweat: thirst; feeling of relief and sense of increased vigour.

Pimenta.

Eugenia pimenta. Myrtus pimenta. Pimenta officinalis. Allspice. Jamaica Pepper. [Pimento, or Allspice, consists of the dried berries of the West Indian Eugenia pimenta and E. acris.] *N. O.* Myrtaceæ. Tincture of the fruit.

Clinical.—Chill. Neuralgia.

Characteristics.—"Allspice" is so named because its odour is said to resemble a combination of cinnamon, nutmeg, and cloves. A tincture was proved by Becket and developed one-sided neuralgias and disturbed sensations of heat and cold.

Relations.—*Compare:* Eucalyp., Eug. j.

SYMPTOMS.

2. **Head.**—Semi-lateral neuralgic lesions.

11. **Stomach.**—Very imperious desire to eat.

24. **Generalities.**—Semi-lateral neuralgic lesions, esp. of head.

27. **Fever.**—Disturbance in calorification and sensibility; parts of body burning hot, others cold.—Peculiar cold sensation as if sponge filled with cold water passed here and there over the surface, succeeded by sensation of heat, as in the reaction after a cold bath.

Pimpernel, *see* Anagallis.

Pimpinella.

Pimpinella saxifraga. Burnet saxifrage. Bibernell. *N. O.* Umbelliferæ. Tincture of the fresh root.

Clinical.—Chilliness. Corns. Epistaxis. Fever. Headache. Lumbago. Stiff neck. Tinnitus.

Characteristics.—The majority of the symptoms of *Pimpinella* were obtained by Schelling from chewing the fresh root. The rest were contributed by Berridge, who proved the 1 x on a man. Chilliness was a marked symptom, chilly in the back even in a warm room, and much < if a window was opened. Sensitive to draughts. Sensation of coldness in occiput as from a cutting wind behind. Cold stream from hip and into right leg. The pains and sensations extended from one part to another, principally from above downward and from before backward (temples to nape; forehead to eyes; nape to shoulders), from within outward; or alternated between different parts. There was rush of blood to head, followed by nose-bleed; whizzing in head, roaring in ears. Sinking sensation in intestines.

Weariness and falling asleep of parts rested on. Frequent yawning and desire to take a long breath, which was difficult. Great drowsiness. The symptoms were < morning (vertigo ; sweat) ; afternoon (heat and rush of blood to head) ; by chewing ; reading ; writing ; reflecting ; rest (weary pain in limbs) ; standing ; stooping ; after stooping ; walking ; by opening window ; in warm room.

Relations.—*Compare :* Rush of blood preceding nose-bleed, Graph. Occipital pains, Hell. n., Nat. s., Glon.

SYMPTOMS.

2. **Head.**—Vertigo : inclination to one side, morning, on rising ; dizzy confusion.—Heat, rush of blood and confusion of head, soon followed by nose-bleed ; afternoon.—Rushing in whole head, esp. down back part, with pressure.—Whizzing in head and sounds as in an empty barrel.—Dulness and heaviness in head, with drowsiness when reading.—Head feels tied up and compressed.—Sticking in forehead, extending to both sides along eyes.—Sticking burning from vertex to both sides and down over temples.—Pressing and pushing from temples to occiput and nape.—Sensation of coldness in occiput as though a sharp draught constantly blowing from behind ; in a closed room.—Tension and pressive pain from occiput into nape.—Pain in occiput, < reading or thinking.—Acute stitches in occiput concentrated in protuberance.—Itching on vertex.—Shivering of scalp, hair bristles.

3. **Eyes.**—Smarting pain in r. eye.—Burning in eyes, esp. upper surface of eyeballs ; disagreeable coolness.—Smarting in lids.—Vision dim, misty.

4. **Ears.**—Fine stitches extending out through r. ear, with roaring.—Roaring in ears as from a distant sound.

5. **Nose.**—Dry, stopped catarrh.

6. **Face.**—Pain as from an ulcer in r. cheek.

8. **Mouth.**—Sore, pressive pain in stump of tooth, l. lower jaw.—Burning aroma on tongue, palate, and throat.—Saliva increased during and after chewing.—Collection of mucus in mouth and fauces, obliging hawking.—Taste : acrid, burning, earthy ; penetrating while chewing, later spreading a warmth through whole body ; mouldy.

9. **Throat.**—Hawking of tenacious whitish mucus from arch of palate, and a crumbly, cheesy, offensive concretion from fauces.

11. **Stomach.**—Eructations : frequent, of gas ; with vertigo and yawning ; tasteless ; acid, after stooping.

12. **Abdomen.**—Fine stitches just above navel.—Rumbling and gurgling.—Sensation as if intestines would sink down from their own weight.

13. **Stool.**—Purging.—Stool dry, harder than usual.

17. **Respiratory Organs.**—Oppression whilst walking, in open air and in house.—Breathing short, difficult ; feeling of apprehension in chest.—Frequently impelled to take a long breath, which is difficult.

18. **Chest.**—The portion of the chest against which he leans becomes painful as if weary.—Transient, needle-like stitches, back and forth in sides of chest, back, small of back, and walls of abdomen.

19. **Heart.**—Sensation of heaviness in præcordial region and abdomen as if intestines would sink down of their own weight.

20. **Neck and Back.**—Stiff neck.—Pressive, tensive pain from nape to shoulder.—Constant, pressive, contractive pain alternately in nape, side of neck, and r. shoulder.—Constant tension and sticking in nape and occiput.—Constrictive, cramp-like pain in small of back, esp. on stooping; on standing upright; on walking.—Tension and tearing in small of back, extending into hips and back.—Burning in loins and small of back.—Pressive stitches in loins.—Tensive pain in back, esp. sacral region.

21. **Limbs.**—Weary pain in limbs while at rest.

22. **Upper Limbs.**—Pressive, sticking pains in r. shoulder; stitches shoot deep into r. chest.—The arm that is resting on the table feels weary and falls asleep.—Fine sticking, drawing from r. upper arm to hand, with a shivering extending through the limb.—Stinging as from nettles on last joint of r. ring finger.

23. **Lower Limbs.**—Pain in hips and pelvis as if broken.—A cold stream, extending into r. leg and foot, with fine stitches now and then.—Painful burning in corns (quite unusual).

24. **Generalities.**—The whole body feels weak and weary.—Weakness and general sick feeling.

25. **Skin.**—Fine stinging as from nettles deeply piercing the skin on last joint of r. ring finger, while writing.

26. **Sleep.**—Frequent yawning; with eructations.—Overpowering sleepiness (for an hour after chewing the drug).—Sleep dreamy.

27. **Fever.**—Unusual chilliness over whole body (in warm room).—Chilliness and shivering of scalp, the hair bristles (in warm room).—Chill runs up middle of back; rest of body warm, and icy cold hands.—Great sensitiveness to every cool temperature, shivering in back when window is opened.—Violent catarrhal fever.—Sweat every morning.

Pinus Lambertiana.

Sugar Pine. (North America.) *N. O.* Coniferæ. Trituration of inspissated sap.

Clinical.—Abortion. Amenorrhœa. Constipation.

Characteristics.—The inspissated sap of *P. Lamb.* makes a sugary substance like manna. A small quantity (from a bit the size of a pea to a teaspoonful) has a decided but gentle laxative action, and in larger quantities emphatically so. It has also an action on the menstrual function, restoring menses when suppressed; and producing abortion in pregnant women.

Relations.—*Compare:* Sabina, Junip., Pin. syl., and other coniferæ.

SYMPTOMS.

13. **Stools.**—Gentle cathartic action.

16. **Female Sexual Organs.**—Used by Indian women to procure abortion.—In suppressed menses restores the flow and removes painful sensations resulting from suppression.

Pinus Sylvestris.

Scotch Fir. Red, Norway, Riga, or Baltic Pine. (The typical pine of Europe.) *N. O.* Coniferæ. Tincture of leaves and young twigs.

Clinical.—Ankles, weak. Anus, itching of. Bronchitis. Constipation. Diarrhœa. Dysuria. Emaciation of lower limbs. Glands, submaxillary and inguinal, swollen. Gout. Hæmorrhoids. Heart, palpitation of. Joints, stiff. Kidneys, pains in. Liver, enlargement of. Rheumatism. Scrofula. Squint. Tinnitus. Urine, increased ; strong. Vertigo. Walking, late. Worms (lumbrici).

Characteristics.—*Pinus syl.* was proved by Demeures in the φ tincture ; and Patzack observed the effects of bathing in an infusion of the leaves. Pine baths may also be made by adding *Oleum pini sylvestris* to an ordinary bath in the proportion of one minim to the gallon. These baths have a reputation in the treatment of rheumatism, gout, paralysis, scrofula, and skin diseases. The provings show that this reputation is founded on a specific relationship. Rheumatic, gouty, and paralytic pains in limbs, bones, and joints ; stiffness ; glandular swellings ; enlarged and painful liver and spleen ; chilliness and sensitiveness to touch. Scalp sensitive. Chest walls sensitive, with a peculiar feeling of *thinness*, as if they would give way at a touch. The kidneys were stimulated ; burning on micturition ; flow increased ; urine strong. Itching of the nose and discharge of round worms was noted. The menstrual function was deranged. Bronchial mucus was increased. Hansen gives "emaciation of lower extremities" and "weak ankles in children" as indications for it, and mentions that the φ tinctures may be used externally, whilst the attenuations are given internally. Chilliness alternating with flushing ; the face is alternately red and pale. Itching in general. The symptoms are < by exertion ; walking ; touch ; in morning ; in evening. In a patient of Cooper's *Pinus syl.* caused "headache < by any movement of the eyes" ; and it cured a case of squint.

Relations.—*Compare :* Tereb., Sabi., Junip., Thuj., Aloe, Pix. Strong urine, Benz. ac. Red margin of eyes, Sul., Bac.

SYMPTOMS.

1. **Mind.**—Anxiety.—Despondency.—Wants to do many things, undertakes all and finishes none.—Mind dull, unable to think ; caused by any exertion.

2. **Head.**—Vertigo, even to falling down.—Dulness ; fulness ; heaviness of head.—Pressive headache.—Tearing in temples.—Scalp sensitive.—Headache < by any movement of eyes.

3. **Eyes.**—Eyes inflamed.—Margins of lids red.—Vision dim ; veiled.—(Squint.)

4. **Ears.**—Sticking in ears.—Roaring in ears.

5. **Nose.**—Violent nose-bleed several days in succession.—Mucous discharge from nose.—Sensation of coryza.—Itching of nose.

6. **Face.**—Face alternately pale and red.—Tearing in face.

8. **Mouth.**—Pain in teeth, with heat of face and pain in head.—Dry mouth with increased thirst.

9. **Throat.**—Uneasiness in throat as if something in the way.—Painful swelling of submaxillary glands.

11. **Stomach.**—Appetite at first decreased, afterwards increased.—Pressure in pit of stomach after eating, with great distension.

12. **Abdomen.**—Distension of hypochondrium, with pressive, burning pains.—Enlargement of liver.—Pressure and fulness in liver and spleen.—Colic with incarcerated flatus.—Pain in inguinal glands with swelling.

13. **Stool and Anus.**—Troublesome itching at anus.—Stool: thin, pasty, with colic and great excitement; bilious.—Discharge of round worms; itching and burning on anus; bloody, slimy, hæmorrhoidal discharge for several days.—Constipation.

14. **Urinary Organs.**—Violent boring-burning pains in kidneys, extending along ureters.—Spasms of bladder.—Burning pains when urinating. —Micturition difficult.—Very greatly increased secretion of urine.—Urine of strong odour.

16. **Female Sexual Organs.**—Menses, usually scanty, became more profuse.—Menses: earlier; delayed.

17. **Respiratory Organs.**—Hoarseness.—Increased bronchial mucus. —Short, dry cough.—Expectoration greater when coughing.—Breath tight, esp. when walking.

18. **Chest.**—Oppression.—Anterior portion of chest painful to touch; it seems as if very thin and ready to give way on the slightest pressure; all evening.—Burning in sides of chest.—In middle of sternum sensation as if a cupping-glass had been applied inside.

19. **Heart.**—Palpitation.

20. **Neck and Back.**—Drawing and stiffness in nape extending into occiput.—Pressive, tensive drawing pain between shoulders and small of back; motion difficult.

21. **Limbs.**—Limbs: stiff; heavy; weak, can hardly walk—Gouty pain in all joints of hands and feet, esp. finger-joints.—Pressive-tensive pains in limbs.—Drawing-paralytic pains in limbs.

23. **Lower Limbs.**—Knees stiff with stinging-burning pains, so that they give out.—Pain in l. tibia when walking, it = sensation as if he would double up on himself (in morning only); next day same pain in r. tibia, with gripings in whole abdomen.—Cramps in calves when stretching in bed at night.—In evening, itching lancinations, crosswise, in fold separating first and second phalanges of r. great toe, > by applying hand.

25. **Skin.**—Nettle-rash.—Itching of whole body, < about joints and on abdomen.—Itching of nose.

26. **Sleep.**—Great sleepiness, esp. forenoon, with restless sleep in evening.—Sleepless.—Dreams which seem when remembered like real occurrences.

27. **Fever.**—Chilliness, esp. towards evening, alternating with flushes of heat.—Perspiration: general; easy.

Piper Methysticum.

Macropiper methysticum. Ava. Kava-kava. Kawa. *N. O.* Piperaceæ. Tincture of fresh root.

Clinical.—Albuminuria. Anus, prolapse of. Brachialgia. Brain-fag. Catalepsy. Cystitis. Dysuria. Eczema. Gonorrhœa. Headache. Head, enlarged feeling. Ichthyosis. Leprosy. Neuralgia. Neurasthenia. Orchitis. Paraplegia. Prostatorrhœa. Rheumatism. Toothache. Urethritis. Uric acid, excess of.

Characteristics.—*Piper methysticum* (it is called *Macropiper methysticum* in most recent botanical works, but I retain the older name by which it is best known in homœopathy) furnishes the root called Kava in Polynesia. The natives use it as a stimulant, either chewing the root or drinking a beverage made of it before undertaking any important business or religious rites. Excessive indulgence in it produces a skin disease like leprosy, called at Tahiti Arevareva. Lutz (quoted *H. W.*, xxviii. 175) describes the disease as observed amongst natives of the Sandwich Islands: "The skin, particularly that of the extremities, assumes the appearance of well-marked ichthyosis, associated with a certain degree of atrophy, such as is observed in senile skin. There is an absence of inflammatory symptoms." The mental symptoms of the "Intoxicating Pepper" (μέθυσις, drunkenness) are the most interesting feature of the drug's action. W. N. Griswold proved the third and second dilutions, and developed a large number of nervous, mental, and brain symptoms, among which are some which have proved to be keynotes. The drug causes a feeling of buoyancy, as if every nerve was strung up to the highest pitch; feels he can work without fatigue, quickly followed by a feeling of tired brain, and over-sensitiveness to all external impressions. Mental tension; feeling as though the head were enlarged even to bursting. The mental symptoms, excitement or depression, and the headache, were > *by diversion of mind*. This is one of the keynotes, and it has served to indicate *Piper m.* in connection with other symptoms. Griswold cured a case having burning in chest, > by diverting mind (*Org.*, i. 229); and three cases having: "Agonising pain, with tossing, twisting, and writhing; patient *driven irresistibly to change position, which generally gives little or no* >." This italicised passage is the second keynote of *Piper m.* These cures were with the 1 x or φ tinctures. Skinner gave fractional doses of φ tincture in water to a highly excitable young girl who had severe toothache and earache, and had worn out her family by the incessant day and night attendance she required. The pains were dragging, heavy, < at night in bed, and after or when eating, "forgets all about her pains if amused with anything, but directly she is tired of it she exclaims, 'Oh, my tooth or ear!'" In addition she had "Agonising pain with tossing, twisting, and writhing; irresistibly driven to change position." The patient slept well that night the first time for a fortnight, and had no more pain. The remaining swelling was removed by *Puls.* 200. Skinner also reports this case: Miss R., 20, has toothache in a decayed molar, > if attention is diverted by anything sufficiently exciting. When pain is at all violent she has no rest in any position, must keep continually changing it. *Piper m.* 500 (F. C.) was given, and there was relief very soon after the first dose. A few doses completely removed the pain (*Org.*, i. 299).—*Piper m.* has much dizziness and vertigo ; > on closing eyes. The forehead was full, " solid with pain ;" this shifted to occiput and cervical spine, where it became a compression, extending as a constricting sensation to stomach and chest. The sensation of enlargement of head was marked and persistent. Farrington says convulsions simulating catalepsy are produced. Cerna (quoted *H. W.*, xxvi. 556) as a result of his investigations found *Piper m.* a general and local anæsthetic. It diminishes reflex action by its action on the cord, and kills by paralysing respiration. Cerna illustrated its relationship to *Cubeba* by citing cases of gonorrhœa, acute and chronic cystitis, gleet, prostatorrhœa, vaginitis, cured with it. The provings give the indications. The symptoms were < before meals (sour eructations) ; reading and thinking ; urinating (burning in urethra) ; walking. Going down stairs = symptoms to rush up. > Moving ; diverting mind ; open air ; closing eyes (vertigo).

Relations.—*Antidoted by :* Puls. and Rhus (partially). *Compare :* Cubeba, Piper nig., Matico (botan.). In > by diverting mind, Ox. ac. > By motion, Rhus. Feeling of buoyancy, Coff. (but with Coff. the reverse condition of brain-fag does not quickly follow). Neurasthenia, Pic. ac., Arg. n., Avena. Unbearable pains, Coff., Aco., Cham.

SYMPTOMS.

1. **Mind.**—Hilarious from 10 a.m. till 1 p.m.—Lively after an emission. —Lively and inclined to work, can dance with more ease than usual.—Agreeable excitement and support against great fatigue.—From increased doses intoxication of a sorrowful, silent, and sleepy character, different from that produced by alcohol.—Faculties sharpened.—(Capable of working more without fatigue or brain-fag.)—Lazy and drowsy.—Deep torpor and irritation from least noise (intoxication from root grown in damp soils).—Want of vigour, timid, apprehensive.

2. **Head.**—From 5 to 9 p.m. very dizzy; swimming sensation and faintness.—Intoxication, with fantastic ideas and desire to skip about, although he cannot for a moment hold himself on his legs.—Vertigo in morning in bed, with frontal pressure.—Brain tired ; in morning on waking, > getting on feet.—Tired feeling in brain at night.—Fulness, sometimes in one part, sometimes in another, < in forehead.—Heaviness of head.—Headache with pressure in upper part of orbits ; with sleepiness.—Shooting : intermittent after 3 p.m., in l. supra-orbital nerve ; in l. temple.—Headache : in l. supra-orbital nerve ; back of eyes ; l. brain from front to back ; over eyes and deep-seated ; at 9 a.m., < 3 p.m. ; in afternoon and evening, with drowsy and stupid feeling ; above eyes at 5 p.m. ; at 7 p.m. ; in l. side and deep in upper part of orbits, with pain on moving eyes ; intermittent in r. frontal eminence, > open air and motion ; above r. eye radiating over eyes, at 10 a.m. ; heavy in forehead and temples, < thinking and reading.—

Frontal brain "solid with pain" ; this ache during day generally moved to base of brain and along medulla, > by slight motion, < by large, continued and active motion ; slight mental effort, passing from topic to topic, for an instant > ; sustained effort <.—Compressive pain and soreness back of head and cervical cord ; disappear later leaving cerebellum sensitive ; parts feel treble their normal size.—Dulness in forehead, with fulness and pressure, and on raising head or moving it to either side vertigo, after the noon meal the pressure shifted to lateral and occipital regions, < lying down, but not amounting to real pain, pressure ; < remaining in one position, > moving, apprehension of pain by rapid movement, but temporary relief from it.

3. **Eyes.**—Conjunctivæ red.—Pain along r. optic nerve when reading at 3 p.m.—Pain deep in l. eye as if ball would be pressed out, in the street at 5.30 p.m.—Dizzy blindness when dressing, vertigo, > closing eyes, directing attention to head and exerting the will, at the same time vertigo, then rush of blood and fulness in forehead, then similar sensation in occipital and basilar regions.

4. **Ears.**—Singular pressure in lobules of pinna of l. ear.

6. **Face.**—Pressure outward in face at 7 p.m.

7. **Teeth.**—Teeth deep yellow.—Teeth sensitive to cold water, cold air, brushing, &c.

8. **Mouth.**—Tongue feels as if covered with velvet or fur at night.—Burning on tongue.—Burning in whole mouth followed by numbness.—Dryness of mouth on waking from afternoon nap, with sweat (in a hot day).—Salivation.—Taste : nauseous ; sweet, then piquant and sharp ; pappy ; everything tasteless ; lost to food, but ravenous haste in eating.—Taste and relish to food not as usual, at noon, but appetite unusually good.

10. **Appetite.**—Appetite : formidable at 8 p.m. ; slight ; hungry at noon, but not able to eat much ; able to eat but little supper.

11. **Stomach.**—Sour eructations, < an hour before meals and at night, at times rolling up and rumbling from stomach to mouth, but generally breaking at throat-pit, and in throat-pit sensation of something that cannot be swallowed, the latter temporarily > by eructations.—Bloating at 11 p.m.—Constriction extending from base of brain.—Crampy pain, > pressure against edge of table.—Warmth in stomach.

12. **Abdomen.**—Pain : every day about 9 a.m. ; in forenoon after first stool, with distressing full sensation ; > motion.—Pain in abdomen, above umbilicus ; in r. groin when walking, then a large stool, the latter part soft.

13. **Stool and Rectum.**—Diarrhœa threatened.—Stool : loose in morning, more difficult in evening ; soft, difficult.—Constipation : stool hard ; large ; light-coloured.—Stool large ; soft.—Urging : all day ; every evening.—Continuous desire, next day forced a large stool, which caused prolapsus ani.—Burning in rectum.

14. **Urinary Organs.**—Micturition at 4.45 a.m.—Burning in urethra during micturition.—Urine nearly neutral at 10 a.m., hot and over-acid at night.—Urine : increased ; scanty in morning.

15. **Male Sexual Organs.**—Shooting in penis.—Erection : in afternoon ; at night ; at 4 a.m. after an emission.—Pain in r. testicle.—Emission early in morning, without dreams.—Amorousness.

18. **Chest.**—Heaviness behind upper part of sternum, as from wind that

cannot be eructated.—Constriction of chest and stomach, extending from base of brain.

19. **Pulse.**—Pulse steadied.

20. **Back.**—Pain in back only felt on pressure.—Soreness about second dorsal vertebra.

21. **Limbs.**—Pain : in r. foot and wrist and l. toe at 10 p.m. ; r. elbow and l. knee, with stiffness ; r. foot and back of l. hand at 11.30 p.m., with heat of them.—Pain in r. arm as if marrow would be affected, changing its location, with paroxysmal paralysed feeling in hands, in toe at 9 p.m.

22. **Upper Limbs.**—Pain : in l. shoulder ; in l. arm in the street, with flushing heat in l. hand.—Excoriating pain in r. arm, as if the marrow would be affected ; paralysed feeling in hands.—Pain in r. arm, running in all directions, with heaviness, soreness, and tired sensation.—Dragging in l. arm at 8 p.m., > 10 p.m.—Tingling as from an electric current from l. elbow to fingers.—Numbness of r. elbow.—Pain in r. wrist, < writing.—Weakness of l. hand.—Pain in joint of l. thumb, < pressure.

23. **Lower Limbs.**—Drunk in his walk, but intellect unclouded, aware of his inability to control the movements of his legs.—Numbness of lower limbs.—Weakness ; all day ; in afternoon ; in thighs as if unable to stand.—Sticking in l. knee at 4 p.m. when walking.—Heaviness of legs when walking. —Pain : in feet ; l. foot and toe ; r. sole ; at outer and under border of l. foot and in r. great toe, with coldness of l. foot.—Sticking : in end of l. toe on waking at 4.45 a.m., in great toe when moving and walking.

24. **Generalities.**—Emaciation and decrepitude.—Trembling.—Pains (esp. of head) temporarily > by turning mind to another topic.—Feeling as if drug descended and impressed lower part of system, causing trembling of abdomen and lower limbs and blood-vessels connected therewith, but on descending stairs the drug seemed to come upward through the circulation, reaching the brain, causing exhilarating dizziness and disposition to swing and stagger, as if under the influence of liquor, felt talkative and happy, after the dizziness felt a "toned-up" condition of brain and nervous system, dizziness returned on beginning to move.—Nervous system strung up to its highest tension.—Stimulating and sedative effects, then sweat.—Vigour ; all day, with exhilaration, next day feelings varying and generally depressed.—Uneasiness and weakness during day, with timidity and apprehension.—Weakness in morning, > rising and moving around.—Want of tone and life in all functions towards night.—< In open air and on motion.

25. **Skin.**—Covered as in leprosy with large scales, which fall off and leave white spots, and these often become ulcers.—Dryness, esp. where it is thick, as on hands and feet, with scales, cracks, and ulcers.—Painful hard swelling in lower corner of l. ear ; red, painful lump, threatening to become an abscess, on forehead above r. inner canthus and on back.

26. **Sleep.**—Sleepiness : at 10 p.m., soon afterwards liveliness and wakefulness ; irresistible.—Hard sleep several times a day.—Stupid sleep.—Heavy sleep with disturbing but unremembered dreams.—Sleepless ; from 12 till 2.30 a.m. ; at 4 a.m., after an emission, then sound sleep, next night wakeful after an emission till I got up for breakfast ; latter part of night, mind working on business problems, next morning tired feeling before and after rising.—Difficult falling asleep.—Restless sleep last part of night.—Fragmentary sleep

last part of night.—Fragmentary sleep from 12.30 till 4.20 a.m., with varied and exciting dreams, then sleeplessness so that I had to get up at 4.30 a.m., did excitedly all kinds of unusual office work.—Dreams : curious, nonsensical, wild ; amorous ; of travelling by rail ; active, vivid, last part of night, alternating with half-conscious waking ; in afternoon, of fighting unknown men, left them to follow an unknown woman, and when she left me found that she had conducted me to a prayer-meeting, which must have changed to a restaurant, for I ordered a Hamburg beefsteak, but woke before it was served ; of a fire, heard the engines and firemen.

27. **Fever.**—Chilliness for the last few hours, at 8 p.m.—Heat : at 9 a.m. ; flush of general heat ; in face and hands, < l. hand ; flushing, in cheeks ; heat in l. ear-flap and l. hand ; over upper part of body in evening.—Hands sought cool places, otherwise no perceptible increase of heat.—Heavy perspiration, with great dryness of mouth on waking from afternoon nap.

Piper Nigrum.

Pepper. *N. O.* Piperaceæ. Trituration or tincture of dried fruits (peppercorns).

Clinical.—Anus, fissure of. Blenorrhagia. Breasts, swelling of ; eruption on. Constipation. Cough. Dysuria. Hæmorrhoids. Headache. Menses, irregular ; scanty. Milk, excessive flow of. Neuralgia. Priapism. Speech, difficult. Teeth, caries of. Tongue, eruption on ; heavy. Toothache. Uterus, cramps in.

Characteristics.—The Peppers are tropical climbing shrubs. *Piper nig.* yields the pepper of commerce. The fruit when ripe is red. It is gathered before it is fully ripe and spread on mats in the sun, when it loses its red colour and becomes black and shrivelled. This is Black pepper. White pepper is the same fruit freed from its outer skin by maceration in water and subsequent rubbing (*Treas. of Bot.*). The symptoms of the proving are Houat's. The only additional symptom is one recorded by Berridge as having occurred in a lady on two occasions from taking a large quantity of pepper : "Feeling as if temples and malar bones were pressed in, < on left side." This confirms one of Houat's symptoms. The full, heavy headache of Houat's provings I can confirm by personal experience : I get the headache whenever I take food highly peppered ; and I know others who do the same. Sensations of *burning* occur almost everywhere. *Pressure* is almost as common : Pressure in nasal bones, in temples and facial bones. Contraction of uterus and sensation as if something about to enter it. Sensation of a foreign round body rising to stomach. The symptoms are < by change of temperature ; in damp weather ; in evening ; by motion.

Relations.—*Compare :* Piper m., Cubeba (botanical ; also mental, genito-urinary, skin, and general symptoms).

SYMPTOMS.

1. **Mind.**—Hot-headed, irascible, and often gay.—Amorousness with hypochondriasis.—Fear of being poisoned.

2. **Head.**—Heaviness and congestion of the cerebellum, with pale face.—Rushing and congestion of blood to head with throbbing.—Brain : empty feeling ; numbness causing swooning ; fluctuation and oscillation in morning.—Pressure on head ; as if bones of cranium and face rested on lower jaw.—Neuralgic pain through whole head at every change of temperature.—Violent headache ; feels as if it would burst at vertex.—Pressing pains at temples as if they would be broken in.

3. **Eyes.**—Eyes inflamed and burning, with sensation of cold in lids.—Lids ulcerated and bleared.—Lachrymation and photophobia.—Dim sight and vertigo, with headache, nausea, and vomiting.

4. **Ears.**—Crusty ulcers in concha of ears.

5. **Nose.**—Frequent sneezing, epistaxis.—Dry and fluent coryza.—Dryness and burning in nostrils ; nostrils stopped up.—Pressure on nasal bones as if being crushed.

6. **Face.**—Feeling as if temples and malar bones were pressed in, < l. side.—Red, burning face.—Drawing faceache ; as if muscles and bones were ranging themselves on one another.—Convulsive closure of jaws.—Eczema on lips.

8. **Mouth.**—Tooth decays.—Violent toothache, < in warmth and evening.—Eruption of little vesicles on margin of tongue.—Painful, heavy tongue ; impeded speech.—Whitish coating on middle of tongue.—Burning dryness of mouth and throat.—Heat and dryness of palate and tongue, as if burned.

9. **Throat.**—Constant accumulation of mucus in throat and expectoration.—Burning in throat with sensation of stiffness as if it were an iron tube.—Burning pains in tonsils, with sensation as if they were being pierced.—Paralysis of muscles of throat ; can cry but not articulate intelligibly.

11. **Stomach.**—Constant, unquenchable thirst.—Vomiting with great exertion ; it seemed as if stomach itself would be vomited.—Sensation of heat and dryness in stomach.—Cramps and drawing in stomach, with desire for coarse and extravagant food.—Gastric discomfort.

12. **Abdomen.**—Burning and lancinating pains in liver, as if a tumour there.—Disposition of abdomen to obesity.—Abdomen swollen, hard, burning.—Tympanites with sensation as if everything in it were in ebullition.—Borborygmi.—Inflammation of intestines with great thirst.—Heaviness, flatulence.—Colic and cramps ; sensation as if intestines would burst.—Painful restlessness and anxiety in intestines.—Sensation of round foreign body rising to stomach, with heavy pain in intestines.—Electrical-like discharges in intestines when he moves.

13. **Stool and Anus.**—Inflammation of rectum, anus swollen and burning ; fear to go to stool on account of the difficulty and pain.—Fissures at anus.—Large flowing hæmorrhoids.—Long-lasting constipation, then involuntary, thin stools.

14. **Urinary Organs.**—Full, swollen bladder, frequent inclination to urinate without success.—Burning pains in bladder as from live coals.—Burning in glans and urethra.—Blennorrhœa, greenish, offensive.—Difficult micturition.—Urine : turbid, brownish ; diabetic ; bloody ; containing sand.

15. **Male Sexual Organs.**—Excessive priapism.—Inflammation and swelling of penis, with priapism and burning pains.—Burning, pricking, excoriating pains in glans.—Strong ejaculation, or almost none, and very difficult.

16. Female Sexual Organs.—Ovaries and uterus congested, with pricking and lancinating pains.—Contraction of uterus with sensation as if something strove to penetrate into it.—Burning and distending pains in uterus.—Menses : difficult, retarded ; capricious, irregular, with colic and black blood.

17. Respiratory Organs.—Ulceration and false membranes thick, deep in larynx.—Voice : low, deep, rough, unintelligible.—Hoarseness with coughing and constant snuffing.—Severe coughing, esp. evening and when going to sleep.—Cough : violent, occasionally spitting of blood ; croupy ; hollow.—Dyspnœa and attacks of suffocation.

18. Chest.—Disposition to obesity of chest.—Painful spots on chest, < coughing, breathing, motion.—At each coughing spell it seemed as if chest would be torn and he would spit blood.—Burning, lancinating pains ; sensation of heat and dryness of chest.—Burning and swollen heat.—Great flow of milk.—Dartrous eruption on l. breast.

19. Heart.—Sensation as if heart were surrounded with water.—Frequent palpitation.

20. Back.—Burning in loins and kidneys, with contractive movements.

21. Limbs.—Inflammation and swelling of joints.

24. Generalities.—Bones brittle.—Motion of carriage deafens and = spasms.—Spasms with tetanic stiffness of limbs.—< From motion ; in evening ; in damp weather.

25. Skin.—Crusty ulcers in ears.—Large pustules on face, leaving scars. —Eczema on lips.—Very tender skin.—Itching, < by scratching, heat, and motion.

26. Sleep.—Irresistible drowsiness.—Lethargic sleep.—Wakens at night without being able to sleep again.—Nightmare.

27. Fever.—Dryness and coldness of skin, heat with biting dryness.—Heat in forehead with heaviness of head and vertigo.—Cold sweat with great heat through whole body.—Sweat which seems to corrode the skin.

Piperazinum.

Piperazine. Piperazidine. Ethylenimine. Diethylene-diamine.
$C_4H_{10}N_2$. Trituration. Solution.

Clinical.—Glaucoma. Gout. Lead paralysis. Renal colic.

Characteristics.—*Piperaz.* is a synthetic product which was intended to replace Spermin (C_2H_5N), and was named Dispermine. It was found, however, to be a different body both in chemical and physiological properties. It occurs in well-defined, colourless, acicular crystals (Helbing), or in lustrous tables (J. Gordon) ; is deliquescent and mostly soluble in water. It readily unites with uric acid, forming a very soluble compound (urate of piperazine). When taken by the mouth it is not entirely oxydised, as part is discoverable unchanged in the urine. John Gordon experimented with *Piperaz.* and found that a 1-per cent. solution in normal urine at body temperature dissolved to a large extent a fragment of uric acid cal-culus, and converted undissolved portions to a granular and pulp condition. The amount of urea is increased in the urine of thos taking it ; and Helbing (*Modern Materia Medica*) says it has been use with success in mental diseases, and in a case of lead paralysis wit "very remarkable results." J. R. Hamilton, of Hawick (*Lance* December 30, 1893), reports success in treating renal colic wit *Piperaz.*; and Walter, of Odessa (quoted *H. W.*, xxv. 10), cleared u two cases of glaucoma, giving one grain daily in carbonated water, a the symptoms disappearing within three weeks. [After a teaspoonfu dose of an effervescing preparation of *Piperaz.*, a patient complained tha he was seized with a bad attack of acute gout, that was quit unexpected (Cooper).]

Relations.—*Compare:* Phloriz., Hydrang., Urt. u.

Piscidia.

Piscidia erythrina. Jamaica Dog-wood. *N. O.* Leguminosæ. Tinc-ture of root bark obtained when the plant is in flower, befor leaf.

Clinical.—Fever. Sleep, sudden. Sweat, profuse.

Characteristics.—The pounded leaves and young branches c *Piscidia eryth.* and some allied species are used, like *Cocculus*, fo poisoning fish—hence the name *Piscidia* (*Piscis-cædere*). The experi-ment recorded in Allen is by W. Hamilton, who took a drachm of th tincture in water for toothache, and went off to sleep with suc suddenness that when he awoke, twelve hours later, he was sti holding the glass and vial from which he had taken the dose.

SYMPTOMS.

8. **Mouth.**—When chewed, unpleasant acrimony in mouth, like that c *Mezer.*

26. **Sleep.**—"A sleep the most profound I ever experienced, arrested m so suddenly that I remained motionless the whole night with the uncorke vial in one hand, and the glass out of which I had taken the dose in th other, until the sun was high above the horizon, a space of twelve hours, whe I first returned to consciousness, free from every pain or ache, and witho any of the unpleasant sensations which invariably succeed an overdose c *Opium.*"

27. **Fever.**—"Violent sensation of heat generally, increasing in intensity the sensation of burning gradually extended to the surface, and while I wa considering what antidote I ought to employ, a profuse diaphoresis burst o from every pore."

Pix Liquida.

Liquid Tar. (A product of dry distillation of various coniferous woods.) Tincture.

Clinical.—Acne. Ardor urinæ. Bronchitis. Desquamation. Diarrhœa. Eczema. Enuresis. Eruptions. Hands, eruptions on. Phthisis. Psoriasis. Vomiting, black.

Characteristics.—In old-school practice Tar is known as a "stimulant expectorant" in chronic bronchitis and phthisis, a stimulant to the skin in psoriasis and scaly eczema. Buckley (quoted by Allen) has recorded severe constitutional effects following the local application of preparations of tar in skin affections. Among these are: High fever; black vomit; black stools; dark-coloured urine; acute eczema; acne. Homœopaths (led by Jeanes) have brought out the special indications for the remedy; and chief among them is a pain at the third left costal cartilage, where it joins the rib. This is really a pain of the left bronchus (Hering), and when associated with offensive muco-purulent expectoration the indications for *Pix* are complete. Cases of phthisis and chronic bronchitis with these characteristics have been cured by it. A case of chronic bronchitis in a merchant, 55, is recorded in *Hom. News* (xxix. 414). The cough was < nights, breath short, copious expectoration, some fever and night-sweats. Ill three years and growing worse. Raynaud's prescription of Wood Tar, a teaspoonful four times a day, after meals and at bedtime, cleared up most of the symptoms.—*Pix* often cures the enuresis somni of children (R. T. C.).

Relations.—*Compare:* Tereb., Pinus syl., Kre., Eupn., Petrol. In chest pains, Illic. (Illic. has pain at third *right* costal cartilage; occasionally also left), Myrica, Therid. Desquamation, Chi. sul.

SYMPTOMS.

2. **Head.**—Fulness and pain in head.

11. **Stomach.**—Pain in stomach.—Vomiting: constant; of blackish fluid (from application to skin).

12. **Abdomen.**—Excessive pain in bowels and loins.

13. **Stool and Anus.**—Dark-coloured stools (from application).

14. **Urinary Organs.**—Ardor urinæ.—Dark-coloured urine (from application).

17. **Respiratory Organs.**—Expectoration of purulent matter, offensive in odour and taste, and accompanied by pain referred to third l. costal cartilage (really in l. bronchus); pain may or may not go through to back.—(Third stage of phthisis.)—Pain at third l. costal cartilage where it joins the rib; râles; muco-purulent expectoration.—Suppuration of l. lung with pain at third rib.—Cough chronic, < night; expectoration purulent; fever at night.

24. **Generalities.**—Great exhaustion.

25. **Skin.**—Acute eczema.—Acne.—Eruptions, esp. on backs of hands,

itching intolerably at night and bleeding when scratched.—Skin cracked, bleeding when scratched, with sleeplessness.—Violent itching.—Desquamation.

27. **Fever.**—Occasionally high fever (from application).

Plantago.

Plantago major. Plantain. Ribwort. *N. O.* Plantaginaceæ. Tincture of whole fresh plant. Tincture of the root.

Clinical.—Ague. Breast, inflammation of. Burns. Ciliary neuralgia. Diabetes. Diarrhœa. Dysentery. *Earache. Ear, inflammation of.* Emissions. Enuresis. Erysipelas. Erythema. Hæmorrhoids. Impotence. *Neuralgias;* of herpes. Polyuria. Rhus poisoning. Snake-bites. Spleen, pains in. Tobacco habit. *Toothache.* Urination, delayed. Worms. Wounds.

Characteristics.—Hale sums up the ancient and modern history of *Plantago maj.* the weed which furnishes food for our cage-birds. (*Plant. m.* must not to be confounded with *Musa*, sometimes called "Plantain," which belongs to a different class, viz., the Endogens.) *Plantago* has had a reputation in medicine from remote antiquity, a reputation which homœopathy has revived. It was used in intermittent fever in remotest times. In A.D. 1558 the *Herbal of Dodoens* commends the juice of leaves or roots for "toothache and bleeding of gums." John Parkinson in his *Theatre of Plants* (A.D. 1640) says "the root taken fresh out of the ground, washed and gently scraped with a knife, then put into the *ear*, cures the toothache like a charm." In Switzerland the leaf fibres are frayed out and put into the ear for the same purpose, and if they relieve the pain they "turn black" (says Reutlinger) and have to be removed, if there is no relief they remain green. In domestic practice, says Hale, it is constantly resorted to as an application in all affections of the skin with irritation, pain, and heat, the bruised leaves being applied to the part. Hale enumerates the following as having been relieved by it: Erysipelas, *Rhus*-poisoning, erythema, burns, scalds, inflammation of the glands (notably the breasts), bruises, incised wounds, bites of animals, chilblains, frostbite. A case is related (*H. R.*, xi. 241) of a man who allowed himself to be bitten by rattlesnakes and cured himself by drinking the juice of the plant and applying bruised leaves to the bites, changing them frequently. The tincture has been extensively proved by F. Humphreys (who wrote a monograph upon it), Heath, and others, and the homœopathicity of its cures was clearly brought out. The neuralgic pains of teeth, ears, and face were especially pronounced. Some new symptoms were brought to light. The very copious discharge of urine along with the thirst suggest diabetes; and the laxity of sphincters has led to the cure of a number of cases of enuresis. Foul breath, sinking and weight in stomach, flatulence, diarrhœa, dysentery, and hæmorrhoids, all appeared in the proving. *Plant.* is one of the most useful of *local* remedies in homœopathy, and one of its local uses is as an application to inflamed and painful piles. In all neuralgic conditions where the suffering part can be reached *Plant.* φ may be painted on without any fear of injury, and often with the most signal relief of suffering. In common with others, I have used it with success in numberless cases of toothache and earache ; but I have also given relief in the painful neuralgia of shingles and in pleurodynia. F. P. Stiles (*Minn. H. Mag.*, v. 225) relates three brilliant cases : (1) Mrs. S., 39, for ten days had terrible neuralgic pain in right side of face, shooting into temporal, superior, maxillary, and orbital regions. *Plant.* φ applied locally to gums, temple, and cheek, removed the pain in a few minutes. Some days later a slight return was promptly relieved in the same way. (2) Mr. R. had neuralgia in left superior maxillary and lower orbital region of long standing. Promptly relieved in the same way. (3) Mrs. N., neuralgia of right upper jaw, pain unbearable, radiating to ear, temple, and cheek. A tooth had been extracted without relief. *Plant.* φ removed all the pain. "Toothache with earache," "toothache with salivation," are leading indications. *Plant.* has a relation to tobacco. It produces disgust for it in chewers ; and it cures neuralgia resulting from tobacco. The pains are tearing, boring, bruised. There is great surface sensitiveness. Pains come suddenly and are apt to be erratic. Unendurable pains. There is darting up and down the urethra. Breath and flatulence are offensive. Some *characteristics are :* Loud noises going through one. *Sudden* discharge of yellowish (or saffron-coloured) water from nose. The *left* side was most affected. The symptoms are < at night. > By eating (colic). < By contact ; mental exertion ; by motion ; heat and cold ; cold air ; sharp wind : heat of room.

Relations.—*Antidote to :* Apis, Rhus, Tabac. *Antidoted by :* Merc. (toothache). *Compare :* In neuralgias, Cham., Merc., Spig., Kalm., Coloc. Unendurable pains, Aco., Cham., Hep. Wounds and bruises, fetid breath and flatus, Arn. Wounds, Calend. Punctured wounds, Led., Hyper. Hæmorrhoids, external and internal use, Ham. Enuresis, Bell., Caust. (Bell. has irregular action of sphincter ; Plant. and Caust. relaxation). Earache with toothache ; intolerance of warm room, Puls.

Causation.—Bruises. Burns. Cuts. Punctured wounds. Snakebites.

SYMPTOMS.

1. **Mind.**—Mind inactive, with dull, muddled feeling in head.—Despondency, confusion of thought.—Irritable, morose ; impatient, restless mood, with dull, stupid feeling in brain.—Great mental prostration, < by mental exertion, which = rapid breathing and anxiety.

2. **Head.**—Twinges of pain in different parts of head, now through r. temple, extending backward ; then through occiput from ear to ear ; then in other parts of head more or less severe.—Severe, lightning-like stitches over l. eye, extending to r. 12.30 to 5.45 p.m., disappearing suddenly, involving whole forehead, and accompanied at the height with nausea at pit of stomach ; > hard pressure with cold hand, < warmth.—Severe pain in l. side of head,

from forehead extending deep into brain, coming on in paroxysms.—Intermittent pulsative pain in vertex and in small spot beneath scalp.—Headache with toothache.—Dull headache.—Oppression deep in head, and sense of something lying in the head, through from one ear to the other.—Itching of scalp.

3. **Eyes.**—Ciliary neuralgia from decayed teeth ; dull, heavy ache in l. eye, with exquisite tenderness of ball ; l. upper incisor decayed.—Eyes red ; dim ; inflamed ; sore.—Aching deep in orbit.—Lids sore, swollen.

4. **Ears.**—Pain in r. ear with pains in teeth and face ; pains sharp, twinging, running.—Earache : neuralgic ; with toothache ; darting, twinging, stabbing pains in lower maxillary branch of trifacial.—Pains often centre in ear (l.).—Hearing : more acute ; least noise goes through one ; ringing in ears.

5. **Nose.**—Frequent sneezing, with sudden attacks of profuse, watery, bland coryza.—Sudden discharge of yellowish (or saffron-coloured) water from (r.) nostril.—Red papules round nose.—Sensation at bridge as if nasal bones being pressed together.

6. **Face.**—Neuralgia l. side of face, pains shooting and tearing, extending from jaw to ear.—Violent bruised, aching pain, r. face.—Drawing in r. malar bone.—Eruption on forehead.—Small, red, rough, scaly erythematous patches size of pea on (esp. l.) face.—L. cheek swollen.—Lips livid, dark, sickly, rough.—Water bladder on upper lip.—Dry, scaly eruption on lower lip.

7. **Teeth.**—Teeth (l.) feel elongated, sore ; pain unbearably severe, boring digging in sound teeth ; < from contact and extremes of heat and cold.—Aching in decayed teeth, or shooting up l. side of face ; face red.—Rapid decay.—Sharp stabbing along upper maxillary nerve, < by contact.—Violent pain in l. upper molars ; sound teeth ; excessive boring, digging pain, profuse flow of saliva ; < by walking in cold air and by contact, by much heat ; partial > lying down in a moderately cool room ; pain unendurable (> by *Merc.* 30).—Teeth sensitive, sore.—Grinds teeth at night.—Gums bleed easily.—Gumboil.

8. **Mouth.**—Tongue coated white, with dirty, putrid, clammy taste.—Food tasteless.—Breath putrid.—Aphthæ in children.

9. **Throat.**—Dry, parched throat.—Scraping in throat.—Profuse secretion of (very tenacious) mucus ; with much hawking.—Soreness and swelling of submaxillary glands on both sides.

10. **Appetite.**—Appetite poor.—Thirst.—Causes disgust for tobacco in chewers.

11. **Stomach.**—Eructations ; frequent, empty ; tasting like sulphur or carbonic acid gas.—Nausea with drowsiness or faint, tremulous feeling.—Sinking sensation.—Heaviness of stomach as from a stone ; even after a light meal.—Heat in præcordia with fulness in abdomen while walking in fresh air.—Coolish, painful sensation, as from over-distension after hearty meal.

12. **Abdomen.**—Gone sensation.—Severe pains in l. (and r.) hypochondrium.—Distension with passage of fetid flatus.—Violent griping, esp. upper abdomen.—Colic : > by eating ; flatulent.—Pain in abdominal muscles ; in l. and r. ilia.

13. **Stool and Anus.**—Stool: brown, fermented, frothy; watery, brown; watery; papescent; excoriating.—Diarrhœa: loose, frequent stools with flatulence; < 8 to 10 a.m.—Before stool: colic, frequent discharge of offensive flatus.—During stool: griping, tenesmus, partial prolapse, weakness, faintness.—(Chronic diarrhœa.—Cholera infantum.—Dysentery.)—Painful blood piles (locally).—Angry, inflamed piles.—Worms.

14. **Urinary Organs.**—Tenderness over region of kidneys on pressure.—Frequent passage of large quantities of pale urine; < night; stools grey; irritable; puffy under eyes; eats heartily; sleeps soundly.—Copious nocturnal enuresis from laxity of sphincter.—Irritable bladder with frequent micturition.—Delayed, dribbling urine.—Urethra: tingling with unpleasant itching in meatus; sudden darting stinging running up; sharp cutting in from within out.—Urine: large quantities, clear, frequent; very dark red, of strong odour; deep orange colour; white sediment.

15. **Male Sexual Organs.**—Sexual debility.—Unconscious emission in sleep.

16. **Female Sexual Organs.**—Erysipelas of breasts.—Mastitis.

17. **Respiratory Organs.**—Hoarseness.—Cough in cold air.—Panting breathing; inclined to sigh.

18. **Chest.**—Orgasm.—Oppression; < reading or talking.—Sharp stitches.—Muscular drawing.

19. **Heart.**—Heat in præcordia when walking in open air.—Violent palpitation; on ascending stairs.—Pulse strong, full, intermittent.

20. **Neck and Back.**—Neck stiff and sore.—Stiffness of sterno-cleido mastoid (< r.), < moving head to side affected, > moving it to opposite side.—Pulsative pain between scapulæ.—Pain in sacrum.

22. **Upper Limbs.**—Stinging, dull pains here and there.

23. **Lower Limbs.**—Hard, white, flattened, isolated papules on inside of thighs, some having red points in centre.—Great pain and stiffness in l. leg and knee, < stooping.

25. **Skin.**—Violent itching, < night.—Pricking, stinging pains.—Tensive sensation.—Burning after rubbing where scratched.—Redness, swelling, and vesicles on hands and face.—Papules which exude yellowish humour and form a crust.—Erythema.—Burns.—Rhus poisoning (local use).—Inflammatory affections of skin and involvement of cellular tissue.

26. **Sleep.**—Excessive and continued yawning.—Insomnia from abdominal trouble.—Grinding teeth during sleep.—Sleep restless; disturbed by dreams.

27. **Fever.**—Chilliness with sensation of heat in chest, with erratic pains in limbs, chest, head; from 1 to 3 p.m. with disposition to stretch and chilliness on moving about; cold hands in a warm room.—Chill: without thirst; with gooseflesh, 2 p.m., running over body, < moving about; fingers cold, coldness of body with shivering; head feels irritable; feet and hands cold even in warm room.—Heat, with thirst; great excitability, mental agony, restlessness; room seems hot and close; oppression of chest, rapid respiration; breathing difficult as if there was no air in room; burning heat of head, face, hands, feet; head hot, painful, dull, stupid; hands hot, clammy.—Sweat: cold over lumbar and sacral region; heat of room unbearable, producing perspiration.

Platanus.

Platanus acerifolia ("the tree commonly grown in and about London as P. occidentalis."—*Treas. of Bot.*). *N. O.* Platanaceæ (of the Urtical alliance). Tincture of young shoots.

Clinical.—Cataract. Ichthyosis.

Characteristics.—Burnett has recorded (*Dis. of Skin*) a case of ichthyosis in an aged lady, in which *Platanus* caused considerable improvement in the condition of the skin. Another case (*Delicate Children*) was that of a girl, 5½, "of the coal-black variety of the strumous, her forehead low and projecting," who was blind from double cataract due to the shock of a fall in the first instance, the lenses having gradually silted up. In this case *Platanus* φ was given (five drops night and morning) for a number of months, "with very evident improvement in the nutrition of the child's lenses." [Burnett names the remedy *Plat occ.*; but his tincture was made from the London tree, which is *Plat. acer.* It sheds its bark annually, which was the signature of its skin action.]

Platinum.

Platinum. An Element. (Also called Platina.) Pt. (A.W. 194·3.) Trituration.

Clinical.—Amenorrhœa. Chlorosis. Constipation. Convulsions. *Delusions.* Dentition. *Depression of spirits.* Dysmenia. *Erotomania. Fear.* Gout. Hæmorrhage. Hæmorrhoids. *Hysteria.* Lead poisoning. Masturbation. *Melancholia.* Menorrhagia. Menses, suppressed. *Mind, affections of. Neuralgia. Neurasthenia. Numbness.* Nymphomania. *Ovaries, affections of.* Pruritus vulvæ. Rheumatism. Sexual perversion. Spasms. Tapeworm. Uterus, induration of. Vaginismus. Yawning, spasmodic.

Characteristics.—The original name of *Platinum* was "Platina," being a Spanish word meaning "like silver" (*Plata* being Spanish for silver). The metal was introduced into Europe from South America in the middle of the eighteenth century. It is always found in association with other metals, chiefly Rhodium, Osmium, Iridium, Palladium. Hahnemann was the first to think of it as a medicine, and his proving in the *Chronic Diseases* is the basis of our knowledge of its action. One characteristic symptom, either when found alone or in association with other conditions, has led to many cures with *Plat.*—lost sense of proportion in both ocular and mental vision. Objects look small or the patient thinks them small. This becomes pride and hauteur in the mental sphere; the patient (generally a woman) looks down on everything and everybody. This is a keynote of *Plat.* Another is the occurrence of cramps, cramping pains and spasms, developing into convulsions. The cramping pains = numbness and tingling in the parts affected. Pains as if nipped, squeezed in a vice, and these pains increase gradually to an acme and then as gradually decline. In the rectum this becomes tenesmus ; in vagina, vaginismus. Another general keynote is the alternation of mental and physical symptoms : as physical symptoms disappear mental symptoms appear, and *vice versâ*. Nash cured a case of insanity of some duration with *Plat.*, being led to the remedy by an alternation of the mental symptoms with a pain the whole length of the spine. This alternating feature is also seen between one mental state and another : Changing moods ; sad and gay alternately ; laughs and cries by turns. There is also a perverse state : Laughs immoderately, but in the wrong place ; laughs at serious things. The mental disorder at times takes a homicidal form. Jahr cured with *Plat.* a woman who had an inspiration to kill her child, and Jules Gaudy recorded (*Jour. Belge d'H.*, quoted *Amer. H.*, xxii. 314) the case of a woman who was tormented with an almost irresistible impulse to kill her husband, whom she loved passionately, and with whom she was perfectly happy. The sight of a knife had an irresistible fascination for her, and she was often obliged to leave the table to free herself from the impulse. A few months before, she had lost a child a short time after confinement, which had been followed by profuse and desperately persistent hæmorrhage. Recovering from this she became restless, irritable, and her whole existence was ruled by this terrible impulse. *Plat.* 6x and 30x relieved and finally cured her. Kent (*Med. Adv.*, xxv. 184) records the case of a middle-aged lady, mother of several grown-up daughters, who complained of a peculiar mental symptom : A fear, in the absence of her husband, that he would never return, that he would die, or be run over. She wept all the time he was away. Kent discovered that she had been treated for uterine displacement, and was then wearing a pessary. This was removed. Menstrual flow was copious, black, clotted. The external genitals were so sensitive that the usual napkin was intolerable. *Plat.* cured the whole case, including the displacement. Almost every symptom in this case was a characteristic. The sensitiveness of the external genitals is often so great as to make coition impossible. Digital examining of such a patient causes great pain. The action of *Plat.* to a large extent centres in and radiates from the sexual organs, male and female. It corresponds to masturbation before puberty, and also to the effects of masturbation. It was one of Gallavardin's remedies for the impulse to pederasty and sodomy. Tendency to uncover completely in sleep is a leading note of it. Excessive desire, especially in virgins. Premature and excessive development of sexual instinct and organs. Nymphomania < in puerperal state. During menses uterine spasms, convulsions. Convulsions of puerperal state. Catalepsy during menstruation. Spasms alternate between convulsive actions and opisthotonos ; full consciousness. Spasms alternate with dyspnœa. Excessive itching in uterus ; pruritus vulvæ. *Plat.* has some characteristic symptoms in relation to the bowels. Its cramping tendency makes it an antidote to lead poisoning ; and it has constipation scarcely less marked than that of *Pb.*, though differing from it. The stools of *Plat.* are tenacious and sticky, adhere to the rectum and anus like putty ; or they may be hard as if burnt ; the constipation comes on whilst travelling ; in emigrants ; during pregnancy. *Peculiar Sensations* and *Symptoms* are : As if her senses would vanish. As if parts of malar bones were between screws. As if everything about her were very small. As if she were constantly growing longer and longer. As if she did not belong to her own family. Vertigo as if torn and pulled with threads. Forehead as if constricted ; screwed on ; as if a board pressed against it. As if temples too tightly bound. Scalp as if contracted ; as if a heavy weight on it. As if head were enlarged. As if throat constricted ; palate elongated ; tongue scalded. As if abdomen, chest, nape, limbs, thigh, great toe, tightly wrapped or constricted. Back and small of back as if broken. Crawling, tingling, numb sensations. Spasmodic yawning. Pains go from right to left. The right side is somewhat more pronouncedly affected than the left. Severe stitches in right ovary. The symptoms are periodic and paroxysmal, as well as alternating. *Plat.* is *suited to* women with dark hair ; thin, sanguine, bilious ; with too frequent and too profuse menses ; sexual organs exceedingly sensitive. Hysterical and hæmorrhoidal patients. The symptoms are : < By touch and pressure. < Fasting. < During menses. < Rest ; sitting ; standing ; bending backward. > By motion. Walking and going upstairs < pressure in genitals ; > hysteric rheumatism. Walking against wind = sudden arrest of breathing. < Evening and night. Headache commences on waking. < In warm room ; > in open air (but open air = fluent coryza and shaking chill on going from room ; heat > cramp pain in legs and irritability and chilliness. Obliged to stretch, which >.

Relations.—*Antidoted by :* Puls., Nit. sp. d. (Teste, who classes Plat. with Thuj., Brom., and Castor, says Colch. is the best antidote to all four). *Antidote to :* Lead. *Complementary :* Pallad. (both affect right ovary, but Pallad. has > from pressure). *Compatible :* Bell., Ign., Lyc., Puls., Rhus, Sep., Ver. *Compare :* Pride, Pall. (Plat. egotistical, despises others ; Pall. easily wounded, attaches importance to others), Lyc. (imperious). Spasms and emaciation from ante-puberty masturbation, Staph. Uterine affections, nymphomania, Aur., Sep. (the nymphomania of Plat. is more intense ; Plat. is intermediate between Aur. and Sep. in weariness of life ; the uterine cramps of Plat. are followed by numbness ; those of Sep. are a clutching as if suddenly seized then suddenly relaxed). Hysteria, indurated ulcers, Tarent. Sees ghosts and demons, Hyo., K. bro. Shamelessness, uncovers, Pho., Hyo. (Hyo. sees things larger ; Plat. smaller). Thinks death near and fears it, Aco., Ars. Dark, stringy hæmorrhage, Cham., Croc. (Croc. has sensation of something alive). Pains come and go gradually, Stan., Arg. n. (Bell. and Lyc., suddenly). Sensitive to coitus, Sep., Bell. (dry vagina), Fer., Nat. m., Apis (with stinging in ovary), Thuj., Kre. (followed by bloody flow), Murex, Orig. Constipation when travelling (Lyc. when from home ; Bry. when at sea). Weak and exhausted feeling for two hours after stool, Sep. Sticky stools like soft clay, Alm. Hysteria, pressure at root of nose, Ign. Excessive sexual development, especially in virgins, K. pho.

Masturbation in girls, Orig., Gratiol. Dark-haired women, Sep. Laughs immoderately at serious things, Anac., Nat. m., Lyc., Pho.

Causation.—Fright. Vexation. Bereavement. Fit of passion. Sexual excess. Masturbation.

SYMPTOMS.

1. **Mind.**—Sadness, esp. in evening, with strong inclination to weep often (every second day) alternating with excessive gaiety and buffoonery.—Involuntary inclination to whistle and sing.—Involuntary weeping.—Loud cries for help.—Thinks she stands alone in the world.—Anxietas præcordium to an excessive degree, with great fear of death, which is believed to be very near, accompanied by trembling, palpitation of heart, and obstructed respiration.—Sensation of dread and horror.—Fear, with trembling of hands and feet and confusion of ideas, as if all persons approaching were demons.—Hysterical humour, with great mental depression, nervous weakness, and over-excitement of vascular system.—Mental symptoms in general : amativeness ; state of madness.—Timorous disposition.—Great irritability, with prolonged ill-humour, after a fit of passion.—Apathetic indifference and absence of mind.—Pride and self-conceit, with contempt for others, even for those who are usually most beloved and respected ; < indoors, > in open air and sunshine.—Impulse to kill her own child ; her husband ; (on seeing a knife).—Distraction and forgetfulness.—Loss of consciousness.—Incoherency of speech.—Delusion of the senses ; feeling as of being too large, and, on the contrary, all other things and persons seem to be too small and too low.—Delirium, with fear of men, often changing, with over-estimation of oneself.—Mania : with great pride ; with fault-finding ; with unchaste talk ; trembling and clonic spasms, caused by fright or from anger.

2. **Head.**—Tensive confusion in forehead, as if head were compressed in a vice.—Pressing headache from without to within the forehead and temples, gradually increasing and decreasing, < in evening from stooping, while at rest, in the room ; > from exercise and in open air.—Transient attacks of vertigo in evening with loss of consciousness.—Vertigo on sitting down or ascending stairs.—Headache which increases gradually, or by fits, until it becomes very violent, and which diminishes progressively in same manner.—Attack of headache, with nausea and vomiting.—Sensation of numbness in head, and externally at vertex, preceded by a sensation of contraction of brain and of scalp ; < in evening and while sitting, > from motion and in open air.—Pain in sides of head, as if caused by a plug.—Constrictive headache, as if a tape were tightly drawn around it, with sensation of numbness in brain, flushes of heat and ill-humour, < from stooping and exercise.—Formication in one temple, extending to lower jaw, with sensation of coldness on that spot ; < in evening and when at rest, > from rubbing.—Pressive, cramp-like, compressive pains in the forehead and temples, esp. in root of nose, greatly < by movement and by stooping, sometimes with heat and redness of face, inquietude, and weeping.—Tingling in temples, as if caused by insects.—Buzzing and noise in head, like that of a mill.

3. **Eyes.**—Pain in eyes after fatiguing the sight by looking attentively at an object.—Tension in sockets, with gnawing pain, as from excoriation in

margins.—Cramp-like pain in edges of orbits.—Compressive tension in eyeballs.—Aching in eyes with sleep.—Creeping tingling in canthi.—Sensation of heat or of coldness and smarting in eyes.—Trembling or spasmodic quivering of eyelids.—Eyes convulsed.—Objects appear smaller than they really are.—Confused sight, as if directed through a veil, often with painless twitchings round the eye.—Quivering and sparkling before sight.

4. **Ears.**—Otalgia with cramp-like pain.—Shocks in ears.—(Sticking jerking in r. outer ear with) sensation of numbness and of coldness in ears, extending to cheeks and lips.—Gnawing tingling in ears.—Roaring, whizzing, and ringing in ears.—Dull thundering and rumbling in ears.

5. **Nose.**—Cramp-like pain, with sensation of numbness in nose and at root of nose.—Ineffectual want to sneeze and tingling in nose.—Dry coryza, often semi-lateral.—Corrosive sensation on nose, as of something acrid.

6. **Face.**—Face pale, wan, and sunken.—Burning heat and glowing redness in face, with ardent thirst and dryness of mouth, esp. in evening.—Distortion of muscles of face.—Sensation of coldness, with tingling and sensation of numbness throughout (r.) side of face.—Cramp and tensive pressure in zygomatic processes.—Benumbing, dull pressure in malar bone.—Pulsative digging in jaws, esp. in evening and during repose, with involuntary weeping.—Lockjaw.—Gnawing, with pain as from excoriation in lips and chin, which compel scratching.—Smarting and lancinating vesicles on lips.—Lips dry and cracked.—Plexus venarum, of a reddish blue colour, on chin.—Sensation of torpor or coldness round mouth and chin.—Cramp in jaw.

7. **Teeth.**—Odontalgia with pulsative and digging pain.—Cramp-like drawing, which recurs by fits, in teeth.—Numb pain in l. lower teeth.—Fissures in gums.

8. **Mouth.**—Sensation of coldness, esp. in mouth.—Crawling sensation on tongue.—Burning pain under tongue.—Sensation in tongue as if it had been burnt or scalded.

9. **Throat.**—Sensation as if throat were raw during (empty) deglutition and at other times.—Cramp-like drawing in throat, like a constriction.—Sensation as if palate or uvula were elongated.—Scraping and accumulation of phlegm in throat.—Hawking up of phlegm.

10. **Appetite.**—Mucous, clammy taste.—Sweetish taste on tip of tongue.—Adipsia.—Loss of appetite after the first mouthful.—Complete loss of appetite.—Repugnance to food, arising from sadness.—Dislike to food.—Bulimy.—Voracious rapidity in eating, with a disposition to find fault with everything (to detest everything around himself).—After a meal, risings, pressure on stomach ; and colic.

11. **Stomach.**—Ineffectual effort to eructate.—Empty, noisy eructations.—Serum of a disagreeable sweetish bitterness ascends throat, and puts patient in danger of choking.—Continued nausea, with lassitude, trembling, and anxiety.—Aching (pressure) in stomach, esp. after a meal.—Sensation of constriction in pit of stomach, extending into abdomen.—Fermentations in epigastric region.—Flatulent soreness towards hypogastrium.—Contractive pain in scrobiculus, as if it were squeezed too tightly.—Pressure or shocks, or else throbbing, shootings, and pinchings in scrobiculus.—Burning sensation in scrobiculus, sometimes extending from throat into abdomen.

12. **Abdomen.**—Pains in abdomen, with dull and jerking pressure.—

Inflation of abdomen, with difficult and interrupted expulsion of flatus.—Pressing and bearing down in abdomen extending into pelvis.—Lead colic.—Constriction in abdomen.—Pinchings in umbilical region.—Shootings in the side of abdomen and in umbilical region.—Gnawing in abdomen.—Drawing in groins, commencing from sacrum.

13. **Stool and Anus.**—Constipation: after lead poisoning or while travelling; sometimes very obstinate.—The stool is discharged with difficulty, seeming to stick to anus and rectum like putty.—Frequent want, with scanty evacuation, which is voided in pieces, and with great efforts.—Evacuations of consistence of pap.—Stool hard, as if burnt.—Tenia and ascarides are discharged from rectum during evacuation and at other times.—After evacuation general shuddering or sensation of weakness in abdomen.—Frequent itching, tingling, and tenesmus in anus, esp. in the evening (before sleep).—Violent and dull lancinations in rectum.

14. **Urinary Organs.**—Red urine with a white cloud, or else which becomes turbid, and deposits a red sediment.—Slow but frequent emission of urine.

15. **Male Sexual Organs.**—Burning pain and gnawing in scrotum.—Unnatural increase of sexual desire, with frequent erections, esp. at night (with amorous dreams).—Voluptuous crawling in genital organs and abdomen, with anxious oppression and palpitation, then painless pressure downwards in genitals with sticking in sinciput and exhaustion.—Flow of prostatic fluid.—Coition of too short duration, with but little enjoyment.

16. **Female Sexual Organs.**—Sensation of bearing down towards genital organs, with aching in abdomen.—Unnatural increase of sexual desire, with painful sensibility and voluptuous tingling from genitals up into abdomen.—Nymphomania, which may occur even during the lying-in period.—Induration of uterus.—Sanguineous congestion in uterus.—Miscarriage.—Metrorrhagia (with great excitability of the sexual system) of thick, deep-coloured blood, with drawings in groins.—Catamenia too early and too profuse (blood dark and coagulated), sometimes with headache, restlessness, and tears.—Menstruation, when the discharge is very abundant, thick and black like tar, and is very exhausting; spasms and screaming at every menstrual period.—Catamenia too long continued.—Before catamenia, cuttings and pains like those of labour in hypogastrium.—Cramps at commencement of catamenia.—Painful sensitiveness and constant pressure in mons veneris and genital organs, with internal chill and external coldness, except face.—Severe stitches in r. ovarian region.—During catamenia, pressure as of a general bearing down towards genital organs, which are very sensitive.—Leucorrhœa, like white of eggs, flowing chiefly after urinating, and on rising from a seat.

17. **Respiratory Organs.**—Aphonia.—Short, nervous, dry cough, with palpitation and dyspnœa.—Short, difficult, and anxious respiration.

18. **Chest.**—Shortness of breath, with constrictive oppression of chest.—Inclination to draw a long breath, prevented by a sensation of weakness in chest.—Anxious oppression of chest, with sensation of heat, which ascends from epigastrium.—Pain in chest, as if a weight were pressing upon it, with want to take a full inspiration, which is hindered by a sensation of weakness.—Tension, pressure, and shootings in sides of chest, which do not permit

lying down on either side.—Aching and dull blows in chest.—Spasmodic pressure in one side of chest.—Spasmodic pain in chest, commencing slightly, increasing to a certain intensity, and gradually diminishing in same way.—Dull lancinations in sides of chest, during an inspiration.

19. **Heart.**—Burning and sticking low down by heart.—A dull pressure in region of apex of heart.—Anxious palpitation of heart.

20. **Neck and Back.**—Rigidity of nape of neck.—Weakness and sensation of tensive numbness in nape of neck (the head sinks forward).—Contusive pain in loins and in back, esp. when pressing upon them, or else when bending backwards.—Pains in back and small of back as if broken, after a walk < bending backwards.—Spasmodic pain in loins.—Sensation of numbness in coccyx, as after a blow.

21. **Limbs.**—Cramp-like jerking and drawing pains in limbs and joints.—Tension in limbs (esp. thighs) as if bound too tightly with ligatures.—Attack of spasmodic rigidity in limbs, without loss of consciousness, but with clenching of jaws, loss of speech, eyes convulsed, and involuntary movements of the commissures of lips and eyelids.—Tingling restlessness, sensation of weakness and trembling in limbs, esp. during repose and in open air.

22. **Upper Limbs.**—Heaviness and lassitude of arms, with paralytic pulling.—Paralysed sensation in l. arm; in both arms.—Aching and spasmodic pain in forearms, hands, and fingers, esp. when grasping anything firmly.—Itching, gnawing, pricking, and burning sensation in arms, hands, and fingers.—Sensation of stiffness in forearms.—Painful throbbing in fingers.—Distortion of fingers.—Numbness of fingers.—Trembling of r. thumb, with numbness.—Numbness of little finger.—Ulcers on fingers.

23. **Lower Limbs.**—Spasmodic pain and tension in thighs, feet, and toes.—Weakness of thighs and knees, as if they were broken.—Pain as from a blow in l. knee.—Shocks and blows in legs.—Lassitude of legs.—Restlessness and trembling in legs, with a sensation of numbness and rigidity.—Lassitude and numbness in feet when seated.—Coldness of feet.—Gnawing, excoriation, and smarting in ankle-bones, greatly < by least touch.—Painful throbbing in toes.—Swelling on ball of toe, with tearing and nocturnal pulsations.—Ulcers on toes.—Pain in great toe as if too tightly enveloped.

24. **Generalities.**—Dark-haired females.—Face changing colour frequently.—Rising in throat.—Tapeworm, other symptoms agreeing.—Contraction of inner parts.—Catalepsy; epilepsy with rigor; tonic spasms.—Very great paleness of skin.—Spasmodic yawning.—Pains like labour pains.—Sensation as of a hoop around parts.—Violent shocks as if from pain.—Sensation of prickling in the outer parts.—Sensation of coldness in outer parts.—Compressive, cramp-like, constrictive, or pressive pains, as if caused by a plug, or by dull blows.—Cramp-like, jerking, and drawing pains in limbs and joints.—Tension in limbs, as if bound too tightly with ligatures.—Pains, as from a contusion, a blow, or a bruise, esp. when pressing on part affected.—Pains, slight at commencement, increase gradually, often at regular intervals, and diminish in same manner.—Sensation of torpor and paralytic rigidity in various parts, often with trembling and palpitation of heart.—Attack of spasmodic rigidity in limbs, without loss of consciousness, but with clenching of jaws, loss of speech, eyes convulsed, and involuntary movements of commissures of lips and eyelids.—The spasmodic attacks manifest themselves chiefly

at daybreak.—Affections caused by fright, by vexation, or by a fit of passion. —Moral and physical affections, appearing alternately.—Excessive weakness (paralytic weakness in limbs).—Dull, pushing, or inward pressing pains, as from dull blows.—Tingling restlessness, sensation of weakness and trembling in limbs, esp. during repose and in open air.—Majority of symptoms < by repose, in the evening; from anger; more in females than males; after lying down and rising again; when sitting; after rising; and > by movement.—The affections which are > in open air are generally < towards evening and in a room.

25. **Skin.**—Tingling gnawing, with pain as of excoriation, and itching or burning, pricking, and shooting pain on various parts of skin, which provokes scratching.—Ulcers (on fingers and toes).

26. **Sleep.**—Convulsive and spasmodic yawning, esp. in afternoon.—Great disposition to sleep in evening.—Prolonged sleep in morning.—Anxious dreams of wars and bloodshed.—Lascivious dreams.—Waking at night, esp. after midnight (with frightful dreams, want of consciousness), or with anxious, sad, and distressing thoughts.—Bewilderment at night on waking.—At night patient lies on back, with arms above head, legs drawn up, with strong inclination to uncover them.

27. **Fever.**—Pulse small, feeble, frequently tremulous.—Constant shivering and shuddering over whole body, esp. in open air.—Shaking chill when going from the room into the open, even warm air.—Chilliness predominates, with low spirits, which ceases during heat.—Heat with sensation of burning in face, without any visible change in colour of face (she thought she was very red, but colour the same as usual).—Flushes of heat, interrupted by chilliness.—Gradually increasing, and in the same manner gradually decreasing heat.—Perspiration only during sleep, ceasing as soon as one wakens.

Platinum Muriaticum.

Chloride of Platinum. $PtCl_4$. Solution.

Clinical.—Caries. Chancre. Condyloma. Laryngismus. Mercury, abuse of. Œsophagus, stricture of. Stomach, cancer of.

Characteristics.—*Plat. mur.* was experimented with by Hofer, of Pau, who applied locally a saturated solution and administered solutions internally. Fever, headache, constricting sensations and fibrillary twitchings were induced by internal doses; the local application produced acute irritation of the skin and glans penis, with an eruption on the latter like commencing chancre. *Plat. mur.* has been used in cases of caries (especially of nasal bones and bones of tarsus); of syphilitic caries; syphilitic rheumatism; chronic gonorrhœa; condylomata; gastric carcinoma; acne.

SYMPTOMS.

1. **Mind.**—Thinks he has been poisoned.

2. **Head.**—Some headache, with slight acidity of stomach.—Severe headache, esp. in occiput, with fever.

8. **Mouth.**—Metallic taste.

11. **Stomach.**—Acidity of stomach with headache.—Warmth and heaviness in epigastrium.—Nausea and inclination to vomit.

15. **Male Sexual Organs.**—[From application of saturated solution to the parts.]—Violent itching on glans and prepuce, with sensation of warmth and very troublesome sticking ; symptoms of acute inflammation of urethra, pain on urinating, slight dysuria ; after some hours an eruption about glans penis, somewhat livid, slightly raised, size of pin head, looks like commencing syphilitic sore, but disappears in twelve hours.

17. **Respiratory Organs.**—Violent constriction of larynx, so that speech and swallowing were decidedly impeded.

24. **Generalities.**—Involuntary movement of fibres of muscles of nape, back, and extremities for several hours.

25. **Skin.**—Skin discoloured yellow, becoming covered with rosy red eruption that disappears after a few minutes (from local application).

27. **Fever.**—Slight shuddering, pulse accelerated, warmth in epigastrium.

Platinum Muriaticum Natronatum.

Chloroplatinate of Sodium. $PtCl_4 2NaCl$. Solution.

Clinical.—Flatulence. Polyuria. Salivation.

Characteristics.—Hofer experimented with *Plat. m. n.* on the same man who took *Plat. mur.* The chief additional symptom was decided by increased secretion of urine and saliva.

SYMPTOMS.

2. **Head.**—Slight headache.

8. **Mouth.**—Decided increase in saliva.

11. **Stomach.**—Feeling of warmth and heaviness in stomach.—Eructation of gas.—Nausea and inclination to vomit.

12. **Abdomen.**—Rumbling in abdomen.—Transient colic.

13. **Stool.**—Emission of flatus.

14. **Urinary Organs.**—Decidedly increased secretion of urine.

Plectranthus.

Plectranthus fruticosus. *N. O.* Labiatæ. Tincture of fresh plant.

Clinical.—Abdomen, coldness of. Cholera. Cramps. Dentition. Diarrhœa. Dysphagia. Fever. Intermittent fever. Lumbrici. Neuralgia. Rheumatism. Shoulder (r.), pains in. Spastic paralysis. Stiff-neck. Sweat, local. Throat, sore. Toothache. Wrists, pains in.

Characteristics.—*Plectranthus* was extensively proved by the Austrian Provers' Association. Severe symptoms were induced in head, throat, intestines, and rectum, limbs and joints. Toothache with swelling of face and difficulty of opening mouth. "Pain near right jaw-joint as if a tooth were coming through" suggests a use for the remedy in difficult cutting of wisdom teeth. Burning sensation extended throughout the digestive tract ; and there was also coldness of abdomen, > in open air. Many pains about the navel. Paralytic pains in joints. Pains of many kinds in right shoulder. Exhaustion, bruised sensation, general discomfort were experienced. Cramps and paralytic pains in joints. Hansen mentions spastic paralysis as having been remedied by it. Among the *peculiar symptoms* are: As if a morsel stuck in throat after swallowing. As though air were piercing the marrow of the bones. Cool sensation followed by burning at root of tongue and palate. Pressure as from a heavy weight in stomach. Discharge of white mucus from anus causing scratching. Pressure on rectum and bladder. Whites of eyes yellow, < left. Sweat of right foot, left foot dry ; of right foot and both hands and no other part ; of scalp. The right side was more affected than the left. The symptoms are < after eating (pressure in stomach ; pain in umbilical region). < By all food and drink (burning in mouth). Chewing = pain in temples. < By motion ; moving head ; turning body ; by swallowing ; whilst urinating, > after. < By warmth of stove. > By application of ice ; by eructations. Many of the pains and symptoms were *sudden*, and came and went suddenly.

Relations.—*Compare:* Urinary symptoms, Ocim. Black stools, Lept. Stitches in chest, K. ca. Pains come and go suddenly, Lyc., Bell. Crumb in throat, Hep., Nit. ac., Arg. n.

SYMPTOMS.

1. **Mind.**—Fretful.—Ill-humoured.—Peevish.—Distracted in mind ; cannot keep his attention on an interesting subject.

2. **Head.**—Head confused, heavy, dull.—Pressure (and stitches) in r. frontal eminence.—(Violent headache in anterior part of skull as far as vertex, becoming intolerable.—Swashing and throbbing with every motion ; not > by cold applications ; thirst and difficulty of swallowing.)—Pressive pain in occiput ; < lying on back ; < out of doors ; tension in cervical muscles.—Profuse perspiration on scalp.

3. **Eyes.**—White of eyes yellow (< l.).—Vision seemed remarkably clear (on a dull day).—Flickering before eyes.

4. **Ears.**—Sticking and stitches in both ears.—Roaring in ears.

5. **Nose.**—Excessive catarrh, frequent inclination to sneeze ; great stoppage with at times discharge of tenacious yellow mucus.—Dryness, mornings.

6. **Face.**—Painful drawing in r. cheek, infra-orbital region ; extending to last upper molars ; continued through the night with fever ; next day r. cheek swollen and very sensitive.—Lips very dry ; burning.

8. **Mouth.**—Violent drawing in upper and lower incisors with swelled cheek.—Periodic drawing in r. teeth extending to temple and ear, < chewing, > going out.—Pressive pain in r. lower sound teeth.—Upper incisors sensitive.—Tongue coated.—Sensation on root of tongue and on soft palate, at first cool, then burning.—Dry mouth.—Burning through mouth and fauces, <

by all food and drink.--Opening the mouth became very difficult ; ulcers on r. side of palate ; digging in r. upper teeth with increased secretion of saliva ; sticking and burrowing extending to r. articulation of jaw as though a tooth erupting.

9. **Throat.**—Scraping in throat ; stitches.—Dryness with thirst, not > by glass of water.—Burning as from pepper, from root of tongue to stomach (6 a.m. to 4 p.m.).—Sensation as if a morsel of food stuck in throat on swallowing.—Tension in pharynx when drinking, with disagreeable tickling in both ears, that obliges frequent hawking.—Acute pressure in pharynx, on swallowing became a burning, not affected by external pressure, increased to 9 a.m., when it became a sensation of swelling.—Dysphagia.

11. **Stomach.**—Appetite great ; eats hastily, though without satiety ; on rising from a meal pressure as from a weight in stomach with desire to drink a great deal ; after taking a few sips a pulling in stomach causing tension in œsophagus.—Loss of appetite.—Great thirst.—Eructations : frequent ; empty ; and hiccough.—Nausea ; vomiting.—Sudden gushing vomiting twice at night without any other symptoms.—Weight on stomach < after eating.—Cutting in epigastrium followed by two thin, frothy stools.

12. **Abdomen.**—Contractive pain in umbilical region always < after eating.—Violent griping at umbilicus with desire for stool.—Rumbling and movement.—Crawling about umbilicus disappearing along rectus muscle towards symphysis pubis.—Cutting low in abdomen with desire for stool.—Coldness through (upper) abdomen in warm room, morning.—Drawing sticking in l. inguinal region.

13. **Stool and Anus.**—Painful pressure in rectum, with constant griping followed by profuse, dark, frothy stool, succeeded by burning and tenesmus in anus ; later sudden desire and painful pressure ; only a little mucus and gas evacuated with burning in anus.—Discharge of white mucus provoking scratching of anus and followed by burning.—Stool : almost black ; pasty, yellowish brown ; watery, mixed with mucus ; first pasty, then liquid ; omitted for five days, then bluish nodular evacuated with great effort.—During stool : griping and rumbling in abdomen ; painful dragging in rectum.—After stool : weakness of lower limbs ; coldness of abdomen ; cold sweat on forehead.—Evacuation of round worms.

14. **Urinary Organs.**—Pressure in bladder, immediately followed by desire to urinate, sudden cutting pain from root of penis to base of bladder compelling to sit still.—Burning in navicular fossa during and after micturition, which was scanty and unsatisfactory.—Frequent, sudden desire, had hardly time to reach the closet, but only a few drops passed, followed by a sensation as though bladder full, afternoon ; in evening copious micturition with great >.—Increased urination.—Urine dark with reddish-yellow sediment.

15. **Male Sexual Organs.**—Transient drawing sticking along r. side of penis and urethra.—Violent erection.

18. **Chest.**—Burning at sterno-clavicular joint.—Stitches : in pectoralis major, arresting breath ; between r. fourth and fifth ribs ; in r. side.—Pain in r. chest extends up to r. scapula and nape of neck, so violent at night was compelled to jump out of bed and cry out ; as though a number of needles sticking into head till head was turned towards the side ; with profuse sweat

painful inspiration, great heat of head; < by application of mustard paste, > gradually by application of ice.—Tension in chest.

19. **Pulse.**—Pulse hard, full with the fever.

20. **Neck and Back.**—Stiffness and pressive tension in nape, < by every motion of the head.—Drawing in nape.—Coarse stitches from without inward between scapulæ, while walking; during expiration.

21. **Limbs.**—Sticking and paralytic drawing in all the joints and limbs. —Sensation of paralysis in joints of fingers and toes.

22. **Upper Limbs.**—Paralysed sensation: in upper limbs; r. shoulder; r. shoulder and wrist, suddenly appearing and disappearing; in both shoulders.—Lameness; sprained feeling; weariness; shaking; drawing tearing in r. shoulder.—Sensation in l. shoulder as if one were beating on it with a knuckle.—Drawing tearing in joints of upper-arms, fore-arms, and fingers, < r.—Sudden pain in outer condyle of l. wrist.—Stitches in r. wrist.

23. **Lower Limbs.**—Weariness in lower limbs.—Painful cramps in calves waking him up, not > by stretching.—Stitches in l. hip-joint; burning in r.—Cramp in adductors; tension in hamstring.—Drawing in fascia of r. thigh.—Tearing beneath r. patella; stitches in l.—Pains in both knees.—Wakened at night by sudden start from a violent sticking in malleoli of ankles. —Burning in periosteum of r. tibia.—Numbness in leg.—Toes painful as if burnt.

24. **Generalities.**—Weariness.—Stitches.—Sensation as though air were piercing the marrow of the bones.

25. **Skin.**—Prickling in l. palm.—Crawling in l. little finger; in ball of l. thumb.

26. **Sleep.**—Drowsiness.—Waked often.—Troubled by confused, unremembered dreams before midnight.

27. **Fever.**—Sudden, violent, shaking chill with chattering of teeth, waking him from sleep, followed by dry heat.—Chilliness through whole abdomen with warm face and hands; < by heat of stove; > moving about in open air.—Coldness over back and heat of hands; could not get warm in heated room.—Sudden heat on scalp lasting a few minutes, followed by profuse sweat; after sweat dried up, forehead cold to touch.—Sour sweat at night.—Sweat on r. foot and both hands; no other part.—Profuse sweat r. foot, l. foot dry.

Plumbago.

Plumbago littoralis (Mure.—Allen says P. scandens corresponds to Mure's figure, and grows in Brazil. Mure says P. lit. is "a creeper inhabiting the shores in the bay of Rio Janeiro"). *N. O.* Plumbaginaceæ. Tincture of leaves.

Clinical.—Costiveness. Eyes, inflammation in. Fever. Kidneys, pain in. Saliva, milky.

Characteristics.—Mure proved this plant. The most *peculiar symptoms* were: Saliva profuse, milky. Ulceration of commissures of lips. Costiveness with red urine. Vertigo after eating. Pain in humerus on lifting anything. Hot arms with cold hands. "Many of the plants of this genus are acrid and caustic in the highest degree. The root of *P. scandens*, the Herbe du Diable of San Domingo, is a most energetic blistering agent when fresh; so also is that of *P. rosea*. The beggars employ *P. europea* to raise ulcers on their body to excite pity; and used internally it is said to be as effectual an emetic as *Ipecacuanha*" (*Treas. of Bot.*). In Mure's proving "Aversion to everything" is noted; also "ulceration of commissures of lips," which is an evidence of its acridity.

Relations.—*Compare:* Costiveness with red urine, Lyc. The Plumbaginaceæ are allied to the Primulaceæ and the Plantaginaceæ (the root of Plumb. europ. is used dried as a remedy for toothache).

SYMPTOMS.

1. **Mind.**—Taciturn.

2. **Head.**—Vertigo; after eating.—Excessive heat about head.—Dartings in head.—Pain in temples.—Frontal headache.

3. **Eyes.**—Heat in eyes.—Inflammation and running of l. eye.

4. **Ears.**—Acute pain l. ear.

5. **Nose.**—Sensitive smell all day.

8. **Mouth.**—Saliva: profuse; milky.—Ulceration of commissures of lips.—Bitter mouth.

9. **Throat.**—Painful constriction of throat.—Sore throat.

11. **Stomach.**—Aversion to everything.—Heaviness at stomach.

12. **Abdomen.**—Pain in iliac region.—Pain behind false ribs when inspiring.

13. **Stool.**—Costiveness with red urine.

15, 16. **Sexual Organs.**—Violent sexual desire.

18. **Chest.**—Pain: at r. ribs; sides of chest.—Prickings in chest.

19. **Heart.**—Pain at heart.—Painful stitch in heart region.—Palpitation.—Pulse hard and small.

20. **Neck and Back.**—Pain in kidneys as if pinched.—Pain in back.

22. **Upper Limbs.**—Pain in r. shoulder; burning and pricking.—Pain in humerus when lifting anything.

23. **Lower Limbs.**—Weakness of joints of lower limbs.

24. **Generalities.**—Prostration.—Darting pains here and there.—Pain in joints.—Acute pains all over for three hours.

26. **Sleep.**—Drowsy.—Dreams of dead bodies.

27. **Fever.**—Chilliness when moving.—Hot arms with cold hands.—Internal heat coming and going.—Very hot internally at night.—Heat in limbs.

Plumbum.

PLUMBUM METALLICUM. The Element. Pb (A.W.206·39). Trituration.
PLUMBUM ACETICUM. Acetate of Lead. Sugar of Lead. Pb $(C_2H_3O_2)_2 3H_2O$. Trituration.
PLUMBUM CARBONICUM. Carbonate of Lead. Pure White Lead. Plumbic Carbonate. Pb CO_3. Trituration.

Clinical.—*Amaurosis. Anæmia.* Anæsthesia. Aneurism. *Anidrosis.* Appendicitis. Asthma. *Atrophy. Bone, exostoses on.* Brain, softening of; tumour of. Bright's disease. *Colic. Constipation.* Cystitis. *Depression of spirits.* Diplopia. Dropsy. Dysmenorrhœa. Dysuria. Emaciation. *Epilepsy. Epulis. Eyes, inflammation of.* Ganglion. Gout. Hæmoptysis. Hæmorrhoids. *Headache.* Hernia, strangulated. Hyperæsthesia. Hypopion. *Ichthyosis.* Intermittent fever. *Intestines, obstruction of.* Intussusception. Jaundice. *Jaw, tumour of. Kidneys, affections of;* granular. Liver, affections of. Lockjaw. Locomotor ataxy. *Melancholia.* Metrorrhagia. *Myelitis.* Nephritis. *Numbness.* Œsophagus, stricture of. *Paralysis;* diphtheritic; agitans. *Perichondritis.* Proctalgia. *Progressive muscular atrophy.* Prolapsus ani. Sciatica. Spine, diseases of; sclerosis of; tumour of. Spleen, affections of. Stricture. *Tabes mesenterica. Tobacco habit.* Tongue; paralysis of. Typhlitis. Umbilicus, abscess of; hernia of. Uric-acidæmia. Vagina, spasm of. Vaginismus. *Veins, varicose.*

Characteristics.—*Plumbum*, the *Saturn* of the Alchemists, has been proved by Hartlaub, Trinks, Hering, and Nenning. To their symptoms have been added those of numberless cases of poisoning among workers with lead and painters, symptoms from drinking lead-contaminated waters, from the use of lead in cosmetics, and from cases of suicide. In the old school metallic lead was seldom used, being considered inert; but Bœrhaave gave it internally reduced to an impalpable powder for leucorrhœa, dysentery, syphilis, and gout (Teste). In the form of plaisters and "Goulard water" the salts of lead have been largely used as external applications in skin diseases, vaginal and urethral injections, and much injury has not infrequently resulted, especially from repelled eruptions. The effect of the three preparations of lead enumerated above have all been included in the Schema, as no attempt has ever been made to keep them separate; nor has any specific difference been noted. Among painters and lead manufacturers the best-known symptoms are the colic and drop-wrist. In addition there are set up conditions of kidney irritation with albuminuria, ending in granular degeneration with attendant heart hypertrophy, optic neuritis, and blindness. There is an excess of uric acid in the blood of persons under the influence of lead, and actual gouty deposits and gouty attacks have been observed. In one case of lead poisoning I saw there was chronic enlargement of the knees and contraction of the lower limbs, completely crippling the patient. In another case there were small aneurisms almost all over the body. In those who have drunk lead-contaminated water the effects vary in intensity according to the amount of contamination and duration of exposure. When the poisoning has been going on insidiously for years a state of anæmia is set up, with dry, inactive, scaly skin, and inveterate constipation. Tunzelmann (*B. J. H.*, xxxii. 17—quoted

C.D.P., where a full collection of cases may be found) reports a number of cases of *acute* poisoning from drinking water containing lead : (1) A cook, ill three weeks. Unable to retain any food on stomach ; constant nausea, and even when no food was taken frequent vomiting of greenish watery fluid, < night. Skin yellowish ; conjunctivæ decidedly yellow. Tongue furred, coat at back very yellow ; horrible taste, fœtor of breath ; bowels confined. Extreme debility. *Hydrast.* 3 gave great relief, but three months later the hands became paralysed, which led to the testing of the drinking-water and the discovery of lead. (2) Youth, æt. 12, had bronchial catarrh with loose cough and consolidation of left apex. As soon as the poisoned water was stopped he rapidly got quite well. (3) An elder brother had hæmoptysis, coughing up half a pint of blood. Nothing was found wrong with the lungs beyond slight feebleness of respiration at apices. Three months later, after a day's rowing, the hæmatemesis returned with epistaxis. Now distinct dulness was found at right apex. Rapid recovery followed stopping the water. Caspar (*C. D. P.*) relates the case of a pregnant young woman who swallowed three ounces of white lead on October 8th. The first symptoms set in some hours later with vomiting. Next morning she was found suffering from inflammatory pain and jaundice. The evening of the 10th she gave birth to a seven-months' child, and died the following morning. The autopsy revealed : Features relaxed ; skin dirty yellow. Bloody, frothy ichor escaped from nostrils in large quantities, and from genitals, saturating the bed ; the mouth also, from which the tongue point protruded, was full of it. Abdomen distended and of stony hardness, genitals swollen and discoloured ; brain markedly bloodless ; pleura contained 8 ozs. of bloody fluid, lungs distended, filled with frothy, decomposed blood ; heart empty, very soft, dirty brown ; trachea dark cherry-colour. Pectoral muscles very soft, brown, the blood exuding from them being greasy. Liver dirty brown, very soft ; spleen filled with black, tar-like blood ; both kidneys very soft and full of blood. Blood in vena cava black, tar-like. Women who work with lead frequently abort ; women who do not work with lead but whose husbands do, abort in even greater proportion. Children born under these conditions are frequently idiotic or epileptic. According to Teste, *Plumb.* is *particularly adapted* to adults, males rather than females ; particularly to persons of a dry, bilious constitution, with somewhat jaundiced complexion, irascible, hypochondriac, or disposed to religious monomania. (But children are by no means excluded. I have seen apparently hopeless cases of marasmus in infants with large, hard abdomens and extreme constipation cured with *Plumb.*, usually in 3rd trituration of the metal or the acetate.) Teste mentions the following cases as having been successfully treated by him with *Plumb.* (1) Chronic cystitis. (2) Stricture after gonorrhœa. (3) Tenacious salivation (mercurial), < in damp weather, saturating pillow in sleep. (4) Excessively painful retraction of testes and penis, which seemed to re-enter hypogastrium (consequence of sexual excesses and repelled tetters). (5) Nightly bone pains (after failure of *Merc*, &c.). (6) Pulling and pressive chronic headache in forehead, < by mental labour ; intolerable in company. (7) Mental derangement from syphilis with obscure paralysis of right arm, paroxysms of religious monomania, erotism without erection, periodic fever without sweat, cramp-like retraction of abdomen from time to time. (8) Nervous disease characterised chiefly by wandering pains in limbs, spasms of facial muscles, paroxysms of screaming, fright without cause, sudden fainting in passing from one room to another or entering a room full of company. (9) Marsh intermittent with quotidian or double tertian type, especially when splenic region is painful to touch. In such cases, says Teste, neither *Ars.* nor *Chi.* can be compared to *Plumb.* These cases bring out some of the keynotes of *Plumb.*, and chief among them is : *Retraction* and *sense of retraction.* "Violent colic, sensation as if abdominal wall were drawn back by a string to the spine." Actual drawing in of abdomen is frequently present and is characteristic. The cheeks are retracted, sunken. Excessive and rapid emaciation. In the same category with colic are : Cramps, spasms, convulsions, paralyses, tremors. Fröhling (*A. H. Z.*, cxxxii. 68—*Amer. Hom.*, xxii. 422) relates the case of N., farmer, 46, who was taken ill in November, 1893, with attacks of colic with vomiting and extreme constipation ; action only obtained by large enemata. Had been constipated in former years but without illness. *Opium* had given only temporary relief. After December, 1893, vomiting was rarer, but colic increased in intensity up to February, 1894, when Fröhling saw him first, and found him *wasted to a skeleton, abdomen drawn in ;* appetite bad, felt ill, mind somewhat affected, unable to give sensible answers to questions. *Constant urgent call to stool*, only *small, hard, black balls* passed. Liver dulness only heard from upper border of sixth to upper border of seventh rib. Lead poisoning was suspected, but as no evidence of it could be found *Plumb.* 6 three times a day was prescribed. In six days colic attacks were less frequent, and less severe ; two stools passed without enema ; mind clearer. Improvement continued in all respects, and in fourteen days N. was able to leave his bed, to which he had been confined since November. By the middle of March he made an hour's journey to see Fröhling, and was hardly recognisable, he had gained so much flesh, and his liver was found of normal size. Wingfield (*M. H. R.*, quoted *Amer. Hom.*, xxi. 426) reported two characteristic cases : (1) Mrs. D., 50, no children, sparely built, very nervous, constipated fifteen years, takes a teaspoonful of Cascara extract every other night. Tongue coated with yellowish white fur. Has constant headaches, and after each motion is thoroughly exhausted, and has to lie down the rest of the day. *Plumb.* 6x gr. iii. twice a day. In two days bowels commenced acting naturally. In three weeks headaches gone, tongue clean, much less nervous. (2) Miss M., 25, florid ; has boils appear on face and arms, and chronic constipation. The constipation had been a trouble since she was twelve years old. Slight spinal curvature. Tongue furred, occasionally has headaches. Suffers much at menstrual periods. *Plumb.* 6x twice daily at once relieved the constipation, and soon the boils disappeared. Patient soon felt quite well. Arriaga (*La Homœopatia*, No. 9, 1893 ; *H. M.*, xxix. 190), of Mexico city, reports the case of a woman, 73, seized with symptoms of intestinal occlusion, violent colic, nausea, obstinate constipation, meteorism, complete anorexia, and no fever. *Nux* relieved the colic, and then *Plumb.* 12, and later 13, gradually brought about recovery in four days. Nash cured a severe case of post-diphtheritic paralysis in a middle-aged man. The leading symptom was *excessive hyperæsthesia*—could not bear to be touched anywhere, it hurt so. *Plumb.* 40m (Fincke), a single dose, cured. Nash tells of a man, 70, attacked with severe pain in abdomen, and finally a large, hard swelling developed in ileo-cæcal region, *very sensitive to contact* or least motion. It began to assume a bluish tint, and on account of his age and weakness the man's life was despaired of. But his daughter, the wife of a medical man, found the symptoms in *Raue* under *Plumb.*, in the chapter on Typh litis, and *Plumb.* 200 cured. Anæsthesia is as strongly marked as the hyperæsthesia of *Plumb.* The excessive emaciation of *Plumb.* and the action on the spine make it a remedy of the first importance in progressive muscular atrophy. Among the spasms are : Vaginismus ; spasm of uterus and expulsion of its contents ; sensation as if there was not room enough for fœtus ; spasm of bladder ; of œsophagus ; strangulated hernia. Clonic or tonic convulsive movements of limbs from cerebral sclerosis or tumour. Epilepsy preceded by vertigo, sometimes sighing, followed by stupid feeling. (In a case cured by Skinner, after a fit the head turned to the right. There was < 8 to 9 a.m.) Paralysed parts lose flesh. Progressive locomotor ataxia. Restlessness ; lassitude ; faintness. Sensation in abdomen at night which causes patient to stretch violently for hours ; must stretch in every direction. Assumes strangest attitudes in bed at night. *Peculiar sensations* are : As if something were working at top of head, with a sense of screwing from behind forward. Eyelids as if paralysed. As of a ball rising from throat into brain. As if a wheat-hull in throat. Cornea as if breathed upon. Eyes as if too large. As of a plug in throat. As if everything were weighted down. As if abdomen and back were too close together ; abdomen drawn to spine with a string. Bowels as if twisted ; constricted ; distended with gas. As if abscess forming near umbilicus. Sphincter ani as if drawn in. As if a bag not quite filled with fluid lay in bowels. As if fluid rolled from one side to other of abdomen. As if thighs pierced with needles. As if feet made of wood.—Pains are wandering or radiating, vague, paroxysmal. Ailments develop slowly and intermit for a time. Alternations are common : Delirium with colic ; diarrhœa and constipation ; jerks of flexors and extensors ; paralysis and colic. Right side is most affected, symptoms go from left to right (throat). In ladies poisoned by cosmetics the vaginismus which resulted increased *pari passu* with paralytic symptoms. With *Plumb.* 6 Theuerkauf cured in six weeks a case of hypopion with great pain (*B. J. H.*, xxxvii. 303). W. H. Woodyatt (*Ibid.*, 205) reports a case of "vaso-motor neurosis" affecting left eye. Mrs. D., 29, had been ill two weeks, and supposed she had caught cold in the eye. The symptoms were : Drooping upper lid, intense photophobia, very profuse lachrymation of hot tears, pericorneal injection, *deep bluish redness of sclerotica*, most marked at corneal margin. Cornea very faintly hazy. *Pupil contracted. Sight misty. Ars.* 6x and *Plant.* 6x failed to relieve. *Plumb.* 6x was then given with immediate improvement, which went on to cure in seven days. The italicised symptoms were the leading indications for *Plumb.* In a case of right-sided sciatica which had been greatly benefited by *Gnaph.* 1, but which had returned, the symptoms being : Stiffness ; soreness from great trochanter and point of exit of nerve to knee ; weakness in thigh ; < by stooping ; walking = sensation as if pushing a knife in thigh, *Plumb.* 6 was given four times a day. Up to the twelfth day there was no change ; on that day the pain suddenly went. The case had lasted nine months. The symptoms are < by touch. > By hard pressure and by rubbing. > At rest. < By motion. Mental exertion <. > Lying down. < Lying right side (swelling in abdomen ; cough). Lying on left side < violent palpitation. Bending back > pressure in stomach ; pain in epigastrium ; pain in back. Bending forward = pressure in stomach ; > pain in back. Bending double > colic. Back sensitive when leaning on it. > Stretching limbs. < At night. < In rough, foggy weather. Open air, coldness in ; sensitive to ; > vertigo. Damp weather = profuse salivation. < In room full of company.

Relations.—*Antidoted by :* Sulphuric acid, diluted, taken as a lemonade, is one of the best antidotes to the chronic effects of lead ; Alcohol is a preventive ; Alumen, Alumina, Ars., Ant. c., Bell., Coccul., Hep., Kreos., Nux, Op., Petrol., Plat., Piperaz., Zn. (Teste, who classes Plumb. with Merc. and Ars., says Æthus cyn. is the best antidote in his experience ; he names also Hyo., Plect., Strm., and Electric.) *It antidotes :* Bad effects of long abuse of vinegar. *Compatible :* Ars., Bell., Lyc., Merc., Phos., Pul., Sil., Sul. *Compare :* Constipation, inertia, hard black balls, Op. (Plumb. has also some spasmodic constriction at anus). Delirium, bites and strikes, Bell. (Plumb. has tremors of head and hands ; yellow mucus about teeth ; colic alternating with delirium). Head and abdominal symptoms alternating, Pod. Brain softening, Zn. (Plumb. has pain in atrophied limbs alternating with colic), Vanad. Constipation from inertia, vaginismus, Plat. (Plat. > these conditions of Plumb.). Irritable piles with drawn-up sensation at anus, Lach. Peritonitis with retracted abdomen, Euphb. Head turns to right, Stram. (to left, Lyc. ; to either, Bufo, Camph.). Globus, Ign., Lach., Lyc. Diseases originating in spine, Pho., Pic. ac., Zn. Weak memory, unable to find right word, Anac., Lac c. Face greasy, shiny, Nat. m., Sanic. Desire to stretch, Amyl. n. Illusion of smell, Anac.

Causation.—Repelled eruptions. Sexual excess

SYMPTOMS.

1. **Mind.**—Silent melancholy and dejection.—Great anguish and uneasiness, with sighs.—Anxiety, with restlessness and yawning.—Weariness and dislike to conversation and labour.—Discouragement.—Weariness of life.—Weakness or loss of memory.—Slow of perception ; increasing apathy.—Unable to find proper word while talking.—Coma.—Imbecility.—Dementia.—Mania.—Delirium ; alternating with colic.—Fury.—Frantic delirium (bites, strikes), sometimes with demented aspect.—Dread of assassination, poisoning ; thinks every one about him a murderer.

2. **Head.**—Head confused and heavy, as from apathy and melancholy. —Dizziness to the extent of falling senseless.—Intoxication.—Vertigo, esp. on stooping, or looking up into the air.—Headache, as if caused by a ball rising from throat into brain.—Heaviness of head, esp. in (cerebellum) occiput and forehead.—Tearing in forehead and temples.—Lancinating headache.—Congestion of blood to head, with pulsation and heat.—Violent pains in integuments of skull from occiput to forehead.—Great dryness of hair.—Hair becomes very greasy.—Falling off of hair of scalp, also of eyebrows and whiskers (moustaches).

3. **Eyes.**—Pressive and very acute pain, as if eyeballs were too large.—Heaviness of eyes when moving them.—Paralysis of upper eyelids.—Contraction in eyes and eyelids.—Tearing in eyelids, with sleep.—Sanguineous congestion in eyes.—Inflammation of eyes and of iris.—Nocturnal agglutination of eyes.—Swelling of eyes.—Yellowish colour of sclerotica.—Spasmodic closing of eyelids.—Eyes convulsed.—Pupils contracted.—Sight confused, as if directed through a mist, which forces the patient to rub eyes.—Hypopion. —Myopia.—Diplopia.—Blindness, as from amaurosis.—Optic neuritis.

4. **Ears.**—Tearing in ears.—Boring and shooting in ears.—Sensibility to noise.—Occasional sudden diminution of hearing.—Deafness; sudden.—Buzzing in ears.—Hears music, with frightful delirium.

5. **Nose.**—Coldness of nose.—Erysipelatous inflammation of nose.—Red, purulent vesicles in nasal angles.—Fetid smell in nose.—Loss of smell. —Obstruction of nose.—Accumulation of tenacious mucus in nostrils, which can only be expelled by way of the nasal fossæ.—Fluent coryza, with discharge of serous mucus.

6. **Face.**—Face pale, yellow, hippocratic.—Bewildered air; distorted countenance.—Bloatedness of face.—Semilateral swelling of face.—Paralysis of lower two branches of r. facial nerve.—Skin shining and greasy to sight and touch.—Tearing in maxillary bones, which is removed by friction, or made to appear in another place.—Boring in lower jaw.—Exfoliation (painless) of lips.—Cramps in jaw.—Lockjaw.—Swelling of submaxillary glands.

7. **Teeth.**—Tearing, jerking pains in teeth, < by cold things.—Teeth coated with yellow slime.—The teeth become black.—Fetid, hollow, carious teeth, which break off in notches.—Looseness and falling out of teeth.—Grinding of teeth.—Gums pale and swollen; purple-coloured thin border on gums nearest teeth.—Painful and hard nodosities on gums.

8. **Mouth.**—Dryness of mouth.—Copious accumulation of sweetish saliva in mouth, with dryness of gullet.—Salivation; tenacious; mercurial; < during sleep.—Froth in mouth.—Viscid mucus in mouth on waking in morning.—Hæmoptysis.—Aphthæ and fetid ulcers in mouth, and purple blotches in mouth and on tip of tongue.—Breath fetid.—Inflammation, swelling, and heaviness of tongue.—Tongue brown and dry, with rhagades.—Tongue green, slate-coloured, or coated yellow.—Paralysis of tongue, preventing speech; cannot put tongue out.

9. **Throat.**—Sore throat, as if caused by a swelling (plug) or foreign body in gullet.—Sensation as if a ball were rising in throat (globus hystericus). —Sensation of constriction in throat (as soon as the least effort is made to swallow, with great urging to do so).—Paralysis of gullet, with inability to swallow.—Drawing in throat when eating, as if œsophagus were being torn

out.—Sensation as if an insect were crawling in œsophagus.—Inflammation and induration of tonsils ; granular sore throat, going from l. to r.—Formation of consecutive, small, exceedingly painful abscesses in tonsils.

10. **Appetite.**—Sweetish, bitter, metallic, or horribly offensive taste.—Sulphurous, acid taste in bottom of throat.—Violent thirst, esp. for cold water. —Anorexia.—Violent hunger, even shortly after a meal.—Great desire for bread and fried things, cakes, rye bread, tobacco.

11. **Stomach.**—Risings, with a taste of food.—Empty risings, sometimes very violent and painful.—Sweetish risings.—Hiccough.—Regurgitation of sweetish or sour water.—Disgust and frequent nausea, with disposition to vomit, sometimes with retching.—Continued and violent vomiting of food, or of greenish and blackish matter, or yellowish, with violent pains in stomach and abdomen.—Vomiting of bile or of blood.—Vomiting of fæcal matter, with colic and constipation.—Very violent pains in stomach.—Sensation of heaviness and aching in stomach, sometimes after a meal.—Dull and anxious pressure in scrobiculus.—Constrictive cramps in stomach.—Shootings from pit of stomach into back.—Cuttings and burning pain in stomach.—Inflammation of stomach.

12. **Abdomen.**—[Drawing pain from before backward, as though abdomen were drawn in and through towards backbone, sometimes making abdomen concave ; sensation as though a string were inside abdomen drawing it in ; generally there is great despondency with this pain.—Painters' colic with this sensation, as though abdomen were drawn in and touching the spine ; pulse may be down very low, 50, or even 40.—Gastralgia with sensation as though abdomen and backbone met.—Great liver remedy ; inner belly in general ; inner region of navel ; sometimes umbilical hernia, and is an excellent remedy for this ; l. side of abdomen generally (H. N. G.).]—Pain in liver, with lancinating pressure.—Hepatic region sensitive to pressure.—Heat and burning in liver and spine.—Sticking and darting in liver, first anteriorly, then posteriorly.—Jaundice.—Cirrhosis ; first enlarged, then contracted.—Affections of spleen.—Very violent pains in abdomen, with retraction of navel.—Inflation and induration of abdomen.—Violent colics, with constrictive pain, esp. in umbilical region, with violent contraction of abdomen (navel and anus are violently drawn in), sometimes forming elevations and depressions, < by slightest touch, and sometimes increased at night to the highest degree.—Large, hard swelling in ileo-cæcal region, very sensitive to contact or least motion ; sneezing or coughing.—Colic and paralysis of lower extremities.—Pinchings and cuttings in abdomen.—Shootings round navel.—Sensation in upper part and in sides of abdomen as if something detached itself and fell down.—Pulsation in abdomen.—Burning sensation or coldness in abdomen. —Inflammation, ulceration and gangrene of intestines.—Hard nodosities in abdomen, as if caused by internal induration.—Soreness of abdominal muscles, < by movement and by touch.—Continued production and incarceration of flatus, with grumbling and borborygmi in abdomen.—Abundant expulsion of very offensive and hot, burning flatus.—In rectum very urgent effort to expel flatus without any result.

13. **Stool and Anus.**—Most obstinate constipation ; stools blackish.—Continued and ineffectual want to evacuate.—Fæces difficult to evacuate, hard, sometimes in round pieces, like sheep dung, and tenacious.—Balls in con-

glomerate masses, discharged with difficulty.—Loose evacuations.—Long-continued diarrhœa, generally of yellow excrement, or else painful, and often very offensive.—Sanguineous diarrhœa.—Watery diarrhœa, with vomiting and violent colic, esp. pain in umbilicus.—Painful retraction and constriction of anus.—Intolerable pain from spasms of rectum, with every evacuation lasting an hour or two ; horrible constriction, much < if stool solid.—(Constipation from anal spasm in children.—R. T. C.)—Prolapsus ani, with paralysis.—Fissures of anus.

14. **Urinary Organs.**—Retention of urine.—Difficult emission of urine, only drop by drop, dark coloured, scanty, albuminous.—Tenesmus of bladder.—More frequent and more copious emission of urine.—Watery, or reddish, fiery, turbid, and sometimes thick urine ; sediment consisting of red blood-corpuscles and cylinders ; all the symptoms of acute nephritis ; with amaurosis and cerebral symptoms.—Discharge of blood from urethra.—Diabetes.

15. **Male Sexual Organs.**—Swelling and inflammation of genital organs (of penis and scrotum).—Contraction and constriction in testes, with jerking in spermatic cord.—Retraction of testes.—Excoriation of scrotum.—Sexual desire excessively increased, with frequent erections and pollutions.—Loss of sexual desire.—Insufficient emission of semen during coition.—(Impotence.)

16. **Female Sexual Organs.**—Retarded menstruation.—Amenorrhœa, chloro-anæmia.—Nymphomania.—Wants to stretch limbs during ovarian pains.—Spasmodic dysmenorrhœa.—Cessation of menses on invasion of colic ; may reappear after paroxysm, or not again until next period.—Metrorrhagia with sensation of strong pulling from abdomen to back ; during climacteric, dark clots alternating with fluid blood or bloody serum.—Strangulation of prolapsed portion of vagina, intense pain.—Mucous discharge per vaginam.—Feels a lack of room for fœtus in uterus ; inability of uterus to expand ; threatened abortion.—During pregnancy cannot pass urine, from lack of sensation ; or from paralysis.—Puerperal eclampsia ; albuminuria.—Pulling, tearing, contractive pains in breasts, uterus, and vagina, with or without colic ; the breasts become momentarily harder, or with the colic they become smaller.—Induration and inflammation of breasts.—Leucorrhœa.—Miscarriage.—Vaginismus.—Hyperæsthesia of genitals.—Obstructed bowels during pregnancy.—Milk scanty and watery.

17. **Respiratory Organs.**—Hoarseness and roughness in throat.—Aphonia.—Constriction of the larynx.—Copious expectoration of mucus from larynx, which is viscid, transparent, or yellowish green, and in lumps.—Dry, convulsive cough.—Expectoration of pus with the cough.—Cough, with expectoration of blood, hæmorrhages from lungs.

18. **Chest.**—Difficult, anxious, oppressed, and panting respiration.—Shortness of breath.—Spasmodic asthma.—Oppression of chest, appearing periodically.—Fits of suffocation.—Pressure on chest, esp. when breathing deeply or laughing.—Shootings in chest and sides, sometimes with obstructed respiration.—Apices of lungs affected.—Small red papules on chest, which desquamate.

19. **Heart.**—Ebullition in chest, with anxietas præcordium, and perceptible palpitation.—Change in muscular structure without coincident disease of valves, with or without atheromatous degeneration of vessels, usually hyper-

trophy and dilatation of l. ventricle, sometimes with parenchymatous nephritis. —Bruit de souffle.—Palpitation, < on ascending stairs or running.—Pulse rapid, jerky, weak.—Tachycardia.

20. **Neck and Back.**—Tension in nape of neck, extending into ear on moving head.—Tearings and shootings in loins, in back, and between shoulder-blades.—Distortion of spine.—Itching on coccyx above anus, going off when scratched.

22. **Upper Limbs.**—Convulsive movements of arms and hands, with pains in joints.—Drawing and tearing in arms and fingers.—Wrist-drop.—Weakness and painful paralysis of arms and hands.—Dilatation of veins on back of hands, arms, and calves.—Ganglion on back of hands.—Wens on hands.—Difficulty in moving fingers.—Red and swollen spots on fingers.

23. **Lower Limbs.**—Drawing in hip-joints when lying down.—Painful sensation of paralysis in hip-joints, and in those of hands and feet, esp. on going up stairs.—Violent pains in limbs, esp. in muscular parts of thighs ; < evening and night.—Sciatica ; walking causes great exhaustion ; with consecutive atrophy.—Cramp in calves, < at night.—Paralysis of thighs and feet. —Numbness outer side r. thigh from hip to knee.—Numbness of legs and feet.—Tearings and shootings in thighs and knees.—Sensation of numbness in feet, with difficulty in putting them to the ground.—Cramps in soles of feet. —Swelling of feet.—Fetid sweat on feet.—Distortion of toes.—Pain in great toe at night.—Ingrowing toenails.

24. **Generalities.**—[Jaundice, where the sclerotica is yellow, face yellow, urine yellow ; vomiting in bed after retiring for the night, restless, sleepless, &c.—Loss of smell ; reddish-yellow face.—Affections in lower teeth ; tongue ; sweetish taste, as in expectoration of cough with sweetish taste.—Obstructed flatus with terrible colic.—Retraction of soft parts in general ; pinching pain with sensation of tearing ; sphacelus ; grey ulcers.—H. N. G.]—Drawing and tearings in limbs, < at night, sometimes shifting their position on the parts being scratched.—Burning sensation in various parts of body.—Violent tingling pains in bones, coming on fitfully.—Cramps and constrictive pains in internal organs.—Numbness, stiffness, pain as from fatigue, and contraction of some of the limbs.—Paralysis ; of the limbs of those who work in lead.—Convulsive trembling and jerking of limbs, convulsions and cramps, sometimes followed by paralysis.—Epileptic fits (without consciousness).—Swooning, esp. in a large company.—Heaviness and torpor of limbs.—Great weakness, with trembling of limbs.—Depression, with want to lie down, and throbbing of arteries in whole body after slight exercise.—Muscles flaccid.—General emaciation, esp. in paralysed parts, followed by swelling of those parts.—Excess of uric acid in the blood.—Anæmia.—Anæsthesia.—Hyperæsthesia.—Arthralgic and neuralgic pains in trunk and limbs.—Dropsical swellings, sometimes of whole body.—Sensitiveness in open air.—The symptoms develop themselves slowly, and sometimes disappear for a time and reappear subsequently.—< In the night ; from rubbing.

25. **Skin.**—Sensitiveness of skin to open air.—Lead coloured, dry, rough, bluish, or yellow skin.—Dark brown spots over whole body.—Tendency to inflammation and suppuration of slight wounds.—Burning pain in ulcers.—Excoriations.—Decubitus.—Sphacelus.

26. **Sleep.**—Great drowsiness during day ; tendency to fall asleep, even

while speaking.—Coma and lethargy, sometimes with dizziness.—Retarded sleep.—Nocturnal sleeplessness, with abdominal spasms.—Jerks during sleep.—Must stretch in every direction.—Assumes strangest attitudes in bed at night.—Many dreams, sometimes lascivious, with erections.—Talking during sleep.

27. **Fever.**—Pulse very variable, generally contracted, small and slow; at times hard and slow, occasionally small and quick.—Predominance of shiverings and coldness, esp. in the limbs and in open air.—Chill predominates, increasing towards evening, with violent thirst and redness of face.—Coldness in open air and when exercising.—Cold or clammy sweat.—Transient, anxious heat (with thirst, redness of face, and sleepiness).—Internal heat in evening and at night, with yellowness of buccal cavity.—Entire lack of perspiration.

Plumbum Chromicum.

Chromate of Lead. Chrome Yellow. $PbCrO_4$. Trituration.

Clinical.—Colic. Convulsions. Cramps. Diarrhœa. Dysphagia. Erythema. Screaming. Tenesmus.

Characteristics.—Several cases of poisoning by Chrome Yellow have been observed. The symptoms present the cardinal features of lead poisoning—cramps, convulsions, retracted abdomen. Characteristic features were a violent diarrhœa of yellow colour. Yellow stools with constipation. Convulsions with terrible pains. Erythematous redness of chest and abdomen. Pupils enormously dilated. The face was red and hot, and there was heat of the body generally. The symptoms were < towards evening. > By drinking warm milk.

SYMPTOMS.

1. **Mind.**—Apathetic, but when questioned knew what was going on around.—Apathetic, almost soporous.

2. **Head.**—Headache with ringing in ears, pains in chest, loss of appetite, inclination to vomit.

3. **Eyes.**—Pupils enormously dilated.—Eyeballs fixed, staring.

4. **Ears.**—Ringing in ears with headache.

6. **Face.**—Face pale.—Face red and hot.—Face livid during convulsions.—Expression of most profound prostration.—Lips violet.—Lips dry.—Jaws firmly closed.

8. **Mouth.**—Tongue coated yellow.—Point of tongue red.—Bad odour from mouth.

9. **Throat.**—Swallowed with difficulty; shortly before death.

11. **Stomach.**—Appetite lost.—Great thirst.—Nausea and vomiting.—Softening of coats of stomach.—Pain in epigastric region.

12. **Abdomen.**—Abdomen hard and forcibly retracted.—Pain in umbilical region.—Violent cramps in abdomen with constipation.

13. Stool and Anus.—Violent diarrhœa.—Yellow diarrhœa.—Constipation with yellow fæces.—Constipation.

17. Respiratory Organs.—Respiration short ; laboured.

18. Chest.—Pain in chest.—Redness of chest and abdomen.

19. Heart.—Pulse tumultuous.—Pulse irregular and intermittent.

20. Back.—Pain in spine.

24. Generalities.—Frequent convulsions, during which face becomes livid.—Frequent screaming.—Convulsions with terrible pains.—Prostration.—Restlessness.

25. Skin.—Skin of chest and abdomen remarkably erythematous.

26. Sleep.—Sleeplessness.

27. Fever.—Whole body hot.

Plumbum Iodatum.

Iodide of Lead. Plumbic Iodide. PbI_2. Trituration.

Clinical.—Arterio-sclerosis. Atrophiæ. Crusta lactea. Glands, enlarged. Paralysis. Pellagra. Scrofula. Spleen, enlargement of. Tonsils enlarged. Ulcers.

Characteristics.—*Plumb. iod.* is used in old-school practice as an external application in cases of enlarged glands, chronic ulcers, and porrigo capitis. It has also been given internally for enlarged glands and chronic enlargement of the spleen. Hansen mentions "arterio-sclerosis ; atrophiæ ; pellagra ; paralyses," as conditions relieved by it. A combination of *Plumb.* and *Iod.* indications will be the chief guide.

Podophyllum.

Podophyllum peltatum. May Apple. Mandrake (American). *N. O.* Berberidaceæ (by some placed in the Ranunculaceæ and closely related to both). Tincture of root gathered after fruit has ripened ; of whole fresh plant ; of ripe fruit. Solution of resinous extract, Podophyllin.

Clinical.—Acidity. Amenorrhœa. *Anus, prolapse of.* Asthma, bronchial. *Bilious attack.* Bronchitis. Cataract. Cholera infantum. Cornea, ulcer of. Dentition. *Diarrhœa ;* camp. *Duodenum, catarrh of.* Dysentery. Dysmenia. Dyspepsia ; from calomel. Fevers. Flatulence. Gagging. Gall-stones. Gastric catarrh. Goître. Hæmorrhoids. Headache, sick ; bilious. Heart, pains in. Hydrocephaloid. Intermittents. Jaundice. Leucoma. *Liver, affections of.* Ophthalmia. Ovaries, pains in ; numbness in ; tumour of. Palpitation. Pneumonia. *Proctitis.* Prostatitis. Pustules. Sciatica. Stomatitis. Strabismus. Taste, lost ; perverted ; illusions of. *Tenesmus.* Tongue, burning in. Urticaria. Uterus, prolapse of. Whooping-cough. Worms.

Characteristics.—*Pod.* grows throughout the United States in damp, shady places in woods, has leaves five to nine-lobed, large white nodding flowers, yellowish fruits, egg-shaped, not unlike a small lemon, hence the plant is sometimes called Wild Lemon. It flowers in May and June, and the fruit ripens in October. Indian tribes use the root to expel worms, and drop the juice of the root into the ear to cure deafness. "All the tribes are fond of the fruit," says Rafinesque, quoted by Hale, who gives a full account of the medicine. The botanic and eclectic practitioners adopted the remedy and used it as the "vegetable mercury." The first homœopathic proving was made by Williamson. An unintentional proving recorded by E. V. Rose (*H. W.*, xxv. 246) brings out the chief characteristics of *Pod.*, and shows that its reputation as a "vegetable mercury" is not undeserved: Mr. J., 26, took at 11 a.m. gr. x of *Pod.* 1 x to "stir up his liver." At 6 p.m. was taken with an indescribable sick feeling all over, and a persistent dry, rough feeling in pharynx and œsophagus, extending along right Eustachian tube, with dull, aching pain in right ear; feeling as though a ball or lump in upper œsophagus. At 8 p.m. dull and stupefying headache, chiefly frontal, < lying down. Fulness in stomach, belching of gas, sour eructations; marked salivation and offensive odour from mouth. Sleep disturbed, full of confused dreams; rolled and tossed about, bed felt too hard; and a feeling as though head and shoulders were lying too low. At 3 a.m. call to stool, which was profuse, watery, dark green. Calls frequent. *Before* stool: peculiar weak, dull, griping pain below umbilicus; fulness in rectum. *During* stool: weak feeling in stomach. *After* stool: tenesmus and faint feeling. These symptoms passed off in two or three days, the diarrhœa being followed by constipation, which was quickly removed by *Nux*. These symptoms are nearly all proved characteristics of *Pod.*: The early morning <; the *profuse* stools, faint, gone sensation; fulness and tenesmus in rectum. *Pod.* is an irritant wherever applied. Externally on the skin it produces a rawness like intertrigo. The dust of the powdered root getting into the eyes sets up intense inflammation, ulceration, and leucoma. These effects have proved leading indications for its internal use in eye affections. The fulness and tenderness of the rectum noted in Ross's case went on to actual prolapse in the provings. I have many times cured with *Pod.* 6 prolapsus ani in children. With *Pod.* 1 x Mr. Knox Shaw relieved "continual urging and straining" in a case of rectal cancer too far gone for operation. The genital organs were involved with the rectum in the tendency to prolapse. "Symptoms of prolapsus uteri with pain in sacrum; with muco-gelatinous stools"; "sensation at stool as if the genital organs would fall out" are keynotes of the provings which have led to many cures. Pains in the ovaries, especially the right, extending down the anterior and inner side of thighs. In the pregnant and puerperal state *Pod.* is frequently indicated: in the vomiting of pregnancy; swelling of labia; severe after-pains with strong bearing-down sensation; hæmorrhoids and prolapsus recti after confinement. A peculiar symptom of pregnancy indicating *Pod.* is: "Can lie comfortably only on stomach (early months)." The irritation of *Pod.* is shown in the brain, but it is then generally reflected even from the abdominal viscera (cholera infantum) or the teeth (dentition). There is moaning and whining during sleep; the head is thrown back and rolls from side to side; the child grates its teeth. "Great desire to press gums or teeth together" is a keynote. The salivation, foul breath, and moist, tooth-indented tongue of *Merc.* are reproduced in the *Pod.* provings, and so also is the congested, sensitive liver, with excess or absence of bile. These, combined with the feverishness and proneness to sweat, make *Pod.* one of the important antidotes to *Merc.* Fevers of many kinds are met by *Pod.*—remittent, chiefly bilious remittent, intermittent. Delirium is not rare, and is apt to be loquacious. Moaning and whining during sleep. Much drowsiness and desire to stretch. *Alternating* conditions are noted: Diarrhœa alternating with constipation; headache alternating with diarrhœa; headache in winter, diarrhœa in summer; inflammation of scrotum *or* of the eyes; not of both. Some *Concomitants* are important: Pains in sacrum, in lumbar region with rectal and uterine symptoms; cramps in calves with stools. The stools may be painless, or may be preceded, accompanied, and followed by colic, tenesmus and other symptoms. The concomitance of diarrhœa with other affections points to *Pod.* Loquacity during chill and heat is a keynote in fevers. Nash cured an obstinate case of intermittent through this symptom: Chills violent, followed by intense fever with great loquacity; when the fever was past patient fell asleep, and on waking remembered nothing of his loquacious delirium. "Burning tongue" is another leading symptom. A case is related by W. A. Burr (*Critique*, quoted *Hom. News*, xxviii. 87) of a young man who had for some weeks a burning sensation along left edge of tongue, occasionally shooting to tip, or through to opposite edge. He had been in poor health, "bilious," for years. With catarrh of stomach, duodenum, and bile ducts extreme discomfort followed even the blandest foods. *Pod.* 3x improved in two days, and the tongue was well in a week. L. M. Barnes (*Hom. News*, xxix. 45) reports these cases: (1) A lady for four months after miscarriage had much ovarian pain, < at night. She was sleepless, nervous, restless. Much bearing down in abdomen and back. She was a large, stout woman, with a pendulous abdomen. *Pod.* cured after *Puls.* and *Act. r.* had only partially relieved. (2) A stout woman, 60, complained of burning, aching, cutting pain in rectum. Was obliged to be on her feet all day. Nervous, cross, irritable. *Pod.* cured. *Pod.* is *suited to* bilious temperaments, especially after mercurialisation. *Peculiar sensations* are: As if strabismus would occur. Pain in head as from ice on occipital protuberance. As if tongue, throat, and palate had been burned. As if a thousand live things moving about in abdomen, or of fish turning over. As if everything would drop through pelvis. As if heart ascending to throat. Ball in upper œsophagus. *Notable symptoms* are: Thirst for large quantities of cold water. Intense desire to press the gums together. Viscid mucus in mouth, coating teeth. Diarrhœa whilst being bathed or washed; of dirty water soaking through napkin; with gagging. Patient is constantly shaking and rubbing region of liver with his hands. Great loquacity during chill and heat. *Pod.* is predominantly right sided—right throat; hypochondrium; ovary. Guernsey mentions that it is often called for in complaints of pregnant and parturient women, with sensation as if intestines were falling down. He mentions also "whooping-cough with costiveness and loss of appetite." The symptoms are < by touch (spot on right hypochondrium); >

by pressure. > Rubbing (inclination to rub liver region with hand) > Lying down ; lying on abdomen ; stretching in bed. Pain in lef leg < by straightening out the limb. < Motion ; walking ; ascend ing stairs ; exertion. < Morning, especially early morning, 2 to . a.m. Some symptoms < night. < Open air ; while washing External heat > pain in bowels. Heat of stove does not > chilliness but wrapping warmly in bed does >. Hot weather, summer, < diar rhœa. < After eating and drinking ; after acid fruit and milk. < By swallowing. < Before, during, and after stool.

Relations.—*Antidoted by :* Lact. ac., Nux, Coloc., Lept. *Anti dote to :* Merc. *Compatible :* After Ipec. and Nux in vomiting ; afte Calc. and Sul. in liver diseases. *Incompatible :* Salt, which increase its action. *Compare :* Morning diarrhœa, Sul., Dros., Bry., Nat. s Rx. c. Hot, yellowish, green, offensive diarrhœa, Cham. (Cham. < evening ; Pod. < morning, in one gush). Cholera morbus, profus stools, Ver. (Ver. has much pain ; Pod. may have absence of pain) Diarrhœa < after eating ; headaches alternating with uterine an bowel affections, Alo. (Plumb. delirium alternating with colic). Pro lapsus ani *before* stool with weakness in abdomen (Alo. *after* stool) Prolapsus uteri < during stool, Stan. (with Pod. the stool is diarrhœi and comes with a rush). Prolapsus recti et uteri, Nux, Sep. Bearing down in hypogastric and anal regions, > lying down, Sep. Prolapsu of rectum, Bell., Æsc. h., Nit. ac., Rut. (especially in children, Chi Chi. s., Pod.). Duodenal catarrh, Berb., Chi., Hydras., Lyc., Merc Ric. c. Diarrhœa immediately after eating, Alo., Ars., Chi., Lyc. Staph., Trbd. (*whilst* eating, Fer.). < After eating or drinking, Dig. Trbd. Headache from over-excitement, Epipheg. Blur before head ache, K. bi., Ir. v. Wants to bite gums together, Phyt. Tongue as i burnt, Sang. Blue tongue, Gymno. As if something alive in abdomen Croc. Regurgitation of food, Sul. Pain under right scapula, Chel Diarrhœa, ovarian pain, ovarian tumour, dysmenia, Coloc.

Causation.—Over-lifting or over-straining (prolapsus uteri) Summer (diarrhœa).

SYMPTOMS.

1. **Mind.**—Conscious during chill, but cannot talk, forgets words.— Delirium, loquacious during heat ; forgetful after of what has passed.— Depression : imagines he is going to die or be very ill ; in gastric affections —Disgust for life ; headache ; biliary disorders.—Over-fatigue of mind fron business ; when in bed he rolled his head on waking and while awake.

2. **Head.**—Vertigo : while standing ; in open air ; with tendency t fall forward ; with sensation of fulness over eyes ; from gastric or biliou disorders.—Momentary darts of pain in forehead, obliging one to shut eyes.— Stunning headache through temples, > by pressure.—Sudden pain in fore head, with soreness of throat, evening.—Pressing in temples, forenoon, wit drawing in eyes as if strabismus would follow.—Throbbing in temples, aching eyes, hot tears, in morning.—After stool, 10 a.m. : Frontal headache wit feverishness ; sensation of great dryness in forehead and eyes, > for shor time by bathing with cold water.—Sick headache accompanied by constipa tion.—Headache alternating with diarrhœa.—Bilious headache, burning a

vertex and over forehead, pain lasts twenty-four hours, ends in vomiting; pale urine during attack; passes much bile next day; < from over-excitement or walking.—Morning headache with flushed face and heat in vertex.—Dull headache with pain behind eyes; liver torpid.—Pain in vertex on rising in morning.—Sick headache most in occiput, preceded by blur before vision, coming suddenly.—Head hot, rolling head from side to side; dentition.—Reflex irritation of brain from disorders of bowels; grinding teeth at night; morning in sleep; eyes half-closed; head sweaty.

3. **Eyes.**—Inflammation of eyes with excruciating, heavy pain, great turgescence of vessels.—Superficial ulceration of each cornea with general congestion of conjunctivæ; ulceration central and extensive, in r. eye its base was densely white, as if lead had been used (after ten days, from the dust whilst grinding the root).—Eyes inflamed in morning.—L. eye sore.—(Arcus senilis lessens and a dribbling of saliva ceases in an old man.—R. T. C.)—Eyes glazed and motionless (from ripe fruit).—Eyes sunken.—Heaviness of eyes with occasional pains at vertex.—Smarting; inflammation of lids.—Pain in eyeballs and temples, with heat and throbbing of temporal arteries.—Drawing in eyes as if squint would follow.—Scrofulous ophthalmia < in morning.—(Cataract has been known to clear after *Pod.* given internally.—R. T. C.)

4. **Ears.**—Aching pain in r. ear, with rough feeling extending from there along r. Eustachian tube.

5. **Nose.**—Nose pinched.—Soreness and little pimples on nose.

6. **Face.**—Corpse-like pallor.—Complexion sallow, dingy.—Hot, flushed cheeks.—Under jaw fallen.

7. **Teeth.**—Great desire to press gums together; jaws clenched; grinds teeth at night; difficult dentition.—During dentition; catarrhal cough; catarrh of chest; cholera infantum; hydrocephaloid.—Teeth covered with dried mucus in morning.

8. **Mouth.**—Total loss of taste, could not tell sweet from sour; sleepless, restless.—Everything tastes sour or putrid; sweet.—Taste of fried liver in mouth at night.—Bad taste after other symptoms had disappeared.—Feeling as if tongue, and sometimes palate and throat, had been burned.—Tongue: furred white with foul taste; white, moist, shows imprints of teeth; dry, yellow; full and broad with pasty coat in centre; red, not bright red; rough with uniformly erect papillæ; dull bluish colour; red, dry, cracked, somewhat swollen and often bleeding.—Offensive breath; at night; perceptible to patient.—Copious salivation.—(Dribbling of saliva in an old epileptic case ceases.—R. T. C.)—Much viscid mucus in mouth (morning).—Mouth and tongue dry on awaking.—Nursing sore mouth; canker.

9. **Throat.**—Dryness of throat.—Burning in throat (from the ripe fruit).—Soreness of throat extending to ears; r. to l.; l. side sore, < swallowing liquids, morning.—Rattling of mucus in throat.—Goître.—Dry, rough feeling in pharynx and œsophagus, extending along r. Eustachian tube with aching pain in r. ear.

10. **Appetite.**—Indifference to food; loss of appetite; smell of food = loathing.—Satiety from small quantity of food, followed by nausea and vomiting.—Appetite variable, at times voracious.—Great thirst for (cold water in) large quantities; moderate thirst during fever.—Increased thirst after eating.

—Desire for something sour.—Thirst towards evening.—After eating : regurgitation of food, sour ; hot, sour belching ; diarrhœa ; vomits food an hour after, craving appetite afterwards ; depression of spirits.—After eating and drinking : diarrhœa.—After acid fruit and milk : diarrhœa.

11. **Stomach.**—Heartburn, waterbrash, heat in stomach.—Eructations : smelling like rotten eggs ; hot ; sour.—Nausea : distressing and extreme ; with attempts to vomit ; motion of gagging is made with mouth but not accompanied with retching ; stomach contracts so hard and rapidly that the wrenching pain = patient to utter sharp screams ; gagging or empty retching.—Gagging in infantile diarrhœa.—Nausea and vomiting with fulness in head.—Vomiting : of milk in infants, with protrusion of anus ; of food with putrid taste and odour ; of thick bile and blood ; of hot, frothy mucus ; with congestion of pelvic viscera during pregnancy.— Acidity in afternoon with unpleasant, sickly sensation in stomach.—Tender over stomach and bowels, < least touch or motion.—Hollow, empty, weak, sinking feeling at epigastrium ; without hunger.—Stitches in epigastrium from coughing.—Dyspepsia from calomel, aching behind eyes, clayey stools.—Gastric catarrh.—Awakened by violent pains in stomach and bowels.—After breakfast and dinner burning in stomach as if caused by hot steam.—Heat in stomach.—Cold water < ; it = oppression and uneasiness ; small quantities of it were ejected, tasting bitter and causing much burning in œsophagus.

12. **Abdomen.**—Acute burning in region of pyloric orifice, with violent retching and vomiting of bile and belching of wind ; constipation ; after attacks, prostration ; slight jaundice and persistent tenderness to touch in one spot corresponding to entrance of common bile duct into duodenum.—Fulness in r. hypochondrium, with flatulence, pain, and soreness.—Twisting in r. hypochondrium with burning.—Stitches in hypochondria, < while eating.—Pain in region of liver with inclination to rub the part with the hand.—Excessive secretion of bile, great irritability of liver.—Hepatitis with costiveness ; tenderness and pain in region of liver.—Gall-stones and jaundice.—Biliousness ; nausea and giddiness ; bitter taste and risings ; tendency to bilious vomiting and purging ; dark urine.—Abdomen swelled almost to bursting (fruit).—Flatulence.—Abdominal plethora : bloated feeling ; soreness, uneasiness ; > after stool ; causing uterine troubles.—Rumbling.—Colic.—Awakened by violent pains in stomach and bowels, griping, stitching, > for short time by pressure ; 3 a.m. (first night).—Pain in transverse colon, 3 a.m., followed by diarrhœa.—Pain in limbs at daylight, > by external warmth and bending forward whilst lying on side, < lying on back.—Heat in bowels with inclination to stool.—Woke 2 a.m. with stitches in bowels and desire to go to stool ; > flexing thighs or abdomen.—Symptoms generally, and esp. abdominal symptoms, < morning, > evening.—Tenderness over hypogastrium.—Pain extended into lower bowels and r. ovary.

13. **Stool and Anus.**—Emission of fetid flatus.—Morning diarrhœa, then no more stools during day.—Diarrhœa early in morning, continuing through forenoon, followed by natural stool in evening.—Diarrhœa immediately after eating and drinking.—Stools in morning, with strong urgings in bowels and heat and pain in anus.—Small, frequent, bilious stools with tenesmus.—Diarrhœa, yellow stools, one every hour for five hours.—Stools of pure blood (produced.—R. T. C.).—Infantile dysentery (cured.—R. T. C.).—

Dysenteric diarrhœa.—Stools : thin, watery, green ; green ; muco-gelatinous with pain in sacrum ; 4 a.m., yellow, undigested fæces, mixed with mucus, offensive ; with violent tenesmus ; burning, acrid, causing much bearing down during and after stool ; with gagging and excessive thirst in children ; gushing, watery, profuse, green, with sudden urging, often painless ; offensive, < in hot weather ; pasty ; yellow, watery, with meal-like sediment ; smelling like carrion ; mucous and blood-streaked ; black, only in morning ; tar-like ; changing colour.—Stool with much pain and deadly nausea.—Diarrhœa and constipation alternating every day or two, for several days after the most prominent symptoms had disappeared.—Diarrhœa with great sinking at epigastrium, sensation as if everything would drop through pelvis, prolapsus ani.—Small stools, yellow, watery, coming after meals with sick feeling, in pregnancy.—Diarrhœa from indigestion after eating canned fruit.—*Before* stool : intense nausea ; sudden urging ; loud gurgling as of water ; rumbling in l. side ; violent colic or absence of pain ; prolapsus ani.—*During* stool : urging in bowels ; heat and pain in anus ; sensation as if genital organs would fall out ; in women bearing down as from inactivity of rectum ; nausea ; gagging, tormina, and pain in lumbar region ; colic or absence of pain ; prolapsus ani ; pains in sacrum ; tenesmus.—*After* stool : extreme weakness and cutting pain in intestines ; exhaustion, even after natural stool ; flashes of heat running up back, cutting in bowels, severe and painful tenesmus ; colic continues ; faintness and pain in lumbar region ; prolapsus ani ; sore anus ; sensation of emptiness in abdomen and rectum.—Aggravation of internal piles ; rectum protrudes more than an inch after every stool, or sudden motion as sneezing, even during mental excitement ; prolapse sometimes persists for days from swelling and congestion.—Prolapsus ani : in infants, stool bloody, or too large ; with uterine displacement.—Secretion of mucus from anus.—External piles, bleeding or not.—(Cancer of rectum.)

14. **Urinary Organs.**—Micturition painful ; scanty with frequent voidings.—Urine : yellow, containing sediment ; very red.—Diabetes mellitus and insipidus ; chalky stool, urination immediately after drinking, frequent, profuse.—Urinary tenesmus.—Enuresis ; (markedly < on lying down, hence at night.—R. T. C.).

15. **Male Sexual Organs.**—Sticking pain above pubes and in course of spermatic cords.—Diseases of prostate gland associated with rectal troubles. —Inflammation either of scrotum or of eyes ; seldom of both.—Inflammation of scrotum is attended with a pustular eruption which suppurates freely.

16. **Female Sexual Organs.**—Symptoms of prolapsus uteri, with pain in sacrum, muco-gelatinous stools.—Sensation as if genital organs would fall out at stool.—After-pains with strong bearing down.—Pain in r. ovary and uterus.—Numb aching in l. ovary ; heat down thigh ; third month of pregnancy.—Pain in ovaries, esp. r. ; extending down limbs.—Pain from r. ovary down anterior crural nerve, pain < as it descends ; < straightening limb.—Shooting pain in r. ovary, before and during menses.—Ovarian tumour : with pains extending up to shoulder.—Prolapsus uteri : with diarrhœa ; from washing ; after over-lifting or straining ; after parturition.—Induration of os uteri.—(Extreme tenderness of uterus, backache, sick feeling and enuresis on lying down.—R. T. C.)—Menorrhagia from straining.—Menses, retarded ; with ovarian, hypogastric, and sacral pains, < from motion, > lying down.—

Bearing down in abdomen and back during menses; ovarian pains running into thighs.—During pregnancy: swelling of labia; can lie comfortably only on stomach, early months; excessive vomiting.—Hæmorrhoids and prolapsus ani after confinement.—Pendulous abdomen.

17. **Respiratory Organs.**—Chronic bronchitis.—Inclination to breathe deep; sighing.—Sensation of suffocation on first lying down at night.—Bronchial asthma; < after catching cold.—Cough: loose, hacking; with remittent fever; dry; loose; rattling in chest, during dentition; from disease of liver.—Whooping-cough, with constipation and loss of appetite.

18. **Chest.**—Catarrh of chest during dentition.—Pneumonia.—Snapping in r. lung like breaking a thread, when taking a deep inspiration.—Pains in chest < by deep inspiration.—Oppression in chest with constant desire to breathe deep, which is prevented by feeling of constriction in chest.

19. **Heart.**—Sensation in chest as if heart ascending to throat.—Sticking (or stinging) in region of heart.—Palpitation: with a clucking sensation rising up to throat, obstructing respiration; from exertion or mental emotion; with heavy sleep and feeling of fatigue on waking; nervous, in consequence of excessive hepatic action.—Pulse: quick and small; slow, scarcely perceptible; pulseless.

20. **Neck and Back.**—Nape of neck stiff, muscles sore.—Pain under r. scapula.—Pain between shoulders, morning: with soreness, < night and morning, < by motion.—Pain in small of back, when walking or standing, with sensation of back bending inward.—Pain in lumbar region with sensation of coldness, < at night and from motion.—Pain in lumbar and sacral regions < during stool, and still < after.—Pain in loins < walking on uneven ground or from mis-step.—Sacral pain.

21. **Limbs.**—Aching in limbs < night.—Weakness of joints, esp. knees.

22. **Upper Limbs.**—Pain in course of ulnar nerve of both arms.—Rheumatism in l. forearm and fingers.—Pains from head into neck and shoulders; fingers numb.—Weakness of wrists, sore to touch.

23. **Lower Limbs.**—Pain and weakness in l. hip, like rheumatism from cold; < by going up stairs.—Sharply defined ache in sacro-ischiadic foramen, with tenderness on pressure.—Slight paralytic weakness of l. side.—Heaviness and stiffness of knees as after a long walk.—Cracking in knee from motion.—Cramps in calves, thighs, and feet, with painless, watery stools.—Sharp pains in outer and upper portion of l. foot.

24. **Generalities.**—Faintness and emptiness after stool.—Prostration with the pain.—Stiffness on beginning to move.—Sudden shocks of jerking pains.

25. **Skin.**—Sallow skin; jaundice; also in children.—Skin moist with preternatural warmth.—Scabs on arms and legs.—Pustules slow in healing.—Rawness and itching of genitals; also pustules.—Cold, clammy skin.—Erysipelas.—Rubefaciant and vesicatory.—Intolerable itching of body and arms.—Urticaria.—Skin has peculiar odour in patients taking *Pod.* (Ussher).

26. **Sleep.**—Sleepiness: in daytime, esp. forenoon; with rumbling in bowels in morning.—Heavy sleep; fatigue on waking.—Drowsy, half-closed eyes, moaning, whining, esp. children.—Great restlessness, tossing about in bed, yawning and stretching, which > completely.—Rising up in sleep without waking.—Drowsiness or restless sleep, with grinding of teeth or rolling of

ead.—Worrying and sleepless early part of night, apparently from nervous ritability.—Sleep disturbed, full of confused dreams.—Rolled and tossed bout, bed felt too hard ; feeling as though head and shoulders lying too w.

27. **Fever.**—Chilliness while moving about during fever, and in act of ing down, with sweat immediately after.—Chilly at first on lying down in vening, followed by fever and sleep with talking and imperfect waking.— hill 7 a.m.—Backache before chill.—During chill great loquacity.—Shaking ıd sensation of coldness continue some time after heat commences.—Heat egins during chill or whilst he is yet chilly.—Chilly with stool.—Pain in owels first attended with coldness, which is followed by heat and warm veat.—Feverish during afternoon, with occasional chilliness, not > by heat stove, but > by covering up warmly in bed.—Heat with violent pains in ead ; thirst ; loquacity.—Flashes of heat running up back during stool.— avenous hunger with thirst during fever.—Bilious fever ; bilious intermit- nt ; remittent ; infantile remittent ; intermittent, quotidian, tertian, quartan. -Sweat : profuse, dropped off prover's fingers ; of feet in evening ; bathed in ɔld ; warm on head and legs.—Sleep during sweat.

Polygonum.

OLYGONUM ACRE. P. punctatum, Ell. P. hydropiperoides, Pursh. Smart Weed. (North America.) And

OLYGONUM HYDROPIPER. Persicaria urens. Water-pepper. (Britain.) Tincture of whole fresh plant. *N. O.* Polygonaceæ.

Clinical.—Amenorrhœa. Antrum, pain in. Blepharitis. Colic, flatulent. ough. Diarrhœa. Dysentery. Dysmenia. Dysuria. Eczema. Epilepsy. onorrhœa. Gravel. Hæmorrhoids. Heart, affections of. Hysteria. Laryngitis. ephritis. Neuralgia. Orchitis. Prostatitis. Sciatica. Spermatic cord, pain in. leen, affections of. Strangury. Ulcers.

Characteristics.—*Polyg.* was proved by W. E. Payne and others. dditions by Ed. Bayard, included by Hering, appear in the Schema. Smart Weed," says Hale, "is a popular domestic remedy throughout .S.A. Applied externally it has the effect of a mustard plaister, and e leaves saturated with hot water are applied to relieve cramps and olic, and as an emollient in inflammation and sprains. The provers ere all men, but clinical experience has shown a definite action in e female generative sphere, amenorrhœa, aversion to coitus, and ngestion of the ovaries having been cured by it. Leading symptoms e : Aching pains in hips and loins, with weight and tension in elvis, and "Tearing in groin, < right." The pains are : Lancinating, itting, pulsating, shooting, wandering, and flashing. One prover escribed them as like aurora borealis, and a case of sciatica with ins of this description was cured with *Polyg.* The left temple was arkedly affected ; left side generally more so than right. Sensations cold were numerous, and alternated or coincided with heat in the me or other parts. Coldness of right side of face when pain in left side was most severe. Burning in chest with cold feeling at pit of stomach. Feet burning, then suddenly cold. Diarrhœa, as with its relations, *Rheum* and *Rumex*, is marked, and also dysuria. There is excessive weakness, trembling, and sensitiveness to cold. Epilepsy and hysteria have been cured with it. The Polygonums are named by Gerarde "Arse-smarts." Burnett (who prescribed *Polyg. hydropiper* under its name *Persicaria urens*) regarded it as a splenic, and as useful in old cases of syphilis. As a splenic he found it often required in cases of gout; and in gouty eczema with much irritation he used it with much benefit in the 6th, 12th, and 30th. *Peculiar Sensations* are: As of sudden rising of scalp. As if whole intestinal contents were fluid. As if hips drawn together. As of galvanic shock through lower extremities. The symptoms are < by cold; damp; change of temperature; this is the most characteristic condition. Warmth >. Pressure of clothing = distress. Lying down = pressure in occiput; dizziness and wavering of sight. Rising = sudden pain in occiput. Bending head down =, and bending head back >, pain in ears.

Relations.—*Compare:* Botan., Fago., Rheum, Rumex. Cough, diarrhœa, Rumex. Burning in mouth and throat, Caps. < Pressure of clothes, Lach. Headache waking him from sleep, Lach. Wandering pains, Puls., K. bi. < From cold and damp, Dulc., Merc., Rhus. > Bending head back, Seneg. Averse to coitus, Nat. m., Plumb. Also Asar., Caulo., Senec., Xanth.

Causation.—Cold. Damp. Sprains.

SYMPTOMS.

1. **Mind.**—Great depression followed by excessive irritability.—Gloomy views of life, dislike of change and excessive dread of death.

2. **Head.**—Dizziness.—Pulsative, acute pain in l. temple.—Under pressure of great weariness or excitement a dull, depressing pain through whole head, causing a sensation of torpor and strong desire to sleep, but inability to do so.—Pressure in back of head on lying down.—Pressure and soreness in head during menses.—Pain on sudden rising in back of head with pain over eyes.—Headache < in damp weather, > in moderately warm temperature.—Sensation of sudden rising of scalp, with extreme irritation and increased dry exfoliation.

3. **Eyes.**—Burning in eyeballs; dry sensation in lids.—Convulsive twitching in lids when closed and when lying down, dizziness and wavering of sight.—Inflammation of edges of lids.

4. **Ears.**—Dull hearing.—Ringing in ears.—Sudden sounds on tympanum, producing momentary cessation of hearing.—Acute pain in ear when bending head down; > bending head back.—Ear symptoms < in damp atmosphere.—Secretion of ears increased.

5. **Nose.**—Inflammation, smarting, raw feeling of Schneiderian membrane.—Tickling in nose.—Frequent sneezing as from cold.—Red, inflamed appearance of nostrils, with swollen sensation.—Feeling of congestion through eyes and nose.—Coldness in external nose.

6. **Face.**—Acute pain in l. face extending to temples, sometimes darting through whole l. side of head.—Excruciating pain and heat in l. side of face

< by cold or damp.—Coldness in r. face when pain most severe in l.—Pain in r. antrum as if proceeding up from a tooth (sound).

8. **Mouth.**—Gums tender.—Cold or cooling temperature in mouth, producing acute toothache.—Tongue : coated yellow ; feels swollen.—Heat and burning : from root of tongue to pit of stomach ; from tip of tongue to mouth and throat (r. upper).—Heat in roof of mouth with excitation of salivary glands.—Increased flow of hot saliva, gives no > to parched condition.—Saliva abundant and thin (before thin and scanty).—Taste : bitter ; pungent, like pepper.

9. **Throat.**—Throat dry, hot, burning, with sense of excoriation.—Glands feel swollen ; < from cold or moist air.—Contracted feeling in throat after swallowing, followed by thirst.

11. **Stomach.**—Appetite : voracious ; lost.—Food tasteless.—Great thirst for cold water, yet drinking = nausea.—Nausea : as if proceeding from small intestines ; with coldness in abdomen.—Acidity.—Weight in stomach.—Burning in stomach.—Cold feeling in stomach : with headache ; with burning in chest.—Pressure of clothes = distress.—Pain on pressure followed by throbbing and distress.—Uneasiness in stomach and abdomen.

12. **Abdomen.**—Burning heat in stomach and bowels.—Tympanites and flatulent colic.—Cutting, lancinating, griping pains, with great rumbling as if whole intestinal contents were in a fluid state and in violent commotion, the movement proceeding from below up, producing nausea and disposition to vomit, with liquid fæces discharged with great force, with pain in loins.—Pain in hypogastric region, rectum, and anus.—Throbbing in l. inguinal glands.

13. **Stool and Anus.**—Copious stool followed by smarting in anus.—Straining at stool with mucous, jelly-like discharges.—Stools : yellowish green ; hard, lumpy ; dark, followed by burning in rectum.—Urging with discharge of much fetid flatus.—Tenesmus ; with nausea ; with pulsative pains in hips and loins.—Constipation alternating with diarrhœa.—Interior of anus studded with itching eminences, as from corrugation without contraction, a kind of hæmorrhoidal tumour.—Hæmorrhoids with itching and burning.—Pruritus ani (used as a wash).

14. **Urinary Organs.**—Inflammation of kidneys from cold.—Cutting pains along ureters to bladder.—Painful cutting and feeling of strangulation at neck of bladder while urinating, lasting long after.—Strangury.—During an attack of gonorrhœa extremely violent pains on urinating, causing him to tremble and cry.—Pulsating pain ; pain ; and burning in prostate on urinating.—Pains in bladder.—Deposit in urine of mucus and phosphates.—Frequent and profuse discharge of clear, light, or straw-coloured urine.—Albumen.

15. **Male Sexual Organs.**—Pain in testicles, spermatic cords, and neck of bladder when urinating.—Itching at orifice of urethra and around glans with desire to urinate.—Itching and stinging of prepuce.—Pain and soreness in l. testis, extending along l. spermatic cord ; occasionally darting at same time in r. cord and testis.—Loss of power and semen, sometimes followed by inflammation of glans.—Extremely convulsive action in the functional uses.

16. **Female Sexual Organs.**—Intense dislike to coition, followed by

perturbation and irritation if approached ; inaction of flow of secretions.—Aching pain in hips and loins, and sensation of weight and tension in pelvis.—Menses : absent ; delayed, with distress and pain ; too copious ; tardy ; fetid.—During menses : pressure and soreness in head ; grinding pain through abdomen.—Congestive weakness and loss of power.—Congestion of ovaries ; tearing sensation in groin, < r.—Burning in vagina.—Acrid, excoriating leucorrhœa.—Shooting pains through breasts, with great soreness, distension, and tenderness.

17. **Respiratory Organs.**—Stifling sensation in larynx ; irritability of whole system ; weakness of sexual function.—Constriction of larynx.—Crowding and pressure about larynx with irritation of bronchi.—Roughness as of adhesion of mucus to larynx, producing spasmodic hacking and hoarseness.—Hacking cough, < by change of temperature.—Dry cough, in night, excited by tickling, prickling-tingling in upper anterior part of chest, behind sternum ; dry sensation in larynx when coughing.

18. **Chest.**—Sharp pain under r. scapula, extending into chest and pit of stomach, with heavy beating of heart and throbbing of carotids.—Pulsative pressive pains about xiphoid cartilage.—Cutting in l. chest.—Burning in chest with cold feeling in pit of stomach and shooting pains.

19. **Heart.**—Sharp, cutting, shooting pains in region of heart, extending to l. scapula.—Increased action of heart with loss of rhythm.

20. **Neck and Back.**—Awoke at midnight with lameness l. side neck to shoulder, making movement painful ; with pulsative, wandering pains.—Pulsative pains in l. loin.—Aching in loins with pain around l. hip-joint.—Pain in back and at lower extremity, acute or drawing, lateral in its action, as if hips being drawn together (kidney affection).—Tearing and drawing in loins on exposure to cold, followed by lameness and soreness.

21. **Limbs.**—Trembling ; bruised feeling ; weakness in limbs.—Shooting pains in arms and back of legs.—Distension of blood-vessels in hands and feet.

22. **Upper Limbs.**—Pains in arms and inability or sense of weakness on lifting slightest weight.—Pains pulsating, intermittent, shooting, wandering, generally shooting down to finger-tips, sometimes shooting up.

23. **Lower Limbs.**—Sciatica ; pain flashing like aurora borealis.—Pulsative pains in hips and loins with ineffectual urging and tenesmus.—Swelling of legs and feet.—Superficial ulcers and sores.

24. **Generalities.**—Pulsating, wandering, flashing pains, like aurora borealis.

25. **Skin.**—Skin dry.—Scarlet eruption round waist ; itching, burning spasm.—Eczema.—Chronic erysipelatous inflammation.—Old and indolent ulcers.

26. **Sleep.**—Sleep, restless, uneasy, full of dreams.—Dreams : unremembered ; laborious and fatiguing ; of headache and wakes with headache.

27. **Fever.**—Alternation of heats and chills and chills and heats.—Feet alternately hot and cold ; burning for an hour, then suddenly cold.—Profuse sweat and trembling of whole body from moderate exercise.

Polyporus Officinalis, *see* Boletus Laricis.

Polyporus Pinicola.

Polyporus pinicola. Pine agaric. *N. O.* Fungi. Tincture of fresh plant.

Clinical.—Anus, prolapse of. Constipation. Hæmorrhoids. Intermittent fever. Liver, affections of. Malar bone, pain in. Prolapsus ani. Rheumatism. Spleen, affections of. Tonsils, enlarged.

Characteristics.—The Pine agaric, *Pol. pin.*, like the Larch agaric, *Polyporus officinalis* (described in this work as *Boletus laricis*, its older and less correct name), was proved by Dr. Burt. The symptoms of the two have a very close resemblance, and many are common to both. Despondency ; aching distress in many parts ; stiffness of back ; of fingers ; enlarged tonsils with dysphagia and constant inclination to swallow ; neuralgic pains in head, face, and temples ; pain in liver and spleen with diarrhœa or constipation and piles—these are the chief features of the proving. Hale says it is a remedy for ague in the Middle and Southern States, taken during the intermission macerated in whisky. Quotidian fevers, he says, are most suited to it. The symptoms are < by motion ; by walking ; > by rest. < In damp air. < After stool.

Relations.—*Compare :* Bol. lar., Bol. lur., Agar.

SYMPTOMS.

1. **Mind.**—Despondency with the pain.—Gloomy ; spells of depression.—Wants to get away out of sight and lie down.

2. **Head.**—Congestion to head and face ; vertigo when walking ; lightness ; fulness.—Severe headache, < reading or walking ; with soreness over eyes.—Sharp, neuralgic, cutting pains in temples.

3. **Eyes.**—Smarting in eyes.—Dull pains in eyeballs.—Agglutination of lids.

5. **Nose.**—Nostrils constantly filled with thick yellow mucus.

6. **Face.**—Face congested.—Severe aching distress in r. malar bone, with neuralgic pains in temples.

8. **Mouth.**—Tongue : coated white ; yellow.—Taste : sweet, flat ; flat, rough ; slimy, coppery.

9. **Throat.**—Throat dry, sore, frequent inclination to swallow.—Tonsils much congested, enlarged ; frequent efforts to swallow, quite painful.

11. **Stomach.**—Sour eructations.—Nausea.—Burning in stomach and dragging in r. hypochondrium.—Constant very severe distress in lower epigastrium, causing faintness ; < by pressure and by walking.—Severe pain in epigastrium all morning.

12. **Abdomen.**—Dull, dragging, drawing, aching, burning in both hypo-

chondria.—Pain and distress in liver; and all dorsal region; < walking.—Distress and colicky pains in umbilical and hypogastric regions.—Rumbling.—Hard, distressing, sickening pain in hypogastrium, causing faintness; followed by stool.—Drawing in r. groin.

13. **Stool and Anus.**—Stool: ran from bowels in deep yellow stream; loose; hard, dry, lumpy, then mushy; lumpy with mucus and bile; costive, hard, dry lumps, brought on piles and slight prolapsus ani.

14. **Urinary Organs.**—Urine scanty and high coloured.

17. **Respiratory Organs.**—Pressing sensation in larynx with dryness of fauces.

19. **Heart.**—Burning distress in præcordial region; sharp pains on full inspiration.—Pulse soft, feeble.

20. **Back.**—Back stiff.—Aching in back; and hips.—Felt ill with aching and sore sensations along spinal column.

21. **Limbs.**—Constant rheumatic, drawing pains in fingers, wrists, knees, ankles, feet.

22. **Upper Limbs.**—Drawing in elbows and flexor muscles of both arms.—Fingers ache; feel quite stiff.

23. **Lower Limbs.**—Hips ache.—Drawing inside r. thigh.—Sharp pain in r. tibia.—Hard, drawing pains in knees and ankles, causing restlessness.—Aching distress, weakness of ankles and feet, walking very difficult.—Soles of feet and heels feel as if pounded; < when boots on.

24. **Generalities.**—Rheumatic pains in every part of the body < in damp weather.

26. **Sleep.**—Sleepy, yawning, and stretching.—Wakeful after 3 a.m.

27. **Fever.**—Paroxysms of chilliness, cold shivering sensations followed by feverishness.—Chills and a shivering sensation.—Face hot, flushed.—Hands and palms hot and dry.—Slight perspiration.

Populus Candicans.

A variety of P. balsamifera. Balm of Gilead. [This name applies especially to the variety P. candicans; but also to all P. balsamiferæ. In England the name "Balm of Gilead tree" is given to the Black Italian Poplar, which abounds in Italy, but the origin of which is not known.] *N. O.* Salicaceæ. Tincture of the resinous buds.

Clinical.—Aphonia. Asthma. Brain, base of, congested. Bullæ. Catarrhal fever. Constipation. Coryza. Dysmenia. Dyspepsia. Dysphagia. Ecthyma. Heart, affections of. Hydroa. Liver, enlargement of. Phosphaturia. Sunstroke. Throat, burning in; paralysis of. Vagina, burning in.

Characteristics.—C. F. Nichols (*H. P.*, viii. 234) gives an account of *Pop. cand.*, the effects of which he observed. "The resinous gum exuding from buds and stalks, deliciously aromatic in perfume, is widely used to heal wounds, open sores, and eruptions, and often suppresses these latter to the harm of the patient." As an application, Nichols says, it is like *Arn.*, dangerous, though most people are not susceptible to its poisonous effect. He has never seen blisters of the size of those of *Pop. c.* produced by any other drug: blisters hang down like bags of water the size of walnuts. Burning was a common symptom—eyes, nose, throat, bowels, vagina. W. C. Stilson (*H. P.*, xi. 88) relates a case of poisoning in a man who one evening drank rum in which Balm of Gilead buds had been placed for making a liniment. A few hours later his wife heard him breathing heavily, and on waking him found he could not speak. Stilson found him only able to speak in hoarse whispers, and he would forget in the middle of a sentence what he was going to say. Face ashy pale; wild look. Tongue and mouth dry. Throat dry, burning, constricted, felt as if spiders had spun webs on it. It was some days before he recovered. Since this occasion Stilson has cured several cases of catarrhal hoarseness and aphonia with *Pop. c.*, and one case of nervous aphonia: Mrs. S. had nervous prostration, and during the attack aphonia. The aphonia remained after the patient got well otherwise. *Pop. c.* φ cured. Among the *peculiar symptoms* observed by Nichols is surface anæsthesia with or without numbness. The finger-ends are actually thickened, horny, insensible to pinching and pricking. There is numbness in back radiating from spine. The skin is harsh, generally dry and cold, with a stinging burning behind the surface as if an eruption would appear; or as if sweat would break out. Other *peculiar sensations* are: Whole body feels swollen, bruised, lame, sore, and painful, exhausted as in dry, sultry weather. Eye feels twisted with the headache. Constipation, bowels feel hot and dry. The menses were at first scanty, later abundant and early, with dysmenorrhœal pain > by application of hot cloths. The symptoms were < on moving. < Before menses. < After food and drink. < Lifting arms. < By contact of clothes. > Hot applications. < After sleep (mind).

Relations.—*Antidoted by:* Rhus. *Compare:* Salix, Pop. trem., Salicylates. < Contact of clothes, Lach.

SYMPTOMS.

1. **Mind.**—Hopeless foreboding < after sleep.—Fear and anguish.—Expectation of death.—Feels as if the will were paralysed.—Loquacity.—Vanishing of thought.—Forgets to finish a sentence.—Voices sound distant and words just spoken seem as if uttered long ago; objects seem multiplied.

2. **Head.**—Vertigo from lifting head.—Vertigo and heat of head as if scorched by sun.—Confusion in head, with expansive fulness, all parts feel lame, swollen, inflamed, thickened, painful, burning, throbbing in head and brain, < cerebellum and cerebro-spinal axis, dulness of the senses as from congestion.—Boring through l. temple.—Weight on vertex.

3. **Eyes.**—Sensation as if l. eye were twisted during the headache.—Burning irritation in eyes, nose, mouth, throat, and air passages.

6. **Face.**—Face yellow.—Burning prickling on face.

8. **Mouth.**—Tongue: white, dry; feels thick and numb.—Tongue and mouth feel burnt and dry, but are moist, wants drink, but can take only a

little, < after food and drink.—Speech thick.—Taste: bitter; sweet in morning.

9. **Throat.**—Distressing burning in throat, as from swallowing hot fat. —Throat red, dry, burning; felt as if spiders had spun webs in it.—Deficient power of deglutition; food stops in œsophagus or is passed with difficulty.

10. **Appetite.**—Appetite lost, loathes meat.—Nothing relished.—Hungry but dares not eat for fear of choking.

11. **Stomach.**—Belching of gas feeling like hot steam.—Nausea with sinking in epigastrium.—Vomits bile.

12. **Abdomen.**—Wears her clothes loose.—Flatulent colic doubling the body forward.—Pain in r. hypochondrium with enlargement.

13. **Stool.**—Stools watery, green, alternating with constipation.—Constipation, bowels feel hot and dry.—Stools small, round, preceded by cramps in abdomen; lack of expulsive power.

14. **Urinary Organs.**—Urine: strong, high coloured, hot, scanty; increased, variously coloured, red, dark, light, phosphates abundant.—Urine dark, straw colour; smoky.

16. **Female Sexual Organs.**—Menses scanty, usually delaying, afterwards absent, then abundant, early, with dysmenorrhœa, > hot cloths.—Vagina burns as if scalded.

17. **Respiratory Organs.**—Hoarseness.—Aphonia.—Dry cough when tired.—Cough caused by "cobwebs" in his throat.—Suffocation.—Breathing dry, asthmatic, with dyspnœa, sits bent forward, < lifting arms.

18. **Chest.**—Pulmonic, cardiac, and capillary circulation oppressed, feels as if death must result, as if there must be fatal organic lesions.

19. **Heart and Pulse.**—Pain in heart, stitches.—Heart's sound irregular, usually muffled, with a systolic murmur, < before menses.—Palpitation when rising or lying on l. side, with vertigo.—Pulse rarely exceeded 60.

20. **Back.**—Numbness in back radiating from spine.—Burning weariness in small of back.

22. **Upper Limbs.**—Finger-ends thickened, horny, insensible to pinching and pricking.—Nails blue as in ague (not thickened).

24. **Generalities.**—Emaciation.—Rheumatic and gouty pains to ends of fingers and toes.—Whole body feels swollen, bruised, lame, sore, and painful, exhausted as in dry, sultry weather, movements heavy, laboured, clumsy, stinging, restless irritation as if an eruptive fever would come to the surface, feeling as if sweat would break out.—Burning irritation of eyes, nose, skin, mucous membrane of mouth, throat, and air passages, and oppression of respiration and circulation.—Catarrhal feverish state of mucous surfaces — Weakness.—Stiffness of muscles, tendons, ligaments, with lameness and with dry feeling in cartilages, as if lame.—Insensibility of surface, < back and abdomen, so that rubbing and pounding were borne without pain and insisted upon for the sake of warmth.—< Morning; < before menses.

25. **Skin.**—Skin harsh, generally dry and cold, with burning-stinging below the surface, as if eruption would appear, rarely blotches and fine papules.—Burning prickling on face, chest, and hands, the parts became dark red and swollen, and there were blisters as large as walnuts, hanging down like bags of water, with watery, acrid, sticky oozing, external heat like coals of fire on skin, at times internal heat, with cool skin, > hot applications, the

eruption returned each year with fear and expectation of death, loquacity, discussing repeatedly her symptoms, vertigo from lifting head.

26. **Sleep.**—Sleepless after midnight, with restlessness, < from early morning till noon.—Dreams: frightful, vivid; fearful after fitful sleep.

27. **Fever.**—Sudden coldness of extremities, with numbness of them and heat of head.—Fever and unrest.—Fever with congestion of brain, fulness, heaviness, dulness, soreness, with expansive pressure, as if swollen, deadening heat in head as if scorched by the sun, vertigo, oppression of vital forces and circulation as if over-heated, fatigue, faintness, and burning, throbbing oppression.—Dry heat.—Heat of cerebellum and neck, with feeling as if the capillary circulation were congested and oppressed.—Sweat on head and neck.

Populus Tremuloides.

Aspen Poplar. (The American Aspen; the British Aspen is P. tremula.) *N. O.* Salicaceæ. Tincture of inner bark. Solution of Populin.

Clinical.—Ardor urinæ. Bladder, catarrh of. Gleet, chronic. Prostatic affections.

Characteristics.—The few symptoms of the Schema were provided by Paine (eclectic), whom Hale quotes. Paine used *Pop. t.* in affections of the bladder, urethra, and prostate. Hale confirms its action in vesical tenesmus and inflammation of the neck of the bladder. He gives this case: A lady had metritis, vaginismus, and cystitis, and was apparently cured. A ride on the cars brought back: Weight, pressure, and aching in pelvis and vesical tenesmus with frequent desire to urinate. *Pop. p.* 3x removed all these symptoms in three days. In the cases cured by Hale he says there was little pain *during* urination, but as soon as the last drops were voided, or a little before, a severe cramp-like pain just behind pubes lasting ten to fifteen minutes.

Relations. — *Follows well:* Cannab., Canth. (succeeded after they had only partially helped). *Compare:* Pop. can., Sal. nig., Gaulth., Salicin, and Salicylates.

SYMPTOMS.

1. **Mind.**—General nervous excitement.

11. **Stomach.**—Nausea and vomiting.—Warm pungent sensation; (or from larger doses) fierce burning sensation in stomach.

13. **Stool.**—Slight purging of bilious matter.

14. **Urinary Organs.**—Very copious discharge of urine; irritation of bladder and urethra.

27. **Fever.**—Warmth in stomach followed by glow of heat on entire surface.

Pothos Fœtidus, *see* Ictodes.

Primula Obconca.

P. obconca. *N. O.* Primulaceæ. Tincture of whole fresh plant.

Clinical.—Chapped hands. Eczema. Eyes, inflammation of. Itching. Liver, pain in. Skin, affections of. Spleen, pains in.

Characteristics.—*Prim. ob.* is an ornamented variety of Primrose. Gardeners, amateur and professional, have discovered after much suffering that it has with some persons a most powerful action on the skin, its action taking place chiefly by contact but partly by effluvia. The Rev. F. H. Brett (*H.W.*, xxv. 496), who was one of the first to notice its poisonous properties, undertook to prove it. He had handled the plants freely up to that time without experiencing any ill effect. He cut up some young plants and added some vigorous fresh leaves of an old one and made a tincture. This he allowed to stand for a week, and then took three or four drops, three times a day for four days. Two days after ceasing to take it symptoms began to develop in the right little finger, and two days afterwards in the right thumb. These became very intense, and ran a chronic course ; and now he could not go near a plant of *Prim. ob.* without setting up an <. When plants were in the room there was < at night. < By rubbing or scratching. At the same time Brett noted that pains in the liver and spleen to which he had been subject now troubled him no more. The right hand was much more affected than the left. His symptoms are marked "(B)" in the Schema. With *Prim. ob.* 3 I cured a chronic psoric dry eruption on the leg of a woman. Cooper relieved a case of severe eczema on the leg with bleeding.

Relations.—*Compare :* Anag., Prim. ver., Prim. vulg.

SYMPTOMS.

3. **Eyes.**—Burning irritation of eyeballs and eyelids, nostrils, and mouth.—Lids greatly swollen, covered with large bullæ ; half closed ; stiff and unmovable.

6. **Face.**—Face, neck, and greater part of body, burning irritation and discoloration of skin.—Urticarial eruption on face—Papular eruption on chin.

12. **Abdomen.**—Pain in region of liver, and a less severe pain in spleen always occasioned by bending from side to side (cured by the proving.—B).

22. **Upper Limbs.**—Elevated mass of points in outer side first joint r. little finger (B).—Heat, itching, and bright-red, tense, solid elevation on outer surface r. thumb ; these coalesced, forming a solid mass over back of thumb like corrugated leather (B).—At intervals for weeks bright red patches appeared on backs, inner sides of, or spaces between the fingers, itching intensely at first and leaving low elevations, flat and smooth like polished leather, stiffness in bending fingers as if skin rigid (B).—Eruptions made their way down thumb to wrist, inner side of which became covered with red patches, as if grains of sand under skin (B).—At outer edge of hand a row of hard lumps under skin (B).—At times whole back of hand would assume a

dark red colour, when excited, bright red; rubbing or scratching < the itching tenfold (B).—Blisters on back of r. thumb and between thumb and index, discharging clear fluid when punctured (B).—Desquamation occurred in about eight weeks (B).—Moist eczema, papular and excoriated, cracked over joints; symptoms < at night when itching is unbearable.—Purple blotches on backs of hands and fingers; deep blisters formed at tip of each finger and above and below each phalangeal flexure; fingers stiff.—Dryness and heat in palms.—L. hand much less affected than r. (B).

25. **Skin.**—Eruptions: eczema; moist eczema; erythema; papules; vesicles; like scales.—Eruption preceded by pricking sensation which gradually changes to a smarting.—Skin diffusely infiltrated and swollen; small bullæ form.—Deep infiltration stiffening parts.—Cracks as from frost over joints.—Desquamation; sometimes furfuraceous; sometimes lamellar; exposing papillary layer.—Intense itching < at night.

27. **Fever.**—At night feverish, hands and face would burn, then intolerable itching.

Primula Veris.

Cowslip. *N. O.* Primulaceæ. Tincture of entire fresh plant.

Clinical.—Apoplexy, threatened. Eczema. Fevers. Migraine. Neuralgia. Vertigo. Voice, affections of.

Characteristics.—The flowers of *Prim. veris* are said to be narcotic (*Treas. of Bot.*). "Cowslip wine" is a favourite remedy in the country for many small disorders. Cooper cured with *P. ver.* ϕ a case of eczema of the hands after *P. obc.* had failed. He also cured with it eczema palmaris of years' duration in a man æt. 70. Schier, of Mentz (*Univ. Hom. Ann.*, p. 99), proved a tincture of fresh plant including root. The duration of action is only a few days in healthy persons. The conditions in which Schier commends it, and which are borne out by the symptoms, are: Threatened apoplexy, arising apart from psychic depression; as an external application when there is no skin lesion, "as this remedy has a certain relation with the skin. Prudence is necessary here, especially for persons with sensitive and easily vulnerable skin." The symptoms are < by bent position; stooping; movement; in room; in closed carriage; travelling by rail. < In open air.

Relations.—*Compare:* P. obc., P. vulg., Cycl., Anag.

SYMPTOMS.

1. **Mind.**—Happy disposition.—Stubbornness.—Heat with anxiety.

2. **Head.**—Vertigo; whirling; sensation of falling backward; as if brain moved, wanted to get out of skull; as of heavy weight on head.—Fear of falling on standing up.—Fulness and heaviness of head.—Head hot with rush of blood to head; red spots on cheeks.—Hammer-like, boring, beating, sometimes dull headache, in both temples, occiput, and above forehead, < r.

temple in morning; > by pressure; < stooping, movement, travelling b rail; > in open air; < indoors.—Sensation as if band across forehead an occiput; cannot keep hat on.—Tension of skin of forehead.—Burning itchin of scalp, in r. temporal region and occiput.

3. **Eyes.**—Flies flying before eyes, violent vertigo as if everythin revolving.—Burning and pricking pains in orbital cavities.—Sensitive t light; > in darkness.

4. **Ears.**—Buzzing and ringing in l. ear.

5. **Nose.**—Pressure at root of nose < r. side.

6. **Face.**—Face hot; pale.

8. **Mouth.**—Tongue clear but imprinted with teeth; papillæ of edge very red.—Salivation.—Dull sensation in r. half of tongue and digestive tract

9. **Throat.**—Burning pains r. side of throat.—Pricking when breathin in r. side of thyroid body.

11. **Stomach.**—Tendency to vomiting.—Sensation of emptiness an burning at orifice of stomach and in duodenum.

12. **Abdomen.**—Rumbling in bowels.

13. **Stool and Anus.**—Painless liquid stools; with malaise < by pres sure on head.—During stool: fever, goose-flesh.—After stool: tenesmus.

14. **Urinary Organs.**—Turbid earth-coloured urine smelling of violets or of strong urine.—Tenesmus, painful irritation of ureter.

17. **Respiratory Organs.**—Dull sensation r. side of larynx, pharynx tongue, and digestive tract.—Cough with burning and pricking in respirator tracts.—Voice remarkably fine, clear, and strong, the high notes easily giver out.—Sensation as if r. half of larynx stopped up.

19. **Heart.**—Palpitation with feeling of weakness.

20. **Neck and Back.**—Stiffness r. side of neck.—Short, intense pai beside insertion of r. sterno-mastoid muscle.

21. **Limbs.**—Weight and lassitude of limbs, esp. shoulders.—Twitchin in throat going to forearm, and in great toe going to calf.

22. **Upper Limbs.**—Burning in r. axillary joint preventing movemen of r. arm > in bed, lying on painful part.—Pricking in fourth and fift finger of both hands.—Itching in palms.—Burning in hollow of r. hand, ir arm, esp. in l side.

23. **Lower Limbs.**—Tearing in l. leg and thigh.—Sensation as if l. leg was swollen with tearing and drawing.—Itching in l. little toe.

24. **Generalities.**—Beating, tearing, burning, and drawing sensations.— Trembling of hands and feet.—Malaise of head > in open air. < In ben position; by movement; in a room; riding in closed carriage.—Weight and lassitude of limbs.

25. **Skin.**—Sensitive, easily vulnerable skin.—Itching.

26. **Sleep.**—Sleeps well with pleasant dreams.

27. **Fever.**—Febrile excitement.—Intense heat with anxiety as if fearing a stroke of apoplexy.—Wants to get cool.—Sweat on forehead, feet and hands cold.—Head hot with red spots on cheeks.—Feet and hands sweat, rest o body cold.

Primula Vulgaris.

Primrose. *N.O.* Primulaceæ. Tincture of fresh plant.

Clinical.—Dropsy; wandering. Heart, pressure at.

Characteristics.—Cooper cured with *P. vulg.* φ a case of wandering dropsy. In a cancer case, one dose caused the disappearance of dropsy from the leg and led to oppression at the heart. "Pressure at heart" Cooper thinks a characteristic aggravation.

Prinos Verticillatus.

Black Alder. *N. O.* Aquifoliaceæ. Tincture of the berries. Tincture of fresh bark.

Clinical.—Diarrhœa. Fever.

Characteristics.—The genus *Prinos* is very closely allied to the hollies. "The bark of *P. vertic.* is bitter, and has been used in the treatment of fever, and in the form of a lotion as an application in cases of gangrene. The berries are tonic and emetic" (*Treas. of Bot.*). The only recorded experiment with *Pri. v.*, the effects of swallowing twenty berries, bears out the last statement: the effect was to cause vomiting (and also an extremely profuse greenish diarrhœa); increased appetite and tense feeling of well-being in spite of great loss of weight.

SYMPTOMS.

9. **Throat.**—Acrimony in fauces.

11. **Stomach.**—Appetite and digestion better than usual after the liquid stools.—Sensation of commotion in stomach, not exciting nausea, ate heartily in spite of it; walking precipitated vomiting of a little bile.

12. **Abdomen.**—Inclination to stool; had natural stool which > all sensations.

13. **Stool and Anus.**—Natural stool; half an hour later, most profuse stool consisting of natural fæces diluted with an immense quantity of greenish liquid; without pain or uneasiness; in another hour and a half similar stool but less in quantity.

24. **Generalities.**—Felt remarkably well after the diarrhœic stool though had lost ten pounds in weight.

Propylaminum, *see* Trimethylaminum.

Prunus Padus.

Cerasus padus. Padus racemosa. P. vulgaris. Bird cherry. *N. O.* Rosaceæ. Tincture of leaves and bark of small twigs collected when in blossom.

Clinical.—Headache. Heart, affections of. Rectum, pains in.

Characteristics.—*Prunus padus* was proved by Lembke. The plant is now classed with the Cherries, but I retain it under its old name. "In Scotland it is known as the Hayberry. The fruit is small, black, and nauseous to the taste. In the North of Europe it enters into the formation of a palatable liqueur ; the juice is also expressed and drunk with milk, while the residue of the fruit is kneaded up into cakes" (*Treas. of Bot.*). Lembke's proving brought out marked symptoms in head, rectum, chest, and heart. Pains were pressive in head, sticking in rectum, pressive beneath sternum. Heart-beats were tumultuous. The symptoms were < by pressure ; sitting ; standing ; stooping, and walking.

Relations.—*Compare :* Heart, Cratæg., Pru. sp., Pru. v., Lauroc.

SYMPTOMS.

1. **Head.**—Dulness, with dull pressure in forehead.—Momentary sensation as if head would sink to r. side.—Head heavy, confused.—Pressure at base of brain.—Pressure ; on forehead with external heat ; in l. temple.—Heaviness of occiput with dull pain extending transversely through occiput.

3. **Eyes.**—Pupils much dilated.

5. **Nose.**—Pulsating feeling under skin at root of nose, with visible trembling movement < by stooping.

9. **Throat.**—Sore throat with frequent swallowing of saliva.

11. **Stomach.**—Great nausea.

12. **Abdomen.**—Drawing pain in hypochondrium and umbilical region, < by pressure.—Abdomen greatly distended by gas.

13. **Stool and Anus.**—Sticking in rectum while sitting and walking ; repeated and lasting all day.—Stitches in rectum.

14. **Urinary Organs.**—Profuse bright-yellow urine.

17. **Respiratory Organs.**—Some dull stitches in larynx compelling to swallow.

18. **Chest.**—Pressure behind sternum with difficult respiration.—Pressure behind lower sternum, as if heavy weight lying on it, no > by deep inspiration ; < walking.—Some sudden violent stitches beneath r. ribs.

19. **Heart.**—Oppression of heart while standing.—Every beat felt in chest while sitting.—Beats tumultuous, felt in neck and actually shake head.—Violent, irregular beats.—Pulse very slow ; and small.

22. **Upper Limbs.**—Weakness in elbow joints.

24. **Generalities.**—Sensation of general weakness ; of weakness extending from side of neck into r. arm, soon followed by similar sensation l. side.

27. **Fever.**—Frequent sensation of coldness in back.—Heat deep in small of back.

Prunus Spinosa.

Blackthorn. Sloe. *N. O.* Rosaceæ. Tincture of buds just before flowering.

Clinical.—*Appetite, lost.* Ascites. Breast, pain in. Choroiditis. Ciliary neuralgia. Cystitis. Dropsy. Dysuria ; flatulent. Earache. *Eyes ; choroiditis.* Glaucoma. Heart, affections of. Hernia. *Herpes zoster.* Leucorrhœa. Menorrhagia. Metrorrhagia. Neuralgia. Sprains. Strangury. Stricture. Toothache. Vitreous, opacities of.

Characteristics.—*Prun. spi.* was proved by Wahle. The symptoms resemble those of *Pru. pd.* in general, but some very strongly characterised ones were produced. The pains were pressive and *out*-pressive, and out-shooting. These pains are felt in skull, eye, root of nose, and ears ; the teeth feel raised out of their sockets. Shooting from within out, from before backward. These pains occurring in and around the eye have led to its successful use in glaucoma, ciliary neuralgia, choroido-retinitis, irido-choroiditis, irido-cyclitis. Spraining pains and pains which take away the breath. A remarkable symptom is : "Breath always seems to remain sticking in pit of stomach." This symptom, with "pain as if sprained in left ankle," led Lippe to make a remarkable cure in this case : A young lady, 16, jumped from a carriage whilst the horse was running away and sprained her ankle. Left ankle and foot much swollen. As swelling abated, breathing became rapid ; great oppression with constantly recurring desire to take a long breath ; *felt as if air inhaled did not reach pit of stomach*, and till she could force air so far down had to yawn and try to take a deep inspiration.—The tightness, stitches, and sticking pains in chest have marked *Prun. spi.* as a remedy in many cases of neuralgic pains with or following herpes zoster. The urinary symptoms are perhaps the most peculiar of all. Pressure of abdominal flatulence on the bladder is not an uncommon symptom, and is met by *Prun. spi.* : "Flatulence presses on bladder and = cramps in bladder so that he is obliged to double up." Strangury of the most painful description was produced, and this symptom, which is quite characteristic : Hurriedly impelled to pass urine, which, however, seems to pass forward into glans penis and then return and cause most violent pain in urethra. Menses are too early ; too profuse ; last too long, and are thin and watery. There is leucorrhœa, which weakens and stains yellow. The right side is much more affected than the left. *Peculiar sensations* are : As if a sharp corner pressing against top of head. Headache as if from sun. As if skull would be pressed outward by a sharp plug. As if inner portion of eye would be torn out. Eyeball as if crushed, or pressed asunder. As if tooth would be torn out. As if tongue had been burned. As if hernia would protrude. Burning as from a wound in rectum ; as from salt in a wound in anus. Sighing as if climbing a steep mountain. As if small of back had been injured. As if right thumb sprained ; as if left ankle sprained ; as if first joint of big toe pulled out. C. M. Boger gives this confirmation of *Prun. spi.* (*Med. Couns.*, xvi. 264) : Man, 60, with enlarged prostate, had frequent urging to urinate, day and night. Shooting pains in neck of bladder unless desire to urinate is at once gratified. Urination delayed if any great amount has accumulated. Spasmodic tenesmus of bladder and rectum at close of urination, with pains in glans. Pulsation in glans from jar of walking. *Prun. spi.* 1 m. (Fincke) removed the symptoms. The symptoms are: < By touch and pressure. Biting teeth together > toothache. > From rest; from doubling up. < Motion; from jarring; must walk carefully. < Night. < From warm food (toothache).

Relations.—*Compare:* Heart, Cratæg., Lauro., Pru. p. Eyes, Bell. Burning tongue, Sang., Polyg. Stool like dog's, Pho. Leucorrhœa staining yellow, Agn. c., Carb. a., Chel., Kre., Nux, Sep., Thu., Nit. ac.

Causation.—Sun. Sprains. Over-lifting.

SYMPTOMS.

1. **Mind.**—Sadness, indifference, moroseness, and ill-humour.—Restlessness, which does not allow one to remain in one place, walks about constantly, with dyspnœa and short breathing.

2. **Head.**—Reeled and staggered back and forth.—Heaviness in head, and vertigo.—Pressure in head, principally in forehead, occiput, and temples.—Pressive pain beneath skull, as if skull would be pressed through with a plug.—Pressing asunder headache so violent that he almost lost his reason.—Sharp pains beginning in r. forehead shooting like lightning through brain and coming out at occiput.—Painful jerks in forehead shooting back.—Violent nervous pains in head, with loss of ideas and of consciousness.—Pressure in head mostly manifests itself from without inwards.—Pressive pain from within out beneath upper part of r. temporal bone; from thence to frontal bone < by external pressure.—Twinging pain: in r. temporal bone to ear, causing earache; extending outward.—Pressive pain r. vertex as if sharp corner pressing against it.—Jerking sticking back part l. frontal bone.—Painful jerking through r. hemisphere of brain, on motion.—Nervous out-pressing pain in occiput and occipital bone (l.).—Headache, as from heat of sun.—Stitches in scalp.

3. **Eyes.**—Pains in the eyes, as if the balls were torn out.—Glaucoma.—Ciliary neuralgia; pain in eyeball as if crushed or pressed asunder; sharp shooting pain extending through eye back into brain, or above eye extending into, around it, or over corresponding side of head; pain commences behind ear and shoots forward to eye, < motion, > rest; pains occasionally periodic, may be < at night.—Pain in r. eye as if it were torn asunder; as if inner portion would be torn out.—Itching in corners of eyes and in edges of lids.

4. **Ears.**—Binding sensations in ears.—Pressing-asunder pain in r. ear, like earache.

5. **Nose.**—Frequent sneezing.—Pressing-asunder pains about nasal bones.

6. **Face.**—Itching sticking in upper part of malar bone.

7. **Teeth.**—Violent nervous or wrenching pains in teeth, or else a sensation as if teeth were raised up, and pulled out.—Pricking pains in teeth.—Toothache > biting teeth together.

8. Mouth.—Shootings, and burning pain, in tongue.—Tongue loaded with whitish mucus.—Itching crawling in tip of tongue and front teeth.—Mucous, clammy, or bitter taste in mouth.

9. Throat.—Rawness, scraping, crawling in throat, causing hacking cough.

11. Stomach.—When eating at times seized with hunger, but a very small quantity of food satisfies the appetite.—Constant nausea, with dislike to all food, and diarrhœa.—Fulness, distension, and oppression in pit of stomach, with shortness of breath (as after a full meal, or from over-lifting).

12. Abdomen.—Aching pains in hepatic region.—Violent spasmodic colic, which hinders lying on back or sides, also walking, except very slowly; > on bending thorax forwards.—Pressive colic in epigastrium, or in r. side of abdomen, even at night.—Colic as from eating much fruit and drinking much water after.—Shootings in abdomen, which interrupt respiration.—Dropsical swelling of abdomen, with loss of appetite, scanty urine, hard and knotty fæces.—Ascites, with loss of appetite, scanty urine, hard, knotty stool, which is difficult to pass.—Incarcerated flatulency pressing on bladder, causing cramps in it, and compelling one to walk stooped.—Incarceration of flatus, with spasmodic colic, and cramps in bladder.—Shootings in r. inguinal region, and pressure, as if a hernia were about to protrude.—Swashing like a bladder full of liquid in fold in r. lower abdomen.—Very painful stitches r. groin, > by pressure with hands.

13. Stool and Anus.—Difficult, hard, and knotty fæces.—Diarrhœa; with colic, and copious evacuation of fæcal matter; fæces consisting of mucus, with burning in rectum as from a wound.—Much offensive water involuntarily discharged from rectum at night by one suffering from ascites; whereupon the swelling in r. abdomen steadily decreased, and disappeared in eight days.—Hard stool, intermitting, looking like excrement of dogs, in small lumps, with stitches in rectum extorting cries.—Cramp-like bubbling in rectum while sitting.—Pressive pain as if an angular body were pressed inward on r. side of rectum an inch above anus.—Cramp-like pains in rectum.—Discharge of blood from anus after evacuation.

14. Urinary Organs.—Cramps in bladder, also at night disturbing the sleep.—Tenesmus of bladder, every half-hour for eight hours.—Burning in sphincter vesicæ.—Pain as from suppuration or ulceration; < taking hold of urethra.—Scanty and brown urine.—Stream of urine like a thread, with pressure to stool.—Stream forked.—Hot, corrosive urine.—Bright yellow urine, with whitish, and sometimes a sky-blue coloured sediment.—Strangury.—Continuous urging to urinate, with burning-biting in bladder and urethra; when the effort is made to urinate, burning in urethra, so that one must bend double without being able to urinate.—Urgent desire to urinate; the urine only reaches glans penis and causes there violent pains and spasms, also with tenesmus in rectum; the pain in bladder is momentarily > as soon as the urine descends in the urethra.—Urine reaches glans penis and then returns.—Spasmodic retention of urine.—Tenesmus of bladder.—Violent burning pains in urethra when endeavouring to urinate. —Pain in urethra, as from excoriation, esp. when it is touched.

15. Male Sexual Organs.—Flaccidity of penis, and retraction of prepuce.—Agreeable itching in the scrotum immediately > by scratching.

16. Female Sexual Organs.—Discharge of a watery and pale blood from uterus.—Tickling, itching in region of ovaries, not > by scratching and rubbing.—Metrorrhagia daily for eight to ten weeks, becoming more and more watery the longer it lasted.—Menses watery and thin.—Catamenia too early, and too copious, with sacral pains.—Corrosive leucorrhœa, staining yellow.

17. Respiratory Organs.—Scraping and roughness in throat, with inclination to cough.—Cough excited by a tickling as with a feather, or crawling in larynx and upper part of trachea; cough renewed by holding the breath.—Wheezing cough.—Breathing difficult, caused by a sensation of heaviness in lower part of thorax.—Oppressed, short, difficult, anxious, and panting respiration.—Respiration is continually arrested at pit of stomach.

18. Chest.—Pain in chest, when speaking, with weak voice.—Sensation of heaviness and oppression in chest.—Pains under sternum, and oppression, with fulness in scrobiculus, and distension of abdomen.—Stitching pains in fleshy parts of l. breast on deep inspiration, extends to every side and even above l. shoulder; while walking and sitting.

19. Heart.—Furious beating, even when at rest, and great danger of suffocation from slightest motion; visible pulsation of carotids; face bloated and purple; lips purple; menses suppressed.—Knocking at heart with laboured breathing.—Even very moderate motion < beats of heart fearfully.—Far advanced œdema of feet in girl, 14, with hypertrophy of heart.

20. Neck and Back.—Pressive pain in nape which involves whole occiput on stooping.—All parts of back and small of back seem stiff as if he had been injured.—Stitches between shoulder-blades on drawing a long breath.—Pain in small of back when sitting.—(Pain in small of back as if all strength had gone.—R. T. C.)—Stitch on r. loin to navel, taking away breath; < lying on back.—Pain, as from ulceration in loins.—Stiffness in back and loins, as if caused by a strain.

22. Upper Limbs.—Pressure on r. shoulder, extending to deltoid muscle, preventing one from raising arm.—Soreness of axillary glands.—Tension, wrenching pains, and paralytic sensation in various parts of arms and hands.—Paralytic pains in l. elbow-joint extending to wrist.—R. wrist: wrenching pain during rest; pain as if bruise would form.—Sensation as if sprained in r. thumb, hindering one from writing; cannot hold the pen.—Itching in fingers, as from chilblains.

23. Lower Limbs.—Pains in hips at night, before midnight.—Pain in hip, < forenoon, and free from it after midnight.—Restlessness in legs, has to change the position continually.—Wrenching pains in knees and feet.—Burning sensation in legs.—Pain as from sprain l. ankle.—Pain in first joint of big toe, as if it were pulled out.

24. Generalities.—Shootings in muscles.—Trembling in whole body.—Uneasiness in body, with shortness of breath and oppression of chest.

26. Sleep.—Sleep after a meal.—Retarded sleep and sleeplessness at night.—Waking too early.—Lassitude in morning, as after unrefreshing sleep.—Sleep full of dreams and phantasies.—Dreams of furunculi; or of salt things.

27. Fever.—Shivering, esp. in evening.—Dry heat over the whole body, esp. in genital organs.—Sweat on face only, during sleep.

Prunus Virginiana.

Cerasus virginiana. Choke-cherry. *N. O.* Rosaceæ. Cold infusion or tincture of inner bark. Solution of concentrated resinous extract, Prunin.

Clinical.—Acidity. Anorexia. Dyspepsia. Heart, weakness of ; hypertrophy of ; irritable. Pyrosis.

Characteristics.—Hale says the cold infusion of *Prun. virg.* has been used from time immemorial for irregular, intermittent action of the heart with deficient impulse. Hale adds cough, sympathetic with heart troubles ; dyspepsia with tendency to acidity ; slow digestion ; loss of appetite and pyrosis. Excessive doses have caused "dull, heavy feeling in head" like that of the other Pruneæ. Seymour Tayler (*H. W.*, xxx. 80) says it is especially useful in dilatation of right heart, whether as a result of chronic bronchitis or of mitral stenosis. Laidlaw (*N.Y. Med. Times*, xxiv. 290) gives as a particular indication : Persistent coughs acquired in winter, < *at night on lying down*. Also : Spasmodic and asthmatic coughs, attacks of wheezing and whistling in trachea and large bronchi ; and cough left behind after an attack of influenza. Laidlaw's first case was this : A delicate girl, 20, took cold, which began with coryza and in a few days passed into a cough with scanty expectoration and soreness under sternum. Cough was persistent and annoying at all times, but < *at night*. After many other remedies had failed *Prunin* (the preparation Laidlaw uses), one grain every two hours, relieved in two days and cured in a week. A recurrence some months later was rapidly cured by the same remedy. Burnett used it for weak digestion especially of elderly people. He regarded it as a mild form of *Hcy. ac.* The ϕ tincture, in 5- or 10-drop doses, has been most commonly used.

Psorinum.

Psoricum. The nosode of Psora. [The sero-purulent matter of a scabies vesicle was used by Hahnemann. The product of "Psora sicca" (epidermoid efflorescence of Pityriasis) by Gross. The salt from a product of Psora by Hering.] Triturations.

Clinical.—Acne. *Adenoids.* Anus, itching in. Asthma. Backache. Boils. Cancer. Cholera infantum. Cough. Constipation. Cornea, ulcers of. Crusta lactea. Crusta serpiginosa. *Debility.* Diarrhœa. *Diphtheria, after-effects of.* Dyspepsia. Eczema ; rubrum. Enuresis. Eruptions ; moist ; itching. Gleet. Gonorrhœa. Gout. Hæmorrhages. Hæmorrhoids. Hair, dry ; tangling. *Hay fever.* Headache. Head, congestion of. Hernia. Hydrocele. **Impotence.** *Influenza.* Injuries. *Itch.* Itching. Leucorrhœa. Lienteria. **Liver, affections of** ; chronic inflammation of. Melancholia, religious. **Nose, redness of.** *Odour of body, fetid.* Ophthalmia, scrofulous. Otorrhœa ; fetid. *Ozæna.* Pediculosis. *Perito-*

nitis, tubercular. Plica polonica. ***Polypus.*** **Quinsy. Sciatica. Scurvy. Skin, affections of.** Spina bifida. **Spleen, affections of; induration of. Sprains. Syphilis.** *Throat, mucus in.* Tinea **capitis et faciei. Tonsils, concretions in. Ulcers.**

Characteristics.—As *Sulphur* has been the chief remedial agent in both schools in the treatment of itch and itch-like eruptions, it is natural to find in the nosode of Psora, or constitutional itch, a close analogue of *Sulph. Psorinum* has been proved entirely in the potencies, and I know of no more trustworthy proving in the materia medica. I have frequently seen *Pso.* develop some of its own symptoms in patients whom it has benefited in other ways. A man who complained of "cloudiness of mind and difficult thinking," and who had among other symptoms, "Left foot colder than right," received *Pso.* 30. It removed these symptoms; but whilst under its influence these new symptoms appeared: Heavy headache across the eyebrows; greasiness of face and forehead. A woman to whom I gave *Pso.* 30 complained that after each dose she had a feeling "as if something in the head were being screwed up and drawn"; one of Hahnemann's symptoms is "Spasmodically contracting headache." A patient who took *Pso.* 500 complained that it had a "filthy taste." From *Pso.* 20m (F. C.) I have seen produced an eruption of boil-like indurations in both axillæ, first (and worst) in left then in right. The general symptoms were very greatly relieved at the same time. One great mark of distinction between *Sul.* and *Pso.* is that the *Pso.* patient is exceedingly chilly, likes to have a fur cap on in summer; whilst the *Sul.* patient is predominatingly hot. H. C. Allen gives another: *Pso.* is indicated in *chronic* cases when well-selected remedies fail to relieve or to permanently improve (in *acute* diseases *Sul.*); also when *Sul.* seems indicated but fails to relieve. *Pso.* is *specially suited to*: (1) Scrofulous, nervous, restless persons who are easily startled. (2) Psoric constitutions; lack of reaction after severe diseases. (3) Complaints of psoric origin; patients emit a disagreeable odour. (4) Pale, sickly, delicate children. (5) Peevish, unhealthy-looking children, who have a disagreeable odour about them. (6) Dirty people in whom the body has a filthy smell which no amount of washing can remove. (7) Those subject to diseases of the glands and skin; and who have had eruptions suppressed. The chief of the keynotes of *Pso.* is: Lack of vital reaction; prostration after acute disease, depressed, hopeless, night-sweats. Hopelessness, despair of perfect recovery is part of the lack of reaction; emaciation and foul body odour may accompany it. "Foulness" may be considered the second keynote of *Pso.* Eruptions have offensive discharges; the otorrhœa is horribly offensive. The diarrhœa (especially of cholera infantum) is profuse, watery, dark brown, and even black, and is putrid—smelling like carrion. The ***Med. Visitor*** (xi. 378) collected a number of cases illustrating the action of *Pso.* (I italicise some of the characteristics): (1) W. A. Hawley reports a case of cholera infantum which seemed to defy every remedy. Stools very ***thin and watery, dirty greenish, smelt*** *like carrion.* Child very fretful, had no sleep for two days and nights. *Pso.* 42m (Fincke), one dose in water. In two hours the child went to sleep; in four days it was well without repetition of the dose. (2)

Another case of Hawley's : Miss N., 20, had an eruption in *bends of elbows and knees*, dry, scaly, with little pointed vesicles round the reddened edges ; *disappeared entirely in summer and reappeared when cold weather set in ;* violent *itching*, < *by warmth of bed or by scratching. Pso.* 42m, two doses at six weeks' interval, cured. No return the following winter. *Pso.* also cured—(3) Headache preceded by dimness of sight or spots before eyes (Haynel). (4) Headache and eruptions, < during changeable weather (W. P. Wesselhoeft). (5) Always very hungry during headaches (W. P. W.). (6) Miss C., convalescing from typhoid fever, reported: "Stationary, no appetite." *Pso.* 400 produced immediate change and ravenous appetite (J. B. Bell). (7) Mr. P., 50, complained of nothing but weakness ; no appetite ; *least exertion puts him into a perspiration. Pso.* 40 cured rapidly (J. B. Bell). Mr. X., 21, was obliged one day to run till nearly exhausted. Though strong and well before he now became *weak, perspiring easily*, severe *pains right side*, < *by coughing, laughing, and motion. Pso.* 40 cured rapidly (J. B. Bell). [I have frequently verified the action of *Pso.* in liver affections with pains as in the last case.] (8) *Extreme dulness ; fears inflammation of brain ;* > *by nose-bleed.* Headache following darkness before eyes. Black spots before eyes. *Pso.* cured (Haynel). (9) *Horribly offensive*, nearly painless, *almost involuntary, dark and watery stool ; only in night and most towards morning* (H. N. Martin). (10) Mr. C., 43, spare, dark. Hypochondriacal. "Nervous" nine months. Had to give up business. Took much *Quinine* and other drugs. Complains of very disagreeable feeling about the head and manifests mental *depression ; thinks he will never recover ;* has *lost all hope.* Cannot apply his mind to business. Seems confused ; cannot reckon. *Numbness of legs and arms*, < *left side ;* < *going to bed*, formication and crawling with prickling and smarting on scalp, and same on extremities. Tongue coated white. After three months treatment was stationary. It was then ascertained that he *sweated very easily on least exertion, and somewhat at night*, and had loss of memory. *Pso.* 400 soon caused improvement, and enabled the patient to return to business (J. B. Bell). G. A. Whippy (*Am. Hom.*, xxiii. 391) cured the following case with *Pso.* 200, a dose every third night : Carpenter, 40, long-standing discharge of reddish cerumen from left ear, < at night. Sensation of valve opening and shutting in left ear, < afternoon. Buzzing in ear, which stopped suddenly and was followed by violent itching. Dull, heavy pain in base of brain in afternoon, with sensation as though skin of abdomen was greatly relaxed and drawn down. Face sallow and *greasy ;* several pustules on chin and neck which itch intensely and bleed when scratched.—Other leading indications of *Pso.* are : Sick babies will not sleep day or night, but worry, fret, cry ; or good and play all day, restless, troublesome, screaming all night. Weakness from loss of fluids ; after acute disease ; with or without organic lesion. Whole body painful, easily sprained and injured. Great sensitiveness to cold air, change, storms ; to sun ; restless for days before a thunderstorm. A symptom not seldom met with in practice and useful to remember is : "Feels unusually well day before attack." Headache > by eating ; from suppressed menses ; > by nose-bleed. Dry, lustreless hair ; plica polonica. Acne < during menses ; from fats, sugar, coffee, meat. Quinsy, throat burns, feels scalded, cutting, tearing, intense pain on swallowing, profuse, offensive saliva ; tough mucus in throat ; must hawk continually ; tendency to quinsy. Profuse sweat after acute diseases, with > of ail suffering. Skin has dirty look as if never washed. *Pso.* has cured more cases of hay fever in my practice than any other single remedy. Many cases have a psoric basis, and when the basic taint is corrected the irritating agents have no effect. Nasal polypus I have also cured with *Pso.* when the general symptoms indicate the remedy. *Peculiar Sensations* are : As if frightened. As if he would lose his senses. As if stupid in left half of head. As if brain had not room enough in forehead. Eyes as if pressed outward. As from heavy blow on forehead. As if brain would protrude. Back of head as if sprained. Right side of occiput as if dislocated. As if piece of wood lying across back of head. As if head separated from body. As if sand in eyes. As if he heard with ears not his own. Cheek-bones as if ulcerated. Condyle of jaw as if lame. Tongue as if burnt. Teeth as if glued together. Plug in throat. Throat as if narrowing. As if intestines hanging down. Everything in chest as if raw, scratched ; torn loose. Arms as if paralysed. Hip-joint as if ulcerated. Joints as if encased in armour ; as if would not hold together. Hands and feet as if broken. The pains of *Pso.* may be erratic and alternate (headache and toothache). The symptoms are < by touch ; pressure (of truss) ; rubbing ; scratching ; riding ; bandage ; blow ; fall. Slight emotions = severe ailments. (*Pso.* cannot bear to have the limbs touch each other at night ; or weight of arms on chest.) > When eating ; < immediately after (rush of blood to head). < After cold drinks (pain in chest). Drinking = cough. > Lying down (most ailments, especially of chest ; but < cough, and = gurgling at heart). < Lying r. side (liver). < Riding in carriage or exercising in open air ; (riding > short breath). > By rest and in room. Overlifting = thoughts to vanish. < Walking ; moving. < Evening and before midnight ; night ; morning on waking. Open air < (> taste ; cough ; itching) ; nose sensitive inhaling. < Before thunderstorm (restless for days before). Winter = cough. Summer = diarrhœa ; itching eruptions. < During full moon (enuresis). < Periodically.

Relations.—*Antidoted by :* Coffee. *Compatible :* Carb. v., Chi., Sul. (if Sul. is indicated but fails to act give Pso.). *Followed well by :* Alm., Borax, Hep. *Complementary :* Sul., Bac. (Bac. is the *acute* of Pso.), after Lact. ac. (vomiting of pregnancy) ; after Arn. (blow on ovary) ; Sul. after Pso. in mammary cancer. *Inimical :* Lach. *Compare :* Sick babies fret day and night (Jalap) ; good all day, screams all night (Lyc. opp.). Effect of thunderstorm, Pho. Headache preceded by dim vision, Lac d., K. bi. Headache with hunger ; > while eating, Anac., K. ph. ; > nose-bleed, Melilot. Plica polonica, Lyc., Bar. c., Sars., Bac. Offensive, cheesy concretions from throat, K. mur. > By sweat, Calad., Nat. m. > Lying down and keeping arms stretched far apart (Ars. opp.). < Mornings on waking and evenings lying down, Pho., Bac. Eruptions easily suppurate, Hep. Drinking = cough (> Caust.). Drinking <, Dig. Teeth stick together (Tub. teeth feel jammed together). Pediculosis, Ped., Bac., Nat. m. Earthy, greasy face, Nat. m., Bry. Erratic pains ; < from fats, < evening, Puls. Tongue as if burnt, Sang. As if parts separated, Ars. (body at waist), Bap. (limbs). Convalescence, profuse sweat, K. ca. (K. ca. has not the hopelessness of Pso.). Despair of recovery, Chi., Lauro. (chest), Caps., Op., Val., Amb. Lack of reaction, Op. (patient not sensitive), Lauro. (over-excitable and nervous), Carb. v. (emaciated, weak pulse ; Pso. psoric diathesis). Hay fever, Gels. (morning sneezing), K. iod. Hunger at night, Chi. s., Pho., Sul., Ign., Lyc. Axillary affections, Jug. c., Jug. r., Elaps. Crusta lactea, Melitagrinum. Explosion in ear, Alo.

Causation.—Emotions. Over-lifting. Mental labour. Repelled eruptions. Stormy weather. Thunderstorm. Injuries. Blows. Sprains. Dislocations.

SYMPTOMS.

1. **Mind.**—Good-humour in morning ; works with pleasure ; enjoys everything.—Excitable before sleep.—Excitable, vexed with everything.—Fear.—Anxiety : when riding in a carriage ; with trembling of hands and restlessness.—Melancholy : religious ; she could commit suicide, then is full of phantasms, peevishness, and lachrymation ; alternating suddenly with liveliness.—Despair : fear of failing in business ; wishes to die in spite of the best hopes.—Driven to despair by excessive itching.—Ill-humour : in morning ; and constant thoughts of dying ; could weep about everything.—Quarrelsome.—Every moral emotion = trembling.—Disinclination to work ; to ride in a carriage, then desire to ride all the time, even in bad weather.—Sentimental.—Inability to rid himself of ideas which first appeared to him in a dream.—Thinking that he understood what he had read he tried to explain it, and found that he did not understand it.—Memory lost ; so that she does not recognise the room after looking out of the window.—Thoughts vanish after over-lifting.

2. **Head.**—Vertigo : mornings ; everything turns around with him ; with headache, confusion, roaring in ears.—Sticking in head, with weakness, had to lie down towards 7 p.m., and soon fell asleep, copious sweat at night, which >.—Thrusts in head.—Tearing in head (which he formerly had) this time with fever and general arthritic pains.—Headache : in evening ; with eructations ; with thirst, coldness, and dryness of mouth and lips ; intermittent ; spasmodically contracting ; as if a hammer were beating in head, esp. unilateral (in a herpetic patient) ; as if everything would protrude through forehead towards evening.—Fulness during mental labour.—Congestion of brain, > nose-bleed.—Cloudy feeling in night on waking, as if he had been intoxicated in evening, with stupor and tumbling about.—Heaviness in morning.—Weakness of head.—Pulsation of blood during mental labour.—Sticking in l. side of forehead ; in r. side extending into eye.—R. side of head and r. eye swollen and painful as if it would burst.—Drawing in forehead extending to nose.—Pinching in upper forehead beginning morning in bed, < morning and evening, with heaviness, sometimes whole sinciput aches and then temples feel pressed in, afterwards it alternates suddenly with pain in molars, < walking in fresh air.—Pain in centre of forehead ; with weakness

of it.—Pain in sinciput, < temples, < steady mental exertion, > motion, esp. in open air, < morning and evening, with heaviness in sinciput, often it suddenly passes off and attacks l. molars.—Pain as if brain had not space enough in morning on rising, > washing and breakfast; contracting pain.—Drawing in sinuses as in coryza.—Stupefied feeling in l. forehead in morning.—Shooting from l. temple into head.—Boring in l. temple.—Pain in temples: after mental exertion; hammering; crampy, in skin of r. at 7.30 p.m.—Fulness in vertex as if brain would burst, with formication in head followed by heavy sleep.—Intermittent pain in a spot in vertex.—Strained pain in r. side of occiput at noon.—Pain in occiput as if a piece of wood lay across from r. to l. —Feeling as of a cord around skin, < about occiput, which feels as if pressed outward.—Always hungry during headache.—Congestion of blood to head immediately after dinner.—Headache < by change of weather; if it changes in night the headache wakens him.—Hair: dry, lustreless; tangles easily; glues together.—Spot of white skin with white lock of hair becomes natural colour under *Pso.*—Sensation as if head separated from body.—Averse to having head uncovered; wears a fur cap in hot weather.—Viscid sweat about head.—Humid eruptions.—Tinea capitis et faciei.—Crusta serpiginosa.—Rawness and soreness behind ears.—Humid, scabby eruption, full of lice.

3. **Eyes.**—Eyes: gummy; surrounded by blue rings; glassy, with pain in them; agglutination in morning.—Swelling of lids and of face.—Inflammation of r. eye.—Pain in r. eye as if it would burst.—R. eye feels melting away. —Ophthalmia, with pain as from sand in eyes, and lachrymation at night.—Sticking: in l. eye; pain in r. eye, < touch.—Pain in eyes with burning, in evening when looking sharply at something, and by candle-light.—Pain as from sand, or foreign body (in r. evening when closed).—Biting in eyes.—Tired in evening as from much reading by candle-light.—Lachrymation: towards evening; on looking long at one object.—Pimples: like hordeola on upper lid; red, like fresh hordeola on margin of upper lids, and sensation as if something were moving before the eyes, as if one were playing with his fingers before them.—Itching: of r. lid; l. lower lid, from one side to other; of canthi; inner canthi, with heat.—Vision of sparks.—All objects in room appear to tremble.—Dazzling in evening when walking in street.—Vision blurred suddenly.

4. **Ears.**—Discharge of fetid pus (l.).—Otorrhœa, with headache.—Discharge of reddish cerumen from l. ear.—Sticking: towards noon; in l. lobe in evening; in l. after the buzzing; in meatus internus, transiently > boring in with finger, frequently returning, < evening during rest.—Intermittent tearing through external meatus, as from temporal muscle to styloid process. —Pain: in r. ear, in morning; ulcerative, in l., and at the same time on r. ear a pimple appearing like healthy skin, but split into four parts by a cross like a wart, in the centre a deep indentation.—L. concha inwardly inflamed, with suppurating pimples.—Sensation as if something burst suddenly when eating or swallowing saliva.—Sensation in l. ear as if breath came from it instead of from respiratory organs.—Feeling as if stuffed with cotton, forenoons.—Biting in l. ear.—Itching in r. ear.—Coldness in r. ear, then sticking.—Ringing: in l. ear, evening; in r. or l., with buzzing in head so that she hears hardly anything, and behind ears in region of sterno-cleido-mastoideus, a sore pain, sometimes heat extending to vertex, < towards evening, when she feels as if

pulled by the hair.—Roaring so that he feels stupefied.—Buzzing in ears.—Feeling in r. ear as if he heard with the ears of another person, evening.

5. **Nose.**—Inflammation of septum, with white pustules.—Sticking in l. nostril when boring in with finger.—Boring in r. nostril, then sneezing.—Drawing extending up to frontal sinuses, with pain in eyes as if coryza would set in, then discharge of fluid from nose.—Dry coryza ; nostrils nearly dry, and sensitive when breathing through them.—Scratching crawling towards root of nose as if coryza would set in.—Stoppage of nose.—Sneezing ; without coryza.—Coryza : with cough and expectoration of yellowish green mucus ; dry ; dry with obstruction of nose ; fluent ; fluent, from l. nostril.—Tough mucus, he can hardly do a minute without his handkerchief, without coryza, with feeling of a plug high up in nose, which nauseates him, > stooping.—Clear, watery fluid pours out, < l. nostril, < stooping.—Nose red.

6. **Face.**—Face pale ; sickly looking ; yellow.—Congestion to head, cheeks and nose red and hot.—Pain in zygoma on touch as if bone were suppurating, in evening.—Sticking in lower jaw.—Pain as if lame in condyle of jaw.—Crusta lactea.—Coppery eruption on face.—Roughness of skin of face ; eruption on forehead between eyes ; offensive stools.—Swelling of upper lip.—Dryness of lips ; and brown and black colour.—Burning of lips ; painful and seem swollen.—Pimple on upper lip.—Vesicles around corner of mouth, and outwardly above them larger sore spots, exuding a fluid which seemed to originate from scratching the vesicles, and cause continual scratching.—Corners of mouth sore, often ulcerated ; sycotic condylomata.—Yellow vesicles on red edge of lower lip sore on touch.—Clear vesicles on inner surface of lower lip.—Painful itching on r. half of upper lip as if swollen.

7. **Teeth.**—Looseness of teeth, < incisors, so that he fears they will fall out, the pain < by touch, > open air, with much mucus of an offensive odour in mouth.—Blood suddenly escapes from a hollow molar.—Sticking from one side to the other, extending to head, then burning pain in r. cheek, which is swollen.—Stitching in teeth on touching them in order to remove something lodged between them.—Sticking in a carious r. upper tooth as if it would be pulled, at dinner, then grumbling and hammering pain in all r. teeth, only in daytime, > fresh air.—Tearing ; jerking in l. molars, sometimes only slight pain alternating with headache.—Teeth seem on edge in afternoon when smoking.

8. **Mouth.**—Ulceration of r. gum after toothache.—Inflammation of gum of a posterior r. hollow lower molar, with swelling and crawling pain, < touch.—Tongue : coated ; white ; yellowish white.—Ulceration of tongue and gums, with sore throat.—Tongue : dry ; at tip, as if burnt, painful ; burnt feeling from tip to middle, so that he has hardly any taste.—Thick, tough mucus from choanæ ; of nauseous taste ; teeth stick together.—Adhesion of tough mucus to posterior wall of soft palate, tasting like old cheese, coming from choanæ. –Scratching in back part of mouth, and when leaning backward asthmatic feeling.—Swollen sensation in palate.—Dryness of mouth.—Taste : bitter mornings before eating, > eating ; when not eating ; > eating and drinking ; bad, finally coppery ; like cat's urine to bread and butter in morning ; oily to the dinner ; flat, insipid ; foul, she drinks to get rid of it ; filthy.—Increase of the nauseous taste after eating and smoking tobacco.—Sticky taste.

9. **Throat.**—Submaxillary glands swollen and painful to touch, also a painful pustule below l. lower jaw.—Angina, on r. side an ulcer, with sore pain deep in throat and burning in palate.—Painful pimple on fauces.—Stitches : in l. tonsil ; in l. sinews on turning head.—Pain in l. tonsil, with swollen feeling.—Quinsy, intense pain to ears on swallowing, profuse, offensive saliva ; tough mucus in throat, must hawk continually ; tendency to quinsy.—Hawks up cheesy balls, size of pea, of disgusting taste and carrion-like odour.—Pain on swallowing saliva.—Intermittent pain and difficult swallowing.—Soreness with difficulty in swallowing ; can take without difficulty only cold food.—Scraping in throat as if she would become hoarse (in a herpetic patient) ; with suffocation, causing dry cough.—Burning in throat ; extending farther downward.—Dryness of throat : in morning, with scraping ; of fauces, with moisture in mouth.—Swollen feeling in fauces.—Sensation of plug in throat, impeding hawking.—Tickling in throat : mornings ; causing cough ; then empty eructations.

10. **Appetite.**—Hunger great ; in afternoon, with thirst for beer ; in evening after a walk : in evening ; for breakfast.—Hunger without appetite —Appetite diminished.—Easily satiated though he has a good appetite.—Loss of appetite, but constant thirst.—Disgust for pork.—Desire to smoke in evening, but when not smoking the desire for it ceased.—Desire for acids.—Aversion to smoking after breakfast, but when he begins smoking is relished —Thirst : during dinner ; after the chill, then heat in mouth ; with dryness and burning in mouth ; for beer.—Eating (dinner) = congestion to head.—Drinking = cough.

11. **Stomach.**—Eructations : tasting like rotten eggs ; sour ; rancid in evening.—Pyrosis ; after drinking water ; when lying down, colic > eating —Hiccough : after eating ; when smoking a pipe after eating.—Waterbrash on lying down, > getting up.—Nausea : during the day, a kind of vomiting of sweet mucus every day at 10 a.m. and in evening ; in morning ; in pit of stomach in morning ; after all food ; after supper, > eating something roasted.—Vomiting : sour ; of sour mucus, so that teeth are on edge, in morning before eating ; of food, then of a sour, slimy fluid.—Bloating.—Sticking in pit of stomach.—Cramp in epigastric region ; cutting.—Oppression.—Contracting pain in epigastric region.—Weakness and pressure.

12. **Abdomen.**—Deep-seated, stitching, pressing pains in region of liver < external pressure and lying on r. side ; pain hinders sneezing, laughing yawning, coughing, deep inspiration and walking.—Sticking : in sides of abdomen ; r. side ; region of spleen ; under last l. rib ; in hepatic region region of spleen, > standing still, renewed by walking, later felt even during rest.—Swollen sensation horizontally across below short ribs when sitting.—Abdomen bloated : after eating ; after eating frozen things.—Constant feeling of emptiness and looseness of abdomen ; sensation as if intestines were hanging down.—Rumbling in morning ; gurgling and roaring.—Foul-smelling flatus.—Cutting in abdomen ; in evening, > passage of offensive flatus ; as from a purge.—Cramps in abdomen in morning in bed.—Griping : when driving ; in women, < pubic region.—Pinching in abdomen in morning, so that he has to run for the closet, > stool.—Pain in abdomen ; towards evening, > eating ; after eating, > emission of flatus, with nausea ; and in lumbar vertebræ, with flatulent troubles, pain in spermatic cords and testicles as i

filled with blood, a soft, difficult stool.—Pain as from canine hunger, < epigastric region, an hour after supper, with accumulation of flatus.—Frequent sticking to l. of umbilicus during rest.—Cutting in umbilical region.—Gurgling in small intestines.—Twitching in r. groin after driving.—Sticking in inguinal glands.—Pain in r. inguinal ring.—Bearing down towards pubes, with tenesmus and painful burning micturition.

13. **Stool and Anus.**—Stool: fluid, dark brown, foul-smelling; thin, watery, dirty greenish, like carrion; horribly offensive, nearly painless, almost involuntary, dark and watery; only in night, < towards morning.—Diarrhœa preceded by colic; green, bilious, mixed with mucus; four times a day, without pain.—Involuntary stools during sleep.—Lienteria.—Soft, difficult stool; and copious.—Obstinate constipation, with severe pains.—Stools: either costive or mushy: of normal consistency, in small balls, almost involuntary, at night, with violent emission of flatus; two in forenoon; four or five a day, preceded by colic; sometimes shooting away as from a syringe, at another time it is mushy, sometimes of normal consistency.—Stool wanting.—Spasmodic pain in rectum.—Burning high up in rectum.—Sensitive hæmorrhoidal pain in rectum.—Chafed sensation in rectum and anus during a drive.—Ineffectual urging.—Burning hæmorrhoids in anus.—Itching in anus.

14. **Urinary Organs.**—Discharge of prostatic fluid before micturition.—Tenesmus urinæ and discharge of a few drops when he thinks he has done.—Frequent micturition at night.—Sticking inwardly from orifice of urethra.—Burning during micturition with cutting.—Urine has a red sediment and a pellicle of fat.

15. **Male Sexual Organs.**—Relaxation of genitals; with indifference to sexual affairs.—Aversion to coitus.—Impotency.—No discharge of semen during coition.—Glans inflamed, with an ulcer on it, testes swollen and heavy.—Burning pain at tip of penis on beginning to urinate.—Chronic painless discharge from urethra, staining linen yellow.—Chronic gleet.—Frequent tightness of penis, with drawing.—Absence of erections; even with lascivious thoughts, afterwards morning erections and pollutions, with satyriasis.—Drawing in testicles, but more steady in small of back.—Painful suppurating vesicle on scrotum.—Hydrocele: from repeated inflammation caused by pressure of truss (*Puls.* cured the inflammation).

16. **Female Sexual Organs.**—Menses too late; and scanty.—Amenorrhœa; in psoric subjects; with phthisis.—Dysmenorrhœa; near climaxis.—Leucorrhœa; large lumps; unbearable in odour; violent pains in sacrum and r. loin; great debility.—Intolerable itching from anus to vagina, with knotty stools, < at night.—Ulcers on labia.—L. ovary indurated from a blow.—Sensitive knotty lump above r. groin.—Cutting in l. groin.—During pregnancy: congestion; fœtus moves too violently; tympanites; nausea, vomiting; obstinate cases.—Breasts swollen; nipples red; burning and itching pimples about nipples.—Mammary cancer.

17. **Respiratory Organs.**—Hoarseness; when talking phlegm sticks in larynx.—Talking is very fatiguing.—Suffocating, crawling sensation in larynx, producing a paroxysmal, dry, hacking cough.—Tickling in trachea, with cough.—Inclination to cough, with sensation of coldness.—Cough in evening, > keeping quiet, with pain in chest and throat, talking = cough.—Cough with weakness of chest; so that he could not remain in bed at night,

with weakness and vertigo.—Dry cough : all day, with nausea and retching and tickling in throat ; from tickling in trachea, as if narrowing ; with soreness under sternum ; with heaviness on chest.—Cough, < morning on waking, and in evening on lying down, with expectoration of green mucus, nearly like matter, with nausea, chest is affected and expectoration is difficult ; with copious expectoration ; sometimes of mucus streaked with blood ; with salivation and vomiting of acid mucus.—Suffocation in larynx when sitting bent backward, with crawling, causing paroxysmal, dry, hacking cough, and at same time contraction and heaviness in chest and pain in upper part of sternum.—Dyspnœa in evening.—Short breath ; in fresh air, > riding and lying down.—Want of breath on walking in fresh air ; < sitting, > lying, with pain in chest.—Whistling respiration on waking, with constriction, again in evening whistling in chest.—Breathes easily when doing some light work, as trimming trees.

18. **Chest.**—Twitching through l. chest, anterior side.—Sticking : in l. chest ; l. mamma ; under l. false ribs ; in r. side on coughing or breathing ; even when not breathing ; in sternum on deep breathing, and on touch a pressing and bruised pain.—Feeling as if everything in it were torn when lifting.—Pain as if a lung had been torn loose and something were pressing it down.—Cutting as with knives ; in evening, with burnt feeling in throat, eructations, then emission of flatus.—Boring in r. chest, with oppressed breathing.—Pain under sternum when coughing as if something would be torn away, extending to throat.—Pain on spots ; ulcerative pain under sternum ; pain as from a load, < bending head forward, with want of breath.—Oppression ; pressure ; contracted feeling in chest.—Dull feeling in chest, with pain in back.—When in bed has to remove the arms as far as possible from chest, otherwise they increase the pain.—Hot sensation in chest.—Suppuration of lungs.—Chronic blennorrhœa of lungs.—Hydrothorax.

19. **Heart.**—Stitches in cardiac region, low gurgling extending to heart, for a moment breathing is impossible.—Pain in heart > lying down ; thinks the stitches will kill him if they continue.—Gurgling in heart region esp. noticeable when lying down.—Pericarditis.—Palpitation ; with anxious oppression.—Pulse : weak ; irritable, indicating a return of abscesses on neck.

20. **Neck and Back.**—Glands of neck swollen, and on touch bruised pain extending to head.—Sticking in neck, with pustules.—Herpetic eruption on side of neck extending from cheek.—Nape excoriated by discharge from eczema capitis.—Tearing in nape.—Boring in nape, with stiffness.—Pain in nape in afternoon, only in the house, when supporting head with hands it feels as if it had no body, as if he could pass through it with the hands.—Pain in muscles of r. neck, in their upper sinewy part, as from sudden tension, on turning head to r. backward or sideways, > pressure.—Tensive pain in nape after waking, as if he had lain in an uncomfortable position.—Drawing pain extending to shoulder, after waking.—Sticking in back ; extending towards chest on coughing.—Boring in vertebræ in morning, with colic, as from rheumatism.—Aching in back ; bruised feeling in evening, cannot straighten it.—Scapulæ : sticking between in morning ; tearing ; rheumatic sticking tearing in and between, down sides.—Boring in dorsal vertebræ ; pain between second and third in afternoon.—Sticking : in loins extending to knee in morning ; in os pubis during bodily exertion.—Cutting in loins so that she

could not walk alone.—Pain in loins; and itching; like molimina hæmorrhoidalia, < motion, so that he could not walk straight comfortably; as if third vertebra from below were wanting or broken.—Drawing in loins, and sometimes in testicles.—Tightness in ischii when walking, extending to knees.—Weakness of loins.—Backache: with constipation; after suppressed eruption.—Spina bifida.

21. **Limbs.**—Trembling of hands and feet.—Stretching.—Tearing: in l. knee and shoulder; intermittent, in joints, in humerus, knee, and toes, > motion.—Wandering pains, < tibiæ and soles, also in finger-joints, at times in r. patella, > motion.—Weakness of joints as if they would not hold together.

22. **Upper Limbs.**—Tearing in l. shoulder in afternoon and evening when resting.—Tearing in arm; intermittent sticking in l. arm.—Arm and shoulder swell up from an old eczema-patch on left wrist, and immediate relief follows dose of *Pso.* (R. T. C.)—Spasmodic pain in bones of l. arm in evening at rest.—Sensation in l. arm, in morning in bed, as if asleep with crawling in fingers; with numbness of three first fingers and half of hand. —Tearing in elbow; r. in evening.—Sticking in l. index.—Tetter on arm, with small, millet-like eruption, exuding a yellow fluid; itches intensely in heat.—Eruption in bends of elbows and around wrists.—Itch-like eruptions on wrists, with rheumatism in limbs.—Trembling of hands.—Swelling and tension of backs of hands and of fingers.—Pustules on hands, near finger-ends, suppurating.—Copper-coloured eruption or red blisters on backs of hands.—Itching between fingers; vesicles.—Herpes on palms. —Sweat on palms, esp. at night.—Warts, size of pin's head, on l. hand and fingers.—Nails brittle.

23. **Lower Limbs.**—Pain in hip-joints as if dislocated, < when walking, with weak arms.—Sciatica: tension down to knee while walking.—Paralysis of legs from suppression of eruption on arms.—Legs, < tibiæ and soles, pain as from too much walking, mornings in bed, > rising, with restlessness of legs.—Leg on which he lies in bed too weak to endure the pressure of the other, he has to change his position continually.—Sensation in r. leg as if it would go to sleep.—Tibiæ and soles feel bruised, as after a tiring walk, mornings in bed.—Sticking in r. ankle in morning on every step with strained sensation.—Feet, trembling; inclination to turn l. inward when walking, with sensation as if he really had turned it the wrong way.—Pain in feet < during rest, with itching.—Gouty pain in l. foot.—Cramp or spasm in toes, < l. great toe, when stretching them or taking off boots.

24. **Generalities.**—Looks pale, exhausted, thin, his clothing is too large for him.—Hot trembling over whole body in morning during rush of business.—R. side of body full of burning pains.—Soreness.—Gouty pains in l. toe, both knees, and back.—Stormy weather affects him, = restlessness in his blood a few days beforehand; makes him sick and = hæmorrhoidal troubles. —Weakness: towards evening, > going to bed; after riding in a waggon; from a little labour.—Sensation when in the sun as if it pushed her down, she had to rest in the shade in order to walk on.—Heaviness of whole body as before intermittent fever.—> Morning; in fresh air; when lying.

25. **Skin.**—Rash: above l. brow and on l. cheek; red, on external throat, beginning with sticking.—Nodules on face, neck, and legs.—Pimples: on

forehead ; on neck and mammæ ; with black points in centre, painful when scratched ; on external throat.—Burning like heat-rash below eyes ; causing itching, smarting pain, burning after scratching, and feeling sore (in a herpetic patient) ; and ulcers, from which watery fluid oozed for hours after being opened, < hands, wrists, and palms.—It < herpes and causes smarting and itching.—A scab on nose which commonly fell off when coughing is now adherent and hard.—Pustules on nape, with sticking.—Boils on chest and loins ; on buttocks, with burning itching, soon disappearing, leaving crusts.—Itch-like eruption on face, hand, back, and leg, and agglutination of eyes.—Vesicles : on face ; quickly filling with yellow lymph, sore to touch on forehead, face, and behind r. ear ; filled with lymph, painful to touch on various parts, some forming itching papules.—An old rhagade near r. styloid process suppurated, itched, and was surrounded by blisters filled with clear water, these soon changed to pustules, which healed under a crust.—Crawling on all limbs, with falling asleep of them.—Itching : on forehead ; tip of nose ; l. arm ; biceps of l. arm ; r. elbow ; soles in evening after a glass of Muscat wine, with tickling and heat ; of face, neck, and hands on touch ; over whole body after rubbing papules and vesicles ; between fingers, and vesicles filled with lymph ; on r. carpus, with red spots ; voluptuous, where a flea had bitten, with white, hard blisters on a red base.—< Of the itching, which he had had for years on knees, < l., and the herpetic eruption begins to become pustular.

26. Sleep.—Yawning : at noon ; and shivering pale blue rings, with tearing and spasmodic pains in umbilical region in evening ; in evening, with early sleepiness.—Sleepy all the time ; in daytime ; early.—Sleeps when she sits down.—Sleep unusually sound.—Cannot fall asleep in evening.—Cannot sleep on the habitual r. side, but sleeps on l.—Gnashing of teeth at night, so that he wakes.—Restless sleep ; and unrefreshing.—Sleep restless but refreshing.—Restless sleep on account of disquiet dreams.—Dreams : anxious in morning, of robbers, travels, and dangers ; uneasy, earnest ; that he is on the closet, and thus nearly soils his bed ; of his business and of his plans.

27. Fever.—Coldness < evening, with hot flashes, debility, and sleepiness.—Coldness with heat, thirst, and sweat.—Internal coldness towards noon, with shivering and horripilation.—Creeping coldness in afternoon, with internal shivering.—Horripilations.—Feet cold all night.—Heat : in afternoon ; in evening when riding in a carriage, with sweat ; of whole body suddenly, at meals and in evening, with trickling sweat all over face, frequent thirst, dryness, and burning in mouth.—Heat in evening, as if she would lose her senses, at night delirium, thirst, and sweat, then she feels well.—Burning : in head ; in forehead ; in nose, transiently > by discharge of mucus.—Burning in nose, then fluent coryza.—Burning in face, then vesicles.—Burning in r. ear with itching.—Sweat : on waking ; in morning when out of doors ; with consequent debility, and taking cold easily ; sweat on palms ; on face ; on palms at night ; perinæum on moving about.—Want of sweat, dry skin.

Ptelea.

Ptelea trifoliata. Shrubby Trefoil. Hop Tree. Wafer Ash. *N. O.* Xanthoxylaceæ of the Rutaceæ. Tincture of bark of root.

Clinical.—Asthma. Constipation. Dysentery. Dyspepsia. Erysipelas. Gall-stones. Gastralgia. Headache, gastric; bilious. Intermittents. Jaundice. Liver, congestion of. Nightmare. Phosphaturia. Rheumatism. Spleen, affections of. Worms.

Characteristics.—*Ptelea* is the Greek name for the Elm, and was applied by Linnæus to a genus of shrubs and small trees, natives of North America and Asia, and included in *Xanthoxylaceæ*. In Canada the young green shoots of *Pte. tri.* are used as an anthelmintic in the form of an infusion. The fronds are bitter and aromatic, and have been used as a substitute for hops (*Treas. of Bot.*). One of the provers of *Pte.* confirmed its anthelmintic powers by "a very copious expulsion of ascarides." The proving was very thorough and extensive, and T. Nichol, Burt, and Cowperthwaite were among the provers. A very marked action was produced on the liver, and Nichol, one of the provers, values it highly (says Hale) in "hepatic difficulties, and in those erysipelatous and urticarious eruptions that are so often concomitant with affections of the liver." Hale says it has not the violent action of *Pod.* or *Ir. v.*, but "a slow, pervading" action, and causes chronic ailments. He has found it useful in "bilious headache, dyspepsia, gastralgia, congestion of the liver, chronic hepatitis, and chronic erysipelas." Others have used it in chronic rheumatism, dysentery, and constipation. Hale says the oily constituent of *Pte.* resembles Turpentine; and one of the most marked symptoms of the proving is: "Pressure as from a stone in pit of stomach," recalling *Abies n.* and the conifers. In the proving the liver was swollen and tender, but there was > lying on right side, and < lying on left. [H. K. Leonard (*H. R.*, xiii. 468) cured a seemingly hopeless case with *Pte.* 1 x on this symptom: Weight, aching distress, dull pain in hepatic region, > lying on right side; turning on left = a dragging as if liver pulling on its ligaments.] The "dull, muddled head" is another liver symptom. J. Preston (*B. J. H.*, xlii. 71) cured with *Pte.* a case of jaundice following gall-stones, with great emaciation.—Aching distress; general aching and soreness; malaise. A number of *alternating* symptoms were noted. Nervous pains alternating from left arm to left eye and temple. Liveliness alternates with sadness. As gastric symptoms improved difficulty of breathing came on. There is the ravenous hunger of the antipsorics; empty sensations in œsophagus, in stomach. Sensitive to light, sound, to open air. Enlarged feelings were noted: head feels large; fingers feel numb, and large and clumsy. Headache with hunger, especially on awaking, may prove a keynote. Right (liver) side most affected. The symptoms are < in hot room; > in cold air. < After sleep; on awaking. After eating, feeling of liveliness. After breakfast: distress in stomach, headache and hunger >; one hour after, <. > After eating acid things. < From cheese ; butter ; pudding. General < after eating. > Morning and evening ; < afternoon. < Lying down ; lying l. side ; > lying r. side. < Walking ; speaking ; mental exertion ; moving eyes ; raising eyebrows, before, during, and after stool. Headache > after stool. Straining at stool < vertigo. Coughing = feeling as if head would burst.

Relations.—*Compare:* Xanthox. Headache at base of brain, Ipec. Congestion of brain with feeling of weight in right hypochondrium and liver enlarged, Mag. m. (Pte. > lying right side). Weak mind, peevish, irritable, sensitive, tenesmus, must lie down, Nux, Bry. (Bry. has large stool, Pte. small, hard balls ; both have > lying right side ; Bry. < least attempt to breathe, Pte. on *deep* inspiration only ; Nux has < lying on painful (r.) side and large stool). Eructations like rotten eggs, aversion to meat, longing for acids, Arn. (with Arn. eating = *fulness;* with Pte. it = epigastric *pain and goneness*). Periodic < of gastric symptoms 3 to 4 a.m., Nux (Nux desires fat, Pte. loathes it ; Pte. predominating *bitter* taste, Nux *sour;* Pte. feels effect of food at once, Nux two hours after ; Pte. dysenteric tenesmus before and *after* stool, Nux tenesmus ceases after stool). Head symptoms < straining at stool, Indm. Headache with cough, Caps., Bry., Nat. m. Noise almost = spasms, Asar. Impressions of sounds remain long in ears (images of objects seen remain long, Lac c., Nic.). Pain like a stone at epigastrium, Ab. n., Bry. Sensation as if abdomen retracted, Pb. (Pb. abdomen *hard*, Pte. *soft*). < After sleep Lach. Dreams of fighting, Nat. s. Scalded tongue, Sang., Pod. Clumsy fingers, Bovist. Liver, &c., Hydrast. ; Berb.

Causation.—Repelled eruption (asthma).

SYMPTOMS.

1. Mind.—Liveliness after eating, followed by depression an hour later.—Depression, anxiety, and tendency to worry.—Irritable ; nervous, sudden noise startles and = headache.—Unusual energy with disposition to hurry.—Thoughts chase each other through the mind, impossible to fix attention.—Dull, stupid, dazed, confused, muddled feeling in head.—Malaise of mind and body ; indisposed to physical or mental exertion.—Sudden shrinking from mental work, with sickness and faintness.—Memory weak : for things ; and names.

2. Head.—Head confused, giddy, weak.—Vertigo : with rumbling and swelling in umbilical region ; < straining at stool ; > slow motion, < sudden motion ; < turning head ; < walking ; on rising ; with piercing pain through brain.—Fits of vertigo, > bending head down and closing eyes.—Head light ; or heavy and full.—Severe dull headache, < motion ; < warm room.—Pressive feeling at base of brain.—Stunning, splitting, bursting, throbbing headache ; < by mental exertion ; by coughing.—Headache with hunger on waking, > after breakfast.—Dull, heavy, frontal headache, < moving eyes.—Head feels enlarged.—Darting pain through l. superciliary ridge, extending deep into brain.—Pressive and piercing pain through temples ; < by chewing.—Hot flushes and pain in vertex.—Pains alternate between r. temple and between front and back of head.

3. **Eyes.**—Pressure over eyes, < lifting eyebrows.—Eyes heavy.—Pains over eyes.—Sensitiveness to light.

4. **Ears.**—Swelling of gland under r. ear ; sharp pain behind ear.—Shooting pains from l. ear down spine.—Intolerance of loud talking ; a pleasant voice sounds coarse ; thought it would produce spasms if obliged to listen ; impression produced by the sound lasts long.—Roaring and singing in ears.

5. **Nose.**—Sneezing.—Influenza.—Nose stopped, sore ; breath burns and irritates nostrils.

6. **Face.**—Face pale, esp. round eyes ; sickly, yellow.—Burning in face. —Pain in r. zygoma.—Nervous twitching of upper lip, extending to l. eye.—Lips cracked ; and sore ; dry.

8. **Mouth.**—Teeth (esp. r. molars) all ache ; feel sore and elongated.—Tongue : swollen ; coated yellow ; papillæ red and prominent, rough at back ; dry ; feels scalded.—Soft palate and uvula inflamed, breath hot.—Mouth dry. —Profuse salivation, drivelling whilst lying on face ; tastes salt.—Taste : in morning everything tastes and smells sour ; bitter ; of medicine returning in gusts ; nothing tastes natural.—Unable to speak for some time on waking.

9. **Throat.**—Throat sore ; ulcerated ; < r. side ; < afternoon.—Burning and pricking pains before rising, esp. in tonsils.—Dryness ; roughness ; heat ; constriction in throat.—Heat, dryness, and distressing feeling of emptiness in œsophagus.

11. **Stomach.**—Appetite : voracious ; at supper followed by pain in epigastrium ; awoke with hunger and headache.—Tired before finishing eating.—Desire for acid food.—Aversion to meat, butter, and rich food.—Thirsty ; drank much water.—Absence of thirst ; with bitter taste.—Eructations : tasting bitter ; of bad eggs ; sour.—Hiccough, 3 p.m.—Severe, persistent nausea ; with fever ; with headache ; < lying down ; < speaking or singing.—Efforts to vomit.—Vomiting without >.—Stomach : sour ; burning distress at ; faint feeling.—Weight at stomach with bloating ; wakening him 1 a.m.—Pressure as of a stone at pit of stomach, < by light meal.—Cutting, griping, squeezing, throbbing aching in epigastric region, < by cheese.—Feeling as of sand in stomach.—Aching and sticking in diaphragm < by speaking.—All gastric symptoms < towards morning ; = awakening.

12. **Abdomen.**—Weight and dragging in hypochondria on walking ; standing ; sitting erect ; > stooping forward.—Liver swollen ; tender to light touch ; clothes feel too tight ; < lying l. side, = dragging pain ; > lying r. side.—Pains shoot from r. hypochondrium downwards.—Throbbing ; stitches ; distress in r. hypochondrium.—Cutting, soreness, distress in spleen ; with pressure in forehead.—Pulsation and tenderness in umbilical region.—Borborygmi and colic.—Involuntary discharge of flatus.—Flushes of heat in abdomen.—Abdomen feels hollowed ; empty ; caved in ; soft as if front walls drawn in to spine.—Distress and griping in hypogastrium and groins.

13. **Stool and Anus.**—Pressure in rectum ; urging to stool.—Smarting in anus : after hard stool ; with diarrhœic stool.—Stool followed by tenesmus and succeeded by itching and smarting at anus.—Diarrhœa, stools dark, sulphurous odour.—Cadaverous smelling stools.—Stools with shivering. —Fæces coated with slime.—Copious expulsion of ascarides.—Black, lumpy stool.—Constipation ; with continued urging.—Hard, difficult stool, with straining and smarting.

14. Urinary Organs.—Strange uneasiness in bladder and prostate.—Heat in prostate.—Tickling, smarting, burning, and sensitiveness of urethra.—Urine increased ; copious white sediment ; phosphatic ; high coloured ; yellowish red ; scalding slightly ; muddy sediment.

15. Male Sexual Organs.—Throbbing in glans and pubic region on lying down at night.—Sexual desire greatly increased at first ; later abolished.

17. Respiratory Organs.—Hoarseness ; inability to speak aloud.—Sensation of foreign body in larynx, morning before rising.—When coughing head feels as if it would burst.

18. Chest.—Uneasiness and difficulty of breathing came on as gastric and hepatic symptoms declined.—Stitching pains in lungs.—Tenderness of sternum.—Pain in back of l. breast near axilla.—Darting under r. breast.

19. Heart.—Awoke from afternoon nap with slight pain near heart, and afterwards shooting from under r. breast.—Severe, cramp-like pains in region of heart.—Pulse quick, full, hard, tense.

20. Neck and Back.—Pain in neck ; feels swollen ; cords lame.—Nape stiff, moving = painful tension.—Awoke with headache.—Lameness of small of back.—Cramp-like pains in sacrum when walking.

21. Limbs.—Aching distress ; weary feeling ; rheumatic pain in all limbs.—Stitches in shoulder and hip.

22. Upper Limbs.—Rheumatic pain in shoulders and arms.—Nervous pain alternating from l. arm to l. eye.—< Nervous trembling of hands.—Prickling numbness of hands, feet cold, enlarged, clumsy, stiff.—Fine pains in fingers and region of spleen.

23. Lower Limbs.—Weakness of lower limbs.—Pain in r. hip.—Darting pains in r. thigh.—Throbbing in gluteal region.—Sticking in l. knee.—Drawing pains in l. heel.

24. Generalities.—Weak, languid, sick, tired.—Gone feeling all over.

25. Skin.—Skin : reddish ; dry ; parched.—Intense itching all over body—Eruptions : vesicles ; red spots ; boil on r. forehead ; desquamation.

26. Sleep.—Constant yawning ; drowsy.—Sound sleep but haunted by frightful dreams.—Dreams : vivid, of armies ; of dead animals ; of fighting ; of food and awoke hungry.

27. Fever.—Shivering : by warm stove ; with hot head ; from hips down ; with chattering teeth ; with sensitiveness to cold air.—A cold streak runs up and down spine.—Feverish heat ; with pains in all limbs and nausea.—Dry heat over whole body, esp. palms.—Burning cheeks and hot flushes.—Sweat : all night ; profuse on waking ; on forehead.

Pulmo Vulpis.

Fox's Lung. A Sarcode. Trituration.

Clinical.—Asthma. Bronchitis. Catarrh. Lungs, œdema of ; catarrh of.

Characteristics.—Recent discoveries in the uses of tissues and organs as remedies have thrown light on many curiosities of ancient medicine. As the fox is probably the longest-winded of all animals, the doctrine of signatures pointed to his lungs as a likely remedy for short breath. Grauvogl has put on record this case (quoted *Hom. News*, xxv. 490): Woman, 65, much reduced in flesh by a persistent condition of humid asthma. It commenced with chronic catarrh and symptoms of œdema of the lungs. Strong, sonorous bubbling, now rattling, now whistling sounds over whole chest, and at some distance away; perceptible also to hand laid on chest. Accelerated short breath amounting to suffocation, even without corresponding heaving of the chest, frequently with cough and inability to expectorate. [Sometimes, in light cases, there is no catarrh present, and only persistent shortness of breath, becoming a paroxysm of asthma on the least bodily exertion.] The patient could only live sitting up, bent forward; constant lividity of face, lips, and extremities, and dropsy of legs. Heart's pulsations irregular, and death seemed imminent. *Pulmo vulpis* 1 x gr. i. was given, and repeated in an hour. Visible improvement set in but without increased expectoration. After a third powder the patient was able to lie down, and fell into a refreshing sleep lasting several hours. In eight days she engaged in her domestic duties.

Pulsatilla.

Pulsatilla nigricans. Anemone pratensis. Pulsatilla pratensis. Pasque Flower. (Sunny, sandy pastures in Central and Northern Europe and parts of South of England.) *N. O.* Ranunculaceæ. Tincture of entire fresh plant when in flower (it flowers in spring and again in autumn).

Clinical.—*Acne.* Amaurosis. Amenorrhœa. *Anæmia. Appetite, depraved. Bladder, catarrh of. Blepharospasm. Breasts, pain behind. Bronchitis.* Cataract. *Catarrh.* Chaps. *Chest, pains in. Chilblains. Clavus. Cold. Cough. Diarrhœa;* of phthisis. *Distension.* Dysmenia. *Dyspepsia. Earache.* Epilepsy. Epistaxis. *Eyes, lachrymal sac, inflammation of; granular ophthalmia. Fear. Feet, soles painful.* Fœtus, mal-position of. Freckles. Gonorrhœa. *Gout. Hœmorrhoids. Hands, pains in. Heart, palpitation of. Heartburn. Hydrocele;* congenital. Hysteria. *Intermittent fever. Joints, synovitis of. Labour, spurious pains of. Lactation, disorders of. Leucorrhœa. Measles. Menstruation, abnormal;* vicarious. Moles. *Mumps. Neuralgia.* Nymphomania. *Ovaries, pain in; inflammation of. Phlegmasis alba dolens. Pregnancy; bladder trouble of; sickness of; heartburn of; diarrhœa of.* Priapism. *Prostate, inflammation of.* Prostatorrhœa. Puerperal convulsions. Puerperal fever. Puerperal mania. Retained placenta. *Rheumatism;* gonorrhœal. *Side, pain in. Smell, illusions of.* Spine, curvature of. *Stye.* Synovitis. Tape-worm. *Taste; depraved; lost. Tongue, coated. Toothache. Urine, incontinence of.* Uterus; inflammation of; prolapse of. *Veins, inflammation of;* varicose. Whitlow.

Characteristics.—As some confusion has arisen as to the *Pulsatilla* of homœopathic use, I will give Jahr's description of the plant: "Stems simple, erect, rounded, 3 to 5 inches high; leaves radical bipennatifid, oblong; flowers solitary, terminal, having folioles of calyx campanulate, bent at the point, the odour of the herb but slightly evident, taste acrid and pungent. The fresh plant contains an acrid and vesicating principle, and furnishes a corrosive oil, as well as a kind of tannin, which colours iron green ; in the dry state it is entirely deprived of this acrid quality. Grows in sandy pasture grounds, on hills and declivities exposed to the sun." He further distinguishes this *Black Pulsatilla* from the *Common Pulsatilla* (*Pulsatilla vulgaris, Anemone pulsatilla*) which "grows only on dry and sterile hills and flowers in spring only, whilst the black-coloured *Pulsatilla* flowers a second time in August and September." *P. vulg.* is much less downy than *P. nig.* : "Its flowers clear violet or pale red, straight and not hanging ; seeds surmounted by a long silky tail." It is called Pasque Flower because it is in bloom at Easter, and its flowers are used for colouring Easter eggs. The Anemone is a medicine of ancient date, and its affinity for the eyes seems to have been noted from the first. Perhaps its tearful propensities gave rise to the legend that it sprang from the tears of Venus. Dioscorides mentions it as a remedy for headache and *ophthalmia*. Stœrck was the forerunner of Hahnemann in the modern use of *Pulsatilla*, which he employed especially in chronic affections of the eyes (catarrh, amaurosis, spots on cornea). A young girl who had had amaurosis of both eyes since infancy he cured in two months, administering an extract internally, and insufflating a dry powder. The latter "caused at first an acute pain and profuse flow of tears ; *after which the pains, which had existed previous to the lachrymation, diminished as soon as it commenced*, and finally disappeared with it" (Teste). Other cures by Stœrck are : (1) Foul ulcers on foot with serpiginous tetters on neck and shoulder. (2) Paralysis of right arm of five years' standing. (3) Paralysis of thighs. (4) White swelling of knees. (5) Melancholia. Hahnemann quotes Stœrck's experiences in the proving of *Puls.* in *M. M. P.* "Of the numerous provings left us by Hahnemann," says Teste, "that of *Puls.* seems to be the one to which he has contributed himself more than any other ; it is one of the most interesting and most characteristic provings of his materia medica." Teste himself has given a very luminous account of the remedy. He puts it at the head of a group with *Silic.*, *Calc.*, *Hep.* as its chief members (*Graph.*, *Phos.* in less degree, with *Fer.*, *Cham.*, and *Gadus* as analogues). These drugs act principally, says Teste, on the vascular apparatus. All the symptoms which they have in common depend upon a small number of primordial symptoms (*e.g.*, impeded respiration, engorgement of air passages, irregular beating of heart), indicating vascular disturbance. Hence arise—(1) Throbbings here and there synchronous with the pulse. (2) Blackness and diminished fluidity of the blood. (3) Swelling of veins, capillary engorgement, a sort of ill-conditioned plethora. (4) Diminished vital heat and action. (5) Congestion of blood to head and engorgement of the sinuses. (6) Sensation of heaviness and fulness of brain ; and (7) the same kind of pain sometimes with apoplectic shocks, in centre or (more usually) on right side of brain. (8) Vertigo and cloudiness as in complete apoplexy, especially *when atmospheric pressure is low*, as at the approach of storms, and on heights. [Others follow from which I make a selection.—J. H. C.] Soft stools, and a passive diarrhœa without colic, which *seems to ease the patient* rather than weaken him, and continues for an indefinite period, *e.g.*, in phthisical patients. Sort of numbness, torpor of the genital organs, with absence of erections and pleasurable sensation (especially among women) during an embrace ; or else permanent sexual excitement, " probably from compression of the cerebellum by the blood which flows to it in excessive quantity and remains there, as is the case in certain forms of asphyxia ; this is the cause of the sexual excitement with which phthisicy persons are so often troubled." Delay of menses in spite of evident symptoms of a flow of blood towards the uterus ; the menstrual blood is black, coagulated, impoverished if menses either too early or too late. One is obliged to lie with the head much higher than the rest of the body. Pains which manifest themselves principally in the parts on which one is not lying, but on changing position aggravated breaking out of those pains on the parts on which one has just been lying.—This idea of vascular engorgement usefully strings together many of the leading characteristics of *Puls.*, which will serve to indicate its use in a great variety of disorders. The leaves of the recent herb have an acrid, burning, and nauseous taste. Its juice draws blisters " to the extent, it is said, of causing gangrene, if allowed to remain in contact with the part for a sufficient length of time ; but these properties are, in a great measure, lost by dessication ; and ruminating animals, such as sheep and goats, eat the dry Pulsatilla, if mixed with other herbs, without aversion or inconvenience." An active principle, *Anemonin*, has been isolated ; it is inflammable and crystallises in colourless, odourless neutral needles. Hahnemann says of *Puls.* : " This powerful plant produces many symptoms on the healthy human body which often correspond to the marked symptoms commonly met with ; hence, also, they admit of frequent homœopathic employment, and often do good. We can therefore unquestionably reckon it as a remedy of many uses (polychrest). It is useful in acute as well as in chronic diseases, as its action, even in small doses, lasts from ten to twelve days. . . . The homœopathic employment of this, as of all other medicines, is most suitable when not only the corporeal affections of the medicine correspond in similarity to the corporeal symptoms of the disease, but also when the mental and emotional alterations peculiar to the drug encounter similar states in the disease to be cured, or at least in the temperament of the subject of treatment." Hahnemann now gives in masterly fashion the picture of the *Puls.* disposition and temperament : " A timid, *lachrymose* disposition, with a tendency to inward grief and silent peevishness, or at all events a mild and yielding disposition, especially when the patient in his normal health was good-tempered and mild (or even frivolous and good-humouredly waggish). It is therefore especially adapted for slow, phlegmatic temperaments ; on the other hand, it is but little suitable for persons who form their resolutions with rapidity and are quick in their movements, even though they may appear to be good-tempered. It acts best where there is a disposition to chilliness and adipsia. It is particularly suitable for females when their menses come on some days after the proper time ; and especially when the patient must lie long in bed at night before he can get to sleep, and when the patient is worse in the evening. It is useful for the ill effects caused by eating pork." Hering gives these additional touches to the *Puls.* type : Sandy hair, blue eyes, pale face, easily moved to laughter or tears ; affectionate, mild, timid, gentle, yielding disposition ; women and children ; women inclined to be fleshy ; the pregnant state. The behaviour of the "Wind Flower," the sport of every gust, has been said to typify the action of the remedy. *Changeableness* is one of its most important keynotes : Erratic temperatures in fevers. Wandering pains shift rapidly from one part to another, also with swelling and redness of the joints. Hæmorrhages apparently stop and in a few hours return. Stools constantly changing colour ; no two stools alike. Alternate pallor and redness of face. When one set of symptoms comes on another vanishes. A patient of mine, after a mental strain and fright, had severe occipital pain. I gave *Puls.* 30. Each dose caused the pain to fly from the occiput to the left leg ; the mental balance was soon restored. Metastasis of mumps to testes or mammæ. Nash says *Puls.* will often clear up those cases which have no "head or tail" to them ; in which the symptoms are always changing and contradicting, pains run here and there. The *Puls.* patient is chilly, but at the same time there is extreme aversion to heat. The chief of all the keynotes of *Puls.* is < by warmth ; in warm, close room ; by warm coverings ; warm applications ; and > in open air ; cold air or cool room ; eating or drinking cold things ; cold applications. Another keynote of *Puls.* is thirstlessness, and Teste gives a useful clue to that in suggesting that it depends on the congestive action of the remedy. The loss of thirst and even aversion to liquid food is "as if one had an instinctive dread of increasing the excessive fulness of the vessels." The wandering pains of *Puls.* are generally *distensive*, again suggesting congested vessels ; and the headaches are congestive ; < on stooping forward ; > by tightly bandaging ; as if the brain would burst and the eyes would fall out of the head. The three characters, "chilly ; < by warmth ; thirstless," serve to define the fever of *Puls.* in whatever form it may be met—measles, mumps, typhoid, bilious, catarrhal, intermittent, rheumatic, &c. The chilliness may be one-sided, and associated with numbness ; it may be *flitting*, in spots now here, now there. With the heat there are distended veins and burning hands that seek cool places, and still there is no thirst. In the rheumatic the pains shift from joint to joint. The sweat is profuse, may be one-sided, sour, sweetish sour, or musty in odour. The last completes the similarity of *Puls.* to the "mousey" odour of measles ; the cough, catarrhal symptoms, and rash giving other strong points of correspondence. The ear trouble which is a common sequela and complication of measles or other fever is frequently met by *Puls.*, which also meets the consequences of suppressed exanthemata and metastases, as of mumps to testes or mamma. As a prophylactic against measles *Puls.* has a reputation almost equal to that of *Bell.* against scarlatina : I generally give *Puls.* 3 three times a day. The generative organs of both sexes are strongly acted on by *Puls.*, which may almost be regarded as an organ-remedy in relation to them. Gonorrhœa, with thick, purulent secretion ; and the effects of suppressed gonorrhœa, orchitis, and cystitis; prostatitis; sarcocele, varicocele, hydrocele—all come within the sphere of *Puls.* In the female *Puls.* ranges over the whole sexual period, from puberty to the climacteric, including disorders of menstruation, pregnancy, the puerperium and lactation—all of which present many points of correspondence with the symptoms of *Puls.* Epilepsy with absence or irregularity of menses has been cured with *Puls.* Bojanus (*B. J. H.*, xxxix. 218) relates two cases: (1) Girl, 18, of good constitution, with no hereditary predisposition, had amenorrhœa for six months, and a fit occurred at the time each period was due. Aura: sad, pale as death; chewing movements. *Puls.* 6 one dose a day. Next month menses returned and there were no more fits. (2) Robust girl, 14, with no hereditary predisposition. Fits twelve months. Exciting cause: non-appearance of menses. One great fit per month, small fits daily. Aura: self-willed, angry, stands on one spot, stares into vacancy, stamps her foot. In fit: cries, deathly paleness, biting tongue, flow of urine, continuing the occupation she was engaged with at commencement of fit. *Puls.* 30 one dose a day. Some weeks after a slight fit. Month later menses came on for first time, no great fits, small ones rare. *Puls.* 30 one dose a week. Month later a great fit. *Puls.* once a day. No more great fits, only a few small ones. Cure permanent. A patient to whom I was giving *Puls.* 3 for some heart affection complained that she could not take it because it caused her to wake up in the night with a dry cough, and she was compelled to sit up in bed to get relief. That is a characteristic cough of *Puls.*, and I have frequently cured it in other patients. *Puls.* has a cough with copious expectoration, and this is the more usual; but they may be alternating conditions. The *congesting* action of *Puls.* is well shown in the respiratory symptoms. Remarking on this symptom, "Pressure upon the chest and soreness," Hahnemann says that in the catarrhal condition they refer to, "the glands of the air passages appear to be swollen and inflamed, and unable to secrete the mucus necessary to moisten them; *hence the sensation of dryness, rawness, painfulness, and the illusory sensation as if the air passages were internally constricted by an excessive amount of tenacious and firm mucus which could not be loosened.*" Commenting on another symptom of *Puls.* ("dyspnœa or vertigo, with weakness of the head on lying outstretched upon the back, wholly disappearing on sitting upright"), Hahnemann elucidates some of its Conditions: "The symptoms of *Puls.* caused by lying down, sitting up, rising from sitting, by walking and by standing, consist of varying alternate conditions, all of which belong to the primary action of the drug, but which vary in their character. Usually the symptoms of *Puls.* which occur while lying still upon the back are > by sitting upright, seldom the reverse; frequently the symptoms that appear while sitting still are > or removed by gradual motion and by walking, seldom the reverse. Yet the *act* of rising, before one begins to walk, = symptoms more numerous and more severe the longer the sitting has continued; so also longer continued and more violent motion = aggravation no less long than sitting still, which, however, are only really felt and noticed after one has sat down and become quiet." Other leading indications of *Puls.* are: First serious impairment of health is referred to age of puberty, "never been well since"—anæmia, bronchitis, phthisis. Secretions (of eye, ear, nose, vagina, &c.) are generally thick, bland, and yellowish green. The pains appear suddenly and leave gradually; or tension much increases till very acute, then "lets up with a snap." Great dryness of mouth without thirst. All-gone sensation in stomach, especially in tea-drinkers. < At twilight; in evening (the wide-awakeness on first going to bed comes within this modality). Suffering parts emaciate. *Peculiar Sensations* are: As if beside himself. As if in a hot atmosphere. As if death were near. As if looking through a sieve. Limbs as if bruised; as if asleep. As if one had turned in a circle a long time; as if he would fall; as if he were dancing. As if brain would burst and eyes fall out of head. As if skull of forehead too thin. As if skull were lifted up. As if one had eaten too much. As if a nail driven into occiput. As if head between screws. As if gimlet piercing skull. As if eyes tightly bound by cloth. As if foreign body pressing in eye; sand in eye; thick body forcibly driven into ear; something crawling out of ear; worm creeping into throat. As if nose would be forced asunder. As if face being drawn tighter and tighter, then suddenly let loose as if a string cut. As if a nerve in tooth put on stretch and then let loose. As if he had to swallow over a lump. As of stone in stomach. As if bladder too full; as if it would fall to side on which he is lying; as of a stone in bladder or in abdomen or chest. As if joints would be easily dislocated. Small of back as if sprained. As if a hand passed through back and everything were constricted. Chill as if drenched with cold water. As if head would burst on coughing. Tongue as if burnt. Pain as from subcutaneous ulceration. As of a hot coal above ulcer. The symptoms are < by touch; > by hard rubbing and pressure (but stomach, bladder, uterus, very sensitive to pressure). > Uncovering. Aversion to and < from meat, butter, fat food, pork, bread, milk, buckwheat, ice cream, smoking. Desire for: sour, refreshing things; herring; lemonade. > From cold, < from warm foods. Rest < (> pain in testes; labour-like pains; weakness in joints). Cannot rest though motion <. The longer he lies in the morning the longer he wishes to lie. > Lying with head high. < Lying on l. side; on sound side. Pains which come on when lying on back are > by turning to either side (also *vice versâ*); must sit up and turn. When rising up the red face turns deathly pale. Great inclination to stretch feet. Gentle motion >, slow walking >. Violent motion <. Misstep < stitching pains in stomach. Intellectual labour, or watching will = headache; meditation will sometimes >. Most symptoms < evening and night. < Twilight: "As evening comes on begins to fear ghosts"; all symptoms < alternate evenings. < Before thunderstorm. Sun <. < Hot food; is vomited immediately; < toothache. < Changes of weather. < Getting wet. Wind <. Draught of air > toothache.

Relations.—*Antidoted by:* Cham. (Cham. and Puls. antidote each other and follow each other well. If either one has over-acted the other will probably neutralise the ill effect and carry on the good), Coff., Ign., Nux (Teste adds Sul., and says when the improper use of

Puls. has affected the air passages Calc. ph. has proved his best antidote). *Antidote to:* Chi., Chi. sul., Fer. (in chlorotic girls who have been damaged by Iron, Puls. has excellent effect), Mag. c., Sul., Sul. ac., vapours of Mercury and Copper, Bell., Cham., Coff., Colch., Lyc., Plat., Gels., Strm., Saba., Ant. t., Whisky, Toad-stool poisoning. *Compatible:* Ars., Bry., Bell., Ign., K. bi., Lyc., Nux, Pho., Rhus, Sep., Sul. *Complementary:* Lyc., Sul. ac., Arg. n. (if Arg. n. flags, give Puls.; Arg. n. follows Puls. in ophthalmia); Stn. (Stn. has menses too early and too profuse). *Compare:* Tearfulness, Sep. (Puls. cries when telling her symptoms, Sep. weeps when questioned about her symptoms; Sep. irritability and anger, indifference to household affairs), Nat. m. (Nat. m. is < by consolation), Ign. (Ign. hides her grief). Varicose veins, varicocele, orchitis, phlegmasia alba dolens, Ham. (Ham. has soreness of affected part). Ophthalmia, Arg. n. Cold, Cycl. (Cycl. has spasmodic sneezing), Cep. (both have < in room, > open air, but Cep. discharge is thin and excoriating, Puls. thick and bland), Pen. sed. (Pen. sed. has rawness in nose and throat; and "constant wet feeling without coryza," later thick and purulent like Puls.). Stinging pains in throat < swallowing saliva and after eating, Apis. Feeling as if food lying in œsophagus, Chi., Abies n. Effect of fat food, Ip., Thuj., Carb. v. Effect of ice-cream, Ars., Carb. v., Ip., Bels. Mixed diet, Nux, Ip., Chi. Desire for lemonade, Cyc., Sabi., Bell. Gastric ailments from pork, Ant. c. (tongue as if whitewashed, vomiting predominates; Puls. stool greenish and slimy), Ip. (tongue clean, nausea predominates). Spasmodic, irregular pains = faintness, Nux. Retained placenta, Canth. After-pains, Cham., Xan., Cup. (in women who have borne many children). Non-appearance of milk, Urt. u., Ric. com., Agn. c. Uterine affections, Caul., Helon., Senec., Alet. f., Cycl., Hydras., Lil. Measles, Morbillin, K. bi. Backache < sitting, Zn., Cobalt., Sep., Can. i. Earache, Borax. Knee-joint affections, Anac. (Anac. chronic). < From wine, Zn. (Puls. from sulphurated wines,) Rho., Glo., Nux, Sel., Lach., Fl. ac., Ant. c., Bov., Sil.. Thick, yellowish, green nasal discharge, Merc. (Puls. bland; Merc. has moist mouth and intense thirst, and Puls. and Nux m. dry mouth without thirst). Sudden vanishing of sight with scanty menses, Sep., Cycl. Diarrhœa from fright, Gels. (Puls. stools greenish, yellow, or slimy, or very changeable). Hypertrophy of heart; > from slow motion, Rhus. Menstrual colic, Coccul. (Coccul. as if sharp stones rubbed together with every movement). Vicarious menstruation, Bry., Pho. Ozæna with thick greenish discharge, gleet, gonorrhœal rheumatism, effects of tea, Thuj. (the gleet of Puls. is thicker than that of Thuj.). Scanty menses, Graph. > Open air, Sul. (Lyc. desires open air, but is < in cold, damp air). Climacteric state, Lach. > Uncovering, Lyc., Camph., Aco., Sec. < From heat, Apis, Iod. Nausea in upper chest and in hypogastrium, Puls. (nausea in hypogastrium, generally with uterine bearing down, Rhus). Nausea when fasting, Calc., Lyc., Silic.; when beginning to eat, Nux, Sul. Nausea in chest, Ant. t. Acid stomach, Chi., Calc., Sul., Sil., Robin. Menstrual pain begins with the flow (opp. Lach., pain subsides as flow begins). Acquisitiveness, Ars., Lyc. Dread of disease, Calc., Lach., Nux. < Lying on left side; > cold food and drink, Pho. Ribbon-like stools (Pho. like dog's). Fears darkness, Am. m., Ars., Bar. c., Berb., Calc., Carb. a Carb. v., Caus., Lyc., Pho., Rhus, Stro., Val., Stram. Fear of ghost Aco., Ars., Bro., Lyc., Ran. b., Sep., Sul., Zn. Piles during mense Am. c., Ars., Carb. v., Coccul., Collins., Graph., Ign., Lach., Mur. a Pho., Sul. Faintness connected with stools, Ap., Nux m., Spi., Ve (with scanty stools, Crot. t., Dulc., Ox. ac., Pet. Sars., Sul.) Stoppa of menses from wet feet, Rhus., Lob. i. Chilblains, Agar. Verti on looking up (Calc. on turning head ; Sul. on looking down). < bed at night, Sul., Merc., Cham. Taste bitter with biliousness of morning, the taste felt chiefly in upper chest, Sul. One hand cold th other hot, Chi., Dig., Ip., Mosch. Metastasis of mumps to teste Bell., K. ca., Rhus (to brain, Bell., Hyo.). Effect of taking cold, feve Aco. (Aco. has great thirst and anguish). Inter-menstrual hæmo rhage, Bov., Ham. < Hair-cutting, Bell. > Lying on painful sid Bry. Erratic temperatures (Zn. nervous high temperatures). Pul is a close analogue of Cycl. in many respects, but Cycl. has profu menses, the flow being < sitting and > walking (Puls. < during day Kre. < lying down) ; and Cycl. has < in open air. Puls. and Nu are in most respects antipodal, though they follow each other wel Puls. has > lying on back, < turning to either side ; Nux has lying on back, > turning to either side. Silica is the *chronic* of Puls and Sul. also in many respects.

Causation.—Chill. Wetting feet. Eating : Pork ; Fats ; Pastry Ice-cream ; Mixed diet. Thunderstorm. Tea.

SYMPTOMS.

1. **Mind.**—[This remedy is particularly applicable for complaints whic are found to occur in patients of a mild, yielding, or good-natured dispositio also in those who by their sickness, or naturally, are very easily excited tears—they are very apt to burst into tears whenever spoken to, or when th attempt to speak, as in giving their symptoms, &c.—Affections of the min in general ; covetous ; mistrustful ; absent-minded ; low-spirited (H. N. G. Melancholy with sadness, tears, great uneasiness respecting one's affairs about the health ; fear of death (tremulous anguish, as if death were near), ca and grief.—Involuntary laughter and weeping.—Great anguish and inquietud mostly in precordial region, sometimes with inclination to commit suicid palpitation of heart, heat, and necessity to loosen the dress, trembling hands, and inclination to vomit.—Fits of anxiety, with fear of death, or of a apoplectic attack, with buzzing in ears, shiverings, and convulsive movemen of fingers.—Apprehension, anthropophobia, fear of ghosts at night or evening, with an impulse to hide or to run away, mistrust and suspicion.— Covetousness.—Taciturn madness ; with sullen, cold, and wandering ai sighs, often seated with the hands joined, but without uttering any complain —Despair of eternal happiness, with continual praying.—Discouragemen indecision, dread of occupation, and obstructed respiration.—Dispositi envious, discontented, and covetous, exhibiting itself in a wish to appropria everything.—Caprice, with desire at one time for one thing, at another tim for something else, either being rejected as soon as obtained.—Hysteric laughter after meals.—Hypochondriacal humour and moroseness, < evenin

often with repugnance to conversation, great sensitiveness, choleric disposition, cries, and weeping.—Ill-humour, sometimes with a dread of labour, and disgust or contempt for everything.—Inadvertence, precipitation, and absence of mind.—Difficulty in expressing thoughts correctly when speaking, and tendency to omit letters when writing.—Giddiness ; patient neither knows where he is nor what he does.—Great flow of very changeful ideas.—Nocturnal raving ; violent delirium and loss of consciousness.—Frightful visions.—Weakness of memory.—Fixed ideas.—Stupidity.

2. **Head.**—Fatigue of head from intellectual labour.—Sensation of emptiness and confusion in head, as after long watching or after a debauch, and sometimes with great indifference.—Stupefaction in evening, in warm room, with chilliness.—Stupefying headache, with humming in head, < when lying or sitting quiet, or in the cold.—Vertigo as during intoxication, or vertigo to such an extent as to fall, and staggering, < evening, or morning when rising up, when getting up after lying down, when sitting, when stooping, when walking in open air, or after a meal, as well as on raising eyes, and often with great heaviness and heat in head, paleness of face, inclination to vomit, sleep, cloudiness of eyes, and buzzing in ears.—Meditation and conversation < the vertigo.—Fits of dizziness and loss of consciousness, with bluish redness and bloatedness of face, loss of motive power, violent palpitation of heart, pulse almost extinct, and respiration rattling.—Pain as from a bruise in brain (as if brain were lacerated, on or soon after waking), as in typhus fever or after intoxication with brandy.—Headache as from indigestion, caused by eating fat food (or from the abuse of Mercury).—Pain in head as if forehead would split, or as if brain were tight, compressed, or contracted.—Headache on moving eyes deep in orbits as if forehead would fall out ; and frontal bones were too thin, with dulness of head, evening.—Semilateral headache as if brain would burst and eyes fall out of head.—Soreness as from subcutaneous ulceration in one or both temples, < in evening, when at rest, and in warm room ; > by walking in open air.—Twitching-tearing in temple on which one lies, and going to the other side when turning on it ; < in evening and on raising eyes upwards.—Congestion of blood to head, with stinging pulsation in brain, esp. when stooping.—Shootings, or sharp drawing and jerking pains, or tingling pulsation, and boring in head.—Headache across eyes like a drawing-up and letting go again.—Roaring, buzzing, and crackling in head ; or painful sensation, as if a current of air were crossing brain.—The headache is often only semilateral, extending as far as ear and teeth, where it affects forehead (generally in one temple) above eyes, penetrating into sockets, or it is experienced in occiput, with painful contraction in nape of neck (with vertigo, ringing in ears, and vanishing of sight).—Appearance or < of headache in evening, after lying down, or at night, or in bed in morning, as well as on stooping, on moving eyes or head, when walking in open air, and during intellectual labour ; compression sometimes >.—Headache > by meditation.—Headache with nausea and vomiting, or with congestion and heat in head, or else with shuddering and syncope, vertigo, cloudiness of eyes, loss of sight, and buzzing in ears, photophobia, and weeping.—Pain in scalp on turning up hair (or on brushing hair backwards).—Tickling and itching in head.—Purulent pustules and small tumours, with pain in scalp as from ulceration (suppurating and affecting the skull, more

painful when lying on the opposite well side).—Tingling, biting-itching on scalp, mostly on temples and behind ears, followed by swelling and eruptions sore pain; < in evening when undressing and on getting warm in bed.—Fetid, frequently cold perspiration, at times only on one side of head and face, with great anxiety and stupor; < at night and towards morning, > after waking and rising.—Disposition to take cold in head, < when it gets wet; sweat of scalp and face.

3. **Eyes.**—Affections in general appearing on the cornea; margins of the eyelids; dim-sightedness, with a sensation as though there were something over the eye which the patient wishes to rub away; amaurosis cataract.—Pain in eyes as if scratched with a knife.—Burning sensation pressive pain as if caused by sand; or sharp or shooting pain in eyes, or else boring and incisive pain.—Burning itching in eyes, chiefly in evening (inducing rubbing and scratching).—Inflammation in eyes and margins of lids (and meibomian glands), with redness of the sclerotica and conjunctiva and copious secretion of (thick) mucus (and nightly agglutination).—Swelling and redness of eyelids.—Trichiasis in eyelid.—Styes, esp. on upper lid.—Crystalline lens clouded and of a greyish colour.—Stye with inflammation of sclerotica, and tensive drawing pains on moving the muscles of the face.—Dryness of eyes and lids, esp. during sleep.—Profuse lachrymation, principally in the wind, as well as in open air, in the cold, and in clear, bright daylight.—Acrid and corrosive tears.—Abscess near angle of eye, like a lachrymal fistula (discharging pus on pressing it).—Nocturnal agglutination of lids.—Pupils contracted or dilated.—Amaurosis; paralysis of optic nerve.—Look fixed and stupid.—Dimness of sight, esp. on getting warm from exercise.—Cloudiness of eyes and loss of sight, sometimes with paleness of face and inclination to vomit; (all objects present a sickly hue).—Loss of sight in twilight, with sensation as if eyes were covered with a band.—Sight confused, as if directed through a mist, or as if caused by something removable by rubbing, principally in open air, in evening, in morning, or on waking.—Incipient cataract.—Diplopia.—Luminous circles before eyes, and diffusion of light of candles.—Great sensibility of eyes to light, which causes lancinating pains (and in sunshine).

4. **Ears.**—Pain in ears, as if something were about to protrude from them.—Shootings with itching, or sharp, jerking pain, and contraction in and round ears; the pains sometimes come on by fits, affect whole head, appear insupportable, and almost cause loss of reason (may be accompanied by high fever, &c.).—Earache with shooting down to teeth of lower jaw, < when warm in bed.—Earache in both ears with violent headache, frontal and occipital, < at night.—Inflammatory swelling, heat, and erysipelatous redness of ear and auditory duct, as well as of surrounding external parts.—Painful swelling of bones behind ears.—The cerumen is hard and black.—Bland, nearly inoffensive discharge of mucus and pus from ear.—Discharge of pus, of blood, or of a thick yellowish humour from l. ear.—Discharge from one or both ears, which may come on after measles or any other disease, or may occur spontaneously.—Otorrhœa with throbbing tinnitus.—Warbling, pulsative murmurs, tinkling, roaring, and humming in ears.—Hardness of hearing, as from an obstruction (esp. from cold, from having hair cut, or after suppressed measles).—(Deafness after washing head.—R. T. C.)—Burning,

gnawing scabs at the tragus (with swelling of glands of neck).—Shootings in parotids.

5. **Nose.**—Pressure and pain as from an abscess in root of nose (near inner canthus, as if a lachrymal fistula would form).—The nose feels sore internally and externally.—Ulceration of nostrils and of the alæ nasi (emitting a watery humour).—Discharge of fetid and greenish or yellowish pus from nose (like old catarrh).—Old catarrh, frequently a profuse discharge every morning, in mild and pleasant persons.—Nasal catarrh accompanied by special discomfort in the house, cannot breathe well in a warm room, and great > by going out into the open air.—Blowing of blood from nose and nasal hæmorrhage (blood coagulated; with dry coryza; with suppressed menses), sometimes with obstruction of nose.—Obstruction of nose and dry coryza, principally in evening and in the heat of a room.—Coryza with loss of taste and smell, or with discharge of thick (yellowish green) and fetid mucus.—Tickling in nose and frequent sneezing, principally in morning and evening.—Constant shivering during coryza.—Imaginary smells.—Constant smell before nose, as from a coryza of long standing, or as of a mixture of coffee and tobacco.—Swelling of nose.—Nasal bones pain as if they would be forced asunder.

6. **Face.**—Face pale (or yellowish, with sunken eyes) and sometimes with an expression of suffering.—Painful sensitiveness of skin in face.—Boring in l. malar bone.—(Neuralgia of r. face, < and then > by warmth, tightness across forehead as from a tight-string, keeps her awake at night.—R. T. C.)—Pallor of face, alternating with heat and redness of cheeks.—Heat and redness of r. cheek only.—Sweat on face and scalp; shuddering or one- (r.-) sided sweat of face.—Face (and nose) puffed and of a bluish red colour.—Convulsive movements and muscular palpitations in face.—Tension and sensation of swelling in face, or painful sensibility of skin, as if it were excoriated.—Erysipelas in face, with shooting pain and desquamation of skin.—Red nodosities in region of cheek-bones.—Lower lip swelled and cracked in middle.—Swelling, tension, and cracks in lips, with desquamation of skin.—Gnawing and smarting around mouth.—Sharp and contractive pain in jaws.—Swelling of submaxillary and cervical glands.

7. **Teeth.**—Sharp, shooting pains in teeth, or drawing, jerking pains, as if the nerve were tightened, then suddenly relaxed; or pulsative, digging, and gnawing pains, often with pricking in gums.—Jerking and stinging in teeth, extending to ears and eyes.—Toothache which affects the sound as well as the carious teeth, often only semilateral, and frequently extending to face, side of head, ear, and eye, on the side affected, being sometimes accompanied by paleness in face, shivering, and dyspnœa.—Toothache < or appears principally in evening or afternoon or at night, as well as in heat of bed or of a room; renewed by eating, as also by partaking of anything hot, and by irritation with the toothpick; > by cold water or fresh air.—Toothache from cold (in the first warm spring days), with otalgia, paleness of the face, and chilliness.—The toothache is also sometimes < by cold water as well as by fresh air or by wind; but these cases are rare.—Sensation of burning or swelling, pain as from excoriation, and pulsation in gums (< by the heat of the stove).—Looseness of teeth.

8. **Mouth.**—Dryness of mouth in morning (without thirst).—Offensive

smell, and even putrid fetor from mouth, principally in morning or at night, and in bed in evening.—Flow of sweetish and watery saliva from mouth, sometimes with inclination to vomit.—Sensation as if tongue were too large. —Tongue feels dry, and clammy.—Painful blister on r. side of tip of tongue. —Sensation in middle of tongue, even when it is moistened, as if it had been burned and were insensible ; at night and in morning.—Edges of tongue feel sore as if scalded.—Tongue greatly swollen, dorsum bright red and covered with network of dilated and congested veins; varicose swelling on l. side of tongue.—Tongue loaded with a thick coating of a greyish, whitish, or yellowish colour (and covered with tough mucus).—Accumulation of tenacious mucus in mouth and on tongue ; these parts are, as it were, coated with a white skin.—Cracks and painful vesicles on tongue.—Sensation as if the palate were swollen, or covered with tenacious mucus.—Constant spitting of frothy, cotton-like mucus.

9. **Throat.**—Pain as from excoriation in throat, as if it were all raw, with scraping, burning sensation and smarting.—Redness of throat, tonsils, and uvula, with sensation as if those parts were swollen, < swallowing.—Difficult deglutition, as from paralysis, or from contraction of throat.—Shootings in throat, with pressure and tension during empty deglutition.—Inflammation of throat, with varicose swelling of veins.—Dryness in throat (in morning) or accumulation of tenacious mucus, which covers the part affected (esp. night and morning).—The sore throat is generally < in evening or afternoon.—Sensation of a worm creeping up into throat.

10. **Appetite.**—Insipid. mucus, putrid taste in mouth, empyreumatic, earthy, or pus-like taste.—Taste : fatty ; lost ; in colds where there is an entire loss of taste.—Sweetish, acid, or bitter taste in mouth, and of food, principally meat, bread, butter, beer, and milk, substances which also often appear insipid or cause disgust.—Bitter or sour taste in mouth immediately after eating, as well as in morning and evening.—Wine has a bitter (beer a sweet or bitter) and meat a putrid taste.—Food appears either too salt or insipid.—Want of appetite and dislike to food.—Hunger and desire to eat, without knowing what.—Ravenous hunger, with gnawing pain in stomach.—Complete adipsia, or excessive thirst, with moisture on tongue, and desire for beer, or spirituous, tart, and acid drinks.—Thirstlessness with all complaints.—Sensation of derangement in stomach, similar to that caused by fat pork or rich pastry.—Repugnance to tobacco smoke.—After eating, nausea and eructations, regurgitation and vomiting, inflation, and aching in pit of stomach, colic and flatulence, headache, obstructed respiration, ill-humour and melancholy or involuntary laughter and weeping, and many other sufferings.—Bread, esp., lies heavy on stomach.

11. **Stomach.**—Frequent eructations, sometimes abortive, or with taste of food, or acid, or bitter, and principally after a meal ; like bile in evening.—Regurgitation of food.—Waterbrash.—Frequent hiccough, principally on smoking tobacco, after drinking, or at night, and sometimes with fit of suffocation.—(Constant hiccough with jaundiced look and burning pains about shoulders.—R. T. C.)—Insupportable nausea and inclination to vomit, sometimes extending to throat and into mouth, with distressing sensation as of a worm crawling up œsophagus.—Morning sickness (during pregnancy).—Attacks of constriction and choking in œsophagus.—Scraping sensation in

stomach and œsophagus, like a heartburn.—Vomitings, sometimes violent, of greenish mucus, or bilious and bitter, or acid matter (esp. in evening and at night).—Vomiting of food.—Hæmatemesis.—The nausea and vomiting take place principally in evening or at night, or after eating or drinking, as well as during a meal, and they often manifest themselves with shivering, paleness of face, colic, pains in ears or back, burning sensation in throat, and borborygmi.—(Persistent indigestion in fits, with great weight on chest and sickish feeling, from mental and physical upset.—R. T. C.)—Cold in stomach from ice-cream and fruit.—Colic, with nausea, ceasing after vomiting.—Painful sensibility of region of stomach to least pressure.—Disordered stomach (digestion) from eating fat food (pork).—Pressive, spasmodic, contractive, and compressive pains in stomach and præcordial region, principally after a meal or in evening or in morning, and often with vomiting or nausea and obstructed respiration.—Tingling or pulsations in pit of stomach, or shooting pain on making a false step, or on uneven pavement.—Pain in epigastrium, which is greatly < when sitting (during pregnancy).

12. **Abdomen.**—Inflammation of abdomen, with great sensitiveness of integuments to pressure.—Drawing tension in hypochondria, or pulsative shootings, as in an abscess.—Hard distension of abdomen, principally in epigastrium, with tension, and sensation as if all were full, hard, and impassable, as if no stool or flatus could be expelled, though a stool does pass slowly but not hard, and yet the flatus is passed with difficulty and in small amounts.—Chilliness extending from abdomen to lower part of back.—Pressure in abdomen and small of back as from a stone ; limbs go to sleep while sitting ; ineffectual desire to stool.—Spasmodic and compressive pains, sometimes at bottom of hypogastrium, with pressure on rectum or cuttings, principally round navel (low down in abdomen, penetrating into pelvis), or sharp and shooting pains in abdomen.—Colic and labour-like pains in pregnant women.—Colic with chilliness, while the menstruation is suppressed.—Sensitiveness and inflammation of abdominal walls.—The colics are often accompanied by vomiting or diarrhœa ; they manifest themselves mostly in evening or after eating or drinking ; and are sometimes > by squeezing the abdomen or by repose, while movement < them.—Annular swelling round navel, painful when walking.—Retraction and soreness of abdomen, with great sensibility of integuments of abdomen, which appear swollen, with pain as from a bruise on touching them, or on yawning, singing, coughing, and at every movement of the abdominal muscles.—Stitches and cutting in abdomen in evening ; < on sitting still.—Flatulent colic, principally in evening, after a meal, or after midnight, or in morning, with pressive pains, produced by incarcerated flatus, tumult, borborygmi, and grumbling in abdomen and escape of fetid flatus.—Painless rumbling of flatulence in upper abdomen.—Constriction as from a stone extending to bladder.—Purulent pustules in groins.

13. **Stool and Anus.**—Constipation and difficult evacuations, sometimes with painful pressure on rectum and pains in back.—Constipation, esp. if fæces are hard and large, after intermittent fever suppressed by *Chininum sulph.*—Frequent want to evacuate, even at night.—Involuntary and unperceived evacuations during sleep.—Stools frequent soft, diarrhœic, consisting of yellow mucus or mixed with blood, preceded by cutting in abdomen, or with pains in small of back.—Nightly diarrhœa, discharges watery or green

like bile, after previous rumbling in abdomen.—Stools consisting only of mucus, or acrid, or bloody, or very offensive, or white.—(Diarrhœa, white, cream-coloured stools, involuntary.—R. T. C.).—(White, clayey liverish stools resume their normal colour.—R. T. C.)—Dysentery, with pain in back.—Loose evacuations, even at night, and sometimes with colic and cuttings, shiverings and shudderings, and pains in anus.—Diarrhœa, particularly when it is very changeable and no two stools are alike ; flatus very fetid, sometimes obstructed, causing much pain.—Diarrhœa during menses, particularly if it comes on at night.—Frequent evacuations of whitish, yellowish, sanguineous mucus, or of greenish, minced, bilious, or watery, and sometimes corrosive matter (may contain tapeworm).—Before and after evacuations, burning, smarting, and pains as from excoriation in anus and rectum.—During stool congestions of blood to anus.—Discharge of blood from anus even when not at stool.—Blind and bleeding hæmorrhoids, with itching, smarting, and pain as from excoriation.—Protrusion of hæmorrhoids.—Hæmorrhoidal tumours with great soreness.

14. **Urinary Organs.**—Urine very scanty ; bloody ; with mucus ; reddish ; complaints before making water and during ; when going to urinate there is a sensation as if it would gush away, and patients can scarcely wait.—Retention of urine, with redness and heat in region of bladder, anxiety, and troublesome pains in abdomen.—Tenesmus of bladder and frequent want to urinate, with painful pressure on bladder and drawing pain in abdomen.—Involuntary micturition ; at night in bed, esp. in little girls.—Involuntary emission of some drops of urine when coughing, walking, sitting down, expelling flatus (or during sleep).—Wetting the bed (at night, esp. in mild-tempered, tearful people, and in children).—Enuresis of old people with distended colon (R. T. C.)—Profuse emission of watery urine, with weakness in loins and diarrhœa, or scanty red or brown urine, sometimes with a violet-coloured froth.—Urine, with sediment, red, or of the colour of brick-dust, or violet, or mucous, or gelatinous.—Sanguineous urine with purulent deposit and pains in loins.—Hæmaturia with burning at orifice of urethra, and with constriction in region of navel.—Hæmaturia in cows and in human beings (R. T. C.)—Discharge (thick) from urethra as in gonorrhœa. —Contraction of urethra with a very small stream of water.—During micturition burning in urethra.—Burning during and after emission of urine. —Pulling and pressure in urethra, neck of bladder, and also in the bladder.—Pressure and constriction in bladder, with soreness (sensitiveness) in that region.—Swelling near neck of bladder, with soreness when touched, intermittent stream of urine, and spasmodic pain in pelvis and thighs after urinating.—Urine watery, colourless ; brown ; bloody.

15. **Male Sexual Organs.**—Itching and tickling in prepuce and scrotum, < morning and evening.—Itching-burning on the inner and upper side of the prepuce.—Inflammatory swelling of testes and spermatic cords (sometimes only on one side), with pressive and drawing pains, extending into abdomen and loins, redness and heat of scrotum (from a contusion or after suppressed gonorrhœa), nausea and inclination to vomit.—Burning in testicles, without swelling.—Testicles hang low down.—Dropsical swelling of scrotum of a whitish blue colour.—Excessive increase of sexual passion, almost like priapismus, with frequent and prolonged erections, ardent desire

for coition, and frequent pollutions.—Flow of prostatic fluid.—Inflammation of prostate gland.

16. **Female Sexual Organs.**—Affections in general of the female genital organs; of the uterus.—Nymphomania.—Drawing, pressive pain extending towards uterus with qualmishness, towards morning.—Contractive pain in l. side of uterus, like labour pains, obliging her to bend double.—Spasmodic pains, or drawing tension in uterus, and pains like those of labour.—A burning (sticking) pain in vagina and pudenda.—Metrorrhagia (discharge now stopping, and then stronger again, of coagulated, clotted blood, or with false labour-pains).—Menstrual blood black, with clots of mucus, or pale and serous.—Catamenia irregular, tardy, or premature, of too short or too long duration, or entirely suppressed (esp. if produced by getting the feet wet), with colic, hysterical spasms in abdomen, hepatic pains, gastralgia, pain in loins, nausea and vomiting, shivering and paleness of face, megrim, vertigo, moral affections, tenesmus of anus and bladder, stitches in side, and many other sufferings before, during, or after period.—Suppression of menses (esp. in elderly women in whom they usually occur at full moon).—Delay of first menses in mild, gentle girls, low-spirited, &c.; diarrhœa during menses.—Leucorrhœa, thick, like cream (esp. frequent in lochial discharges where the flow looks like milk), or corrosive and burning, principally at period of catamenia (before, during or after), and sometimes with cuttings (< when lying down; with swollen vulva).—After-pains in females of a mild disposition.—False pregnancy.—During pregnancy: nausea, morning sickness; varicose veins, bluish, < towards evening.—Lame pelvis, < warm in bed, must change position frequently; threatened abortion, flow now ceasing, now returning.—During labour: intense inertia; weeps because she is not delivered; malpositions of fetus; post-partum hæmorrhage; convulsions, following sluggish or irregular pains; lochia scanty, milky, or suppressed; puerperal fever; phlegmasia dolens.—Labour-pains too weak, spasmodic, or ceasing.—Swelling of breasts, with tensive pain as if the milk rushed into them and caused pressure, while nursing.—Lumps on breasts of girls before puberty; or escape of thin, milk-like fluid.—Scanty supply of milk.—Affections of nipples.—Weeps every time child is put to breast; pain extends into chest, neck, or down back, changes from place to place.—Milk suddenly suppressed, lochia becomes milky white.—Galactorrhœa esp. in women who do not nurse their children.—After weaning, breasts swell.

17. **Respiratory Organs.**—Hoarseness, which does not permit one to speak a loud word.—Breathing, groaning, or rattling.—Catarrh, with hoarseness, roughness, dryness, scraping, and pain as from excoriation, in larynx and chest.—Attacks of constriction in larynx, principally at night, when lying in a horizontal posture.—Dyspnœa, esp. when lying on back at night, with giddiness and weakness in head.—Difficulty of breathing when walking.—Short, dry cough as soon as he gets warm.—Dry cough whenever he wakens from sleep, disappearing while sitting up in bed, and returning as soon as lying down again.—Dry, severe cough, mostly in morning, with retching and desire to vomit, and sensation as if stomach were turned inside out.—Violent spasmodic whooping-cough, in two consecutive coughs, caused by itching, scraping, with dryness as from vapours of sulphur in larynx and chest.—Shaking cough, principally in evening, at night, or in morning, excited by a

sensation of dryness or a scraping and tickling in throat, < when lying down, and often accompanied by an inclination to vomit, with retching and vomiting, or by a choking, as from the vapour of sulphur, with bleeding of nose and rattling respiration.—Cough, with shootings in chest or sides, and palpitation of heart.—Moist cough, with expectoration of white, green, tenacious mucus, or of thick, yellowish matter of a bitter, greasy, salty, or putrid taste (loose cough; with expectoration in morning, without expectoration in evening; with expectoration in day, without expectoration at night).—Expectoration of black and clotted blood during cough (during suppression of menstruation).—Shootings in r. shoulder or in back when coughing.

18. Chest.—Respiration accelerated, short, and superficial (during the fever), or rattling and anxious.—Dyspnœa, as from spasmodic tension in lower part of chest, below false ribs.—Tickling on sternum.—Attacks of burning in chest.—Respiration impeded, shortness of breath, choking as from vapour of sulphur, and fits of dyspnœa and of suffocation, with anxiety, spasmodic constriction of chest or larynx, violent hiccough, cough, headache, and vertigo; principally in evening, after a meal, or at night when reclining horizontally.—Movement, quick walking, the open air, and cold < the asthmatic symptoms.—Cramp-like and constrictive tension in chest, principally on breathing (on drawing a long breath), and sometimes with internal heat and ebullition of blood.—Pain as from (subcutaneous) ulceration, or sharp and incisive pain in chest.—Acute suppuration of the lungs.—Shootings in chest and in sides, principally at night and when lying down, and sometimes with difficulty in drawing a full inspiration, inability to remain lying on the side affected, short cough, and paroxysm of suffocation.—(Pain in l. side under heart as if a string were pulling there.—R. T. C.)

19. Heart.—Congestion of blood to chest and heart, esp. at night, with anxious dreams (*e.g.*, of being immured), with starting up and anxious cries.—Catching pain in cardiac region; > for a time by pressure of hand.—Stitches in præcordial region, > while walking, with pressure and anxiety, impeding respiration.—Burning in region of heart.—Frequent and violent fits of palpitation, principally after dinner and after moral emotions, or provoked by conversation, and often with anguish, clouded sight (vanishing of sight), and impeded respiration, esp. when lying on the l. side.—(With menstrual irregularities, chlorosis, &c.; the beat of the heart is felt in the pit of the stomach.) —Anxiety, heaviness, pressure, and burning sensation in heart.

20. Neck and Back.—Rheumatic, tensive, and drawing pains in nape of neck and in neck, sometimes semilateral, and often with swelling of the parts, and pains as from subcutaneous ulceration when they are touched.—Cracking in cervical vertebræ and shoulder-blades on moving those parts.—Itching pimples on neck.—Swelling of glands of neck.—Pains in sacrum and in back, as from having remained some time in a bent posture, or with rigidity, as from the pressure of a belt.—Sacral pains like those of labour.—Pains in back and chilliness from suppressed menstruation.—Shootings in back, in loins, and between shoulder-blades.—Curvature of spine (upper part).

21. Limbs.—Redness and swelling of joints, with stinging pains.—Anxious, tremulous sensation in limbs.—Drawing, sticking, < in joints, which are painful to touch.—Weakness in limbs morning after rising, with relaxation without feeling weary.—Drawing, tearing pains in limbs, shifting rapidly from place to place ; < at night, from warmth ; > from uncovering.—Pain in limbs in morning in bed, < in joints, forcing him to stretch, with general heat.—On waking the parts on which he has lain are asleep, with crawling and tingling.—Coldness of hands and feet ; they seem dead.

22. **Upper Limbs.**—Sharp, jerking, and drawing pains in shoulder-joint, as well as in the arms, hands, and fingers.—Paralytic pains in scapular joint when lifting and moving arms.—Burning sensation in arm in evening or at night, with sensation of dryness in fingers.—Burning heat in hands and arms and in trunk with perspiration down spine (agg.—R. T. C.)—Pressive heaviness in arms, with sensation of numbness, esp. in hands.—Sensation of tension and swelling and wrenching pain in joints of elbows, hands, and fingers, with rigidity.—Swelling of elbow after a contusion.—Swelling of veins on forearm and hands.—Easy numbness of fingers, principally in morning and at night.—Vesicles between fingers, with pricking pain.—Pain as if caused by panaritium in index.—Itching chilblains on hands.

23. **Lower Limbs.**—Pain as from a bruise or from ulceration in the psoas.—Wrenching pain in coxo-femoral articulation, with painful jerks, as in a wound, extending as far as knee, < during repose.—Pulling and tension in thighs and legs, < in calves of legs, as if tendons were too short.—Pain as from a bruise, with sensation of paralytic weakness in bones and muscles of thighs and legs.—Pain as from subcutaneous ulceration in legs and soles of feet.—Cracking in knees.—Swelling of knees, sometimes chiefly above patella, and often with heat, inflammation, sharp drawing and shooting pains.—Enlargement of knee with local varicosis (relieved.—R. T. C.)—Weakness and yielding of knees, with tottering gait.—Pulling and great fatigue in legs, esp. knees, with trembling.—Swelling of veins and varices in legs.—Numbness in legs when remaining long standing.—Pain in tibia as from a bruise.—Tension and drawing in calves of legs.—Hot swelling of legs, or only of the back or of soles of feet, sometimes with shooting pains when the parts are touched, and during movement.—Painful sensation of numbness in soles of feet and in balls of the toes.—Red-hot swelling of feet, extending up to calf, with stinging pain.—Swelling of top of foot.—Œdematous swelling of feet, < in evening.—Piercing shootings and incisive pains in heels (towards evening).—Shootings in soles of feet and extremities of toes.—Chilblains.—The complaints are < when one allows the feet to hang down.

24. **Generalities.**—[Affections in general, and of any kind, appearing in r. abdominal ring ; r. chest ; r. upper and lower extremity ; tongue ; increase of saliva ; larynx ; trachea ; nape of neck ; heart and region of heart ; palpitation of heart, also with anguish : small of back ; shoulder-joints ; fingers ; legs ; shin-bones ; calves, particularly when they are swollen, red, and hot ; heel ; sole of foot ; ball or under part of toes ; knee-joint ; bones of lower extremities ; inflammation of bones in general.—Strong desire for open air, which makes patient feel better in every way, headache, toothache, earache, cold in head, &c., are all > in open air, can breathe better, &c.—Bleeding from inner parts ; congestion of blood to single parts ; apparent deficiency of blood.—Chlorosis (in persons of mild, quiet, &c., dispositions).—Secretion of mucus increased ; nervous debility.—Varicose veins, even when inflamed, esp. when blue, particularly in pregnant females ; feel more comfortable when walking about.—(Phlebitis of single veins.—R. T. C.)—Symptoms < :

in afternoon; from mental affections; on waking; when blowing nose (produces pain in chest, nose, head, or somewhere else, or a cracking in ears); before falling asleep; during expiration; after taking cold; from coughing; from change of position (particularly applicable to the female organism); from loss of fluids; from being frostbitten; lying on l. side; on painless side; lying with head low; having measles, after measles; before and during menstruation; on beginning to move; from taking bread; butter; buckwheat; fat food; fruits; ice; pancakes; warm food; abuse of Peruvian bark; can't bear pressure on the well side if it be made towards the diseased side; from derangement of stomach; during stool, particularly in dysentery if it gives great pain in small of back; while suckling child; in the sun; in the twilight; before, during, or after urinating; women in confinement; from having a tapeworm; from surgical injuries in general; from tobacco; during pregnancy.—Symptoms >: in open air; in a cold place; from cold air; by lying on r. side; with head high; from cold things; from washing; on wetting the affected parts; after discharge of flatus.—H. N. G.]—Sharp drawing and jerking pains in muscles, < at night, or in bed in evening, as well as by heat of a room, > in the open air, and often accompanied by numbness, paralytic weakness, or hard swelling of parts affected.—Shootings and sensation of coldness in parts affected on a change of weather.—Tension in some of the limbs as if tendons were too short.—Shifting pains which pass rapidly from one part to the other, often with swelling and redness in joints.—Sensation of hollowness; of pulsations, knocking, or throbbing in inner parts; of extension in size, as if one part, or every part, were growing too large; of a band around the parts; of buzzing or humming in any part of the body.—Shocks in tendons.—Fitful pains with shivering, labouring respiration, paleness of face, and trembling of legs.—The shiverings increase as the pains become <.—Pain as from a bruise or subcutaneous ulceration on touching parts affected.—Semilateral pains and affections.—Symptoms are < and renewed when seated after long-continued exercise; or on rising after having been seated a long time, as well as during repose, esp. when lying on side or back.—The symptoms which appear when lying on back are > by turning on side or by rising up, and *vice versâ*.—Movement, walking, pressure, external heat, and the open air, equally > many of the symptoms, while they < others.—Symptoms generally most violent in evening or at night before midnight, sometimes also in morning and after a meal.—The symptoms are < every second day in evening.—Agitation and uneasiness throughout body, with inability to sleep or to enjoy repose, and constant inclination to stretch limbs.—Frequent and troublesome pulsations over whole body, < during movement.—Great tendency of limbs to go to sleep.—Frequent trembling of limbs with anxiety.—Sluggishness and heaviness of limbs, with paralytic weakness, painful sensibility of joints, and tottering gait.—Weariness in morning, which is < by a recumbent position.—Fainting fits with deadly paleness of face.—Epileptic convulsions, with violent movements of limbs, followed by weakness, eructations, and inclination to vomit (after suppression of catamenia).—Great sensibility and repugnance to open air.—Great desire to remain lying down or sitting.—Pain as from a bruise in bones of extremities.—Emaciation.

25. **Skin.**—Pale skin.—Itching, mostly burning or pricking (as if caused

by stings of ants), principally in evening, and at night in heat of bed, < by scratching.—Red spots, like morbilli, or nettle-rash.—Frequent redness, even when the parts are cold.—Eruptions from eating pork, itching violently in bed.—Eruptions like measles.—Rhagades.—Suppurating wounds, pus thick and too profuse.—Pus copious and yellow.—Moles or freckles in young girls. —Eruptions similar to varicella coniformis, with violent itching in bed.—Chilblains, particularly when they turn blue.—Exanthema, chapped.—Blue-black swellings.—Chilblains with bluish-red swelling, heat, and burning, or pulsative pains.—Phlegmonous erysipelas, with hardness, burning heat, and shooting pain on touching or moving parts affected.—Furunculi.—Shining redness, hardness, and itching round ulcers, with ready bleeding, and shooting, burning, and gnawing pains.—Deep or fistulous ulcers; where there is much swelling around.—Inflamed or putrid ulcers.—Varices.

26. **Sleep.**—Constant sleepiness and comatose sleep, with agitation and disquieting fancies, day or night.—Great tendency to sleep during day, principally in evening or afternoon.—Irregular sleep, too early in evening or too late in morning, and sometimes with nocturnal sleeplessness.—Sleep retarded, sometimes until two hours after midnight, and often followed by early waking. —A great flow of ideas hinders sleep in evening and at night.—Agitated sleep, with frequent waking; and general numbness on waking.—Inability to sleep except when seated with head inclined forwards or to one side.—During sleep, chattering, talking, delirium, convulsive movements of mouth, eyes, and limbs; tears, cries, and moans, nightmare; starts from fright; shocks in body and jerking in limbs.—Wakes up frightened and confused, knows not where he is, cannot collect himself.—At night great agitation and tossing, inquietude and anguish of heart, ebullition of blood, dry heat, itching, incoherent talking, with fixed ideas.—When sleeping patient lies on back with knees raised and arms placed over head or crossed over abdomen.—Fearful, frightful, anxious, confused, vivid, disgusting, voluptuous dreams, of quarrels and of business of the day, of spectres, and of the dead.—Frequent yawning.

27. **Fever.**—Chilliness of one side only; chilliness without thirst, often followed by fever without thirst (accompanied by vertigo and stupor); heat on one side; perspiration on one side only; want of thirst; febrile symptoms . side.—Continuous internal chilliness even in warm room.—Thirst before chill or heat, seldom during hot stage.—Chilliness (4 p.m.) without thirst, accompanied by anxiety and dyspnœa; this is followed by a drawing pain extending from back into head, three hours later heat of whole body without any thirst, with sweat on face, drowsiness without any sleep and unconsciousness; in morning perspiration over whole body.—Coldness, shiverings, and shudderings, principally in evening or afternoon, and sometimes with paleness of face, vertigo, and dizziness, pain and heaviness in head; anxiety and oppression of chest, vomiting of mucus (when the cold stage comes on), desire to lie down, and flushes of heat.—Partial coldness and shivering, principally in back, arms, legs, hands, and feet, often with heat in head or face and redness of cheeks.—Semilateral coldness with numbness of the side affected. —Dry heat (internal), principally at night, in evening in bed or in morning, and often with fits of anguish, headache, face red and bloated, or perspiration on face, shivering on being uncovered, burning in hands, with swelling of

veins, lamentations, sighs, and moans, profound or agitated sleep, anxious an quick respiration, fainting fits, with cloudiness of eyes, inclination to vomi and loose evacuations.—Partial heat, principally on face, with redness c cheeks, hands, face, &c., often semilateral, with coldness and shivering in th opposite parts.—Heat of face or heat of one hand, with coldness of the othe —Febrile paroxysms composed of heat, which are preceded by shivering with adipsia, and mixed with, or followed by, perspiration; quotidian, tertia or quartan type; < in evening or afternoon; remission in morning durin apyrexia, nausea and loss of appetite, headache, painful oppression at ches moist cough, bitterness in mouth, constipation or (mucous) diarrhœa.—Febri symptoms with loss of consciousness, delirium, tears, and despair, or wit gastrico-mucous or bilious symptoms or with comatose sleep (or consequer upon the abuse of *Quinine*, with bitter taste of food and constipation).- Repugnance to external heat.—Pulse weak and small, but accelerated.—Puls quick and small; or full and slow; or feeble and almost suppressed.—Pe spiration, principally at night or towards morning; profuse and fetid sweat semilateral or partial sweat (on head and face), and sweat with cramps o arms and hands, weariness, comatose sleep, dreamy reveries, and redness face.—Perspiration during sleep, soon ceasing when waking.—Perspire easily during the day.—Night-sweat with stupor.—Smell of perspiratio sour, musty, like musk.—Perspiration at times cold.

Pulsatilla Nuttaliana.

American Pulsatilla. Pasque Flower (American). Anemone Ludo viciana. A. nuttaliana. *N. O.* Ranunculaceæ. Tincture o whole plant.

Clinical.—Amenorrhœa. Clavus. Cold; liability to. Deafness. Diarrhœ Dyspepsia. Feet, fidgety. Home-sickness. Knees; rheumatism of. Liver, pain in. Measles; prophylaxis of. Menses, retarded. Ptosis. Rheumatism; wande ing. Sciatica. Shoulder, r., pain in. Tinnitus. Uterus, pains in.

Characteristics.—The American *Pulsatilla* approaches mor nearly to *P. vulgaris* than to *P. nig.* in its botanical characters. I flourishes especially in the dry and sandy bluffs which form the be of the Mississippi. The flower is pale purplish. "The odour of th *dried* plant is rather faint, being slightly *camphoraceous*, the taste c the dried flowers simply sweetish and herbaceous, that of the leave more astringent with very slight acrimony. The *taste* and to som extent the odour of the fresh plant are both acrid and irritating (Hale). A. W. Miller, a pharmaceutist (referred to by Hale), analyse *P. nutt.* The extracted substances had an acrid, almost caustic taste and well-marked camphoraceous odour. When volatilised they pro duced an irritating, pungent vapour, affecting the eyes and causin sneezing. The analysis revealed the following constituents: (1 Organic—Grape-sugar, gum, resin, an alkaloid and anemonic acid (2) Inorganic—Sulphate of potash, carbonate of potash, chlorate o potassium, carbonate of lime, magnesia, and "a proto-salt of iron.

r. W. H. Miller (brother of A. W. M.), an allopathist, claimed to ave used *P. nutt.* with success in many chronic eye affections, parcularly catarrh, amaurosis, and corneal opacities, cutaneous erupons, and secondary syphilis. Hale instituted the first homœopathic esearch, and Burt was the first prover. The symptoms have a strong esemblance to those of *P. nig.*, and cases cured with *P. nutt.* are aostly such as would be amenable to *P. nig.* A patient of mine was ncidentally cured of a tendency to catch colds by taking *P. nutt.* for ome weeks as a prophylactic against measles. Burnett cured with it case of deafness and œdema of left upper eyelid. The proving howed a powerful effect on the menstrual function, and Hale reports nany cures of retentio mensium : (1) A young lady, formerly subject o retardation of menses, had : Constant chilliness, cold hands and eet, loss of appetite, sour eructations, nausea after meals, hemicrania, oothache, melancholy, general malaria. Menses two weeks late ; ook a chill at the time they were due, when she had precursory ymptoms ; no symptoms of menses now. *P. nutt.* 1 in water every wo hours. After the first dose the menses came on and the contitutional symptoms cleared off. (2) Plethoric, usually healthy young voman, had menses delay two weeks. Continual severe headache, a leaviness and fulness, < moving or stooping ; sight dim, complete lindness on stooping or rising suddenly ; weight in uterine region evere aching extending to back, < evening. Hands and feet cold ; veakness in lower limbs. *Act. r.* failed to relieve. *P. nutt.* 1 x, ; drops every three hours, brought speedy improvement. Next day nenses came on profusely but without pain, two days before the xpiration of the eighth week. The *Puls.* flying pains were very noticeable in the proving. Hale reports this case : Strong, healthylooking man had wandering rheumatic pains chiefly in dorsum of right foot, loins, thighs, chest, arms, head. The head pain was a dull, heavy pressure in vertex, nearly constant, with occasional sharp pains. Some fever but no local inflammation of joints or muscles. Urine scanty, depositing lithates. Acidity of stomach. Appetite good. Bowels normal. *P. nutt.* 1 x cured in three days. Some *Peculiar Symptoms* are : Home-sick feeling. Trembling weakness, weariness, heaviness. Snapping noise in ears. Fidgety feet. Colic before and after stool. Colic after eating a pear. Stiffness of fingers. Hands hot and dry (a constant symptom). The symptoms are < coming in from open air ; after eating ; eating a pear ; at night ; by warmth ; by reading ; on urinating ; on walking. > Walking in open air ; rubbing with flesh-brush ; scratching.

Relations.—See Puls. *Antidoted by:* Ant. c. *Compare:* In fidgety feet, Zn., Caust.

SYMPTOMS.

1. **Mind.**—Sad, gloomy ; with frequent eructations.—Home-sick, despondent.—Anxiety ; at night.—Irritable ; quick, nervous motions.—Dull, disinclined for work.

2. **Head.**—Dizziness on entering house from open air ; sudden, in afternoon with fulness of head.—Dull, heavy headache, mornings ; > by

active exercise before breakfast.—Flying pains in head and feet.—Dul oppressive, frontal headache; on waking.—Hard pains in upper forehead pas in a wave to occiput, involving whole brain.—With headache cutting pain in epigastrium.—Hard pain over l. eye; as if a nail being pressed into fore head.—Pain over r. eye, afternoon, > walking in open air, < in warm room with sense of heat, fulness in head, and dryness of eyes.—Sharp, shootin pains through both temples; in r. temple.—Dull pain in r. temple; in verte —Severe throbbing on vertex.—Full, hot feeling at cerebellum.—Headach arising from nape of neck and upwards.

3. **Eyes.**—Profuse secretion of mucus from eyes.—Dull pain deep i eyes, with smarting.—Dryness; smarting; profuse flow of tears.—Twitching of l. brow and upper lid for half an hour after going to bed; r. lids < reading.—Paralysis of lids.—Œdema of l. upper lid.—Tarsal edges red, dry irritable.—Lids agglutinated; profuse secretion of soft, yellow, or whit matter.—Profuse lachrymation with dull pains in eyeball extending to mala bone.—Neuralgic pains in eyeballs, while walking, < r.

4. **Ears.**—Hard, drawing pains along r. Eustachian tube.—With th pains in head and eyes, frequent drawing pains in ears from within out.— Sharp pains in r. ear and temples.—L. ear feels closed; later both.—Snappin noises in ears; fluttering in r.—Deafness, with œdema of l. upper eyeli (cured).

5. **Nose.**—Dryness and heat in nose.

6. **Face.**—Face red, hot, flushed.—Complexion at first rough; late very clear after disappearance of rash.—After eating, flushed, pressure o blood in face.—Painful drawing in l. cheek-bone and jaw.—Lips dry.

8. **Mouth.**—Tongue: coated white, with flat, pappy taste on rising; covered with tough slime, red, rather dry and swollen, teeth indented, yellowish coat along centre; unusually red after eating.—Breath offensive, to self and others; after eating.—Mouth and lips dry.—Smarting of velum palati.—Mouth filling with saliva.—On awaking, dry, pappy taste in mouth, as if tongue thickly coated (which it was not).—Taste: flat; flat bitter; flat rough; sweetish; bad.—Awoke after afternoon sleep with vinegar-like acidity in mouth and dull, pressing pain in stomach.

9. **Throat.**—Frequent inclination to clear throat.—After eating slight irritation in throat, with easy expectoration of white, tough mucus.—Throat dry, smarts on waking, contains much tough mucus hard to dislodge.— Scratchy, husky feeling in throat.—Sensation of plug in lower throat.

11. **Stomach.**—Great hunger; rapidly returned after eating.—Loss of appetite.—More thirst than usual; cold water extremely grateful.—Eructations: tasting of *Puls.*; while riding belches up food hot and tasteless; of hot, tasteless wind; of sour air.—Thick gulping.—Heartburn.—Nausea; and dull headache, then faintness at stomach; on entering house.—Fulness in stomach preventing eating in spite of appetite (cured in the proving).— Painful emptiness, pressure, then rising towards œsophagus like heartburn.— Emptiness: after action of bowels; after eating.—Gnawing, empty sensation. —Weight and pressure in stomach; after eating; with faintness.—Distress: with severe cutting pains in epigastrium.—Feeling as if needles being pressed through stomach.—Heat in stomach gradually increasing to pain, < in spots under sternum; burning; pricking burning.

12. **Abdomen.**—Dull pains in r. hypochondrium; in l.—Severe pain in nbilicus 6 a.m., with desire for stool, stool dark, covered with mucus, severe ains for half an hour after.—Rumbling; after dinner of wind in distended odomen moving from epigastrium to hypogastrium.—Aching in one spot < y moving.—Colicky pains after eating a ripe pear.—Aching in l. groin; above iliac crest on moving or bending.—Dull pains: in whole abdomen; by oells in hypogastrium.

13. **Stool and Anus.**—Evening and afternoon, feeling as if must go stool immediately, with constant distress in lower epigastrium and mbilicus.—Sudden attack of diarrhœa whilst riding on horseback.—Stools: ark, thin, pap-like; watery, light yellow, painless; mushy; dark, slightly overed with mucus; dry, hard, lumpy.—Constipation.

14. **Urinary Organs.**—Pain on urinating; at end of urethra.—Frequent micturition.—Tenesmus, extending up ureters; uneasiness in kidneys. -Urine: pale; albuminous; excess of water; skunk-like odour.

15. **Male Sexual Organs.**—Distressing erection, soon subsiding.—ain in penis on waking, < on micturating.—Hard, sticking pains in (l.) ermatic cord and testes.—Dull pains in testes, < r.—Emission.

16. **Female Sexual Organs.**—Stinging, darting pains passing through erus from side to side.—Leucorrhœa, bland but so profuse, and with so great epression that the prover refused to take more of the drug although it moved a pleuritic pain.—Leucorrhœa, painless, 4 p.m.—Feeling as if enses coming on.—(Menses became more regular.)—Menses weak, too soon ever before; but discharge, which had been formerly too dark and with ain, was this time natural in colour and painless).—Menses, always copious, ecame increased to flooding and lasted three days.—In morning on waking found menses had returned first time since weaning babe (two onths).

17. **Respiratory Organs.**—Coughed much.—Constant inclination to ough.—Small sore spot in upper trachea.

18. **Chest.**—Sharp, stabbing pain in pectoralis major muscle, followed y burning distress therein.—During evening severe pain under l. arm nearer ck.—Aching pain in chest all forenoon.—Itching blotches on r. breast; r. de chest.

19. **Heart.**—Audible pulsation of heart.—Pulse accelerated.

20. **Neck and Back.**—Stiffness r. side neck, morning.—Backache.—ameness in back, esp. loins.—Woke frequently with backache.—Weakness loins; feeling as if menses coming on.

21. **Limbs.**—Aching in limbs and loins wakes him frequently.—Frequent ing pains in hands, feet, toes.

22. **Upper Limbs.**—Rheumatism of r. shoulder.—Lameness in muscles r. upper arm.—Muscles stiff.—Frequent momentary pains in wrists and gers.—Fingers stiff.—Hands dry and hot all day.

23. **Lower Limbs.**—Sharp neuralgic pains along sciatic nerve from p-joint to middle of thigh.—Drawing in (l.) sartorius muscle, when walking. Pain in both knees; < l.; severe, dull in r. for two hours in bed; rheuatic.—Legs heavy while walking; trembling weakness; nervous pains, < l. Cramp.—Dull pain in ankles; flying pains.—With desire to urinate, afteron, and at night, nervous sensation is felt, irresistible fidgets, < night.—

Elevated eruption on ankles and half-way up leg, several large blotches back, dark red; itches all the time, < night.—Very cold feet, evening.

24. Generalities.—Great debility; on rising; in evening.—Langu feverish, depressed.

25. Skin.—Elevated blotchy eruption on legs and back.—Slight rash back and shoulders.—Itching scattered pimples r. side of chest; light r rash-like blotches on r. breast, itching severely at night; < when heated Red rash on body, face, neck, back, chest, abdomen, limbs, < chest a abdomen; later erythema; later nodules, turn white after scratching *Ant. c.* 200).—Itching: intense all over; < night before bedtime; > ru bing; < riding in cold air; returned repeatedly throughout the winter.

26. Sleep.—Sleepy; sleep not refreshing.—Sleepless: for an hour 4 a.m for several hours; from over-eating.—Restless, with frontal headache.—Ma dreams; confused.

27. Fever.—Chilly; with full, uncomfortable feeling in stomach; w inclination to yawn; with papescent stool; shaking.—Heat; feverish; w debility; skin hot, flaccid; > cool, blustering wind.—Hot face, cold fe hands hot and feverish.

Pyrethrum Parthenium.

Chrysanthemum parthenium (Bern.). Feverfew. *N. O.* Composit
Tincture of fresh plant.

Clinical.—Convulsions. Delirium. Dysentery. Fevers. Loquacity. Rheumati

Characteristics.—*Pyr. p.* "has bitter tonic properties like th of Chamomile (*Anthemis nobilis*); and is a popular remedy in slig fevers (whence the name 'Feverfew'). The smell of the whole he is said to be particularly offensive to bees" (*Treas. of Bot.*). So popular "insect powders" are made of the dried flowers of *Pyrethr roseum. Radix pyrethri*, or Pellitory of Spain, which is used as irritant and as a toothache cure, is the root of *Anacyclus pyrethri* The roots of the genus have a hot taste, whence the name Pyrethr (πῦρ, fire). One observation has been recorded with *Pyr. p.* A b 3½, took 50 minims of the tincture. It nearly proved fatal, caus diarrhœa, convulsions of a tetanic nature, twitchings, loquaci delirium, restless, rapid, and weak pulse, and profuse sweat at nig Some observations of Cooper's will be found in the Schema. Coo has also cured cases of subacute rheumatism with *P. roseum.*

Relations.—*Compare:* Cham., Cin., Absin., Artemis, and ot Compositæ.

SYMPTOMS.

1. Mind.—Very excited, talked incessantly for four hours.—Lying state of stupor; easily roused but quickly relapsing.

8. Mouth.—Soreness of tongue.

13. Stool.—Diarrhœa, 5 a.m., with pain; at first profuse and exhausti with tenesmus; afterwards involuntary evacuations of mucus slightly tinged with blood; better next morning.

19. **Heart.**—Pulse very rapid (120 to 130) and feeble; became normal the fifth day.

21. **Limbs.**—Old subacute rheumatism of hands and small bones relieved.—R. T. C.)

24. **Generalities.**—Twitching of muscles of limbs (not those of face); subsided by morning of third day.—At 12.30 violent convulsions lasting an hour and leaving the child apparently moribund, but he gradually recovered.—Convulsive movements like those of tetanus.—Restlessness.—Feet, legs and body, which were swollen, decidedly reduce, and next menstrual period is dark and deficient (in a gouty woman, 50.—R. T. C.)

27. **Fever.**—Profuse perspiration; and restlessness (first night).

Pyrogenium.

Pyrogen. Pyrexin. Sepsin. A product of the decomposition of chopped lean beef in water, allowed to stand in the sun for two or three weeks. Dilutions; (which should be made, according to Burnett, direct and *without* glycerine).

Clinical.—Abscess. Anus, sweating near. Bed-sores. Bright's disease. Constipation. Diarrhœa. Dysentery. Eczema. *Enteric fever.* Fistula. Headache. Heart, rapid action of; consciousness of; failure of. *Hectic fever.* Indian continued fevers. Influenza. Intestines, ulceration of; obstruction of. *Labour: puerperal fever. Ovary, abscess of.* Peritonitis. Phthisis pulmonalis. Ptomaine poisoning. Puerperal fever. *Pyæmia.* Sepsis. *Spine, Pott's curvature of.* Tabes mesenterica. Tuberculosis. Typhilitis. Ulcers, varicose; obstinate. Varicosis.

Characteristics.—John Drysdale was the first, in 1880, to suggest the use of this substance as a medicament (*On Pyrexin or Pyrogen as a Therapeutic Agent*, Baillière, Tyndale & Cox). Burdon Sanderson has stated (*B. M. J.*, February 13, 1875) that "only liquids which contain bacteria or have a marked proneness to their production" are capable of setting up pyrexia. This remark struck Drysdale, and though, of course, he could not endorse the "only" of the statement—many drugs known to homœopaths set up fever—he saw that the fact might be turned to account. Sanderson further defines *Pyrogen* as "a chemical non-living substance formed by living bacteria, but also by living pus-corpuscles, or the living blood- or tissue-protoplasms from which these corpuscles spring." In Sanderson's experiments with *Pyro.* the following effects were observed. (1) From a non-fatal dose: The animal shivers and begins to move about restlessly. The temperature rises from 2° to 3° C., the maximum being reached in three hours. Thirst and vomiting come on, followed by feculent and thin mucous, and finally bloody diarrhœa and tenesmus. In five hours these symptoms begin to subside, and the animal recovers with wonderful rapidity. When death occurs it is from heart failure. In *non-fatal* cases with gastro-enteric symptoms the temperature gradually rises for four hours, and as gradually subsides : in *fatal* cases it rises rapidly to 104° F., then rapidly declines to below normal. (2) From a fatal dose : There is intestinal hæmorrhage, purging, collapse, and death. After death extravasations of blood are found in heart, pleura, and pericardium ; the spleen is enlarged and full of blood. Mucous membrane of stomach and small intestines is intensely injected with detachment of epithelium and exudation of bloody fluid, which distends the gut. The blood is dark, the corpuscles being in clumps instead of rolls, and many being dissolved in the liquor sanguinis. White corpuscles partially disintegrated. Drysdale prepared a tincture of *Pyro.*—which he preferred to call *Pyrexin*, since it is not a mere fever-*producer* : others have called it *Sepsin* ; but this is too close to *Septicæmin*, a name given to a related and perhaps identical nosode : I have chosen to retain the name *Pyrogen*, by which the remedy is best known in homœopathy—and put his own suggestion into practice. His success was very encouraging, but as he continued to use the ϕ tincture and lowest attenuations the difficulty of keeping the preparation was not small ; and the remedy did not come into extensive use till Burnett published his pamphlet on *Pyrogenium in Fevers and Blood-poisoning* in 1888. Burnett used chiefly the 6th centesimal dilution, which is perfectly harmless, and which will keep indefinitely. Heath, who made one of the preparations used by Burnett, gave some of it to Swan, of New York, who ran it up into the high infinitesimals. Much of the American experience is with Swan's attenuations, including a proving by Sherbino (*Med. Adv.* xxv. 369), whose symptoms I have marked (S) in the Schema. The remainder of the symptoms of the Schema are for the most part clinical. Yingling (*H. P.*, xiii. 402) collected symptoms from many reported cases, and arranged them with the symptoms of the proving (Yingling erroneously describes *Pyro.* as prepared from "pus from septic abscess." This is *Septicæmin.* He refers, however, to Burnett's pamphlet and to cases cured with *Pyro.*, leaving the actual substance referred to not in doubt. H. C. Allen, who published the proving and most of the cases in *Med. Adv.*, rightly describes *Pyro.* as a "Product of Sepsis"). Drysdale's original cases include a number in which threatened typhoid was averted, a case of tabes mesenterica cured, and one of ulceration of the colon greatly benefited. Burnett's were cases of fully developed typhoid all cut short at the height by *Pyro.* 6 given every two hours. In his pamphlet is included a successful experience of Dr. Shouldham's with *Pyro.* 6 in two cases of diphtheritic sore throat. I have had ample opportunity of observing the power of *Pyro.* over typhoid fever, and typhoid and hectic states including one of discharging abscess connected with Pott's disease of the spine. T. M. Dillingham reports (*Med. Adv.*, xxvii. 367) the case of a young German Jewess who had been under treatment at various hospitals for Bright's disease, and at the *Hahnemann* Hospital of New York among others. To this she was readmitted on March 14, 1890 when she first came under Dr. Dillingham's care. The urine showed an enormous amount of albumen and a variety of casts. Feet and legs greatly swollen, face puffy. Throbbing headache, often accompanied by profuse nose-bleed, nausea, and vomiting ; < motion an light; abnormally bright eyes, widely dilated pupils. *Bell.* gave temporary relief; but on May 31st the condition was desperate. Dillingham then learned that the trouble dated from a large abscess resulting from a lanced, badly cared-for felon of the left thumb. She was ill six weeks with this abscess, having, as her doctors said, "blood poisoning." Soon after this her face and feet began to swell. On May 31st the condition was this: Feet, legs, and genitals greatly swollen. Frightful throbbing headache, > by tight band constantly worn. > By heat; very fond of the *hot bath.* Headaches had terrible aggravations lasting two to four days, during which time she could neither lie in bed nor sit up, but was in constant motion, groaning and crying piteously for help. *Pyro.* cmm, Swan, one dose was given, and no other medicine, although the patient on one occasion begged for something to stop the pain. In the course of June she began to mend, and on October 20th was discharged cured. In Sherbino's proving he was cured incidentally of a consciousness of the heart and its working, and palpitation from least excitement or anxiety, < beginning to move; congestion to head as if apoplexy would ensue. *Cactus* had done no good. Sherbino cured: (1) a case of puerperal fever with *Pyro.*, being led to its selection by the very high pulse rate. (2) Relapse of typhoid, pulse 140, temperature 102° F.; both were normal in twenty-four hours. (3) Young lady, 17, fever, aching bones, bed felt very hard. Numb, paralytic feeling. *As the fever left the pulse kept mounting up. Pyro.* cmm, Swan, repeated as often as effect ceased, cured.—*Pyro.* is one of the *germinal* remedies of the materia medica. When once the idea of its essential action is grasped an infinity of applications become apparent. As Drysdale put it, "The most summary indication for *Pyro.* would be to term it the *Aconite* of the typhous or typhoid quality of pyrexia," and wherever poisoning by bacterial products (*e.g.*, in the hectic of phthisis) is going on *Pyro.* will be likely to do good. *Sepsis* is the essence of the action of *Pyro.* H. C. Allen gives this indication for its use in septic states: "When the best selected remedies fail to relieve or permanently improve"—analogous to the action of *Pso.* and *Sul.* in other conditions. Also: "Latent pyogenic process, patient continually relapsing after apparent simillimum." As *Pyro.* is a product of carrion, the carrion-like odour of bodily emaciations, secretions, and excretions is a keynote for its use. Other leading indications are: Restlessness; must move constantly to > the soreness of parts. "Constipation, from impactum of fæces in fevers; stool large, black, carrion-like." "Chill begins in back, between scapulæ." "Severe general chill of bones and extremities." "In all cases of fever commencing with pains in the limbs," Swan. "Pulse abnormally rapid, out of all proportion to temperature." *Pyro.* 5, five drops in water night and morning, assisted in the cure of a case of anal fistula in a case of Burnett's (*On Fistula*, p. 66). Under its action a sweating at the seat which the man had had for many years disappeared; and the skin of his hands, which were subject to dry eczema, assumed a much cleaner aspect. J. S. Hunt (*H. W.*, xxxi. 54) reports five cases of varicose ulcers, all of which healed quickly under *Pyro.* Bellairs (*H. W.*, xxxiv. 298) gave *Pyro.* 200 to an elderly woman who suffered for years with an ulcerated leg, which was riddled with deep, burrowing wounds, extremely painful and discharging freely. *Hep.*, *Sil.*, *Ars.*, *Ham.*, did no good. Under *Pyro.* once or twice a day "a large boil" formed on the calf of the leg and discharged its contents, after which the various ulcers healed up directly. The symptoms are > by heat (drinking hot water; hot bath). > Tightly binding head. > Stretching out limbs; walking about; turning over or changing position. Heart's action and cough < by motion. Eyeball < moving eye. Cough < motion and in a warm room. < Sitting up in bed; rising. (Cough > sitting up; < lying down.)

Relations.—*Compare:* Septicæmin (B. Sanderson says bacteria and pus cells produce the same chemical result; Pyro. and Sept. may therefore be identical, but I think it best to keep them distinct); Malar. (the *vegetable* Pyrogen); Lach. In typhoid with soreness, bed feels hard, Bap., Arn., Rhus. > Motion and stretching limbs, Rhus. Cough < by motion and in warm room, Bry. Uterine hæmorrhage, Ipec. ("if Ipec. fails when indicated give Pyro.," Yingling). Offensive diarrhœa, Pso. Black stools, Lept. Constipation, Op., Sanic., Pb. Lochia thin, fetid, Nit. ac. Vomits water as soon as warm in stomach, Pho. Throbbing headache, Bell. Varicose, offensive ulcers of old persons, Pso. Skin ashy, Sec. Suppuration, Hep.

Causation.—Blood poisoning. Ptomaine poisoning. Sewer-gas poisoning. Typhoid fever (remote effects of). Dissecting wounds.

SYMPTOMS.

1. **Mind.**—Loquacious; can think and talk faster than ever before (S). Irritable (S).—Delirious on closing eyes; sees a man at foot of bed.—Whispers; in sleep.—Sensation as if she covered the whole bed; knew her head was on pillow, but did not know where the rest of her body was.—Feels when lying on one side that she is one person, and another person when turning on the other side.—Sensation as though crowded with arms and legs.—Hallucination that he is very wealthy; remaining after the fever.

2. **Head.**—Staggers as if drunk on rising in morning (S.)—Dizziness on rising up in bed.—Pains in both mastoids, < r.; dull throbbing in mastoid region (S).—Great throbbing of arteries of temples and head; every pulsation felt in brain and in ears; the throbbings meet on top of brain (S).—Painless throbbing all through front of head; sounds like escaping steam (S).—Frightful throbbing headache > from tight band.—Excruciating, bursting, throbbing headache with intense restlessness (often accompanied with profuse nose-bleed, nausea, and vomiting).—Sensation as if a cap were on.—Rolling of head from side to side.—Forehead bathed in cold sweat.

3. **Eyes.**—L. eyeball sore, < looking up and turning eye outward (S). —Projecting eyes.

4. **Ears.**—Loud ringing, like a bell, l. ear (also r.) (S).—Ears cold.—Ears red, as if blood would burst out of them.

5. **Nose.**—Nose-bleed; awakened by dreaming it and found it was so. —Sneezing: every time he puts hand from under covers; at night.—Nostrils closing alternately (S).—Cold nose.—Fan-like motion of alæ nasi.

6. **Face.**—Face: burning; yellow; very red; pale, sunken, and bathed in cold sweat; pale, greenish, or chlorotic.—Circumscribed redness of cheeks

8. **Mouth.**—Tongue : coated white in front, brown at back ; yellowish brown, bad taste in morning (S).—Tongue : coated yellowish grey, edges and tip very red ; large, flabby ; yellow brown streak down centre.—Tongue clean, smooth, and dry ; first fiery red, then dark red and intensely dry ; smooth and dry ; glossy, shiny ; dry, cracked, articulation difficult.—Taste : terribly fetid, as if mouth and throat full of pus (produced by dose of *Pyro.* cm, Swan) ; sweetish.—Breath horrible ; like carrion.

9. **Throat.**—Diphtheria with extreme fetor.

10. **Appetite.**—No appetite (S) ; or thirst.—Great thirst for small quantities, but the least liquid was instantly rejected.—> Drinking very hot water.—Thirst and vomiting (dog).

11. **Stomach.**—Belching of sour water after breakfast (S).—Nausea and vomiting.—Vomiting : persistent ; brownish, coffee-ground ; offensive, stercoraceous ; with impacted or obstructed bowels.—Vomiting and purging.—Vomits water when it becomes warm in stomach.—> By vomiting.—Urging to vomit ; with cold feet.—Stomach feels too full (S).

12. **Abdomen.**—Full feeling and bloating of abdomen (S).—When lying on l. side bubbling or gurgling sensation in hypochondria, extending back to l. of spine (S).—Pain in umbilical region with passage of sticky, yellow stool.—While riding in a buggy aching in l. of umbilicus ; < drinking water ; > passing flatus downward.—Soreness of abdomen so severe she can hardly breathe, or bear any pressure over r. side.—Very severe cutting pains r. side going through back, < by every motion, talking, coughing, breathing deep ; > lying on r. (affected) side ; groaning with every breath.

13. **Stool and Anus.**—Feculent and thin mucous, and finally bloody diarrhœa and tenesmus (dog).—Two soft, sticky stools, 8 to 9 a.m.—Involuntary escape of stool when passing flatus (S).—Profuse watery, painless stools, with vomiting.—Stool horribly offensive, carrion-like.—Stool very much constipated, large, difficult, requires much effort ; first part balls, last part natural, with streaks of blood ; anus sore after (S).—Constipation : hard, dry accumulated fæces ; stool large, black, carrion-like ; small black balls like olives.—Congestion and capillary stasis of gastro-intestinal mucous membrane, shedding of epithelium bloody fluid distending intestines (dog).—(Sweat about anus removed ; fistula relieved.)

14. **Urinary Organs.**—Urine scanty ; only passed twice in twenty-four hours (S).—Urine : yellow ; after standing, cloudy with substance looking like orange peel ; red deposit on vessel hard to remove ; deposits sediment like red pepper (S).—Got up three times in night to urinate (S).—(Bright's disease of kidneys.)—Urine albuminous, containing casts ; horribly offensive, carrion-like.—Frequent calls to urinate as fever comes on.—Intolerable tenesmus of bladder ; spasmodic contractions, involving rectum, ovaries, and broad ligaments ; [cured in a case of Yingling's with *Pyro.* cm Swan (and higher) ; patient's next period came on naturally and painlessly, whereas before menses had been painful and extremely offensive.]

15. **Male Sexual Organs.**—Testes hang down relaxed ; scrotum looks and feels thin.

16. **Female Sexual Organs.**—Puerperal peritonitis with extreme fetor ; a rotten odour.—Parts seriously swollen (Bright's disease).—Menses horribly offensive ; carrion-like.—Menses last but one day, then a bloody leucorrhœa,

horribly offensive.—Hæmorrhage of bright red blood with dark clots.—Septicæmia following abortion ; fœtus or secondines retained, decomposed.—(Has cured prolapsus uteri, with bearing down, > by holding the head and straining, as in the act of labour.)—Abscess of l. ovary, acute throbbing pain, great distress, with fever and rigors (*Pyro.* cm, Swan, produced an enormous flow of white creamy pus with general >).—Lochia : thin, acrid, brown, or fœtid ; suppressed, followed by chills, fever, and profuse fetid perspiration.

17. **Respiratory Organs.**—Wheezing when expiring (S).—Cough : with large masses of phlegm from larynx ; < by motion ; < in warm room ; cough = burning in larynx and bronchi ; = pain in occiput ; = stitching in small of back, only noticed in the chair ; coughs up yellow sputa through night (S).—Cough > sitting up, < lying down.—Expectoration : rusty mucus ; horribly offensive.

18. **Chest.**—Pain in r. lung and shoulder, < talking or coughing.—Neglected pneumonia : Cough, night-sweats, frequent pulse, abscess had burst discharging mucn pus of mattery taste (rapid recovery under *Pyro.* cm. three doses).—Chest sore, purple spots on it.—Severe contracting pain within lower sternum, sometimes extending to rib-joints and up to throat, as if œsophagus being cramped.—Ecchymoses on pleura (dog).

19. **Heart.**—Pain in region of l. nipple, as if in heart ; increased action ; pulse 120 (S).—Heart tired as after a long run ; increased action < least motion (S).—Every pulsation felt (painlessly) in head and ears (S).—Sensation as if heart enlarged ; distinct consciousness of heart (S).—Sensation as if heart too full of blood.—Feels as if the heart were pumping cold water (Yingling).—Violent, tiresome heart action.—Palpitation or increased action without corresponding increase of temperature.—Palpitation < by motion —Loud heart-beats ; audible to herself and others.—Could not sleep for whizzing and purring of heart ; when she did sleep was delirious.—Cardiac asthenia from septic conditions.—Ecchymoses on heart and pericardium (dog).

20. **Neck and Back.**—Throbbing of vessels of neck running up in wave from clavicles.—Weak feeling in back ; stitching pain on coughing (S).

21. **Limbs.**—Aching : in bones ; all over body as from a severe cold with soreness of flesh, head feels hard ; > motion (S).—Cold extremities.—Numbness of hands, arms, and feet, extending over whole body.—Automatic movement of r. arm and r. leg, turned the child round from r. to l. till feet reached the pillow : repeated as often as she was put right (cerebro-spinal meningitis).

22. **Upper Limbs.**—Pain in shoulder-joint ; in front, passing three inches down arm (S).—Hands and arms numb.—Hands cold and clammy.—Dry eczema of hands.

23. **Lower Limbs.**—Aching above knees, deep in bones, while sitting by a hot fire ; > by walking (S).—On going to bed aching in patella ; > flexing leg (S).—Aching above l. knee as though bone broken (S).—Aching above knees in bones, > stretching out limbs (S).—Tingling in r. little toe as if frost-bitten.—Feet and legs swollen (Bright's disease).—Numbness of feet.

24. **Generalities.**—Cannot lie more than few minutes in one position > change (S).—Debility in morning, staggered on trying to walk (S).—Nervous, restless (S).—Aching all over, bed feels hard.—Great muscular debility ; rapid recovery in few hours (dog).

25. **Skin.**—Skin pale, cold, of ashy hue.—Obstinate, varicose, offensive ulcers of old people.

26. **Sleep.**—Slept awhile; woke to roll and tumble in every conceivable position (S).—Unable to sleep for brain activity and crowding of ideas (S).—Restlessness > after sleep.—Cries out in sleep that a weight is lying on her.—Whispers in sleep.—Kept awake by purring of heart.—Dreams: of various things; of business.

27. **Fever.**—"In all cases of fever commencing with pains in the limbs" (Swan).—Shivers and begins to move about restlessly; temperature rises gradually and as gradually subsides (dog).—Temperature rises rapidly to 104° F., and sinks rapidly from heart failure (dog, fatal dose).—Chilly at times and a little aching; a little feverish (S).—After dinner, ache all over, chilly all night, bed feels hard (S).—After getting into bed, chilly, teeth chatter; woke 10 p.m. in perspiration on upper part of body; > motion (S).—Feels hot as if he had a fever, but was only 99° F., feels like 105°.—Cold and chilly all day.—No fire would warm; sits by fire and breathes the heat from it; chilly whenever he leaves it; at night when the fever came on he had a sensation as if lungs on fire, must have fresh air, which gave >.—Frequent calls to urinate as soon as fever came on; urine clear as water.—Every other day dumb ague.—Perspiration horribly offensive, carrion-like; disgust up to nausea about any effluvia arising from her own body.—Cold sweat over body.

Pyrus Americana.

Mountain Ash (American). (Swamps and mountain woods from Maine to Pennsylvania.) *N. O.* Rosaceæ. Tincture of fresh bark.

Clinical.—Bladder, irritation of; prolapse of. Chills. Clairvoyance. Dyspepsia. Gout. Heart, affections of. Hysteria. Rectum, constriction of. Rheumatism. Sciatica. Tongue, paralysis of. Uterus, prolapse of.

Characteristics.—*P. amer.*, the American Mountain Ash (the British is *P. aucuparia*), was proved by Gatchell on himself, a married woman, and two lads. Gatchell's only symptom was "irritation of the eyes." Another prover had a similar symptom. By far the greatest number were induced in the woman; though hers were largely confirmed by those of the boys. Neuralgic, rheumatic, and gouty symptoms were very severe. The emotional balance was disturbed and a kind of clairvoyance induced. Labour-like or spasmodic pains were frequent—in uterus; in bladder like prolapse; constrictive at base of lungs and round waist; like spasm of heart; as if left leg drawn up. *Peculiar Sensations* are: As if full of cold water; as if stomach full of cold water; coldness extends up œsophagus under sternum. As if she were outside of herself and could see into herself. As if rectum were shrunken and dried up. As if left leg drawn up and would never straighten again. The symptoms were < by moving about (pains and chilliness); < by exposure to cold.

Relations.—*Antidoted by:* Camph. *Compare:* Neuralgic and gouty pains, Pru. sp. Heart, Cratæg. Chilliness, Camph.

SYMPTOMS.

1. **Mind.**—Feels like crying.—Sad, weeping mood; tears will come (in a lad).—Feels gloomy and discouraged but cannot cry.—Feels resolute; full of gloomy determination.—Hypochondriac, not nervous; lazy, would like to lie in bed and bc waited on.—Thinks she is clairvoyant, can read character and understand motions, see into herself.—Seems to be able to go out of herself for a short distance, to walk round and return into her body; seems to her that fundus of stomach is depressed in abdomen, and pyloric end on fire, a red spot like raw beef there as if stomach burnt up with raw whisky.—Cries, feels babyish apprehension; fears something terrible going to happen.—Feels weak as if about to die, moans, groans, calls for help.—Brain active, intellect clear, thoughts vivid, whole being intensified.—Indolent, indifferent, no inclination to read.

2. **Head.**—Headache begins over eyes; pains knife-like; l. side of head aches terribly, like a toothache.—Headache extends to r. side.—Head feels as if it would burst.—Great weight at vertex.—Shooting pains in forehead.—Headache penetrating in temples.

3. **Eyes.**—Irritation of eyes.—Eyes feel as if they had been crying a long time; smart.

8. **Mouth.**—Tongue partially paralysed, cannot direct it.

9. **Throat.**—Throat feels obstinate.

11. **Stomach.**—Craves hot tea.—Wants soft food, feels as if meat would not digest.—Stomach feels weak as if nothing would digest; it feels dry and wrinkled.—Feels as if stomach full of cold water.—Thinks mucus accumulated in cold stomach.—Feeling of coldness extends up sternum and œsophagus.

12. **Abdomen.**—Feels constricted round waist; obliged to loosen clothes at once.

13. **Stool and Anus.**—Sensation as if rectum were shrunken and dried up.

14. **Urinary Organs.**—Irritation of bladder and urethra.—Sensation as if bladder prolapsed.

16. **Female Sexual Organs.**—Sense of prolapse of womb.—Bearing down and pressing out as if swollen and burning all over.

17. **Respiratory Organs.**—Hoarseness.—Dry cough, as if pharynx stuffed with cotton.—Can hardly breathe, as if cold water in stomach.—Can't talk loud; voice gone.—Some cough.—Spasmodic breathing as of nervous women (in a lad).

18. **Chest.**—Feels as if lungs congested, esp. at base; and constricted.

19. **Heart.**—Aching at heart.—Oppression about heart as if it had stopped beating, as if going into convulsions.—Sense of spasm at heart; as if blood too thick to circulate (> *Camph.*).—Heart aches as if from some great sorrow.

20. **Neck and Back.**—Sick feeling under r. scapula.

21. **Limbs.**—Twinging pains in arms, legs, and toes.—Joints all feel constricted and sore.

22. **Upper Limbs.**—Some pain in finger-joints.

23. **Lower Limbs.**—Pains drawing, rending along backs of thighs to oes, < l.—Feels as if l. leg drawn up and would never straighten again.—Tight feeling of patella.—Knees and toes feel as if immensely swollen and ache.—L. great toe feels as if torn from its socket.—Toes burn.—Pain in knees subsides and is followed by pain in tendons and along calves; drawing, cutting pain.—Unendurable aching of bones of toes.

24. **Generalities.**—Aches everywhere, in every joint; pains acute, ntense, like inflammatory rheumatism.—Feels as if full of cold water.—< Motion; dreads to move on account of joints.—< Cold; sensitive to cold and air.—Pains seem to move in meandering lines.

25. **Skin.**—Clammy feeling of skin.

27. **Fever.**—Chilly when air strikes him.—Chilly down back and both legs.—Very cold, shivering internally; thinks she must look blue.—Cold creeping all over.—Glow all over; hands sweat.—Chilly and with a very tranquil feeling, esp. of consciousness.

Quassia.

Picræna excelsa (Jamaica) and Quassia amara (Surinam). *N. O.* Simarubaceæ. Tincture or cold infusion of the wood.

Clinical.—Intermittent fever. Worms.

Characteristics.—The *Quassia* now found in the shops in th form of "Quassia chips" is the wood of Picræna, the Jamaica Quassia The name "Quassia" was given by Linnæus to Quassia excelsa, o Surinam, from the name of a negro, Quassi or Coissi, who employe its bark as a remedy for fever. The wood of this tree was formerl employed in this country under the name of *Surinam Quassia*. Th wood is very bitter, and yields its properties best to cold distille water. In the old school the infusion is used as a bitter tonic i dyspepsia, and as a clyster for clearing the rectum of threadworms There is a short homœopathic proving: J. O. Müller took a singl dose of the tincture; Eidherr four doses of 30x. Lembke took th extract. The most peculiar characteristic symptoms were: Drawin in hypochondria and sensation as if abdomen were empty an retracted; with sensation as if he would have a stool; stool at firs hard, with effort, later pasty (Eidh.). Sticking in liver and abdome (Mül.). Peculiar beating through abdomen, extending into extremitie (Mül.). Eidherr had "coldness running over back, with constan inclination to yawn and desire to stretch out the feet," which gives clue to its action in fevers.

Relations.—*Compare:* Cedron, Botan. Fevers, Cedron. Worms Cina.

SYMPTOMS.

1. **Mind.**—Awoke with great anxiety 1 a.m., unable to sleep or read next day could not perform any mental labour from absence of thought.

2. **Head.**—Constant dulness of head.

11. **Stomach.**—Qualmishness.—Drawing in stomach, with sensation a if stomach full of hot water.

12. **Abdomen.**—Slight drawing in both hypochondria, with sensation a if abdomen empty and retracted to spinal column; < by deep breathing with sensation as if he would have a stool.—Very acute sticking in hepati region; followed by dull pain.—Sticking pains between umbilicus an stomach.—Abdomen hard and distended.—Peculiar beating through abdome extending into extremities, with general nervous troubles.

13. **Stool.**—Stools at first hard, with great effort, afterwards pasty, once very thin.

14. **Urinary Organs.**—Secretion of urine increased, solid constituents diminished.

20 **Neck and Back.**—Severe drawing pains in cervical muscles.

23. **Lower Limbs.**—Drawing pain in calves.

24. **Generalities.**—General discomfort.

27. **Fever.**—Sensation of coldness running over back, with constant inclination to yawn and stretch out the feet.

Quebracho.

Aspidosperma quebracho. White Quebracho. *N. O.* Apocynaceæ. Tincture and trituration of the bark. Trituration and solutions of the alkaloid Aspidospermine and its salts.

Clinical.—Asthma. Cardiac asthma. Fever.

Characteristics.—*Quebracho* is a Brazilian fever remedy from which the alkaloid *Aspidospermine* has been isolated. This is in small, very brilliant, white crystals, sparingly soluble in water, readily soluble in alcohol and ether. Hale says *Queb.* produces in animals respiratory paralysis, slowed heart, and paralysis of extremities. It relieves dyspnœa in phthisis and pleurisy, but without influencing the fever. The 1x relieved asthma *with livid face;* and dyspnœa with cyanosis is frequently relieved by it. Hale gives these cases as relieved by it: (1) Mitral incompetence and stenosis with *severe nocturnal dyspnœa.* (2) Fatty heart (*Queb.* had no influence on the œdema, which was removed by *Dig.*). Jos. P. Cobb (quoted *A. H.*, xxvii. 74) records a case of heart affection of some duration in a man, 24. There was some enlargement, especially of right side, much dyspnœa, and a slight mitral murmur. Following this were signs of emphysema and severe attacks of asthma. Râles were heard, and "pearls" of rounded gelatinous masses were expectorated. *Aspidospermine* 3x gave more relief than any other remedy.

Quercus.

Quercus robur (var. pedunculata and sessilifera). English Oak. *N. O.* Corylaceæ or Cupuliferæ. Tincture of acorns (peeled and crushed or shredded). Spirit distilled from the tincture (Spiritus glandium quercus). Water extract of acorns with addition of alcohol (Aqua glandium quercus.)

Clinical.—Alcoholism. Breath, offensive. Constipation. Diarrhœa. Dropsy (splenic). Fistula. Giddiness. Gout. Intermitting fever. Leucocythæmia splenica. Spleen, affections of.

Characteristics.—*Quercus* is one of Rademacher's splenic remedies. It was introduced to homœopathic practice by Burnett, who published in his *Diseases of the Spleen* a translation of Rademacher's account of the remedy, and how he came to learn about it. Rademacher gave the tincture of acorns to an old brandy drunkard who had long suffered from the spleen, which was at times very painful, and who was at that time "sick unto death" with ascites and dropsy of the legs. The urine at once increased, but the patient complained that each dose of the medicine caused constriction of the chest. This led Rademacher to prepare the Distilled Spirit, and finally the Aqua, as milder preparations, which they proved to be; for the remedy completely cured the patient without causing further constriction of the chest. In the course of cures of spleen cases Rademacher noticed that not only was the flow of urine increased, there was also, especially in old spleen engorgements, an eliminative diarrhœa, with > of the symptoms generally. Another observation was this: "Certain few people feel, as soon as they have taken it, a peculiar sensation in the head, lasting barely a minute or two, which they say is *like being drunk*." This put Burnett on the track of another use of this remedy, which he has elaborated in his *Gout and its Cure*, in the treatment of alcoholism and its effects. Here are some of his cases. (1) Military man, 64, broken down with gout and alcoholism and pretty severe chronic bronchitis. Heart irregular. Liver and spleen enlarged. Complained bitterly of gnawing at pit of stomach. Gait tottering, hands quivered. He had lost his wife and had to keep himself up with nips of spirits, for which he had a constant craving. *Quer. gland. spir.* ϕ, ten drops in water, three times a day, completely revolutionised his state and took away his abnormal craving for spirits. (2) In a merchant of 57, given to nips of sherry, *Quer. g. s.* ϕ threw out a gouty eczema on scalp, poll, and backs of hands, which took three months to cure, after which *Quer. g. s.* was again given and completed the cure. (3) An officer who drank too much had foul breath; eyes yellow, puffy underneath. *Quer. g. s.* ϕ cured. (4) Hunting man, 40, free liver, gouty, had varicose veins of legs, originating apparently in enlarged spleen, left by typhoid fever. *Quer. g. s.* ϕ cured. The patient said it kept his "bowels very regular." (5) A country squire, 60, bachelor, appeared in a hopeless condition. Was unable to state his own case. Flushed, much pain over the eyes and in both rib regions. Stooping caused great pain, < left hypochondrium. Liver and spleen much enlarged. Nervous, depressed, glum, taciturn, easily moved to tears. Could not walk without support *on account of his great giddiness*. Breath in highest degree disgustingly stercoraceous, nearly caused Burnett to vomit when examining him. That smell of breath, says Burnett, is an unmistakable sign of the chronic tippler, indicating undigested alcohol in the *primæ viæ*. Burnett subsequently ascertained that he was quite a sober man, but took frequent nips, particularly when confined to the house by wet weather. The (*a*) Pain in left side; (*b*) Giddiness; (*c*) Flushed state indicated *Quer.*, which was given. In a week the *breath was normal;* giddiness a little better; tenderness of rib region much diminished. In six weeks quite well. Burnett does not find *Quer.* a remedy for the liquor habit, it stops short at that; but it diminishes the craving and *antidotes the alcoholic state.* On the other hand, *Quer.* is by no means a remedy for alcoholic effects only. Giddiness with spleen trouble is met by it; and I have given it with good result to a young lady for extreme whirling vertigo, a sequel of influenza. The patient was greatly relieved when she took it in a severe attack; but if she took it when the giddiness was only slight it caused severe aggravation. Patients to whom Cooper gave it complained that they "felt as if in a vice; dared not move for fear of a fit of apoplexy, or an attack of giddiness." "Deafness with noises in the head" is another effect observed by Cooper. Palestine missionaries who used *Quer. g. s.* on Burnett's indications in spleen affections found it no less effective in the intermittent fevers which gave rise to the enlarged spleens. Powdered Oak-bark is an excellent dry dressing for ulcers and discharging wounds. The Schema is made up of clinical symptoms (*i.e.*, symptoms either caused or cured in patients).

Relations.—[The Oak is a near ally of the Willow, and the febrile and vertiginous properties of Salicin and its compounds are analogous to those of Querc. Tannin, Tannic acid, and Gallic acid are obtained from the bark of the oak and the "galls" or oak apples, produced by the puncture of gall-flies.] *Antidote to:* Alcohol. *Compare:* In giddiness, Coccul., Gels., Chi., Nat. m., Nat. sal., Dig. In spleen affections, Cean., Scill., Cedr., Urt. ur., Rubia tinct., Thuj. In alcoholism, Nux, Ars., Chi.

Causation.—Alcohol.

SYMPTOMS.

1. **Mind.**—Nervous, depressed, glum, taciturn, easily moved to tears; not quite capable of stating his own case.

2. **Head.**—Wheeling vertigo.—Vertigo with affections of spleen and l. side.—Afraid to move for fear an attack of apoplexy or giddiness would come on.—Peculiar sensation in head, feel as when drunk; sensation lasts a minute or two.—Gouty eczema of scalp, poll, and backs of hands.

3. **Eyes.**—Eyes yellow; puffy underneath.

4. **Ears.**—Deafness and noises in the head.

6. **Face.**—Flushed.

8. **Mouth.**—Foul breath; stercoraceous.—Tongue foul.

11. **Stomach.**—Removes craving for alcohol.—Gnawing at pit of stomach.—Flatulent dyspepsia.

12. **Abdomen.**—Pain in splenic region.—Ascites.—Enlarged liver and spleen.—Pain in hypochondria, < l., much < by stooping.

13. **Stool and Anus.**—Diarrhœa (eliminative, with > of symptoms; and not weakening).—"It keeps his bowels open."—Fistula in alcoholics.

14. **Urinary Organs.**—Increased flow of urine.

18. **Chest.**—Constriction of chest; in præcordia.

19. **Heart.**—Fluttering, irregular heart.

22. **Upper Limbs.**—Gouty eczema of backs of hands.—Hands tremble.

23. **Lower Limbs.**—Dropsy.—Tottering gait.—Varicose veins.

24. **Generalities.**—Flushed state.—Exceedingly nervous.

Quininum, *see* Chininum Sulphuricum.

Ranunculus Acris.

Ranunculus acris. Buttercup. Goldcup. Crowfoot. *N. O.* Ranunculaceæ. Tincture of whole plant.

Clinical.—Erysipelas. Fever. Gangrene. Lumbago. Neuralgia. Rheumatism. Ulcers.

Characteristics.—*Ranunculus acris* is distinguished from *R. bulbosus* by its slender cylindrical flower-stalk, that of *R. bulb.* being furrowed. Both are common "buttercups," and have acrid and poisonous properties. *R. acris* was proved by Franz and Lembke, and the chief skin symptoms were observed in a woman of seventy who applied a handful of the herb to her limbs, with the result of setting up violent constitutional symptoms and fever and intense inflammation, going on to gangrene of the skin of the legs. In the provers a pain of a rheumatic character was experienced in the muscles and joints, especially ankles and wrists, which occurred when walking and also when at rest. Lumbar pains < on bending or turning the body. Heat, faintness, and fever.

Relations.—*Compare:* Ran. bulb.

SYMPTOMS.

1. **Mind.**—Anxiety.

2. **Head.**—Headache.—Tearing in forehead, in face.

3. **Eyes.**—Eyes contained a quantity of fluid blood and showed several livid spots of hard texture (in dog poisoned with the juice).

6. **Face.**—Red face.—Violent tearing in r. cheek, towards temples, evening.—Skin of r. cheek has peculiar feeling as though touched here and there with a cold, thin body; later in l. cheek.

9. **Throat.**—Continuous scraping taste in throat.

11. **Stomach.**—Frequent eructations of tasteless flatus.—Nausea; with much saliva.

13. **Stool and Anus.**—Copious fluid stool without pain at 5 p.m. and at 7 p.m.—Two loose stools, morning.

14. **Urinary Organs.**—Frequent micturition during night; urine normal.

18. **Chest.**—Tearing in muscles, r. side of chest behind nipple, < during inspiration; next day similar pain r. chest.—Lungs red and congested (dog).

19. **Heart.**—Pulse small and rapid.—Heart contained coagulated blood (dog).

20. **Back.**—Pain several times in lumbar muscles on bending and turning the body ; and in joints ; also when sitting or in motion.

21. **Limbs.**—Joints sore.—Boring and drawing pain in r. tibia and in elbow.—Violent pressing pain in joints of elbow, ankle, and knee when sitting ; > motion.—Tearing in wrists, ankle, and thumb, in walking and resting.—Tearing in joint of wrist, ankle, and shoulder, in forehead and in muscles of r. chest.—Tearing in hip, shoulder, and ankle-joint.—Wandering pains in limbs, in joints of hands, knees, feet, and toes.

23. **Lower Limbs.**—Heaviness and weakness in legs on walking ; also in bed in morning.—Tearing in front of tibiæ and in temples.—Drawing pains in ankle-joints ; tearing in l., walking and at rest.

24. **Generalities.**—Tremulous, faint, anxious, restless, small, rapid pulse, red face.—Awoke at night with most violent pains.

25. **Skin.**—Obstinate ulcers.—Skin (of legs) hot, red, painful, blistered in places ; next day gangrenous.

27. **Fever.**—Violent erethistic fever, with intolerable pains in legs and feet, which were burned, blistered, and gangrenous.—Intolerable heat and faintness.—Head hot and heavy.—Heat in head.—Skin somewhat moist in morning.—Forehead damp.

Ranunculus Bulbosus.

Ranunculus bulbosus. Buttercup. Bulbous Crowfoot. *N. O.* Ranunculaceæ. Tincture of whole plant.

Clinical.—Alcoholism. *Breast, pain below. Chest, pains in.* Chilblains. Corns. Delirium tremens. Diarrhœa. Dropsy. Dyspnœa. Eczema. Epilepsy. *Feet, pains in.* Gastralgia. Hay-fever. Herpes zoster. Hiccough. Hydrocele. Jaundice. *Liver, pain in. Neuralgia.* Nyctalopia. Ovaries, neuralgia of. Pemphigus. Pleuritic adhesion. *Pleurodynia.* Rheumatism. Spinal irritation. Warts. Writer's cramp.

Characteristics.—The caustic and pain-producing properties of the Ranunculaceæ reach their highest expression in the Buttercups themselves. *R. bulb.* forms a constituent of some arsenical plaisters used to disperse cancers. *R. bulb.* was proved by Franz, and some effects of its external application have been observed, and results of inhaling the fumes whilst preparing the plant, or when it has been burned. The last caused headache, and in one instance epilepsy, followed by cachexia, nodous gout, headache, and death. In a child who was cured of ague with subsequent dropsy and hydrocele by applying *R. bulb.* to the wrist, ulcers of the fingers penetrating down to the flexor tendons were produced. In one prover the effect of expressing the juice with the fingers was to cause a long-lasting and recurrent eruption of vesicles on the fingers, a characteristic feature of which was the *blueness* of the vesicles and the *horny* nature of the scabs : "Small, deep, transparent, dark blue little elevated blisters of the size of an ordinary pin's head, crowded together in oval-shaped groups of the size of a shilling, with intolerable burning itching, emitting when opened a dark yellow lymph, afterwards becoming covered with a herpetic, *horny* scurf" ;—a complete picture of herpes. The pains as well as the appearance of herpes are met with in the pathogenesis of *R. bulb.* —pains in nerves, serous membranes, muscles, tendons, joints, eyes, and internal organs. The pains are lancinating, pressing and out-pressing, jerking and sticking, as if bruised with external sensitiveness. From the acrid vapour arising whilst the juice of the plant was being prepared these symptoms arose : "Smarting from eyes as from smoke in evening. Smarting in eyes, nose, and fauces ; the eyes run and are very painful, so that he has to stop using them for half an hour because he cannot see anything ; whites slightly inflamed ; mucus runs in torrents from nose ; fauces painful as if sore *during an inspiration*, less during deglutition "—symptoms which have led to many cures of hay-fever with *R. bulb.* The " < during inspiration " is part of the general sensitiveness of *R. bulb.* to air, to cold air, and to change, which is the grand keynote of the remedy, and which will serve to indicate it in a large number of the cases to which it is otherwise appropriate. Another keynote is sensitiveness to touch : sore, bruised sensation ; soreness of parts affected. These symptoms make *R. bulb.* an important vulnerary. Hering mentions "hemeralopia" as having been cured with *R. bulb.* in a woman during pregnancy, and in her three-year old son. The word "hemeralopia" has been used to denote both *day*-blindness and *night*-blindness. Hering uses it in the latter (and rarer) sense, for he says of the woman, she " can see well during the day." H. C. Allen speaks of " day-blindness " as an indication, probably translating " hemeralopia " literally. The concomitant symptoms were : Heat, biting, and pressure in eyes ; redness of conjunctiva and lids, especially inner surface of lower lids ; lachrymation ; pus in canthi ; pustules on eyes ; eyes look weak ; pupils dilated ; candle-light appears as a bright circle ; can see well during day." With the concomitant symptoms *R. bulb.* would probably cure either day- or night-blindness. " Pressure and smarting in eyeballs " is very characteristic. *R. bulb.* causes a very painful form of indigestion : White-coated tongue ; bitter, sour, or sweetish taste, with accumulation of saliva ; scraping burning in throat ; spasmodic hiccough ; spasmodic feeling in œsophagus and pharynx, ascending ; eructations ; nausea, pressure on sternum with laboured breathing ; violent burning in cardiac end of stomach ; hunger early in morning, thirst in evening." Conversely *R. bulb.* has proved one of the most effective agents for removing the bad effects of alcoholic drinks : hiccough ; epileptiform attacks ; delirium tremens. In the last case the quarrelsome, angry mood on the one hand, and the abject fear of ghosts on the other, further point to its appropriateness. Pains in liver and spleen region < by touch. In pleurisy, pleurodynia, intercostal neuralgia and spinal neuralgia and herpes the pains are—sharp, stitching, shooting, come in paroxysms, are induced by atmospheric changes, sudden exposure to cold or heat, < in wet, stormy weather ; from touch, motion, or turning the body. The chest is particularly the seat of these pains. " Muscular pains about margins of shoulder-blades in women of sedentary employment, often burning in small spots, from needlework, typewriting, piano playing" (H. C. Allen).

"Jerks and shocks; and sudden tearings in right forearm and between thumb and index finger while writing," point to *R. bulb.* as one of the remedies in writer's cramp and professional neuroses. *Sensations* of *R. bulb.* are: Confusion of head as if intoxicated. As if head would be enlarged. As if head pressed asunder. Hypochondria in lowest ribs painful as if bruised. As if everything in abdomen sore and bruised. As if there were subcutaneous ulceration. Burning in left side of chest; in region of short ribs. As if something tearing in chest. As if cold wet cloths applied. As if a full breath could not be drawn. As of a knife thrust through side and into back. Muscles as if pounded. The "cold-water feeling" occurred in a patient of Burnett's (quoted by A. C. Pope in a lecture reported *H. W.*, xviii. 308). A woman, 30, had had a fall two years before Burnett saw her, and ever since had this peculiar sensation: *Whenever she goes out of doors* she feels as if wet cloths were applied to three different parts of the anterior walls of thorax—both infraclavicular fossæ, and under left breast. Never felt indoors, but constant as long as she is out. Guided by this symptom, "Unusual chilliness of outer parts of chest when walking in open air," with the general "< in open air" and "< walking in open air," Burnett gave *R. bulb.* In two days the patient was better; in three weeks the sensation had completely gone and the general health very much improved. Dudgeon reports this case (*B. J. H.*, xxiv. 160): Lady, 27, three weeks after confinement went for a drive. The day was cold, and an accident occurred to the carriage which frightened her. In the evening she had a slight rigor, and complained of pain in left side about sixth and seventh ribs. < Slightest movement; > sitting rather bent forward and leaning a little to the left. Pulse 120, no heat of skin. No signs of lung or pleural involvement. *Bry.*, and later *Arn.*, gave no relief, and for two days the symptoms grew worse; the patient having to be propped up with pillows, leaning forward and to the left, her head resting on her breast, not daring to breathe at all deeply. *R. bulb.* 1 relieved her in ten minutes, when she "felt a wrench in her side and the pain was gone." She was able to lie down, slept all night, and made a rapid recovery. There were some slight returns of pain, now on one side, now on the other, but *R. bulb.* soon removed them. The symptoms are < by touch; by pressure (consequence of falls). < Motion; walking; lying down; lying on side (affected); sitting up; change of position; < evening and morning. < Change of temperature; sudden exposure to cold or heat; open air. < Inspiring. < When temperature becomes lower; draught of air; rainy, stormy weather. < After eating. < From anger.

Relations.—*Antidoted by:* Bry., Camph., Puls., Rhus. *Incompatible:* Sul., Staph., Nit. sp. d., Alcohol, Wine, Vinegar. *Compare:* R. acris, R. scl. Smarting and pressure in eyeballs, Pho. Burning in spots in back, Aga., Pho. Spinal irritation, Agar. Exposure to cold or heat, Aco., Arn. Corns sensitive, smart, burn, Sal. ac. < Touch and motion, Bry. (Bry. > lying on painful side, R. bulb. <). < Wet, stormy weather, Rhus. Effects of alcohol, Querc. Headache at vertex as if pressed asunder; < evening; < going from cold to warm air, and *vice versâ*; tearful mood; acidity; sore spots in chest after pneumonia, feeling of subcutaneous ulceration, Puls. Pain along inner edge left scapula, at times extending below inferior angle and through left chest, Chel. Diaphragmitis, Cact. Zona, Rhus, Mez., Ars. Eczema with horny scabs, Ant. c. (Act. c. callosities on feet). Hay-fever, Pso., K. iod., Saba., Sil., Ars. Fear of ghosts, Aco., Ars., Bro., Carb. v., Coccul., Lyc., Pho., Pul., Sep., Sul., Zn. Hunger in early morning, Aga., Ant. c., Asar., Calc., Carb. a., Chi., Lyc., Mur. ac., Rhus, Saba., Zn. Sleeplessness from dyspnœa, Cad. s., Grind., Lach.

Causation.—Anger (slightest fit of, = trembling and dyspnœa). Change of temperature or weather. Injury. Alcohol.

SYMPTOMS.

1. **Mind.**—Pusillanimity and inquietude, esp. in evening.—Fear of ghosts in evening; dares not be alone.—Hasty, irritable, and quarrelsome humour, esp. in morning.—Oppression, with much weeping.—Loss of ideas. —Difficulty in meditating.—Vanishing of thought on reflection.—Obtuseness of intellect.

2. **Head.**—Weakness, giddiness, and confusion of head; as if intoxicated.—Whirling vertigo, to such an extent as to cause falling, when passing from a room into open air.—Headache with anxiety and weakness during a meal.—Semilateral headache above eye, with dejection and desire to weep.—Compression and expansive pressure in sinciput and vertex.—Sensation of puffiness all over head (as if head were too large and distended).—Tearing and pressure in temples.—Blows in occiput.—Rush of blood to head.—Pressing headache (neuralgic) in forehead and on vertex, as if pressed asunder, with pressure on eyeballs and sleepiness.—Headache with nausea and sleepiness.—The headache is induced or < by a change of temperature.—The headache, for the most part, appears when passing from a hot to a cold place, and *vice versâ*.—Crawling, creeping, or burning-sticking in scalp.

3. **Eyes.**—Itching in eyes.—Aching in eyeballs.—Pressure in eyes.—Balls sore on moving them.—Pupils insensible.—Burning, soreness, and smarting in lids.—Smarting and burning pain in canthi, as from excoriation. —Smarting and sore feeling in r. outer canthus.—Smarting in eyes as from smoke.—Mist before eyes.—Nyctalopia.—Inflammation of eyes and lachrymation.

4. **Ears.**—Shootings in ears, esp. in evening.—Cramp-like sensation in and on ears.

5. **Nose.**—Troublesome and painful tingling in nose.—Nose red, swollen, and inflamed, with tensive pain and many scabs in interior.—Hay-fever.—Obstruction of nose, esp. in a room, with pain as from excoriation.—Copious discharge of viscid mucus from nose.—Blood flows from nose.—Internal tingling and upward pressure.

6. **Face.**—(Dry) heat in face, with bright redness of cheeks.—Vesicular eruption on face as from a burn; smarts as if scalded; eruption in clusters. —Tingling in face, principally in chin and nose.—Spasmodic and whirling neuralgic pains in face and jaws.—Cramps (spasms) in lips.

8. **Mouth.**—Toothache on waking in morning.—Incisive pains in molars

as if being torn out.—Accumulation of much water in mouth.—Salivation.—White saliva with metallic taste (like copper).

9. **Throat.**—Accumulation of much (tough) mucus in throat.—Spasmodic sensation, of something which ascends œsophagus and passes into throat.—Inflammatory burning pains (scraping burning) in throat and palate.

10. **Appetite.**—Mawkish, sweetish taste, or taste of a sour bitterness.—Butter tastes too sweet.—Bitter, empyreumatic taste while eating, or after having eaten dry food.—Thirst augmented in afternoon.—Feeling of hunger and rumbling in stomach early in morning.

11. **Stomach.**—Frequent risings.—Spasmodic hiccough.—Frequent nausea in afternoon or evening, sometimes with headache.—Pains in stomach.—Pressure on scrobiculus.—Pain as from excoriation and burning sensation in pit of stomach, as also in cardiac orifice of stomach, esp. when the parts are touched.—(Inflammation of stomach.)

12. **Abdomen.**—Contusive pain in hypochondria, sometimes when touched ; evenings ; pain in back and ill-humour.—Pain as from excoriation in l. hypochondrium, principally on moving the trunk.—Lancinations (stitches) in hepatic region, arresting the breathing, with stitches and pressure on top of r. shoulder.—Stitches in l. side of abdomen.—Pinching colic, sometimes alternating with pain in chest.—Immediately after eating violent stitches from l. lumbar region transversely through abdomen, esp. below umbilicus and towards r. groin.—Intestines painful when abdomen pressed upon ; pains as from subcutaneous ulceration.—Pulsations in l. hypochondrium.—Dull pains in abdomen, with sensibility of intestines during a walk.—Pinching (colic) pains in abdomen (sometimes alternating with pains in chest), with rotatory movements, and a sensation, on external pressure, as if contents of abdomen were bruised and ulcerated.—Burning pain in abdomen as from excoriation, as in chronic inflammation.—Frequent expulsion of very fetid flatus.

13. **Stool.**—Slow and hard evacuations.—Frequent, easy, and profuse evacuations ; natural stool in afternoon.

14. **Urinary Organs.**—Frequent urging to urinate.—The scanty urine soon becomes turbid and cloudy.—Dysuria.—Ulcers in bladder.

15. **Male Sexual Organs.**—Frequent erections towards morning and dizziness in head.—Emissions towards morning.

16. **Female Sexual Organs.**—Acrid and gnawing leucorrhœa.—Ovarian neuralgia always excited by atmospheric changes.

17. **Respiratory Organs.**—Short and obstructed respiration, with oppression of chest, as after grief or vexation, with want to take a full inspiration and to weep much.

18. **Chest.**—Aching in chest.—Rheumatic pain in chest, or pain as of subcutaneous ulceration.—(Rheumatism of either side of chest with pains in circumscribed areas.—Pain with some constriction of entire chest, with some bronchial catarrh in an old gouty subject.—Rheumatism of l. chest which sets in suddenly, < on inspiration, with headache over l. eye and in vertex.—R. T. C.)—Burning pressure on chest.—Lancinations in chest and in r. side of chest, frequently deeply seated, and extending to liver.—Painful external sensibility of lower parts of chest and of epigastrium.—Painful sensibility of all the external parts of chest, intercostal muscles, pleura, &c., which manifests itself or is < esp. by movement, touch, and stretching the

body.—Pain in chest as from adhesion of pleura.—Adhesion of the lungs after inflammation).—Immediately she goes out of doors a sensation as if she had cold wet cloths applied to three different parts of front of chest, viz., both infraclavicular fossæ and just under l. breast ; sensation remains as long as she is out, and disappears as soon as she re-enters the house ; prevents conversation while out (from a fall two years before).—Acute pain principally in shoulder, axilla, and breast, so severe in breast she dreaded cancer.

20. **Back.**—Contusive rheumatic pains in whole trunk and between shoulder-blades.—Pain along whole inner edge of l. scapula, at times extending behind inferior angle and through l. chest.

22. **Upper Limbs.**—Spasmodic (rheumatic) tearing, shooting, and jerking pains in arm (stitches in the arms and hands).—While writing he feels sudden tearings (stitches, jerkings ?) in r. forearm and between thumb and index finger.—Rheumatic pain in both elbow and shoulder-joints early in morning.—(Chronic stiffness of r. wrist with shoots up arm and down to thumb, which is also stiff. — R. T. C.)—Visible spasmodic contraction in region of styloid process of l. ulna.—Coldness of hands.—Itching in hands and fingers.—Crawling in single parts of fingers.—Tetters on palms of hands. —Tingling in fingers.—Tetters, blisters, and ulcers on fingers ; penetrating down to flexor tendons.—Shining red, loose swelling of fingers, with inflammation, &c., changing to flat, spreading ulcers.—Cauliflower-like wart on outer side of terminal phalanx of r. thumb.—Pain under nail of r. index finger as from a splinter.

23. **Lower Limbs.**—Drawing pains along thighs (extending downwards).—Spasmodic, piercing pains, and itching in middle of thighs.—Great weakness in lower limbs when walking, forenoons.—Cracking in knee-joints. —Painful stiffness in joints of feet.—Cramps in instep.—Pulsative lancinations in heels (l., when standing).—Pain in heels as if pinched by boots (when boots were off).—Violent stitches in l. fourth toe.—Sore pain and stitches in tips of toes ; between the toes ; on dorsa of toes.—Pains as from excoriation and lancinations in toes.—Corns sensitive to touch, smart or burn.

24. **Generalities.**—[Biting or pungent pain ; pain as if parts would burst, were pressed or pushed asunder.—Waking too early in morning.—Affections of external angles of eyes ; hypochondrium, particularly about spleen ; lower region of abdomen ; palms of hands.—Contusive pains ; shootings, or tearing, rheumatic, and arthritic pains in limbs and muscles.—Jerking of muscles.—Shocks throughout the body.—Epileptic fits.—(Indurations.—Icteric affections.)—Pains excited by touch, movement, stretching, or change of position, esp. in trunk and extremities.—Many symptoms appear also on a change of temperature, also in morning and evening, and after a meal.—< On entering a cold place ; from spirituous liquors ; with drunkards ; when stretching the limbs ; at changes of temperature, whether from hot to cold, or *vice versâ*.—H. N. G.]—Lassitude, and pain as from having been beaten, in all the limbs.—Trembling in limbs (with dyspnœa) after the slightest fit of passion.—Sudden weakness, as if about to faint.—Fainting with the pains in stomach.

25. **Skin.**—Frequent and violent itching in different parts of skin.—Lancinations in skin, which change to itching.—Vesicular eruptions, like blisters after a burn.—Deep blue vesicles, small, deep, transparent, thickly grouped, with burning itching and hard and tettery scabs.—Horny excrescences.—

Flat, corrosive ulcers, with sharp edges, and burning and lancinating itching. —Callous and other excrescences.—Tetters over whole body.—Chilblains; of amputated stump of leg.

26. **Sleep.**—Inclination to sleep during the day.—Retarded sleep and nocturnal sleeplessness, frequently from oppression of chest (dyspnœa), heat, and ebullition of blood, but mostly without any assignable cause.—Frequent awakening in night and remaining long awake.—Waking early in morning.—Inability to remain lying on side.—Anxious dreams of danger (on the water), or vivid and lascivious dreams.

27. **Fever.**—Pulse : full, hard, and rapid in the evening; slower in the morning.—Attacks of fever after a meal or in evening, characterised principally by chilliness, with pains in abdomen and other distressing symptoms.—Heat in head, with coldness in hands.—Shivering in evening, with heat in face.—He feels the chilliness, esp. in the open air, and on the well-covered chest.—The fever consists only of a chill.—Heat in evening, esp. on face; frequently only on r. side, with cold hands (and feet).—Heat, with internal chill at same time.—Perspiration very scanty, and only in morning on waking.

Ranunculus Ficaria.

Ficaria ranunculoides. Scrophularia minor. Lesser Celandine. Pilewort. *N. O.* Ranunculaceæ. Tincture of whole fresh plant.

Clinical.—Hæmorrhoids.

Characteristics.—The "Lesser Celandine" is not botanically related to the true Celandine, *Chelidonium magus*, or to the Figwart tribe (*Scrophularia*), though it is named in the old books *Scrophularia minor*. *R. ficaria* is in all respects a true Crowfoot except that it has three deciduous instead of five persistent sepals, and nine petals instead of five. "It groweth in medows, by commonwaies, by ditches and trenches, and it is common everywhere, in moist and dankish places. It cometh forth about the Calends of March, and floureth a little after : it beginneth to fade away in April, it is quite gone in May, afterwards it is hard to be found, yea scarcely the root" (Gerarde). Gerarde's cut of the plant shows whence the idea of its use in piles was derived—the cluster of small tubers growing around the crown of the root bears a striking resemblance to a bunch of piles. Sir J. Sawyer, of Birmingham, has recently (*Chem. & Drug.*, May 25th, 1901) confirmed the old signaturists in these observations. He has successfully used an ointment prepared by macerating in lard at 100° F., for twenty-four hours, the whole plant, gathered when in bloom, and cut up. The proportions are one part of the plant to three of lard. Homœopaths would do well to give it internally at the same time.

Ranunculus Flammula.

Ranunculus flammula. *N O.* Ranunculaceæ. Tincture of whole plant.

Clinical.—Ulceration.

Characteristics.—*R. flam.* has produced gangrene of the arm down to tendons and bone, in the case of a female, from applying the plant to the wrist. It produces in horses who eat much of it distension of abdomen, and inflammation and gangrene of abdominal organs. But (according to *Dic. des Sc. Med.*, quoted by Jahr) it is only hurtful to horses if eaten in excess ; it promotes digestion when eaten moderately.

Ranunculus Glacialis.

R. glacialis. Carlina or Cacline (mountaineers of Viq). *N. O.* Ranunculaceæ. Tincture of whole plant.

Clinical.—Apoplexy. Cerebellum, pain in. Dyspnœa. Headache. Night-sweat. Thighs, sweat on.

Characteristics.—Dr. Coddé, of Spoleto, proved the φ tincture, and 3rd and 9th dilutions of this plant. It produced an enormous weight in the head with vertigo and feeling as if apoplexy were impending, > by Coffee ; a right-sided early morning headache > by rising ; dyspnœa < lying down, and compression of chest ; intolerance of weight of coverlet (the < by touch and pressure of *R. bulb.*) ; coldness of thighs ; general copious night-sweat, especially abundant on thighs.

SYMPTOMS.

2. Head.—Towards 9.30 a.m., when walking in open air, enormous weight in head, vertigo ; as if seized with incipient apoplexy ; > *café au lait.*—Behind head in region of cerebellum, sense of *tension.*—Just before daybreak, headache, < r. side, ceased on getting up.

17. Respiratory Organs.—When lying in bed breathing became difficult.

18. Chest.—On turning in bed, internal pain in infero-posterior chest.—Compression in whole chest, evening.—A little before midnight could not endure coverlet on chest.—Stitches r. chest.

26. Sleep.—Sleeplessness at night.—Broken sleep.

27. Fever.—Coldness, even on thighs.—General and copious nocturnal sweat, < on thighs.—At daybreak, slight general sweat.

Ranunculus Repens.

Ranunculus repens. Creeping Buttercup. *N. O.* Ranunculaceæ. Tincture of whole plant.

Clinical.—Back, pulsation in. Eyes, smarting of; inflammation of. (Feet, weakness of.) Sleep, short but refreshing.

Characteristics.—Franz reports a number of symptoms experienced from preparing the juice of this plant. The symptom of phantasmagoria appears in brackets as though there were a doubt about it, and I therefore leave it so. There is quoted in Jahr an account of the effects of eating *R. rep.* observed in a flock of sheep. Several fell down as if struck by lightning; eyes rolled; breathing hurried. Some reeled and died with their heads bent towards left groin. Mucous membranes of eyes injected; mouth dry; abdomen slightly distended; ruminations ceased. Some raised themselves, reeled, fell down again, bleated piteously; most were in profound coma. Bleeding <; ether in milk gave much >. Great weakness in feet remained behind. *R. rep.* has furrowed flower-stalks like *R. bulb.*, but it has a spreading calyx and creeping scions.

SYMPTOMS.

1. **Mind.**—(In evening, in bed, he dreams while yet awake that he is in a large city, and sees well-dressed people, masquerades, Turks, &c.)—Profound coma (sheep).

2. **Head.**—Evening in bed, crawling sensation on forehead and region of hair, > sitting up.

3. **Eyes.**—Smarting in eyes; profuse lachrymation.—Eyes rolled; conjunctiva injected (sheep).

8. **Mouth.**—Mouth dry (sheep).

12. **Abdomen.**—Abdomen sligthly distended (sheep).—Reeled and died with heads bent towards l. groin (sheep).

20. **Back.**—Evening in bed, beating like full, strong pulsation in sacral region.

23. **Lower Limbs.**—Great weakness of feet remained behind (sheep).

24. **Generalities.**—Fell as if struck by lightning (sheep).—Died with heads bent towards l. groin (sheep).—Raised themselves, reeled, fell again, bleated piteously (sheep).

26. **Sleep.**—Wide awake and feeling extremely well in morning, though he slept only a few hours.

Ranunculus Sceleratus.

Ranunculus sceleratus. Marsh crowfoot. Celery-leaved crowfoot. *N. O.* Ranunculaceæ. Tincture of whole plant.

Clinical.—Aneurism. Anus, itching in. *Chest, sternum, pain behind.* Corns. Coryza. Diphtheria. Earache. Glossitis. Gout. Hæmorrhoids. Herpes; zoster. *Liver, pain in.* Neuralgia. Nose, ulceration of. Pemphigus. Quinsy. Sternum, pains in. Stomatitis. Toes, affections of. *Tongue, peeling, mapped.* Varicosis.

Characteristics.—The best-known characteristic of *R. sc.* (which is a well-proved drug) is the mapped or peeled tongue, and when this is associated with smarting, burning, and rawness *R. sc.* will be the remedy. *R. sc.* has the acridity of all the Ranunculi, causing burning in mouth, throat, stomach, chest, urethra, and other parts. It causes blisters on the skin which leave a raw surface with acrid discharge. It has cured pemphigus in a three-months old infant, with continual thirst, weak, intermitting pulse, trembling, with anxious features. After *Ars.* 4 had caused improvement, *R. sc.* 3 healed up the resulting ulcers. External sensitiveness is a leading feature of *R. sc.*, especially of region of chest and sternum. These symptoms with others have led to the cure of many chest affections, including aneurism. A leading Concomitant of *R. sc.* is arrest of breathing: pains in liver, spleen, chest, or heart, < on deep inspiration and associated with external soreness calls for *R. sc.* Gnawing and boring are common sensations with the remedy, and most of the symptoms are right-sided; but there is one left-side symptom that is peculiar: continual gnawing in left palm. The right toes, especially the right big toe, are the seat of many acute pains, giving the remedy a high place in acute attacks of gout, and also painful corns. Among the *Sensations* of *R. sc.* are: As if head were too full and too large. As if face covered with cobwebs (this proved a keynote in a case of aneurism which was much relieved by *R. sc.*). As if a plug were lodged in umbilicus. Pressure as from a dull instrument. As if diarrhœa would set in. As of a needle thrust deep into big toe. With pains in stomach there is fainting. Convulsive twitches of limbs. The effects of *R. sc.* (which German shepherds call "cold fire") on horned cattle is: Loss of appetite; trembling and shivering; distention of abdominal veins. A dog poisoned with it became anxious, howled, tossed about, bent double, was very restless at night. He was killed, and after death the stomach was found contracted, inflamed in several parts, surface corroded; papillæ prominent; swelling, pale redness and contraction of pylorus. Mahoney (*M. A.*, xxvi. 110) cured with *R. sc.* 3 in an aged woman subject to gout aching in dorsa of feet, especially the right, with wakefulness at night. *K. ca.* 30 had previously removed pain passing downward over the glutei. The symptoms are: < By touch; pressure; blow. < By motion; deep inspiration; walking; letting limb hang down. < Evening; after midnight; morning. < In open air. < After a meal.

Relations.—*Antidoted by :* Puls. Wine and Coffee antidote only partially. The ulcers were somewhat relieved by Peruvian Balsam. *Follows well :* Ars. in pemphigus. *Followed well by :* Lach. in diphtheria with denuded tongue. *Compare :* R. bulb. (R. sc. more irritative). Headache, gnawing in small spot at vertex, Puls. Mapped tongue, Nat. m., Ars., Rhus, Tarax. (R. sc. has more burning and rawness than any). Cobweb sensation, Alm., Bar. c., Bor., Bro., Bry., Calc., Con., Graph., Mag. c.

SYMPTOMS.

1. **Mind.**—Indolence, and aversion to (mental) labour, in the morning.—Sadness and melancholy in the evening.

2. **Head.**—Vertigo, with loss of consciousness.—Headache, as if head were compressed in a vice.—Gnawing, drawing, spasmodic, dull pressure, often affecting only a very small spot on vertex (or temples).—Compressive and expansive pressure in temples.—Heaviness and sensation of fulness in head, which seems to be swollen and increased in size.—Contraction of integuments of head.—Smarting and itching in scalp.

3. **Eyes.**—Pain in eyes on moving eyeballs quickly.—Biting-gnawing in eyes and corners of eyes.—Frequent aching (painful pressing) in eyeballs.—Smarting in canthi, from time to time.—Eyes convulsed.—Lachrymation.

4. **Ears.**—Otalgia (r. ear), with pressure (or gnawing pain) in head, and drawing in teeth.—Drawing, shooting, and boring at exterior of auditory duct.

5. **Nose.**—Smarting and tingling in nose.—Pricking in point of nose.—Frequent sneezing.—Much serous mucus in nose.—Ulcers or large sores on r. side of nose.

6. **Face.**—Face as if covered with cobwebs.—Drawing in face, with a sensation of coldness.—Spasmodic twitchings in facial muscles and extremities, risus sardonicus.—Sensation of quivering round commissures of lips, and lower lip.

7. **Teeth.**—Toothache, with shooting pains, and bluntness of teeth.—Jerking and shooting drawings in teeth.—Red and painful swelling of gums, which bleed easily.

8. **Mouth.**—Dryness of mouth.—Frothy salivation.—Tongue coated white.—Shooting in tip of tongue.—Inflammation of tongue, with burning sensation, and redness.—Desquamation and rhagades on tongue.

9. **Throat.**—Contraction, with choking in throat, < by eating bread.—Burning sensation in throat.—Scraping in throat.—Swelling of tonsils, with lancinations.—Smarting and shootings in gullet.

10. **Appetite.**—Sweetish taste in the morning, with white and loaded tongue.—Anorexia.—Violent thirst with the fever-heat.

11. **Stomach.**—Risings, with taste of the food, after a meal.—Frequent, empty risings.—Sour, rancid risings, in evening.—Nausea, esp. after midnight, or in morning, with inclination to vomit.—Pain in stomach, with fainting fits.—Violent pains in stomach, with uneasiness.—Sensation of fulness, of pressure, and of tension in epigastrium, < by external pressure, with < in

the morning.—Constrictive pains in stomach.—Lancinations in epigastrium. —Pain as from excoriation, and burning sensation in epigastrium.—(Inflammation of stomach.)

12. Abdomen.—Dull aching in hepatic region, < by taking a deep inspiration.—Lancinations in hepatic region.—Pressure and shootings in splenic region (in liver and kidneys), < by breathing deeply.—Shootings, shocks, and pressure in lumbar region.—Pains in abdomen, with syncope.—Dull pressure, as from a plug, or a sensation of twisting behind navel, at night, or in morning.—Spasmodic pains in abdomen.—Pinching and cutting in abdomen.—Jerks in abdomen (in abdominal integuments).

13. Stool and Anus.—Itching, tickling, burning of anus.—Fine stitches into rectum.—Moisture in anus.—Itching and pressing-out sensation at anus, as if premonitory of hæmorrhoids, < walking.—Great urging after a meal; only flatus passes.—Retarded evacuations.—Frequent and urgent want to evacuate, with soft fæces.—Serous, fetid diarrhœa.

14. Urinary Organs.—Strangury.—Burning in fore part of urethra a short time after urinating.—Tickling crawling at meatus.—Drops pass after urinating, wetting sheet.—Frequent desire.

15. Male Sexual Organs.—Pullings in penis.—Lancinations in glans. —Smarting in scrotum.—Pollutions.

17. Respiratory Organs.—Small dry cough, seldom recurring, and without effort.—Obstructed and deep respiration.—Involuntary sighs.

18. Chest.—Pain in chest as if beaten, with sensation of fatigue in that part, esp. in evening.—Oppressive pressure on chest.—Pinching and shootings in chest, and region of heart, sometimes with suspended respiration. esp. in evening, or at night.—Stitches in chest and intercostal muscles.—Gnawing behind sternum, which suspends respiration.—Painful sensibility of exterior of chest, esp. of sternum.—Burning soreness behind xiphoid cartilage.—Painful drawing in pectoral muscles.—Constant pressure as of a dull instrument below r. false rib, < inspiration.—Painful sticking in r. chest.—Very painful pinching around l. nipple.

19. Heart.—Pressure as from a blunt piece of wood in region of heart. —Stitches in region of heart.—Sticking-contracting pinching in heart-region causing tightness of breath.

20. Back.—Pain in loins, as if bruised or paralytic.—Pricking and tingling in back and chest.—Aching between scapulæ.—Sudden violent jerks in loins during walk in open air, arresting breathing.

21. Limbs.—Gout in fingers and toes.

22. Upper Limbs.—Soreness under r. arm in armpit.—Boring shootings in forearms, extending to fingers.—Gnawing in r. elbow-joint.—Stitch in elbow.—Boring in bones of hands.—Gnawings in palm.—Gnawing, boring, and shooting jerks in bones of fingers.—Swelling of fingers.

23. Lower Limbs.—Gnawing and boring throughout legs and feet, esp. in toes.—Gnawing pains in l. heel.—Burning and smarting on dorsum of r. foot.—Jerking shootings, and tingling in great toes.—Sudden stitches in forepart of r. big toe as if needle thrust in deep, causing him to cry out.—Sudden stitches in r. big toe, passing into a burning.—Lancinations and burning pains in corns.

24. Generalities.—Under this drug the symptoms usually appear on e r. side ; on crown of head ; toes.—Boring sensation ; gnawing pains in ner or outer parts ; prickling in outer parts.—< Evening ; before midnight. (Arthritic affections.)—Piercing, gnawing, shooting, tingling pains, which anifest themselves, or are <, towards the evening.—Pressive and drawing ins.—Periodical affections.—Convulsive jerks (twitches of the limbs).—ncope.—Fainting with the pains.

25. **Skin.**—Vesicular eruptions, with acrid, thin, yellowish discharges.—bstinate ulcers.—Itching, boring, biting, tingling, gnawing in various parts body, now here, now there, < evening.—Pemphigus.—Large isolated isters which burst and leave ulcers.

26. **Sleep.**—Sleeplessness after midnight, with anxiety, heat and thirst ; with restlessness and tossing about.—Imperfect sleep after midnight ; with xious, frightful dreams, of corpses, serpents, beetles, &c.—Early waking a.m.), with prolonged watchfulness.

27. **Fever.**—Pulse quick, full, but soft, with heat at night.—Chill and illiness (shivering) during meals.—Heat in the evening in the room after alking in the open air.—Dry heat at night, with violent thirst and ebullition, ostly after midnight.—Waking after midnight, many nights in succession, ith heat over whole body, violent thirst, pulse accelerated, full, soft.—Heat edominates.—Perspiration after the heat, towards morning, mostly on rehead.—Intermittent fever, after midnight ; heat and violent thirst, with ll, soft, quick pulse, followed by general perspiration, mostly on forehead.

Raphanus.

aphanus sativus. Radish. (And R. raphanistrum. Wild Radish.) *N. O.* Cruciferæ. Tincture from fresh root immediately before flowering in spring. Tincture of whole fresh plant.

Clinical.—Alcoholism. Amblyopia. Axilla, inflamed gland in. Breasts, pains neath ; between. Catalepsy. Cough. Diarrhœa. Dysmenorrhœa. Emaciation. istaxis. Faintness. Fever. Flatulence. Flushings. Headache. Heart, palpita-n of. Heel, pain in. Hernia. Hysteria. Insomnia. Lienteria. Liver, affec-ns of ; abscess of. Menorrhagia. Metrorrhagia. Myopia. *Numbness.* Nympho-ania. Œsophagus, affections of. Olecranon, pain in. Pemphigus. (Priapism.) egnancy, toothache of. Seborrhœa. Tonsillitis. Toothache. Yawning.

Characteristics.—Nusser proved both the Garden Radish and e Wild Radish (the former probably only a cultivated variety of the tter), and of the Garden Radish he took tinctures of the long, round, d black (the favourite in Germany) varieties, and ate the different dishes themselves. The Schema contains his symptoms, with others om effects of eating radishes ; and provings by Curie made on a oman with 15th and 30th dilutions. These provings developed many mptoms which have proved to be characteristics. *Rap.* affords a arked example of a common article of diet being at the same time a oison and a medicine. A patient of mine, a man, has these symptoms henever he eats even a single radish : "Burning sensation in epigas-ium, followed by hot eructations, lasting a whole day and ending in a headache." Turnips (*Brassica rapa*) produce in him a simila effect, but in less degree. The leaves of *Rap.* are said to antidot its roots, and the *arum* root is said to antidote the effects c Radish leaves (Cooper). The hysterical, mental, and uterine sym toms of Curie's prover were very well marked ; a state approachin catalepsy was induced : "On returning a little to herself she wa unable to speak or stir." The "globus" symptoms are as marked a with any other remedy : "A number of balls ascend from abdomen t throat." "A hot, foreign body goes up like a ball from uterus *an stops at the beginning of the throat*, where it feels like a morsel too larg to be swallowed, thence descends to the stomach, causing a sensatio of something hard to digest, leaving an empty sensation with hunger. Many of the symptoms of *Rap.* seem to make for the throat, and a cas of mine bears on this. A man, 43, after taking *Lyc.* reported this condi tion : "Good deal of pain in back, sides, and body, < after eating Cannot lie on either side. *Very sinking at 4 a.m.* Bowels confined. Pass ing wind after severe pain." *Rap.* 30 every three hours was prescribec His next report, a week later, was this : "He felt the first dose of *Raj lie at his throat all night* ; it gradually passed down and the pains go better. After two or three days his water became thick like soap suds [Turbid urine with yeast-like sediment is characteristic of *Rap.*] Ca lie on sides better. Bowels less confined. Wind less." *Rap.* is one c the most flatulent of remedies. Wind accumulates so that it almos stops the breathing. The most characteristic feature is when th flatus cannot be passed either up or down. Such a condition occu ring after abdominal operations has been relieved by *Rap.* Many symp toms, physical and mental, seemed to rise from the uterus, culminatin in a very pronounced attack of nymphomania. With these was aver sion to her own sex and to children, especially girls. Other menta symptoms were : Capricious manner, stupefaction, sadness, tears ; an this at times alternated with hopefulness. Brain excitement. On prover had sense of intoxication on waking in the morning. Anothe felt intoxicated after dinner, though only water was drunk. Thi should give *Rap.* a place in some forms of alcoholism. Extrem anxiety, with feeling of impending death. The following case fron Allen's Appendix is fairly typical of *Rap.* poisoning. A man ate freel of radishes. Thereafter he began to feel nausea and drawing pains extending from sternum to middle of abdomen. This went on fo about a fortnight, when at 7 p.m. on May 26th he began to feel ver ill. The pains became <, and spread to back, but did not go lowe than umbilicus. He took half an ounce of Castor oil ; during th night he became < ; pain still very severe. A 8 a.m. bowels relieved when pain and nausea became < than ever and he was admitted to hospital, and soon after put in a warm bath. While in the bath h vomited dark, slimy matter. Vomiting went on till the 29th. Tym panitic swelling and great (writhing and twisting) pain in region o ascending and transverse colon, and in left groin. Pain < by pres sure. Small enema brought away lumps of fæces with > of pai and sickness. Convalescent, June 2nd. Among the *Peculiar Symptom* of *Rap.* are : Œdema of lower eyelids. When she turns her eyes i the direction of the ear she feels a pain in the ear, temple, and parieta one. Vertigo with loss of vision. Eyes filled with blood, sight lost. ,oss of vision and hearing just before vomiting. Stopped sensation ı ears. Teeth feel as if made of papier mâché. Appetite without unger 4 a.m. in bed. Constant, violent thirst. ("Woke between 3 nd 4 a.m. with headache and drank much water.") "Drinks more han he micturates." Also "Pains more severe when he drinks liquid." ensation as if she had put her cold feet into very hot water. Cough = jarring of head and chest ; seems to come from epigastrium ; can- ot get low cough to loosen phlegm ; from laughing. Expectoration f a very large amount of tenacious white mucus from pharynx and esophagus with sensation of stricture in throat. On breathing, pain nder breasts and in back. Heavy lump and coldness in centre of chest between mammæ preventing sleep. Sensation of an iron band ound waist. Sensation of stiffness. Numbness in hands ; in soles of feet and buttocks ; of the parts near the painful bones. Sensation of swelling of bones ; of hands, arms, eyes ; yet feet feel small. Swell- ng of abdomen. Sensation of a hot foreign body like a ball going up rom uterus to throat. Hot breath ; hot eructations. Sensation of a number of balls rising from abdomen to throat. Many symptoms ascend : Pain in vertebral column as if a foreign body passed through it from top to bottom and was stopped at certain points by obstacles causing pain. Acute pains in coccyx ; sensation as if an abscess forming. Sensation as of an abscess in liver. Pressure in hypogastrium as if a hernia would protrude. Throbbings in the body that became lancinations. Chilliness along the back and posterior surfaces of arms. Icy cold knees. Feverish sensation as if a cold coming on. Many symptoms besides those of globus appear to have their seat in the œsophagus, including the pains in the back on swallowing. There are few remedies with a greater proportion of distinctive symptoms than *Rap.*—E. T. Blake reports (*M. H. R.*, xxxi. 7) two cases of sexual insomnia cured with *Rap.*, one of which shows that *Rap.* has an influence on the male sexual sphere analogous to that it has on the female. A young man suffering from reflex epilepsy had had a generally adherent prepuce removed. Healing was delayed by furious priapism, which caused dragging at the sutures. *Rap.* 1 x given each night cured. Blake's second case was in a woman of 40, with old pelvic troubles. *Orig.* had failed, and *Plat.* had helped only slightly. *Rap.* cured. The symptoms are < in night and morning on waking. < 3 to 4 a.m. < By touch (gland in axilla, abdomen, uterus—cannot bear touch of clothes ; pain in bones). < By jarring : jar of walking = soreness and tenderness of bowels and brain. Cough = painful shock in brain ; efforts to vomit ; pain in chest. Walking = efforts to vomit ; pain in heel. Walking in open air > the symptoms. Lying down = nausea and faintness ; > the symptoms. Can only lie on back. Motion < pain in belly. Throwing back head > pain in occiput. Laughing = cough. < By eating and drinking ; but drinking > pain in chest. After breakfast, pain in heart. (Riding in carriage = pain in heart.) Strangulation when she begins to eat or drink. Cold water held in mouth > dryness of throat. Everything swallowed = pain in back. Must keep mouth open in order to breathe ; the air entering pains and burns. Epistaxis > (headache). Vomiting > (blindness and deafness).

Relations.—*Antidoted by:* Copious draughts of cold water. (Milk and water < the pains in abdomen.) *Follows well:* Lyc. Botan., Armor., Brassic., Cheiran., Thlasp. b. p., Matthiol., Sinap. *Compare:* In flatulence, Carb. v. Accumulation and retention of flatulence, Lyc. (Rap., flatus does not pass away; bowels move, but no flatus passes). Pressure above root of nose, K. bi. Headache > by epistaxis, K. bi. Meli., Mill., Pso. Masturbation in females, Grat., Orig. Swallowing = pain in back, Rhus, Globus, Ign., Asaf. Alternation of mental states, Ipec. < By jar, Bell., Nit. ac. < 3 to 4 a.m., K. ca., K. bi., Thuj., Med. Extreme sensitiveness, K. iod. Sensitiveness to electric states, Rhod., Merc., Pho. Icy coldness of knees, Carb. v. Burning in tongue, Sang. Laughing = cough, Arg. n. Coughing jars head; skin greasy, Bry., Nat. m. > Bending head back, Seneg. Uterine affections, Thlasp. b. p., Sep. As if intoxicated, Querc. Toothache in pregnancy, Rat., Mag. c. Sexual insomnia, K. bro.

SYMPTOMS.

1. **Mind.**—Nymphomania with aversion to her own sex; the touch of a woman's hand caused weariness, disgust, and fury.—Capricious mania, stupefaction with sadness and tears, alternating with hopefulness.—Excitement of brain; sense of intoxication on waking; at dinner, though she only drank water.—Sadness, irrepressible tears, melancholy, and numbness.—Fatigue of mind and body; loss of memory; effort to pursue a train of thought = confusion of head.—Aversion to children, esp. to girls (in a woman).—Want of spirit, it seems to her as if she were dead, as if she could not bestir herself to drive away the flies that settle on her face.—Great anguish, with fear of death, which is believed to be so near that the patient desires religious consolations.

2. **Head.**—Head, bewildered on awakening in morning, with dull pain (pressure) in forehead.—Vertigo: with dim sight; in evening, head feels tightly bandaged.—Headache, waking him from sleep; 3 to 4 a.m.—Headache after dinner.—At 11 a.m. violent rush of blood to head and chest, causing cough, preceded by burning.—Headache; pressure on eyes from without inward, extending to behind ear.—When writing feels a shock in brain; when sitting down suddenly, sensation in ears as when drowsy.—Headache and confusion in forehead and vertex in morning succeeded by flushes which end in coolness of whole surface.—Severe headache in temples, eyes, and root of nose.—Brain feels tender and sore from least jar.—Violent pain in forehead.—Aching in (skin of) forehead, sometimes throughout night, or with confusion in head.—Aching (pressure) above eyes, with obscuration of sight, which disappears after a fit of vomiting.—Aching above root of nose.—Lancinating pains in vertex.—Tightness in skin of vertex.—Dull pain in occiput, > throwing head back.—Gnawing in occiput followed by numbness.—Sweat on head, after rising.

3. **Eyes.**—Blue rings round eyes.—Eyes deeply sunken.—Redness of eyes.—Œdema of lower lid; pupils slightly dilated.—Pricking in eyes; heat when shutting them; coldness when opening them.—Itching of l. eye with deep stitches.—Coldness in l. eye.—Eyes filled with blood, sight lost.—Sight

tronger, and longer in a myopic patient.—Congestion with dim vision on waking.—Pressure above eyes ; with loss of vision, > after vomiting.

4. **Ears.**—In l. ear tearings and shootings, which seem to be in the one.—Lancinations in r. ear.—Loss of sight and hearing just before vomiting, ollowed by vomiting with great effort.—Itching in concha of l. ear, which is ainful to the touch.

5. **Nose.**—Nose pointed.—Epistaxis of deep red blood ; > head.—Dull ain in root of nose extending to occiput.—Pressure, as from a weight, on back f nose.—Breath feels burning hot in nose.—Smell as of bad oil burning, seems come from interior of head or root of nose, where is a gnawing sensation as om a sore place.—Stoppage of nose.—Smell of horse-radish.—Frequent ieezing ; or at least frequent want to sneeze.

6. **Face.**—Face, red, sombre.—Cheeks burn, are red ; whole head and ce red.—Face disfigured, with pointed nose and yellow cheeks, or else ith hollow eyes and livid complexion, so that the patient becomes alarmed his own looks.—Face pale, with expression of anxiety, great feebleness, and uch suffering.—Yellow complexion, esp. in morning, on rising.—Tearing in malar bone ; and zygoma.—Gland of lower jaw hard and swollen.

7. **Teeth.**—Lancinating toothache in (l.) molars.—Incisors become loose; ıms ulcerated.—Gnawing pains in teeth and gums ; teeth feel as if made of pier mâché.—Abscess on gums.—Gums turn black.—Gums feel as if parated ; painful, inflamed ; ulcerated.—Toothache < during pregnancy ; ening ; lying down ; > walking about.

8. **Mouth.**—Tongue : white ; covered with a thick white coating.—ongue pale and bluish red, with a deep furrow, and minute pale red spots in e centre (when the improvement commences).—Heat at root of tongue.—equent burning in fore part of tongue.—Must keep mouth open to breathe ; entering = pain, burns as if everything was alive ; uvula swollen and red ; igue rather white, red on edge.

9. **Throat.**—Heat and burning in throat, at times, chiefly in tonsils, with cinations.—Swelling, redness and pain in tonsils, as if raw.—Accumulation mucus in throat, as in bronchial catarrh, copious expectoration of white d very viscid mucus, which becomes detached from gullet and œsophagus morning, after heavy sleep, with pain of excoriation in throat.

10. **Appetite.**—Taste : of horse-radish ; mawkish ; bitter ; very disagree-e ; of pepper.—Voracious appetite, after eating feels smaller and less tight n before.—After dinner hollow, empty sensation ; her stays feel too large. Appetite, without hunger, 4 a.m. in bed.—Anorexia.—Repugnance to food. pugnance to tobacco (in the case of one habituated to its use).—During the orexia, longing for boiled milk.—Violent and constant thirst.—Drank much re than he wanted.—Everything swallowed = pains in back.—Burning in ophagus and chest.

11. **Stomach.**—Frequent eructations of air from stomach, having a rid taste.—Burning in epigastrum followed by hot eructations lasting whole and ending with a headache (from eating a single radish).—Fits of nausea, f about to faint, of such a kind that the patient is obliged to sit upright, ıg unable to lie down, although extremely weak.—Relaxation of stomach. ıclination to vomit ; frequent, sometimes momentary ; with loss of sight hearing, or with obscuration of sight, and dulness of hearing ; with regur-

gitation of water and of mucus, which is sometimes streaked with bloo
when coughing, with pressure on chest, and regurgitation of acid, colourle
mucus.—Vomiting: violent, of food; of food, mingled with white muci
sometimes with extreme nausea, great pressure on chest, and coldness;
mucus and of bile; at first of a green and very bitter liquid, afterwards
clear water; each time before vomiting, shuddering over back and arm
heaving of the chest and coldness.—Black vomit.—Vomiting of fæcal matt
—Pains in stomach, which urge continual eating.—Great pressure in stomac
and pit of stomach; lancinations and pricking in those parts.

12. **Abdomen.**—In hepatic region, lancinations, or else aching, wi
pain of excoriation.—Violent pain in r. lobe of liver, like tightness.—Pinchin
in abdomen, esp. in umbilical region, sometimes with shootings, and pressu
at r. of navel.—Violent cuttings and lancinations in umbilical region, esp.
r. side, after breakfast.—Sensation of heat in abdomen, esp. in umbili
region.—Burning below navel.—Inflation and fulness of abdomen, follow
by pinching, as if preceding a stool.—Borborygmi in abdomen, esp. at nig
or else when about to vomit.—Emission of wind upwards and downwar
with odour of the medicament, esp. after drinking water.—No emission
wind takes place for a long time, either upwards or downwards (chara
teristic).—Abdomen greatly swollen, very hard, painful to pressure, e
hypogastrium; it seems she will choke with the swelling.—Great swelling
abdomen commencing at stomach.—In morning woke with cramping, s
pains in hypogastrium, distension and great tenderness, could not bear
clothes to touch her; no < before nor > after stool; pains constant,
much < on motion; bowels sore and tender from least jar in walking.—Pa
from incarcerated flatus, coming in paroxysms; colon and other intesti
project in little tympanitic tumours all over abdomen, which is flaccid
interval; diarrhœa of yellow-brown fluid, with no passage of flatus by mo
or anus for a long time (22 days after ovariotomy).—When she leans on
side, loins immediately >, but at same time a pressing pain in lower bow
and sensation as of a round body, impelled from beneath, rises suddenly a
stops in throat, where it feels like a morsel too large to be swallowed; the
it seemed to descend into stomach, where it = a sensation of something h
to digest and left an empty sensation with hunger and lancinations in lo
abdomen; each lancination = flushing as if blood rushed to eyes; e
burn; dizziness; ebullition of blood throughout body; cold feet w
pricking; sensation as if she had put her cold feet into very hot water; t
great heat.—Pain in hypogastrium and kidneys as before menstruation; la
tude in groins and top of thighs; pain with heat in sides almost with ev
breath.—Feeling in hypogastrium as if a hernia would protrude.—Hea
lower abdomen, < l.

13. **Stool.**—Frequent want to go to stool, esp. at noon.—Frequent, liq
and copious evacuations, sometimes ejected violently, of a yellowish brov
or else, brown and frothy (characteristic).—Chronic diarrhœa, green, liq
mingled with mucus and blood.—Loose stools of undigested substance
Nine stools, mostly in morning, yellowish-brown liquid, rather copiou
Hard stool.—No stool.—Constipation; bloating of abdomen; no emissio
gas up or down; prompt satiety when eating; sedentary life.

14. **Urinary Organs.**—Tearing in region of kidneys, esp. on stoopin

)esire to urinate with pain in region of mons veneris, like a pressure in fundus f bladder.—Urine scanty ; or else more in quantity than the drink swallowed. —Want to urinate, with scanty emission ; it is necessary to wait a long time or the appearance of the urine.—Pale urine, of a dirty yellow, with sediment ike yeast.—Turbid urine.—Burning in (forepart of) urethra when urinating.

15. **Male Sexual Organs.**—(Priapism.)—Drawing and tearing pains in . testicle, afterwards in sole of r. foot also.

16. **Female Sexual Organs.**—Pain in uterus, in groins when touched nd in abdomen ; pain with inflammation ; pains in bones, joints crack ; veakness of vertebral column.—Sensation of a round foreign body, which ises from fundus of uterus and stops at entrance of throat.—Much pain in vomb and groins ; much heat, urging to urinate every moment and inability o do so.—Burning pain starts from uterus, stops at pit of stomach, when it hanges into nervous contraction and = sensation as if she would have convulsions.—Constant titillation in genitals, increasing till 1.30 a.m., when it bates with an abundant flow of mucus.—Nervous irritation of genitals, of litoris, impelling to onanism.—Great flow of vaginal mucus without desire. —Every day between 3 and 4 p.m., a little blood flows from vagina, like rose-coloured water, and a very small quantity of it for about a minute, a little while fter.—Menses very profuse and long-lasting ; blood in clots as in abortion.—Abundant menses from beginning of period ; flushes ascend from uterus to ead, pass into loins and spread throughout the body, occasioning a sensation s if about to perspire ; pricking in legs and under soles ; vanishing of hought, faintness ; great difficulty in speaking ; these flushings occur three r four times an hour.—Nymphomania, beginning in morning, continuing nceasingly till 11 p.m. ; ceases after a very severe paroxysm, which lasts 2½ ours.—Great sexual excitement, violent desire.

17. **Respiratory Organs.**—Cough, with accumulation of mucus in hroat, as in bronchial catarrh.—Breath of the smell of the medicament.—Tickling in larynx, as if in epiglottis.—Hoarseness.—Cough and hoarseness ; hest feels squeezed as if in a vice ; can scarcely breathe or speak.—Cough ; t seems as if something came from epigastrium ; also when she laughs ; tick-ing at bottom of larynx, nevertheless it seems to start from epigastrium.—Sensation as if viscid mucus at bottom of throat which cannot be coughed up ; ough does not seem to reach it.—After coughing, acid risings, as of bitter vater.—Hawking = irritation which excites a dry cough, producing a painful hock in head and sides of chest.—Sputa : sticky ; easy expectoration f round masses of mucus.—Uneasy respiration ; cannot continue in any osition.—During expiration, pains between shoulders and in each side of hest ; during inspiration only a tightness of chest.—Drawing pains in whole hest, as if stretched fibres returned to their place which = great pain etween shoulders and in each side of chest.—Uneasy breathing, oppression, ome difficulty in swallowing, it seems as if water would return through the ose ; intense burning in œsophagus and chest ; bad in morning ; > noon ; nuch < evening ; > walking in open air ; everything she swallows = pain n back.—Strangulation when she begins to eat and drink.—Must keep mouth open in order to breathe.—Expired air feels very hot.

18. **Chest.**—Painful weariness in chest and under ribs.—When she reathes severe pain under breasts and in back.—Pain in chest gradually

extending to spinal column.—Pressure and sticking, extending from pit stomach to pit of throat; and to back; < eating; coughing; somewhat by drinking.—Heavy lump and coldness in centre of chest, between breas preventing sleep.—Acute sticking and lancinations in a small spot on lar, pectoral muscles externally near axilla.—Lancinations in chest on coughi or breathing deep.—Sticking in middle of sternum.—Pressure in middle chest.—Rattling sensation in one or other side of chest almost under arms if something about to be loosened, during respiration.—As if a band of ir round waist.—Superficial lancinations in or near sternum.—Frequent burni in r. chest.—Severe cramp in (clavicular portion of) sterno-cleido-masto muscle, followed by long-lasting pain.—Violent stitches in l. chest.—Extern heat in r. breast.—Little painless blisters on breasts.

19. **Heart and Pulse.**—Violent, rapid beating (palpitation) of heart.- Pain at heart: in evening; after breakfasting on chocolate; and headacl when riding in a carriage.—Pulse: accelerated; feverish; slow; sma jumping.

20. **Back.**—Numbness of muscles of neck near l. ear; coldness in l. ey —Cracking in nape of neck.—Painful lassitude throughout body, esp. back head, neck, and loins.—Weak back, must wear stays as a support; feels as middle of back crushed, waist hollow, shoulders uneven; could not keep he balance.—Tearing and tension along crest of r. scapula.—Spine weak: i dorsal region; in loins.—Acute pains in coccyx; as if an abscess forming.- Pain in vertebral column as if a foreign body passed through it from top t bottom, and was stopped at certain points by some obstacle which = pain i chest and any part it passes through.—Burning itching on the back.—Tearin in lumbar region, on stooping, pricking pains in l. arm-pit.

21. **Limbs.**—All bones crack, esp. in nape of neck.—Weakness an bruised feeling in limbs after a short walk, as after a long one.—Sensation i arms and legs as if garters too tight.—Trembling of limbs.

22. **Upper Limbs.**—Tearing on top of l. shoulder.—Sticking pains in shoulder.—Gland in r. armpit, swollen and tender to touch.—A small, blac mark appears on shoulder, and some reddish spots on chest.—Pulling an tearing in l. arm and in joint, with weakness of elbow-joint as if carrying heavy weight.—Burning lancinations in r. elbow-joint, as if in tendon c biceps.—Sticking in l. olecranon process.—Lancinations in l. elbow-joint, a if in the bone.—Weakness, tearing and pricking pains immediately above r wrist.—(Transient) numbness in hands; and slightly all over, sometimes i one place, sometimes in another.—Pain in fingers; nails painful, esp. of hand; pains under nails as of burns or pin stuck in.

23. **Lower Limbs.**—Lancinations in l. hip-joint, back of trochanter.— Numbness of buttock (< r.).—Burning in small spot on thigh in upper oute part.—Legs heavy, as if paralysed; knees weak as if they would be dislocated —Tibia painful to touch; burning on spot as if hot coal held near tibia.— Numbness of soles and buttocks.—Lancinations under soles, feet at first cold later warm.—Itching lancination in r. sole.—Violent pains in heel wher walking, > at rest, and esp. when boot off.—Corns began to pain.—Sensation of paralysis of l. leg on lying down.—Coldness of knees and feet, with disposition to sleep, head confused, dull pain in forehead, and inclination to vomit.—Cramp in calf, at night, in bed.—Tearing pains in side of r. foot.—

Lancinations and tingling in sole of r. foot.—Redness and swelling of r. heel, with violent pinching pains on planting foot on the ground, and on walking; afterwards a blister forms there, full of clear and reddish water, which disappears after getting up.

24. **Generalities.**—Great lassitude and depression, sometimes with contusive pain in all limbs.—A child lies down during the day in consequence of feeling ill.—Perceptible emaciation.—Hysterical attack; on returning to herself is unable to speak; pain like a hot ball rises from uterus to chest.—A number of balls seem to rise from abdomen to throat.—Hysterical attacks preceded by cramps starting from uterus to chest.—Sensitive to electricity of atmosphere, and it = painful feeling and low spirits.—Sensation of swelling; eyes, hands, and arms seem swollen, but feet appear smaller; wrists feel as if lashed with a whip.—Numbness, heaviness, paralytic pains.—Pains in bones when touched; numbness in parts near painful bones.

25. **Skin.**—Skin, generally moist; a burning sensation passes from one part to another; odour of horse-radish from all parts of body.—Skin greasy.—Itching and heat of skin; fever; pimples under skin; a plaister on leg draws out a tetter.—Itching of whole body; scratching = burning.—Itching in different parts, esp. inner canthi, r. wrist, r. thigh, scrotum, anus, back, and scalp.—(Painless pemphigus.—Hansen.)

26. **Sleep.**—Nervous yawning.—Inclination to sleep; drowsiness, during nearly the whole day, with mumbling while dreaming.—Agitated sleep, with frequent awakening, cephalalgia, nausea, and pinching in umbilical region.—Sleep, with dreamy reveries.—Sleeplessness from 11 p.m. to 2 a.m., after which agitated sleep, with confusion in head.—Coldness of knees and feet with disposition to sleep.—Sleep which terminates at 3 a.m., with uneasy dreams.—Awakening at 3 a.m., with violent shuddering of back and arms.—During sleep, copious perspiration, or else low whispering, as if in conversation with friends, or quarrelling.—Lascivious dreams.

27. **Fever.**—Shuddering, esp. along back and at posterior surface of arms and feet, chiefly after drinking cold water.—Frequent shuddering with heat in interior of head, and over whole skin; after the shuddering, internal heat, or else alternation of shuddering with heat.—Woke 3 a.m. with violent shivering over back and arms.—Icy coldness of knees and feet at night, preventing sleep.—Coldness, evening, in bed, with weakness of joints, esp. elbows, and followed by profuse sweat.—Internal coldness, with skin hot and moist, the patient constantly complains of cold, while the skin is constantly burning to the touch.—Sweat having the odour of the medicament (likewise the breath).—Profuse perspiration during sleep, esp. towards morning.

Ratanhia.

Rhatany Root. Ratanhia. Mapato. Pumacuchu. The root of several species of Krameria, especially Krameria triandra. *N. O.* Polygalaceæ (or Leguminosæ according to some). Tincture of the root.

Clinical.—*Anus, fissure of.* Breath, offensive. Constipation. Diabetes. Dysentery. Dyspepsia, atonic. Epistaxis. *Eyes, pterygium.* Fissures. Gonorrhœa.

Hæmorrhages. Hæmorrhoids. Hiccough Hydrothorax. Infra-mammary pain. Itching. Metrorrhagia. Miscarriage. Nipples, fissures of. Pimples. Pleurisy. Scurvy. Snoring. Speech, arrested. Stomach, distension of; ulceration of. Throat, contraction of. Tinnitus. Worms.

Characteristics.—"*Krameria triandra*, remarkable for its entire, obovate, acuminate leaves, covered on both sides with silky hair, is one of the species most known as yielding the Rhatany root of commerce, but all the species (of *Krameria*), as far as known, are intensely astringent. In Peru an extract is made from this species which is a mild, easily assimilated astringent medicine, possessed of great power in passive, bloody or mucous discharges; it acts as a tonic in weakness of digestive organs and muscular debility, and is even useful in intermittent and putrid fevers. It is also styptic and restores tone to relaxed parts, and when applied as plaisters is said to cure all kinds of ulcers. An infusion is used as a gargle and wash, and the powder forms with charcoal an excellent tooth-powder. The colour of the infusion of the root of the *Krameria* is *blood-red*, on which account advantage is taken of it to adulterate port wine" (*Treas. of Bot.*). Teste (who puts *Rat.* in his Sulphur group), writing of its pre-homœopathic use, says, "There is perhaps no plant the properties of which have been so well indicated by chance as this. Used as an astringent and tonic, this root sometimes arrests passive hæmorrhages (*epistaxis*, *hæmoptysis*, *metrorrhagia*, &c.). It was successfully used against *scurvy*, *mucous discharges*, such as *chronic catarrh of the bronchia*, *vagina*, *large intestines*, &c., against various forms of *incontinence of urine*, *chronic œdema of the skin*. Dr. Tournel, who, no doubt, did not suspect that *Ratan.* produced abortion, had the happy idea of prescribing it as a tonic in cases of incipient miscarriage, and thus preventing that accident in delicate and nervous females who had never yet been able to go their full time." All these uses are really homœopathic, as is also the cure of a case of fissure of the rectum by Bretonneau, whom Teste quotes from Trousseau and Pidoux: A lady suffered from constipation and fissure of rectum, which caused her horrible pains and had damaged her health. Bretonneau ordered a daily injection mixed with one-fourth of *Rat.*, and in a short time constipation and fissure were cured. Other like cases were cured; and then the same treatment was given in cases of fissure without constipation, and again with the same success. The provings (Hartlaub and Trinks chiefly) bring out the keynotes of *Rat.* in rectal cases: "Straining, stool so hard she cried out, with great protrusion of hæmorrhoids; *followed for a long time by burning in anus*." The burning persisting for a long time after the stool is very characteristic of *Rat.*; and it occurs when the stool is diarrhœic as well as hard. Burning also precedes and accompanies the stool. Another peculiarity in connection with the stool is a bursting headache, which accompanies and follows a straining at stool. Dry heat with sudden stitching like knife-stabs. Oozing at anus. Dropping of blood from anus. One patient cured by *Rat.* of fissure had > by application of hot water; he sat in a sitz-bath as hot as he could endure; the relief only lasted while in the bath. In connection with the rectal symptoms is an important head symptom:

"Pains in middle of forehead, as if brain would fall out," and a similar pain after stool. The head pains are also < on bending forward. The eye symptoms are striking: burning, smarting, twitching of lids, obscured vision. This symptom has led to the cure of cases of pterygium: Inflammation of whole of eye; a membrane seemed to extend to central point of eye, which burned. The old use of *Rat.* in nose-bleed, scurvy, and as a tooth-powder are justified by the symptoms of the proving: Violent nose-bleed; bleeding gums; toothache < lying down. A curious symptom in the aching molars is a sensation as if coldness rushed out of them. Toothache of pregnancy compelling the patient to get up at night and walk about. "Tasteless water collects in mouth" may meet another condition of pregnancy; and *Rat.* both causes and prevents abortion, metrorrhagia and leucorrhœa. It also meets fissure of the breasts in nursing women, as well as fissure of the anus. Contractive sensations (*Rat.* is "astringent") are numerous: in stomach; groins; anus; eyes; neck; muscles; throat; "painful spasmodic contraction of throat during which she could not speak a loud word." *Peculiar Sensations* are: As if intoxicated. As if head in a vice. As of a white speck before eyes; skin before eyes. As if coldness rushed out of molars. As if rectum and anus were all twisted up. As if splinters of glass in rectum and anus. As if rectum protruded and then suddenly went back with a jerk. As if abdomen (and chest) cut to pieces. Movement as if something alive in abdomen. As of cobwebs about right side of mouth. Jerkings and quiverings. *Eyelids feel stiff.* Right side is most affected.—Cushing, who made a proving of *Rat.*, says (*Med. Cent.* quoted *H. R.*, XI. 142) it caused great itching in the rectum; and he has cured with it since nearly every case of pin-worms in his practice. In a woman, old and feeble, he cured with *Rat.* 3x internally, and a *Rhatany* rectal suppository each night, frequent discharges of mucus, blood and pus from the bowels night and day with great pain and burning in rectum almost wholly preventing sleep. Cushing considers that, next to *Sang. nit.*, *Rat.* meets more rectal cases than any other remedy. Rummel (quoted *H. R.*, i. 140) relates the case of a servant girl who had rapid twitching of the lids of right eye to such an extent as to hinder her seeing. There seemed to be also a rotary motion of the ball. *Bell.* and *Calc.* failed to relieve. *Rat.* 12 relieved quickly. The symptoms are: < By touch (teeth). Pressure > pain in chest. < Lying down; > by motion. < Straining at stool; sitting bent over (headache); stooping. Stepping = pain in ribs. Sitting = weariness and heaviness in right thigh; pain in right knee and great toe. Bending arm <; extending it >. Eating <; emission of flatus >. After dinner, hiccough; before dinner, abdominal distension. > Hot-water applications. > Open air; moving about in open air. < Night; "most symptoms come in evening, night and morning. They are > by exercise and in open air, very much < by uneasiness of mind" (Teste).

Relations.—*Follows well:* Sul., Bovis, Sep. in uterine affections (Teste). *Compare:* Botan.; pleurisy, Seneg. Fissure of anus, Nit. ac. Anal symptoms, Sul., Ir. v., Canth., Pæon., Graph. (Graph.

is nearest, but has not the constriction of *Rat.*). Splinters of glass in rectum, Thu. (Sticks, Æsc. h.). Pain in head from straining at stool, Indm., Pul., Sil. Hiccough, Cycl. Burning on tongue, Rap. Ran. s., Sang. Toothache of pregnancy, Rap., Mg. c., Cham. Alive sensation, Croc., Thu. Cobweb sensation, Ran. s., Bar. c.

SYMPTOMS.

1. **Mind.**—Irritable, peevish, and quarrelsome humour.—Apprehensive depression when alone, > in company.—Woke with a start, 2 a.m., with trembling apprehension and fear—Changeable mind.

2. **Head.**—Dulness of head as if intoxicated.—Bruised pain in small spots on head.—Jerking in small spot r. temple.—Pains in head, as if cranium were about to burst, esp. when sitting with body bent forwards.—Long-lasting headache as if screwed in a vice.—Jerking, smarting, and shooting in head.—Congestion in head, with heat and heaviness.—Dull, deep stitches on vertex.—Painful tearing and burning on vertex, even at night, > in open air, during menses.—Pain in middle of forehead, as if brain would fall out while straining at stool.—Pains in head as if it would burst after stool.—Tearing from occiput to vertex.—Sensation as if scalp from root of nose to vertex were stretched.—Stiff feeling in forehead < knitting brows.—Itching of scalp not > by scratching.—Itching l. occiput, where small glandular swellings were found.

3. **Eyes.**—Pains in eyes as if compressed in a vice, and could not be moved.—Sensation in r. eye as if screwed in, or as if there were an impediment so that it could not be moved, still she could move it easily.—Contractions and burning sensation in eyes, esp. in evening.—Inflammation of sclerotica; a membrane seemed to extend to central point of eye that burned.—Sensation as if a cuticle were placed before eyes.—Agglutination of eyes at night, and lachrymation in morning.—Jerks and quivering of eyes and eyelids.—Twitching in r. eye and r. upper eyelid.—Stiffness of upper lids with soreness of upper tarsal edges.—White spot before eye, which obstructs the sight (in evening, by candle-light, with constant urging to wipe the eyes, and > after wiping).—Vision dim for distant objects.—Myopia.

4. **Ears.**—Tearing in ears.—Itching and shooting in ear.—Violent stitch in r. ear; chirping in r. ear; crawling as if insect in r. ear.—Nocturnal tinkling, and ringing in ears.

5. **Nose.**—Itching in nose.—Violent itching on tip of nose > by rubbing.—Nostrils inflamed and scabby, with burning sensation.—Epistaxis.—Violent nose-bleed, three times a day, for five days in succession.—Dryness of nose, with frequent sneezing.—Dry coryza, with complete stoppage of nose.

6. **Face.**—Heat in face.—Tearing pain in face and jaw bones.—Violent tearing in l. malar bone, evenings.—Sensation of cobwebs above r. side of mouth.—Tearing in inner surface of lips in a small spot.—Tearing in l. side of lower jaw and corresponding teeth.—Burning vesicles on the red part of upper lip.

7. **Teeth.**—Toothache in evening, esp. after lying down (compelling one to rise and walk about); or in morning, generally with tearing or jerking,

or at times with digging pains.—Pulsative pain in teeth.—Bleeding of teeth.—Painful sensation of coldness and elongation in the molars, and as if coldness rushed out of them.—(Violent pain in one l. upper incisor, which is painful to the touch.)—Acid blood from gums on sucking them.—Burning at tip of tongue.

8. **Mouth.**—Dryness of mouth at night.—Tension and burning sensation on tongue.—Tasteless water collects in mouth.—Breath offensive.

9. **Throat.**—Sore throat, generally felt during empty deglutition.—Painful spasmodic contraction in throat, which stops the voice (unable to speak a loud word).

10. **Appetite.**—Mawkish taste in morning, in bed.—Thirst ; in evening.—Anorexia, with dislike to food and drink.—Constant desire to eat.—Risings, with taste of food ; empty.

11. **Stomach.**—Violent hiccough, which causes pain in stomach.—Long-continued hiccough after dinner.—Nausea and disgust, esp. at night (1 a.m.), with retching and vomiting of food (> in open air).—Vomiting: of water ; of mucus streaked with blood.—Pains as from ulceration in stomach.—Excessive distension of stomach.—Stomach feels too full.—Digestion more difficult.—Rolling and constriction in stomach.—Painful constriction of stomach, which is sometimes removed by risings.—Sensation in stomach, and above scrobiculus, as if abdomen had been cut to pieces, < deep breathing.—Heat and burning sensation in stomach and epigastrium.—Sudden painful bursting in pit of stomach.

12. **Abdomen.**—Repeated violent sticking in r. (and l.) hypochondrium.—Pullings, and a sensation of coldness, in umbilical region.—Pinchings in abdomen, and sides of abdomen, sometimes with a burning sensation.—Movements in sides of abdomen as of something alive.—Shootings, pinchings, and contraction of groins.—Pinching in both groins > by emission of flatus, morning on waking.—Griping in lower abdomen, externally violent itching.—Constrictive pain in small spot in groins ; in r. groin.—Sticking in groins, in afternoon while sitting.—Dragging downward in both groins, as before menses, with discharge of mucus from vagina.

13. **Stool and Anus.**—Hard and broken evacuations, with urgent want to evacuate (with straining) and protrusion of hæmorrhoidal excrescences.—Ineffectual want to evacuate, with troublesome pains in loins.—Straining ; so hard that she cried out ; great protrusion of hæmorrhoids, followed for a long time by burning in anus.—Sudden stitches.—Fissures ; excruciating pains immediately after stool, if costive.—Fissure with constriction.—Dry heat, with sudden stitches, like stabs with pen-knife.—Oozing from anus.—Burning in anus before and during a diarrhœa-like stool.—Very urgent desire for normal stool.—Diarrhœa with evacuation of some drops of blood, accompanied by dragging in groins and rumbling in abdomen.—Stool yellow, diarrhœa-like, with burning like fire in anus.—Sensation as if splinters of glass sticking in anus and rectum in every direction ; as if rectum protruded and went back with a jerk ; > in hot sitz-bath.—Severe itching about anus.—Pin-worms.—Soft loose evacuations, preceded by cuttings, with burning pains in anus, before and after.—Thin, fetid stools, burning like fire in anus.—Sanguineous diarrhœa.—Discharge

of blood from the rectum, with or without stool.—Pains in head, as if it would burst (during and) after evacuation.

14. **Urinary Organs.**—Frequent and urgent want to urinate, with scanty emission.—More frequent and more abundant emission of urine, even at night.—Pale urine.—Urine more scanty, which soon deposits a cloud, and becomes turbid.—Burning in urethra (and root of penis) when urinating.

15. **Male Sexual Organs.**—(The chronic gonorrhœa became much worse.)—Burning in root of penis while urinating.—Itching in scrotum not > by scratching.

16. **Female Sexual Organs.**—Pressure in groins, as of a general bearing down towards genital organs, followed by leucorrhœa.—Leucorrhœa with itching in rectum and discharge of bloody mucus.—Catamenia too early and of too long duration, and too copious, with pains in abdomen and loins.—Metrorrhagia.—Miscarriage.—Uterine pains following retrocession of eruption on loins.—Menses suppressed, with swelling of abdomen and breasts, simulating a pregnancy of several months, accompanied by profuse leucorrhœa and constant pain in kidneys.—Menses delayed.—Fissure of nipples in nursing women.

17. **Respiratory Organs.**—Dry cough, with tickling in larynx, and pain of ulceration in chest.—Some tight mucus evacuated with great difficulty.

18. **Chest.**—Pressure at chest on the least exertion, with shortness of breath.—Violent pressure in chest as from a stone, with short breath, on slight exertion.—Rush of blood and heat to chest, with difficult breathing.—Ulcerative pain in chest during and after coughing.—Burning stitch in last ribs near back on stepping.—Pain as if cut to pieces in small spot in upper sternum.—Coarse stitch as with a knife in sternum, felt at every breath on ascending steps, takes away breath.—As if pointed instrument sticking in sternum just above ensiform cartilage.—Sticking burning cutting beneath l. chest, along one rib, evening.—Sticking and drawing along l. clavicle as if skin drawn in.—Stitch in l. ribs, so violent it = her to cry out.—Several fine stitches beneath l. breast, on ribs, extending downward.—Throbbing-burning, cutting and ulcerative pains beneath l. breast near pit of stomach < motion, > pressure.—Painful constriction in both sides of chest.—Shootings in chest, esp. when going up stairs, with obstructed respiration.—Congestion (of blood to) chest, with heat, and impeded respiration.

19. **Heart.**—Sharp sticking in præcordial region, rather external.—Pulse full.

20. **Neck and Back.**—Drawing tension, from nape of neck to the bottom of spine.—Stiffness in nape on turning head, > on violent motion.—Tearing in nape of neck, with heaviness of head.—Pain in loins and back, as if they had been beaten.—Bruised pain in whole spine.—Bruised pain in loins and hips, morning rising, > on motion.

21. **Limbs.**—Tearing in limbs.—Contraction of flexor muscles.

22. **Upper Limbs.**—Tearing in shoulder, arms, forearms, and wrists.—Spasmodic and painful contractions in elbows and fingers.—Pain in bend of elbow (r.) when flexed, > when extended.—Violent tearing in r. wrist.—Jerking, tearing, and stitches in thumbs.

23. **Lower Limbs.**—Drawing and tearing in thighs, knees, legs, feet and

toes.—Tension and burning sensation in thighs.—Jerking in thighs, calves, and feet.—Tearing from l. tendo Achillis up.—Sprained pain in last joint of big toe, while sitting, > on motion.—Sticking and burning tearing in l. big toe.—Tickling on heels and soles.—Voluptuous itching in l. sole.

24. **Generalities.**—Weakness and prostration with anxiety and sweat over whole body.—Malaise with frequent yawning, repeated and laboured attempts to draw a long breath and distressing constriction across chest.—Sore pain frequently mingled with fine sticking now in chest now in shoulders, &c.—Shooting pains, as from excoriation.—Jerking in different parts.—Hæmorrhage.

25. **Skin.**—Sickly skin.—Small red and white pimples which do not suppurate, esp. between shoulders and on loins, remaining a long time.—Pimples; itching and burning after scratching.—Formication and itching eruption on back.—Itching: in nape and between scapulæ; on scrotum; front of thigh; bends of knees, &c.

26. **Sleep.**—Disposition to sleep, esp. after dinner.—Violent yawning.—Retarded sleep.—Frequent waking, and prolonged wakefulness.—Waking with a start, with trembling, inquietude and fear.—Snoring.—Dreams: of battles; sick people; quarrels, anger, vexation; funerals, death of friends; earthquakes.

27. **Fever.**—Predominance of coldness, and of shivering, esp. in evening. —General chill 8 or 9 p.m.—Chilly even in warm room.—Heat of whole head with heaviness.—Heat and puffiness of face.—Dry heat in anus with cuttings. —Woke 1 a.m. with sweat, thirst, and dry mouth.—Nocturnal perspiration.

Rhamnus Catharticus.

Rhamnus catharticus. Buckthorn. *N. O.* Rhamnaceæ. Tincture or fluid extract of ripe berries.

Clinical.—Appendicitis. Colic. Constipation. Diarrhœa. Tympanites. Typhlitis.

Characteristics.—The common Buckthorn produces black, shiny, four-sided berries, with an acrid taste. From these a syrup is made, and forms the *Rhamni succus* of the old school. It produces "copious watery stools and occasions a good deal of nausea and severe tormina. Was formerly given in dropsy, but owing to the severity of the drug is now little used" (Milne). The Schema is made up of symptoms observed in a boy poisoned by eating the berries. The ileo-cæcal symptoms seem to point to it as a possible remedy in cases of appendicitis. Homœopaths have found *Rham. cath.* φ in doses of a few drops a useful palliative in cases of constipation.

Relations.—*Compare:* Cascara, Cean. In appendicitis, Ir. t.

SYMPTOMS.

3. **Eyes.**—Eyes glistening and injected.
6. **Face.**—Trembling of lips.—Commencing trismus.

8. **Mouth.**—Coated tongue.—Extremely bitter taste.

9. **Throat.**—Scraping in throat.

11. **Stomach.**—Complete loss of appetite.

12. **Abdomen.**—Violent rumbling and griping, esp. cutting pains in ileo-cæcal region and in transverse colon.—Colic.—Abdomen hard; tympanites.

13. **Stool.**—Diarrhœa.—Liquid stools.

14. **Urinary Organs.**—Urine highly coloured.

17. **Respiratory Organs.**—Respiration short, anxious.

19. **Heart.**—Pulse variable.

21. **Limbs.**—Weakness and prostration in all limbs.

24. **Generalities.**—Unable to rise; seemed to desire to press his head against the wall.

27. **Fever.**—Violent chilliness.—Skin at one time warm, at another cold.

Rhamnus Frangula.

Rhamnus frangula. Alder Buckthorn. *N. O.* Rhamnaceæ. Tincture and trituration of the bark gathered in spring from the younger branches. Tincture of bark of root. Tincture of ripe berries.

Clinical.—Anus, itching of. Appendicitis. Ardor urinæ. Cæcum, gurgling in. Diarrhœa. Flatulence. Urethritis. Vomiting.

Characteristics.—All parts of *Rh. fr.* appear to produce irritant and cathartic properties. The majority of the symptoms of the Schema were the result of the root bark, but the leaves were no less active. Stools of a dark-green colour were observed, copious, thin or pasty. With the stools there was much rumbling in the ileo-cæcal region and along the transverse colon with weakness after stool. (*Rh. ca.* has rumbling, griping, and cutting pains in ileo-cæcal region.) There was more vomiting with *Rh. fr.* than with *Rh. ca.*, and the former was abandoned as a cathartic because it so frequently produced vomiting instead. "Burning in urethra while urinating and frequent micturition" may prove an indication in gonorrhœa.

Relations.—*Compare:* Rh. ca., Cean., and Cascara (botan).

SYMPTOMS.

1. **Mind.**—Depression of spirits.

2. **Head.**—Vertigo.—Dulness of head.—Frontal headache.

8. **Mouth.**—Dry tongue.—Salivation.—Coated tongue.—Taste bitter (after stools).

9. **Throat.**—Burning scraping taste and irritation along throat.

11. **Stomach.**—Thirst.—Diminished appetite.—Aversion to food.—Eructations and efforts to vomit.—Nausea, with increased salivation.—Frequent vomiting instead of diarrhœa.—Sourish vomiting.—Constant inclination to vomit.—Warmth in stomach and abdomen.

12. **Abdomen.**—Distension.—Profuse emission of flatus.—Rumbling.—Increased sensitiveness.—Increased peristalsis.

13. **Stool and Anus.**—Itching in anus.—Violent tenesmus.—Thin pasty stools.—Fifteen thin stools with violent rumbling and gurgling, esp. in ileo-cæcal region and along transverse colon, followed by distension of abdomen, thirst, coated tongue, bitter taste and weakness.—Stools without great urging, thick, pasty, dark green, copious.—Stools hard, scanty.—Constipation at first followed by diarrhœa.

14. **Urinary Organs.**—Slight burning in urethra, while urinating.—Frequent micturition.

19. **Heart.**—Accelerated pulse.

24. **Generalities.**—General exhaustion.—Weakness; after stools.

26. **Sleep.**—Great sleepiness.

Rheum.

Rheum officinale. R. palmatum. Rhabarbarum. Rhubarb (though called "Turkey-rhubarb," the root comes from China, the exact species yielding it not being certainly known). *N. O.* Polygonaceæ. Tincture and trituration of the dried root. [A tincture of the fresh leaves and young stalks should be investigated.]

Clinical.—Ardor urinæ. Breath, offensive. Constipation. Deafness. Dentition, difficult. *Diarrhœa.* Duodenum, catarrh of. Dysentery. Ears, thickening in. Frowning. Headache. Jaundice. Kidneys, affections of. Ménière's disease. Milk, abnormal. *Mouth, mucus in.* Nipples, pain in. Nose, pain in. Nurselings, affections of. Œsophagus, constriction of. Rheumatism. Salivation. Screaming, of children. Snoring. Stomach, disordered. *Taste, bad.* Tongue, numbness of. Urination, difficult, of childbed. Urine, red.

Characteristics.—Hahnemann's proving of *Rheum* has confirmed many of its traditional uses. In the form of Compound Rhubarb Powder (*Pulv. Rhei. Co.*—Gregory's powder) along with *Magnesia* and *Ginger*, most of us can remember it as one of the terrors of the nursery. In its homœopathic form it has no terrors, but it remains a great remedy of sucklings and children, especially during dentition, to whom as well as to pregnant and nursing women it is *particularly suited*. Milne well summarises its action from the traditional point of view: "Tonic, cathartic, and a feeble astringent, the latter property being overborne by the cathartic and only coming into play afterwards" [*i.e.*, the constipation which follows Rhubarb purgation]. "In small doses, it improves digestion and appetite, and renders the renal secretions more healthy. In larger doses it is an excellent cathartic, acting on the whole bowel and especially the duodenum, and increasing the peristaltic action. It is well suited for the early stages of diarrhœa, as a laxative in constipation from debility of the digestive organs, and in disorders of children, such as flatulence and irritation of the alimentary canal. It renders the serum of the blood yellow, the urine is almost of a blood-red colour." In connectio with the last observation it must be remembered that *Rheum* contain a large amount of *Chrysophanic acid* (named from its brilliant yellow crystals). Among its many other constituents is *Oxalate of Lim* (*Calc. ox.*) and *Rheo-tannic* acid. Milne's observations agree in the main with homœopathic experience, but it is the latter alone which brings out the distinctive characters of the medicine. The grand keynote of *Rhe.* is *sourness:* The stools are sour; the taste is sour the whole body has a sour smell. No amount of washing will wash the sourness out of a characteristic *Rheum* baby. Such a condition may occur in sucklings, or at the period of dentition; and it may be associated with another characteristic *Rhe.* symptom, night-screaming and yet another sopping-wet hair. The *Rhe.* child is as acid in temper as he is in body: peevish, impatient; screams for things dislikes even his favourite playthings. "Screaming of children with urging and sour stools" is characteristic. With a few drops of *Rhe.* φ I have relieved severe constipation in an acid child who was intoleran of almost all remedies in the attenuations. But *Rhe.* is by no means exclusively a children's remedy. Its symptoms are good for any period of life. The stomach disorders calling for *Rhe.* are charac-terised by: Sour, flat, slimy taste; or insipid or nauseous. Food tastes bitter, even sweet things (there is no bitter taste independently of food). The mouth is covered with offensive mucus after sleeping; and after sleeping there is bad taste and offensive breath. There is hunger for various kinds of food and the first few mouthfuls nauseate. The effects of eating plums or unripe fruit. There is nausea in abdomen. Colic is severe, compelling one to bend double, < stand-ing; < just before stool; not > after; < at once by uncovering an arm or leg. The evacuations are *accompanied by shivering* and followed by renewed urging. "Shivering with stool" should draw attention to *Rhe.*—That there is much yet to be learned of the action of *Rhe* is evident from the following: (1) Two cases (in men) of severe skin eruptions are quoted, *H. W.*, xxvii. 17, from the effects of Rhubarb root taken for constipation. The first symptoms in one case were rigors and pains in the legs. Soon lips, face, and tongue began to swell and became livid. A rash developed involving lips, beard, eyelids, and scalp, scabs mixed with abundant bloody pustular exudations. Hæmorrhages and pustular eruptions then appeared all over the body; blebs with clear fluid on backs of hands. Lymphatic glands swollen and painful. Removal of scabs left shallow dirty ulcers. Blood passed freely from urethra, but sometimes the urine was wholly free from it. Urine brownish yellow; free from albumen or sugar. Temperature 103·3° F. The second case was similar to the above. The patient had taken the powdered root. He woke one morning with burning sensation in face and found it covered with blisters and pustules. These were brownish red, irregular, size of pea or bean, deeply infiltrated at bases. Both surfaces of hands were also affected. The eruption, which closely resembled pemphigus, disappeared in a few weeks without treatment, leaving bluish pigmentation, but no cicatrices. There was no fever in this case. (2) From these cases given me by Cooper (*a*) A lady suffering from characteristic symptoms of Ménière's disease, feeling of things spinning round with extreme giddiness and noises in the head, was cured by a chemist giving her 10 grains of powdered rhubarb, on the idea it was due to the liver. Before this great suffering had been endured without any relief. (*b*) In vertiginous symptoms due to brain exhaustion with flushings followed by perspiration and awful muffled and discordant tinnitus, great relief followed the sniffing of 3x trit. of *Rheum palmatum.* Among the *Peculiar Sensations and Symptoms* of *Rhe.* are : Tendency to frown. Sensation as if brain moved when standing. Dull stupefying headache with bloated eyes. Sweat on hairy scalp, constant and very profuse ; whether asleep or awake ; in motion or quiet, hair always sopping wet ; may or may not be sour. Stupefying drawing in root of nose extending to tip, where it tingles. Bladder weak, must press hard to urinate. *Sensations :* as if in a dream. As of a lump around navel. As of a load on upper part of chest. Cutting as if in lumbar vertebræ. Heaviness as on waking from a heavy sleep. Coldness in teeth. Blunt feeling in teeth. Constriction of stomach ; of gullet. Crackling, crepitation, or bubbling in muscles and any part of body. Tongue numb, numbness of part of limb lain on. Symptoms are mostly left-sided or go from above down or from right to left. *Localities* are : Left loin ; brain ; upper part of body (sweat). "*Rhe.* has the property of setting up pains in old disease depôts, in the seat of old cellulitis and old psoriasis patches, producing hot burning pains therein as well as in the unaffected veins of the thighs and other parts. Its good effect in old middle and internal ear thickenings seems due to the creation of tissue-activity in dormant structures" (R. T. C.). Forcing pains are felt in dartrous patches. The symptoms are : < Night ; and morning after sleep. < Uncovering ; from cold. Uncovering arm or leg < colic. > Wrapping up ; from warmth. In open air : eyes full of water. Hot weather < colic. > Lying doubled up ; takes the queerest positions in order to rest awhile. Lying on limbs = them to go to sleep. Motion <. Walking <. [On the indication "Diarrhœa only during active exercise," Hurndall (*H. W.* xxxvi., 28) cured a horse of a diarrhœa which only came on when he was at work.] Standing < (vertigo as if brain moved ; colic ; uterine bearing down). < After eating ; after eating plums. < Before, during, and after stool (colic > or not > after stool).

Relations.—*Antidoted by :* Camph., Cham., Coloc., Merc., Nux, Puls. *Antidote to :* Canth., Mg. c. "May be given after abuse of Magnesia, with or without Rhubarb, if stools are sour" (H. C. Allen). *Complementary :* After Mg. c. when milk disagrees and child has sour odour. *Compatible :* Ipec. *Followed well by :* Bell., Puls., Rhus, Sul. *Compare :* Botan., Polyg. h., Rumex, Lapath. Constituents : Chrys. ac., Calc. ox., Silic. Foul breath, Querc., Arn. < After sleep, Lach., Nat. m., Sul. Sour stools, Hep., Mg. c., Calc. (Rhe. has twitching of muscles of face and fingers during sleep ; also puts arms over head). Queer positions, Plb. Head sweat, Calc., Sil., Sanic. < Uncovering, Rx. c. (Rhe., colic ; Rx. c., cough). Screaming children with diarrhœa, Jalap. Bubbling sensation, Berb. Difficult dentition, Kre., Cham. Sour body smell, Hep., Mg. c. (Mg. c. is deeper acting than Rhe.).

Impatience, Cin., Stp. Children cry and toss all night, Pso. As if in a dream, Ambr., Anac., Calc., Can. i., Con., Cup., Med., Strm., Val., Ver., Ziz.

Causation.—Eating prunes. Eating unripe fruit. Dentition. Spasms. Dislocations.

SYMPTOMS.

1. **Mind.**—Indifference.—Indolence, and dislike to conversation.—Peevish disposition, with tears.—Restlessness, with desire to weep.—Impetuous desire for particular objects.—The child demands various things with vehemence and weeping; even its favourite playthings.—Screaming of children with urging and sour stools.—Unable to collect her senses for long after waking.—State of mind as if half asleep (or in a dream).—Delirium.—Incoherent talk.

2. **Head.**—Stupefying cloudiness of head, as after intoxication, with prominent (bloated) eyes.—Vertigo, which occasions falling sideways, when standing.—Giddy headache, with anxiety.—Pressive headache, esp. in sinciput, temples, and vertex.—Pressure as with a finger at point where head joins neck.—Heaviness of head, with heat and tearings.—Dull and cramp-like tension in head.—Throbbing in head, sometimes proceeding from abdomen.—Movement of brain when stooping.—Sweat on forehead and scalp after slight effort.—Hair *always* (awake or asleep, active or still) sopping wet, may or may not be sour.

3. **Eyes.**—Eyes weak and downcast, with aching pain, esp. when looking steadily at any object.—Pressure and pullings in eyelids.—Smarting in eyes, as if caused by dust.—Painful throbbing in eyes.—Convulsive starting in lids.—Lachrymation (swimming eyes, full of water), esp. in open air.—Pupils contracted.

4. **Ears.**—Otalgia with itching in ear.—Pressure (at meatus as from a finger) and throbbing in ears.—Dulness of hearing, as from relaxation of tympanum, with rumbling in ears, > by violent swallowing but only for a moment.—Crackling and bubbling in ear and in muscles on side of neck.—(Ménière's disease).—(Old-standing and frequently recurring deafness with cicatricial membrana tympani gets well after single dose of *Rhe.* ϕ.—R. T. C.)

5. **Nose.**—Stupefying drawing from root of nose to tip, where it tingles.—Sensation of heat in nose.

6. **Face.**—Face pale; or one cheek red, the other pale.—Tension of skin of face.—Frowning and contraction of muscles of forehead.—Itching rash on forehead and arm.—Cold perspiration on face, esp. on mouth and nose.—Twitching at commissures of lips.

7. **Teeth.**—Digging pains in teeth which are carious.—Painful sensation of coldness in teeth (with accumulation of much saliva).—Difficult dentition of children.—Teeth feel blunt.

8. **Mouth.**—Sensation of numbness and insensibility in tongue, with loss of taste for whole day (from chewing the stem).—Tongue swollen, articulation affected (poisoning case).—Salivation with colic or diarrhœa.—Mouth covered with offensive mucus after sleeping.—Offensive breath (after sleep).—Dryness and sensation of dryness in mouth.

9. **Throat.**—Contraction of gullet.

10. **Appetite.**—Loss of taste.—Mawkish, clammy, or sour taste.—Bad taste after sleep.—Food has a bitter taste.—Appetite for different things, which, however, changes to disgust at the first mouthful.—Dislike to fat and insipid food.—Repugnance to coffee (not sweetened with sugar).—Hunger without appetite.

11. **Stomach.**—Nausea, as if proceeding from stomach, with colic.—Fulness in stomach, with pressure, as if overloaded.—Contractions in stomach.—Shootings and throbbings in pit of stomach.

12. **Abdomen.**—Distension of abdomen, with tension.—Pressure in umbilical region.—Cutting and rumbling in abdomen as from flatulence.—Nausea in abdomen.—Cuttings in abdomen, which force a curving of the body, often shortly after a meal, < by standing ; < from eating.—Colic : < at once by uncovering an arm or leg ; not > by stool ; before and during stool, > after ; with very sour stools in acid children.—Incarceration of flatus, with aching and tension in chest.—Palpitation and jerking (swelling-bubbling sensation which seemed as if it could be heard) in abdominal muscles.—Itching stitches in inguinal gland.

13. **Stool and Anus.**—Urgent and frequent want to evacuate, without any result, < by movement, and walking.—Diarrhœa only when exercising.—Desire for stool after a meal.—Loose evacuations, generally of a sour smell, liquid, or of the consistence of pap, preceded and followed by tenesmus, with constrictive pinching in abdomen, and shuddering during the evacuation.—Stools frequent, soft, semi-liquid, evacuated with great pain in back and burning in rectum.—Stools : brown, slimy ; loose, thin, curdled, sour-smelling ; corroding anus ; mucous and fecal ; whitish, curdy, turning green on exposure on diaper ; pea-green ; fetid ; frothy.—Liquid, slimy stools as if fermented, with pale face, ptyalism ; child draws up legs ; smells sour.—Greyish or brown diarrhœa, mixed with mucus ; followed by tenesmus, pain in back, and great burning in anus and rectum.—Profuse diarrhœa, with vomiting, and great weakness.—Diarrhœa of lying-in women ; of children.—Constipation after the proving.

14. **Urinary Organs.**—Increased secretion of urine.—Urine red ; or greenish-yellow.—Blood flows freely from urethra (poisoning case).—Weakness of bladder : the urine cannot be discharged without effort.—Burning sensation in bladder.—Burning urine.—Urine has agreeable benzoic odour.

15. **Male Sexual Organs.**—Unusual emissions.

16. **Female Sexual Organs.**—Bearing down in uterine region while standing.—Drawing burning in l. ovarian region.—Urinary complaints after abortion.—Milk yellow, bitter.—Diarrhœa after confinement.—Stitches in nipples.

17. **Respiratory Organs.**—Cough : dry in evening ; with expectoration of mucus.—Snoring inspiration during sleep.

18. **Chest.**—Dyspnœa on breathing deeply, as from a weight on (upper part of) chest.—Lancinations in chest.—Rush of blood to chest.—Crackling bubbling (even audible) in r. then l. pectoral muscles.—Palpitation of muscles of chest.—Pains and lancinations in breasts.—Milk of nursing women bitter and yellow ; the infant refuses the breast.

20. **Back.**—Violent cutting, as if in lumbar vertebræ, < from stool.—

Cutting-drawing in l. lumbar region beneath short ribs, and in front of l. lower abdomen, just above pubes, or cutting in intestines.—Tension in back and small of back.—Rigidity in loins and hips, which does not permit standing upright.

21. **Limbs.**—Simple pain in all joints during motion.—The limbs on which he lies fall asleep.—Lameness of wrists and knees after spasms and dislocations.

22. **Upper Limbs.**—Lancinations in arms.—Tearing in arms, forearms, and joints of fingers.—Jerking in arms and hands.—Muscular palpitation (bubbling sensation) in joints of elbows.—Veins (on hands) swollen, and hands hot.—Perspiration, sometimes cold, on palms of hands.—Jerking in fingers.

23. **Lower Limbs.**—Great lassitude in thighs.—Jerking in muscles of thighs.—Numbness of legs when crossed.—Muscular palpitations in hams, legs and toes.—Stiffness of ham, with pain during movement.—Shootings in knees and legs.—Bubbling sensation from bend of knee to heel.—Stiffness in bend of knees with pain on motion.—Intermittent burning as from glowing coals between internal malleolus and tendo Achilles.—Sticking itching in hollows of soles.—Bubbling-crackling sensation in ball of l. big toe.

24. **Generalities.**—[We use this remedy most particularly for sour-smelling children; stools, vomit, breath, all smell sour. Before or during stool there are colicky pains about umbilicus; straining before stool, which is finally voided with ease; infants who cry a great deal with colic in the night; tenesmus without stool.—H. N. G.].—Affections of l. side of body.—Perspiration on upper part of body.—Soreness of the joints during movement.—Pulsative pains.—Palpitation in muscles, esp. round joints.—Numbness of the limbs upon which patient has been lying.—Lassitude and heaviness in whole body as after waking from deep sleep.

25. **Skin.**—Pemphigus on face, scalp, and hands; face, lips, and tongue swollen; face livid (poisoning cases).—Itching rash on forehead and arms.

26. **Sleep.**—Sleep and yawnings.—Disturbed sleep at night, with tossing, cries, moaning and snoring, or with convulsive quivering of eyelids, muscles of face, and of fingers, esp. in children.—The hands are passed over the head when going to sleep, and during sleep.—Nocturnal raving and moving about in bed, although eyes are closed.—After sleep, headache and dizziness; or fetid mucus, of a putrid smell and taste, in mouth.—Anxious, sad, vivid dreams.

27. **Fever.**—Shuddering, without external coldness.—Alternate shivering and heat, with anxiety, and repugnance to everything.—Heat in hands and feet, with coolness of face.—Perspiration easily excited by the least exercise, esp. on forehead and scalp.—Sweat stains yellow.

Rhodium Oxydatum Nitricum.

Nitrate of the Oxide of Rhodium. (Rhodium Rh. A.W. 103.)
Solution.

Clinical.—Anus, itching of; burning in. Constipation. Ears, pains in. Hæmorrhoids. Headache. Hearing, illusions of. Impotence.

Characteristics.—The metal *Rhodium* is found in association with *Platinum*. The preparation of it used by Hering was thus obtained : " A small quantity of Rhodium sponge, hydrate of potassa and nitre were exposed to the action of the blowpipe until oxidised. After having the oxide well washed and boiled in nitric acid for a few minutes and exposed to a gentle heat for an hour, the nitrate was obtained from the oxide : a fluid of a golden colour, and of the consistency of syrup." Dilutions of this were made, and the 4th was proved for Hering by Dr. Pehrson, the 2nd and 3rd by Dr. Negendank. The bowels were affected in both, constipation with piles being relieved in one, and constipation with itching of the anus being caused in the other. Some *Peculiar Symptoms* were : Headache on being waked up in the night. Headache alternating with faintness. Faintness > by passage of stool. Heat preceding chill and alternating with it. Sensation as if teeth blunt ; as if sand between them. Scraping or harsh noise = disagreeable sensation in teeth. Hearing more acute ; illusion that he hears whispering.

SYMPTOMS.

1. **Mind.**—During whole day very unusual hilarity and gladness.—Illusions of whispers.—Irritation of the mind making regular meditation impossible, and causing a sense of dissatisfaction.

2. **Head.**—On being disturbed at night aching in forehead, preventing further sleep.—Tearing in forehead on being awakened ; and at other times.—Headache alternating with diarrhœa.

3. **Eyes.**—Everything appeared as if the degree of light was lessened, principally the point (print ?) whilst reading, which continued during the following day.

4. **Ears.**—Stitches in membrana tympani ; hearing more acute.—In evening unnatural irritation of sense of hearing, a constant whispering being heard as illusive as if caused by human beings ; a few times he went to see if there was not some one there.

5. **Nose.**—Eruptions on nostrils temporarily removed.

6. **Face.**—Heat and sweat over face.

8. **Mouth.**—Teeth feel blunt ; every scraping and similar noise = most disagreeable sensation in them.—Teeth feel as if sand between them.

11. **Stomach.**—Stinging pain in pit of stomach, which after two hours changed into a griping pain in integuments of bowels.

13. **Stool and Anus.**—The usually large stool passes with less difficulty than usual ; piles improved.—Stool in small round balls like cockles, with burning in anus during and for some time after.—Much odourless flatus passed.—Tenesmus as if stool would come, but only flatus passes.—Loud emission of flatus.—Diarrhœa with much wind, stool bubbling out ; from 6 to 9 a.m., when it ceased and a headache commenced.—Passage of stool > faintness.—Foul stool.—Itching of anus, as if caused by the piles, stools tardy.

14. **Urinary Organs.**—Burning in urethra towards head of penis.

15. **Male Sexual Organs.**—Lack of desire, power, and pleasure.

21. **Limbs.**—Aching on inside l. thigh and on l. little finger.

22. **Upper Limbs.**—Aching in upper joint of r. middle finger, evening.—Intense aching l. wrist, evening.—7 p.m. aching in r. wrists.

23. **Lower Limbs.**—Burning, sticking pain rushing downwards in l. leg.

24. **Generalities.**—From 4 to 7 p.m., after mental exertion, faintness, not > by eating, drinking, rest, &c.; at 7 as this began to diminish r.-sided headache began and was still felt on waking, 5 a.m.; during the faintness urging to stool with inability, stool felt in l. side of rectum; by pressure around anus round balls were evacuated, causing intense burning in anus; faintness ceased instantaneously the moment the stool had passed.—Constipation lasting several days.

27. **Fever.**—Fever with sweat over face, 3 p.m., followed by chill; fever and chill alternated till 6 p.m.

Rhododendron.

Rhododendron chrysanthum. Siberian Rhododendron. Yellow Snow-rose. *N. O.* Ericaceæ. Tincture of fresh leaves.

Clinical.—Amenorrhœa. Asthenopia. *Bone, pains in. Bunions.* Chorea. Ciliary neuralgia. Coryza. Delirium. Diarrhœa. Diphtheritic paralysis. Earache. Epistaxis. Eyes, affections of. Fever. Flatulence, incarcerated. Gums, itching of. *Hydrocele.* Lienteria. *Lumbago. Memory, weak. Neuralgia.* Nightmare. Ovary, cyst of. *Rheumatism.* Spleen, pain in. Sprains. *Stiff-neck.* Testes, affections of. Tinnitus. Toothache. Vagina, cysts in. Wrists, pains in.

Characteristics.—The golden-flowered *Rhododendron* is not much known in general medicine, but the *Treasury of Botany* says of it that "it is narcotic in its properties and is used medicinally." Growing among the fogs and storms of the Siberian mountains, its provings (by Seidel, Wahle, Herzog, Helbig, and others) show that it produces sensitiveness to storms and weather changes; and this gives the grand keynote of its use in medicine. *Rhod.* disturbs all parts of the economy, producing delirium, fever, headache, neuralgias (earache, toothache), rheumatism, and inflammations, but the chief determining characteristic is that the symptoms come on or are < on the approach of a storm; during a storm; or in wet weather. Sensitiveness to electric changes. It is *suited to* nervous persons who dread a storm, and are particularly afraid of thunder; < before the storm; affections which come on in the spring and autumn, the seasons of change. This is the chief modality, and will be found in some degree present in a large number of cases requiring *Rhod.* But *Rhod.* has other characteristics. Among these is loss of memory: Words are omitted while writing; sudden disappearance of thought; forgets what he is talking about, has to think awhile before he can recall it. Vertigo and confusion, "brain feels as if surrounded by fog." The narcotic reputation of *Rhod.* is borne out in the provings, for it produced actual intoxication, and also made the provers extraordinarily sensitive to the action of wine. Vertigo occurs whilst lying in bed, and is > by moving about. An intense degree of tinnitus aurium was caused by it, and this, associated with the vertigo, gives *Rhod.* a place in Ménière's disease. A *Peculiar Symptom* is: "Loud sounds re-echo long in ears." Like the other Ericaceæ, *Rhod.* has a strong effect on the kidneys, producing increased urine, with offensive smell, clear, brown red, or of greenish tinge, and, whatever colour it may be, of offensive smell. This offensive smell reappears in the axillary sweat. But the general sweat may be aromatic in odour and not unpleasant. "Formication with sweat" is characteristic. *Rhod.* sets up diarrhœa; and also a paralytic condition of the rectum, so that an effort is required to expel a soft stool. Pains in rectum extend to genitals; and the male generative organs experience the most intense action of the drug. The scrotum shrinks; testes are retracted; or else they swell (especially at night), and are the seat of a bruised pain, as if they had been crushed violently. These pains are < by touch; < sitting; > moving about. They may be so violent as to arrest breathing. The menses are too early and too profuse; the menses are always accompanied by fever and headache. Menses reappear soon after they have ceased. In one prover *Rhod.* restored the menses after six months' absence. It has cured cysts in the vagina, and has caused the rupture of an ovarian cyst. Chorea of left leg, arm, and face, < on approach of a storm, has been cured by it. The paralysing effect of *Rhod.* was exemplified by the poisoning of a flock of sheep from eating the leaves. A number of them died immediately after the administration of stimulants, and the autopsy showed that cause of death was paralysis of the swallowing muscles (T. C. Collings, quoted *H. W.*, xxix. 158). Cooper cites a parallel case of death from post-diphtheritic paralysis affecting the throat muscles, occurring a few minutes after drinking tea. In both instances the fluid entered the trachea instead of the gullet and caused suffocation. Both sides are affected by *Rhod.* Symptoms frequently alternate: left and right nostril; burning in uterus and pains in limbs; chilliness and heat. Pains go from within outward. H. S. Budd (*H. R.*, xv. 300) relates the case of Mrs. X., 44, married ten years, three children. Neuralgia for three years. Attacks occur usually on Friday or Saturday and last till Monday or Tuesday, but are induced any time by high winds, damp weather, or an approaching storm. *Ammonol*, *Phenacetin*, *Antikamnia*, had all failed, and *Passif.* only partly relieved, sometimes enabling patient to get sleep. The pain was < after hard work; during any movement; in very cold weather; from hot applications. Intense soreness all over right half of head. Cannot rest on pillow or endure even lightest hairpins when pain is worst. < At night. *Intensely* nervous and hysterical at being *touched*, even by accident. During pain increased activity of kidneys, ceasing when pain ceases. Pain greatest in right lower jaw. Sometimes > for an hour by chewing gum or eating. Afraid of thunder. Omits words when writing. *Rhod.* 16x every hour was given on May 12th. Each dose caused immediate <. Next morning pains stopped suddenly and did not return. On June 7th there was a premonitory twinge, and a powder of *Rhod.* 1m was given, after which there was complete immunity. E. V. Moffat (quoted *Am. H.*, xxiii. 268) treated a girl, 10, for neuralgia, which had existed for several years. The patient was of marked gouty heredity, and had been treated by leading old-school doctors in

New York. She was well during the summer, but suffered intensely during winter. Pains general and shifting, sometimes intercostal, sometimes sciatic ; in bad weather never absent. The last form was prostrating headache, incapacitating her for school work. The eyes were normal. *While the sun shone she was comfortable.* If it stormed or threatened she was miserable. If she had a headache on a stormy day and the sun came out, in ten minutes she was relieved, and it returned at once if snow or rain came on. A cold day, especially if damp, was almost as bad as a storm. *Rhod.* φ, in repeated and increasing doses, cured in three weeks. Colour, spirits, strength returned, and she no longer minded the weather or missed her school. *Peculiar Sensations* are : Brain as if in a fog. Scalp as if bruised. As if a worm in ear. As if water rushing into ear. As if throat lined with mucus. As from tension under short ribs. Testicle as if violently contused or crushed. As if a fist pressed forcibly against stomach. As if blood ceased to circulate in arms. As if arms asleep. As if feet and legs asleep. As if heavy weights hanging to feet. As of subcutaneous ulceration. Undulating sensation arising from abdomen. Warm undulations in heart. Bruised pains. Pains flying about. Crawling sensations. A *Peculiar Symptom* in the eyes is : One pupil dilated, the other contracted. There is a splenic stitch on walking fast. The incarcerated flatus is felt in the hypochondria and small of the back. It is not at all unusual to meet this symptom, " Flatus felt in the back," in cases of flatulent indigestion. " Increased warmth of hands even in cold weather " is another peculiar symptom. The symptoms are < by touch (toothache, testicles, chest—this sensitiveness is general). Rest < ; motion (especially *commencing motion*) >. (Walking = stitches in spleen ; motion < pain in ears ; and prosopalgia). Rheumatic pain in shoulder on which he rests ; goes off on turning. < Sitting. > Rising. < Standing. < When writing. < Wind ; east wind ; rough weather ; wet, cold weather ; getting wet. < Before a storm (ciliary neuralgia ; pains through eye from head ; toothache ; diarrhœa ; dysentery ; pain in deltoids ; paroxysmal chorea). > Warmth. > Wrapping up. (But heat in bed < formication of anus ; and toothache.) Dry heat >. < Change. < Thunder. Toothache > whilst and after eating and from warmth. Pain in left side > by eating. Drinking cold water = pressure at stomach. < Drinking wine ; easily intoxicated. Belching >. General sweat >. < Night ; morning in bed and on rising.

Relations.—*Antidoted by :* Bry., Camph., Clem., Rhus. *Compare :* Arbut., Kalm., Led., Uva ursi, and other Ericaceæ. < Wet weather ; < weather changes, < rest, > motion, Rhus (Rhus affects periosteum more than Rhod. ; Rhod. > *commencing* motion, Rhus <). < During thunderstorm, Nat. c., Phos., Pso., Sil. < From wine, Zn. Heat in heart, Croc., Lchn., Op. Orchitis become chronic, indurated testicle, Clem., Puls. (Rhod. has tendency to atrophy ; and crushed feeling in testes). Orchitis, crushed sensation, Aur., Cham. Wandering rheumatism < in wet and stormy weather ; right side neuralgia, Kalm. . Fibrous deposits in great toe, Colch., Led. (Led. has > by cold). < In stormy, wet weather, Dulc., Nat. s., Nux m. (Rhod. most *before* the storm). Diarrhœa from fruit, Rhe. > Wrapping up head,

Sil. Sensation of subcutaneous ulceration, Pul., Ran. b. Bruised pains, Arn., Con. One pupil contracted the other dilated, Cad. s., Phys. Hydrocele, Bry. Intoxication, Querc. Sounds re-echo, Caust., Pho., Ph. ac., Sars.

Causation.—Stormy weather. Thunder. Sprains. Eating fruit. Getting wet. Catching cold.

SYMPTOMS.

1. **Mind.**—Delirium ; staggers ; falls asleep on his knees ; starts and appears terrified in sleep but awakes cheerful.—Mental derangement.—Frightful visions.—Sombre, morose humour.—Excessive indifference, with dread of all kinds of labour.—Nervous persons who dread a storm, and esp. thunder.—Excessive forgetfulness.—Sudden loss of ideas.—Leaves out whole words when writing.—While talking forgets what he is talking about.

2. **Head.**—Reeling sensation in head ; brain feels as if surrounded with a fog.—Head bewildered in the morning after rising, with sleepiness.—Intoxication.—Vertigo with anguish.—Whirling vertigo in bed, as if the head were about to be turned backwards.—Headache (in forehead and temples) excited or < by wine or by cold, damp weather (> after rising and moving about).—Tension in the forehead.—Drawing pressure in sinciput and temples, principally in bones.—Violent drawing and tearing in bones and periosteum of cranial bones ; < when at rest, in morning ; > from wrapping head up warmly, from dry heat and from exercise.—Aching in l. half of forehead, spreading to l. temple, continuous, < by wine.—Tearing boring in l. temple.—Lancinations in the sinciput and sides of the head.—Throbbing in head.—Painful sensibility of the exterior of head as from subcutaneous ulceration.—Pain as from contusion or blows in the occiput.—Violent pain r. occiput as if a foreign body had been forced in.—Gnawing itching (biting and burning) in scalp, esp. in evening.—Hair stands up as if electrified (R. T. C.).

3. **Eyes.**—Pressive shootings in the margin of orbits, with spasmodic contraction of eyelids.—Darting like arrows through eye from head < before a storm.—(Severe r. keratitis with aching in r. side of head and forehead, < in thunder.—R. T. C.).—Aching in eyes, commencing on one side of face.—Sticking pain in r. eyeball, as with a red-hot needle darting from within outward.—Sensation of dryness and burning in eyes from time to time, esp. in bright daylight and when looking steadily at an object.—Suppuration of lids at night.—Irritation of lids (agg. R. T. C.).—Swollen lids which become easily red.—Agglutination of lids.—Quivering jerks in lids.—Contraction of one pupil while the other is dilated.—Clouded sight when reading and writing.—Eyes tire easily (agg. and cure.—R. T. C.).

4. **Ears.**—Otalgia (r. ear) with jerking tearings.—Tearing and boring in and near the ears.—Sensation as of a worm in ear.—Continued dull humming in ears, < by swallowing.—Loud sounds re-echo long.—Continued buzzing in ears, feeling as if water rushing into them.

5. **Nose.**—Epistaxis.—Diminished smell.—Semilateral obstruction at root of nose, esp. in morning.—Fluent coryza with obstruction of one nostril (l. nostril, sometimes alternating with r., > in open air), and loss of smell and taste.—Increased secretion of nasal mucus in open air.—A bright red spot on nose, sensitive to touch, lasting several days.

6. **Face.**—Shuddering chilliness over face.—Violent tearing, jerking faceache, < in wind and changes ; > while eating and from warmth.—Prosopalgia extends from temple to chin ; spreads over r. side of face.—Lips dry and burning.—Vesicles on the lips (on inner side of under lip), with pains as from excoriation when eating.

7. **Teeth.**—Toothache with drawing tearing in molars, in cold, damp weather ; or on approach of or during a storm ; < by touch.—Rheumatic toothache radiating from r. lower jaw to teeth.—Nocturnal odontalgia with otalgia.—Itching in the gums.—Swelling and pain as from excoriation between lower gums and cheek.

8. **Mouth.**—Copious accumulation of saliva in mouth, with dryness of gullet and smarting vesicles under tongue.—Greenish coated tongue with bitter, putrid taste.

9. **Throat.**—Scraping in throat ; sensation as if lined with mucus.—Constriction and burning sensation in throat.

10. **Appetite.**—Dulness of taste.—Food has no flavour.—Augmented thirst.—Gnawing, hungry sensation before a meal.—Speedy satiety, with good appetite, followed by uneasiness.

11. **Stomach.**—Nausea, with inclination to vomit, pressure in stomach, and waterbrash, > by eructations.—Gulping of rancid or bitter fluid.—Empty eructations.—Vomiting of green, bitter substances.—Vomiting after anything fluid, esp. cold water.—Aching (and heaviness) in stomach at night, or after drinking cold water.—Contractive pressure in scrobiculus with obstructed respiration.—Pressive shootings in pit of stomach and hypochondria.

12. **Abdomen.**—Spasmodic pains in hypochondria.—Pain as from tension under short ribs.—Tension in the region of the spleen (when or) after stooping.—Shootings in spleen on walking quickly.—Distension of abdomen, esp. in upper part, with sensation of fulness, which hinders respiration, morning and evening.—Painful incarceration of flatus in hypochondria and loins.—Grumbling and borborygmi in abdomen, with risings and expulsion of fetid flatus.—Drawing pain in r. and (slighter) l. inguinal ring while sitting.

13. **Stool and Anus.**—Urgent want to evacuate, with slow evacuation.—As soon as he gets out of bed diarrhœa comes on.—Difficult evacuation, even of soft fæces.—Fæces of consistence of pap.—Mucous evacuations.—Diarrhœa after eating fruit or in cold, damp weather ; food passes undigested.—Diarrhœa which does not weaken.—Shooting pain in rectum extending to just below ribs.—Crawling in anus as from ascarides.—Throbbing in anus.—Drawing from rectum to genital organs.

14. **Urinary Organs.**—More frequent want to urinate, with drawing in the region of the bladder and in the groins.—Pain in urethra as from subcutaneous ulceration.—Increased discharge of a fetid urine.—Urine clear, greenish, hot.—Twitching and stitches at urethral orifice between acts of micturition.

15. **Male Sexual Organs.**—Pain as from excoriation between genitals and thighs.—Throbbings and shootings under glans.—Drawing and pain as from a bruise in testes extending into abdomen and thighs.—Testes, esp. epididymis, intensely painful to touch.—Testes swollen and retracted.—Itching, sweat, and shrinking in scrotum.—Transparent swelling of the scrotum, as from hydrocele.—Swelling of the testicles after gonorrhœa.—Induration of

testes; induration and swelling of l. testicle.—Contusive pain in first one then in the other testicle.—Drawing pain in r. testis and cord, > by motion; sometimes pricking, beginning r. testis, spreading in zigzag manner along perinæum to anus, so violent it arrested breathing.—Crawling pain in testes. —Increased desire.—Aversion to coitus and want of erections.—Profuse emission with amorous dreams.

16. **Female Sexual Organs.**—Suppressed catamenia.—Premature and too profuse catamenia.—Fever with headache at each menstrual period.—Pain in ovaries; < in change of weather.—Caused rupture of cyst in r. ovary. —Serous cysts in vagina.—After parturition, burning in uterus alternately with pains in limbs, fingers flexed.

17. **Respiratory Organs.**—Catarrh and hoarseness of trachea.—Dry, shaking cough, with oppression of chest and roughness of throat, esp. night and morning (in paroxysms from tickling in the trachea).—Scraping cough with scanty expectoration of mucus.

18. **Chest.**—Transient, dull pain from chest to l. hypochondrium when walking fast.—Pressure at chest with obstructed respiration.—Dyspnœa from constriction of chest.—Warm undulation in chest and about the heart.—Rush of blood to chest.—Bruised pain at chest externally.—Knife-like cuttings in l. chest when bending to r. and backward.

19. **Heart.**—Boring pain in region of heart.—Warm undulations at heart.—(Heart irritable, pulse weak and quick.—R. T. C.).—Heart beats stronger.—Pulse: slow; feeble, small, and slow.

20. **Neck and Back.**—Rigidity of nape.—Rheumatic tension and drawing in muscles of nape and of neck.—Stiff-neck, gums and teeth sore, pains fly about everywhere.—Pain in sacrum, becoming intolerable on stooping.—Wrenching or contusive pains in back and loins (< at rest and in rainy weather).—Small of back painful when sitting as if back had been bent too long, or as if he had been lying on it too long.—Rheumatic drawing and tearing in back and shoulders.

21. **Limbs.**—Rheumatic and arthritic drawing and tearings as if in the periosteum of limbs, excited by rough weather and < by repose.—Wrenching pain and searching drawings in joints, with redness and swelling.—Chronic rheumatism affecting the smaller joints and their ligaments.—Restlessness, tingling, weakness, and sensation of paralytic stiffness in some of the limbs.

22. **Upper Limbs.**—Drawing pains in arms in rough weather.—Sensation as if the blood did not circulate in arms.—Weakness with tingling and heaviness in arms, extending to tips of fingers during repose.—Pulling and tearing in forearms and hands as if in periosteum (during wet, cold weather), < during repose.—Wrenching pain in joints of hands.—Sensation as if the wrists were sprained.—On small spot of metacarpal bones painful sensation as if an exostosis would form.—Increased heat in hands, even in cold weather. —Itching of r. middle and ring fingers with erysipelatous redness.

23. **Lower Limbs.**—Wrenching pain in joints of hip and knee.—Sensation of soreness in thighs near the genitals.—Itching of inner surface of thighs.—Sensation as if skin were cold and shrivelled in certain parts of the legs.—Perspiration on legs.—(Dropsical) swelling of legs and feet.—Feet and legs as if asleep.—Drawing and tearing in legs and feet as if in periosteum, esp. during repose.—Excessive coldness of feet, even in a warm room; can-

not be got warm in bed ; prevents sleep.—Pain in tendo-Achillis on stepping. —Rheumatic enlargement of great toe mistaken for bunion.—Gout with fibrous deposit (not urate of soda).—Sensation as if heavy weight were hanging to feet.—Corns on feet with shooting pain.

24. **Generalities.**—We think of this remedy chiefly for the sufferings that are < in windy weather, even if the patient be not exposed to it ; he may be in bed or in a warm, comfortable room, but the blowing of the wind < the symptoms.—Tendency to faint in young girls of phthisical tendency who grow rapidly and are upset by thunderstorms (R. T. C.).—Affections in general of the r. upper extremities ; r. abdominal ring ; l. side of nose ; testes ; r. lower extremity ; inner surface of thigh.—Serous cysts in vagina.—Induration or swelling of the testicles, particularly of the r. one.—Diarrhœa after eating fruit ; flatulent colic.—Arthritic nodes.—Dragging up or rooting sensation ; crawling of the skin or over the skin like ants ; toothache which ceases suddenly, beginning again in two or three hours ; feeling of heaviness in stomach after drinking cold water.—Great dejection and painful weariness after the least exercise.—Dropsical swellings. —Frequent remission of sufferings, and appearance of them generally in morning.—Sufferings excited or < by cold, damp weather, or by the approach of a storm, as also during repose.

25. **Skin.**—Eruptions.—Burning and tearing with erysipelas.—Itching burning, and creeping.

26. **Sleep.**—Strong disposition to sleep during day, with burning sensation in eyes.—Profound sleep before midnight, after having gone to sleep early in evening.—Sleeplessness after midnight.—Sleep in morning, disturbed by bodily agitation and pain.—During sleep oppression of chest, a sort of nightmare.

27. **Fever.**—Pulse slow and weak.—Chilliness in morning in bed and during day if cold air blows on him.—Shivering alternately with heat.—Augmented heat, esp. in hands.—Fever in evening with heat in head, coldness of the feet (after lying down, continuing long), burning sensation in eyes and nose, painful weariness and adipsia, followed by nocturnal heat and sleeplessness.—Sensation of heat, esp. in hands, although they feel cold to the touch. —Profuse debilitating perspiration, esp. when exercising in the open air.—Offensive-smelling perspiration in the axilla.—While perspiring the skin itches and tingles, like formication.—Perspiration with tingling and itching in skin. —Perspiration of an aromatic smell.

Rhus Aromatica.

R. canadensis. R. suaveolans. Betula triphylla. Lobadium aromaticum. Turpinia glabra. Fragrant Sumach. *N. O.* Anacardiaceæ. Tincture of fresh root bark. (Pharmacop. of Amer. Inst. says of fresh leaves.)

Clinical.—Atony. Bladder, hæmorrhage from. Diabetes. Diarrhœa, chronic. Dysentery, chronic. Enuresis. Hæmorrhages. Kidneys, hæmorrhage from. Uterus, hæmorrhage from ; atony of.

Characteristics.—Hale quotes J. T. McClanahan's account of *Rhus arom.*: "It is a shrub, growing from two to six feet high, on high, rocky soil; stems straight, branching near the top; flowers yellow, fruit clustered, red, seedy, and acid. When the bush is fractured it emits a strong odour. The bark of the root is the proper medicinal part." McClanahan's grandfather, Dr. John Gray, used *Rh. a.* as a remedy in diabetes, and his father, Dr. F. McClanahan, in other genito-urinary diseases. J. T. McClanahan records these cases: (1) Mr. A., 27, cadaverous, emaciated, haggard, had diabetes insipidus. *Rh. a.*, teaspoonful doses of the powdered root bark in sweet milk, three times a day, completely cured in four months. (2) Mrs. B., 37, had diabetes mellitus. First noticed increase of urine ten months before; became so weak she had to abandon house-work. Pain in back; thirst; appetite, now ravenous, now deficient. Skin sallow, doughy. Temperature 101·5° F. Cough and night-sweats occasionally. Diarrhœa at times. Specific gravity of urine, 1032. *Rh. a.*, half-teaspoonful doses every four hours. Quantity of urine diminished next day, and as this diminution progressed the doses of *Rh. a.* were given at increasing intervals, and in three months it was discontinued, proper diet having been observed in the meantime. Cod-liver oil and hypophosphites were given after the *Rh. a.* was discontinued. (3) Mr. C. had incontinence of urine more than a year, constant dribbling. *Rh. a.* φ gtt. x, three times a day, improved at once, and cured completely in eight weeks. (4) Girl had enuresis during day and night for two years. *Rh. a.* φ, one part to glycerine three parts, a teaspoonful three times a day, cured. (5) Boy, early in summer had diarrhœa, stools pale and thin, running from him like water; no particular pain or fever. Pale, emaciated, limbs trembling, scarcely able to stand. Abdomen flabby. *Rh. a.* φ gtt. iii, in water after each stool, cured rapidly. (6) A labourer had "chronic dysentery" two months. On the average five stools a day, sometimes copious and painless, sometimes scanty and with pain. Stools consisted largely of blood and mucus or clear blood. Patient thin, anxious, bowels (abdomen) flabby. Skin sallow. *Rh. a.* φ in ten-drop doses, with boiled milk diet, cured. McClanahan also mentions hæmorrhage from kidneys, bladder, and uterus; menorrhagia and other excessive discharges accompanied by a relaxed condition of the uterus as indicating the remedy; also atonic conditions generally. These experiences have been confirmed by others. J. A. McKay (*Hom. News*, quoted *Am. H.*, xxii. 394) relates the case of Mrs. S., 45, who had severe, profuse uterine hæmorrhage for eight days, which three old-school doctors failed to arrest. The condition was becoming desperate, large clots passing away, and the patient fainting from the loss. *Rh. a.* φ gtt. x, every six hours, was given. The first dose checked the flow, which ceased entirely after the second.

Relations.—Rh. a. is closely allied to Rh. g. They are both non-poisonous, and have terminal flowers, instead of the axillary flowers of the poisonous varieties.

Rhus Diversiloba.

R. diversiloba. Californian Poison Oak. *N. O.* Anacardiaceæ.
Tincture of fresh leaves.

Clinical.—Chicken-pox. Eczema. Erysipelas. Skin, sensitive.

Characteristics.—Murray Moore observed the effect of *Rh. d.* on three persons : (1) Miss M., 25, of brown hair and fair complexion, walked up a hill one warm morning, and whilst perspiring gathered ferns which grew among the *Rh. d.* trees, the leaves of which she must have touched, though she did not pull any. The result was a very severe poisoning, which provided the majority of the symptoms of the Schema. (2) J. W., light-haired, robust Englishman, 23, lay down whilst sweating among the bushes and was smartly poisoned. *Ver. v.* ϕ internally and a lotion of *Magnesia sulph.* externally checked the spread of the disease. (3) Boy, 10, pure blond type with thin, freckled skin, plucked some of the leaves, and in eighteen hours the poisoning symptoms came on, facial esysipelas with extreme œdema, closing both eyes, itching and burning. The symptoms became general. M. Moore relates also the case of a man who was poisoned in California in September and returned to the Eastern States and there had an annual eruption for six successive years. During the seventh attack he was carried off with pneumonia, which Moore thinks would not have been the case but for the *Rhus* complication. (*C. D. P.*)

SYMPTOMS.

2. Head.—Dull frontal headache.—Head hot.

3. Eyes.—L. eye closed entirely by swelling ; r. partially.

6. Face.—Vesicular erysipelatous rash with great œdema and swelling of glands in neck ; vesicles dried into a crust so dense that movements of mouth and face were painful.

11. Stomach.—Loss of appetite ; nausea ; vomiting.—Whole digestive system deranged for three weeks.

13. Stool.—Bowels costive.

14. Urinary Organs.—Urine scanty, high-coloured ; felt hot when passed.

15. Male Sexual Organs.—Heat and itching of scrotum and adjacent surfaces of thigh, < on hairy parts.

21. Limbs.—Stiffness of limbs ; of all joints on first moving them.

24. Generalities.—Extreme languor.—On rising from bed fainted ; again later in day.

25. Skin.—Eruption very like chicken-pox.—After the erysipelatous condition of the skin subsided extreme irritability (to flannel) remained, and hypersensitiveness to cold air.—Five months after the poisoning there was a recurrence (without fresh exposure) shortly after taking a bath rather too hot.—The day after he had been among the bushes heat and itching commenced on scrotum and adjacent surfaces of thighs, < on hairy parts ; next day ɔules on red œdematous base appeared on forehead and neck, rapidly eading in all directions, with heat, itching, and burning, but very little 'exia ; itching > by cold ; < by heat, warmth, rubbing, or scratching.

27. **Fever.**—In afternoon chills and feverishness by turns, and general laise.—Slight pyrexia.

Rhus Glabra.

carolinensis. R. elegans. R. virginica. Common Smooth Sumach. Pennsylvania Sumach. Upland Sumach. (Rocky or barren soils in North America.) *N. O.* Anacardiaceæ. Tincture of fresh bark ; of root ; of berries.

Clinical.—Debility. Diarrhœa. Dreams, annoying. Dysentery. Epistaxis. ɛmorrhages. Headache. Mouth, ulcers in.

Characteristics.—*Rhus glabra*, *R. tryphina*, and *R. coriaria* have id fruit and astringent bark, which is used in tanning. *Rh. g.* is a ciduous shrub with stem 2 to 12 feet high, and has terminal flowers, d fruit clothed with acid crimson hairs, like the other non-poisonous ɪoes. The tincture of the bark was proved by Dr. A. V. Marshall himself with very substantial doses. The symptoms of the Schema : his, and they bear out the traditional uses of the remedy. One of ɛse is, "profuse perspiration arising from debility" (Scudder) ; and arshall had "profuse sweat during sleep" and such a degree of bility that he was obliged to leave off the proving. Hale mentions ɪt an infusion of the *root* has a popular repute in diarrhœa and sentery, especially when the discharges are fetid ; and that the *rries* are used for chronic cough, wheezing cough, and laryngeal thma. A tincture made of the whole pannicle ("Sumach-bobs") red a patient of his who had every spring an attack of laryngeal ugh with dyspnœa and almost complete loss of voice. Farmers ɪce "bobs" in the mangers of horses who have "heaves." Cooper served an aggravation in a case of psoriasis : the patient felt irri- ɔle and despondent, and the skin became irritable. In the proving ere were dull, heavy headaches, > by exercise. (Hale says it has red *occipital* headaches.) There was < of stomach symptoms by her food or drink. < By touch (abdomen ; ulcers in mouth). < ter sleep. > By movement.

Relations.—*Compare :* Rh. a. and other Anacardiaceæ, and the ɪnthoxylaceæ, which are an allied order.

SYMPTOMS.

1. **Mind.**—Distaste for society.—Stupid ; forgetful ; indifferent to sur- ɪnding objects.

2. **Head.**—Dull, heavy headache on waking, > by exercise.—Dull, avy pain in front and top of head.

5. **Nose.**—Bleeding from l. nostril and mouth.—Bloody scabs in l. stril.—L. nostril hot and dry.

8. **Mouth.**—Tongue furred white.—Several small, very sensitive ulc on mucous membrane opposite the bicuspids.—Taste flat, alkaline.—Taste drug remains long.—Bleeding from mouth.

9. **Throat.**—Expelled two clots of blood from throat soon after waki

11. **Stomach.**—Loss of appetite (3rd d.).—Hunger (4th d.).—At bre fast could eat but little though feeling as if he had fasted many days (6th —Distress in stomach, disturbed, very restless.—Pain in stomach much < all food or drink.

12. **Abdomen.**—Sharp cutting in umbilical region and abdomen Umbilical region tender to pressure.

13. **Stool and Anus.**—Diarrhœa in afternoon, < towards evening d.) ; later dry, hard stool ; then first part dry, later moist ; then natural ; again diarrhœa of short continuance.

14. **Urinary Organs.**—Scanty, high-coloured urine.

20. **Back.**—Pain in small of back.

23. **Lower Limbs.**—Aching and fatigue of lower limbs, can har stand.

24. **Generalities.**—Lost two pounds weight in three days.—Exhaust and painful fatigue compelled him to relinquish the proving.

26. **Sleep.**—Sleep : disturbed by annoying dreams ; very restles Dreams of flying through the air.

27. **Fever.**—Sense of coldness while there is actual increase of heat the skin.—Skin hot, dry, with thirst.—Sweat, profuse during sleep.

Rhus Radicans.

POISON IVY.

Rhus Toxicodendron.

POISON OAK.

[Under the name *Rhus* Hahnemann published his proving of "*R. ra cans*, also called *Toxicodendron*." Botanists agree in recognis no distinction other than that of habit between the two. Mi paugh (*American Medicinal Plants*) tells in his masterly acco of the plant that he has seen the two varieties springing fr the same root-stock. He advises that the tincture should made from specimens of both. *Rhus tox.* is a shrub with er stem from two to four feet high. The stem is devoid of ro lets. *Rhus r.* has more or less tortuous stems, four to thirty f high, profusely studded with dark-coloured rootlets, by wh it clings to its support.—Our own Ivy (*Hedera helix*) in same way may run along the ground, rooting at intervals i cannot find a support, and growing to a great height if it ca and it may be an erect shrub with no rootlets and no tende to climb.—The two forms have been proved independently, a when necessary to distinguish them I shall name them *Rh. r.* and *Rh. t.* When reference is made to both or either in this work I use the term *Rhus* without distinction. All other varieties of Rhus will be distinguished.] *N. O.* Anacardiaceæ. Tincture of fresh leaves gathered at sunset just before flowering time.

Clinical.—Abortion. *Acne rosacea.* After-pains. Amenorrhœa. Anus, fissure of. Appendicitis. *Appetite, lost.* Beri-beri. Bones, pains in. Cæcum, inflammation of. *Chilblains. Circulation, feeble. Cyanosis. Dengue fever.* Diarrhœa; chronic. Diphtheria. *Dysentery.* Dysmenorrhœa. Dyspepsia. *Ear, eczema of. Ecthyma. Enteric fever. Erysipelas. Erythema nodosum.* Exostosis. *Eyes, inflammation of; choroiditis; sight, weak. Feet, pains in.* Gastro-enteritis. Glands, inflammation of. *Gout.* Hæmorrhages. Hæmorrhoids. *Hands, pains in.* Hernia. *Herpes. Herpes zoster. Housemaid's knee.* Hydrocele. Influenza. Intermittents. *Jaw, cracking in.* Liver, abscess of. *Lumbago. Measles.* Menorrhagia. Metrorrhagia. Neuralgia. Ovary, tumour of. *Paralysis.* Paraphimosis. *Pemphigus.* Periosteum, pains in. Pleurisy. Pleurodynia. Pneumonia; typhoid. Ptosis. *Pyæmia. Redgum. Relapsing fever. Rheumatism. Scarlatina. Sciatica. Sleep, restless.* Small-pox. Spine, diseases of. *Sprain.* Strictures. *Tongue, affections of. Typhus fever.* Urticaria. Warts. Wens. *Yawning.*

Characteristics.—The Poison Ivy grows in thickets and low grounds in North America, flowering in June. It was introduced into England as a plant in 1640. In 1798 Dufresnoy of Valenciennes first used it as a medicine. It was brought to his notice by the cure of a young man of an herpetic eruption (*dartre*) of six years' duration, through his being accidentally poisoned with the plant. Dufresnoy used it successfully in eruptive diseases, paralysis, rheumatism, and amaurosis. The milky juice, which turns black on exposure, is used as a marking ink (like *Anacard.*) and as an ingredient of varnishes for finishing boots. The tincture contains Rhoitannic acid ($C_{18}H_{28}O_{13}$) and Toxicodendric acid, a poisonous, volatile principle. A peculiarity of the plant is that it is *more poisonous during the night*, and when bursting into leaf, or at any time in June or July *when the sun is not shining upon it.* Absence of sunlight, *together with dampness*, seems to favour the exhalation of Toxicodendric acid. "An acrimonious vapour, combined with carburetted hydrogen, exhales from a growing plant of the Poison Oak during the night. It can be collected in a jar, and is capable of inflaming and blistering the skin of persons of excitable constitution who plunge their arms into it" (Porcher, quoted by Millspaugh, from whose work I take the above facts). Those who care for Signatures will not fail to connect the cardinal aggravations of *Rhus*—at night and from damp —with the increased virulence of the plant at night and in damp atmosphere. (One prover of *Rh. ven.* was not influenced by contact with the leaves *when his skin was dry*, but only when perspiring; and the worst poisonings with *Rh. divers.* happened to persons when moist and heated.) Millspaugh relates instances of *Rhus* poisoning: Out of ten men employed to clear a piece of land of shrubs among which the Poison Vine greatly predominated only four escaped: "Most of the men soon began to show signs of being tired, and at the end of the fourth day six of them were flat on their backs too sick for anything." Actual contact with the plant is not necessary in order to produce its effect. One sultry day in June a young lady drove a croquet ball across a lawn to a clump of Poison Ivy that grew beside it. Knowing her susceptibility she reached under the plant and drew out the ball without touching a leaf. During the evening of the same day her face began to itch and burn, and in the night it swelled so that the eyes were not merely closed, the lashes even disappeared in the swelling. It took nearly two weeks for her to recover. Millspaugh summarises the effects of *Rhus* (the majority of poisonings have been caused by *Rh. rad.*) as follows: First redness and swelling of the affected part, with intolerable itching and burning, followed by vertigo, weariness, and a sort of intoxication. Infiltration of face and eyes, and agglutination of the lids after sleep; great restlessness, pain, thirst, and fever. The surface of the skin becomes after a time studded with confluent bullæ where the cellular tissue is loose, then a dermatitis follows resembling erysipelas; this may spread rapidly and finally be communicated to the mucous membranes. This is followed by swelling of the mouth and throat, cough, nausea, and vomiting. Rheumatoid pains develop about the joints, and a painful stiffness asserts itself in the lumbar region, while the legs and arms become numb. Confusion of mind and delirium may then set in, during which the patient may become so ill-humoured, restless, and anxious that he will jump out of bed. Concomitants are: Inflammation of eyes, dilation of pupils, weak vision, sometimes diplopia; epistaxis; brown-coated tongue with triangular red tip; swelling of parotids; difficult swallowing; griping; diarrhœa; profuse urination; oppression; rapid pulse; prostration; soreness of muscles, < by rest; > by exercise; sleepiness; chilliness followed by fever and copious sweat.—The American provings were made with *Rh. rad.*, and the majority of the poisonings have occurred from this plant. Though it is not certain that Hahnemann used *Rh. tox.* at all, or exclusively, Jahr gave a separate presentation of the *Rh. rad.* symptoms. H. C. Allen (quoted *Critique*, vi. 409) notes in *Rh. rad.* a periodicity which marks it as a great antipsoric. It is, he says, on deeply psoric or tubercular constitutions that its toxic effects are most felt and longest lasting, and these constitutional effects "seem ineradicable without the antipsoric." One case of his showed a return of symptoms at 12.45 a.m. on July 5th, each year during sixteen years, except the year 1898, when the previous use of *Tuberculinum*, a dose once each month, prevented an attack; and modified the 1899 attack. Guernsey considers *Rh. rad.* deeper acting than *Rh. tox.*, being indicated in phlegmonous erysipelas, especially where it begins in ankles and moves gradually up the leg, moving in the deeper tissues, no fever; and for axillary glands when the swelling is very deep and hard. Farrington gives as distinctive indications for *Rh. rad.*: Occipital headache with rheumatic stiffness of nape. Drawing tearing pains in legs. Pleurodynia when the pains shoot into the shoulders. Mahony (*M. A.*, xxvi. 109) reports a case of eczema on perineum and scrotum with *sweat in cleft of nates*, both relieved in a week with *Rh. rad.* 12, twice daily.—Hahnemann quickly perceived the keynote of the *Rhus* symptoms: "We observe," he says, in his preface to the proving, "this curious action (which is found in few ther medicines, and in these never to such a great degree), viz., *ıe severest symptoms and sufferings are excited when the body or the limb is t rest, and kept as much as possible without movement.* The opposite of ıis, namely, an increase of the symptoms by movement, is much ıore rarely observed." He contrasts *Rhus* with *Bry.*, which has lmost identical rheumatic pains with the opposite Conditions. Neid-ard adds a note in Hempel's *Jahr* which brings out a modification f this " < by rest " which is of the greatest practical importance, as can testify. Neidhard says that the disease in which he has made ıost use of *Rhus* is a form of rheumatism common in North America, nd characterised by the following symptoms : " Rigidity, paralytic 'eakness of the joints, with stinging pain along the tendons and ıuscles. Swelling and redness on or near the joints. Rheumatism f the hip-joint and wrist seem to be most effectually controlled by s action. *The greatest rigidity and pain is experienced on first moving ıe joints after rest, and on waking up in the morning.* After the joints re moved for a while the pain is lessened." Contrasted with *Bry.*, *hus* has : " The more he moves the > he is " ; whereas *Bry.* has The more he moves the < he is." It is necessary to bear mind this distinction or a wrong prescription will often be ıade. *Rhus* has not only < *during* rest, but < *after* resting also. lowever, *Rhus* and *Bry.* complement each other : it is not unusual for ıe Conditions of a case to change under one of these remedies, and ıen the other will be required. Hahnemann says " these two antago-istic sister remedies "—each in its place—successfully met the typhus hich prevailed in the countries desolated by the war which raged om the summer of 1813 and onwards. Of 183 cases treated by 'ahnemann in Leipzig not one died. This *restlessness* of *Rhus* will be ound to qualify the symptoms in a large proportion of the cases in 'hich it will be called for. It is as restless as *Acon.* and *Ars.*, but in different way from either. With *Rhus* it is due to the pain and reness temporarily > by movement ; or a nervous internal uneasi-ess which makes the patient want to be on the move when there is particular pain present (Nash). The presence of restlessness is a ading indication for *Rhus* in fevers, typhoid and other. Other indi-ıtions are—clouded sensorium, stupefaction, muttering delirium, dry ngue. The characteristic tongue of *Rhus* is dry or dark coated, ith triangular red tip. In intermittents a characteristic is " Cough ıring the chill." Hahnemann pointed out another keynote of *Rhus :* Multiplied experience has taught me that *Rhus* is the most efficacious ıd the specific remedy for the frequently fatal effects of over-lifting, ordinate exertions of the muscles, and contusions." He was, of urse, led to this inference by the " bruised and sprain-like pains " ıd " stiffness " of the provings. *Rhus* is in the front rank of vul-raries. It meets threatened abortion from a sprain ; and also pro-nged after-pains and other effects of the strain of a severe labour ; illary abscess from this cause has been cured with *Rhus.* Straining, eumatic coughs. Ailments from straining a single part, muscle, or ndon ; over-lifting, particularly from stretching high up to reach ings. There is an analogy to this in the dreams—dreams of great ertion ; rowing, swimming, working hard at his daily occupation.

Rhus has cured many forms of paralysis : Rheumatic paraplegia from getting wet, lying on damp ground ; sleeping in damp sheets ; after exertion ; after parturition, sexual excess, or fevers. Ptosis. Paralysis of single limbs. Numbness of parts paralysed. Facial neuralgia, lumbago, and sciatica (esp. of left side), with restlessness ; coming on after a wetting or after a bath are cured by *Rhus*. The neuralgic pains and eruptions make *Rhus* a perfect simillimum in many cases of herpes zoster. Fever-blisters round mouth. Howard Crutcher relates (*M. A.*, xxii. 38) how after standing on a wharf with his right side exposed to a cold wind from the river he began to have severe pains shooting up the ulnar nerve, a steady ache uniform throughout arm and forearm, but extremely severe in structures beneath deltoid. The pain was much < in a warm place ; it did not interfere with movement. At 8 p.m. Crutcher took *Rhus* 30 dry on the tongue, and almost immediately he was called into the open air again. In thirty minutes the pain was decidedly better ; in ninety minutes it was gone. A case of *Rhus* poisoning reported by Morey (*Med. Cent.*, February 1898 ; *H. W.*, xxxiii. 309), showed an effect on the menstrual period and was remedied by *Crocus*. Miss M. was severely poisoned by *Rh. rad.* (it is called " Ivy ") in July, 1895, during her menstrual period. She was treated with *Bell.* and *Rhus* internally, and an *Oxide of Zinc* ointment externally, and appeared to make a rapid recovery. On September 1, 1897, without further known poisoning, another similar attack developed during the menstrual period, and frequent minor attacks had occurred in the two years, always at the time of the menses. Later on she had another attack which developed rapidly and greatly alarmed her. The menstrual flow commenced a week before she came to Morey, was very scanty, *dark, and clotted*, as had been the case for some time. The flow had scarcely well begun when it ceased suddenly and the eruption appeared. *Croc.* was given, and the first dose re-established the flow, which was normal in appearance and quantity, and the eruption at once disappeared. *Peculiar Sensations* are : As if intoxicated. As if asleep. As of a weight behind right orbit. As of a band strapped across forehead. As if head were swelling out. Brain, as if loaded ; as if torn ; as if loose ; as if fluctuating ; as if a quantity of blood shot into it when stooping. As if muscles of back of head screwed together. As if a hundredweight on nape of neck. As if a veil before eyes. As of sand in eyes. As if lids difficult to move. As if jaw would break. Teeth as if being torn out ; too long ; loose. As if tongue had been skinned. As if a hernia about to protrude. As if pharynx inactive or paralysed. Stomach, as if overloaded ; as if a stone in ; as if pit of stomach swollen or drawn together. Hypochondria and abdomen as if beaten. Digging as if caused by a worm. As if a knife in right abdomen. As if something torn loose in abdomen, chest, and inner parts generally. As if a lump lay like a pressing heavy weight in abdomen. As if one side of rectum grown up. As if everything would come out of rectum. As if breath were stopped at pit of stomach. As if sternum were pressed inwards. As if sprained or dislocated : back, jaw, arms, wrist, hip, knee, ankle. As if one had been lying in an uncomfortable position. As if bruised in right side of lumbar vertebræ and in small of back. As if flesh all of back had been beaten. As if back were broken. As if some : were pressing on left shoulder. As if hand were held in hot ter. Hand, as if withered ; as if lame ; as if pins pricking points 1 palmar surfaces of first phalanges of fingers. Rectus cruris scle as if bruised. As if hamstrings and tendons of limbs too short. if knee too short. Legs (and right foot) as if made of wood. Feet 1 ankles as if asleep. Heels as if stepping on pins. As if running ls under skin of heels. As if walking on needles. Joints as if ised. As if bones ached. As if sinking through bed. As if some-ng forced him out of bed. Bones, as if being scraped ; as if flesh ng torn loose from them. As if whole body was burning. As if d water poured over him. As if blood ran cold through veins. As subcutaneous ulceration. As if inner parts grown together. *Pecu-r Symptoms* are : Craving for cold drink and laborious dreams. rpes alternating with asthma and dysentery. Chokes easily on allowing. Swallowing = pain in middle of back. Anorexia in late and throat. Nausea in chest. Taste of blood with cough (no od being raised). Coldness in left tibia. Scalp sensitive, < turn-; hair back. Hour-glass contraction of abdomen. The symptoms : < By touch ; > by rubbing. < From riding ; blows ; jars ; ains. < By rest ; and commencing motion ; > continued motion. ying down > colic and diarrhœa.) Lying on hard floor with low under back > pain in back. Must hold head to > weight in Bending head back > pain in occiput ; = pain in head and down ne. Limbs lain on fall asleep ; no sweat on them. < Side lain . Lying on left side = palpitation and pain in heart. Swallowing pain in back. Inclination to stretch. Stretching = cracking in ees ; soreness in abdomen. Unwonted exercise = paralysis. er-exertion = palpitation ; < coxalgia. < Evening ; night ; orning after sleep. Sensitive to cold open air ; raw north-east nds. Effects of drinking cold water ; getting wet, especially after ing heated, cold bathing ; sea bathing. > By warmth and hot plications. < Warmth of bed. Sciatica is > by warmth from ercise. < Change of weather ; damp, stormy weather ; before a rm ; snowstorm ; in autumn ; in winter. Nausea < after eating. aves cold water, which is vomited immediately.

Relations.—*Antidoted by :* Bry., Bell., Camph., Coff., Crot. t., ind., Merc., Sang., Sul., Verb. h. *Antidote to :* Bry., Ranunc., Rhod., t. t., Sapon. (Ars.). *Complementary :* Bry. *Inimical :* Apis, before after, especially in skin affections. *Compatible :* Arn., Ars., Bry., lc., Calc. ph., Cham., Con., Lach., Ph. ac., Puls., Sul. *Followed well :* Calc., Bell., Graph., Nux, Pho., Pul., Merc., Sep., Sul., Ars., Bry. *mpare :* The other Rhoes and Anacardia. Eye symptoms, > by tion, Comoc. (Rhus > by warmth ; Comoc. <). Rheumatic ralysis from exposure to damp and cold, Caust. (Rhus restless, > motion day and night ; Caust. restless only at night). Parotid nd, Am. c. (Rhus left ; Am. c. right). Result of working in water, lc. Granular ophthalmia, Arg. n. (Rhus has more spasm ; if lids forced open scalding tears gush out and cause pimples round the e). Cough excited by cold drink, Sil. (> Caust.). Sweat of body, ad dry (Sil. sweat of head, body dry). Nose-bleed at beginning of typhoid, Ph. ac. (with Rhus it >, not with Ph. ac.). Enables pers to withstand muscular fatigue, Fl. ac., Ars., Coca. Hypertrophy heart from over-exertion, Bro., Arn., Aco. Ulcers on legs in drop Ars., Lyc. (Lyc. in dropsy from liver disease). Fear of being poison Glo., K. bro., Hyo., Bap. Profuse gushing tears excoriating che Euphr. (Rhus < right eye ; pus thinner). Ptosis or any oc paralysis, Gels. (Rhus rheumatic patient, from wetting ; Gels. w sluggish thought and suffused face). Scarlatina, erysipelas, &c., w drowsiness and œdema, Apis (Rhus dusky red, bodily restlessne Ap. rosy red, fidgetiness. Rhus itching preponderates ; Ap. less t dency to form pus). Enteritis, peritonitis, typhlitis, Lach. He affections with numbness of left arm, Aco. (tingling in fingers), Kal Puls. (numbness, especially about elbow), Act. r. (as though a tightly bound to body), Phyt. (right arm). Dreams of business of d Bry. (Rhus and Bry. have opposite Conditions ; and Rhus me state is hopeless and despondent, Bry. fretful, peevish, irritab Typhoid, Pho. (follows Rhus well ; pneumonia ; stools yell and blood-streaked, at times like "flesh water"), Ars. (irritable a anxious in spite of prostration), Bapt. (face dark red, besotted ; st dark, fluid, very offensive ; drowsy, stupor ; tossing about with de sion that limbs are scattered about ; bed feels hard), Arn. (compl apathy ; involuntary stool and urine ; bloody sputa if lungs affecte Empyema and induration of axillary glands, Bell. (Bell. at clima Rhus after labour). Eczema, Mez., Jug. r. (favus). Cough < fr evening to midnight, Mez. (Rhus also from uncovering). Colic bending double, Coloc. (Rhus also > moving about). Conjunctiv from getting wet, Calc. Glaucoma, Caust. Cracking and breaki pain in jaw, Ign., Petr. Paralysis from rheumatic meningitis (fr rheumatic myelitis, Dulc.). Acute spinal paralysis of infants, S (complementary). Averse to be uncovered, Ars., Hep. Bearing do in hypogastrium, Puls. Flesh feels beaten off the bones, Th Aversion to darkness, Am. m., Bar. c., Calc., Carb. a., Stro., V Stram. Averse to be washed, Ant. c., Clem., Hep., Sep., Spi., S Effects of raising arms high to lift things, Pho. Bloody urine d charged in drops, Pul. Phimosis, Cann., Merc., Sul., Nit. ac., Se Thuj., Sabi. Hunger in early morning, Aga., Ant. c., Asar., Ca Carb. a., Lyc., Ran. b., Saba., Zn. Semilateral coat of tongue, Dap Lob. (Rhus white). Hot breath, Calc., Carb. s., Sul. Nocturnal sali tion, Cham., Nux, Pho. Difficult swallowing of solids, Atrop., Be Bar. c., Calc., Chi., Dro., Lyc., Plb., Sil. Parotitis, Aur., Merc., Pil metastasis to testes, Rhus, Pul., Bell., K. ca. Yearly returns, A Cold from wetting head (Bell. from hair-cutting). Sensation of s cutaneous ulceration, Ran. b., Pul. Chokes easily when swallowi K. ca. > Warm food, Lyc. Epistaxis at night, (Bry. mornin Punctured wounds as if stepping on nails, Hyper., Led. Backac > lying on hard floor, Nat. m. Hydroa, Nat. m. Acne from getti wet, or ice-cold drinks, when heated, Bellis. Desires cold drink a vomits it immediately, Ars. Ailments from spraining *a single p* muscle, or tendon, Calc., Nux. Vertigo < lying down (Apis >) ; rising from lying or stooping, Bry. Jelly-like stools, Colch., K. bi.

Causation.—Slightest anger. Cold. From wetting head. Da

sheets. Bathing, in fresh or salt water. Getting wet when heated. Strains. Over-exertion. Over-lifting. Raising arms high to lift things. Drinking ice-water. Beer (headache).

SYMPTOMS.

1. **Mind.**—Anxious sadness and excessive anguish, esp. (at twilight) in evening and at night, with wish for solitude and inclination to weep.—Restlessness which will not suffer the patient to remain seated; and compels him to throw himself about in bed.—Anguish with fear of death and sighs.—Fear of being poisoned.—Suicidal mania (desire to throw himself into the water).—Irritability and ill-humour, with repugnance to labour.—Moral dejection with anthropophobia.—Helplessness and profound despondency.—Uneasiness respecting one's children, affairs, and the future, with want of self-confidence.—Weakness of memory and forgetfulness (cannot remember the most recent events).—Want of ideas and of mental energy.—Difficult comprehension.—Slowness of conception and mental dulness.—Delusions of the imagination and visions.—Mild delirium; with insensibility.

2. **Head.**—Head bewildered as from intoxication.—Stupefaction; with tingling in head and pain in limbs, > on motion.—Staggering gait without vertigo.—Staggers to r. when walking.—Vertigo and staggering as if about to fall; esp. when getting out of bed (chilliness and pressure behind eyes).—Vertigo as if he were held up high, while sitting.—Emptiness in head.—Vertigo, with fear of death, on lying down in evening.—Headache (< in the morning, while lying; from cold) immediately after a meal or after drinking beer, and also on moving the arms (> by heat and when moving about).—Headache < morning, r. side, with vertigo as if she would fall back on getting out of bed, acute darting pains in both temples, can hardly hold up, and a mist comes before sight when doing anything quickly or getting up in a hurry (produced.—R. T. C.).—(Incito-motor function defective).—Attacks of headache with need to lie down; every vexation and exercise in the open air renews the attacks.—Periodical headache.—Pain in head as if brain were bruised, esp. in morning, < by moving and lifting up head.—Passive congestion of head > by repose.—Heaviness and pressive fulness of head (esp. in forehead; as if a weight were falling forward, with heat in face), with sensation, on stooping, as if the brain were about to burst.—Head so heavy obliged to hold it upright to > the weight pressing forward into forehead.—Sensation of compression or expansion in head.—Drawings and tearings in head, and esp. in temples, principally in evening and at night.—Lancinating headache day and night, extending as far as ears, root of nose, and the cheek-bones, with the teeth set on edge.—Beating and pulsations in head, esp. in occiput.—Pains, esp. in occipital protuberances.—Sanguineous congestion in head.—Burning sensation, esp. in forehead (when walking) and occiput.—Occipital headache with rheumatic stiffness in nape (*R. rad.*).—Painful tingling in head.—Sensation as if a quantity of blood shot into brain when stooping.—Rush of blood to head with burning-tingling and beating in brain, bright redness of face, great restlessness of body in morning when at rest, < after eating.—Liability to take cold from having head wetted.—Buzzing and noise in head.—Balancing and sensation of fluctuation in head

at every step, as if brain loose, also when shaking head.—Painful sensibility of exterior of head, as from subcutaneous ulceration, esp. on turning up hair and on touching it; < on side on which he does not lie, and from becoming warm in bed.—Contraction of the scalp as if the hair were pulled. —Drawing and tearing in scalp.—Swelling of head.—Erysipelatous swelling of head and face with vesicles drying up and forming itching scabs.—Gnawing tingling in scalp.—Dry herpes on scalp.—Periodical scald-head, reappearing every year.—Scald-head with thick scabs, which destroy the hair, with greenish pus (offensive smell), and violent itching at night.—(Eczema of entire hairy scalp, causing loss of hair.—R. T. C.).—Small, soft tubercles on the scalp.—Wen of many years' duration cured with *Rh. t.* φ, which caused erysipelas at same time (*H. W.*, xxxi. 199).

3. **Eyes.**—Pains in eyes on moving ball of eye.—Pressure and burning sensation in eyes.—Eyes fixed, dull, and downcast.—Smarting in eyes and lids.—Affections of internal surface of eyelids.—Inflammation of the eyes and lids, with redness and nocturnal agglutination.—Profuse lachrymation (eyes full of water, blear-eyedness) with œdematous swelling round eyes.—Meibomian glands enlarged, cilia fall out.—Photophobia.—Bladder-like swelling of the lids, closing the eyes.—Swelling (erysipelatous) of whole eye and of surrounding parts.—Rheumatic ophthalmia, particularly of r. eye.—Gouty keratitis, < in damp, rainy weather, sight dim.—Paralytic rigidity of the eyelids.—Jerking and quivering of eyes and eyelids.—Blue colour about the eyes. —Heaviness of the eyelids.—Styes; on the lower eyelids.—Veil before eyes and weak sight; all objects appear pale.

4. **Ears.**—Otalgia.—Painful throbbing in ear at night.—Swelling of ears. —Discharge of sanguineous pus from ears, with deafness.—Whistling, squeaking, or ringing in ears when walking, changes to low resonance when lying down, as if membrana tympani were burst.—Swelling and inflammation of parotids with fever.—Suppuration of parotids.

5. **Nose.**—Redness of point of nose, with pain as from excoriation on touching the part.—Hot swelling of the nose.—Breath seems so hot it burns the nostrils.—Dryness of the nose.—Discharge of greenish fetid pus from nose —Epistaxis also at night and on stooping or hawking; blood dark; scabs about nares.—Frequent violent and almost spasmodic sneezing.—Abundant discharge of mucus from nose, without coryza.

6. **Face.**—Face pale, sickly, wan, with eyes surrounded by a blue circle and nose pointed.—Drawing and burning in superciliary region and in cheekbones.—Face disfigured and convulsed.—Face red, with burning heat.—Erysipelatous inflammation and swelling of face, with pressive and tensive shootings and burning tingling.—Vesicular erysipelas, with yellow serum in the vesicles.—Humid eruption and thick scabs on face, with running of fetid and sanguineous serum.—Acne.—(Acne rosacea; impetigo on the face or on forehead.)—Commissures of lips sore and ulcerated.—Herpetic, crusty eruption round mouth and nose, with itching, jerking, and burning sensation.—Exanthema on cheeks, chin, and around mouth.—Desquamation of skin of face.—Incisive contractions and burning spasmodic pains in cheeks (which are red and hot).—Cold sweat on face.—Eruptions of burning pimples round lips and chin.—Cramp-like pain in jaw-joint when at rest and when moving the jaw, with cracking on least movement, > by strong pressure from without

and by taking warm things.—Spasms in the jaw.—Constant desire to yawn until it seems as though the jaw would break.—Hard and painful swelling (pressive digging) of the parotid and submaxillary glands (with sticking on swallowing).—Lips dry and brownish.

7. **Teeth.**—Toothache as from excoriation, or with tearings, shootings, jerkings, digging, and tingling, frequently at night, or < in open air and > by external heat (and in warm room), sometimes also in consequence of a chill.—Looseness of teeth.—Teeth feel elongated.—Looseness of lower incisors, cannot bite with them.—Fetid exhalation from carious teeth.—Burning pain in gums as from excoriation, also at night.

8. **Mouth.**—Dryness of mouth with violent thirst.—Copious accumulation of saliva in mouth.—A yellow, and sometimes also a sanguineous, saliva flows from mouth at night.—While sitting asleep in afternoon saliva runs from mouth.—In morning in bed mouth full of salt water.—In morning mucus and tongue are salt.—Copious accumulation of viscid mucus in mouth and throat, with frequent expectoration.—Offensive smell from mouth.—Tongue : dry, red or brownish, and cracked ; triangular red tip ; yellowish-white at root.—Tongue white ; often on one side.—Sensation as if tongue covered with a skin.

9. **Throat.**—Sensation of dryness of throat.—Sore throat, as if caused by internal swelling, with pain as from a bruise even when speaking, and with pressure and shootings during deglutition.—Sensation in throat as if something were torn out of it.—(Sore throat after exertion in speaking.)—Difficulty in deglutition and pain in swallowing solid food as from contraction of throat and œsophagus ; difficult swallowing of liquids as from paralysis.—Brandy causes an extraordinary burning sensation in throat.—Copious accumulation of mucus in throat, with frequent hawking in morning.—Pulsative pain in bottom of gullet.

10. **Appetite.**—Putrid taste, esp. in morning and after a meal.—Insipid, clammy, acrid, bitter, sour, or metallic taste.—Greasy taste in mouth but food tastes all right.—Taste as if stomach had been deranged with putrid meat, but food tastes right.—Sweetish taste in mouth.—Bitter taste of food, esp. of bread, which appears rough and dry.—Anorexia with repugnance to all food, esp. bread, meat, coffee, and wine.—Anorexia in palate and throat with empty feeling at stomach, and at same time ravenous hunger, which goes off after sitting for some time.—Sensation of fulness and satiety in stomach, which takes away all appetite.—After a meal strong disposition to sleep, pressure and fulness in stomach and abdomen, nausea with inclination to vomit, lassitude, vertigo, and shuddering.—When eating sudden vomiting.—Bread lies heavy on stomach.—Want of appetite with unquenchable thirst.—Hunger without appetite.—Pain and heat of head after drinking beer.—Thirst most frequently from a sensation of dryness in mouth, also at night or in morning, with desire chiefly for cold water and cold milk.—Craving for dainties ; for oysters.

11. **Stomach.**—Risings with taste of food.—Empty risings after a meal or after drinking.—Eructations from stomach, which seems to be transferred to r. side of chest, as if it settled there.—Violent risings with tingling in stomach, > by lying down, < on getting up.—Pituita in the stomach.—Pain in stomach and nausea from drinking ice-water.—Nausea and disposition to vomit, principally after a meal and after drinking, as also in night or morning

after rising, > by lying down.—Vomiting immediately after eating.—Pains in stomach as if there were a stone in it, esp. after a meal ; and when standing. —Pressure at stomach and scrobiculus, often with obstructed respiration.— Beating and shooting in epigastric region.—Squeezing, sensation of swelling, and pain as from ulceration in pit of stomach.—Sensation of coldness in stomach.—Sensation in pit of stomach as if something were torn away from it, esp. on stooping or making a false step.

12. **Abdomen.**—Distension of abdomen, esp. after a meal.—Pressive drawing from below upward, in l. hypochondrium.—Soreness, as if beaten, in hypochondria, and still more in abdomen ; < on side lain on when turning and when beginning to move.—Pressive heaviness in abdomen, as from a weight.—Contractive spasms in abdomen, which force patient to remain bent double.—Hard and visible contraction of abdomen across navel ; abdomen distended above and below this stripe.—(Pain in abdomen with tightness across forehead and sleeplessness.—Violent and continuous pain round navel, caused by retching.—R. T. C.).—Digging turning in abdomen, as if caused by a worm.—Incisive tearings, jerks, and pinchings in the abdomen (esp. after eating ; > after stool).—Pain in region of ascending colon.—Burning sensation in the abdomen.—Relaxation of the abdomen, with internal shaking at every step.—Violent colic, often at night, or < by all kinds of food or drink, sometimes with sanguineous evacuations.—Sensation in abdomen as if something were torn away.—Scarlet colour of abdomen.—Soreness in integuments of abdomen, as if they were ulcerated, esp. on stretching in morning.—Swelling of inguinal glands.—Pressure in groins towards exterior as if a hernia were about to protrude.—Bloated abdomen, esp. after eating.— Great flatulence, with grumbling, fermentation, and pinching movements in abdomen.—Exceedingly offensive flatus.

13. **Stool and Anus.**—Constipation, sometimes alternating with diarrhœa.—Hard and slow evacuations.—Tenesmus, sometimes with nausea, and tearing or pinchings in abdomen.—Painful tenesmus without stool.—Evacuations loose, bloody, watery, or mucous, frothy, gelatinous, red, or streaked with white and yellow.—Dysentery ; jelly-like, odourless stools, more frequent after midnight, preceded and followed by much pain with great restlessness.— Obstinate or dysenteric diarrhœa.—Fæces perfectly white.—Nocturnal diarrhœa, with violent colic, headache, and pains in all limbs (> after an evacuation or when lying on abdomen).—Chronic painless diarrhœa, only in morning preceded by marked commotion in the bowels.—Diarrhœa with tearing pains running down back of the leg with every stool.—Involuntary stools when asleep at night.—Short respiration during stool.—Tingling and itching in anus and rectum.—Sense of constriction in rectum, as though one side had grown up.—Protrusion of hæmorrhoids from anus after a soft evacuation, with pain as of excoriation.

14. **Urinary Organs.**—Retention of urine.—Frequent and urgent want to urinate, day and night, with profuse emission.—Incontinence of urine, esp. during repose (at night or when sitting).—Urine emitted in a divided stream. —Emission, drop by drop, of blood-red urine, with tenesmus.—Diminished emission of urine, although much drink may be taken.—Deep-coloured, irritating urine, which soon becomes turbid.—White, turbid urine.—Urine clear as water with a snow-white sediment.—Swelling of urethra.

15. **Male Sexual Organs.**—Profuse eruption on genital organs (closing the urethra by swelling).—Inflammation of the glans.—Running vesicles on the glans.—Swelling of the glans and prepuce ; prepuce dark red.—Paraphimosis.—Red spots (blotches) on the interior of prepuce.—Swelling and thickening of scrotum (with intolerable itching).—Erysipelas of scrotum.—(Hydrocele ; from over-lifting).—Scrotum flaccid and hanging low.—Moist eruption on scrotum.—Frequent erections at night, with want to urinate.—Strong sexual desire in morning.

16. **Female Sexual Organs.**—Catamenia premature and too profuse.—Menstrual flow light-coloured and acrid, causing biting pain in the vulva.—Erysipelatous inflammation of the external genitals.—Soreness of vagina soon after (or hindering) coitus.—Catamenia of too long duration.—Menstrual discharge = violent pain in vulva.—Membranous dysmenorrhœa.—Menorrhagia from strains ; from wetting.—Discharge of blood during pregnancy.—Pain as from excoriation and shootings in vagina.—(Uterine polypus with metrorrhagia.—Relieves shooting pains of cancer uteri.—R. T. C.).—Bearing-down pain ; when standing.—After-pains of too long duration, after severe labour, with much and excessive straining.—Discharge of blood and clots of blood from uterus, with labour-pains.—After labour, vitiated discharge from vagina, with shootings upward in the parts and a bursting sensation in the head.—For weeks after delivery pain in r. limbs with numbness from hips to feet (varicose veins).—Abortion from strain.—Axillary abscess after delivery.—Breasts painfully distended, red in streaks, rheumatic state.—Amenorrhœa from getting wet ; with milk in breasts.—Milk-leg, typhoid metritis after delivery.—Diminished secretion (or suppression) of milk ; with burning over body.

17. **Respiratory Organs.**—Hoarseness and roughness of throat, with a sensation of rawness in chest.—Sensation of coldness in throat on taking an inspiration.—Tendency to be choked when swallowing.—Burning exhalation from larynx.—Sensation of constriction in throat-pit after a short walk.—Cough excited by a tickling in air-passages ; generally short and dry, with anguish and shortness of breath, and principally in evening before midnight.—Dry, fatiguing cough.—Dry, teasing cough coming on just before the chill and continuing during the chill.—Cough with vomiting of food, esp. in evening, and when lying on back.—Cough after waking in morning.—During the cough gets a taste of blood in the mouth but does not cough up blood.—Short cough with bitter taste in mouth, in evening after lying down and in morning after waking.—Cough with stitches in chest and profuse general perspiration.—Whooping-cough ; spasmodic, violent cough, caused by tickling in larynx and chest, with expectoration (except in evening) of acrid pus or greyish-green cold mucus of putrid smell ; or of pale, clotted, at times brown blood.—Putting hand out of bed brings on a cough.—Pneumonia with typhoid symptoms, often after re-absorption of pus.—Cough with pain in stomach, or with shaking in chest and head.—Terrible cough which seems as if it would tear something out of chest.—Cough with expectoration of a bright-red blood and sensation of faintness in chest.

18. **Chest.**—Difficult respiration after a moderate walk.—Anxious oppression of chest, even at night.—Nausea in chest ; < stooping.—Respiration impeded by a pressure and squeezing in pit of stomach.—Shortness of breath in evening with tension in chest.—Frequent want to take a full inspiration.—

Weakness in chest, which renders speech difficult after a walk in open air.—Sensation of constriction in chest.—Shootings and lancinations in chest and sides of chest ; esp. when sitting with body bent forwards, when speaking, when breathing deeply, when sneezing, seldom when walking or when using vigorous exertion.—Inflammation of lungs, also pneumonia nervosa.—Pleurodynia, chest pains shoot into shoulders (*Rh. rad.*).—Tingling in chest, with tension of muscles of chest, < by repose.—Rush of blood to chest.

19. **Heart.**—Weakness and sensation of trembling in heart.—Violent palpitation of heart while sitting quietly.—Shootings in region of heart, with painful sensation of paralysis and numbness of l. arm.—Pulse rapid, small, compressible.

20. **Neck and Back.**—Rheumatic stiffness of nape and neck, with painful tension during movement.—Painful swelling of axillary glands.—Rheumatic tearing between scapulæ, not affected by movement, < by cold, > by heat.—Tearing between shoulders, drawing together from both sides.—Transient coldness in back.—Contusive pain in loins, esp. on touching the parts, and during repose.—Pain in small of back when sitting still or when lying ; > when lying on something hard or from exercise.—Bruised pain in sacrum when he lies still on it or sits still ; feels nothing of it when moving.—Painful rigidity in loins.—Painful exostosis on sacrum.—Distortion of the vertebral column.—Pains in loins, in back, and nape, as from lifting too great a weight.—Drawing and stitches in back, esp. when seated and on stooping.—Opisthotonos.

21. **Limbs.**—Swelling, stiffness, and paralysed sensations in joints, from sprains, over-lifting, or over-stretching.—Lameness, stiffness, and pain on first moving after rest, or on getting up in morning ; > by constant motion.—Trembling or sensation of trembling in limbs.—The limbs on which he lies, esp. arms, go to sleep.—Rheumatic tension, drawing, tearing in limbs, during rest.—Excessively cold hands and feet all day.

22. **Upper Limbs.**—Burning shooting under l. axilla, on the arm.—Tearing and burning sensation in shoulder, with paralysis of arm, esp. during the cold season, during repose, and in heat of bed.—Coldness, paralysis, and insensibility of arm.—R. arm weak ; rheumatic paralysis.—Exostosis in arm, with burning sensation and ulcers, which discharge a sanious pus.—Erysipelatous swelling and pustules, with burning itching in arms, hands, and fingers.—Red spots on arms.—Violent stitches in r. upper arm from without.—Jerks, shootings, and tearing in arms.—Tension in elbow-joint.—Jerking tearing in elbows, wrists, and joints of fingers.—Digging in bones of the forearm.—Weakness and rigidity of forearm and fingers during movement, and trembling of those parts after the least exertion.—Hot swelling of the hands in evening.—Swollen veins on hands.—Vesicular eruption in clusters on wrist.—Rhagades ; smarting of back of hands.—Back of hand covered with chaps and hot ; skin hard, rough, and stiff.—Tearing in all the finger-joints.—Warts on hands and fingers.—Hang-nails.—Swelling of fingers.—Jerking in thumbs.—Contraction of fingers.

23. **Lower Limbs.**—(Eruption with sweat in cleft of nates.)—Aching pains in legs ; must change position every moment.—(Pains in l. lower limb, thigh chiefly, from septic absorption in old abdominal disease, with vesical irritation.—R. T. C.)—Shootings and tearings in hip-joint, extending to ham,

sp. when resting on foot; or with dull drawings and burning sensation luring repose, and painful sensibility of joints on rising from a seat or on going up stairs (or other over-exercise; involuntary limping).—Tension nd stiffness of the muscles and joints of hips, thighs, legs, knees, and eet.—Paralysis of the lower extremities.—Cramp in calf after midnight, when lying in bed, and when seated after walking; it goes off on bending he knee.—Cramps in buttocks, thighs, and calves, esp. at night, in bed, r when seated after walking.—Spasmodic twitching of the limbs when tepping out.—Tension in the knee as if the tendons were too short.—Painful welling above knee.—Drawing and jerking tearing in the thighs and legs.—Lancinations in the thighs, legs, knees, feet, and toes.—Heaviness in legs, esp. n hams and calves.—Tingling pain in shafts of tibiæ at night when the legs re crossed, with constant necessity to move, preventing sleep.—Coldness in . tibia.—Paralysis of legs and feet.—Shootings and wrenching pain in ankle-bones when resting on foot.—Inflammatory swelling of instep, sometimes with pustules and miliary pimples on part affected.—Swollen round ankles fter sitting too long, particularly in travelling.—Erysipelatous swelling of eet.—Swelling of feet in evening.—Numbness and paleness of feet (feet lead).—Distortion of toes.—Corns on feet, with burning sensation and pain as rom excoriation.

24. **Generalities.**—[We are led to think of this remedy where we find n irresistible desire to move or change the position every little while, ollowed by great relief for a short time, when they must again move, and xperience the same relief for a short time; this condition is usually < at night.—After resting for a time, or on getting up from sleep, when first moving about, a painful stiffness is felt, which wears off from continual motion; but relief is experienced from continual motion—*e.g.*, a nursing mother may have sore nipples, and when the child begins to nurse, the nipple hurts exceedingly, but on continued nursing it becomes much easier.—Pain n chest (often rheumatic), < by using arms—as in making a bed, sweeping, &c., stiffness of nape of neck; sensation as if flesh were beaten off the bones, or as if a dog were gnawing it off; as if any part were contracted; as if a part were increased in size; as if certain parts were grown together; of heaviness in outer or inner parts; jerking pains in outer parts; darting and rending pains; of tension or tightness in outer or inner parts; arthritic pain in the joints; trembling sensation in inner parts; dyspeptics often complain of trembling in the stomach; of scraping along the periosteum.—For any troubles or complaints, whether acute or chronic, resulting from a sudden and a thorough drenching by a shower of rain; by getting wet in any way; there may be troubles of very long standing, which were so caused.—Troubles in general affecting the r. abdominal ring; l. chest; l. arm; l. lower extremity; l. side of body; of scalp, as in erysipelas when it runs up to the scalp; glands about the neck, particularly if they are swollen or inflamed with red streaks, as often are in scarlet fever; joints of the jaws, particularly when they are < on beginning of motion, and get > from continued motion; of the abdominal cavity in general; mons veneris, there may be a great deal of itching, sometimes a hard blue boil is found there; shoulder-blades; small of the back, as, *e.g.*, when one stoops his back hurts so that he cannot straighten up without help—this may result from an old sprain, or from a

sudden "crick" in the back; sacrum; buttocks; forearm; shoulder, back of hand; fingers; joints in general; shoulder-joint; elbow, wrist, bones of the arm; calves; joints of the leg; hip-joint, knee, and ankle; weakness of joints.—Coagulated blood from the nose; cough bloody, blood being coagulated; face covered like erysipelas; increase of saliva; difficulty in swallowing, it hurts so in the back; fluent catarrh of the nose.—Inability at first to move the parts affected.—One is very easily sprained by lifting; palsy of the limbs; staggering when walking.—Strictures after inflammation, and hence may sometimes be used for strictures resulting after gonorrhœa; swelling in general, with inflammation and without; debility; aversion to washing; wounds, with sprained muscles.—Axillary glands where the swelling is very deep and hard.—Symptoms < before a storm of rain; after midnight; in the morning; before falling asleep; from bathing; can't bear cold water; complaints coming on in autumn; on taking a deep breath; on inspiration; from cold in general; in cold air; in cold and wet weather; from coughing; while chewing; from drawing up the limbs; from exertion of the body; after drinking; after fatigue; on uncovering the head; from surgical injuries; from sprains; from lying down; from lifting; from cold food; cold water; anything cold; during perspiration; from wet poultices; while resting; on first rising; while sitting; while talking; after undressing; in foggy, or foggy and wet weather; from getting wet; in winter; from getting wet while perspiring; women in confinement; small-pox; after-effects of syphilis.—H. N. G.]—Epidemic diseases with œdema of fauces threatening œdema glottidis, vessicles stud pharynx and voice is hoarse; rawness and roughness of pharynx (Dunham).—Rheumatic and arthritic drawings, tension, and tearings in limbs, increased to the highest degree during repose, as well as in bad weather, at night, and in the heat of the bed, often with sensation of torpor and numbness in the part affected after moving it.—Cramp and tension in different parts as from contraction of tendons.—Contraction of some of the limbs.—Tensive shootings and stiffness in the joints, < on rising from a seat, and in open air.—Paralytic rigidity in limbs, esp. on beginning to move the part after repose.—Ready benumbing of parts on which patient reclines.—Torpor of some parts with tingling and insensibility.—Tingling in parts affected.—Wrenching pain in limbs.—Paralysis, sometimes semilateral.—Red and shining swellings, with shooting pain as from excoriation when touched.—Contusive, or else a sensation in some places as if the flesh were detached from the bones.—Pressive drawing in periosteum as if the bones were scraped.—Sensation in internal organs as if something were torn away.—Swelling and induration of glands.—Icterus.—Jerking in muscles and limbs.—Convulsive movements and other sufferings, resulting from a cold bath.—Semilateral affections.—< And appearance of pains and symptoms during repose or at night, as also on entering a room from the open air; > obtained by movement and walking.—The cold, fresh air is not tolerated; it seems to make the skin painful; (a keynote on rheumatism.—Dunham).—Reproduction or < of many sufferings in unfavourable weather.—General excitability of nervous system, < by slightest indulgence of anger.—Drawings in all the limbs when lying down.—Trembling of limbs after the least fatigue.—Unsteady gait.—Great lassitude and weakness with want to lie down.—Syncope.—Inability to bear the open air whether it is hot or cold; it makes a painful impression on the skin.

25. **Skin.**—Vesicular erysipelas where the vesicles are large.—Exanthema on face in general—on chin, face, cheeks, mouth, nose, forehead, causing much burning itching.—Pustulous chilblains.—Exanthema in general; burning; burning itching; pustulous; with swelling; blotches; like milk-crust; moist; like nettle-rash; blue with erysipelas; scurfy; tensive or tight feeling in; pock-shaped; black; purulent; zona or shingles; petechiæ; prickling; tickling; blisters which will sometimes spread up the limb, and are sometimes circular in form, spreading with a red edge in the advance, which gradually turns to a blister, the red border still keeping in advance (if the edges be black, *Arsen.*); itching < after scratching.—Tetters in general.—Ulcers burning; with corroding pus; with ichorous pus.—Rash itches a great deal, in scarlet fever, small-pox, &c., with the peculiar restlessness.—Phlegmonous erysipelas, esp. where the erysipelas begins in the ankle, and moves gradually up the leg, running up in the deeper tissues, no fever.—Itching over whole body, chiefly in hairy parts.—Stinging and tingling on skin, burning after scratching.—Humidity of skin.—Hardness of skin with thickening.—Swelling (hard) of affected parts.—Erysipelatous inflammations.—Nettle-rash.—Eruptions, generally vesicular, scabby, with burning itching, appearing esp. in spring and autumn.—Eruption of small pustules on a red bottom, like zona.—Gangrenous ulcers resulting from small vesicles, with violent fever.—Petechiæ, with great weakness, amounting to entire prostration.—Black pustules.—Herpes, sometimes alternately with asthmatic sufferings and dysenteric looseness.—Warts, esp. on hands and fingers; large jagged, often pedunculated, exuding moisture and bleeding readily.—Rhagades on hands.—Panaritium.—Tingling or shooting or else burning smarting in ulcers, esp. at night.—Chilblains.—Corns on feet, with burning sensation, and pain as of excoriation.

26. **Sleep.**—Frequent, violent, and spasmodic yawnings.—Spasmodic yawning without inclination to sleep, and with stretching of limbs and pain as from dislocation of articulation of the jaw.—Yawning in general; with violent stretching of the limbs; falling asleep late; lying on the back during sleep.—Strong disposition to sleep during day, and also in morning in bed.—Somnolency, full of distressing and broken dreams.—Sleeplessness, esp. before midnight, generally caused by a sensation of heat, ebullition of blood, and uneasiness which does not permit patient to remain lying down.—Disturbed sleep, with anxious and frightful dreams.—Coma somnolentum, with snoring, murmurs, and carphology.—Sleep hindered by gloomy ideas.—Waking caused by bitterness and sensation of dryness in mouth.—Sleep at night hindered by a pressure at stomach, digging pinchings in abdomen, and nausea, with inclination to vomit.—Inability to remain lying on side at night.—Starts with fright and jerking of body during sleep.—Incomplete and agitated sleep, with tossing and many troublesome thoughts.—Vivid dreams of the business of the day, with talking during sleep.—Weeping while asleep.—Dreams of fire.—Sleep, with open mouth and short breathing.

27. **Fever.**—Pulse irregular; generally accelerated but weak, soft; sometimes it cannot be felt or is intermittent.—Shivering and coldness, generally in evening, and accompanied by paroxysms of pain, and other accessory symptoms.—External coldness along skin · coldness, but does not mind cold air.—Shivering and shaking in open air, with violent thirst.—Con-

tinual transient shiverings, as if cold water had been thrown over body.—Sensation of coldness on moving even but a little.—Chill in back and heat in anterior portion of body.—Coldness and paleness of face, alternately with heat and redness.—Shiverings and heat intermixed, either general and simultaneous (internal shivering with external heat, and *vice versâ*), or in different parts.—General heat, as if hot water were thrown over him, or as if the blood were flowing hot through the veins.—General perspiration, frequently already during the heat, and then often not in the face.—Fever in evening, first shivering, then heat and thirst, (and perspiration) accompanied or followed by cuttings and diarrhœa.—First headache (throbbing in temples); afterwards chilliness, with thirst and tearing pains in limbs as from fatigue; afterwards general warmth, with slight chills during motion and livid face; finally profuse, sour-smelling perspiration.—Tertian or quotidian fever.—Tertian fever with nettle-rash, which disappears after the attack; during the apyrexia burning and redness in sclerotica.—Double tertian fever; first shivering and thirst, then general heat, with shivering on least movement, lastly perspiration.—During the shivering pain in limbs, headache, vertigo, pulsative toothache, accumulation of saliva in mouth, and inclination to vomit.—During nocturnal heat drawing in all limbs.—Transient heat with perspiration, commencing from umbilical region, and rapidly alternating with shiverings.—During or after the fever, jerks, tingling in ears, deafness, dry coryza, sleeplessness, with restless tossing, jaundice, and nettle-rash, pressure in pit of stomach, palpitation of heart with anxiety, colic, diarrhœa, and other gastric affections, and nocturnal thirst.—Malignant fever with loquacious delirium, violent pains in all limbs, excessive weakness, dry or black tongue, dry, brownish, or blackish lips, heat and redness in cheeks, carphologia, pulse quick and small, coma somnolentum, with snoring and moans.—Sweat during the pains.—Perspiration in general; with heat; offensive.—Perspiration when seated, often with violent trembling.—Nocturnal sweat, sometimes with miliary and itching eruption.—Sweat in morning, sometimes of an acid smell.—Sweats from warm drinks.—Constant perspiration.

Rhus Venenata.

Rhus venenata. Poison Elder. Poison Sumach. Swamp Sumach. —It is frequently named "R. Vernix," and it is given under this name in Hempel's *Jahr.*, but the name belongs properly to the allied Varnish-tree of Japan. (North America, in swampy ground.) *N. O.* Anacardiaceæ. Tincture of fresh leaves and stem.

Clinical.—Boils. Chilblains. Diarrhœa. Dyspepsia. Dysphagia. *Eczema.* Eruptions. *Erysipelas.* Erythema nodosum. Glands, cervical, ulceration of. Hæmorrhoids. Herpes. Hydroa. Impetigo. *Irritation. Lips, swollen; sore.* Lumbago. Measles. Menorrhagia. Ophthalmia. Paraplegia. Prurigo. *Purpura.* Scabies. Stiff neck. *Tongue, cracked.* Urticaria.

Characteristics.—*Rhus ven.* is one of the most actively poisonous of the Rhoes. P. B. Hoyt, who (according to Hale) first drew attention to it, and made the first provings, says it is more poisonous than *h. t.*, which he can handle with impunity, whilst he was violently ffected by *Rh. v.* in spite of extreme caution. Further, he considers . more actively curative ; in a case of *Rhus* sore throat, when *Rh. t.* ailed *Rh. v.* acted with excellent effect. Another observer, Butman, ays that persons who have been poisoned by *Rh. t.* are more liable han others to *Rh. v.* poisoning, the *Rh. v.* is "set to work" by the *h. t.* On the other hand *Rh. v.* in the attenuations is credited with he cure of *Rh. t.* poisoning. Hoyt's experience is interesting. Vishing to prepare a tincture he went to a swamp and procured ome sprouts. In doing this he had on a pair of buckskin gloves, nd kept carefully to the windward side of the plant. Nevertheless n an hour and a half a most intense itching and burning (more urning) set in in scrotum and penis. The glans was very painful ; light friction > for a moment the itching but not the burning. The ymptoms continued next day. At 11 a.m. he made the tincture, ising great caution in manipulating the plant. At 3 p.m. itching and urning began on back of right hand. A restless night followed. Awoke in morning with itching, especially on palmar surface of wrists. This spread all over body, symptoms steadily advancing. Dizziness ; eyes and ears became affected, fever set in. When the symptoms passed off it was found that some chronic dyspeptic symptoms and inflammation of the eyes had been much benefited.—I have frequently used *Rh. v.* with good effect in skin diseases. Bayes told me of a case of universal eczema with intense distress in an old man which he cured in a fortnight with *Rh. v.* A case of pemphigus in a young man of 27 came under my care after years of treatment under allopathic specialists who had given him *Arsenic* until they could give no more, telling him at the same time that nothing but *Arsenic* could do him any good. *Rh. v.* 3x and 30 completely cured in a few months, and the cure enabled the patient to marry. I have found *Rhus* an excellent remedy for arsenical overdosing. A minor use of *Rh. v.* is as a topical remedy in itching, burning chilblains. The φ tincture painted on relieves almost instantly and practically cures the chilblains in a large number of cases. *Rh. v.* has many symptoms referring to the bones ; and according to Hering it affects those parts where the bones are directly covered with skin, as the forehead, backs of fingers, &c. There is a "pain half way down the œsophagus" which is probably a variant of the *Rhus* "Pain between the shoulders on swallowing food." *Peculiar Sensations* of *Rh. v.* are : Sensation as if mouth and throat had been scalded. As if sand on lips ; in mouth. Sensation in arm as if the bone would break. Pains wander about ; upward and downward along the periosteum ; come and go suddenly ; chill runs up back. Butman observed that *blondes* are more susceptible to *Rh. v.* poisoning than brunettes. When once affected persons are liable to a renewal of the affection (without further poisoning) each year at the same time. Persons poisoned by *Rh. t.* and *r.* are more liable to be poisoned by *Rh. v.* Children are more readily poisoned than adults. Hale records a case bearing on the comparative action of *Rh. v.* with *Rh. r.* and *Rh. t.* : A lady had several times every year a sore mouth, with intense redness of mucous membrane of tongue, cheeks, and fauces in small vesicular points ; intense burning and feeling as if mouth and throat had been scalded. If unchecked every mucous membrane including those of rectum and vagina became involved. No remedy helped till *Rhus* was tried. *Rh. r* and *Rh. t.* only slightly relieved, but *Rh. v.* 3 always removed the affection quickly. Under the name *Rhus vernix* E. F. Beckwith relates (*M. A.*, xx. 369) the poisoning of Mrs. T. Williams, 32, sandy hair, light complexion, good general health. Twelve years before she had worked all day over a stove in which the wood of Swamp Sumach was burned. She was badly poisoned, was unable to see for four or five days, and was treated with lotions of sugar of lead and butter-milk. Ever since then she had a rash just before the menses, or if she took cold. At the time Beckwith saw her she had a lump in centre of left breast, a dense mass occupying nearly one-half the gland substance, which she believed to be cancer, a sister having died of what was said to be cancer of the breast. She had first noticed it, the size of a hazel-nut, six years before when nursing her last child. The symptoms connected with this were also < before menses and had *Rhus* characteristics. The symptoms from this patient I have marked (B) in the Schema. The symptoms were < by touch and pressure. > Gently rubbing and scratching. < Before stools. < Damp days. < Hot weather. < Rest. > Moderate exercise or open air. > Hot bath. Chills in warm room. Washing with cold water or snow > itching on back. < Mental exercise. Motion < pain in elbow. Walking < frontal headache. Eating raw things < burning of lips. All symptoms < morning after waking. Diarrhœa 4 a.m. "Pain as if sprained" shows the relation of this *Rhus* to sprains. It is most poisonous on hot days in summer; to persons immediately after a meal; and to those in a state of perspiration—"if my skin was perfectly dry when collecting the juice of *Rh. v.*, it had not the slightest effect on me" (Bigelow, quoted by Hale).

Relations.—*Antidoted by:* Pho., Bry.; Clem. (itching on hands and genitals, anus, lips, mouth, and nose); Ranunc. (rheumatic pains < on taking cold); Nit. ac. (sprained pain in r. hip). Blue clay applied externally > itching and burning entirely (Hering). Coffee had no effect on the symptoms. *Follows well:* Rh. t. *Compare:* Skin and botan., Anac., Comoc. Rh. r., Rh. t. Stitching pains, K. ca. Wandering pains, Puls. Pains come and go suddenly, Lyc. Pain at root of tongue, K. iod.

Causation.—Sprains.

SYMPTOMS.

1. **Mind.**—Great sadness, no desire to live, or do anything, everything seems gloomy.—Apprehensive, restless, variable feeling; sometimes cheerful, then hypochrondiacal.—Cannot connect ideas or concentrate mind; forgetful; dull; stupid.

2. **Head.**—Dizzy when first getting out of bed (B).—Whirling vertigo, much < evening.—Head enormiously swollen, eyes closed. — Dull, heavy stupefying headache.—Sharp pains in parietal bones.—Jerk-like drawing here and there in nerves of head.—Dull frontal headache < by walking and stooping.—Headache as though brain squeezed. < Stooping (B).—Tearing

in r. temple extending from forehead upwards into l. half of head, always seated in the bone ; thence to l. occiput and down to nape.—Jerk-like headache in occiput.—Skin of forehead rough ; pimples ; herpes phlyctenuloides.

3. **Eyes.**—Eyes nearly closed with great swelling ; red.—Eyes feel as if being pressed out of head.—Eyes ache as though pressed on (B).—Eyes feel as if sand in them (B).—Smarting, burning irritation and acridity about eyes ; profuse lachrymation.—Blear-eyes, < night ; cannot read by candle-light (B).—Photophobia.—Sharp pain in r. eye, extending to supraorbital region.—Constant dull aching pains in eyeballs.—Sight dim.—It becomes black before eyes while looking.—Flashes of light before eyes (B).

4. **Ears.**—Transient stitches in r. concha.—Jerk-like tearing in bone behind r. ear.—Much earache ; hammering-throbbing deep in ear after dark (B).—Jerk-like cutting stitches in ear.—Vesicular inflammation of ears, exuding a yellow watery serum.—Very troublesome deafness.—Ringing, rustling, and noises in r. ear.

5. **Nose.**—Nose red and shiny, redness not removed by pressure.—Erysipelas.—Profuse secretion from r. nostril of thin ichorus fluid ; l. stopped.—Both nostrils filled with tenacious mucus.—Nose dry ; sore.—Loss of smell.—Nose sore internally coming on a few days before menses, lasting three or four days after (B).

6. **Face.**—Nose and r. side of face much swollen, esp. under r. eye.—Skin of face dry, rough, scurfy, seems thickened and indurated. Face red, swollen, shining, glistening ; desire to rub constantly ; hot water > and = peeling.—Face more swollen l. side than r.—Heaviness in swollen face.—Boring in r. upper jaw.—Drawing pains in r. upper and lower jaw.—Sensation as if sand on lips.—Face and esp. upper lip swollen.—Lips sore, swollen, blistered, cracked.—Cannot get lips cool.—Itching of upper lip and chin 4 p.m.

8. **Mouth.**—Drawing in r. upper teeth.—Gums swollen.—Eruption on gums of upper incisors.—On drinking anything warm, slight irritation on inner lips, gums, and tip of tongue.—Tongue . coated white in middle, back and edges red ; red on tip ; red and cracked in middle ; cracked in middle and covered with little vesicles ; several vesicles on under side.—Sensation as if tongue were being pulled out by the roots.—Distress in root of tongue and fauces. — Scalded feeling in tongue ; while at dinner it extends to mouth and fauces, causing dryness.—Tongue and mouth as if burnt with an acid.—Itching of tongue and roof of mouth.—Tongue and lips feel cracked. — Breath hot, feverish, offensive. — Breath hot, and not offensive ; feels like steam.—Fever sore on mouth.—Mouth feels rough as if sand under mucous membrane when touched.—Saliva increased ; viscid.—Hot water runs from mouth when lying down, with sickness at stomach < at night (B).—Slimy, nasty, putrid taste (B).—Taste : lost ; slimy ; flat, rough.—Cannot speak distinctly, palate fallen and feels as if something in mouth impeding speech, unchanged by hawking and clearing throat.

9. **Throat.**—Soreness l. side throat, swelling extending downwards.—Throat sore, swollen.—Irritation and acridity about throat and eyes.—Tonsils red, congested, dull aching distress in them.—Irritation ; dryness ; burning in throat.—Pharynx and œsophagus irritable and sensitive, painful and difficult

to swallow, food caused pain and seemed to stop mid-way to stomach; col
water produced the same effect as very hot tea, and an aching such as is fel
after drinking ice-water, though thirst was great.—Frequent desire to swallow
—Swallowing difficult.—Feels as though hairs in throat *way back;* lastin
several days at a time (B).—Difficulty in swallowing solid food, throat feel
as though it were drawn up (B).

11. **Stomach.**—Appetite: improved; lost.—Thirst very great.—Eruc
tations.—Nausea and loathing.—(Dyspepsia and belching relieved.)—Sever
pain in stomach 2 a.m.; sudden call to stool two hours later.—Much distres
and pain in (cardiac end of) stomach.—Sudden vomiting when at tabl
eating (B).—Pressure in stomach after eating, and I can pound lightly o
stomach and throw up any meal (B).—Pressure in pit of stomach (B).—
Creeping or crawling sensation in stomach (B).—Stomach feels bad in evenin
(B).—Pork = vomiting instantly (B).

12. **Abdomen.**—Hard beating or throbbing a little below pit o
stomach (B).—Distress in umbilicus with dry, lumpy, dark stools.—Abdome
bloated, very sensitive to least pressure.—Swelling of abdomen, in mornin
have to rub it down with my hand before I can button my clothing (B).—
Sharp cutting pain in umbilical and hypogastric regions.—Colic, rumbling
and soreness to touch.—Pain in hypogastrium before every stool; very littl
warning.—Pain in bowels < mornings.

13. **Stool and Anus.**—Bleeding hæmorrhoids with extensive itchin
and burning.—Discharge of blood from rectum after a stool.—Neuralgi
pains in anus.—Most intolerable burning and itching in anus.—Diarrhœ
2 to 5 a.m., stools nearly white.—At 4 a.m., large watery stool passed wit
great force and attended with violent colicky pains; during next two hour
there were similar profuse stools, after which pains ceased.—Stool: ver
dark; dark and partly undigested; dark, hard, and small in quantity.

14. **Urinary Organs.**—Burning in urethra.—Urine increased.—Desir
to void urine often, but in small quantities.

15. **Male Sexual Organs.**—Groins and penis affected in morning.—
Scrotum red, swollen, much corrugated, covered with vesicles; prepuc
swollen; glans swollen and very sore; cuticle of penis and scrotum peel
off in patches as large as a sixpence.

16. **Female Sexual Organs.**—Menses (which were near at hand
came on immediately in very large clots like pieces of meat.—Every mont
dull heavy pain in l. ovarian region (B).—Hard, labour-like pains for one da
before menses (B).—Soreness of vagina during menses (B).—Menstru
discharge regular, rather scanty, always bright pink in colour.—Terrib
lancinating pains through l. breast < for three days before menses (B).–
Burning in l. breast and l. side of body (B).—Sometimes sensation as if
thousand small needles were sticking in l. breast (B).—Breast symptoms
< moving l. arm forward and across body; by pressure; just before an
during menses; at night and when lying down; > by motion; continuo
work (B).—Breast must be supported; it aches when it hangs down (B).–
Eruptions just before menses (B).

17. **Respiratory Organs.**—Dryness and pains in larynx.—Hoarsenes
—Harsh, dry cough, lasting more than two weeks.—Sense of oppression as
the air was too heavy.

18. Chest.—Violent stitches through chest with great suddenness.—Violent stitches in l. lung causing anxiety, esp. on breathing.—Stitches in both lungs; in apices.—Rush of blood to chest with anxiety.—Stricture in chest.—Pain over sternum; lancinating in sternum and r. leg.—Drawing pain in lower l. side.

19. Heart.—Stitches in heart.—Palpitation with stitches in heart.

20. Neck and Back.—Stiff neck or crick-in-neck.—Ulceration of cervical glands, which discharged a very offensive dark-coloured pus; dark red areola round ulcers.—Dull pain in cervical, dorsal, and lumbar regions.—Back very stiff.—With rumbling of flatus in bowels, pains in back extending from lumbar region to umbilicus.—Sharp pain under l. scapula, extending through to ribs.—Rheumatic pains between scapulæ.—Dull, heavy pains in lumbar region < stooping or walking.—Drawing in lumbar muscles extending into hips.—Drawing in l. loin.—Dull, aching pain and weakness across loins.—A little pain in sacrum.—Lumbago from a strain or a cold.

21. Limbs.—Trembling of limbs with twitching of muscles.—Swelling of all the limbs with redness, and thirst.—Wrists, ankles, feet ached so severely he could not sleep.

22. Upper Limbs.—Tearing in l. arm, extending up from elbow; a sensation as if the bone would break.—Pain from l. breast extends into l. arm (B).—Drawing in l. arm, forearm, and last three fingers; arm feels paralysed.—Paralytic drawing in r. arm, esp. wrist, extending to tip of fingers.—Jerking pain in muscles of both arms.—Crawling in l. arm, esp. when resting it upon anything.—Severe pain in l. elbow-joint preventing moving it.—Rheumatic pains in l. elbow and shoulder-joints < on motion.—Weakness of forearm and fingers, which are cold.—When hand becomes numb and goes to sleep it feels as if puffed up (B).—L. hand becomes numb on sitting or lying down (B).—Dull, drawing pains in wrists and fingers.—Wrists and fingers very stiff.—Dark-coloured ganglion on wrist.—Drawing pressing pain in r. wrist, extending through the bones to elbow.—R. hand swelled without redness.—Constantly aching dulness in hands and fingers.—Drawing in r. fingers.—Backs of hands swollen and puffy.—Blue finger-nails.—Hands swelled and clumsy.

23. Lower Limbs.—Paralysed and bruised sensation in legs.—Pain as if sprained or dislocated in r. hip. (> by *Nit. ac.*).—Drawing, cramp-like pain in l. thigh.—Crop of boils on r. thigh.—Paralytic drawing with pains in bones of left leg.—Streaks of pain run down l. leg (B).—Great weakness of knees and ankles, they ache constantly.—Jerk-like drawing in leg.—Wandering drawing pains.—Drawing in knees.—Cramp-like pain and tension in calves.—Ankles and feet ached so that it was painful to stand or walk, < afternoon.—Throbbing in both feet as if distended with blood.—Jerk-like drawing in r. foot, extending from ankle to heel, and shooting up with pains in the bones.—Crawling and crackling in r. foot.—Pulsation in r. foot.—Eczema of (l.) foot.—Swelling of feet < at night; sensitive to touch (B).

24. Generalities.—Great lassitude; stretching.—Great restlessness.—Swelling of whole body with intolerable irritation.—Numbness and lameness of l. arm, side, and leg (B).—Bruised feeling in all the limbs.—All muscles stiff, esp. back of r. leg.—Stiffness and soreness.—Rheumatism before a storm (B).—Lying on l. side = shortness of breath (B).—Sensation as though blood hot and rushing along the vessels (B).

25. **Skin.**—A fine white rash keeps under the skin.—Ulcers, cuts, and other lesions surrounded by a miliary whitish rash.—Nightly itching, and an eruption very like erythema nodosum.—Within twenty-four hours itching with swelling, which gradually extends over body assuming erysipelatous appearance.—Red indurated elevations, esp. on face, neck, and chest.—Redness, swelling, and vesicular rash on skin of eyes, nose, cheeks, lips, ears, behind ear and front of neck.—Boils on forehead, neck, and arms.—At night much itching of face and sexual organs.—Rash-like pimples appear under skin just before menses, esp. on head, face, back, and hands; burning, but not quite like burning in breast and side (B).—Rash appears also if she takes cold (B).—Fine vesicular eruption on forearm, wrist, back of hands, between and on fingers; vesicles are situated on an inflamed erysipelatous base, and accompanied with most intolerable itching, esp. in evening in a warm room and in bed; after scratching and rubbing (which cannot be resisted) the itching is intolerable; large quantities of serum run from each vesicle after it is scratched.—Clusters of vesicles.—Boils on r. thigh.—Desquamation.—Itching and complete desquamation of skin of hands.—Deep, corroding phagedænic ulcers with cadaverous-swelling pus.—Itching and creeping sensation, < by warmth.

26. **Sleep.**—Restlessness with dry, hot skin.—Sleep disturbed by many dreams: of death and near future; lascivious; with wild fancies.—Bad dreams which impress her much next day (B).—Sleep bad till after midnight on account of nausea and pressure in stomach and chest; restless, tossing (B).—Starts on falling asleep (B).

27. **Fever.**—Chills: over whole body; run up back even when warm and in a warm room.—Feeling of coldness when moving (B).—Shivering down the back.—Skin hot, dry, burning, at night with restlessness.—Intermittents without sweat.—Frequent attacks of ague (B).—Dry, burning.—Flashes of heat as though a stream of hot air was passing over body, with throbbing and tearing pains from each temple back to occiput and down neck to each shoulder.—Hands constantly very dry and hot.—Slight moisture behind r. ear.

Ricinus.

Ricinus communis. Palma Christi. *N. O.* Euphorbiaceæ. Tinctur (made with *hot* alcohol and water) or trituration of fresh seeds Tincture of fresh plant.

Clinical.—Albuminuria. Aphthæ. Cholera. Cholera infantum. Diarrhœa. Duodenum, catarrh of. Dysentery. Eruptions. Gangrene. Gastro-enteriti Jaundice. Lactation. Peritonitis.

Characteristics.—The castor-oil plant is a native of India. I the tropics it is a small tree growing to the height of eight c ten feet. Under the name of Palma Christi it is cultivated as a annual in this country, its stems reaching from three to five fee The oil of medicine is obtained from the seeds. The blandes which is in common use is "cold drawn," *i.e.*, expressed with out the aid of heat, and contains the smallest amount of the acrid principle. A decoction of the seeds, which is used in the East and West Indies, contains a much larger proportion. The homœopathic preparation should be made in such a way as to secure the full properties. The leaves have an especially powerful action on the breasts and female generative organs. Hale made the first collection of the pathogenetic effects of *Ric.*, and pointed out its analogy to cholera, which Salzer (*On Cholera*) confirmed. Cases of poisoning, some of them fatal, have been recorded from the ordinary oil, but the greater number of the pathogenetic effects have resulted from eating the seeds. Fatal effects have followed eating three seeds, and one seed has caused violent effects. After twenty seeds gastro-enteritis and death preceded by general convulsions and collapse occurred. The most detailed case is that of a sergeant who ate seventeen seeds (two years old) as a purgative. Four hours later he had several loose stools, pyrosis, cramps in the stomach, nausea and vomiting, the vomit containing fragments of seeds and drops of oil. The stools became more numerous and more copious of serous liquid mixed with mucus, and were passed without tenesmus or colic. Later the diarrhœa was accompanied with cramps and chilliness. Other symptoms were: Pale face; forehead covered with cold sweat, features drawn, eyes convulsed and turned up, conjunctiva injected, copious lachrymation. Intelligence quite clear. Headache, vertigo, buzzing in ears, and *sensation as if a bar were laid over his stomach, with profound anguish.* Burning thirst; pyrosis, vomiting fluid lightly coloured with bile, and containing some glairy filaments. Epigastrium very sensitive, pains *radiate* therefrom to navel and hypochondria, not < or > by light or strong pressure. At the same time he felt a sensation of violent constriction in intestines. Diarrhœa became colliquative, stools like cholera - stools. Complete anuria. Voice veiled. Profound adynamia. Next day severe fever followed. A small quantity of dark, thick urine was passed, and was found to be highly albuminous. On the fourth day *pronounced jaundice* appeared. On the sixth day the urine had ceased to be albuminous, and the patient was discharged. Salzer gives to *Ric.* the same importance in cholera *with diarrhœa* that *Camph.* occupies in relation to *spasmodic* cholera. The stools of *Ric.* correspond exactly to the rice-water stools in cholera, whilst those of *Ver. a.* do not. *Ric.* also has *painless evacuations* which are met with in many cases of cholera. *Ric.* therefore corresponds to the diarrhœic stage of cholera, and also to the collapse stage if vomiting and purging still continue. Salzer quotes B. L. Bhaduri as having observed "rice-water stools, cramps, and suppression of urine brought on by eating the seeds." Hale says that before he had learned to use *Ric.* as a homœopathic remedy he had often been discomfited by seeing aphthous diarrhœa cured with small (half-teaspoonful) doses of castor oil, repeated three or four times a day, by old nurses or impatient mothers. Such diarrhœa often arises in improperly-fed children. It begins with sickness, frequent and griping evacuations, greenish yellow to dark green, becoming more liquid and more or less mixed with slimy or gelatinous mucus or blood. Each stool is accompanied with pain and tenesmus, mouth dry and aphthous, anus inflamed, belly tumid and painful, child becoming more and more feverish and somnolent. Hale later gave a 1 x trituration of the oil with sugar. In acute and chronic dysentery, and in those cases in which there is impaction of fæces, Hale has seen the oil promptly curative. Post-mortem examination in the fatal poisoning cases has shown the gastro-intestinal mucous membrane abraded and inflamed. In one case the whole intestinal membrane was coated with blackish blood and that of the stomach reddened and softened. Hering remarked that puerperal fever had become much less common in Philadelphia (where it used to be very common) since homœopaths interdicted the use of castor oil in confinements. *Ric.* has great power over lactation. O. McWilliams (quoted by Hale) observed in the Cape Verde Islands that the leaves of the plant were applied to the breasts to increase the flow of milk if it were delayed, and even to produce it in women who had never borne children or who had not suckled for years. In increasing the flow of milk in nursing women the breasts were fomented with a decoction of the leaves of the plant, the boiled leaves being afterwards thinly spread on the breasts. For producing milk in others more vigorous measures were resorted to. The women had to sit over a boiling decoction of the leaves, care being taken to prevent the escape of steam. When the decoction was sufficiently cool the parts were bathed with it, and also the breasts, to which the leaves were applied as in the other case. Women with well-developed breasts are more easily influenced. When the breasts are small and shrivelled this treatment acts more on the uterine system, bringing on the menses long before their time or causing immediate flow if the time is near. Tyler Smith experimented with the leaves. In his cases the application produced: Swelling of the breasts, throbbing and other pains in them; swelling of the axillary glands, with pains running down the arms. *Pains in the back like after-pains were caused in every case.* Leucorrhœa was increased. Soon discharges from the breasts became milky, and menses came on too soon. The *radiating* pains; bar sensation; constricting and cramping pains are the most peculiar.

Relations.—*Compare:* Croton., Jatr., and Euphorbiaceæ. In cholera, rice-water stools, Agar. ph., Jatr. Bar sensation, Hæmatox. Galactogogues, Agn. c., Asaf., Puls. Duodenal catarrh, Berb., Chi., Hydrs., Lyc., Merc., Pod.

SYMPTOMS.

2. **Head.**—Vertigo.—He cannot go into open air after a dose of *Castor Oil* as the brain seems exhausted and easily overpowered (R. T. C.).—Headache; severe.—Acts on base of brain (R. T. C.).—Sudden pain as if seized by something in occiput extending round to backs of ears, eyes, and forehead with rush of blood to head and shocks which come and go as from electricity, thirty times in five days (agg.—R. T. C.).

3. **Eyes.**—Eyes convulsed and turned up; conjunctivæ injected, copious lachrymation; pupils only moderately dilated.

4. **Ears.**—Buzzing and humming in ears.

6. **Face.**—Features drawn.—Face slightly congested.—Face pale; features strongly contracted.—Twitchings of mouth.

8. **Mouth.**—Tongue: coated white; and dry; furred.—Salivation.

9. **Throat.**—Burning pain in gullet accompanied the vomiting.

11. **Stomach.**—Anorexia.—Thirst, great; burning.—Pyrosis.—Nausea and vomiting persistent; vomited mattery liquid, slightly coloured by a little bile; contains only a few mucous threads in suspension.—Vomiting profuse; with burning in gullet and all the symptoms of Asiatic cholera.—Vomiting and purging.—Painless vomiting.—Vomits pultaceous substances.—A kind of bar across stomach, which caused profound anguish.—Pit of stomach very sensitive; pains radiate from this centre, shooting to umbilicus and hypochondria.—Cramps; burning, in stomach.

12. **Abdomen.**—The different segments of the recti muscles can be seen successively and individually contracting under the skin.—Rumbling.—Feels as if all the intestines violently drawn together.—Violent colic; and yellowish-green vomiting.—Cramps with the diarrhœa.—Pain over abdomen < by pressure.

13. **Stool and Anus.**—Violent purging with the diarrhœa.—Bloody diarrhœa.—Diarrhœa without pain.—Diarrhœa almost incessant, colliquative, like cholera.—Rice-water stools.—Stools serous liquid mixed with mucus.—Diarrhœa incessant, with cramps and chilliness.—Complete confinement of bowels for five days; this made him uncomfortable, and caused headache.

14. **Urinary Organs.**—Complete anuria.—Passes a little dark, thick, highly albuminous urine (lasted four days).

16. **Female Sexual Organs.**—Menses too early; excessive.—Leucorrhœa.—Breasts thick, swell, with swelling of axillary glands and pains running down arms.—Thin discharge from breasts becomes milky.—Brings milk in breasts of virgins and women who have not suckled for years.

17. **Respiratory Organs.**—Voice altered; veiled.

19. **Heart.**—Pulse: extremely small, scarcely perceptible, though normal in frequency; very frequent.

20. **Back.**—Pains in back like after-pains.

21. **Limbs.**—Prurigo on wrists and bends of knees.

23. **Lower Limbs.**—Gangrene of one foot necessitates amputation.

24. **Generalities.**—Pale and listless.—Anæmia.—Profound adynamia.—Collapse.—Convulsions.—Muscular contractions.—Very painful cramps in trunk and limbs.

25. **Skin.**—Pronounced jaundice; skin saffron yellow.—Pruriginous eruptions, or redness and itching, at wrists and bends of knees.

26. **Sleep.**—Great desire for sleep.

27. **Fever.**—Chilliness with the diarrhœa.—Perspiring freely.—Skin moist and cool, esp. lower limbs.—Forehead covered with cold sweat.

Robinia.

Robinia pseud-acacia. Common or False Acacia. North American Locust. *N. O.* Leguminosæ. Tincture of fresh root bark. Tincture of fresh bark of young twigs. Trituration of the beans.

Clinical.—Acidity. Coryza. Dyspepsia. Flatulence. Headache, gastric. Hyperchlorhydria. Indigestion, nocturnal. Intermittents. Neuralgia. Pyrosis. Stomach, affections of. Urticaria.

Characteristics.—The roots of *Robinia* (says *Treas. of Bot.*) "have the taste and smell of liquorice, but are a dangerous poison, and accidents have occurred from their being mistaken for liquorice roots." The poisonings that have been recorded have been due to eating the beans or chewing the bark. Of thirty-two boys so poisoned (*H. R.*, iv. 72) in the mildest cases there occurred—Vomiting of ropy mucus, dilatation of pupils, dry throat, flushed face. In the severest the vomit was more copious and mixed with blood; with retching, epigastric pains, debility, stupor, cold extremities, dusky pallor, heart's action feeble, intermittent, extremities pulseless. Recovery took place in two days. The provings of Burt and Spranger have developed the symptoms which have led to the chief clinical uses, but some of Houatt's symptoms have also been confirmed. The chief keynote of *Rob.* is *acidity*, especially if the time of aggravation is *night*. Cooper has observed improvement which was going on under *Rob.* cease at night-time. Sour stomach; vomiting of intensely sour fluid which set the teeth on edge. Eructations of a very sour fluid. Clinical experience has added to these: Sour stools of infants, with sour smell of body and vomiting of sour milk. Heartburn and acidity coming on when lying down at night and preventing sleep. Halbert (*Clinique*, March, 1899, *H. W.*, xxxiv. 373) relates a case of hyperchlorydria treated with *Rob.*: Mrs. S., 40, had had stomach troubles many years, for which she had had bitter tonics, stomach douchings, electric massage. She had acid eructations and vomitings of intensely sour food; extreme appetite, but gastric pains an hour or two after meals; stomach and bowels distended with gas almost constantly, and flatulence was extremely irritating. Craved meats, but could not tolerate vegetables; craved solid food, but did not dare take it. Emaciated and cachectic. Meat, eggs, and milk was the diet prescribed. Lavage was performed every alternate day, and after it the patient was directed to eat a full meal; *Rob.* 3x was given every two hours, and steady improvement occurred in all particulars, till health was practically restored. Burt had a severe neuralgia in left temple, preventing sleep from midnight to daylight. He had also a "dull, heavy aching in stomach," and a "constant dull, heavy frontal headache, much < by motion and reading. The combination of gastric and head symptoms has placed *Rob.* among the chief remedies in migraine and sick headaches. Among Houatt's symptoms was a facial neuralgia spreading to eyes, forehead, with contraction of the jaw and features; and also a sensation as if the jaws would be dislocated or fractured. Hering gives this case of neuralgia as having been cured with *Rob.*: "Jawbone feels as if disarticulated; intensely sour taste and vomiting." The paralytic symptoms were very marked in one of the poisoning cases. Flatulence and diarrhœa were produced, and also constipation, with constant ineffectual urging. Among the *Peculiar Sensations* are: As if brain revolved. As if head were full of boiling water. As if brain struck against skull. Jawbone as if disarticulated. Stomach as if scalded. As if whole body would pass away with stool. The left side was most affected. A sleepy, dull feeling in head and limbs changed from right to left. A. L. Fisher (quoted *H. R.*, iv. 27) has relieved with *Rob.*, when everything else failed, the intensely acid vomiting in four cases of gastric cancer. Millspaugh points out that *Trifol. prat.*, which is a domestic remedy for cancer, is a near botanical ally of *Rob.* The symptoms are < by touch (neuralgia from contact of food), < by motion. < By reading (headache), < Lying down (heartburn and acidity). < Being raised from the horizontal (nausea and vomiting). < Night. < From fat, gravies, flatulent food, cabbages, turnips, new bread, ice-cream, raw fruit, &c.; they = gastric headache.

Relations.—*Compare:* Laburn. In acidity, Rhe., Calc., Æth., Mg. c., Puls. In neuralgia, Ars., Chi. Flatulence, Chi., Carb. v., Lyc. Ineffectual urging to stool, Nux. Gastric headaches, Ir. v. Jawbone as if dislocated, Rhus. Changing sides, Lac c. (Rob. right to left). Heart, Phaseol. Dilated pupils, dry throat, and flushed face, Bell.

SYMPTOMS.

1. **Mind.**—Very low-spirited.—Excessively irritable.—Tried to write but could not (agg.—R. T. C.).—Can hardly tell what she is doing (agg.—R. T. C.).

2. **Head.**—Vertigo and dulness of head in whatever position it is placed.—Sensation as if brain revolved, < lying on r. side.—Vertigo with unsteadiness and nausea.—Unable to hold his head upright; on eighteenth day could hold it up for a time, but it dropped if the effort was long continued (in a child who ate locust beans).—Constant dull, heavy, frontal headache, much < by motion and reading.—Dull headache: with profuse nasal discharge and frequent sneezing; with sharp stitches in temples.—Steady headache with sensation as if head full of boiling water; as if brain struck against skull when moving.—Sick headache, with sour stomach; from fat meat, gravies, flatulent food, cabbage, turnips, warm bread, pastry, ice-creams, raw fruits, &c.—Severe neuralgic pain in l. temple, preventing sleep from midnight to daylight.

3. **Eyes.**—Eyes sunk.—Eyes sore, watery; with rough throat.—Pupils contracted (in poisoning cases dilated).

4. **Nose.**—Profuse continual discharge from nostrils, with sneezing and dull headache.—Wax-like tumour on nose.

6. **Face.**—Neuralgic faceache, spreading to eyes, forehead, ears, and teeth, changing the whole features.—Spasmodic pains in jaws, feels as if they

would be broken or disarticulated; intensely sour taste in mouth.—Face flushed (in mild poisoning cases); dusky pallor (in severe cases).

8. **Mouth.**—Burning, lancinating pains, esp. in carious teeth, spreading to cheeks, eyes, and temples, < at night or on contact of food, esp. if cold or spiced; teeth become loosened from the spongy and easily bleeding gums.—White coating on tongue, with red tip.—Tongue covered with whitish-brown fur, smooth and slimy.—Mucous membrane of mouth pale.

9. **Throat.**—Dry scratching in throat.—Dryness of throat, with flushing of face.—Rough soreness.—Roughness, with sore eyes.

11. **Stomach.**—Thirst.—Constant eructations of a very sour fluid.—Heartburn and acidity of stomach at night on lying down.—Regurgitation of acid and bitter substances, everything turns to acid.—Nausea for three hours, followed by vomiting of an intensely sour fluid.—Nausea and attempts to vomit when placed in sitting posture.—Water taken before eating, at night, returned in morning green and sour.—Vomiting of intensely sour fluid, setting teeth on edge.—Vomiting of ropy mucus; tinged with blood; retching and epigastric pains.—Vomiting, with slight convulsions.—Sour stomach.—Dull, heavy, aching dulness in stomach.—Very severe, sharp pains in stomach all day and night.

12. **Abdomen.**—Constant dulness in epigastric region, with cutting pains in stomach and bowels and a good deal of rumbling.—Burning distress in stomach and region of gall-bladder.—Bowels greatly distended with flatulence, seemed to fill up whole abdomen; tympanites; > passing flatus.—Soreness in bowels when moving or by pressure.

13. **Stool and Anus.**—Desire for stool, but only flatus passes; finally constipated stool.—Sour stools of infants, with sour smell from body and vomiting of sour milk.—Diarrhœic stools, yellow, green, burning, with nervous agitation, weakness, cold sweat, dyspnœa.—Stools: loose, black, fetid, with great tenesmus; watery, whitish, excessively frequent and generally involuntary, with sensation as if whole body would pass away with stool; heat and pressure in epigastrium; cramps.—Sudden attacks of purging and vomiting.—The daily motion has a slimy look and bilious tinge.—Bowels costive, with frequent ineffectual desire for stool.

14. **Urinary Organs.**—Urine scanty and painful; or profuse and turbid.

16. **Female Sexual Organs.**—Nymphomania; whitish, greenish, yellowish, thick, and acrid, purulent leucorrhœa, with tumefaction and bruised feeling in neck of womb and general prostration; ulcerative pains in vagina, with acrid, yellowish leucorrhœa of most fetid smell.—Hard swelling of womb.—Cramps in womb.—Menses too late, black.—Hæmorrhage between the periods, accompanied by purulent leucorrhœa.—Eruptions and ulcers like herpes on vagina and vulva.

17. **Respiratory Organs.**—Voice reduced to a whisper and efforts to cry exceedingly feeble, suddenly ceasing with a slight sigh, as if from exhaustion.—Feeble respiration.

19. **Heart.**—Heart's action very feeble; embarrassed when moved from horizontal position.—Almost pulseless.

21. **Limbs.**—Could not move in slightest degree fingers, hands, arms, or legs; later could move fingers of r. hand a little; later could stir legs, but not draw them up; tickling feet caused much distress (from the beans).

24. **Generalities.**—Features and limbs shrunken as if from excessive liarrhœa (but there was none).—Faintness < when raised from horizontal osition.—Child cried when its arms were laid hold of.—Improvement which vas going on ceases at night-time (R. T. C.).

25. **Skin.**—Covered from head to foot with the worst form of rticaria.

26. **Sleep.**—Sleepiness and dulness in limbs and head (with stinging ain in temples), changing from r. to l. side.—Restless sleep all night on ccount of frequent sneezing; from indigestion.

27. **Fever.**—Hands and feet cold.—Paroxysms of pain late in afternoon, asting till 3 to 4 a.m., face hippocratic, much flatulence.—Hectic fever with ight-sweats.

Rosa Canina.

Dog-rose. *N. O.* Rosaceæ. Tincture of the hairy excrescence of insect origin called Cynosbati. Tincture of ripe fruits.

Clinical.—Bladder, affections of. Dysuria.

Characteristics.—Hips are used for making the very pleasant Confection of Roses used in general medicine as a basis for pills and electuaries. *Cynosbati* has been used in ancient times as a remedy in urinary difficulties. Burnett has confirmed this to some extent. A proving made by himself only evoked a somewhat increased flow of urine and a little heat in the urethra.

Rosa Damascena.

Damask or Damascus Rose. *N. O.* Rosaceæ. Tincture of the flowers (?).

Clinical. Hay-fever.

Characteristics.—Farrington mentions that *R. dam.* was introduced by Jeanes as a remedy at the beginning of rose-cold when the Eustachian tube is involved, with some degree of deafness and tinnitus.

Rosmarinus.

Rosmarinus officinalis. Rosemary. *N. O.* Labiatæ. Tincture of whole plant.

Clinical.—Abortion. Baldness. Menses, too early.

Characteristics.—The most violent of the symptoms of *Rosm.* were observed on a woman who took a strong infusion for eight days, with the result that miscarriage occurred. In another woman it brought on the menses four days too soon. Chilliness predominated, the chill not being followed by heat. Oil of Rosemary has an ancient reputation as a remedy for baldness, headache, and flagging mental powers. Hence it has been called "Herb of Memory." This Shakespere alludes to when he makes Ophelia say, "There's Rosemary, that's for remembrance."

Relations.—*Compare:* Hedeo., Menth. pul.

SYMPTOMS.

1. **Mind.**—Anxiety.—(Memory deficient.)

2. **Head.**—Vertigo.—Headache.—Heaviness and dulness of head.—Weight and tension round head.—(Baldness.)

16. **Female Sexual Organs.**—Violent pains followed by uterine hæmorrhage and miscarriage, succeeded by faintness, spasms of chest, cold hands and feet, small, rapid, irregular pulse.—Menses four days too early.

17. **Respiratory Organs.**—Oppression of breathing.—Spasms in chest.

26. **Sleep.**—Overpowering sleepiness with yawning.—Sleeplessness.

27. **Fever.**—Coldness so that she could not leave the bed.—Chill over whole body, legs icy cold, no thirst and no subsequent heat.

Rubia Tinctorum.

Rubia tinctorum. Madder. *N. O.* Rubiaceæ. Tincture of the root.

Clinical.—Anæmia. Bones, affections of. Spleen, affections of.

Characteristics.—The bones of young animals fed on Madder become tinged red. Burnett has found *Rub. t.* an excellent remedy (in ten-drop doses of the ϕ) in anæmia and under-nourished conditions, especially in splenic anæmia.

Relations.—*Compare:* Chin., Coff., Galium (bot.). In anæmia, Ferr.

Rumex Acetosa.

Rumex acetosa. Sorrel. *N. O.* Polygonaceæ. Tincture of the leaves.

Clinical.—Convulsions. Gastritis. Œsophagus, inflammation of. Paralysis. Throat, sore. Uvula, elongated.

Characteristics.—*Sorrel* was at one time cultivated in this country as a salad, and the Buckler-shaped, or French Sorrel, is still cultivated in France, where it is considered as a powerful antiscorbutic. The leaves contain a large quantity of Binoxalate of Potash (*Kali oxal.*). The symptoms of the Schema were observed on three men who ate largely of the leaves. In one very violent convulsions were induced of a peculiar kind, the limbs being thrown reciprocally backwards and forwards and the head from side to side ; the hands being alternately clenched and unclenched, the eyes prominent. Other remarkable symptoms were : Swelling of lower eyelid. Elongated uvula. Pain all down œsophagus < by swallowing. Persistent short, dry cough. There was complete paralysis of bodily powers ; copious green vomit ; constipation.

Relations.—*Compare :* Kal. ox., Lapath. In persistent cough, Rx. c.

SYMPTOMS.

1. **Mind.**—Unconscious.

2. **Head.**—Distress in head and an inch and a half below tip of sternum.

3. **Eyes.**—Eyes sunken.—Lower lid puffed ; pupil sluggish.—Eyeballs fixed, glassy, prominent.

6. **Face.**—Features collapsed.

8. **Mouth.**—Tongue : moist and furred ; white and furred and rather swollen ; furred in middle, tip and edges red.

9. **Throat.**—Pharynx congested, anterior part covered with limpid secretion, uvula much elongated ; constant pain from throat and throughout œsophagus to cardiac orifice of stomach, < when swallowing.

11. **Stomach.**—Appetite lost.—Great thirst.—Vomiting ; thick, pulpy, dark-green matter.—Continued retching.

12. **Abdomen.**—Soreness at epigastrium and fulness of abdomen.—Very severe pain at epigastrium with occasional exacerbations.—Violent and universal pain in bowels, so intense he pressed them firmly and rolled, vociferated loudly, with a pallid, haggard countenance, and, as it were, thrust out his eyes.

13. **Stool.**—Constipation.

14. **Urinary Organs.**—Deficient urine and alvine evacuations.—Urine increased, phosphatic, turbid, and whey-like.

17. **Respiratory Organs.**—Unremitting short cough, unattended with expectoration (persisted ten days).—Perpetual groaning or moaning.

19. **Pulse.**—Pulse : feeble ; small and weak ; small and frequent.

24. **Generalities.**—Lay on his back in a paroxysm of general convulsions, with arms elevated reciprocally, casting them forward and bringing them backward, doing the same with his legs, opening and reclosing his fists, and alternately throwing his head from r. to l. ; eyeballs fixed, glassy, prominent ; rattling and grinding of teeth without foaming at mouth ; absolutely senseless (fit lasted a quarter of an hour).—About 3 p.m. suddenly fell from his seat exhausted ; was lifted up and taken into the air ; legs again lost power and he fell, and when down vomited a diffluent, raw, greenish mass ; was again raised, but could only support himself feebly.—Bodily powers prostrated.

26. **Sleep.**—Sleeplessness.

27. **Fever.**—Heat and rigors.—Linen saturated with cutaneous exudation.

Rumex Crispus.

Rumex crispus. Curled Dock. Yellow Dock. *N. O.* Polygonaceæ. Tincture of fresh root.

Clinical.—Abortion. Aphonia. Asthma. *Borborygmi. Bronchitis.* Catarrh. Corns. Coryza. *Cough. Diarrhœa.* Dyspepsia. Epistaxis. Feet, tender. Gastralgia. Heart, pain in; affections of. Indigestion. *Irritation. Lichen.* Mouth, ulceration of. Phimosis. Phthisis. Prurigo. Rheumatism. Throat, sore; ulcerated. Trachea, affections of. Urticaria.

Characteristics.—The "Yellow Dock" or "Curled Dock" is a common British weed, introduced and growing wild in North America, where the provings were made. The common Dock of our fields and roadsides, *Rumex obtusifolia*, has a reputation among children as the best antidote to the nettle's sting; a reputation which is very well deserved, as I can testify. *Rumex crispus*, according to Joslin, quoted by Hale, was used by allopaths internally and externally for the cure of itch. This points to one of the leading actions of *Rx. c.* as developed in the provings. Among the constituents and salts of *Rx. c.* are *Sulphur* and *Calc. ph.* (Hale); and *Sul.*, *Calc.*, and *Pho.* are strongly represented in its action. *Rx. c.*, again, is a close ally of *Rheum*, and has analogous purgative and other properties. The provings were made by Houghton, Joslin, H. M. Paine, Bayard, Rhees, &c., both with the tincture and with attenuations, and its characteristics were well defined. A keynote of many *Rx. c.* cases is sensitiveness to cold air. The cough and skin symptoms are < by uncovering or exposure to air. Guernsey thus describes the cough of *Rx. c.*: "Cough caused by an incessant tickling in throat-pit, which tickling runs down to the bifurcation of the bronchial tubes; touching the throat brings on the cough; by covering up all the body and head with the bed-clothes there is no cough." Correspondingly this symptom of Paine's has led to many cures of skin cases: "*While undressing*, and for some time after, considerable itching of surface of lower limbs"—where *exposure to air* is again the exciting cause. The characteristic diarrhœa of *Rx. c.* occurs in the early morning, driving the patient out of bed; it comes on after catarrh, and is often associated with the characteristic cough of the remedy. The *Rx. c.* cough causes expulsion of urine; and it may even cause expulsion of the fœtus in pregnant women. P. P. Wells relates this case (Hale): Mrs. X. had had eight miscarriages in the early months, each miscarriage being attended with a dry, shaking, spasmodic cough in paroxysms of great violence, which was regarded as the cause of the abortions. At the beginning of the ninth pregnancy she came under homœopathic treatment. The cough came on—very dry, harsh, loud, shaking, < at night, preventing sleep, excited instantly by pressure on the trachea. *Rx. c.* 30 promptly relieved. Wells also cured with *Rx. c.* 200 (Lehrman's preparation) the following in a man: Cough beginning with tickling behind top of sternum, sometimes in paroxysms lasting for five to ten minutes. Trachea sore to external pressure; feels excoriated through its whole extent, as also do the fauces. Cough is excited by pressure on throat-pit ; violent with scanty difficult expectoration ; shakes head as if it would fly to pieces and chest so that he feels he might raise blood any minute. Paroxysms exhaust him ; headache during cough. Joslin pointed out the *left* chest had more verified symptoms than any other region. Further Conditions of *Rx. c.* are < lying on left side ; > lying on right side. < At 11 p.m. and 4 a.m. Another Condition of the cough is that it is induced or < by any *irregularity of respiration*, such as a little deeper breath than usual or a little more rapid. Cough when eating. Joslin reports a number of cases of gastric derangement cured with *Rx. c.* (1) A young lady had shootings from pit of stomach into chest in various directions ; sharp pains in left chest ; dull aching in forehead and slight nausea. One dose of 30th removed all her symptoms and restored her appetite. (2) A lady, 50, had had for three weeks pain in pit of stomach, aching in left chest, flatulence, eructations, pains and distension in stomach after meals. *Rx. c.* 200, one dose, cured in two or three hours. (3) Young lady had sensation of *fulness and pressure in pit of stomach extending up towards throat, carried down on swallowing and rising again to throat*. *Rx. c.* 200 cured. (4) A gentleman not used to tea took a cup, very weak, of the black kind ; then followed aching in pit of stomach and aching above it in chest, and especially on each side of lower end of sternum. *Rx. c.* 30 cured in a few minutes. The flatulence and rumbling of *Rx. c.* are well marked, and I have found it the best general remedy for the painless but annoying borborygmi frequently complained of by women. The left side is more markedly affected than the right. The circulation is much disturbed, violent palpitations of the heart and throbbing throughout the whole body being noted. Carleton Smith points out (*H. P.*, x. 275) that in a case of cough cured by Cardoza with *Rx. c.* the characteristic was "cough only during the day, not at all at night." This gives *Rx. c.* a place beside *Fer.* and *Mang.* Smith has cured with *Rx. c.* many cases of indigestion in which this symptom was present : "Lump in throat, not > by hawking or swallowing ; it descends on deglutition, but immediately returns." *Peculiar Sensations* are : Eyes pain as if from dryness. Tongue as if burned. Lump in throat ; it descends on deglutition, but immediately returns. Hard substance in pit of stomach. Bunch in throat or behind sternum. Pressure of a stick in rectum. As if urine could not long be retained. As if she could not get another breath. As if air did not penetrate chest. As if a feather swaying to and fro in bronchi. As if head would fly to pieces (with cough). As if he might raise blood any minute. As if cough did not reach low enough to raise phlegm. As if heart suddenly stopped. Sternum feels sprained. Raw feeling under clavicles. Hands cold when coughing. The symptoms are < by touch ; pressure ; riding. < By cold ; > by warmth. < Change : warm to cold or cold to warm ; changing rooms. < Lying down (pain in pit of stomach > lying perfectly quiet). < Lying on left side ; burning in left side. > Lying right side. < Talking. < Deep inspiration ; or irregularity of breathing. < Walking. < Evening and night ; and morning on waking, 3.30 and 11 p.m., 2 to 5 a.m < When eating and after meals. > Discharge of offensive flatus.

Relations.—*Antidoted by :* Camph., Bell., Hyo., Con., Lach., Pho. *Compare :* Hard, dry, tickling cough, < reading, < touching larynx, Cin. Asthma of consumptives < 2 a.m., Meph., Sticta. Pains in left lung < moving ; cough from change of temperature, Bry. (Bry. more when change is to warm air ; Rx. c. more when to cold). Tickling cough from suprasternal fossa excited by speaking, Sil. Morning diarrhœa hurrying patient out of bed, Sul. Annoying, tickling cough on lying down, Hyo., Con. Urticaria, morning diarrhœa, Apis (opposite Conditions). Dry cough from tickling in suprasternal fossa < least cool air or deep inspiration, Bell. Effects of tea, Thuj. Stitching pains in chest, pulsations over whole body, K. ca. Tough mucus, K. bi. Cough when eating, Calc. Burnt sensation in tongue, Ran. b. Stick in rectum, Æsc. h. Cough < changing air, Spo., Pho. < Lying left side, Pho., Pul. Raw sensation in larynx and trachea when coughing, Caust. Spurting of urine with cough, Caust., Pul., Scil. Early morning diarrhœa, Alo., Nat. s., Pod., Sul. Skin symptoms < uncovering, Hep., Nat. s., Oleand. Cough starting in throat-pit (Bell. more in fauces ; Pho. more in bronchi). Incessant cough and botan., Rx. ac. Diarrhœa and botan., Rhe. Botan., Fago., Polyg., Lapath. Cough only during day, Fer., Mang.

SYMPTOMS.

1. **Mind.**—Low-spirited : with serious expression of face ; with suicidal mood.—Irritable ; disinclined to mental exertion.—Indifference to surroundings.—Stagnation of ideas, lassitude, and uneasiness.

2. **Head.**—Headache after waking in morning, preceded by a disagreeable dream.—Dull (and bruised) pains : on r. side ; in occiput ; in forehead with bruised feeling, < on motion.—Darting pain or sharp piercing in l. side of head.—Catarrhal headache with great irritation of larynx and trachea, clavicular pain and soreness behind sternum.—Bruised sensation on waking, continued till noon, disappeared suddenly after dinner.—Headache < in open air.—Pungent drawing in l. occiput with a similar pain in l. nostril and feeling as if coryza would ensue.

3. **Eyes.**—Pain in eyes as from dryness ; lids inflamed, < evening.—Sore feeling in eyes without inflammation.—Deep-seated pain in r. eye.—Sharp, shooting pain in (and over) l. eye.

4. **Ears.**—Ringing in ears.—Itching deep in ears.—Pain, throbbing, stopped sensation in ears.

5. **Nose.**—Great desire to pick nose.—Nose obstructed ; dry sensation, even in posterior nares.—Sudden, sharp, tingling sensation in Schneiderian membrane, followed by violent and rapid sneezing five or six times in succession, with watery discharge.—Violent sneezing with watery coryza and headache), < evening and night.—Accumulation of mucus about posterior nares.—Yellow mucus discharged through posterior nares.—Epistaxis, violent sneezing, and painful irritation of nostrils.—Influenza with violent catarrh, followed by bronchitis.

6. **Face.**—Great paleness of face while standing.—Heat of face ; redness < evenings ; dull headache ; with pulsations over whole body.—Pain in side of face, including r. temple and ear ; also l. side of upper lip.—Pain in r.

jaw, morning.—After retiring late at night, lancinating pains in lower jaw at root of l. canine teeth.

8. **Mouth.**—Pain in teeth of both sides, morning.—Toothache : entirely > after eating dinner ; > by rinsing mouth with cold water.—Grumbling stinging toothache in r. upper molars, while riding in a cold wind ; with pain in forehead.—Tongue coated : white ; yellow ; yellowish-brown, or reddish-brown.—Dryness of anterior part of tongue, with sense of repletion in stomach and as if one had eaten spice.—Sensation of excoriation at edges of tongue.—Front of tongue dry and hot.—Soreness of r. edge of tongue.—Sensation as if tongue and mouth burnt.—Ulceration of mouth and throat.—Taste : bitter (mornings) ; nasty ; flat (on rising).—Flow of saliva.

9. **Throat.**—Scraping in throat ; excoriated feeling with secretion of mucus in upper part.—Sensation of a lump in throat, not > by hawking or swallowing ; it descends on swallowing, but immediately returns.—Sensation of a lump in œsophagus.—Aching in pharynx with collection of tough mucus in fauces.—Catarrhal affections of throat and fauces.—Throat dry, swallowing difficult ; pain in l. side on swallowing.

11. **Stomach.**—Appetite : much increased ; lost.—Thirst.—After meals : flatulency ; heaviness in stomach or epigastrium ; aching in l. breast ; pressure and distension in stomach.—Nausea in night before diarrhœa.—Sensation of hard substance in pit of stomach.—Fulness and pressure in pit of stomach extending toward throat-pit ; descends with every empty deglutition but immediately returns. — Tight, suffocative, heavy ache in epigastrium, through to back ; clothes seem too tight ; weak feeling in epigastrium, all < when talking ; frequently takes a long breath.—Shooting from pit of stomach to chest ; sharp in l. chest ; slight nausea ; dull aching in forehead.—Aching and shooting in pit of stomach and above it on each side of sternum.—Eructations ; empty ; tasteless.—Hiccough.—Pyrosis.—Nausea ; > by eructations. —Nausea and vertigo while dressing in morning, compelling him to lie down again.—Sensation of undigested food and upward pressure in throat-pit.—Severe pain in digestive organs on waking.—Pain in stomach with the pain in the lungs.—Burning and cutting in stomach.

12. **Abdomen.**—Pain in hypochondrium from walking or deep inspiration.—Griping near navel partially > by discharge of offensive flatus ; flatulent colic soon after a meal.—Pain occurring or < during inspiration.—Sensation of heaviness and fulness in abdomen with rumbling.—Borborygmus.—Pain in abdomen in morning, followed by a stool.—Colic from a cold, with cough.

13. **Stool and Anus.**—Stools : painless, offensive, profuse ; brown or black, thin or watery ; preceded by pain in abdomen.—Before stool : sudden urging, driving him out of bed in morning.—Morning diarrhœa, with cough from tickling in throat-pit.—Diarrhœa 6 to 10 a.m.—Copious diarrhœic stool with colic pain just above hypogastrium, and a very disagreeable rumbling in bowels together with nausea and loss of appetite ; these sensations continued throughout the day with four or five evacuations which passed away in a stream as if a large quantity would be discharged ; nevertheless each discharge was suddenly arrested, and the inclination passed away entirely for a short time ; but on rising the urgency returned, and on returning to the closet a new stream poured forth as before.—Fæces black ; scanty.—Constipation for several days, followed by a dry, hard stool.—Itching at anus with dis-

charge of offensive flatus.—Sensation as from pressure of a rough stick forced up rectum, painful on walking.—Hæmorrhoids protrude; much heat and itching at anus, and sensation as if a foreign body there.

14. **Urinary Organs.**—Sudden urging.—Frequent inclination with feeling as if urine could not long be retained.—Involuntary micturition with cough.—Copious colourless urine in afternoon.—Urine less copious, flocculent deposit, oily surface; marked brick-dust sediment.

15. **Male Sexual Organs.**—Tendency to phimosis.—During evening feeling of soreness and excoriation, with redness of end of prepuce.—Itching of prepuce.—Sexual desire diminished; lost.

17. **Respiratory Organs.**—Hoarseness < evenings; voice uncertain.—Voice: changes suddenly; on two consecutive days at 2 p.m. rose several notes; higher with catarrh; nasal.—Aphonia after exposure to cold.—(Reflex aphonia from tubercle of l. apex.)—Tenacious mucus in larynx, constant desire to hawk.—Violent irritation to cough in larynx while eating (at three meals).—(Cough all day, > lying down at night.)—Pain in top of larynx; mostly l. side.—Dry, spasmodic cough, like beginning of whooping-cough; in paroxysms; preceded by tickling in throat-pit, with congestion and slight pains in head, and wrenching pains in r. chest; began a few minutes after lying down at night (11 p.m.); lasted 10 to 15 minutes, after which he slept all right; a less severe paroxysm in bed on waking and throughout day; this lasted two weeks, when he began to expectorate adhesive mucus in small quantities, detached with difficulty.—Hacking cough.—Cough < by any irregularity of breathing.—Hoarse, hacking cough 11 p.m. and 2 to 5 a.m.—Cough with pain behind mid-sternum.—Pressure on throat = cough.—Dry, tickling, spasmodic cough, with tenderness in larynx and trachea, rendering cough quite painful.—Teasing periodical cough, < in cool air or by anything which increases the volume or rapidity of inspired air.—Cough < from changing rooms.—Cough originally caused by inhaling extremely cold air during winter, < lying down, esp. 11 p.m.—Cough provoked by change from cold to warm or warm to cold.—Cough < lying l. side; > lying r.; > covering up mouth; > wearing respirator.—Sensation of breathlessness; as if air did not penetrate chest; or as when falling or passing rapidly through the air.—Frequent feeling as if she could not get another breath.

18. **Chest.**—Clavicular pain; raw pain just under each clavicle while hawking mucus from throat.—Pain in chest: in both sides; dull aching in anterior part, with headache and belching.—Sharp stitching or stinging through l. lung.—Acute stitch along l. margin of sternum.—Burning stinging: in l. side near heart; in whole l. chest suddenly when taking a deep inspiration while in act of lying down in bed at night.—At 3.30 p.m., while writing at desk, stitches in substance of l. lung.—Burning, shooting pain in r. chest.—Sharp pain near l. axilla.—Pain in centre of l. lung.—Sternum feels sprained—Great pressure and sense of depression in upper part of breast.—Very sharp pain in breast running r. to l.—Sharp cutting pain in l. breast at noon lasting an hour.

19. **Heart.**—Heart feels as if it suddenly stopped beating; followed by a heavy throbbing.—Dull pain in region of heart, with dull pain and heaviness in l. upper arm, esp. elbow.—Dull pain in heart on deep inspirations.—Burning in region of heart.—Severe stinging in region of heart, extending

through chest to apex of l. scapula, with frequent desire to take a deep breath, which < the pain (afternoon for two or three hours).—Sharp pain in l. side of heart.—Palpitation : after supper ; < going upstairs ; violent with throbbing carotids.

20. **Neck and Back.**—Sensation as if a thread were tightly tied round neck just below ears, with a slight roaring in the ears.—Pain : in back of neck ; running down back.—Aching between scapulæ.—Stinging burning just below inferior angle of l. scapula ; followed and accompanied by stinging, almost itching pain l. chest just below nipple.—Pain under r. scapula.—Pain in l. scapula.—Burning pain in small of back near tip of r. sacro-iliac joint.—Sore pain in l. sacro-iliac joint, lame as from over-lifting ; < by sudden motion ; followed by pulsation in nates.—Aching and sense of great fatigue in loins.

21. **Limbs.**—Twitching of r. arm and leg.—Pain in upper and lower limbs of same or opposite side.

22. **Upper Limbs.**—Pains in shoulder down to elbow, arms feel strained.—Hands cold when coughing,—Bruised aching and stinging pain in arms, hands, elbows, and r. wrist.

23. **Lower Limbs.**—Stitching in back of r. hip ; limping walk.—Legs ache.—Stitch-like pain in knee-joint when standing.—Legs covered with small red pimples.—Feet cold.—Feet sensitive, stinging in corns.—Tender feet.

24. **Generalities.**—Lassitude and weariness.—Restless in evening.—Pains not fixed or constant anywhere.—Throbbing through whole body.—Unusual sensitiveness to cold or open air.

25. **Skin.**—Itching in various parts, < on lower limbs.—Eruption covered uniformly several regions of skin, with exception of face ; itching more of a pricking than a burning ; < by cold, > by warmth.—Contagious prurigo or "army itch."—Stinging-itching or prickling itching of skin.—Vesicular eruption, itching when uncovered and exposed to cool air.—Periodic itch.—Urticaria ; < in open air.

26. **Sleep.**—Sleep : disturbed ; wakeful, restless ; short naps and unpleasant fancies, even when awake.—Unpleasant dreams ; of danger and trouble ; early in the morning ; of being naked in the street ; of murders ; of autopsies.—Wakes early with headache.

27. **Fever.**—Chilly, < on back ; colic, nausea, stitches near middle of chest.—Increased frequency of pulse and afternoon fever.—Sensation of heat, followed by that of cold, without shivering.—Flushes of heat, < on cheeks.—Sweat on waking from a sound sleep.

Rumex Obtusifolia, *see* Lapathum.

Russula.

Russula fœtens. *N. O.* Fungi. Tincture of the fresh mushrooms

Clinical.—Blindness. Chorea. Convulsions. Enuresis.

Characteristics.—Some species of *Russula* are edible, and are much esteemed as a food on the Continent. Alphonse Barrele observed the effects of eating cooked *Russula fœtens*, which produced a very severe poisoning. Hallucinations, muscular tremors, and clonic spasms recall the effects of *Agaric*. The eye symptoms were even more pronounced, complete blindness lasting many days occurred, with this peculiarity of the pupil, that it was sometimes normal, sometimes dilated, and sometimes contracted.

SYMPTOMS.

1. **Mind.**—Unconsciousness.—Muscular spasms, deathly anxiety, dyspnœa.—Hallucinations constant for three days after spasms ceased.

3. **Eyes.**—Pupils at one time normal, at another dilated, at another contracted.—Consciousness returned on third day, patient could hear but was completely blind.

6. **Face.**—Cyanosis.

11, 12, 13. **Stomach, Abdomen, and Stool.**—Nausea, colic, vomiting, diarrhœa, cold extremities.

14. **Urinary Organs.**—Involuntary micturition.

17. **Respiratory Organs.**—Dyspnœa.

19. **Heart.**—Pulse small and contracted.

24. **Generalities.**—Constant trembling of muscles, at times interrupted by tonic contractions, increasing to general clonic spasms with complete loss of consciousness.—Patient recovered after two or three weeks.

25. **Skin.**—The attack was followed by pseudo-erysipelas on elbows and painless furuncles over whole body, esp. on scapulæ and small of back.

Ruta.

Ruta graveolens. Rue. *N. O.* Rutaceæ. Tincture of whole fresh plant.

Clinical.—*Amblyopia.* Anus, prolapse of. *Bone, bruised; pains in. Bruises.* Bursitis. Cartilages, bruises of; pains in. *Chest, sternum, pains in.* Constipation. Dislocations. Dyspepsia. Enuresis. Epistaxis. Exostosis. *Eyes, sight weak*, pains in. Facial paralysis, from cold. Fevers. *Fractures. Ganglion.* Hæmorrhages. *Hands, pains in.* Paralysis. *Perichondritis.* Periostitis. Rectum affections of; prolapse of. Restlessness. *Rheumatism. Sciatica.* Spleen, affections of. *Sprain.* Stammering. Tongue, cramp in; swelling of. Urination difficulty of. Varicocele. Veins, swollen; varicose. Warts.

Characteristics.—The common Rue of our gardens is a native of Southern Europe. It was formerly in great repute in medicine epilepsy, hysteria, hydrophobia, weakness of sight (from excessive reading), ozæna, epistaxis, foul gumboils, flatulent colic (in hysteric females), inertia of the bowels, having been cured with it empirically (Teste). It was also supposed to be a kind of universal antidote: "Even in our own time the Roman ladies imagine that the most odoriferous flowers may be left in their rooms without the least danger provided a bush of garden rue be amongst them" (Teste). Practitioners (says *Treas. of Bot.*) have perhaps been deterred from employing it by the symptoms of acrido-narcotic poisoning induced by an overdose. Locally applied *Rue* is a powerful irritant, and one species, *Ruta montana*, is dangerous to handle even with gloves. *Ruta* is "useful in feverish complaints, promotes perspiration and removes noxious material; in headache, nervous and hysteric complaints, weakness of the stomach and pains in the bowels, suppressed menses, and if taken for a long time it benefits epilepsy. The expressed juice benefits nightmare" (Green's *Herbal*). In large doses it causes violent gastric pains, excessive and sometimes bloody vomiting, profuse salivation and swelling of the tongue, great prostration, confusion of mind, and convulsive twitchings, with, in pregnant women, abortion (M. Hélie). In olden times it was used to ward off plague, and is at the present day the great remedy for pip or roup in fowls: a disease which affects the throat and causes chokiness and turns the comb of the fowl black; it is due to impure water and is contagious. "It certainly acts strongly on deposits of scirrhous material in both the breasts and in the vagina and sometimes lessens the size of these" (Cooper). Hahnemann's proving shows how largely the old uses were founded on a homœopathic relationship. The vulnerary remedies indicate in symptoms of their provings the peculiar form of injuries for which they are adapted; there are the *sprained* pains of *Rhus*, the *bruised* pains (in skin and muscles) of *Arn.*; *Ruta* also has bruised pains, but these are more particularly manifested in *bones*. *Ruta* is one of the chief remedies for injured bones, and especially *bruised* bones. This power of *Ruta* does not appear to have been known before the provings were made. But impaired sight due to straining the eyes was an old use of the remedy; and here are symptoms from the provings: "His eyes feel as if he had strained the sight too much by reading;" "Weak, pressive-like pain in right eye, with dimness of surrounding objects, as if from having looked too long at an object that was fatiguing to the eyes;" "A feeling of heat and burning in the eyes, and pain in them when he reads (in the evening and by candle-light)." Each of these symptoms was experienced by a separate prover. Another effect of bruising is seen in prolapse of the rectum *after confinement*. But *Ruta* has, independently of this, a powerful action on the rectum, and caused prolapse in the provers and many severe symptoms. Tearing stitches in rectum when sitting. The prolapse is $<$ by stooping, and especially by crouching together; it comes on immediately on attempting a passage. Rushmore (*H. P.*, x. 516) cured with one dose of *Ruta* 900 (Fincke) a case of prolapse *preceding a very difficult stool*.—Tearing in rectum and urethra while urinating. Constipation; from inactivity of rectum or impaction of fæces following mechanical injuries. A curious clinical symptom is a sensation of nausea located in the rectum. Among the general symptoms are: Great weakness after a short walk; limbs feel bruised; small of back and loins painful. Tottering as if thighs were weak; limbs pain when walking. Does not know where to lay his legs on account of uneasiness and heaviness; lies now in one place, now in another, and turns from side to side. All parts of the body on which he lies, even in bed, are painful as if bruised. Facial paralysis from catching cold, in robust, sanguine persons. Rheumatic paralysis of wrists and ankles. *Ruta* is *specially suited* to robust, sanguineous persons; and corresponds to hæmorrhages from nose (with pressure at root), gums, rectum. *Peculiar Sensations* are: Pain as if from a fall in periosteum. As if a nail were driven into head. Head as if bruised or beaten. Eyes, as if strained; as if a shadow flitting before them; as after looking too long and intently at an object; as if eyes were balls of fire. As if one were digging about in the ear with a blunt piece of wood. As of a lump in throat. Bladder as if constantly full. Spine as if beaten and lame. Wrists as if sprained. As if pain were in marrow of bone, or as if bone were broken. Thighs as if beaten; as if weak. As if there were an ulcer on ankle. All parts of body bruised at night, feeling as if it were time to rise. Restlessness is a very frequent *Concomitant* of *Ruta* conditions. A peculiar symptom is cramp in the tongue with embarrassed speech. A prolonged use of *Ruta* 3x has cured ganglion in front of left wrist (Oran W. Smith, *H. P.*, ix. 308). Slow pulse, contracted pupil, salivation and swollen tongue are features of its action. The symptoms are: < By touch. Pressure < sore spot on sternum; > pain below r. scapula, and stitches in small of back. Backache > lying on back. [This is characteristic, and has led to many cures; and the relief of a case of malignant disease of kidneys and bladder (Rushmore, *H. P.*, x. 516). This is important in connection with a use Cooper has made of *Ruta* ointment, prepared by extracting the plant in warm vaseline as an application in broken cancer of the breast.] Walking or riding = chafing. Dyspepsia from straining stomach by carrying heavy weights. Scratching >. Rubbing >. Rest <. Motion >. Lying down = parts lain on to be sore; > pain below right scapula; > stitches in small of back. Sitting <. Stooping <. Bending over = fæces to escape. Exertion <. Ascending <. Going up and down stairs = hamstrings to feel shortened and weak. < At night. < Morning. (Vertigo on rising. Rheumatic pain in back < before rising. Sweat in bed.) Warm stove = chilliness. Indoors = yawning and stretching. Open air = vertigo. Cold applications <. Cold wet weather <. < Reading and straining eyes. < During menses.

Relations.—*Antidoted by:* Camph. *Antidote to.:* Merc. *Complementary:* Calc. ph. in joint affections. *Compatible:* After Arn. in joint affections; after Symphyt. in bone injuries; Calc., Caust., Lyc., Ph. ac., Puls., Sul., Sul. ac. (diseases of bone). *Compare:* In diseases of bone, Angust. (also botan.), Conchiol. Restlessness, effects of cold and damp, Rhus. Eye-strain, Nat. m., Onos., Seneg. Prolapse of rectum, Æsc., Bell., Chi. s., Nit. ac., Pod. Pain in back < in morning before rising, Pet. Sore as if bruised in parts lain on, Arn., Bap., Pyro. Constipation after injuries, Arn. Warts on palms, Nat. c.,

Nat. m. (on backs of hands, Dul.). Chafing. *Compare also:* Arg. n., Con., Euphras., Lyc., Cham., Sep.

Causation.—Bones, injuries of. Bruises. Fractures. Sprains. Carrying heavy weights. Over-exertion of eyes.

SYMPTOMS.

1. **Mind.**—Anxiety, as from a troubled conscience.—Disposition to quarrel and to contradict.—Unfitness for labour.—Cross and suspicious, imagined he was always being deceived.—Patient dissatisfied with himself and others, and disposed to weep.—Melancholy and moral dejection (towards evening).—Slowness of conception.—Frequent absence of mind.

2. **Head.**—Head bewildered, as from too little sleep.—Whirling vertigo, which causes falling when rising in morning, also when seated, and when walking in open air.—When sitting, sudden vertigo : all turned round him in a circle ; thereafter glowing cheeks.—Headache as from stunning pressure on whole brain, with great inquietude.—Headache as if a nail were driven into head.—Headache after excessive use of intoxicating drinks.—Throbbing or tearing pain in forehead, with confusion in head, in evening before lying down, and in morning on waking.—Heat in head (with much restlessness).—Intermittent boring stitches in r. side of forehead.—Shooting, drawing pain from frontal to temporal bone.—From temporal bones to occiput, in the periosteum, pain as from a fall.—(Occipital headache < during menses, with pains in backs of eyes (< in l. eyeball), with dyspepsia ; cannot bear a bright light, eyes tire, ache and prick and turn bloodshot when she uses glasses—R.T.C.)—Tensive drawing or lancinating pains in exterior of head, as from a blow or contusion, esp. in periosteum.—Gnawing itching in scalp.—Nodes and abscesses on scalp, with pain as from excoriation when touched, formed after a tearing pain had been felt in the part which they occupy.—Biting itching (ulcers) on scalp.—Small ulcers and running sores on scalp.

3. **Eyes.**—Pains in eyes when viewing an object minutely.—Itching smarting in canthus.—Aching in eyes.—Eyes hot like balls of fire ; ache ; feel strained.—Burning sensation in eyes when reading by candle-light.—Burning under l. eye.—Itching in inner canthi and on lower lids, which becomes smarting after rubbing them, whereupon the eye becomes filled with water.—Lachrymation in open air (not in room).—Speck on cornea.—Red areola round candle in evening.—Quivering and jerking in muscles of eyebrows.—Spasms in (lower) lids ; the tarsus is drawn hither and thither, and when it ceases water runs from both eyes for an hour and a half.—Tendency to stare.—Contraction of pupil (Aitken).—(Detachment of retina.)—Asthenopia.—Astigmatism (?).—Sight confused, as if directed through a mist, and complete cloudiness at a distance.—Obscuration of sight from reading too much, with clouds, or like a veil before eyes.—A green halo around the light in evening.—Bad effects from over-straining eyes, from reading too much, esp. fine work at night.—Dancing spots before eyes.

4. **Ears.**—Earache with scraping pressure ; as if a blunt piece of wood were pushed about in it.—Itching lancinations in ear.—Pain in cartilage of ear and under mastoid process as from a bruise.

5. **Nose.**—Acute and hard aching in root of nose.—Perspiration on back of nose.—Epistaxis with pressure at root of nose.

6. **Face.**—Pains in face, in periosteum, as if caused by contusion or blows.—Spasmodic tearing in cheek-bone.—Itching and gnawing at face and on cheeks.—Erysipelas in forehead with swelling.—Eruption of pimples on lips.—Lips dry and sticky.—Acne.

7. **Teeth.**—Toothache with digging pain (in the lower teeth).—Painful sensibility and ready bleeding of the gums.

8. **Mouth.**—Mouth dry and glutinous.—Cramp in tongue, with embarrassed speech.—Profuse salivation and swelling of tongue (Taylor, *Med. Juris*).

9. **Throat.**—Sore throat, as if a tubercle were in bottom of gullet, during empty deglutition.—Sensation as from excoriation and pressure on velum palati when swallowing.

10. **Appetite.**—Mawkish and dry taste of food, like wood.—Violent thirst for cold water in afternoon.—Disgust at first mouthful with a sensation of fulness and satiety in abdomen, although the appetite is good.—Sudden nausea when eating, with vomiting of food.—Pains in stomach after eating bread, or crude and indigestible food.

11. **Stomach.**—Empty risings or with the taste of food.—Hiccough when smoking.—Putrid risings after eating meat.—Risings like those of hysterical women.—Nausea at pit of stomach.—Vomiting, even of food.—Pains in stomach after having eaten uncooked or indigestible food.—Pinchings in stomach after eating bread.—Gnawing (sensation as from emptiness or hunger), burning, or pressive pains in stomach.—Tearing shootings in epigastrium.

12. **Abdomen.**—Gnawing pressure in hepatic region.—Gnawing and eating pain about navel.—Sick feeling in abdomen followed by soft stools.—Pulsation and pricking in l. hypochondrium.—Painful swelling of spleen.—Pain in abdomen as from a bruise, with digging in lumbar region.—Pressive pinchings in hypogastrium.—Incisive pinchings in sides of abdomen.—Shooting pains, which pass into abdomen, when sitting down.—Sensation of coldness or of heat, and burning sensation in abdomen.—Gnawing in abdomen.—Colic with burning or gnawing pain.—Colic as from worms (in children).—Lancinations in muscles of abdomen, which compel retraction of abdomen.

13. **Stool and Rectum.**—Difficult fæces, as from inactivity of rectum (or impaction following mechanical injuries), evacuated only with straining.—Constipation alternating with mucous, frothy stools.—Fæces scanty, hard, knotty, like sheep-dung.—Slimy diarrhœa alternately with constipation.—(Chronic and obstructed diarrhœa.—R. T. C.)—Frequent want to evacuate, with scanty but soft evacuations.—Ineffectual want to evacuate, with prolapsus recti.—Prolapse of rectum immediately on attempting a passage ; from slightest stooping ; after confinement ; frequent unsuccessful urging.—Prolapsus recti at every evacuation (whether hard or soft stool).—Discharge of blood with stool.—When sitting, tearing stitches in rectum.—Pruritus ani with smooth appearance of skin round anus.—R. T. C.).—Tearing in rectum and urethra when not urinating.—Nausea felt in rectum.

14. **Urinary Organs.**—Want to urinate, sometimes very urgent, with pressure on bladder and scanty emission of green urine.—Pressure on bladder

(as if continually full), sometimes also after emission of urine and at other times.—Frequent and profuse emission of urine, even at night.—Continued want to urinate, even immediately after an emission.—Retention of urine.—Involuntary emission of urine at night in bed and by day during movement (walking).—Urine charged with gravel.

15. **Male Sexual Organs.**—Increased sexual desire.—Pollutions.

16. **Female Sexual Organs.**—Sterility.—Catamenia very irregular.—Symptoms < at menstrual period.—Catamenia of too short duration, preceded and followed by leucorrhœa.—Corrosive leucorrhœa after the catamenia.—(Pruritus pudendi.—Vaginal pruritus with irritation of skin elsewhere.—Pruritus vulvæ, very severe, affecting external lips, which are swollen, began in vagina with pain under l. breast and dimness of sight.—R. T. C.)—Metrorrhagia as a forerunner of miscarriage.—Bearing-down pains.—Miscarriage; at seven months.—Lameness and soreness all over; with feeble contractions during labour.

17. **Respiratory Organs.**—Bruised pain in larynx.—Cough in evening after lying down, with copious expectoration of viscid mucus, and heaving as if about to vomit.—Croaking cough at night with scraping in chest.—Cough, with copious expectoration of purulent matter.—Expectoration of thick, yellowish mucus, almost without cough, but with a sensation of fatigue in chest.—Wakened about midnight with a choking cough.

18. **Chest.**—Breath very short, with dyspnœa.—Aching at chest with sensation of fulness.—Nocturnal compression in lower part of chest.—Lancinations in chest, often with suspended respiration, principally when going up stairs.—Sensation of coldness or of heat in chest.—Gnawing in r. chest with corrosive burning.—Gnawing sensation in (l.) chest.—Phthisis after mechanical injuries of chest.—A place in region of sternum is painful when touched.

19. **Heart.**—Palpitation of heart with anxiety.

20. **Neck and Back.**—Drawing in nape of neck and in the shoulder-blades.—Pressure on inside of r. scapula.—Pricking itching between scapulæ, not > by rubbing.—Contusive pains in back and loins, often with oppressed respiration.—Pain in loins and sacrum as from contusion.—Shootings in loins when walking and when stooping, or only when seated, > by pressure and when lying down.—Backache > lying on back.—Pain in lumbar vertebræ as if bruised.—Bruised pain in spine; and in iliac bones.—Pain from coccyx to os sacrum as from a fall or blow.

21. **Limbs.**—Pains in the limbs, joints, and bones as if beaten, or after a blow or fall.

22. **Upper Limbs.**—Wrenching pain in the shoulder-joint, esp. when permitting arms to hang down or when resting on them.—Shocks in arms as if in bones.—Dull tearings in bones of the arm and joints of elbow.—Pain as from contusion in joint of elbow.—Pain in forearms as well as in bones and joints of hands as if they had been beaten.—Pressive and spasmodic drawing and tearing in forearms, hands, and fingers.—Paralytic stiffness of wrist.—Wrenching pain or shootings in wrists.—Sensation as from a sprain and stiffness in wrist.—Bones of wrist and back of hand painful as if bruised when at rest and when moving.—Pain in wrist (as from a sprain) on lifting a weight.—Numbness and tingling in hands after exertion.—Spasmodic contraction of

fingers.—Swollen veins on hands; after eating.—Warts; with sore pains; flat, smooth, on palms of hands.

23. **Lower Limbs.**—Falling from side to side when walking, legs will not support him, no power or steadiness in thighs.—Legs give out on ascending or descending stairs.—Sciatica; < by cold applications, and in cold, wet weather.—Spasmodic drawing in thighs, extending into the hip-joint and sacrum.—Contusive pain in hip-joint and bones of the legs, esp. on touching and stretching them.—Weakness in thigh-bones on rising from a seat, as if they had been broken.—Weakness, trembling, and paralytic heaviness of knees and legs, which prevent standing firmly, fatigue and heaviness of legs after walking.—Sensation of contraction in tendons of knee (as if they were shortened, and weakness in them, esp. on descending).—"Rue pounded with honey and salt helps swelling of knee."—Culpepper).—Fistulous ulcers in legs.—Flexion of knees, esp. when going down stairs.—Lameness and pain in the ankles after a sprain or dislocation; as if ulcerated.—(Pain and tenderness in soles, aching in ankles and very acute shooting in back of l. heel, sometimes of r. with pinkish discoloration of it; and shootings up through limb settling in one spot (sacro-sciatic foramen), with aching and heavy drawing across back of neck as if being dragged down; patellæ stiff and snap on bending knees.—R. T. C.)—Burning, gnawing pain in bones of the feet, which does not permit standing or walking.—Paralytic stiffness of instep.—Small epithelial swellings on joints of toes.

24. **Generalities.**—[We are led to the use of this remedy for injuries of the periosteum (as when a fall or an accident injures the periosteum), making it very sore and causing a bruised sensation; when the rectum protrudes from the anus after confinement; prolapsus ani, which may come down every time the bowels are moved; pain as if bruised in the outer parts and in the bones; wounds where the bones are injured; gnawing in the inner parts; affections in general of l. side of head; of the bladder; wrist-joints; lumbar region; bones of the lower extremity; < from lying on painful side; looking fixedly at an object, as in cases of those who have looked closely at watch-making, fine sewing, &c.; from taking uncooked food—H. N. G.].—Contusive pains in limbs, joints, and bones, esp. when touched.—Burning or gnawing pains in periosteum of limbs.—Sensation of soreness of the parts on which one lies.—Pain in long bones as if broken.—Pressive, spasmodic tearings, and drawings in the limbs.—Sensation of fulness in whole body, with obstructed respiration.—Lassitude, weakness, and heaviness in all limbs, esp. when seated, with great restlessness in legs.—Lameness after sprains, esp. the wrists and ankles.—Tottering, unsteady gait, from weakness of thighs.—Sensation in all limbs as if severely beaten, with painful sensibility of sacrum and loins when sitting down after a short walk.—Sensation in head and body as if he had not slept enough.—Knows not where to put his legs on account of restlessness and heaviness, puts them first in one place, then in another, and turns his body from side to side.—Whole body feels as if stuffed full, whereby breathing is impeded.—Cannot bend his body, all joints and hip-bones painful as if bruised.—On touching the painful parts, and esp. hips and thigh-bones, they are painful as if bruised.—Acts specially on yellow elastic tissue (R. T. C.).

25. **Skin.**—Gnawing itching on skin.—Erysipelatous inflammation.—Tendency to excoriation in children, either when walking or riding on horse-

back.—Inflamed ulcers.—Anasarca.—Warts; with sore pains; flat, smooth on palms.

26. Sleep.—Frequent yawning and stretching.—Strong disposition to sleep in evening and after a meal, waking with a start, and piercing cries on least touch.—Nocturnal agitation, with tossing and frequent waking.

27. Fever.—Pulse only accelerated during heat.—Coldness running over one side of head.—Chilliness principally in back and running up and down.—Heat over whole body, mostly in afternoon, without thirst, but with anxiety, restlessness, and dyspnœa.—Heat in face, with red cheeks and cold hands and feet.—Cold perspiration on face in morning in bed.—Perspiration all over when walking in open air.—Shuddering, coldness, and shivering, even when near the fire.—Coldness in hands and feet, with heat in face, confusion in head, and thirst.—General heat with agitation and excessive uneasiness, feeling of suffocation, and pressive headache.—Frequent flushes of heat.

Sabadilla.

Asagræa officinalis. Veratrum officinale. Sabadilla officinarum. Cebadilla. Cevadilla. *N. O.* Melanthaceæ (of the Liliaceæ). Tincture of seeds.

Clinical.—Coryza. Debility. Diphtheria. Dyspepsia; of pregnancy. Earache. Epistaxis. *Hay asthma.* Headache. *Head-lice.* Imaginary diseases. Influenza. Intermittents. Mania. Melancholia. Neuralgia. Œsophagus, stricture of. Rheumatism. Tapeworm. Throat, sore. Toothache. Uvula elongated. Vertigo. Worms.

Characteristics.—*Asagræa* is a Mexican genus belonging to the Colchicum family, Melanthaceæ. It has only one species, *A. officinalis*, which furnishes the Cebadilla seeds from which *Veratrine* is prepared. The seeds were formerly used to destroy vermin (*Treas. of Bot.*). *Saba.* first appears in homœopathic literature as one of Stapf's additions, Hahnemann being one of the provers. Stapf's *Additions* forms a kind of appendix to the *Materia Medica Pura*. The plant, says Stapf, was first described by Monaides about the year 1572. At first it was almost exclusively used for destroying lice, and also worms in putrid ulcers and in the intestines. Stapf points out that the provings reveal remarkable febrile symptoms. *Saba.*, he says, is "not only specific to a certain kind of very bad angina, and to a rare kind of pleurisy where no inflammatory fever nor thirst is present, where the patient complains of coldness mingled with isolated flushes of heat; but also to some forms of fever and ague, where the chilliness sets in with nausea and inclination to vomit, recurs frequently, and sometimes alternates with flushes of heat; where the heat is more perceptible in the face and on the hands than on the rest of the body, with absence of thirst both in the chilly and hot stage." The same authority says that *Saba.* has a long period of action; the primary symptoms develop in the first five days, then recur after the lapse of some time. Symptoms are periodical and paroxysmal. The periodicity of *Saba.* may be as clock-like as that of *Cedr.*, and renders it a leading remedy in intermittent fevers and neuralgias. *Saba.* is a chilly remedy, the symptoms, especially the coryza, being generally < in the open air. The catarrhal symptoms are very severe, and correspond to many cases of hay asthma. I have often relieved cases with *Saba.*, though it does not cure the diathesis. Sore throats characterised by a sensation of a lump or foreign body in the throat, and a *constant necessity to swallow*, I have frequently cured with *Saba.* Kent (*Med. Adv.*, August, 1894) says it is suited to "old, chronic sore throats that are < from cold air. The patient is sensitive to cold air. Every time he takes cold it settles in his nose and throat. Tonsillitis going from left to right." The desire for hot drink distinguishes *Saba.* from *Lach.* The traditional use of *Saba.* as a destroyer of parasites is depicted in the provings: "Violent itching of hairy scalp, compelling her to scratch till blood comes." "Itching of the vertex as if a quantity of vermin had collected there, obliging him to scratch incessantly." "Itching of anus and rectum as from ascarides." "Itching of anus alternating with itching of alæ nasi and meatus auditorius." Kent gave *Saba.* to a pet dog which had great irritation of anus, and soon afterwards he passed a very large number of worms. *Saba.* has an extreme amount of giddiness in its pathogenesis; it may cause staggering and even fainting. Objects seem to whirl round, or to whirl round each other. Stapf had "Vertigo early in the morning after rising." After a dose of *Saba.* in high potency I astonished myself by falling back on the bed with giddiness on rising the following morning. Among the characteristic mental symptoms are: Tendency to be startled. Erroneous impressions as to the state of his body. Imaginary diseases: imagines parts shrunken, &c.; if there is distension from flatus imagines she is pregnant, &c. *Saba.* is intolerant of mental exertion; thinking = headache. Digestion is disordered and the tongue loaded, sinking at stomach and gnawing hunger. *Saba.* corresponds to many forms of indigestion, including that incident to pregnancy. *Peculiar Sensations* are: As if things were turning around each other. As if she would fall if she did not hold on to something. As if eyes went round with the whirling sensation. Lips as if scalded. Tongue as if full of blisters. As if uvula were down. As if œsophagus would be closed. As of a body in throat which he must swallow down. As of a lump in throat. As if a morsel of food had lodged in throat. As of a worm in œsophagus. As if a sore spot was pressed upon. As of a lump in abdomen. As if a ball of thread were moving and turning rapidly through abdomen. As if knives were cutting abdomen. As if abdomen were shrunken; were empty. Croaking as of frogs in abdomen. As of something alive in abdomen. As if stomach were gnawed. As of a thread or string in throat. As if throat were tied with a string. As if articulation were suspended. As if tape prevented circulation in chest. As if interior of bones were scraped out with a sharp knife. As if hot breath came out of his mouth and nose. As if everything were in motion. As if the air itself were in tremulous motion. As if he had taken wine. Shaking as if in a severe chill. As if something sharp in throat. As if a soft body in throat must be constantly swallowed. Pressure on larynx = throat sore. Scratching > itching of scalp; = burning of anus. Lying perfectly still > vertigo. Lying down = cough immediately, < expectoration. Sitting < vertigo. Rising from seat = vertigo. Opening mouth wide = cracking of jaw-joint. Walking = vertigo and afterwards headache; pain in stomach. Getting into sweat when walking < itching of scalp. > Afternoon. Chill 3 p.m. < Morning; and evening. Gastric symptoms < morning. < At new or full moon; at regular periods. Alternating: canine appetite and disgust for meat and sour things; thirstlessness and bulimia with aversion to food. Hot drinks : < toothache ; mouth intolerant of ; craved in sore throat, more easily swallowed. Cold < all symptoms ; < cough. Cold drinks < toothache. Walking in cold air < toothache. Open air : > vertigo ; feels > in ; = lachrymation and spasmodic sneezing. Warm stove > chilliness. When over-heated itching of scalp <. Mental exertion <. Fright = hysterical paroxysms. < From wine. *Saba.* is *suited to :* Persons of light hair, fair complexion, with a weakened, relaxed muscular system. Children. Old people.

Relations.—*Antidoted by :* Camph., Puls., Con. *Follows well :* Bry. (pleurisy). *Followed well by :* Ars., Bell., Merc., Nux. *Compare :* Botan., Verat. alb., Verat. v., Helon. Congestion, Verat. v. Feels > in open air, Puls. Ovaritis, Coloc. Chill in afternoon, Lyc. < From 4 to 8 p.m., Lyc. Imaginary diseases, Thuj. Sensation of something alive in abdomen, Croc., Thuj. ; of machinery, Nit. ac. Effect of mental exertion, Nux, Pic. ac. Fever without thirst, Puls. (with unquenchable thirst, Nat. m.). Attacks at same time every day, Ars., Ced. Hunger in early morning, Aga., Ant. c., Asar., Calc., Carb. a., Chi., Lyc., Mur. ac., Ran. b., Rhus, Zn. Nausea at sight of food, Colch., Lyc. String sensations ; coryza, Cep. (Cep. coryza > out of doors ; Saba. <). Easily startled by noises, Borax. < From wine, Zn. Nervous diseases from worms, Cin., Pso. Worm affections of children, Con., Sil., Spi. Delirium during intermittents. Complaints go left to right, Lach., Lac c. Illusions about his body, Bap. Alcaloid, Veratrin.

Causation.—Fright. Mental exertion. Thinking. Worms.

SYMPTOMS.

1. **Mind.**—Uneasiness and anguish, with great agitation.—Disposition to be frightened.—Startled by noises.—Hysteric paroxysms after fright.—Ill-humour and passion.—Dislike to labour.—Rage.—Difficulty in thinking.—Thinking = headache.—Delusions of the imagination with respect to oneself; the body seems to be collapsed, like that of a corpse, the stomach to be eaten away, &c.—Imaginary diseases.

2. **Head.**—Vertigo, with nausea, > by supporting head.—Vertigo : as if things were turning around him; as if all things were turning round each other; in morning after rising; had to rest his head on the table the whole afternoon to keep off the fainting; more sitting than standing; when going to bed.—Vertigo with fainting and cloudiness of eyes (everything becomes black) on rising from a seat.—Headache with vertigo, > while eyes are fixed steadfastly on an object, and while patient is thinking of one subject.—Headache as if a thread had been drawn from middle of forehead to occiput above temples, leaving a burning sensation behind.—Stupefying headache with coryza, itching, and burning of scalp and general heat of whole body; < in forenoon.—The headache begins in r. side, whence it extends more and more to l.—Corrosive burning point on top of head.—Headache with tensive pain, esp. during intellectual labour.—Headache, esp. after every walk; after eating.—Hemicrania with tænia.—Pressive and stupefying headache in forehead and temples.—Painful heaviness of head.—Boring pains in head after taking exercise.—Pulsative and painful throbbing in head.—Burning, tingling, and

pricking in forehead and scalp (as from lice).—Burning, crawling itching on hairy scalp and forehead, > from scratching, < from getting into a sweat when walking.—Forehead covered with cold sweat.

3. **Eyes.**—Burning smarting in eyes.—Pressure on eyeballs, esp. when looking up.—Redness of margins of eyelids.—Lachrymation, esp. during exercise in open air, when looking at anything bright, when coughing, yawning, and on feeling the slightest pain in other parts.—Weakness of sight.

4. **Ears.**—Otalgia with troublesome pressure; with snapping as of electric sparks before ears.—Tickling in ears.—Itching at anus alternately with itching at meatus auditorius externus.—Burning itching and shootings in tips of ears.—Deafness as if there were a band over ears.—Humming, gurgling, and detonation in ears.—Boring in parotids.

5. **Nose.**—Itching tingling in nose and contractive smarting.—Epistaxis.—Great sensibility to smell of garlic.—Sensitive dryness of upper part of nose.—Violent spasmodic sneezing (shaking the abdomen, then lachrymation).—Obstruction of nostrils, alternately.—Fluent coryza with altered features and bewildered head (influenza; hay-fever).—Great masses of white and transparent mucus are blown from nose, without coryza.—Bright red blood comes from posterior nares and is expectorated.

6. **Face.**—Heat of face with fiery redness, esp. after drinking wine.—Blue circles round the eyes.—Marbled and herpetic skin on the face, burning sensation, pain as from excoriation, pricking and itching tingling in lips.—Beating and jerking in muscles of l. upper jaw, with itching.—Boring in lower jaw and submaxillary glands.—Cracking of the articulation of the jaw on opening mouth wide.

7. **Teeth.**—Toothache with drawing and pulsative pain.—Shooting pains in molars.—Caries of teeth.—Gums bluish.—Pricking in gums.

8. **Mouth.**—Sensation in mouth and on tongue as if they were burnt and excoriated.—Cannot bear anything hot in mouth.—Tongue feels sore as if full of blisters.—Pricking (soreness) in tip of tongue.—Tip of the tongue bluish.—Tongue loaded with a thick yellowish coating (more in middle and at back).—Dryness of the mouth without thirst.—Copious accumulation of (sweetish) saliva in the mouth.—Jelly-like saliva.

9. **Throat.**—Pain in the throat as if caused by a plug or an internal swelling during deglutition and at other times.—Constantly obliged to swallow, with pain in mouth and behind larynx as if something lodged there, with scratching roughness; hawks constantly, < morning and during and after eating.—Sensation of a skin hanging loosely in throat, must swallow over it; as if uvula were down.—Much tough phlegm in throat, must hawk.—Feeling of constriction in the throat (in fauces as from an astringent drink).—Can swallow warm food more easily, in sore throat.—Pressure and burning sensation in throat during deglutition and at other times.—Dryness in throat.—Roughness and scraping in throat, with continued want to swallow or to hawk.—Inflammation of uvula.

10. **Appetite.**—Taste bitter (or of a sickly sweetness).—Violent thirst for cold water, milk, or beer, also in morning.—Hunger, with dislike to all food, esp. meat (coffee, wine, and acids).—Bulimy esp. in morning and evening (principally for honey, pastry, and farinaceous food).—Thirstlessness or thirst only in evening for cold water.—Craves hot things, hot tea (in sore throat).

11. **Stomach.**—Risings, generally empty, and sometimes with shuddering.—Painful and imperfect risings.—Pyrosis.—Corrosive burning pain in stomach and œsophagus; when walking.—Coldness in stomach.—Empty feeling in stomach.—Nausea with inclination to vomit, often with shuddering, > by eating.—Nausea; with constant spitting of insipid water.—Nausea, retching, and feeling of worm in œsophagus.—Vomiting of lumbrici.—Softness, uneasiness, and coldness in stomach.—Digging in epigastric region, with pains as from excoriation (as if a sore spot were pressed below pit of stomach), when pressing upon it (and on inspiration).—A frequent sudden sensation of obstructed respiration in scrobiculus, with anxiety.—Sensation of heat in scrobiculus and burning in stomach.

12. **Abdomen.**—Pressive scraping in hepatic region.—Digging drawing in liver, with pain as from excoriation when pressing upon it.—Sensation of heat in hepatic region.—Colicky pain in abdomen as if caused by worms (or from actual worms).—Constriction in abdomen.—Turning and twisting through whole abdomen as from a lump.—Cuttings as by knives.—Colic: with sensation as if a ball were moving and turning through abdomen, cries out, "Oh! my bowels, they go like a wheel"; with violent urging to stool and borborygmus; from worms.—Violent shootings in sides of abdomen, which force the patient to bend double.—Boring, digging, and rolling in abdomen.—Rumbling in abdomen, as if empty.—Croaking as of frogs in abdomen.—Sensation of coldness or burning in abdomen.—Spasmodic contraction of muscles of abdomen; of l. side, with burning pain; he bent double on l. side.—Red spots and specks on abdomen.

13. **Stool and Anus.**—Constipation.—Broken, hard, scanty stools.—Very difficult stools with much burning in abdomen and sensation as if something alive in abdomen.—Urgent want to evacuate, with scanty evacuation.—Loose brown or fermented fæces, mixed with mucus and blood (floating on the water).—Pinchings, tearing, and tingling in rectum.—Crawling in rectum and anus as from ascarides.—Itching of anus, violent burning after scratching.—Itching of anus, alternating with itching of nose or ear.—Discharges of worms (lumbrici, tapeworm).

14. **Urinary Organs.**—Urgent want to urinate, esp. in evening, with tenesmus and scanty emission.—Increased secretion of urine.—Turbid, thick urine, like clay-water.—Burning in urethra when urinating.

15. **Male Sexual Organs.**—Digging and pressive pain in testes.—Diminished sexual desire.—Tensive and painful erections, without desire for coition.—Pollutions, with flaccidity of penis.

16. **Female Sexual Organs.**—Catamenia: retarded but profuse, and of longer duration; flow by fits and starts; painful bearing down a few days previous.—Cutting pain as from knives in ovary (ovaritis).—Nymphomania from ascarides.

17. **Respiratory Organs.**—Hot breath.—Hoarse, rough voice.—Hawking up of bright red blood, which comes from the nasal fossæ.—Short, dry cough, also at night, provoked by a scraping in throat.—Cough dry, with perspiration and water in the eyes.—Cough with vomiting, shootings in vertex, and pain in stomach.—Dull cough, sometimes with hæmoptysis.—Cough immediately on lying down.—Cough with expectoration and lancinations in chest.

18. **Chest.**—Respiration obstructed, as if there were a stone in the chest. —Short, difficult respiration.—Wheezing respiration.—Pressure on the chest. —Burning sensation in the chest.—Pain from r. (sometimes l.) shoulder into chest as if circulation of blood arrested by a tight bandage; not > by unastening dress; < in open air.—Shootings in sides of chest, esp. when drawing breath and coughing, which disturbs the sleep at night and does not permit lying on the side.—(Inflammation of pleura.)—Red spots and points on chest.

19. **Heart.**—Palpitation of heart with pulsation throughout body.

20. **Back.**—Contusive pain in back and loins, esp. when seated.—Burning-ingling stinging sensation between scapulæ.—Stitches in rapid succession in . side of back.

21. **Limbs.**—Weariness and heaviness in all the limbs, < towards evening, obliging her to lie down.—Coldness of the limbs.—Painful drawings n limbs as if in marrow of bones, with inclination to stretch limbs, > by epose.—Painful sensation of paralysis of the limbs, esp. in knees.

22. **Upper Limbs.**—Convulsive movements of arms.—Trembling of arms and hands.—Red spots, bands, and points on arms and hands.—Pricking ancinations in forearms.—Dryness of skin of hands.—Distortion of fingers.—Yellow spots on fingers.—Desquamation of skin round nails.

23. **Lower Limbs.**—Shootings in thighs and knees.—Weakness and lexion of knees.—Tearing and tension in calves of legs, also at night.—Heaviness of feet.—Swelling of feet, with painful sensibility of soles.—Profuse perspiration on soles.

24. **Generalities.**—[Intermittent complaints which come every week, or wo weeks, or four weeks apart.—Esp. suited for children who are disposed o worms; worms discharged with stool, whether lumbrici or tapeworms.—Sweetish taste.—No thirst during chill; heat often internal.—Troubles ppearing on the r. side; on toenails.—Sensation of knocking, throbbing, or pulsation in the outer parts; great sleepiness in the forenoon.—< in forenoon; before midnight; from cold in general; while resting.—> From moving; while swallowing something; while getting warm; from warmth in general.—Many complaints appear, esp. during the new and full moon.—H. N. G.]—Pricking, pressive, and dull lancinations in different parts.—Tingling in the imbs.—Twitchings, convulsive tremblings, or catalepsy from worms.—Nervous diseases from worms or deeply seated abdominal irritation.—Great debility; n intermittents; paralytic debility in pleuritis.—Convulsions.—Heaviness of head and of movements generally.—Lassitude and heaviness in all limbs, < evening, or towards noon, at which times the pains in the limbs are also <.—n general, < at same hour every day.—Pains in the bones, as if caused by ome one cutting and scraping inside with a knife, esp. in the joint; < by ouch, > by a quick movement of the part affected.—The patient feels better when lying down than when walking or standing; in the open air.—Several symptoms appear first on the r. and then on the l. side.—Great sensibility to cold air, which < the uneasiness and pains.

25. **Skin.**—Parchment-like dryness of skin.—Tingling and burning hootings under skin.—Red bands, spots, and points in different parts of skin, ppearing with greatest intensity in cold air.

26. **Sleep.**—Great inclination to sleep during day, with continued yawn-

ing and stretching.—Sleep retarded by a multitude of thoughts.—Imperfect sleep in evening, with mental fatigue from wandering thoughts.—Agitated and unrefreshing sleep at night, with anxious dreams.—In the morning he starts up from his sleep as from a fright.

27. **Fever.**—Pulse small but spasmodic.—Sensation as if the circulation were suspended.—Chilliness in evening always at same hour; frequently not followed by heat; the chills run up the body.—Heat principally in head and face, often interrupted by chilliness, always returning at same hour.—Fever without thirst, manifested only by chilliness, with intermittent heat, which is more perceptible in the face and hands than in other parts of body.—Hot perspiration in face with coldness of rest of body.—Intermittent fever which returns at same hour; chill, then thirst, then thirst with headache.—Shivering or external coldness and trembling of limbs without shivering, and with more violent thirst or complete adipsia; afterwards heat with moderate thirst, accompanied or followed by perspiration.—In the morning hours perspiration.—During the shivering pain in upper ribs, dry, spasmodic cough, and tearing in all the limbs and bones.—Delirium, yawning, and stretching during the heat.—Sleep during the perspiration.—Quotidian, tertian, quartan fever at regular intervals, with anorexia, pressive inflation of stomach, pains in chest, cough, shivering, weakness and thirst between the shiverings and the heat.—Thirst only between hot and cold stage.—Fever where the gastric symptoms prevail, with dry, convulsive cough in cold stage (quartan ague).—During the apyrexia painful weariness of the limbs without any other symptom.

Sabal Serrulata.

Serenoa serrulata. Saw Palmetto. (Sandy soils of sea coast South Carolina to Florida; most luxuriant nearest the sea.) *N. O.* Palmaceæ. (1) Tincture of fresh ripe berries and seeds, all crushed and macerated in 90 per cent. alcohol for fourteen days and decanted (Hale). (2) Fluid Extract, "probably four times stronger than the tincture" (Hale). [C. S. Estep (*Am. Hom.*, xxvi. 133) uses a dark-green Fluid Extract which is made from the fresh green berries, and is "almost as green as grass and has an oily surface." He makes his dilutions from this. Other preparations have disappointed him.] (3) Oil (prepared from the expressed juice of the fruit by allowing it to stand a few days). (4) Saccharated Oil (one part of the oil to seven parts of cane sugar). (5) Malted Sabal (one part of the Oil to seven of Maltine). (6) Aqua Olei Sabal (a preparation suggested by Hale made by triturating gtt. xvi. of the Oil with Mag. carb. ʒj, gradually adding a pint of distilled water and decanting. For use as a spray).

Clinical.—Appendicitis. Asthma, catarrhal. Atrophic pharyngitis. Atrophic rhinitis. Atrophy. Backache. Breasts, inflamed; painful; atrophy of. Bronchitis. Catarrh. Cystitis. Dysmenorrhœa. Dysuria. Enuresis. Glands, affections of. Gleet. Gonorrhœa. Headache. Hoarseness. Impotence. Innutrition. Iritis. Lactation, defects of. Laryngitis, catarrhal. Lumbago. Menses, delayed.

Jeuralgia. Neurasthenia. Obesity. Ovaries, affections of. Peritonitis. Phthisis. Proctitis. *Prostate, enlarged;* affections of. Puerperal fever. School-headache. Sterility. Strangury. Testes, atrophy of. Throat, sore; catarrhal. Urine, incontinence of. Uterus, affections of; misplacements of; tumours of. Whooping-cough.

Characteristics.—In his little book entitled *Saw Palmetto*, Hale has put together most of our available knowledge respecting his plant. It is a dwarf palm with creeping (or leaning), branching tem, the edges of leaf and petioles serrate, roots fibrous, large, half exposed. The fruit (so-called "berry") is a one-seeded drupe about the ize of an olive, dark purple when ripe, and ripening in October and November. The branching spadices form large pendulous panicles. When eaten the taste is at first exceedingly sweet, but in a few econds this is followed by an acrid, pungent sensation that spreads o fauces, nasal mucous membrane, and larynx. This is in turn succeeded by a feeling of smoothness as if the parts had been coated with oil. The seeds are enveloped in a tough, fibrous membrane, are ery hard, and when cut show a white, oily substance, which burns with a blue flame, giving off an odour of roasted coffee. The fruit is icher in sugar than sugar-cane, and contains two oils, one volatile nd one fixed. The volatile oil is considered to possess the most haracteristic properties of the medicine. Hale describes it as yellow," but he quotes John Uri Lloyd, of Cincinnati, as writing to im, "The principal constituent is a volatile oil. This oil possesses a *eep green* colour." And he goes on to say that the colour is not ue to chlorophyll nor to the copper of the worm used in condensing . This agrees with Estep's contention that the preparation of *Sabal* hould be *dark-green* or *grass-green*. The preparation Estep used was a 'luid Extract prepared by Burrough Brothers, of Baltimore, from the fresh green berries." (Hale directs that the fresh *ripe* berries should e used.) The preparation used by Dr. Mullin's prover was made by Boericke and Tafel. All are agreed that preparations of the dried ruit and of the root-bark do not possess the curative powers of the emedy. While on a hunting trip through the wilds of Florida Hale bserved the great fattening properties of the berries on animals. During summer food is scanty, and the wild animals become very hin, but as soon as the Palmetto fruit ripens they improve rapidly, nd in a few weeks have put on so much fat that they become an asy prey to the hunter. This fat, says Hale, "consists principally of lein, and will not make lard." *Sabal serrulata* was introduced into medicine by J. B. Read and A. A. Solomons, both of Savannah, Georgia. Read gave a "Saccharated oil," of which he says: "By its peculiar oothing power over the mucous membranes it produces sleep and elieves the most troublesome coughs, promotes expectoration, improves digestion, and increases fat, flesh, and strength. It has been sed with benefit in cardiac asthma, phthisis, especially laryngeal, hronic bronchitis, and dilatation of the bronchial tubes. Its action n catarrhal affections is rapid and permanent. A cold in the head may be checked with two or three doses (of the saccharated oil) mixed with boiling water, and used by inhalation it has been found eneficial in chronic ozæna." Dr. Will Scott Mullins, of Louisville, Kentucky, published the first proving made for him by a former student of his, Miss Annie Roask. This prover is described as a very intelligent lady of twenty-three, mediumly developed, small breasts, red hair, blue eyes, 5 feet 7 inches in height, weight, 109 pounds, bust measure 32 inches. These details are important, as this prover developed some of the most characteristic effects of the drug, especially those of the mammary glands, and at the end of the proving (from December 8th to March 1st) her breasts had increased fully one-third in size, and her bust measure was $33\frac{1}{2}$ inches, and her weight $119\frac{1}{2}$ pounds. This prover had also many symptoms in the head and ovaries. Her symptoms are for the most part not distinguished from the others in the Schema, but when I have wished to distinguish them I have appended the letter (R). Another remarkable proving by a woman is that of Dr. Freda M. Langton, of Omaha, Nebraska. Her symptoms, when distinguished, have the letter (L) appended. Mind, bladder, ovaries, and uterus were all strongly affected in her case. One symptom she developed was an irritability and depression ; and sympathy did not merely < as with *Nat. m.*, it *made her angry.* (This condition of mind was present in one of the prostatic cases cured by *Sbl.*) Dr. Langton relates that she was unable to find an antidote, and suffered for three months after the proving before she found one. In searching for a remedy for a case of dysmenorrhœa she found the leading symptoms under *Silic.*, and it struck her that the symptoms of *Silic.* corresponded to her own symptoms. She took it twice daily, and was better in two hours. In three days all the bladder and ovarian trouble was gone. *Sil.* was also given to the dysmenorrhœa patient, but only partially relieved. *Sbl.* was then given, and quickly and permanently cured. *Sbl.* was proved by two men, Dr. R. Boocock, and an unmarried prover whose symptoms are given by Hale (*H. R.*, xiii. 103). Both experienced well-marked symptoms in the genito-urinary sphere, including increased sexual power. I have marked some of Boocock's symptoms (B). Hale's prover had this urinary symptom, which he justly says may prove a valuable indication : " Fears to fall asleep lest something should happen ; starts up with this fear as he is dozing." In all the provings the ϕ tincture, or Fluid Extract, were used in from 5- to 10-drop doses, repeated two or three times a day ; and in the clinical use of the remedy a similar dosage has been adopted. *Sbl.* is an organ remedy of great power, selecting the uterus and prostatic gland (which is the male analogue of the uterus), ovaries and testes and bladder. But the provings are sufficiently detailed to warrant closer homœopathising, and Dr. Langton says that though she gives 5-drop doses four times daily in cases of over-worked brain and school-headache for the " tonic, nutritive, and stimulating" effect of the remedy she gives the 1 x as soon as relief has been obtained, and she finds that the dilution often gives greater relief in the headaches than the larger doses. Mullins also says (*H. R.*, xii. 68) : " I now found the use of the drug in the 3rd and 6th attenuation curative in nearly all of the diseases of the uterus and appendages. Also in headache from reflexed uterine troubles, in mammary abscess, mental irritations, and nervous debility. It is indeed an anti-lean, and well deserves the name of "The Homœopathic Catheter." But, he adds, it must be given on its individual indications. W. E. Reily published (*Hahn. Adv.*, December, 1898) these cases illustrating the prostatic action of *Sbl.*: (1) Mr. J., 56, very despondent; irritable. Sympathy seemed to anger him. Great tenesmus in neck of bladder, with heavy, aching pains, with *sense of coldness extending into external genitals.* Occasional sharp pains extending up into abdomen and down into thighs. Appetite capricious. Constipation chronic. Urination too frequent, disturbing sleep. *Sbl.* ϕ was given, five drops night and morning. Steady improvement followed, and in eight weeks all the symptoms had gone, and with them an annoying eczema of the hands. (2) Mr. M., 45, for a year had gradually increasing frequency of micturition. Despondent; distressed. Appetite capricious. Vertex headache and gastric catarrh. Little sexual desire; coitus followed by digging pain in back and tenesmus of bladder with difficulty in commencing to urinate. Genitals cold, dull aching in region of prostate, extending to abdomen and thighs. *Sbl.* ϕ gradually relieved and cured in three weeks. (3) Mr. E., 35. Frequent urination for 1½ years. Heavy, dragging pains, extending into back and thighs; *back pains much* < *after coitus.* Considerable loss of prostatic fluid at times. Sexual desire much impeded. Severe headache on vertex and gastric catarrh. All symptoms removed by *Sbl.* ϕ. Hale says E. S. Evans, of Columbus, Ohio, considers *Sbl.* "almost specific in iritis when the prostate gland is involved. I have cured cases with the 3x which could not be relieved in any other way." (This is a noteworthy observation. The connection between gonorrhœa and syphilis and the eye is well known, and I have known several cases of ophthalmia develop in patients who were taking another prostatic remedy, *Solidago virgaurea*, for their trouble.) A. L. Davidson (*H. R.*, x. 525) relates a case of impotence in a man, 51, who had difficult micturition, tenderness of prostatic portion of urethra, loss of power, testicles shrunk, penis shrunk and cold. *Sbl.* ϕ, gtt. xv., four times a day, was prescribed. At the end of the first week he complained of drawing pains in spermatic cords, there was freer flow of urine; he slept better and felt better. At the end of the second week the testes were gradually increasing in size, tenderness of urethra had nearly disappeared, and erections were established. In two weeks more the cure was complete, the testes were even larger and firmer than normal. J. Martin Kershaw, of St. Louis, treated a young lady of twenty-three who had had great difficulty in controlling her urine all her life. Undue exertion, lifting, straining, laughing, caused it to dribble away. Unless she rose several times in the night she was sure to wet the bed. *Sbl.* ϕ, gtt. i., four times a day, was given. In one month she was much improved, and under the same remedy she gradually got quite well. Elias C. Price reports these cases. (1) Very nervous lady with chronic inflammation of bladder, frequent painful urination, ten to twelve times in the night and every fifteen to thirty minutes during the day. Spells of pressing pain on rectum, > by warm water enemas, which generally brought away hardened fæces. *Lil. t.* 3x removed this temporarily. Rectal examination disclosed a hard fleshy tumour the size of half a hen's egg on the posterior aspect of the uterus. *Sbl.* (Fluid Extract) gtt. v., thrice daily, diminished the tumour by half in two months, and removed it entirely in three more. (2) Mrs. X., primapara, had, five days after confinement, irritation of kidneys, and a week later symptoms of pelvic peritonitis. Uterus much enlarged, very tender. Did not urinate very often, but when she did the pain was so excruciating that she fainted away, and sometimes did not come to for an hour. For three days no remedy did any good. Then she had violent pain right side of head above and behind the ear, and paralysis of left arm and leg; became unconscious and could not be aroused; at times would talk of things which had occurred before her illness; insensible to external impressions. She remained thus ten days. *Sbl.* (Fluid Extract), gtt. xx., every two hours, relieved the pain on being raised to urinate after the second dose. Recovery from the other condition was very gradual. (3) Miss X., 22, had had irregular menses for years, having once gone nine months without a period. When she came to Price she was three months past her time; *one breast was much smaller than the other*. *Sbl.* (Fluid Extract), gtt. v., thrice daily. In about a month the menses came on freely, lasted four days instead of the usual two. Breasts began to increase in size. In three months one was as large as the other. The following year she again missed her time, and *Sbl.* brought it right in a week. Price has cured with *Sbl.* cases of pelvic cellulitis, peritonitis, puerperal fever, inflammation of uterus, tubes, ovaries, and even appendicitis; and proctitis, especially if the prostatic gland is involved. Showerman gave Hale a summary of his experience with *Sbl.*: (1) A lady who had been for two years unable to rise in the morning without a cup of coffee and something to eat was cured with *Sbl.* in a week. (2) An impotent man was cured in thirty days. (3) Man, 76, enlarged prostate, had to use catheter for three years. Cured in four months. (4) Man passing blood with urine for six months: cured in two weeks. (5) Cases of incontinence. (6) A lady to whom he gave *Sbl.* for nervous debility had to discontinue it because "her sexual passions made her almost furious" from its use. (7) In catarrhal affections he found it very efficacious, and he cured himself with it in four months of a bronchial trouble of seven years' duration which no medicine had relieved before.—Mullins confirms the value of *Sbl.* in catarrhal states, which is one of the uses the remedy was put to by Read, who introduced it. Mullins says: "In chronic bronchitis, with a wheezing, hard cough, < on lying down till 6 a.m., < in damp, cool air and cloudy weather, it is promptly curative." The fattening properties of *Sbl.* have been utilised in medicine. For this purpose it has been given in the form of *Saccharated oil* (gr. x. to gr. lx.) or *Sabal Maltine*. The *Aqua Sabal* Hale found useful as a spray. The symptoms are < in early morning; from rising to bedtime. < By motion. > After sleep. Backache < after coitus. Catarrhal symptoms are < in cold, damp weather. Cough < on lying down at night. < Before menses (depression). Stinging pains appear to be characteristic. Wandering, radiating, and cramping pains were also prominent. *Sbl.* has several groups of associated regions of pain: pains affecting head and ovary; ovaries and breasts; lower back and right temple; prostate and eye.

Relations.—*Antidoted by:* Sil. (Sbl. grows on the sandy shore);

Puls. (delayed menses ; Puls. also grows on sandy soils). *Compare :* Stinging pains in ovaries, Apis, Merc. Pain in right ovary and thigh, Apis. Breasts painful, Con., Calc. School-headaches ; < by sympathy, Nat. m. (Sbl. is most fruitful nearest the sea ; compare Sil. marina). Prostatic affections, Fe. pic., Cham., Arg. n., Dig., Solid. Prostate and eye, Solid. < From coition, K. ca. Wandering pains, K. bi. (the roots of Sbl. are very rich in potash salts). Over-worked women, Mg. c. Hale classes *Sbl.* with remedies "primarily aphrodisiac"—Pho., Turn. aph., Nux, Orig., Coca, Aur., Can. i., Plat., Lil., Santal. ; "primarily anaphrodisiacs" according to him being—Con., Sal. n., Salicin., Agn., Nuph., Ars., Pic. ac., Calad., Camph., Iod., Lupulin.

SYMPTOMS.

1. **Mind.**—Unusual, full, confused sensation ; thinking difficult ; cannot grasp or remember what is read.—Irritability ; impatience ; fretfulness.—Immutability with indifference to wants of others ; mind self-concentrated on her own sufferings, wants to be left alone.—Broods on her symptoms.—Sympathy makes her angry.—Wants to go away and die alone.—Fearfully blue and low down before menses.

2. **Head.**—Vertigo with headache (from fumes of oil).—Severe headache with giddiness and dim vision.—Sharp, darting pain coming and going suddenly (like *Bell.*), now here now there in sides, top, and back of head, through eyes and in temples.—Shooting pains in temples and across forehead.—Soon after rising a very sharp pain in l. temple ; pain across forehead to both temples, < r. ; vague aching on vertex ; pain r. temple running across vertex to l.—Sharp pain in either r. or l. temple, running up across forehead, with pain in l. ovary and uterus ; severe pain in l. temple and a sharp pain on vertex.—Dull, aching pain in r. temple and on vertex, almost unbearable by 3 p.m.—Pain running up from nose and centring in forehead.—Pain and irritation at base of brain and upper third of cervical spine (like that of *Gels.*).—Sensation as if something tightening in brain.—(Neuralgic pains before and after catarrhal attacks.)

3. **Eyes.**—(Iritis when the prostate gland is involved.)

4. **Ears.**—(Chronic inflammation of middle ear.)—Fulness in nose and ears, only bits of dry crumbling wax got away on picking.—Frequent sharp, stitch-like pains inward from ears.—Hearing diminished ; voices seem far off (B.—proving discontinued in consequence).

5. **Nose.**—Pain running up from nose and centring in forehead.—Sneezing and lachrymation, coughing and gagging.—Fulness in nostrils compelling him to pick them, only dry crumbs came away.

6. **Face.**—Papular eruption on l. temple and about mouth.—Slight neuralgia in r. temple and r. jaw.—Pallor.

8. **Mouth.**—Pungent burning sensation in mouth and fauces, extending up and down and causing sneezing, coughing, and gagging ; afterwards smooth, numb feeling, as if mouth coated with fat.—Burning on tongue as if scalded.

9. **Throat.**—Sharp pain in l. side of throat.—Pungent, burning sensation in fauces ; followed by smooth sensation, as if coated with oil.

11. **Stomach.**—Appetite good throughout proving.—Appetite poor and capricious.—Constant desire for milk (usually disliked).—Belching and acidity.—Sharp pain running through stomach; severe pain in l. side of stomach.—Irritation of stomach.—Acute gastritis; fearful burning as from *Sulphuric acid;* could not take meat, vegetable, or pudding, only bread and milk; > by *Robin.* 3 (B).

12. **Abdomen.**—Suddenly most intense, cramp-like pain through abdomen; soon radiated in different directions, to legs, stomach, then to ovaries, where it settled.—Stinging pains running up l. side of abdomen.—Sharp pains running up and down front of abdomen, and also r. side.

13. **Stool and Anus.**—Stools unusually easy; free from hæmorrhoidal troubles (to which the prover—Boocock—was subject).—(Some return of hæmorrhoids with dryness of stool and pressure from within out.—Stools dark, almost black—B.)

14. **Urinary Organs.**—Painful urination; connected with ovarian pain (L).—Tenesmus as in cystitis, a few drops of blood voided on one or two occasions (L).—Feeling as if bladder too full; starting the flow was painful as if forced through very narrow meatus (B).—Feeling as of a stricture about two inches down urethra (B).—Pain extending from bladder up above pubes, with a radiating pain across epigastrium, stitching in region of l. kidney, severe headache with giddiness and dim vision (B).—Scalding on passing water, burning smarting after; slight gluing of meatus and twisted stream (all removed in the proving, stream larger and stronger, no longer required to rise at night—B).—Pain or irritation in region of kidneys; later a trace of albumen and a few renal cells.—Excruciating pain and fainting on being raised up to urinate (cured in a puerperal case).

15. **Male Sexual Organs.**—Slight irritation of prostate.—Some increase of sexual power.—Great excitement first two days and throughout proving; discharge of prostatic fluid.—Amorous feelings, firm erections but fully under control; testes very warm; slight itching deep in perinæum (sperm ducts ?), > by deep pressure.—Increased power and enjoyment in coitus.—Semen feels thick and flows slowly, but causes a hot feeling along the cord.—Testicles tightly drawn up, almost painfully (one of the most prominent and constant symptoms—B).—Sense of coldness extending into external genitals; sharp pain extending up into abdomen; tenesmus, frequent micturition; despondent, irritable, sympathy = anger; constipation, enlarged prostate (*Sabal* φ cured and removed at same time a distressing eczema of hands).—(Coldness of external genitals, dull aching in prostate extending into abdomen.)—(Pain in back much < after coitus.)—Drawing pains in spermatic cords; shrunk testes increase in size.—Hard erection, slight twisting chordee as if stretched from the root.

16. **Female Sexual Organs.**—Furious sexual passion.—Awakened by stinging pain running up from l. ovary into abdomen, and also a sharp pain in r. ovary.—Slight stinging pain in l. ovary at 2 p.m.—Sharp pain in r. ovary, running down r. thigh.—Stinging pain in uterus.—Stinging pain in r. ovary.—A tense, slightly heavy feeling over womb.—Pain in l. ovary, running down the thigh.—Menses delay four days; nine days.—Sore feeling in l. ovary.—Pain in l. ovary after going to bed.—Slight pain low down over womb.—Awakened by a most distressing itching of labia majora.—Pain in l. ovary

nd uterus, coming and going between 2 and 7 p.m.—Sore, heavy feeling in terus until bedtime.—Intense pain through abdomen radiated down into gs, up towards stomach, then to ovaries, where it settled ; never knew the xact location of the ovaries before ; painful urination was added on awaking ext day ; mental indifference with irritability (L).—(Uterine tumour.)—reasts increase in size ; pains in.—(Defective lactation.)—In nursing woman, or four months after confinement, stinging pain in both breasts, < r., commencing at nipple and extending into and pervading entire gland about fteen minutes after child had been at breast ; caused excessively nervous ate and affected whole body ; *Helon.* relieved somewhat, *Sabal* ϕ cured in vo days.

17. **Respiratory Organs.**—Voice changed, throat feels husky.

18. **Chest.**—Sharp pain in l. side of chest, running through l. mamma.—reasts quite tender from pressure, stinging soreness after cold bath.—reasts feel swollen and sore for many days.—Very sharp pains in mammary lands.—Itching of breasts (l.).—Breasts increased fully one-third in size (in ss than three months—R.)

20. **Back.**—Aching across lower part of back.—Deep pains in back, low own.—Fearful backache, low down, before and at commencement of menses. -Pain in back much < after coitus (prostatic case).

22. **Upper Limbs.**—(Annoying eczema of hands.)

23. **Lower Limbs.**—Sharp pain running down right thigh ; third day. -Sharp pain in r. thigh ; fourth day.—Pain running down l. thigh ; second ay.—Sharp pain in r. thigh ; second day.—Aching in calf of r. leg ; seventh ay.—Aching in l. knee and calf of leg ; first day, which continued until bedme.—Pains frequently in l. thigh ; fourth day.

24. **Generalities.**—A feeling of buoyancy all the time notwithstanding e pains.—Increased feeling of vitality and strength all the time the medicine as taken, and for a week after felt as if a stimulant had been taken from her).—Much nervous erethism, cannot keep quiet.—Weakness.—(Poorly ourished women.—Neuralgia of all kinds.—Feeble patients.—" Anti-lean.") -All pains were < in early morning ; or from noon until bedtime.—Pains in aries or uterus, < on motion.—Character of pains mostly sharp and stinging. -Most pains > by sleep.—An uncomfortable feeling all over the body ; third ay.

25. **Skin.**—Papular eruption on face.—(Annoying eczema of hands.)

26. **Sleep.**—Fears to fall asleep lest something (undefined danger) should appen ; starts up with this fear as he is dozing.—Awakened by stinging ains in both ovaries ; second day.—Awakened at 5 a.m. by a severe stinging r. ovary ; fifth day.—Awakened at 1 a.m. by a most distressing itching of bia majora ; eighth day.

Sabina.

Juniperus sabina. Savin. *N. O.* Coniferæ. Tincture of the youn
fresh tops of the branches. Tincture of the oil.

Clinical.—Abortion ; after-effects of. After-pains. Boils. *Condylomata.* Cy titis. Dysmenorrhœa. Gonorrhœa. *Gout.* Inter-menstrual flow. *Leucorrhœ. Menstruation, excessive. Miscarriage.* Moles, promotes expulsion of. Nephriti Nymphomania. Ovaries, affections of. Penis, cartilaginous swelling on. Phimosi Retained placenta. *Rheumatic gout.* Strangury. Sycosis. Toothache. *Uteru bleeding from.*

Characteristics.—Stapf made the first collection of the sympton of *Sabina*, and Hahnemann and his son were among the provers. number of observations on women who had taken the drug to brin on the menses or procure abortion have also been added ; and som cases of fatal poisoning are on record. *Sbi.* acts as a widesprea irritant, inflaming the pyloric end of duodenum and causing patch of inflammation in other portions of the intestines, especially the upp intestines, the omentum and peritoneum (R. T. C.). The action of *Sb* on the generative organs of both sexes is pronounced. It produces fi warts with itching and burning of the external genitals, phimosis the male, swelling of the dorsum of the penis, gonorrhœa ; in th female uterine hæmorrhages, and in the case of pregnant wome abortion. The hæmorrhage is partly pale red and partly clotted, from the least motion ; but may be > by walking. The flow is paroxysms, and is accompanied by labour-like pains. A gra characteristic of *Sbi.* is a pain from sacrum to pubis, and this will a guiding symptom in a large number of the uterine cases requiri *Sbi.* Other characteristics are : (1) discharge of blood between th periods with sexual excitement ; and (2) obscure abdominal pains d to inflammatory states of the peritoneum. In the mental sphere the is much irritability, hysteria, and hypochondriasis, and a peculi feature of it is that music is intolerable ; it produces numbness ar goes through bone and marrow. A close botanic ally of *Thuja*, *S* is yet not too close to be complementary to that great anti-sycoti broad condylomata, fig-warts with much itching and exuberant gran lations are characteristic. Like *Thuja*, it removes wart-like growt from the muco-cutaneous surfaces. It is *suited to :* chronic ailmen of women ; arthritic pains ; tendency to miscarriage ; to the gou diathesis. *Peculiar Sensations* are : As if she would fall. As if parts temporal eminence were pressed asunder. As if skin had grown fa in forehead. As if eyes would be pressed out. As if tooth wou burst. As if he had to swallow over a foreign body. As of a lun in throat. As if vomiting would come on. As if something alive abdomen. Right shoulder-joint as if sprained. *Sbi.* is one of th remedies which affect the heels. Farrington says it is *suited* "plethoric women who suffer from what they call rheumatic infla mation" of the heels. There is an "intermittent aching" in the sol part of the heels. Intermittence and a paroxysmal character a a leading feature with *Sbi.* Pains are paroxysmal and labour-like Hæmorrhage comes in gushes. Suddenly increasing and slowly disappearing pain. The symptoms are < by touch, though pressure >. The dysmenorrhœa pains were > lying on flat of back with limbs extended. < Stooping ; sitting bent ; letting limbs hang down ; motion. Walking > metrorrhagia. Lies on left side during sleep. < Evening, night, and morning. Sleepless and restless after midnight. < In warm air or room. < Warm in bed. > In open air. (Warmth > pain of dysmenorrhœa). Cold applications > wandering pains in joints. < By music. < Taking a deep breath ; > exhaling.

Relations.—*Antidoted by :* Puls. *Complementary to :* Thuj. *Compatible :* Ars., Bell., Rhus, Spo. *Compare :* < By music, Ambr., Thu., Sep. Inter-menstrual flow, Ham., Ambr. Condylomata, Thu., Nit. ac. Hæmorrhage < from least motion, Sec. Menses partly fluid, partly clotted, Fer. Retained placenta, Caul., Sec. Promotes expulsion of moles or foreign bodies from uterus, Canth. > In fresh air, Puls. Affections of the heels, Am. m., Led., Puls., Caust., Mang., Ant. c., Grap., Nat. c., Cep. Desires lemonade, Puls. Clotted hæmorrhage, Millif., Plat. (Plat. dark ; Sbi. bright red). Miscarriage at third month, Croc., Kre. Sensation of something alive in abdomen, Croc., Thu. Suddenly increasing and slowly disappearing pain (Sul. ac. slowly increasing, suddenly disappearing). < In foggy weather, Hyper. < In bed at night, Sul., Merc., Puls., Cham. (toothache), Bry. (rheumatism). Phimosis, Cann., Merc., Sul., Nit. ac., Sep., Thu., Rhus. Tympanites, Tereb. Rheumatism > by cold applications, Led. Menses only when lying down (only at night, Bov., Mg. c.).

SYMPTOMS.

1. **Mind.**—Dejection, discouragement, and sadness.—Hypochondriacal mood.—Great anxiety and apprehension.—Irritable nerves ; music intolerable.—Moroseness with dislike to conversation, esp. when exercising in open air.—Irascibility, with tears and sobs.—Listlessness.—Weakness of memory.

2. **Head.**—Stupefying vertigo, which occasions falling, with cloudiness of sight.—Giddiness, with congestions to and heat in head.—Attacks of megrim.—Heaviness and distressing pressure in head, often extending from sinciput to nape.—Splitting sensation in forehead and temples.—Circumscribed pain in temples.—Painful constriction in temples.—Drawing pains in head, esp. in forehead and temples.—Shooting pains in head, with smarting or aching, often in entire brain.—Digging and boring in head.—Pulsative headache with heaviness and stupefaction.—The headaches (esp. in temporal eminences, r. side) often appear suddenly, diminish slowly, and return frequently.

3. **Eyes.**—Tensive pain in eyes, as if muscles too short.—Eyes dull and downcast.—Heat in eyes.—Smarting tears.—Jerking quivering of lids.—Clouds before eyes.

4. **Ears.**—Pinching in ears.—Hardness of hearing.—(Gets deaf in foggy weather, or any change of weather ; also when tired.—R. T. C.)

5. **Nose.**—Dry coryza.

6. **Face.**—Face pale, with blue circles round eyes.—Black pores in cheeks and round nose.—Paralytic pain and pressure in zygomatic process.—Lancinations (drawing pain in r. angle of jaw) from the lower jaw to cheek-bone (< on touch).

7. **Teeth.**—Drawing toothache during and after a meal and mastication.—Toothache only when chewing.—Aching and throbbing in teeth, esp. in evening and at night, with sensation as if a tooth were being pulled out, < by drinking, smoking, and by heat of bed, > after rising.—Drawing in teeth in consequence of drinking, eating, and contact with air.—Tearing in roots of molars.—(Toothache after gouty pain in great toe had been driven away by external applications.)—Painful sensibility and white swelling of gum round a carious tooth.—Ulcer in gums.

8. **Mouth.**—Dryness in mouth.—Putrid exhalation from mouth.—Reddish or white saliva, which becomes frothy when speaking.—Tongue loaded with a white or brownish coating.

9. **Throat.**—Sore throat during deglutition, as from a foreign body or an internal swelling in gullet, with pressure and choking.—Dull lancinations in throat.—Dryness in throat with drawing pain.

10. **Appetite.**—Taste in mouth and throat as from an inveterate coryza.—Mawkish, fat, or bloody taste in mouth.—Bitter taste in mouth and bitter taste of food, esp. of milk and coffee.—Desire for acids, esp. for lemonade.—Acidity in stomach after a meal.—Poor appetite.

11. **Stomach.**—Empty risings (and heartburn).—Nausea with fulness in stomach.—Vomiting of bile or of (undigested) food eaten the previous day.—Fulness and inflation of region of stomach.—Stomachache.—Lancinations from pit of stomach across back.

12. **Abdomen.**—Aching in hepatic region.—Tympanitic distension of abdomen.—Quivering in abdomen as if something alive were there; resembling fœtal movements.—Contractive pains in abdomen.—Pressive pinchings in abdomen as from a chill or diarrhœa.—Labour-like pains in abdomen to groins; with sensation as if vomiting would come on, without nausea.—Pressing down towards genitals.—Inflammation of intestines.—Pain as from a bruise in abdominal muscles in bed in evening.

13. **Stool and Anus.**—Evacuations at first soft, then hard.—Loose, soft fæces, with noise, and abundant expulsion of flatus.—Discharge of sanguineous mucus from anus.—Discharge of blood from anus after a hard evacuation.—Bleeding hæmorrhoids; excessive discharge of bright red blood or blood and mucus.—Painful hæmorrhoidal pimples in anus.—Tingling in anus.

14. **Urinary Organs.**—Retention of urine, with emission drop by drop, and burning sensation and pain in vesical region.—Vesical irritability with gouty diathesis.—Nephritis with retention; ardor urinæ.—Urgent want to urinate, with scanty emission.—Frequent violent urging to urinate, with profuse discharge.—Profuse emission of urine, even at night.—Painful inflammation of urethra, with discharge of pus, as in gonorrhœa.

15. **Male Sexual Organs.**—Inflammatory gonorrhœa, with discharge of pus.—Sycotic excrescences with burning soreness.—Burning sore pain in glans.—Hard (cartilaginous) swelling on dorsum of penis.—Shootings in glans.—Deep redness of glans.—Painful sensibility of prepuce, with difficulty in

etracting it.—Frænum swollen and tight.—Pain in condyloma as from xcoriation.—Increased sexual desire, with violent and prolonged erections.

16. **Female Sexual Organs.**—Almost insatiable desire for coition vith corresponding gratification.—Sexual desire greatly increased (almost mounting to nymphomania).—Contractive pain in region of uterus.—Stitches leep in vagina.—Sanguineous congestion in uterus.—Hæmorrhages of partly ale red, partly clotted, or of very thin, discoloured, offensive-smelling blood ; < on least motion ; has to lie perfectly quiet to avoid a profuse discharge fter miscarriage.—Metrorrhagia with discharge of clotted or bright-red lood, and pains resembling labour pains in the sacrum and in the groins.—Metrorrhagia, bright blood, < at night.—Catamenia too early and too copious. —Menses continue too long.—Menstrual discharge partly fluid, partly clotted nd offensive ; it may be either bright red or dark and coagulated ; flows nostly in paroxysms, which are brought on by slightest motion ; or flow ceases vhen walking about (menses only when lying down).—Suppressed catamenia vith very offensive-smelling leucorrhœa (like meat washings).—Miscarriage esp. in the third month).—Perceptible swelling of mammæ.—Tingling in nammæ.—Leucorrhœa, itching, yellowish, fetid, and thick, like starch.—Inlammation of the uterus after parturition.—Retained placenta.—After-pains vith sensitiveness of abdomen.

17. **Respiratory Organs.**—Dry cough, excited by a tickling, or ollowed at a later period by expectoration of mucus streaked with blood.—Dry, hacking cough, and tickling in the trachea.—Hæmoptysis.—Tensive, ressive pain in sternum, not affected by respiration.

18. **Chest.**—Pressure on chest.—Pressive, spasmodic tension in chest, rincipally in middle of sternum.—Stitches in l. nipple.—Shooting and pain s from excoriation in xiphoid cartilage, < on taking a full inspiration and on ouching the part.—Trembling in the lungs, with dull rattling and crackling.—ancination (intermittent) in the outside of chest and in clavicles.

19. **Heart.**—Augmented and extended beating of the heart.—Throbbing n all the blood-vessels.—Pulse unequal ; generally quick, strong, and hard.

20. **Neck and Back.**—Contusive pain in the muscles or vertebræ of eck.—Pressive drawing (labour-like pains) in loins, as far as the inguinal egion and down thighs, followed by a bloody, slimy discharge from the agina.—Paralytic pain in small of back, > (or <) bending backward.—Drawing pains in small of back, extending into pubic region.—Pressive tearng and shootings in spine.—Pain in back obliging him to bend inward.—Paralytic pain in back.

21. **Limbs.**—Drawing, tearing pains, esp. at night ; most in wrist-joints nd toes, with red, shiny swelling ; < from motion and touch.—Stitches in lbows ; in heels, extending outward.—Limbs convulsed.—Cracking in joints.

22. **Upper Limbs.**—Wrenching pain in the joints of the shoulder and ands.—Pain as if sprained in r. shoulder-joint, even during rest.—Paralytic earing along r. upper arm as far as hand.—Sticking pains on outer condyles f both elbows.—Aching in r. radius, < motion or touch.—Pressive tearings nd shootings in arms, forearms, and fingers.—Arthritic rigidity and swelling n joint of wrist, with tearing and shootings ; made almost insupportable when he hand hangs down.—Drawing and tearing in bones of hands.—Weakness f hands (when writing).—Distortion of fingers.

23. **Lower Limbs.**—Furunculus with shooting pain in buttock.—Shooting pains in coxo-femoral articulations when resting on the foot.—Stinging pains in hip-joints in morning and when breathing.—Pressure and drawing in thighs and knees.—Middle of anterior surface of thighs feel bruised and painful; only when walking on the level or stepping down, not when stepping up.—Tearing tension in thighs, with sensation when squatting as if the muscles were too short.—Purulent and lard-like ulcer on tibia.—Intermittent aching on l. heel, lower part where it joins the sole.—Sharp stitches from within out on r. and l. heel.—Pressive tearing in bones of feet.—Red and shining swelling of great toe (gout), with boring and lancinating pain.

24. **Generalities.**—[A marked characteristic is a pain which is felt all the way between the sacrum and pubis, from one bone to the other—not particularly in front or behind, but right along from the sacrum to the pubis; this pain may be found in labour pains, after-pains, occurring in dysmenorrhœa, &c.; in hæmorrhage (particularly uterine) where the blood is in fluid and clots together—as, the liquid blood would flow, then will come a clot, and the blood may be flowing rapidly.—Bleeding from the nose, blood being pale.—Bleeding from inner parts in general.—Menstruation too early; too profuse; blood of light colour; bright-red colour; discharge of blood before the proper period.—Affects particularly the uterus; lower part of chest; wrist; heel; toes; arthritic pain in joints.—Cough with expectoration of pale blood.—In threatened abortion.—< On inspiration; taking a deep breath; affections in general during pregnancy; in a room; in a warm room; on getting warm in bed; women in childbed; after parturition.—> In open air; while breathing out, exhaling.—H. N. G.]—Chronic ailments of women.—Twitching pulsation in the blood-vessels.—Shooting and tearing, arthritic pains, esp. in joints, and sometimes with red and shining swelling of the parts affected.—Gouty nodosities.—Lancinating drawing in hollow bones.—Burning, pressive sensation in periosteum, which is swollen.—Hæmorrhage.—Jerking throbbing in all the arteries.—Great weakness and weariness in all limbs, with despondency.—General uneasiness, as from long watching.—Heaviness and indolence of body, obliging him to lie down.

25. **Skin.**—Itching in skin, with excoriation and ulceration, or scabby places after scratching.—Burning sensation in parts affected when they are touched.—Black pores in skin.

26. **Sleep.**—Sleeplessness and restlessness after midnight.—Disturbed sleep with frequent waking, ebullition of blood, heat, and perspiration.—Anxious dreams.—Continued dreams, full of fanciful images, and intellectual efforts.—Talking and loud snoring during sleep.—Tendency to lie on l. side when sleeping.

27. **Fever.**—Shuddering and shivering, with cutis anserina and cloudiness of sight (followed by sleepiness).—Chill in the evening, with attacks of chilliness.—Great chilliness through the day.—Burning heat over the whole body, with great agitation.—Sensation of coldness in whole r. leg.—Heat in face, with icy coldness of feet and hands.—Fever in evening; first shivering, then heat, and lastly perspiration.—Perspiration every night.

Saccharum Lactis.

Milk-sugar. Lactose. $C_{12}H_{22}O_{11}$.

Clinical.—Amblyopia. Angina pectoris. Body-odour, offensive. Diabetes. Dyspepsia. Earache. Gout. Headache. Hysteria. Labia, soreness of. Nervousness. Neuralgia. Ovaries, affections of. Over-exertion. Ptosis. Sciatica. Sighing. Stye. Umbilicus, inflammation of.

Characteristics.—Hahnemann chose globules of *Saccharum lactis* as the chief vehicle of his remedies, because he considered it the most inert substance he could find. But his method of attenuating remedies had shown that no substance is inert in attenuations, and experience shows that no substance is *absolutely* inert in any form. H. A. Hare says of *Sac. l.*: "Scientific and clinical studies have shown it to be possessed of very great diuretic powers when given in full doses." He says further, that its direct action on the kidneys and its slight action elsewhere indicate it in renal dropsy and renal inactivity; that it acts best in cases where albuminuria is absent, and that it causes profuse diuresis in infants fed on it. I have frequently met with patients who could not take *Sac. l.* either unmedicated or as a vehicle without inconvenience. One patient when taking pilules of *Sac. l.* three times a day complained that they made his "eyes ache and feel weak." One of Swan's provers had this symptom: "Sight fails; eyes tire very easily." Swan is the authority for *Sac. l.* as a homœopathic remedy. He has published (*Materia Medica*) a full pathogenesis of *Sac. l.*, proved in the potencies from 30th upward, together with confirmed and cured symptoms. Eleven provers and observers contributed. I have bracketed the cured symptoms in my Schema. *Sac. l.* causes sensations of both coldness and heat. One of the cold sensations is this: "Sensation of extreme cold passing in a fine line from centre of pubes to a point two or three inches above." Swan regards *cold pains* as a keynote, and records this case: Mr. S. had an excessively cold neuralgic pain in cartilage of both ears, the right being the worst, with tingling as if frost-bitten; rubbing with difficulty restored the warmth. Lancinating, neuralgic pains in forehead; in occiput; extending from region above ears down through ears into muscles of neck; in both eyes; < by least breath of air; skin sensitive to touch as in inflammatory rheumatism. These pains were *icy cold*, as if produced by an extremely fine *ice-cold* needle. As *Sac. l.* has "fine cold pains" and pains passing in all directions, *Sac. l.* 1m was given, and relieved all the pains within an hour. (*Sac. off.* has "cold expectoration.") The symptoms are < before a storm; in damp room or basement; morning and evening; by blue and yellow colours; exertion; mental excitement. > By warmth of fire; by red colour; after 4 p.m.

Relations.—Camph. < effects of Sac. l. *Compare:* Sac. off., the Lacs. Right cheek bone, Mg. c. Roof of mouth, Mang. Ball sensation in rectum, Sep. < From sound of running water, Hdfb. Radiating pains, K. bi. Kidney ache, Santal, Sac. off. Fatigue, Pic.

ac., Mg. c. Heat in heart, Lachn. > Lying left side, Lil. t. < From damp, Dulc. Sensitiveness, K. iod., Mg. c.

Causation.—Mental excitement. Over-fatigue.

SYMPTOMS.

1. **Mind.**—Sensation as if it were only by a great effort that she kept together.—Loses her way in well-known streets.—Imagines : that there is a large hole in her back just above sacrum ; that her mother wants to kill her ; that some one is behind her.—Extremely nervous, jumps from her seat at least unusual noise.—Was taken suddenly with fear and trembling of whole body, as from fright.—Longing and melancholy as if homesick, with oppressed breathing.—Her heart aches as if it would burst, yet she cannot weep.—Great fear of death during paroxysm of pain in heart at night.—Inclined to be sarcastic and fault-finding.—Cross and fault-finding, could not speak a pleasant word to any one.—Hysteria in evening, laughing and crying, jumping up and lying down, but could not stand, fell to r. side.—Laziness.

2. **Head.**—Pain about middle of r. lambdoidal suture, through to same point on l. side.—Sharp jumping pains behind r. ear.—Burning like fire, and a thick feeling in a lengthwise strip of two fingers' breadth extending from r. frontal eminence to r. side of vertex for fifteen minutes.—L. side of head felt all drawn up.—Pain in l. eyebrow.—Pain passing from front of l. ear deep into brain.—L. temple sore to touch.—Sensation as of pressure on frontal bone at inner canthi of l. eye ; felt very sore.—Sharp darting pain on l. side of head from temple to occiput.—Forehead feels very heavy, with a tendency to fall forward.—Sharp pain in forehead passing back and forth from one temple to the other.—Head aches all over top and feels drawn up.—Head feels large, and as though all the blood in the body had gone into the head.—Head feels confused, and as if it were tossing on a rough sea.

3. **Eyes.**—Pain through r. eye inwards.—Severe pains in both canthi of r. eye.—Dryness of eyeball so that the lid would stick to it as if it wanted lubricating, preventing opening and shutting of eye or winking.—Swelling of r. upper lid, which increased to a large stye, the lid and all round eye being swollen and red ; on third day it broke in two places and discharged copiously.—Washing eyes in cold water causes a sensation as if needles were sticking into them.—Eyelids feel swollen, which is not the case.—Can only elevate upper lids half way.—Looking at bright light dazzles and makes her close eyes ; no pain.—Sight fails ; eyes tire very easily.

4. **Ears.**—Pain in r. ear and underneath it.—Painfulness of r. external ear (concha), with burning like an ulcer, also when touched.—Pain passing from r. ear to shoulder.—Pain from r. ear to lower part of inferior maxillary bone.—Pain in l. ear and sensation as if there were a gathering.—Shooting pains in and behind ears and all over face.—Pains in external ears and behind them.—Sharp pain inside both ears.—Reverberation of voice when speaking.—Buzzing sound in r. ear.—Sensation as if she could not hear, but she could.

5. **Nose.**—Pain in r. (and l.) side of nose.—Pain in end of nose.—Ridge of nose extremely sore ; it feels sore to touch or from the least movement of facial muscles ; the l. side is the worst and somewhat swollen.

6. **Face.**—Pain passing from corner of mouth to forepart of r. axilla.—

Face feels as if there were one large pain that covered the whole of it.—Burning in cheek-bones towards temples and lower jaw.—Pain all over face, then centring in r. ear.—(Darting, shooting pain, centred in about middle of r. cheek, extending thence up to eye, esp. r. inner canthus, to ear, and up into r. temple, most severe at centre of cheek, considerably decreasing the further it extends from the centre.)—(Swelling of face with pain in head extending down neck and back to feet.)—Wretched appearance, sad expression of face; eyes look as from weeping, though she has not wept.—Great pallor of face with dark places under eyes.—Corners of mouth smart and burn.—Symphysis menti smarts.

8. **Mouth.**—Sore on l. side of tongue.—Tongue coated: yellow on each side, but none on middle or edges; white; yellow.—Lips feel very sore and raw.—Lips dry, with great thirst.—Taste: putrid in mouth after eating; fine spicy taste; like fresh nuts.—Thick bitter mucus in mouth during morning; food tastes fresh, as if there were no salt in it.—Burning in whole mouth.—Roof of mouth sore.—Soreness like blisters in mouth and on tongue.—(Sensation of coolness as of ice in mouth and throat.)

9. **Throat.**—Sensation when swallowing as of a fish-bone in throat.—Spasmodic stricture in œsophagus.—Globus hystericus after lunch at noon, with dull, sick headache.—Throat very sensitive to external pressure; the least pressure causes a feeling as if she were choking.

10. **Appetite.**—Hungry all the time.—Desire for dainties.—When first getting out of bed feels faint for something to eat.—After eating: feeling of distension.—Great thirst; wanted large quantities of very cold water.

11. **Stomach.**—Nausea like sea-sickness.—Nausea does not affect appetite.—Violent sickness, going on all day (agg.—R. T. C.).—Dyspepsia after eating hot pie-crust.—Pressure in stomach as if she had eaten something indigestible.—Heartburn, with sweet taste coming from stomach, without waterbrash.

12. **Abdomen.**—Feeling as if ulcerated anteriorly over r. short ribs, < from touch and when stooping; slight swelling there; also all next day till towards evening.—Pain about length of finger above l. hip, which would come when leaning back, lasted two days, followed by severe pain in forehead.—Sharp pain passing across bowels just above navel and all round body.—Inflammation and soreness of lower half of navel, passing off by morning, with greenish yellow discharge, staining the clothes.—Abdomen sore to touch, painful from the jar caused by walking.—Pain commencing at waist and passing to top of r. breast.—Pain in l. hypochondrium passing under l. breast.

13. **Stool and Anus.**—Severe pain passing through abdomen during stool; felt very sore inside.—Stool preceded by shooting pains across abdomen, which are > by stool.—Before stool pains in breasts and upper abdomen.—Before stool hands and whole body exhaled a fæcal odour, which passed away after stool.—Urgent inclination to stool; felt as though there were a great ball in rectum, much straining, and some flatulence, but no stool and no > from the flatulence.—Stools smell like rotten eggs.—Great soreness round anus, extending three inches up rectum inside.—Constant pressure and soreness at anus, waking her at night.—Creeping, itching, and crawling round anus, extending three inches inside rectum, > for a short time by rubbing.—Shooting pains in rectum.

14. Urinary Organs.—Urination followed by a thick yellow discharge. —Soreness of urethra during urination.—Very severe pain in r. side of abdomen before urination, and sometimes, but not often, lasting during urination, ceasing with it.—Constant and urgent inclination to urinate, with cutting pain streaking up urethra after each passage.—Frequent and violent urging to urinate, with passage of a large quantity each time.—Urine causes intense pain when coming in contact with the labia, which are very sensitive. —Sound of running water produced urination; no power to restrain it.—Urinates very frequently large quantities.—(Involuntary urination in large quantities several times during night.)—(Delay of urination for some time, though desire and opportunity occur.)—Urine stains a dark yellow.

16. Female Sexual Organs.—Menses commenced too early; no pain. —Menses very dark.—Profuse greenish-yellow leucorrhœa.—At times bloody leucorrhœa.—Pain in region of r. ovary.—L. (and r.) ovarian region very weak and painful when walking.—Dragging-down sensation in pelvic region. —Lobulated growths on each side of vagina, nearly filling it; extremely sore and sensitive to touch, or from the pressure caused by sitting; coming on gradually and lasting more than three months.—Itching of labia.—Extreme soreness and rawness of labia and entrance to vagina, with profuse greenish-yellow leucorrhœa.

17. Respiratory Organs.—Sharp pain passing into upper r. breast, about an inch deep; very sore to touch after the pain.—Pain in r. breast.—Constant pain under l. breast, < when bending forward.—Lancinating pains under l. breast, which took away the breath.—Severe pains under l. breast at every inspiration.

19. Heart and Pulse.—Sensation in heart as if a fire were there, with a feeling as if heart would burst, or at times as if a heavy weight were lying on it, all of which spreads from this region over whole inner and outer chest. —Awoke at midnight with severe pains about heart, which seemed as if it had almost stopped beating, with a numb pain about heart, lips, and tongue; great fear of death; when the pains passed off they left great soreness round heart; tingling in lips and tongue; could not lie on l. side; felt numb and strange all over; pulse intermittent.

20. Neck and Back.—Pain passing up and down along r. side of neck. —Hot flashes all over back of neck and shoulders.—Pain with soreness at upper vertebral border of r. scapula.—Pain in r. side of back between scapula and sacrum.—Pain in l. side of back from scapula to sacrum.—Pain in sacrum. —Pain each side of sacrum.—Pain in sacral region, < when taking a long breath.—Pain in back from sacrum to scapulæ.—Pain passing up back from sacrum.—Pain passing up and down from tip of coccyx to r. shoulder.—Sharp pain passing from middle of scapula down outside of arm to end of middle finger, and sometimes to end of little finger.—Pain below l. scapula.—Severe pain under l. scapula.—Pain running up back from waist, l. side.—Constant pain all day in region of l. kidney.—Pain in back part of waist, passing from r. to l.—Pain in lumbar region.—Pain or aching in small of back < by leaning backward, for three or four days.—Pain passing from lumbar vertebræ to half way up dorsal, and then shooting off into both scapulæ.—Dull ache all over back and in r. arm; cannot bend body far forward as it causes intense pain in coccyx; when stooping, as in picking anything from floor, has to incline body to one side or other.—Back aches the whole length of spine.

22. **Upper Limbs.**—Swelling in r. arm below elbow, sore to touch, and pains when she moves arms in certain directions.—Pain in forepart of r. upper arm.—Pain from top of r. shoulder to nape of neck.—Pain from r. shoulder passing down to waist.—Pain in r. shoulder passing a short distance down back.—Pain in top of r. shoulder passing to back and upper part of neck.—Pain passing from r. shoulder to elbow.—Pain in back of r. shoulder.—Pain from r. shoulder to l. breast.—Pain in axillæ.—Sharp pain in all r. fingers except little finger.—Pain in both hands passing to ends of fingers.—Skin under nails looks dirty, it cannot be washed or scraped off for two days.—Pain in dorsal surface of r. hand.—Pain in palm of r. hand.—Itching in palm of r. hand.—Pains all through r. hand.—Grasping anything with r. hand causes pains to pass from all the fingers into palm.—Violent itching of a liver spot on r. hand.—Pains in hands passing in all directions.—Pain in palmar surface of r. wrist passing into thumb.—Pain passing from tip of r. little finger to elbow.—Pain in r. wrist.—Pain passing from r. wrist to elbow.—Pains in both wrists, encircling them.—Pain with slight stiffness in both wrists.

23. **Lower Limbs.**—(Inflammation and awful pain extending down whole trunk of r. sciatic nerve.)—Pains in thighs and hips.—Soreness of gluteal muscles on pressure.—Soreness in streaks, extending from anus down back of legs to heels; can feel a rigidity (not raised) where the soreness is.—Hot flashes in lower limbs.—Pain from forepart of r. knee to anterior-superior spine of r. ilium and passing back to middle of sacrum.—Pain in r. instep when bending foot.—(Pain like gout in r. toe, sometimes slight pains upwards in r. limb; toe will not bear contact of any shoe; pain always the same standing, walking, or lying down; continued exercise < it.)—Balls of feet covered with little corns, which are very painful when walking.—All her corns become painfully sensitive.

24. **Generalities.**—Sensitive in every part of body.—Small shooting pains all over her in morning.—Throbbing in various parts of body.—(Short flying, darting stitches in different parts of body, quite painful, but bearable, appearing in head, ears, and face, as well as in extremities, not confined to any especial locality.)—(Great physical exhaustion, caused by overwork, completely relieved; repeatedly verified by Swan and others.)—The pains during the proving were < by a coming storm, the approach of which was felt some twelve hours previously.—Pains were < in damp room or basement, but > if there was a fire.—All symptoms > after 4 p.m.—Pains were generally < morning and evening.—Symptoms < by blue and yellow colours; > by red.—Prostration from mental excitement (Rushmore).

25. **Skin.**—Very restless at night from itching all over body as soon as she is covered in bed.—Itching of both shoulders.

26. **Sleep.**—Continual yawning all day.—Sleeplessness after midnight.—Cannot sleep on r. side.—Cannot go to sleep without putting arms over head.—Impossible to lie straight in bed, finds herself continually lying diagonally across bed.—Has to lie on l. side as she is comfortable in no other position.—Awoke with the impression that she had dreamed of dreadful pains in chest; does not know whether it was a dream or a reality.—Fatiguing dreams all night.

27. **Fever.**—Great coldness as if a chill were coming on; hands, particularly fingers, feet, toes, icy cold; could not keep warm in bed covered with clothes, and during day sat near a stove but could not get warm.—Hot flashes inside body pressing from below upward.—Strange restlessness at night, feeling of great heat all over, body covered with a light perspiration, just enough to feel uncomfortable.

Saccharum Officinale.

Sugar. (Including Saccharum album, White Sugar.) Saccharose. $C_{12}H_{22}O_{11}$. Trituration. Solution.

Clinical.—Ascites. Cataract. Chlorosis. Cornea, opacity of. Diabetes. Dropsy. Dyspepsia. Hair, rapid growth of. Headache, periodic. Hoarseness. Liver, affections of. Ranula. Rheumatism. Rickets. Scurvy. Spleen, affections of. Tabes mesenterica.

Characteristics.—Like so many other articles of diet, Sugar may be a poison and a medicine as well as a food. Sugar preserves food, as salt does; and both sugar and salt have produced scurvy. Cases of scurvy-rickets in bottle-fed children have been traced to excess of sugar in their food; and the exclusion of sugar from the dietary of the gouty, rheumatic, and the diabetic, shows the pathogenetic power it is credited with among practitioners of the present day. Acidity of the stomach and itching at the anus are common effects of taking too much Sugar. Lippe published "Fragmentary provings and clinical observations obtained principally from S. Bœnninghausen and S. E. Bute, who proved the 30th potency on himself" (Allen). To these symptoms have been added others observed by Swan on a patient who accidentally discovered, after twenty-five years of suffering, that the cause of his trouble was *Sugar*. All the symptoms disappeared when he abstained from sugar in food or drink, and only reappeared when he took it again by way of experiment. Then, from two to four days after taking sugar, the same train of symptoms invariably occurred in this order: (1) A burning at pit of stomach. (2) A white coat on tongue, so thick as to cause stiffness of it. (3) Sharp burning pains run up from kidneys to shoulders, passing under scapulæ. (4) Pains in bones from head to foot, causing a rigidity of the muscles so that it was impossible to rise from bed till he had been rubbed. (5) Chill commencing in small of back and spreading up and down. Severe headache and occasional vomiting with the chill. Fever followed with headache, morbid hunger, and a hectic flush. (6) Increased urine, strong odour, white sediment. (7) Great pain in kidneys. (8) Constipation. (9) Sleeplessness. (10) Œdema of feet and ankles. (11) Weakness of legs, as if paralysed, causing staggering. (12) Painful jactitation of feet and legs during the burning in the stomach. (13) Oppression, slight cough, profuse cream-like expectoration, very offensive, cold. *Sac. a.* 10m and 5m cured him of some remaining symptoms, and the 41m enabled him to eat sugar with impunity. Swan also reports (*Org.* iii. 342) this case: Miss L. was continually eating candies, of which she was very fond, till her digestive organs were affected. A few doses of *Sac. a.* 30m changed her taste so that she ate no more, and could not even bear the sight of them. This case was also cured with *Sac. off.*: "Vomiting bile, < in night and at 1 a.m.; old-standing dyspepsia, milk, eggs, and bread being the only food tolerated; great longing for sugar, which > the symptoms." Farrington traces a great similarity between *Sac. off.* and *Calc.* *Sac. off.* is indicated, he says, in children who are large-limbed, fat, and bloated, with a tendency to dropsy. It has produced opacity of the cornea, and ought to cure it. The children are dainty and capricious; care nothing for substantial food, but want little "nick-nacks"; always cross and whining, and, if old enough, are insolent, and do not care to occupy themselves in any way. Everything too much trouble. H. C. Allen relates (*H. P.*, x. 478) a case of opacity of cornea cured with *Sac. a.*; and with the same remedy in 2m potency he cured swelling round the ankles following rheumatism. According to Lippe, black-and-tan terrier dogs that eat sugar go blind. The cataract and amblyopia of diabetics are well known. Here, again, Salt and Sugar meet: Burnett has shown in his *Supersalinity of the Blood* that excess of salt in food has been an important factor in the production of cataract. The symptoms are < in early morning. < From anger. > In erect position (dyspnœa).

Relations.—*Compare:* Sacch. l. In rickets, acidity, fat children, Calc. Craving for sweets, Arg. n., Sul. Rickets, Sil. Diabetes; swelled ankles, Arg. n. Kidney-ache, Santal.

Causation.—Anger.

SYMPTOMS.

1. **Mind.**—Violent temper; irritable; quarrelsome.—Bilious, sanguineous temperament.—Increased modesty of women.—Melancholic mood with the chilliness.—Dainty, capricious; cross and whining; indolent.—Low-spirited, hypochondriacal mood; peevish.—Indifference; as from home-sickness.—Disinclined to talk; want of interest.—Stupid.

2. **Head.**—Giddiness from indigestion.—Severe headache with the chill.—Headache every week the same day.—Hair grows rapidly.

3. **Eyes.**—Eyes closed by swelling (and inflammation) of lids.—Varicose distension of vessels of eyes.—Ophthalmia.—Sight dim.—Cataract.

4. **Ears.**—Discharge of pus from ears.

5. **Nose.**—Sneezing; dry coryza.

6. **Face.**—Changed expression.—Face: pale; deathlike; bloated; œdematous.—Twitching of muscles of r. cheek over malar bone.

8. **Mouth.**—Dulness of teeth (with sour vomiting).—A white coat on tongue, so thick as to cause stiffness in it.—Rhagades, cracks on the tongue.—Ranula.—Inflammation of salivary glands of lining membrane of mouth.—Aphthæ of children.

9. **Throat.**—Ulcers in throat.

11. **Stomach.**—Morbid hunger with the fever.—Nausea early in morning.—Violent retching.—Vomiting of white, viscid, tough mucus.—Periodical

vomiting.—Vomiting: of blood; acid, making teeth dull; occasional, with the chill.—Stomach bloated.—Stomach overloaded with sour mucus.—Disordered stomach.—Digestion: impaired; weak, with acidity.—Burning at pit of stomach.—Heat in stomach.—Coldness of stomach.—Pressure in stomach, morning, fasting.—Painful constriction of stomach.—Painful sensitiveness of pit of stomach.—Pain in stomach with hypochondriacal persons.

12. **Abdomen.**—Liver: swollen; indurated.—Bile increased.—Spleen swollen.—Pain in liver and spleen.—Abdomen: swollen; dropsical; hard as a stone (in children).—Tabes mesenterica.—Swelling and induration of mesenteric glands.

13. **Stool and Anus.**—Congested and painful hæmorrhoids.—Itching at the anus.—Diarrhœa, stools watery and debilitating; of mucus and blood; bilious.—Constipation alternating with mucous diarrhœa.—Constipation; stools difficult.

14. **Urinary Organs.**—Sharp burning pains run from kidneys to shoulders, passing under scapulæ.—Great pains in kidneys.—Increased urination; strong odour; white sediment.—Urine diminished.

15. **Male Sexual Organs.**—Enormous swelling of scrotum; r. genitals.—Increased desire.—Frequent involuntary emissions.

16. **Female Sexual Organs.**—Menses diminished.—Menstrual blood pale.—Suppressed leucorrhœa.

17. **Respiratory Organs.**—Irritation of larynx, causing a slight hacking cough, with yellow, saltish sputa, which floats on water.—Dry rawness in larynx.—Hoarse, catarrhal voice.—Hoarseness from reading a short time.—Dry cough.—Cough with children.—Expectoration very offensive.—Breathing oppressed, cold expectoration.—Suffocative attacks, must be bolstered up.

18. **Chest.**—Chest muscles wasted.—Pneumonia.—Swelling of lower part of sternum.—Fulness > by expectorating.—Stitches in l. chest.

19. **Heart.**—Rheumatic pain in heart region.—Pulse weak and irregular.

21. **Limbs.**—Tingling in limbs.—Emaciation of hands and thighs.

22. **Upper Limbs.**—Œdema of arms.

23. **Lower Limbs.**—Œdema of lower limbs; hard as stones.—Paralytic weakness of legs.—Painful jactitation of legs during burning in stomach.—Cramps in calves.

24. **Generalities.**—Emaciation with great appetite.—Chlorosis: with dropsy; after anger.—Plethora.—Fainting attacks.—Scurvy rickets in children.—Pains in bones from head to foot.

25. **Skin.**—Dry skin; perspiration suppressed.—Scurvy.—Pale and red blotches over body.—Panaritium.—Proud flesh in the ulcers.—Old herpes.

26. **Sleep.**—Sleeplessness.—Starts in sleep.

27. **Fever.**—Chilliness from 10 a.m. till evening with melancholic mood.—Chill commencing in small of back, spreading up and down; severe headache and occasional vomiting; fever, followed by headache, morbid hunger, and hectic flush in cheeks; no sweats except when weakened by repeated attacks; before and during the paroxysm burning in stomach and back was simply intolerable; no thirst.—Chilliness alternates with perspiration.—Cold in the head.—Intermittent fever every one, two, or three days, irregular in its type.—Chill followed by profuse sweat.—Sweat on head (neck and shoulders).

Salicinum.

Salicin. $C_{13}H_{18}O_7$. Trituration and Solution.

Clinical.—Deafness. Influenza. Ménière's disease. Tinnitus.

Characteristics.—*Saln.* is an active principle (glucoside ?) obtained from different species of Willow. It has been used largely in the treatment of rheumatism in ordinary practice. It has had some fragmentary provings, and Ringer experimented with it on three boys. The characteristics of the *Salicylic acid* compounds were prominent—giddiness, confusion of the head, flickering before the eyes, and tinnitus. The stomach was disordered, vomiting occurred. There was also great instability of temperature. Chilliness, high temperature, and low temperature were induced. *Saln.* has been commended in influenza by Stephen Mackenzie as less irritating than the *Salicylates* and more effective.

SYMPTOMS.

1. **Mind.**—Dulness, does not seem to understand questions.—Dulness and heaviness.

2. **Head.**—Giddiness.—Confusion of the head.—Headache.

3. **Eyes.**—Flickering; fog and sparks before eyes.—Slight congestion of conjunctiva.

4. **Ears.**—Tingling in r. ear.—Persistent ringing in ears.—Deafness.

6. **Face.**—Face flushed ; and dull.—Slight tremor of lips on speaking.

11. **Stomach.**—Vomited twice.

14. **Urinary Organs.**—*Salicin.* is excreted in the urine in the form of *Salicylic hydride*, which sinks to the bottom of the urine as a fine crystalline cloud.

17. **Respiratory Organs.**—Thick, husky voice.—Breathing rather laboured.

22. **Upper Limbs.**—Slight spasmodic movements of upper limbs.—Trembling of hands when held out.

23. **Lower Limbs.**—Slight jerks of lower limbs when they are raised from the bed.

24. **Generalities.**—Muscular twitches.—Much irritability of the muscles on percussion.—Muscular weakness ; grasping power diminished.

27. **Fever.**—Malaise and chilliness evening ; returned 10 a.m. next day with headache, fugitive pains and fever (101° F.).—Lowered temperature.—Temperature rises from 9 a.m. to 1 p.m., and falls from 4 p.m. to midnight.

Salicylicum Acidum.

Salicylic acid. $C_6H_4(OH).CO.OH$. Found in Spiræa blossoms, Gaultheria, &c. Artificially prepared from Phenol. Trituration.

Clinical.—Bone, caries of. Climacteric. Coryza. Diarrhœa. Diphtheria. Dyspepsia, flatulent. Flatulence. Flushes. Foot-sweat; suppression of. Gastritis. Intestines, ulceration of. Iritis. Necrosis. Pharyngitis, herpetic. Puerperal fever. Rheumatism. Rheumatoid arthritis. Scarlatina, anginosa. Sciatica. Stomatitis. Tapeworm. Throat, sore.

Characteristics.—*Salicylic acid* is found in nature in the leaves and barks of Willows, in Oil of Wintergreen (*Gaultheria*), which is one of the chief sources of its supply, and is obtained synthetically from *Carbolic acid.* Like *Carbol. ac.* it has been largely used as a disinfectant, and as it is supposed to be non-poisonous it is used for mixing with and so preserving foods. MacLagan, of London, and Senator, of Berlin, introduced it into medicine as a remedy for rheumatism. Over-dosings led to the discovery of its power to set up the phenomena of Ménière's disease (auditory nerve vertigo), gastric disturbances and delirium, and these form the nucleus of the homœopathic Schema, which has been filled out by fragmentary provings and clinical use. Among the uses of *Sal. ac.* recommended in the general text-books are these: "*Sal. ac.* dissolved in Collodion flexile (gr. xxx to ℥i) is very useful for corns and warts; also to hasten the peeling of palms and soles after scarlet fever" (Brunton). "A mixture of 2 parts with 100 of tallow, applied directly to the feet, not to the stockings, has been found most useful in preventing sweating and soreness of the feet in soldiers after a long march" (Brunton). The property of preventing foot-sweat is by no means an unmixed boon, and serious illness has resulted from it. Consequently in homœopathic practice *Sal. ac.* has been found an excellent remedy for affections following suppression of foot-sweat. *Sal. ac.* has a specific relation to rheumatism, but the massive doses given in ordinary practice have been attended with so many unpleasant symptoms—vital depression, fainting, flatulent dyspepsia, delirium, &c.—that the ingenuity of chemists has been devoted for years past to finding a compound which shall be innocent as well as effective. *Aspirin* (Acetyl-salicylic acid), *Salophen* (Acetyl-para-amidophenol salicylate), and *Salol* (Phenol salicylate), are supposed to fulfil these conditions more or less completely. *Salol* has had an accidental proving which has led to some homœopathic uses. It is the "unpleasant symptoms" which so many practitioners wish to avoid, which are of especial value to homœopaths. Like *Carbolic acid* and other disinfectants, *Sal. ac.* produces fermentative dyspepsia, and diarrhœa with putrid-smelling stools, and it meets dynamically blood-poisoning conditions, such as puerperal fever and septicæmia. Hering says: "Pieces of spongy bone become soft as leather in a few days when placed in a ½ per cent. solution, while compact bone tissues are very slowly softened; enamel of teeth is very slightly affected by it, but the dentine, when it is exposed by caries, is rapidly destroyed. The increased amount of the salts of lime in the urine soon after *Sal. ac.* has been taken shows that the acid deprives living as well as dead bone of its lime salts." He adds that it causes necrosis, especially of the tibia. The symptoms are < by touch. < By motion. < At night. < By cold air or touch of anything cold. > By hot applications, especially by dry heat.

Relations.—*Compare :* Salicin., Nat. sal., Salol. In rheumatism and subsequent weakness, Colch. Piercing in temples ; throat ; diarrhœa ; ulcers ; antiseptic properties, Kre. Antiseptic properties, dyspepsia, fever, urine, Carbol. ac. Tinnitus, Nat. sal., Chi., Chi. s., Carb. s. Bones, Pho., (and throat), Lact. ac. As if blood forced through contracted vessel, Coc. cact. Foot-sweat and suppressed foot-sweat, Sul., Sil. Loquacity, Lach.

Causation.—Suppression (foot-sweat).

SYMPTOMS.

1. **Mind.**—Anxiety ; worrying, restless, yet mild.—Melancholic, wants to be quiet ; feels faint.—Excited mood.—Delirium ; stupid, can hardly collect his ideas, then laughed without cause, talked incessantly and disconnectedly, frequently looked about him with apparent hallucinations (lasted 24 h. ; from 11 grains).

2. **Head.**—Dulness of head ; stupefaction.—Vertigo ; inclines to fall to l., surrounding objects seem to fall to r.—Ménière's disease.—Rush of blood to head.—Severe headache, piercing in both temples.—Headache commencing on top or back of head, running down sterno-mastoid (more r. side), which is tender to touch.—Buzzing sensation in interior of brain as if blood were forced violently through a contracted vessel.

3. **Eyes.**—Diminished acuteness of vision.—(Plastic iritis following acute rheumatism ; pain temporarily > by hot applications.)

4. **Ears.**—Hearing diminished.—Nervous deafness.—Deafness with noises (roaring) in ears.—Roaring in ears and difficult hearing ; hears music ; swarm of bees or buzzing of flies ; rush of blood to head, excited mood.—Tinnitus dependent on hyperæmia.—Auditory nerve vertigo (Ménière's disease) ; a troublesome nausea accompanying the head symptoms.

5. **Nose.**—Wants to sneeze.—Sneezing.—Incipient catarrh ; patients, esp. children, sneeze all day.

6. **Face.**—Dull, heavy aspect ; face flushes quickly on slight excitement.

8. **Mouth.**—Burning in mouth and epigastric region.—Burning and scraping in mouth and throat.—Redness of mouth and fauces.—Stomatitis, mouth hot and dry, tongue covered with burning vesicles.—Foul breath and offensive expectoration.—Mouth dotted with white patches, burning, scalded feeling ; ulcers on tip of tongue.—Canker-sores with burning soreness and fetid breath.—Taste : extremely disgusting ; as of something burnt ; bitter ; bitter bilious, that cannot be got rid of ; food has no taste.

9. **Throat.**—Burning in throat.—Scraping in throat causing cough.—Hæmorrhagic pharyngitis with difficulty of swallowing.—Tonsils red, swollen, studded white.—Violent efforts to swallow, with difficulty in swallowing,

woke him from sleep ; the pain and difficulty became confined to r. side, with sticking along Eustachian tube into ear : swelling of r. tonsil, noticeable externally, with sensitiveness to touch and increased temperature in vicinity ; mucous membrane of throat and posterior fauces red, swollen, with ulcers size of head of a pin, after a while a small lump of cheesy matter of strong odour was expectorated.

11. **Stomach.**—Nausea, gagging, waterbrash.—Frequent vomiting.—Ecchymoses.—Erosions and ulcers in stomach and bowels.—Burning in epigastric region.—Weak, nervous sensation in stomach.—Flatulent and fermentative dyspepsia ; putrid belchings.

12. **Abdomen.**—Abdominal distension.—Ulceration of bowels.—Violent, constant pressure in abdomen, with feeling of incarcerated flatus ; associated with constipation.

13. **Stool and Anus.**—Diarrhœa : stools green ; flushes easily as in hectic ; acid, sour, or putrid smelling.—Costive : stool dry, hard , then diarrhœa, watery, sour, yellow, with great weakness.—Cholera infantum with peculiarly putrid eructations.—Caused expulsion of tænia.

14. **Urinary Organs.**—Diabetes mellitus.—Albuminuria, rheumatic diathesis.—Urine : scanty, clear, brown ; three hours after passage has a green tinge, and a feathery deposit of crystal of *Salicyluric acid;* if these are removed the urine at once becomes putrid ; if left, urine remains fresh for a week.

16. **Female Sexual Organs.**—Leuco-phlegmatic woman, frequent hot flushes, irritability, forgetfulness, dull, heavy pain in cerebellum.—Septic puerperal fever.

17. **Respiratory Organs.**—Respiration hurried, sometimes deepened, sometimes shallow or sighing and almost panting, as if laboured, but no complaint of difficulty of breathing.—Dry cough of a hard, racking, spasmodic character, < at night in old people.

18. **Chest.**—Spasmodic, flatulent asthma ; fetid bronchitis ; gangrene of lungs.—Firmly seated pressure at side of sternum as large as the hand, with feeling as if the bone was sore.

19. **Heart.**—Pulse small, rapid, weak.

21. **Limbs.**—Heat, redness, soreness, and swelling about joints ; < in knees, with acute, piercing pains ; < on motion ; > from dry heat.—Soreness and pain in r. deltoid and r. gastrocnemius, changing next day to l. wrist and forearm ; < touch and movement.

22. **Upper Limbs.**—Rheumatic pain or rheumatoid arthritis, occurring in some women during climaxis ; the pains disappeared, the engorgements of fingers subsided, and the hands could again be used.

23. **Lower Limbs.**—After suppressed foot-sweat, rheumatic pains ; < at night ; after an hour's sleep forced to get up ; pain in course of l. sciatic nerve, drawing burning ; "as if foot were in an ant-hill" ; as if it would like to perspire.—Necrosis of tibia.—Copious foul-smelling foot-sweats.—(Applied locally it brings away corns.)

24. **Generalities.**—Weakness, faintness.—Deprives bone of its lime salts.

25. **Skin.**—Skin red, points like flea-bites.—Skin red and sensitive.—Urticaria.

26. Sleep.—Yawning.—Frequently waked from sleep thinking he heard music

27. Fever.—Slight chill, crawling in spine ; yawning ; chill in finger-tips.—Fever continuous, burning, then sweat with relief ; fever again till exacerbation of symptoms.—Weak, faint after fever and sweat.—Flushes easily as in hectic.—Profuse sweat ; as sweat increased strength declined.

Salix Mollissima.

Salix mollissima. *N. O.* Salicaceæ. Tincture of fresh leaves and young shoots.

Clinical.—Rheumatism. Sciatica.

Characteristics.—Cooper has used *Sal. mollis.* with success in rheumatic affections, especially in sciatic neuritis in nervous subjects, in whom the capillary cutaneous circulation showed up visibly, and there was some tenderness and swelling of the limb.

Salix Nigra.

Salix nigra. Black Willow. *N. O.* Salicaceæ. Tincture of fresh bark.

Clinical.—Diarrhœa. Emissions. Fevers. Gonorrhœa. Impotence. Masturbation. Night-sweats. Nymphomania. Prostatitis. Satyriasis. Spermatorrhœa.

Characteristics.—The Black Willow of North America has a reputation as a purgative and febrifuge. A proving by E. D. Wright, who took half an ounce of the tincture in a day, is given in Allen's *Appendix*. It developed soreness of muscles ; a tired, sleepy state ; loose bowels, sore gums, and fever. *Sal. n.* has been largely used by eclectics in a great variety of affections of the genito-urinary system. W. B. McCoy (*Hom. News*, xxviii. 72) relates a number of cases illustrating this action. (1) Man, 35, lost control of his sexual appetite, and the more he indulged the worse the craving became, and indulgence made him a physical wreck. *Sal. n.* ϕ, in teaspoonful doses thrice daily, cured in five weeks. (2) Youth, 23, had masturbated since he was a boy. *Sal. n.* ϕ, gtt xx., four times a day, was given for a fortnight, the quantity being gradually diminished, until in a few weeks the young man was quite cured. (3) A teacher, 21, five years before had a spell of fever which left him with a tendency to seminal emissions, which had become very frequent, and had reduced him to a very low condition : Extremely thin, sallow, nervous ; cold hands and feet even in heat of summer. Extremely cross and irritable. *Sal. n.* ϕ, gtt. lx., four times a day, was given, with speedy improvement. Later on the dose was reduced to thirty drops. The losses ceased, and in three months the patient had gained 41 pounds in weight. (4) A negro, 53, had sexual desire but without ability; yet during the night he would have emissions without erections. *Sal. n.* φ, gtt. xlv., four times a day, cured in three weeks. McCoy also used *Sal. n.* successfully in gonorrhœa, but other remedies were given as well. A decoction of the fresh bark has proved (*H. R.*, xii. 447) a specific for excessive night-sweats in pulmonary cases.

Relations.—*Compare:* Con., Agn., Pic. ac. In gonorrhœa, Salol, Petrosel.

SYMPTOMS.

2. **Head.**—Skin on temples sore to touch.

8. **Mouth.**—Gums sore.

13. **Stool and Anus.**—Looseness of bowels.

24. **Generalities.**—Muscles sore and lame.—Disposition to lie down and sleep.

27. **Fever.**—Fever (2nd d.).

Salix Purpurea.

Salix purpurea. Red or Purple Willow. *N. O.* Salicaceæ. Tincture or infusion of fresh bark.

Clinical.—Diarrhœa. Fever. Parotitis. Vertigo.

Characteristics.—T. C. Duncan and his wife proved *Sal. purp.*, taking drachm doses of the infusion of the bark. The chief symptoms produced were: Giddiness; loose stools; fever; swelling of the right parotid gland. The fever was marked by heat preceding chill and perspiration. Duncan chewed the bark on one occasion, and this caused the astringent effect on the mucous membrane of the mouth. The only rheumatic symptom was aching in right acetabulum.

SYMPTOMS.

1. **Mind.**—Very nervous, irritable, and despondent all day.—Dulness of intellect.

2. **Head.**—In a few minutes dizzy feeling commencing just in front of ears and passing up to vertex, like a wave; compelled to sit down.

6. **Face.**—Swelling of r. parotid gland.

8. **Mouth.**—Peculiar astringent taste, puckering mucous membrane and closing Steno's duct.—Taste of undigested food.

12. **Abdomen.**—Flatulence.—Pain in abdomen.

13. **Stool and Anus.**—Bowels loose; two stools in one day; with griping.

14. **Urinary Organs.**—Urine slightly acid; excess of triple and earthy phosphates and epithelium; less uric acid crystals (?).

19. **Heart.**—Pulse feeble; circulation torpid.
23. **Lower Limbs.**—Aching in r. acetabulum.
26. **Sleep.**—Rested poorly; waked often; first too hot, then too chilly.
27. **Fever.**—First too hot, then chilly, and at last, towards morning, in a
ɔfuse perspiration.

Salol.

Salicylate of Phenol. $C_6H_4 \left\{ \begin{array}{l} OH \\ COOC_6H_5. \end{array} \right.$ Trituration.

Clinical.—Diarrhœa. Dysentery. Fever. Gonorrhœa. Headache. Influenza. uralgia. Rheumatism. Small-pox.

Characteristics.—*Salol* was primarily used as an anti-rheuatic, especially in the treatment of acute cases. It was given as an tipyretic, in 30 to 45 grain doses, in powders or tablets. It is luble in ether and petroleum spirit; very sparingly, if at all, in ater. It does not disturb digestion because it passes through the ɔmach unaltered, being decomposed in the duodenum, by the fer-ents of the pancreas, into *Salicylic acid* and *Phenol* (it contains 38 r cent. of *Phenol*). These are excreted by the kidneys, and the con-ion of intestinal digestion has been estimated by the length of time quired, after the ingestion of *Salol*, for them to appear in the urine. ɔon this property also has been based the use of the remedy in ute diarrhœa, dysentery, cholera, and other diseases where intes-al asepsis is indicated, and also in affections of the bladder and ethra as a substitute for ordinary mechanical irrigations and injec-ns. Its internal use in gonorrhœa (in 5-gr. doses three times a day) s met with much success (Helbing). The only proving of *Salol* ublished by me, *H. W.*, xxxiii. 118) was made incidentally on a emist from making up powders of *Salol*. He experienced very vere symptoms from inhaling the odour, and possibly also some of powder. The experience was repeated on more than one casion, and I have confirmed most of the symptoms in prac-e, using the 12th attenuation chiefly. Rheumatic pains in joints th soreness and stiffness were marked, especially pain and soreness the buttocks, knees, and wrists. The prover was subject to head-hes, but he never had so violent a headache as that produced by *lol*, and conversely, after the proving, *Salol* 12 immediately relieved n when threatened with one of his usual headaches. The first nptom he noted was that his urine smelt of violets; and it was ly when this passed off that the other symptoms came on. The nts felt stiff, "as if they wanted oiling." C. Begg (*B. M. J.*, January , 1901) refers to the use of *Salol* in small-pox, and other skin affec-ns attended with burning and itching. The relief of itching in all-pox was, he says, a constant and most satisfactory result. When ministered early it prevented maturation. The symptoms were < lking. < Raising eyes. < Sitting on hard stool (pain in buttocks). By touch. < Evening. < Ascending stairs.

Relations.—*Antidoted by:* Bry. *Compare:* Sal. ac., Saln., N[a]. sal., Carbl. ac. Wrist rheumatism, Act. sp., Led., Viol. od. Uri[ne] smells of violets, Tereb. Gonorrhœa, Naphth., Petrosel. Small-p[ox], Carbl. ac. Sarr. Variol.

SYMPTOMS.

2. **Head.**—Dreadful headache, esp. over eyes, could hardly walk [or] hold head up for pain (relieved by *Bryon.* φ, three drops, and a wet compres[s]. —Dull aching in head and all over body; headache continued two days b[ut] was < at intervals.

14. **Urinary Organs.**—Urine smelt strongly of violets; after th[is] passed off the rest of the symptoms came on.

21. **Limbs.**—Feeling of stiffness in joints as though they want oiling. Extremities sensitive to touch.—Rheumatic pains in l. knee-joint, thighs, a[nd] arms, the pain being on the inner side of the joints.

22. **Upper Limbs.**—Pain in shoulder.—Pain in r. arm in evening. Slight pain in l. arm.—Pain in wrists.—Cramp in hand on writing.—Hur[ts] even to carry a book in hand.

23. **Lower Limbs.**—Buttocks sore.—Pain in l. buttock, esp. on walkin[g].

24. **Generalities.**—Dull aching in head and all over body.—Can hard[ly] go up stairs, and it is dreadfully painful to sit on a hard stool.—During th[e] whole time of the proving the hands shrunk when cold, and he could n[ot] straighten the little fingers without much pain.

25. **Skin.**—(Burning and itching eruption.—Small-pox.)

Salufer, *see* Natrum Silicofluoricum.

Salvia.

Salvia officinalis. Common Sage. *N. O.* Labiatæ. Tincture of fresh leaves and blossom-tips.

Clinical.—Cough, tickling. Phthisis. Night-sweats.

Characteristics.—*H. R.* (xii. 408) translates from *Leip. Pop. Z.* [f.] *H.*, August, 1897, an article on the use of *Salvia* as a gargle in sor[e] throat, and as a mouth wash in affections of the gums, but mor[e] especially in affections of the respiratory organs. The tickling coug[h] of consumptives and the night-sweats were entirely relieved by dose[s] of 20 to 40 drops in a tablespoonful of water. The *H. R.* translato[r] adds this case: Mrs. X. had had for three weeks an irritating coug[h] following an attack of pneumonia. The irritation being particularl[y] great, he gave her, fresh from the garden, some Sage to chew, and th[e] irritation was instantly relieved.

Sambucus Canadensis.

.mbucus canadensis. S. humilis. S. glauca. S. nigra (Marsh). Elder-bush. *N. O.* Caprifoliaceæ. Tincture of buds, flowers, tender shoots, and leaves.

Clinical.—Albuminuria. Angina pectoris. Asthma. Blotches. Larynx, dry. ımbago.

Characteristics.—The indigenous North American Elder grows rich alluvial soils, flowers in July, and fruits in September. The ecies, says Millspaugh, is not sufficiently distinct from the European lder (*Samb. nigra*, Linn.), differing only " in being less woody, and ıving more loose cymes, larger flowers, and more compound leaves." has, however, been proved separately by A. Uebelacker, whose mptoms are given in the Schema. The severe chest symptoms and otched face recall symptoms of *Samb. nig.*, with which it is probably entical in action. The chief *Conditions* were : < Lying down. > etting out of bed. > By sweat.

SYMPTOMS.

1. **Mind.**—Depression and dread of undefined danger.

2. **Head.**—Severe drawing in head with fulness ; motion = sensation if water were undulating in it.—Head heavy, confused, with drawing and .rting pains.

6. **Face.**—Face flushed and broken out in blotches ; he looks ill.

8. **Mouth.**—Mouth parched, dry ; desire for drink.

9. **Throat.**—Pharynx and larynx felt dry and swollen, impeding free spiration.

14. **Urinary Organs.**—Pressure in kidney region, followed by profuse w of clear urine.—Frequent urination.—Urine albuminous.

17. **Respiratory Organs.**—Breathing laboured, asthmatic ; wheezing. Had to sit up in bed to get breath.

18. **Chest.**—Heaviness and constriction in chest, as from a heavy load ; .lpitation.—Aroused from sleep by a terrible constriction of chest and eart ; had to jump out of bed to get breath ; could not lie down for fear of ıoking.

19. **Heart.**—Sharp pain in heart (region of valves) with palpitation, at nes visible through the clothes.—Constriction of chest and heart ; must mp out of bed, lying down = choking.—Heart labours heavily.—Pulse rose 100, but became normal at end of perspiration.

20. **Back.**—Back felt sprained.—Pain (pressing) in lumbar region.

21. **Limbs.**—Sharp, darting rheumatic pains in hands and feet.

24. **Generalities.**—Exhaustion.—Uneasiness ; unrest.—Recurrence of mptoms.—All symptoms > by sweat.

27. **Fever.**—Sweat, soon becoming profuse, which gradually > all other mptoms (except exhaustion).—Head perspired less than rest of body.

Sambucus Nigra.

Sambucus nigra (Linn.). Elder. *N. O.* Caprifoliaceæ. Tincture of fresh leaves and flowers.

Clinical.—Angina pectoris. Asthma. *Chest, oppression of.* Coryza, dry. *Coug Croup.* Emaciation. Headaches, catarrhal. Hoarseness. Hydrocele. Ileu Laryngismus. *Perspirations.* Phthisis. Scurf. "Snuffles." *Starting.* Whoopin cough.

Characteristics.—The leaves of *Samb. n.* have an unpleasar odour when bruised, which is supposed to be offensive to mo insects, and a decoction of them is sometimes used by gardeners t keep off caterpillars from delicate plants. By village herbalists th inner bark as well as the leaves are employed for making an ointmen and the flowers serve for fomentations, or are made into a medicina tea; while the berries are the principal ingredient in Elderberr wine (*Treas. of Bot.*). If sheep that have the rot can get at th bark and young leaves they will soon cure themselves (Green Millspaugh says of *Samb. canad.* that a decoction or ointment of th flowers and leaves was used as an application to large wounds "t prevent deleterious consequences from flies." He also says that th bark contains *Viburnic acid*, which is identical with *Valerianic acia* This no doubt accounts for the odour, and suggests a relationship i action between *Sambucus*, *Valerian*, and the *Viburnums.* "Spasm will be found common to all. In *Samb.* the spasm affects mainly th respiratory system—larynx, chest, and nasal passages. *Samb. n.* wa proved by Hahnemann, and appears in *M. M. P.* One of the chie notes of the remedy is œdema: dropsical swellings in various parts o the body, especially legs, instep, and feet. This œdema, when i affects the nose, may give rise to obstruction, as in the "snuffles" o infants with dry coryza, preventing breathing and nursing. When i occurs lower down in the tract it causes dyspnœa: the child awaken suddenly nearly suffocated, face livid, blue, sits up in bed; turns blue gasps for breath, which it finally gets; attack passes off but is agai repeated; child inspires but cannot expire; sleeps into the attack The breathing is rattling. Croup, whooping-cough, asthma, may al manifest this group of symptoms. Nash once relieved with th 200th a very bad case of asthma, having attacks of suffocation o the above kind. The patient was an old lady. The relief wa accompanied by a profuse flow of urine, which carried off a larg amount of dropsical effusion in her legs and abdomen.—It wa mentioned above that the croupy attack "passes off but is again repeated." This tendency of attacks to recur is another note o the remedy. Another grand characteristic is: Profuse sweat during waking hours; dry heat when asleep. This feature marks *Samb.* as the remedy in some phthisical cases and many febrile conditions. Other fever peculiarities are: Deep, dry cough precedes the fever paroxysm; fever without thirst; dreads uncovering. The *Sensations* of *Samb.* are: As if head were filled with water. Skull as if stretched. As if suffoating. The symptoms are > by pressure and being tightly bound. eaning against a hard edge = painful pressure in abdomen with ausea. Contusions = dark red swelling. Rest <. < Lying down ; bed ; on left side. Head low < ; must sit up to regain breath. lotion < generally. Motion of head = tension and dizziness. leep <. < About midnight ; after midnight ; 2 to 3 a.m. (roused ith sense of stoppage of air tubes). < Uncovering. < Dry, cold r. < Cold drink while overheated. < From fright or mental notion. Fright = suffocative attack. *Samb.* is *suited to* diseases of crofulous children which affect the air passages especially ; to ersons previously robust and fleshy suddenly become emaciated. ffects of mental emotion, anxiety, grief, excessive sexual indulgence.

Relations.—(Samb. c. may be regarded as practically identical ith Samb. n.) *Antidoted by :* Ars., Camph. *Antidote to :* Ars. (relieves lments from abuse of Arsen.). *Compatible :* Bell., Con., Nux, Pho., hus, Sep. *Follows well :* Op. (effects of fright). *Compare :* In Millar's thma, Ar. dracont. Dyspnœa ; inspires, cannot expire, Chlorum, eph. Sleeps into the attack, Lach. Peculiarities of sweating, Chi. id Con. (sweats as soon as he closes his eyes to sleep—opp. of amb.), Thuj. (sweats on uncovered parts), Puls. (one-sided sweats). reads uncovering, Nux (must be covered in every stage). Fat people naciate suddenly, Iod., Tub. Effects of excessive sexual indulgence, ho. ac., K. ph. Tenacious mucus in larynx, K. bi. Sleepy but can-ot sleep, Bell. Effects of cold drink when over-heated, Bels. (Bels. acne ; Samb. = phthisis). Effects of dry cold, Aco. Snuffles, n. c., Nux. Plants containing Valerianic or Viburnic acid, Valer., b. o., Vib. t.

Causation.—Fright. Grief. Anxiety. Injury (hydrocele). Ex-ssive sexual indulgence.

SYMPTOMS.

1. **Mind.**—Great tendency to take fright (trembling, anxiety, and rest-sness).—Fright followed by suffocative attacks, with bluish, bloated face.—evishness (constant fretfulness), during which everything makes a disagree-le impression.—Periodical delirium, with frightful visions (and hallucina-ns).

2. **Head.**—Dizziness and confusion in the head, esp. during movement ; rising.—Headache as from intoxication.—Tension in head during move-nt as if it contained water.—Pressure and expansion in head.—Pressive, ring headaches in forehead and temples.—Sudden shocks in the brain.—dden jerks through head.—Digging pain in vertex.—Tearing stitch through alf of occiput, frequently returning and lasting a long time, with a dull sation in the intervals.—The head is bent backwards.—Erysipelas l. side head, ear much swollen.—Scurf on head with intolerable itching.—Skull ls as if stretched.

3. **Eyes.**—Pupils at first contracted, then greatly dilated.

4. **Ears.**—Sharp stitches in (r.) inner ear with cramp pain in it.—Itch-creeping in ears and in throat.

5. **Nose.**—Sensation of numbness in nose, with itching on bridge.—

Sanguineous congestion in nose, with sensation of heaviness in point of no —Obstruction of nose, with accumulation of thick and viscid mucus nostrils.—Snuffles of children.—Dry coryza of children.—Child starts suddenly as if suffocating.

6. **Face.**—Face bluish (or dark blue) and bloated or pale and earthy Circumscribed redness on cheeks.—Sensation of numbness and tension cheeks, as from being swollen.—Red, burning spots on cheeks and nose Gnawing pressure in bones of upper jaw.—Great heat of face.—Heat a perspiration in face.

7. **Teeth.**—Odontalgia with tearing and lancinations in all the tee and with a sensation as if cheeks were swollen.

8. **Mouth.**—Dryness of the mouth and throat, with thirstlessness.

9. **Throat.**—Itching tingling in throat.

10. **Appetite.**—Thirst without relishing the drinks.

11. **Stomach.**—Vomiting in morning, first of milk (or food), that been taken, and of mucus, afterwards of bile.—Pressure in stomach.—Ac lancinations under the stomach, < by pressing upon it.

12. **Abdomen.**—Pinchings (colic pain) in abdomen as from a chill, w (much flatulence and) expulsion of flatus.—Shootings in the l. side of hy gastrium.—Pain in abdomen as from a bruise.—Spasmodic tearings, sho ings, and pinchings in abdominal muscles.—Pressive pain in abdomen, w nausea, when resting it against a hard (edge or) body.

13. **Anus.**—(Irritable anus with piles.—R. T. C.)

14. **Urinary Organs.**—Frequent want to urinate, with copious em sion, also at night.—Deposits a heavy sediment.—Urine of deep yellow Emission of urine in too small a stream.

15. **Male Sexual Organs.**—Swelling of scrotum.

16. **Female Sexual Organs.**—Catamenia too profuse, like metr rhagia.

17. **Respiratory Organs.**—Hoarseness from accumulation of vis mucus in larynx.—Inflammation of larynx and trachea; croup; accumulati of mucus in larynx.—Whooping-cough; suffocative, hollow, deep cou caused by a spasm in chest, with expectoration only during the day small quantities of tough mucus.—The cough is < at or soon after midnig during rest, when lying in bed, or with the head low, from dry, cold air Deep, hoarse, hollow cough, with agitation and thirst.—Continued cough w abundant expectoration of a salt taste, or of sweetish mucus.—Attack suffocating cough, with cries, in children.—Cough with cries, as from a p in the gullet.—Wheezing and quick respiration.—Obstructed respiration wh lying down.—Spasmodic paroxysm of suffocation at night, with tears, gr agitation, and tossing of the hands (when waking after midnight out o slumber, with half-open eyes and mouth, with bloated blue hands and fa and heat without thirst).—Great difficulty in breathing.—Quick, wheezi crowing breathing.

18. **Chest.**—Oppression at the chest, with lancinations in (l.) side (bel nipple); or with aching under sternum.—Pressure on sternum, with counter-pressure from spine to sternum.—Oppression of chest, with press in stomach, nausea, and weakness.—Pressive pain in chest.—Sudden sensat of contraction in sides of chest.

19. **Heart.**—Orgasm in whole body.—Occasional omission of heart-beat. Angina pectoris where pressure proceeds from spine in individuals formerly and robust, now emaciated from mental emotions, sexual excesses, or ninal losses.—Pulse generally very frequent and small; sometimes slow, l, sometimes intermitting.

20. **Neck and Back.**—Pressive heaviness in nape.—Deep, incisive ıcinations in muscles of neck.—Sweat on throat and neck with children.—ins in loins with drawing pressure.—Incisive blows in loins.—Aching in ddle of spine during repose and movement.—Lancinations in scapulæ.

21. **Limbs.**—Hands and feet bloated and blue.

22. **Upper Limbs.**—Drawing in forearms and bones of hands.—Dark ıe bloatedness of the forearms and hands.—Paralytic heaviness in elbow-nt.—Lancinations in wrists.—Trembling of hands (when writing).—Tear-;s in joints of fingers.

23. **Lower Limbs.**—Spasmodic drawings and shootings in thighs.—nsion in tendons of ham as if they were too short.—Acute (deep) lancina-ns in tibia.—Sensation of coldness, numbness, and deadness in the middle (r.) tibia.—Œdematous swelling of feet as far as knees.—Tearing in legs l ankles.—Icy-cold feet with warmth of the body.

24. **Generalities.**—We are often led to this remedy when we find a at deal of perspiration, occurring with any other trouble, which may last the time, or it may come and go in paroxysms; it is sometimes found in thisis; perspiration with disinclination to undress or be uncovered; heat h inclination to be covered (H. N. G.).—Asthma with suffocative attacks breathing; patient may be well enough while awake, but sleeps into the ıble; loud respiration with no mucous rattle.—Babies with snuffles; can't athe well through nose.—Asthma Millari (H. N. G.).—Symptoms < covering; while lying down; while resting.—> From moving; on rising; ile walking; from wrapping up warmly.—General ebullition of blood in ning after lying down, with sensation of trembling.—Sudden drawing over ole surface of body, frequently recurring when seated.—The majority of symptoms manifest themselves during repose and are dispersed by move-nt.—Dropsical swelling of whole body.—Great emaciation.

25. **Skin.**—Bloatedness and dark red swelling, with tension after contu-ıs.—Œdema; anasarca.—Blotches on face.—Red spots on cheeks here l there with burning sensation.—Tingling itching of skin.—Sudden painful wing in all points over surface while sitting.

26. **Sleep.**—Disposition to sleep without being able to sleep.—During p dry heat, after awakening profuse perspiration.—(Sleeps with arms ve head.)—Frequent waking with a start, with anguish, trembling, and tructed respiration, amounting almost to suffocation.—Incomplete sleep, ı mouth and eyes half open.—Lascivious dreams.

27. **Fever.**—Shuddering, with shivering, icy coldness of hands and feet, pricking tingling in skin.—Shivering and shaking before going to sleep. ısupportable heat without thirst, with dread to be uncovered.—Fever with essive perspiration, esp. at night.—Profuse perspiration day and night, but when awake; first breaking out in the face.—Very debilitating perspira-.—Night-sweats, except on head, < towards morning.—Continued perspi-on while awake, changing into dry heat as soon as one goes to sleep.—

Intermittent fever: chills over whole body, with cold hands and fe followed by intolerably dry heat, without any thirst, accompanied by dr of being uncovered, afterwards copious sweat, without any thirst; the sw even continues during the apyrexia.—Pulse generally small and very quick times intermitting.

Sanguinaria.

Sanguinaria canadensis. Blood-root. Puccoon. *N. O.* Papaverac Tincture of fresh root. (The resin, leaves, seeds, seed-vess powdered root, and expressed juice have also been use Acetum.

Clinical.—Alcoholism. Aphonia. Asthma. *Breast, tumour of. Bronch Cancer. Catarrh. Chest, pains in.* Climaxis. *Cold.* Croup. Deafness. Di theria. Dysmenorrhœa. *Dyspepsia. Ear, polypus of.* Flushes, climacteric. Gl Granular lids. Hæmoptysis. *Headache. Influenza.* Keratitis. Liver-cough. *M struation, breasts painful during.* Nails, ulceration of. Neuralgia. Œde glottidis. Ophthalmia. Pharyngitis. Phthisis florida. Physometra. *Pneumo acute. Polypus.* Pregnancy, affections during. Pyrosis. Quinsy. Rheumati Rhus poisoning. Shoulder, rheumatism of. *Smell, illusions of; loss of.* Stom neurosis of. Syphilis. Tinnitus. Tumours. Vomiting. Whitlow. Whoop cough.

Characteristics.—The Blood-root, or Puccoon, commonly fo throughout the United States and Canada, is the sole representat of the genus *Sanguinaria* of the Papaveraceæ. It is herbaceous, a thick, branching root stock, which creeps along undergrour and in early spring sends up from the ends of the little side branc a single long-stalked leaf, and another stalk bearing a solitary flow The leaf is wrapped round the flower-bud when it rises from ground, and is bluntly five to nine-lobed, roundish at first, but aft wards kidney-shaped. The American Indians formerly used orange-coloured juice of the root for smearing their bodies, and staining various domestic articles. The plant has also been succe fully used by American and French dyers (*Treas. of Bot.*). Hale s of the root: "It is succulent, and when cut or broken emits fr numerous points on the transverse surface a light orange, or rat dark vermilion-coloured juice, which has a bitterish, acrid peculiar taste, which remains long in the mouth and leaves a p sistent burning in the throat. The juice of the stem is between a colour and a yellow, as that from the stem of *Chel. maj.* is p yellow, and that from *Papaver somnif.* [*Opium*] is white." It is v to bear in mind the parallelism observable between these th Poppies, no less in their medicinal than in their physical prop ties. The time for collecting the root is early spring or autumn. An alkaloid, *Sanguinarin* (identical with *Chelerythrin Chelidonium majus*), has been isolated, and the *Nitrate* of this been studied separately. Hale refers to a paper by Dr. Tully, p lished in 1813, in which *Sang.* is described as being analogous in action to *Squills, Senega, Digitalis, Guaiacum,* and *Ammonia,* wh shows an accurate conception of its range. In doses of from eight to twenty grains of the powdered root, *Sang.* is an active poison producing : Nausea ; burning in stomach ; tormenting thirst ; faintness ; vertigo ; indistinct vision ; violent, spasmodic efforts of the stomach, free vomiting, followed by alarming prostration. S. L. Mitchell has recorded fatal poisoning of four workmen who drank the tincture in mistake for brandy. They were all soon seized with severe racking and burning pains in the stomach and bowels with intense thirst. "Burning" is one of the leading notes of the remedy, and is found in many different parts. Winterburn has published (*H. M.*, vii. 532) two cases illustrating this indication in the region of the stomach : (1) Mr. F., 48, of sanguino-bilious temperament, energetic, refined, had been ill with pains in the stomach several months. A clairvoyant had recommended "a decoction of blood-root and bone-set in tablespoonful doses." Each dose produced "intense burning pains in the stomach lasting for hours," and it had to be discontinued. Several weeks later Winterburn was consulted, and this is the condition he found : Burning in epigastrium, with pressure, < at night, but coming on soon after lying down and compelling patient to arise. Eructations gave no >. Appetite great ; bowels torpid, an unsatisfactory relief each morning, leaving a sense of discomfort. Peculiar drawing pain in shoulders and arms during sleep, so that when she woke the fists were tightly clenched and flexed on the sternal end of clavicle ; lameness and weariness of the muscles followed. *Sang.* 200, chosen after careful comparison with *Nux*, *Graph.*, and others, was given every night at bedtime. After the first dose the symptoms disappeared "like magic," and the patient was soon well. (2) Mrs. S., 30, a chronic inebriate, had been drinking steadily for three weeks when sickness and diarrhœa set in. *Nux* 1 x aggravated the nausea. *Ars.* 6 checked the diarrhœa and relieved the intense thirst, but did nothing to allay the vomiting. Patient was irritable, angry. Everything she took, even water, was instantly ejected. About every twenty minutes she had a spasm or cramp of the stomach, with gagging and coughing, bringing up some frothy mucus. The straining caused great pain in chest and abdomen. There was, besides, the most intense burning, extending from the stomach up the œsophagus to pharynx, which felt swollen and dry. The only tolerable position was lying slightly turned on her left side. Lying on right side was impossible. Rising from lying = vertigo. Cheeks and hands livid. She believed she would soon die, and was unwilling to be left alone. *Sang.* 200 was given every two hours. By evening the nausea had ceased, but the burning pain remained as before. The smallest particle of food gave great agony ; it seemed as if a spot the size of a florin was ulcerated, and any contact with this was excruciating. She slept better, but awakened next morning in a fright. Next afternoon she was able to take a little solid food, and from that time recovery was rapid. *Burning* is a leading note of *Sang.* Burning of eyes ; of ears. Tongue and throat feel as if they had been burnt or scalded. Burning palms and soles. Burning in chest ; between breasts, streaming from breasts to abdomen. Leonard (*Min. H. Mag.*, ii. 295) says "a circumscribed burning in the chest, commonly followed by heat through abdomen and diarrhœa," is a strong indication for *Sang.* in pneumonic conditions. *Sang.* has also the circumscribed hectic flush on the cheeks, as in phthisis, in which it is frequently indicated. (*Sang.* has also the "hopefulness" of phthisical patients.) The flushed face, at times dark red or livid, is also a prominent feature of *Sang.*, as it is of *Op.* *Sang.* affects the whole respiratory tract, irritates the nasal mucous membrane, and causes coryza, with pain at root of nose, lost or perverted sense of smell, and sensitiveness to the odour of flowers. Influenza, hay-fever, ozæna, and polypus have all come within its range. Laryngitis and membranous croup have been cured by it; and I have found it meet a greater proportion of the tracheal and bronchial coughs of epidemic influenza than any other remedy. The chief features are: Violent, dry cough; wheezing, whistling, metallic; sputa almost impossible to raise. I have seen several cases of this kind rescued from apparently imminent death by *Sang.*, the relief comes by the expectoration of a thick plug of mucus which was causing suffocation, and which the patient was too weak to dislodge. Like *Chel.*, *Sang.* is a right-side medicine, and affects especially the right lung; and is suited to pulmonary affections with liver involvement. After influenza children often get a cough scarcely distinguishable from whooping-cough. I have found *Sang.* the chief remedy for this. It is also the remedy for severe cough *after* whooping-cough—the cough returns with every fresh cold. *Sang.* also acts powerfully on the outer chest, sternum, and mammæ. Like *Chel.*, it has a reputation for curing cancer, polypi, and new growths. I have seen breast tumours diminish under its action. Offensiveness and acridity characterise the discharges of *Sang.*; and the breath and flatus are also offensive. Menses offensive, flow bright red; later blood darker and less offensive. Before menses itching of axillæ. Eruption on the face of young women, especially during scanty menses. Climacteric disorders: flashes of heat; leucorrhœa; painful enlargement of breasts. The headaches of *Sang.* are of great intensity, and have some striking characteristics. They are (1) periodic—every seventh day; (2) begin in the morning, increase to noon, and then diminish; (3) are bursting, or as if the eyes would be pressed out; (4) begin at occiput, spread upwards and forwards, and settle over right eye; (5) like a flash of lightning in occiput; (6) > by sleep; (7) return at climacteric. Hering described the headache of *Sang.* as the "American sick-headache"—rush of blood causing faintness and nausea, pains lancinating or throbbing. Can neither bear light nor odours nor least jar, as any one stepping across the floor; at height of headache vomiting of food and bile; pain so violent patient goes out of her mind or seeks relief by pressing head against pillow or with the hands. Cooper gives as a keynote: "If he goes without food, gets bilious headaches." *Sang.* has also neuralgia of the face > by kneeling down and pressing head firmly against the floor; pain extends in all directions from the upper jaw. The ears are strongly affected by *Sang.* Cooper gives me this case: Girl, 19, had her throat bad three years from scarlatina, and lately increasing deafness; noises all over head, and vertigo and sudden flushings in daytime; menses too frequent, and profuse leucorrhœa; it pains her to walk from backache; had to give up teaching from this; appetite poor from the headaches and tinnitus; *often has pain behind angles of lower jaw* and swellings of gland. All disappeared after a single dose of *Sang.* ϕ, though at first the leucorrhœa was increased. "Fulness and tenderness behind angle of jaws" is, according to Cooper, a keynote. *Sang.* causes many symptoms of rheumatism, but the most characteristic is a rheumatic pain in right arm and shoulder; cannot raise the arm, < at night. Pains in places where the bones are least covered. *Peculiar Sensations* are: As if paralysed. As if forehead would burst. As of a band across forehead. As if head were drawn forward. As if electric current shooting through head. As if temples and scalp were alive with irrepressible pulsation. As if eyes would be pressed out. As if hairs were in eyes. As if she was in a railway car which was moving and jarring her, and as if all about her moved rapidly and confusedly. Pain like drawing a rope on a windlass as tight as possible. Tongue as if burnt. Tip of tongue as if scalded. Tongue as if in contact with something hot. Throat as if swollen. Throat so dry it seems as if it would crack. Pharynx as if burnt or scalded. As if some hard substance in stomach. Constriction in pit of stomach as if suffocating. As of a mass in lower part of rectum. As if upper part of chest were too full of blood. Larynx as if swollen. F. Nichol in giving Hale his experience with *Sang.* in croup, says he used (following Paine, eclectic) a solution of *Sanguinarin* in vinegar, and he found that the most effective preparation. The symptoms are < by touch. [A painful sensitiveness is very characteristic of *Sang.*: Temporal veins painfully sensitive; head and eye very painful; nipples sore.] Hard pressure >; (must kneel down and press head hard to floor in neuralgia). Slightest jar <. Lifting = lumbago. Lying down > rheumatism and headache; but < cough and most other complaints. Cough <. Lying with head low < cough. Lying on left side >. < Lying on right side. Sitting up and passing flatus > cough. Motion; turning head quickly; turning in bed; stooping; coughing; exercise <. Cannot raise arm from side but can swing it to and fro (in rheumatism). Eating <. Going without food = headache. > Eructations (mind confused). Swallowing <. Vomiting > (nausea; headache). Smoking = hiccough. < At night. > After sleep. Headache < by day, sunrise to sunset. Cold open air >. Cold room < cough. Damp weather <. The right side is more affected than the left. Symptoms go from right to left. Periodicity is very marked.

Relations.—*It antidotes*: Opium. *Compatible*: Bell. (scarlatina). *Compare*: Botan., Chel., Op. In rheumatism of right deltoid, Mg. c. (of left, Fer., Nx. m.). Headache extending forward from occiput and settling over (right) eye, Spi. (left eye), Sil., Sep. (both eyes); extending forward, Gels., Lac c.; (backward, Anac., Bry., Chi. s., Naj., Nux). Headache > by hard pressure, Chi., Indg., Mg. m. Paroxysms of headache ending in profuse urination, Ign., Gels., Ver. Menstrual headache, Sep. (Sep. scanty flow; Sang. profuse). Offensive breath with cough, Caps. Faint from odours, Pho., Ig., Val., Nux. Right-side, throbbing, congestive headache, < light and noise, Bell. (Bell.

has "cold feet, hot head," and is > sitting propped up; Sang. headache has more of the gastric form, and is > lying down), Meli. Periodic sick headaches, Ir. v. (Ir. v. every eighth day; every seventh, Saba., Sang., Sil., Sul.). Pneumonia, Ver. v. (more marked arterial excitement), Pho., Ant. t. (face livid, blood carbonised, rattling cough), Sul. (resolution imperfect)—(Sang. has sputa very offensive, even to patient). Rheumatism of right ankle, Chel. > Lying left side, Lil. t. Painfulness to touch of parts where pain has been, Lcprs. Sensitive to sudden sounds, Brx. Jerking or jumping as from something alive in stomach, Croc. Physometra, Lyc., Bov. Liver-cough (Scil. spleen-cough). Pain in bones covered only with skin, Rh. ven. Laryngeal and nasal polypi, Sang. n., Pso., Teuc. Eruption on face of young women during scanty menses, Bels., Calc., Jamb., Pso. Right-side complaints; right to left, Lyc., Chel. > By sleep, Pho.

SYMPTOMS.

1. **Mind.**—Angry irritability; moroseness.—Anxiety and dread preceding the vomiting.—Mind confused, > by eructations.—Mental torpor, stupor, heaviness, sleepiness.—Hopefulness, sanguine of recovery.—Disgusting ideas.—Dreamy state with eyes open.

2. **Head.**—Vertigo: terrible; when moving head rapidly and looking upward; with nausea, fainting, and headache; with ringing in ears; on rising from a sitting or stooping position; on quickly turning the head; with dim vision; with dull, heavy feeling in stomach as if caused by some hard substance there; in cold weather; during sleep; at climaxis.—Head swims on lying down suddenly; gets pain l. side of back near waist, as from spleen; bowels confined; complexion spotty (cured in woman, 32.—R. T. C.).—Sensation of heaviness in head.—Determination of blood to head, with whizzing in ears; flushes of heat; accumulation of water in mouth.—Headache over whole head from 5 p.m. to midnight; then free; and then sickness (vomiting) from 5 p.m. to midnight (agg.—R. T. C.).—Headache, with rheumatic pains and stiffness of limbs and neck.—Periodical sick headache; with vomiting of bile; begins in morning, < during day, lasts till evening; < from motion, stooping, noise, and light; only endurable when lying still, and > by sleep or after vomiting; esp. severe over r. eye.—Headache returns periodically.—Heaviness in head from vertex to centre of forehead, with pressing in glabella and buzzing in head; eyes dull.—Terrific headache as if caused by approaching coryza which does not come, in forehead and middle of vertex, with pressure in eyes, which burn and are moved with difficulty.—Terrific headache during the fever.—Dull, pressive frontal headache.—Headache as if forehead would burst, with chill and burning in stomach.—Frontal headache extending into cheek-bones.—Headache or neuralgia over r. eye.—Headache as if it must burst, or as if eyes would be pressed out; > walking in open air.—Headache with shuddering.—Headache begins in occiput, spreads upward, and settles over r. eye.—Pain in head in rays drawing upwards from neck.—Headache with nausea and chilliness, followed by flushes of heat, extending from head to stomach.—Headache with flushed face.—Pains in head in spots.—Pains in head, which pass rapidly from one

place to another, like electric shocks.—Pulsations in head (throbbing headache), with bitter vomiting, < from motion.—Headache rising up from neck. —Feeling as if head were drawn forward.—Distension of veins on head, esp. on temples, perceptible to the touch and sore.—Sensation of mobility in the scalp.—Head very painful to touch ; where pain has been.—Distension of veins in temples ; sore when touched.

3. **Eyes.**—Neuralgia in and over l. eye.—Burning and watering of r. eye, which is painful to the touch, followed by coryza.—Acute conjunctivitis with ecchymoses, tending to trachoma.—Blepharitis.—Burning dryness in eyes ; followed by copious lachrymation.—Retinal congestion with flushed face and congestive headache.—Yellow sclerotica, jaundice.—Catarrhal ophthalmia, granular lids.—Redness of eyes in morning.—Hard swelling like scirrhus over eyebrows.—Dim eyes, with sensation as if hairs were in them.—Pain in eyeballs on moving them.—Balls sore, with darting through them and dim vision.—Violent twittering before eyes.—Vapour or cloud before eyes.

4. **Ears.**—Burning of ears, with redness of cheeks.—Earache, with headache, with singing in ears and vertigo.—Humming and roaring in ears with painful sensitiveness to sudden sounds in women at climaxis.—Cracking in r. ear while stroking cheek.—Every stroke of a hammer heard near a blacksmith's shop is painful to r. ear.—Vein on r. temple swells up in woman, 50, subject to neuralgia and old vascular deafness ; after *Sang.* φ, one dose, hearing improves for six days strikingly, and then reverts (R. T. C.).—Throat affections causing deafness and earache.—Acts strongly on l. Eustachian tube (*Hydrast.* on r.) ; acts on ethmoid cells specially (R. T. C.).—Increased redness of external ear, with humming and roaring in ears from increased circulation of blood through aural structures.—Burning ears, cheeks red.—Aural polypus.

5. **Nose.**—Fluent coryza with frequent sneezing ; < r. side.—Heat in nose ; coryza, rawness in throat, pain in breast, cough, and finally diarrhœa. —Coryza, watery, acrid ; with tingling ; with heavy pain at root of nose and stinging in nose.—Dry coryza, as from a sudden cold.—Alternately fluent and dry coryza.—Smell in nose like roasted onion.—Rose-cold, with subsequent asthma ; sick and faint from odour of flowers.—Loss of smell and taste.—Dislike to odour of syrup.—Nasal polypus.

6. **Face.**—Circumscribed redness of one or both cheeks.—Paleness of face, with disposition to vomit.—Pain in cheek.—Stitches l. side of face with pains in forehead.—Neuralgia in upper jaw, extending to nose, eye, ear, neck, and side of head ; shooting, burning pains ; must kneel down and hold head tightly to the floor.—Face bloated, with sensation of rigidity and fulness.—Veins distended, feel stiff and sore to touch.—Twitching of cheeks toward eyes.—Stiffness of articulation of jaws.—Fulness and tenderness behind angles of jaw (a keynote.—R. T. C.).—Red cheeks : with burning ears ; with cough.—Lips feel dry.—Under lip burns, is swollen, hard, and blistered ; blisters dry up and form crusts which fall off.

7. **Teeth.**—Pain in hollow teeth, esp. when touched by food.—Toothache from picking teeth.—Pain in carious teeth after cold drinking.—Looseness of teeth (with salivation).—Bleeding, spongy, fungoid gums.

8. **Mouth.**—Pricking on the point of the tongue.—Tongue feels as if burned or as if sore ; is coated white.—White coated tongue with slimy, fatty

taste.—Red streak through middle of tongue.—Tip of tongue burns as if scalded.—Pricking in tip of tongue.—Stitches in l. side of tongue.—Crawling on tip of tongue followed by astringent sensation of whole tongue, on waking. —Dry, acrid sensations, beginning r. side and extending over whole tongue.—Prickling on tongue and hard palate as after chewing *Mezereum.*—Sweet things taste bitter, followed by burning in fauces.—Loss of smell and taste; with a burnt feeling on tongue.—Sore on gums and roof of mouth.—Fetid breath, clammy mouth, sticky teeth.—White patches on mucous membrane.

9. **Throat.**—Ulcerated sore throat, as if raw and denuded.—Feeling of swelling in throat on swallowing, < on r. side.—Throat feels swollen as if to suffocation, aphonia.—Tonsillitis, promotes suppuration.—Throat so dry, seems as if it would crack.—Feeling of dryness in throat (with tickling cough), not > by drinking.—Sensation in pharynx as if scalded by hot drink.—Uvula sore and burning.—Burning pharynx and œsophagus.—Heat in throat > by drawing in cold air.—Inflammation in throat.—Warming sensation in fauces, esp. soft palate.—Burning in fauces extending to centre of sternal region.

10. **Appetite.**—Craving for he knows not what, with loss of appetite; wants piquant, spiced things.—Loss of appetite with great weakness of digestion.—Aversion to butter, which leaves a sweetish taste.—Sugar tastes bitter and = burning.—Tormenting thirst.—Sweet things <, = burning.—Soon after eating: feels empty; difficult breathing, nausea, waterbrash, lassitude almost to fainting, cold sweat to 12 p.m., after a little food.—If goes without food, gets bilious headaches (keynote.—R. T. C.).

11. **Stomach.**—Burning in stomach, with headache.—Inflammation of stomach.—Sensation of emptiness in stomach soon after eating (faint, feverish feeling).—Soreness and pressure in epigastrium; < after eating.—Hiccough whilst smoking.—Spasmodic eructation of flatus.—Frequent fetid eructations with disposition to vomit and pale face.—Pyrosis.—Nausea, which is not > by vomiting.—Extreme nausea with great salivation and constant spitting.—Nausea with headache, and with chill and heat.—Vomiting preceded by anxiety.—Vomiting: of bitter water; of sour, acrid fluids; of ingesta; of worms; with craving to eat in order to quiet the nausea.—Vomiting and diarrhœa.—Sudden attacks of constriction in pit of stomach as if suffocating. —Goneness with sick headache.—Jerking or jumping in stomach as if from something alive.—Neurosis of stomach.—Pain in stomach-pit extending down into bowels, causing rumbling.

12. **Abdomen.**—Hot streaming from breast towards liver.—Sensation as if hot water poured itself from breast into abdomen, followed by diarrhœa. —Dull burning in r. hypochondrium and chest.—Awoke with severe pain in region of spleen.—Violent stitches in spleen.—Pain in l. hypochondrium; < by coughing, > by pressure and lying on l. side.—Jaundice.—Liver-cough.—Colic, with torpor of liver.—Beating and spasms in abdomen.—(Flatus, cough and sneezing.—R. T. C.).—Flatulent distension of abdomen, evening, with escape of flatus from vagina (the os uteri being dilated).—Beating in abdomen.—Indurations in abdomen.—Cutting bellyache from r. to l. of iliac fossa, thence to rectum.—Throbbing in abdomen.—Shooting pains through bowels extending to lower limbs, afternoon.—Knife-thrusts in abdomen followed by watery stools.—Cramp extending from place to place.

13. **Stool and Anus.**—Ineffectual urging to stool. then vomiting.—

Urging to stool, afternoon, but only discharges of flatus.—Distressing, cutting, spasmodic sensation in rectum in evening; recurred several days.—Ineffectual desire with sensation of thick mass in anus; repeated several times in the day without stool.—Diarrhœic stools with much flatulence.—Copious apple-green stools with flatus (offensive) and sudden urging (agg.—R. T. C.).—Frequent discharges of very offensive flatus.—Colic followed by diarrhœa.—Diarrhœa with disappearance of coryza, catarrh, or pains in chest and cough.—Stools undigested.—Dysentery.—Alternate diarrhœa and constipation.—Constipation; stools in hard lumps.—Hæmorrhoids.

14. **Urinary Organs.**—Dull, heavy pain across kidneys.—Pain from kidneys penetrates r. iliac fossa, then shoots through sigmoid flexure to rectum.—Frequent and copious nocturnal urination, urine as clear as water.—(Retention of urine consequent on gravel and calculus.)—Urine is thick and white next day (agg. from 200th.—R. T. C.).—Copious urination goes on all night with much > to chest symptoms (in a lady.—R. T. C.).—Very copious urine at night, with pain in l. hypochondrium; < from coughing; > from pressure and lying on l. side.—Urine: dark yellow; high-coloured, red sediment.—Ardor urinæ.

15. **Male Sexual Organs.**—Burning in glans.—Emissions two nights in succession; after which he felt very well.—Gleet; old cases.—Cheesy secretions from glans (syphilis).

16. **Female Sexual Organs.**—Climacteric disorders, esp. flushes of heat and corrosive, fetid leucorrhœa.—Burning of palms and soles at climaxis compelling to throw off clothes.—Painful enlargement of breasts at climaxis.—Abdominal pains as if menses would appear.—[Delaying menses, chilliness followed by flushes of heat and occasional palpitation, faintness, vertigo, nausea, and violent vomiting, burning in œsophagus, neuralgia in r. temple, in l. chest (mamma) and lower extremities, occasional hacking cough and gastralgia.—Carmichael.]—Menstruation too early, with a discharge of black blood.—Menses: more profuse than usual; with headache r. side; at night time, very offensive, putrid, bright red, clotting, becoming darker towards end and less offensive.—Amenorrhœa.—Metrorrhagia.—Dysmenorrhœa of feeble, torpid subjects, with tendency to congestion of lungs, liver, or head.—Burning pain between breasts in afternoon, < on r. side.—Shootings in bosom and pain in mammæ as from excoriation.—The nipples are sore and painful.—Stitches in nipples, esp. r.—Sharp, piercing pain in r. breast, just beneath nipple; < deep breath, some dyspnœa.—Pain in r. breast extends to shoulder, can hardly place hand on head.—Threatened abortion, pains in loins extending through epigastric and iliac regions and down thighs.—Hydrops uteri.

17. **Respiratory Organs.**—Dryness in throat and sensation of swelling in larynx; with expectoration of thick mucus.—Aphonia with swelling in throat.—Œdema of larynx.—Tickling in throat, evening, after lying down, with dry, hacking cough and headache.—Crawling sensation extending down behind sternum.—Tracheal irritation secondary to heart disease.—Croup: hoarse, muffled cough; complete aphonia; spasmodic cough, painful crowing, stridulous breathing.—Cough dry, tickling in throat-pit.—Distressing, spasmodic, exhaustive cough.—Dry cough, awakens him from sleep, which did not cease until he sat upright in bed, and flatus was discharged both

upwards and downwards.—Continual severe cough, with circumscribed redness of cheeks, with pain in chest; with coryza, then diarrhœa.—Coughs in old men with l. earache, and pains going from l. throat to ear.—Expectoration: tough; difficult; rust-coloured; extreme dyspnœa; hepatisation.—Breath and sputa smell badly even to patient.—Pulmonary consumption, expectoration and breath exceedingly offensive.—Whooping-cough.—Severe cough after whooping-cough; the cough returns every time patient takes cold.—Asthma: excessive dyspnœa; esp. after "rose-cold," < from odours.

18. **Chest.** — Hydrothorax. — Hæmoptysis. — Pneumonia: catarrhal; chronic; r. side; l. side, with heart disease.—Typhoid pneumonia, with very difficult respiration, cheeks and hands livid, pulse full, soft, vibrating, and easily compressed.—Severe dyspnœa and constriction of chest, with inclination to take deep inspirations.—Sharp stitches in r. chest.—Stitches in lower part of l. breast to shoulder.—Pain in breast with periodic cough.—A shooting, sticking pain beneath sternum.—Persistent pain beneath sternum and in r. breast.—Intense burning between breasts, < r. side.—Sharp, piercing, neuralgic pain half-way between sternum and nipple.—Hot, burning streaming from r. chest to liver.—Pain under l. clavicle on waking.—Constriction across both breasts.—Violent stitches under short ribs.—Burning and pressing in breast, followed by heat through abdomen and diarrhœa.—Pain in r. chest to shoulder; can only with difficulty place hand to head.

19. **Heart.**—Painful stitches or pressive pain beneath præcordial region. Surging of blood and racing palpitation, with dry and burning skin.—Weak feeling about heart.—Metastasis of rheumatism (or gout) to heart from outward applications.—Palpitation of heart.—Irregularity of heart's action and of the pulse, with coldness, insensibility, &c.—Pulse slow, irregular, feeble.

20. **Neck and Back.**—Soreness of nape on being touched.—Rheumatic pain in nape, shoulders, and arms.—Pain in r. side of neck as if strained; in l. side.—Soreness down muscles of back; pains shifting about; feels pain more when drawing long breath.—Pain in inner border of r. shoulder-blade.—Pain in sacrum from lifting; the pain in sacrum is > on bending forward.—Pain in sacrum and bowels.

21. **Limbs.**—Rheumatic pain in limbs, esp. in shoulders, arms, and thighs, and < at night.—Burning in hands and feet < night.

22. **Upper Limbs.**—Itching in axillæ before menses.—Rheumatic pain in r. arm and shoulder, < at night in bed; cannot raise arm; motion (turning in bed) much < it.—Pain in top of r. shoulder.—Pain in r. deltoid.—R. arm hung helpless.—Coldness in body and r. arm.—Burning of palms.—Stiffness of finger-joints.—Aching in ball of r. thumb.—Fungoid growth between second and third metacarpal bones, protruding about a quarter of an inch out of palm.—Ulceration at roots of nails on all the fingers of both hands.—Panaritium, first r. then l. finger.—Shooting pains from r. thumb to symphysis menti.

23. **Lower Limbs.**—Rheumatic pain in l. hip.—Rheumatic pain inside of r. thigh.—Bruise-like pain in thigh, alternating with burning and pressure in chest.—Stiffness of knees.—Burning of soles, < at night.—Rheumatic pains in limbs; pain in those places where the bones are least covered with flesh, but not in the joints; on touching the painful part the pain immediately vanished and appeared in some other part.—(Have seen ulcers connected

vith carious ankles and shins change almost visibly after *Sang.*—Gutteridge). –Sharp pain in r. ankle and great toe-joint.—Cold feet, afternoon.

24. **Generalities.**—Great debility and weakness in limbs (esp. in morn-ng on waking), whilst walking in the open air.—Paralysis of r. side.—General orpor and languor.—An uncomfortable, prickling sensation of warmth preading over whole body.—Weakness and palpitation of heart; fainting veakness.—Convulsive rigidity of limbs.—We find this very useful where here is a pain rising from the back of the neck over the top of the head, unning down into the forehead; this symptom may occur alone, or in con-ection with some other trouble (H. N. G.).—Often useful for troubles occur-ing in females at the climacteric period of life—such as flashes of heat, &c. H. N. G.).

25. **Skin.**—Heat and dryness of skin.—Itching and nettle-rash before the ausea.—Old, indolent ulcers, with callous borders and ichorous discharge.—Iasal polypi; fungus excrescences.—Jaundice.—Eruption on face of young vomen with menstrual troubles, esp. deficiency.—Scaly eruptions, carbuncles. -*Rhus* poisoning.

26. **Sleep.**—Drowsiness causing mental and bodily indolence.—Sleep-ssness at night; awakens in a fright as if he would fall.—Can't sleep ithout brandy.—Slightest noise disturbs, yet is sleepy and dreamy. R. T. C.).—Dreams: of sea voyages, with sensation of being rocked; of usiness matters; frightful.

27. **Fever.**—Pulse too frequent and full.—Coldness of feet in afternoon, ith painful, sore tongue; stiffness of knee and finger-joints.—Chill and ivering in back, evening, in bed.—Shaking chill.—Chill with nausea, head-che.—Heat flying from head to stomach.—Fever heat and delirium.—Burn-g heat rapidly alternating with chill and shivering.—Intermittent fevers; arsh fevers; nervous fever.—Fever from pulmonary, hepatic, or gastric flammation.—Copious sweat; cold sweat.

Sanguinarinum.

Sanguinarinum. $C_{19}H_{17}NO_4$. Trituration. Solution in vinegar.

Clinical.—Croup.

Characteristics.—*Sanguinarin.* is a pearly white substance. In nallest physiological doses it acts as "expectorant," in large it causes iusea, and still larger vomiting. In repeated doses it lowers the ilse rate (Thomas, quoted *C. D. P.*). T. Nichol gives in Hale's work s experience with a solution of one grain of *Sanguinarin.* in two inces of vinegar in cases of pseudo-membranous croup. (He does ot say how much of this he gave or how frequently he repeated: obably the dose was a few drops in water given frequently.) He lates this case: W. G., 5, had been ill some days. Nichol found m with a hoarse, muffled cough, complete aphonia, pulse 132. Soft ılate and fauces covered with pearly, fibrinous exudation; a hissing und was heard on auscultating larynx. Great dyspnœa. The child stretched back his head and grasped his throat in agon Features swollen and dark. *Sgn. acet.* was given, and in fifteen hou there was notable improvement. In forty-eight hours the boy w out of danger.

Sanguinarinum Nitricum.

Nitrate of Sanguinarin. $C_{19}H_{17}NO_4HNO_3$. Trituration.

Clinical.—Adenoids. Asthma. Borborygmus. Bronchitis. Catarrh. Cory Deafness. Eustachian catarrh. Hay-fever. Headache. Influenza. Laryngi Polypus. Post-nasal catarrh. Quinsy. Stiff-neck. Throat, sore. Tinnitus.

Characteristics.—*Sang. nit.* is a very fine brownish-red powde pungent, acid, bitter, and inodorous. It is soluble in alcohol, ethe water, and oils, but not in the same proportion in all. Pure *Sa guinarin.* is a pearly-white substance, but when combined with any the acids the result is a salt of some shade of red, crimson or scarl The colour of the blood-root may thus be due to the presence some native salt of *Sanguinarin.* (Hale). *Sng. n.* was proved in trituration by Professor Owens (*C. D. P.*), of Pulte Medical Colleg and some very striking symptoms were elicited. The catarrh symptoms of *Sang.* appear in great intensity—nose, eyes, throat, ar bronchi being affected. Lachrymation, pains in eyes and head, so scalp, obstructed nose, and burning pains throughout all regions we experienced. A sense of *obstruction* is very characteristic : Sensati of obstruction and fulness in the head ; accumulation of muc obstructing nose ; awakes frequently with dry mouth, the nose bei obstructed. Accumulation of mucus behind centre of sternum ; sen of suffocation ; feeling as if air-passages lined with thick, stiff muc or pus. Heat and tension behind sternum is characteristic ; and so expectoration of quantities of sweet-tasting mucus. There is al expectoration of thin, frothy, very tenacious mucus. The sympto of influenza are very completely depicted, even to the loss or perve sion of taste. *Sng. n.* appears to have the nasal symptoms of *Sang.* an enhanced degree. "Sensation arising to nostrils as if he had eat strong horseradish," is present. Hale gives these verifications. (Mr. B., 40, dark, had for eight years, in spite of continuo old-school treatment, chronic post-nasal catarrh, bronchitis, a laryngitis. Voice altered, deep, hoarse ; speech with effort, as from chest. Severe pressure from behind sternum. Mucous me brane dry, raised only a few balls of grey mucus. He spent t winters on the St. John's River, Florida, and was > there, but again on his return north. *Sng. n.* 6 trit. was given every two hou In one week he was better ; there was more moisture in his thr than there had been for two years. Voice markedly better. *Sng.* was now given every four hours. In ten weeks he had regained pounds of his lost weight, and strength in proportion. The voice n having improved in the same degree, *Caust.* 6, and afterwards *Dros.*

ere given, and in sixteen weeks he was perfectly well. (2) Mrs. S., ty missionary, 49, had constant hacking cough, raw, sore feeling in roat, sore aching and pressing behind sternum. She was much posed to cold winds of winter, which set up coryza and irritation. *ig. n.* 6. trit. gr. i., every two hours, enabled her to follow her occupa- on without suffering, and in ten weeks she was completely cured.) O. W., 55, subject to frequent attacks of cold in head, throat, and iest. After a long drive in open trap contracted a severe cold in ead, throat, lungs. Sore and lame all over ; frequent sneezing, chrymation. Next day sore throat very marked, constant tickling throat-pit, exciting cough, at first short and hacking, but in two ays it became violent and convulsive. *Bell.* and *Dros.* did little good. ressure behind sternum became very severe. *Sng. n.* 6 was given very two hours. In four hours copious perspiration came on with equent sneezing. Next day sore throat appeared after waking from troubled and restless sleep ; constriction of throat with difficult wallowing ; tension across chest radiating from behind sternum. *ng. n.* every hour. In one hour free discharge from nose set in ; in iree hours moisture and relaxation of constriction across chest. The ischarge was yellow and sweetish-tasting, continued all day. Slept ell and woke next morning feeling quite free. But little cough or oryza during the day. The following morning he was quite well.— Iering gives this case cured with *Sng. n.* 2 trit. : Troublesome cough or number of years ; excited by an irritation in region of bifurcation f bronchi ; coughs a long time to raise a little whitish-yellow phlegm, ometimes streaked with blood, after which she feels great > ; cough ay and night ; is greatly emaciated. Owens (*M. A.*, xvii. 31) relates hese cases : (1) Mrs. B., 55, widow, fair, catarrhal constitution. hronic cough many years. Asthmatic on taking cold, great accumu- ation during attacks, occasionally raising frothy, viscid mucus tinged vith blood. Gastric catarrh. Great epigastric tenderness. On)ctober 26, 1883, seized with severe catarrhal symptoms, sneezing, urning in nostrils, fluent, watery, mucous discharge from nose, ching in forehead. Cough dry, hollow. *Sng. n.* 3x, gtt. xx., in ix ounces of water, two teaspoonfuls every hour. Complete relief in our hours ; usually took three days. (2) Dr. G. had hay-fever, at its ieight on August 21st. Sensation of cobwebs across nose ten days efore attack is fully established. Nose feels large, tingles, trickling vater ; mucous membrane very sensitive to cold air, causing frequent neezing. < Light. < Rising in morning. Eyes itch, could almost ub them out. *Sng. n.* relieved this attack somewhat. Next year he ommenced taking it in June, and passed through the season without ny attack. C. Wesselhœft regards *Sng. n.* as the simillimum or "New England colds." Adenoids and polypi have been cured vith it. There is great craving for air. Bathing with warm water > ieat in forehead. Touch <. Pressure < soreness of eyes. Head- che is > by discharge of much mucus from nose. < At night.

Relations.—*Compare:* Sang. Burning in nostrils, Ar. t. Tena- cious mucus, K. bi. Hay-fever, Pso. Sweet expectoration, Stan.

Causation.—Driving in cold wind. Winter weather. Exposure.

SYMPTOMS.

1. **Mind.**—Restless from feverish and irritable condition.

2. **Head.**—Slight dizziness all through the proving; with discharge mucus from nose and air passages.—Uncomfortable feeling about the hea all day; decidedly < at night.—Pain in supra-orbital region, proceedir from pain in r. eyeball, of a sore, aching character; soon extended acro forehead and seemed deep in above root of nose.—Burning pain in forehea and root of nose, with aching and soreness in eyeballs < on pressure; th pain became < on l. side of head, through l. temple.—Heat in forehead bathing with warm water.—Pain in l. side of head extended to parietal ridg and back to mastoid process, with stiffness in muscles of l. side of neck an top of l. shoulder as from a draught.—Sensation of obstruction and fulness i head, > by discharge of a large quantity of thick, yellow, sweet-tastir mucus.—Slight aching sensation with soreness all over head and scalp.

3. **Eyes.**—Sore, aching pain in r. eyeball, extending to supra-orbit region.—Pain in l. eyeball extending over orbit and l. side of head.—Redne and soreness of inner canthi, they feel swollen.—Severe heat and burning (eyes.—Burning, pressing aching, and sore pains in eyes.—Profuse lachryma tion; tears gush out.—Redness of lids and conjunctiva.—Sight dim, as looking through gauze, or as if film of mucus spread over sight.

4. **Ears.**—Obstruction of Eustachian tube.—Difficulty in distinguishin sounds.—Roaring in r. ear.

5. **Nose.**—Water trickles from r. nostril (15 m. after first dose).– Watery mucus from both nostrils, sneezing every few minutes, profus lachrymation.—Sensation rising to nostrils as if he had taken strong hors radish.—Burning pains in both nostrils.—Accumulation of mucus obstructin nose and bronchi.—Dry, sore, raw feeling in nostrils.—Free discharge fro posterior nares (esp. l.), tinged with blood.

8. **Mouth.**—Slight acrid, burning sensation on tongue.—Roughness an dryness in mouth and throat.—Heat in mouth as if pepper had been taken.– Awoke frequently with dry mouth and throat from breathing with mout open, nose being obstructed.—Increased flow of mucus and saliva wit sneezing and burning in forehead.

9. **Throat.**—Roughness and dryness in mouth and throat with sense c constriction in throat.—Soreness, roughness, and rawness on r. tonsil, painfu with difficulty in swallowing; red, irritable spot seen on inspection.—I morning raised great quantities of thick, yellow, sweet-tasting mucus; thi continued all day.—Great accumulation of mucus in throat and bronchi.

10. **Appetite.**—Bitter taste extending back to root of tongue.—Every thing tastes dry like chips.—Coffee did not taste natural; wanted somethin succulent—not pungent—but soothing to mouth and throat, which was ho dry, parched, and raw.—Little appetite.

11. **Stomach.**—Sensation of burning in stomach and œsophagus.– Belching up of putrid-smelling gas though she had eaten nothing sinc morning.

12. **Abdomen.**—Borborygmus and pains in abdomen, as if diarrhœ would set in, with sharp, cutting pains.

14. **Urinary Organs.**—Passed urine every hour during the night (28 oz

weight), depositing a white sediment.—Urine had bright yellow sedi-
nt.

17. **Respiratory Organs.**—Short, hacking cough arising from sensa-
n of tightness in chest.—The cough became harsh, leaving soreness and
vness in throat and chest, with scraping, raw sensation in pharynx.—As
on as she began to move in morning coughed up large quantities of thick,
low, sweet-tasting mucus during the day.—Cough became deeper and
tling, the pressure extended to both lungs, greatly increasing the sense of
focation.—Feeling as if air passages lined with thick, stiff mucus or pus.—
ises thin, frothy mucus, which is very tenacious.

18. **Chest.**—Tightness in chest.—Heat and tension behind centre of
rnum.—Tension, burning, and accumulation of mucus behind centre of
rnum.—Strong desire for fresh air.—Pressure in chest extending to both
gs, increasing the sense of suffocation.

20. **Neck.**—Stiffness in muscles of l. neck and shoulder.

22. **Upper Limbs.**—Stiffness in muscles of l. shoulder and neck.

26. **Sleep.**—Sleep poor ; restless from feverish and irritable condition.

Sanguinarinum Tartaricum.

Tartrate or Sanguinarin. $C_{19}H_{17}NO_4C_4H_6O_6$. Trituration.

Clinical.—Exophthalmos. Mydriasis. Stool, bilious. Vision, dim.

Characteristics.—Tully and Terry (*C. D. P.*) experimented with
g. tart. in considerable doses. Tully says he has repeatedly wit-
ssed "all the effects of Sanguinaria root, save the neuralgic pains
d the convulsive affections," from the use of *Sng. tart.* The most
culiar of the symptoms he mentions are: Staring, and protrusion of
eyes ; extreme mydriasis ; haggard expression, and cold surface
d cold sweats.

SYMPTOMS.

2. **Head.**—Vertigo.

3. **Eyes.**—Pupils dilated.—Mydriasis very great ; strongest sunlight
s to contract.—Cloud before sight.—Eyes protruded, staring.

6. **Face.**—Haggard expression.

11. **Stomach.**—Nausea.—Epigastric uneasiness.

13. **Stool.**—Very large quantity of bright yellow bile passed in stool
h. after dose).

19. **Heart.**—Pulse rate diminished ; irregular.—Pulse preternaturally
flowing, without bounding, hardness, or sign of irritation.

27. **Fever.**—Cold surface, esp. of extremities.—Cold sweat.

Sanguisuga.

Hirudo or Sanguisuga officinalis. The Leech. *N. O.* Hirudine:
Tincture of the living animal.

Clinical.—*Anus, bleeding from.* Hæmorrhages.

Characteristics.—Burnett was the first to use *Sanguisuga* a homœopathic medicine. Dangerous hæmorrhages have not un quently followed the application of leeches, and it has been asc tained that the leech does not merely bite, it poisons the bitten p in such a way as to render the blood in it watery. Having a case persistent bleeding from the rectum, the blood being watery, and the usual hæmorrhagic remedies having failed to arrest it, Burn thought that *Sanguisuga* might prove the simillimum. He had tincture made and attenuated, gave the 5th attenuation, and mad brilliant cure. I have had frequent opportunity of confirming value of *Sngs.* in cases of the kind.

Sanicula.

Sanicula aqua. A Mineral Spring Water of Ottawa, Ill., U.S (Containing, approximately, in grains per gallon—Nat. m. Calc. m. $23\frac{1}{2}$, Mag. m. $23\frac{1}{4}$, Calc. bicarb. $14\frac{1}{4}$, Calc. sul. $9\frac{1}{2}$ sul. 5, Nat. bicarb. 1, Nat. bro. $\frac{1}{3}$, Fe. bicarb. $\frac{1}{10}$, Nat. iod. Sil. $\frac{1}{2}$, Alumina $\frac{1}{100}$, and traces of Lith. bicarb., Nat. ph., Bor Dilutions of the spring water. Triturations of the evapor: salt. [This remedy has sometimes been confounded with *plant* Sanicula Marylandica, Black Snake-root.]

Clinical.—Amenorrhœa. Anterior crural neuralgia. Asthma. Bee-st Boils; blind. Borborygmus. Coccyx, soreness of. Condylomata. Conjuncti Constipation; of children. Cornea, ulceration of. Coryza. Cough. Dan Debility. Diabetes. Diarrhœa. Digestion slow. Dropsy; during pregna Eczema. Emaciation. Enuresis. Excoriations. Foot-sweat. Gastritis. (boil. Headache. Indigestion. Influenza. Intermittents. (Intestinal sand.) suppressed. Itching. Leucorrhœa. Liver, soreness of. Lumbago. Melanc Milk, thin. Mouth, sore. Neuralgia. Neurasthenia. Night terrors. Nose, c in. Ophthalmia; tarsi. Os uteri, dilated. Ossification, too early. Ozæna. spiration, excessive. Pot-bellied children. Pregnancy, sickness of; drops Rectum, cramp in. Rheumatism. Rickets. Scurvy. Sea-sickness. Shoul rheumatism of. Throat, sore. Tongue, ringworm of; burning. Tooth Uterus, prolapse of; soreness of; (tumour of). Vomiting, of milk; of water. V boils on.

Characteristics.—The water of *Sanicula* spring is without o or colour, and has an agreeable and slightly alkaline taste. It proved by J. G. Gundlach, who, with his family, drank it for r than a year. Writing in *H. P.*, September, 1890, Gundlach s "Though some five years since the proving was made, we all (tha ıy family) still suffer from the effects, and I fear never will fully get ver them, as nearly all the symptoms still recur." Sherbino proved *anic.* in the potencies, and a large number of the symptoms of both rovings have been confirmed. We have in *Sanic.* one of the best-roved remedies of the materia medica, a polychrest and antipsoric f wide range. My Schema is taken from the arrangement of Frank V. Patch in *Med. Adv.*, xxviii. 161. Brackets indicate cured symp-oms. The cachexia of *Sanic.* is its most pronounced feature—veakness, emaciation, itching, ill-nourished skin, pimply face, "dirty, greasy, and brownish" appearance of body, scrofulous ophthalmia nd scrofulous eruptions, cold, clammy hands and feet, foul-smelling oot-sweat, profuse sweat of back of head and neck, hair dry and ustreless, thick dandriff on scalp and eyebrows, slow digestion, con-tipation, or else diarrhœa, stools turning green, pot-bellied, rickety hildren. On the other hand, when taken by a pregnant woman, *anic.* has caused premature closing of sutures and fontanelles prior o birth. The mental state of the *Sanic.* cachexia is characterised by ack of energy, with no stability of purpose; jumping from one work o another, never finishing anything. There is also much depression, vith sense of impending misfortune. Children are stubborn, wilful, get angry and throw themselves backward. Digestion is slow. Chil-lren vomit milk or thick curds soon after nursing. The menses are rregular, delayed, scanty, and attended with pain. Nervous sensi-bility is exaggerated, and there is general and local intolerance of least ar. This has led to its successful use in train-sickness and sea-sick-ness. The low vitality of *Sanic.* is evidenced in the cold clamminess of other parts besides hands and feet. Sherbino [*J. of Hcs.* (Hitch-cock's), ii. 147] relates this case: Mr. F. had neuralgia of coccyx, acrum, and lumbar region, < by any movement, turning in bed, ising from chair, stooping; > keeping still. Parts sore to touch. *Cold sensation in lumbar and sacral regions as if there were a cold cloth here.* Feet cold and clammy. *Sanic.* 10m cured after other remedies ailed. The foot-sweat occurs between the toes, making them sore, as well as on the soles, which are as if one had stepped in cold water On the other hand, there may be "burning of the soles, must uncover or put them in a cool place," and "child kicks off clothing even in coldest weather." The *odours* of *Sanic.* are characteristic. The stool has an odour of rotten cheese, and no amount of washing will get rid of it. The flatus has the same odour. Vaginal discharges and con-lylomata of penis have an *odour of fish brine.* This has led to a number of cures. The digestive tract is greatly disordered by *Sanic.* Food has a long after-taste; turns sour. Children vomit milk looking ike "Schmierkäse." Appetite is increased—hungry before meals—or disordered. Craves salt; craves fat bacon, which <. Eating = lesire for stool; must leave the table. Great thirst; drinks little and often; vomits as soon as it reaches the stomach. Incontinence of urine and fæces. Urging from flatus, must cross legs to prevent fæces escaping. *Sanic.* is as great a remedy in constipation as in diarrhœa. There is no desire for stool till a long accumulation has occurred. After great straining stool partially expelled recedes. Large evacuation of small, dry, grey balls, which have to be removed mechanically. Stool square, as if carved with a knife. The diarrhœ is changeable in character and colour: Like scrambled eggs; frothy grass-green; turns green on standing; like scum of frog-pond. Ther is excoriation of skin about anus, perinæum, and genitals. As well a weakness of rectum and bladder, there is uterine weakness and bear ing down as if contents of pelvis would escape; must place hand t vulva to prevent it. Walking, misstep, or jar < this, and also sore ness of the uterus. Sherbino (*M. A.*, xxvi. 133) relates the case c Mrs. X., who had been in poor health a number of years. Tal anæmic. Has to urinate too often and too profusely, rises severa times in night. Urine clear, pale. Has leucorrhœa, profuse, change able in colour, at times milky, then yellow, < during stool. Weal and prostrated, rumbling in bowels before meals, > after eating an when stomach is full. Hands cold, clammy; also feet, < in col weather; stockings always damp. Two doses of *Sanic.*, 10m an then 50m, cured all the trouble. H. C. Morrow regards *Sanic.* as th chronic of *Cham.* (*H. P.*, ix. 253). He records the case of a baby wh had been ill through a summer with diarrhœa. Morrow cured it wit *Sanic.* 50m (F.), a peculiar symptom in the case being that the bo *wanted to lie on something hard*, thin as he was. Morrow had himsel suffered since a boy from effects of suppressed itch. Among hi symptoms were—"felt as if he had on cold, damp stockings," an "sweat about the head and neck when asleep, wetting the pillow fa around." *Calc.* gave no relief. Sherbino advised *Sanic.*, and after takin it Morrow was in better health than he had been for twenty years Morrow also relates these cases (*M. A.*, xxiv. 47): (1) A lady was con stipated a year. Had to *strain* very hard to expel the stool; at time fæces so large, hard, and dry, she was compelled to pick it out wit the fingers. *Sanic.* relieved. (2) A fig-wart on glans penis, with discharge from its surface which *smelled like fish brine*. *Sanic.* cured Gundlach relates (*M. A.*, xxvi. 97) these cases: (1) Mrs. K. felt a attack of fever impending. Sad and despondent. Had fever th previous night with headache, but no thirst. Mouth dry, tongu coated, bad breath; inside lips and cheeks many little aphthou ulcers; no appetite; bowels constipated; tired, numb, lame feelin in all limbs; chilly, craves warmth, yet head feels better in open ai *Sanic.* 10m, every three hours, cured. (2) Mr. C. complained that th roof of his mouth felt scalded, < taking anything warm in mouth especially hot drink. Smokers have this kind of sore mouth, bu patient was not a smoker. Gundlach remembered his own simila symptoms of the proving, and gave *Sanic.* 10m, which promptl removed the condition. (*Sanic.* causes a burning of the tongue s intense that it must be put out to cool: here again is the "< b warmth" of the mouth). (3) Gundlach's horse was out of health would not eat, bowels constipated, stools dark and scant. Tired rubbed his tail at every opportunity till nearly all the hair was rubbe off. A veterinarian diagnosed "lampers," and said the gums would b found swollen and sore, and would need scarifying. The gums wer found sore and swollen, mouth slimy, tongue coated. *Sanic.* 10m wa given thrice daily, and no scarifying was needed. He was well in few days. Sherbino (*M. A.*, xxvi. 135) removed with *Sanic.* 10m an

50m these symptoms in a man suffering from the after-effects of influenza and much drugging: Soreness through stomach and liver region. Liver enlarged, great tenderness to pressure or jar. Could not laugh without supporting stomach and bowels. > When stomach full, < when it was empty. G. M. Chase (*M. A.*, xxiv. 336) relates a case of acute gastric catarrh. Patient had had repeated attacks lasting three to seven days. Two doses of *Sanic.* cured. The mental symptoms were the chief guides: Irritable, least word or action would "upset" her. Misconstrues everything. Melancholy, sad, depressed, no energy. Fever but *no thirst.* Headache, cannot bear light or noise. Offensive breath, but not from teeth. *Rheumatic pains in shoulders,* < left, extending to chest. Only > from heat; patient sat with back to the fire. Gundlach (*M. A.*, xxiii. 381) relates this similar case: Mrs. W., 55, after a violent cold two days before, had great pain in muscles of neck, shoulders, and upper back, pain constant, but made sharp by attempts to put her hands to her head or behind her. Could not look round without turning whole body. < From cold or motion; > from warmth and rest until she gets tired of holding head and body in one position, when she would have to move it. *Sanic.* 30 made a rapid cure. C. M. Boger (*M. Couns.*, xvi. 265) relates the case of a light-haired carpenter, 35, who had hacking cough from trachea after rising in morning, also in evening. Sneezing occasionally during day. Crusty sores in right nostril. Dull pain in frontal sinuses, < stooping. Aching in muscles of whole back, stitches upward, < from motion. Foot-sweat, making feet sore, stiffens stockings, destroys shoes. Itching eruption over sternum. Itching pimples on coccyx. *Sanic.* 10m (F. C.) cured. Gundlach (*M. A.*, xxiii. 382) relates these two cases of constipation. (1) Mr. A., always accustomed to take pills. No stool, nor desire, for five days. Dull frontal headache with vertigo; stooping or getting up suddenly = vertigo. When walking gets blind and dizzy, has to stand still till it passes off. Poor appetite; tongue large and flabby, coated yellowish. Bad taste in morning; at times stomach full and oppressed after eating; accumulation of gas. Stool scanty and requires great effort to expel. "Not done" sensation after stool. *Sanic.* 10m cured promptly and completely. (2) Miss R., 20, constipated all her life. Goes a week without desire. Great effort required to expel stool, which would at times slip back. *Sanic.* 30 helped at once. W. J. Guernsey (*M. A.*, xxiii. 382) relates several cases of bowel disorder in children. (1) R., aged one month, has sore mouth. Jumps on waking from sleep. Stool difficult with straining. *Sanic.* 10m cured in a few days. Three months later same child had swelling about eyes. Discharge of water from nose. Rubs nose constantly, looking frightened. *Sanic.* 10m cured in five doses. (2) B., four months, stools loose, green. Restless at night. Losing flesh. Eyes look very heavy. Has had sore mouth removed by the mother with *Borax* wash. *Sanic.* 10m, 50m, and cm, gradually cured. (3) S., aged seven months, stool loose and copious. *Stool becomes pale on standing.* Urinates much. Vomits large chunks of milk. Wakens screaming in fright. *Sanic.* 10m. All symptoms disappeared, but a large carbuncle appeared on right buttock, which, however, was less painful than its size would indicate, opened in five openings and discharged within a week, rapid recovery following. Guernsey chose *Sanic.* on the italicised symptom, being the *direct opposite* of the special *Sanic.* condition, and as it is noted under no other remedy. Opposites as well as similars may serve as indications. Gundlach (*H. P.*, xiii. 158) reports these cases: (1) Printer, 40, suffering for some weeks from results of overwork. Dull pain in forehead over eyes; feels as if eyes being driven back into head; < in warm, close room; by application of mind; > in open air. Mind wanders when trying to apply it. Cannot keep at any one thing. No appetite. Bad taste, tongue coated white, < morning. Dry mouth, no thirst. Fears he will lose his reason. *Sanic.* 10m cured. (2) Mrs. H., 45, constantly chilly mingled with flushes of heat. Chills < moving, even turning in bed; > by external warmth. Chills at irregular times; spread from below up. During chill wants to be covered; during heat wants covers off. Pains and aching in limbs, feels sore and bruised, both flesh and bones; can't put hands to head or behind for pain in shoulders. Head dull, heavy. Warmth > pains, but < head. Bad taste; wants sour things; some thirst with fever; urine dark, scanty. *Sanic.* 10m cured. J. V. Allen (*H. P.*, ix. 380) observed that in the eye cases of *Sanic.* there is marked photophobia without much inflammation. The cases he cured had these symptoms: Must close eyes continually; with this an awful discharge of thick, yellowish, greenish matter, excoriating any part it touches. In one child there was as well greenish nasal discharge, excoriating nostrils and lips. *Peculiar Sensations* are: Head as if open and wind went through it. Of cold cloth round brain. Of scalp all drawn up to vertex. Coldness in throat. Throat as if too large. Back as if in two pieces. Lumbar vertebræ as if gliding past each other, especially when rocking in a chair. Feeling of distraction. There is great fear of the dark; constant desire to look behind her. Dreams of robbers. "Stool full of jagged particles" suggests the condition known as "intestinal sand." Square stool is also peculiar. The symptoms are < by touch. Child cannot bear to be approached. In bed one cannot bear to lie near or touch another. Cannot bear to have one part touch another; sweat where parts (as crossed thighs) touch. Part lain on sweats. Must loosen clothing. Slight pressure < more than hard. < From strain; from riding in cars. < Descending. < Motion; raising arms; putting arms behind back; working. < Misstep, walking, jar. Cough = bursting in vertex. > Rest. < Leaning head forward; > leaning it back. Awakes at night with arms under head. On waking child rubs eyes and nose with fist. Light and noise <. Eating <; urging to stool whilst eating. Also < before eating (hunger); and > after breakfast; and when stomach full. Swallowing <. > Vomiting. < At noon. > In open air. < Warm room (head and skin symptoms chiefly). > Warmth; wraps up head in cold weather. < Becoming cool after running (pain in jaw). < From draught of air, especially cold air. Cannot bear cold wind on back of head or neck. < Change, especially to damp weather. Periodicity, chills every other day. Symptoms of the proving recurred repeatedly during five years. Smoking < eructations, > nausea. Pains go right to left; front to back; and back to front; shift much.

Relations.—W. J. Guernsey considers Sanic. the chronic of Cham. *Compare:* The constituents of the water, especially Nat. m. and Calc. Dread of downward motion, Brx. Head sweat, Calc., Sil. Soreness behind ears, viscid discharge, Graph., Pso. Ringworm on tongue, Nat. m., Ran. sc., Tarax. Drinks little and often, vomits as soon as it reaches stomach, Ars. Symptoms change constantly, Lac c., Puls. Sphincter not under control, Alo. Stool recedes, Sil., Thu.; must be removed mechanically, Sel.; crumbling at anus, Mg. m. Odour of stool follows despite bathing, Sul. Excoriation about anus, Sul., Lyc., Cham. Places hand on vulva for support, Lil. t., Murex. Offensive foot-sweat, Graph., Pso., Sil. Burning soles, Lach., Med., Sang., Sul., Calc. Kicks off clothing in coldest weather, Hep., Sul. Skin of neck wrinkled, hangs in folds, Abrot., Iod., Nat. m., Sars. Vomits "Schmierkäse"; falls asleep after vomiting, Æthus. Fish-brine odour, Calc. (rectum), Graph. (scab of ulcer), Med. (moisture from anus), Tell. (ear discharge), (Trimeth.). Stool when eating, Fer., Trombid. Cough from laughing or talking, Pho., Arg. n. Sweet expectoration, Sang., Stan, < Lifting arms, Bar. c., Con., Cup., Fer., Led. Symptoms increase to noon and decrease after, Sang., Spig. Dreams of robbers, Nat. m. Cries before urinating, Lyc. Fears darkness, Grindel., Stram. Fears touch, Cin., Ant. t., Arn. Seasickness and train-sickness, Arn., Cocc., Tab. Headache from nape to eyes, Sil., Sang. Wraps up head, Mg. m., Sil., Pso. Mental restlessness when reading, Dros. Depression with feeling of impending misfortune, Calc. Irritability, Cham., Con. Child rubs nose and eyes on waking, Scil. Hair lustreless, Alm., K. ca. Clinkers, K. bi.

Causation.—Strains. Jarring.

SYMPTOMS.

1. **Mind.**—Instability of purpose.—Constantly changing his occupation.—Want of energy.—Forgetful.—Depression; mind wanders from one subject to another, even when conversing.—Nervous irritability.—Misconstrues actions of others.—Child headstrong and obstinate, crying and kicking, esp. 9 p.m. to 12.—Headstrong crossness quickly alternating with laughter and playfulness in children.—Intense depression; feels no one admires her, every one hates her, wants nothing to do with any one, most trifling cares unbearable.—Fear of impending misfortune.—Restless desire to go from place to place; great aversion to darkness.—Constant irresistible desire to look behind her.—Feels like cursing (intermittent fever).—(Child wants to be in constant motion night and day.)—Averse to be touched.—Restless; no > from moving.—Easily upset by slight word or act.—Forgets common details of recent occupation.—Dreads work on account of weakness and exhaustion.)

2. **Head.**—Queer, mad, crazy feeling in head.—Vertigo: on rising from stooping; while sitting at table or desk; after eating; with nausea, must lean head against something to keep from falling.—Giddy while kneading with rush of blood to head and desire for cool air.—Faint, smothering sensation with great desire for open air.—Seasick sensation after riding on horseback in the dark.—Nervous, drunken sensation.—(Blindness and dizziness when walking.—Downward motion of elevator = feeling of everything

giving way under her, and as if top of head would fly off.)—Dull, heavy feeling in head; rising from nape and extending to forehead and eyes; on waking.—Sensation on waking in morning as having lain on a hard board.—Dull frontal headache with sharp, shooting pain from r. side of occiput to r. forehead and eye, ending in a sensation that the eye was clutched and pulled back for a moment.—Dull frontal headache, < leaning head forward (reading or writing), or in warm, close room; > leaning head back and in cool, open air.—Headache changes r. to l.—Pain in head < from draught of air, esp. if cold.—Sensation that the head was open and the wind went through it.—Sometimes wraps head up, even in summer, to protect it from wind.—Headache < lying down; > riding in open air.—Dull, constant ache in frontal bone, < over l. eye.—Pain shifts from forehead to back of head.—Cold feeling in brain.—Sensation of cold cloth round brain.—(Headache every week, lasts two or three days, with nausea and vomiting.—Headache from vertex down to occiput.—Pain from upper portion of spine around under jaws to throat, with contracted feeling, < r. side and from swallowing.—Neuralgic pains about head and face after exposure to warm or cold winds.—Pain from back of head to face, at times from as far down as shoulders, < r. side.—Headache < from light or noise.—Neuralgic pains over r. eye.)—Scalp feels contracted from back and forepart to vertex; skin of forehead contracted, frowning, causing desire to raise eyebrows and lean head back; < towards noon, > evening; < motion, leaning head forward, noise, jar, misstep; > rest, lying down, sleep.—Occiput sensitive to pressure.—Great accumulation of dandriff on top of head, with itching on getting head warm; cannot endure cold wind about back of head or neck.—Child sweats profusely about back of head and neck during sleep, wetting pillow all around.—Hair thin, scanty, dry, lustreless.—Hair electric, crackling when combed.—(Falling out of hair.—Small boils on head that do not mature.)

3. **Eyes.**—Sight dim, sometimes sees double, or letters run together.—Sensation as though a white cloud passed over eyes, with loss of sight and faintness.—Eyes feel weak and sore on waking in morning, light painful at first.—Eyes burn, exuding a sticky fluid, which in a few hours dries on the margins of the lids, forming white scales.—Burning and smarting of canthi.—Lids red and inflamed.—Small reddish ulcers on r. lower lid, which burn after removal of the yellow scabs.—Ulceration of margins of lids, also extending over half r. upper lid, with photophobia, itching, and burning.—Awakes with dryness of whole eye and sensation that eyeball is sticking to lid.—Catarrhal ophthalmia, with profuse yellow discharge; first l. eye, then r.—Lids agglutinated in morning.—Eyes sore on motion.—Cornea ulcerated.—Photophobia.—Eyes < at night.—Catarrhal conjunctivitis, lids swollen, eyeballs red.—(Chronic sore eyes.—Scrofulous ophthalmia.—Eye symptoms > morning, < noon, still < as day advances.—Lachrymation in the wind, in cool air, or from cool application.—Great swelling of lids, great effort required to keep them open.)

4. **Ears.**—Eustachian catarrh.—Stuffed feeling in l. ear.—(Soreness behind ears with discharge of white, gluey, sticky substance.)

5. **Nose.**—Nose sore and stuffed with yellow scabs.—Discharge: thin, acrid drops; thick, yellowish, green, profuse; thick, honey-like scabs; white, tenacious, stringy; clots of black blood; bloody ichor; copious, yellow; <

ıdoors and after eating.—Sneezing and itching of nose.—Soreness, tender-ess, or ulceration of alæ.—Squeaking from before backward after blowing ose.

6. **Face.**—Small red pimples, mostly on l. cheek.—Constant dull pain long superior maxillary bone, extending to l. temple, > from warmth, < om cold.—Dull ache in upper r. jaw on becoming cool after running.—Con-ant dull pain on side of face and temple ; drawing of muscles.—Faceache, side, in upper jaw and teeth, extending to temple, < cold or hot drinks, nd least wind about head or face.—Acne about eye and cheek.—Excoriation f upper lip.—(Profuse, scaly dandriff on eyebrows ; and beard.—Large scabs n upper lip, constantly picking them till they bleed.)—Itching eruptions in eard, esp. under chin ; < when warm.—Vesicular eruption on lips and chin.

7. **Teeth.**—Teeth sensitive to cold air, as if they were very thin.—ums sore and painful ; < from eating.—Gumboils.—(Teeth feel too long.—ain in r. dental nerve extending to head and neck ; feels that if she could ick the teeth out and cause bleeding they would improve : < at night and om lying down ; must get up and walk about ; momentary > clenching ıws.)

8. **Mouth.**—On awaking, dark brown streak down centre of tongue, hich is furred and dry like leather.—Sides of tongue turn up.—Tongue lheres to roof of mouth.—Thick yellow coating on back of tongue.—Dis-greeable pappy taste in mouth in morning.—Under surface of tongue a mass f painful ulcers.—Bread tastes dry and flat.—Tongue large, flabby.—(Burn-ıg of tongue, must protrude it to keep it cool.—Ringworm on tongue.)—Roof mouth feels raw ; < from warm or hot drinks, food, &c.—Large, painful lcers on centre of roof of mouth.—Mouth and inside of lips a mass of painful lcers ; child can take no food.—Great dryness of mouth and throat, without ıirst.—Swelling of sublingual glands, with occasional discharge of a tea-oonful of salt liquid.—Breath offensive.—(White aphthæ on lips and in outh, which can be scraped off with finger.—Scurvy with profuse salivation daytime ; < night.—Profuse flow of white, clear, transparent, stringy liva when cutting teeth ; < when awake and in day ; > when asleep and night.—Burning in mouth ; better from cold water or drawing in cool air. -Sore mouth of children, with atrophy, white appearance like curdled milk.)

9. **Throat.**—Ulcers with yellowish base on tonsils.—Soreness on both des of uvula, passing up posterior nares, with pains on swallowing.—Throat ıd posterior wall of pharynx of a purple colour.—Grey exudate on posterior all of pharynx.—Coughing out of large clinkers in morning that had clogged osterior nares for forty-eight hours ; tough, like boiled cartilage streaked ith blood.—Fluent catarrh from posterior nares during day, dry at night.—reyish catarrhal secretion, < in morning after eating, must leave table to ear throat.—Cold sensation in throat, as though a piece of ice had been held ere.—Throat feels too large.—Hoarseness following sore throat ; must clear roat before speaking.—Dryness of throat ; > swallowing saliva or water.—ryness and roughness after sleeping in a draught.—Constant desire to oisten the parts, but cannot.—Can swallow solid better than fluid.—(Sensa-on in pharynx and uvula as though he had inhaled peppermint.—Choking nsation in throat as from a breadcrumb.)

10. **Appetite.**—Great longing for the spring water.—Child wants to

nurse all the time, yet loses flesh.—Child craves meat, fat bacon, &c., which <.—Craving for salt.—Loss of desire for bread, unless fresh baked.—Splendid appetite; gets very hungry before mealtime.—No appetite for breakfast.—Child frantic when it sees the glass of water; drinks large quantities greedily.—(Thirst for small quantity very often, which is vomited almost as soon as it reaches stomach.—Loss of appetite, no desire for anything but water.)—Feels better after eating.

11. **Stomach.**—Bloating of stomach on beginning to eat.—Feels terribly stuffed after a meal.—Shortly after nursing food all comes up with a gush, and child drops into a stupid sleep.—Fulness and bloating of stomach soon after eating, esp. supper, or after taking acids; must loosen clothing.—Cannot taste food for hours after eating.—Food turns sour and rancid, with burning desire for water, which > for short time only, then <.—Eructations, sour, rancid, burning, < after smoking, of tasteless gas, which gives some relief.—Nausea after eating with sick feeling, > from smoking.—Sudden nausea while eating, vomits all the food taken.—Vomiting >.—Child vomits milk looking like "Schmierkäse"; falls asleep after vomiting.—Vomiting of large, tough curds, like the white of a hard-boiled egg.—Vomiting of milk soon after nursing.—Child vomits after drinking cold water.—(Nausea and vomiting from riding in cars or close carriage, with desire for open air.—Seasickness.)—Nausea and cramp in stomach on awaking at night or in morning, or after rising in morning, like "morning sickness"; > after breakfast.—Bloating of stomach on beginning to eat.—Sensation of a lump in stomach.—(Soreness through stomach, sensitive to pressure and jar, cannot laugh without holding his stomach and bowels, < when stomach is empty.)

12. **Abdomen.**—Gurgling in l. hypochondrium, passing down descending colon; < before meals.—Sore, sensitive pain beginning at l. of umbilicus, going around to spine in three days; < from touch; at point where pain ceased, appearance of a vesicular eruption which gradually worked back to umbilicus, with burning and stinging.—Soreness through hepatic region.—Enlargement of liver, sensitive to pressure and jar.—Rumbling in l. side of abdomen at 9 p.m.—Gurgling like distant thunder along course of large intestine.—Bowels bloated as if they would burst.—Sore pains in groins beneath Poupart's ligaments, after walking.—(Rumbling in bowels before meals; > after eating.—Pot-bellied children, abdomen is the largest part of them.)

13. **Stool and Anus.**—No desire for stool for three or four days.—After intense straining the stool, which was nearly evacuated, recedes.—Even soft stool requires great effort to expel.—Large evacuation of small, dry, grey balls; must be removed by fingers lest it rupture the sphincter.—Great pain in perinæum while at stool as though it would burst; whole perinæum sore and burning for some hours after stool.—Slim, yellow stool at least ten inches long, not requiring much effort.—Stool feels full of jagged particles, very painful, lacerating anus and causing soreness and bleeding.—Stools small and infrequent, first part hard and dry, latter part soft.—Constipation with ineffectual urging.—Impossible to evacuate the stool, which is of greyish-white balls, like burnt lime, hard and crumbling, with odour of rotten cheese; it must be removed mechanically.—Yellow, soft, wedge-shaped stool, like an almond nut, without power to expel.—Stool of large lumps of undigestible

caseine, ragged or shaggy, smelling like rotten or limburger cheese.—Stool resembling scrambled eggs.—Thin portion of stool frothy and of a grass-green colour ; whole mass turns green after standing.—Stools green, frothy, watery, like the scum of a frog pond.—(Child's stools changeable ; watery, yellow, green.)—At 9.30 p.m. copious diarrhœa with urging and haste ; stool yellow and fetid as after eating onions.—Soft, sticky, mushy stool twice each day.—Stools as often as food is taken, must hurry from table after each meal.—Cramping pain in colon and rectum.—Urging from flatus, must cross legs to prevent stool from escaping.—(Persistent odour somewhat resembling that of decaying cheese about the child, not removed by bathing ; diarrhœa.—Pain before stool, some > after it.—Pain during stool.—"Not done" sensation after stools.—Stool becomes pale on standing.)—Stool square, as if carved with a knife.—(Excoriation of skin about anus, extending out on each side of nates, genital organs, and groins ; skin very raw, like beef, with watery discharge.—No control over sphincter, often soils himself while standing, running, at play, or even at night.—Stool escapes when passing flatus.)

14. **Urinary Organs.**—Frequent desire for urination with profuse discharge, comes suddenly with sensation that urine was at meatus.—Great effort necessary to retain urine, at times impossible, yet if the desire is resisted the urging ceases.—Cramp-like pain along course of l. ureter, when trying to retain urine, compelling him to stand, although he cannot stand erect on account of the pains.—Sensation that a hard body like a lead pencil were being forced upward and backward from bladder to kidney ; it gradually passes away some fifteen minutes after urination.—Voids large quantities of pale urine of low specific gravity.—Urgent calls to urinate as if bladder would burst.—Child strains to urinate while at stool.—Urine of child scanty, voided at long intervals.—Child cries before urinating.—Urine stains diaper red.

15. **Male Sexual Organs.**—Increased sexual desire at first, then much decreased.—Discharge of semen too early with little sensation.—A few hours after intercourse an odour of fish brine about the glans, sometimes lasting a day or two.—Child's parts smell of fish brine even after bathing.—Scrotum relaxed, clammy sweat about parts.—(Fig-wart on glans penis, sycosis, with discharge from its surface smelling like fish brine.—Copper-coloured, syphilitic sores.)

16. **Female Sexual Organs.**—A few hours after intercourse appearance of a slight watery discharge from vagina with odour of fish brine, lasting about twenty-four hours ; not removed by bathing.—Leucorrhœa with strong odour of fish brine.—Menses irregular.—Menses always late, come on with grinding or dilating pain in lower abdomen, with soreness of womb ; pain in back > when flow established ; tumour size of hen's egg, l. side of womb just above cervix, come on since the passing.—Menstrual blood first pale red thin, and watery, then dark and clotted.—Cramp-like pains like "after-pains' in uterine region before menses, ceasing after flow.—Pain just above sacrum < before the flow and from motion ; > from rest.—Weakness in lower part of abdomen with bearing down as if contents would escape ; < from walking, motion, misstep, or jar ; > from rest and lying down.—Womb sensitive to jar.—Desire to support the relaxed parts by placing the hand against vulva.—(Shoots : from l. side of pelvis across pelvic region, also to under l.

breast.)—Soreness of womb.—Menses suppressed with morning sickness.—Vagina feels large.—Cannot stop menstruation.—(Leucorrhœa profuse changeable in colour; milky, yellow, &c., < during stool.)—During pregnancy: swelling of lower limbs at third month, < evening; swelling and stiffness of hands and feet, particularly of l. side during pregnancy; feet pit on pressure; sad, tearful disposition; after standing, sensation that the os uteri is opening or dilating, with drawing at inside of thighs.—Os uteri dilated to size of half dollar three weeks before labour.—Child's head hard and compact when born, with no sign of suture or posterior fontanelle.—Milk thin, watery, acid reaction.

17. **Respiratory Organs.**—Larynx sensitive to pressure, esp. l. side, with dry, tickling cough.—Stuffed feeling on awaking in morning; unable to speak for a time.—Hoarseness.—(Complete aphonia, must speak in a whisper—Raw feeling in trachea, < after expectoration of large clumps of mucus.—Sensation in trachea on swallowing as though a hard substance were present, like a stone.)—Cough: deep, hollow cough, with loud rattling, caused by tickling under sternum.—Tickling on lying down at night and on awaking.—Irritation to cough felt worst at r. of middle chest.—Rattling cough, child gags and vomits a mouthful of tough, stringy matter.—Cough from laughing or talking; < in warm room; in morning; > in open air.—Cough = bursting feeling in vertex.—Expectoration: yellow; sweet; of large cheesy masses that sink in water; profuse in morning and after meals; of shaggy lumps; loose and lasting all day.

18. **Chest.**—Asthmatic breathing, < after supper.—Wheezing, rattling under sternum, < during or after eating.—Tickling under sternum.—Great soreness of upper chest, when coughing must hold it with hands.—(Burning from throat to lungs.)—Sudden attack of a terrible sensation of a burden on chest; for a few moments it seems as if she would burst, gradually followed by an intense depression of spirits.—Eruption on chest over the ensiform appendix, size of a shilling, with intense itching.

20. **Neck and Back.**—Small, painful boil on l. side of back of neck, not inclined to suppurate.—Neck so weak and emaciated that child cannot hold its head up.—Muscles of back of neck seem too short; weakness and all-gone sensation in small of back.—Skin about neck wrinkles and hangs in folds.—Dull, aching pains between scapulæ on awaking in morning, as if he had lain in a cramped position all night.—Deep-seated pain in muscles of spine, esp. toward l. side.—Soreness and stiffness in back, which is not affected by breathing; > from motion.—Rheumatic pains in shoulders, esp. l., the only > is from heat, patient sits with back to fire.—Pain < from moving shoulders or lifting arms up; cannot place arms on head or behind body.—Sharp pain from least turning; must hold himself stiff and turn whole body in order to look around.—Inclines head forward to ease pain in muscles at back of neck.—Sharp pain at inner angle of l. scapula on putting head back.—L. scapular region very sore.—Weak, tired, broken sensation in lumbar region, coming on just after rising in morning, and gradually increasing till noon, then decreasing till its disappearance, about 6 or 7 p.m.—Sensation in lower lumbar region that the vertebræ were gliding past each other, felt esp. when rocking in a chair.—A dislocated sensation in last lumbar vertebra.—Backache, with burning sensation across lumbar and sacral regions; > from

ntle exercise or lying flat on back; < when sitting.—Region of coccyx re, as if excoriated.—Coldness along spine; < on going into cool air or hen sitting still; > from external warmth and motion.—Back very painful noon.—Sensation that the back is in two pieces.—Back becomes tired and eak from walking over snow.—After a strain, lameness and stiffness of back morning; > after moving about.—Catch in back on reaching or straining. -Gooseflesh on back.—Small boils on back that do not mature.

21. **Limbs.**—Restlessness with pains in joints.—Stiffness and pain in mbs when rising in morning; < on first beginning to move.—(Numb feeling limbs).—Cold, clammy sweat on limbs.

22. **Upper Limbs.**—Constant pain in r. shoulder-joint; < from motion. -Constant dull pain in r. arm and shoulder, with a sense of coldness from bow up.—Sore, bruised feeling on outer side of l. forearm and hand; < by ight pressure more than by hard.—Drawing pain on outside of upper arm to bow on lifting arm; < on rising in morning and from a change to damp eather.—Cannot raise arm or put it behind him on account of sharp pains.— arge oval spot on ulnar side of l. arm, of dusky colour, attended with itching; turns red after scratching.—Gooseflesh on arms.—Boils on wrist that do not ature, hard and painful, but not very red; pain extends to axilla.—Profuse veat in axilla.—Excoriation in axilla.—Hands swollen and stiff on awaking morning.—Cracks on hands exuding blood and watery fluid and forming usts.—Eruption on hands of small vesicles exuding a watery, sticky fluid.— ching eruption on hands.—Eczematous eruption appearing on outside of rst joint of thumb on l. hand, spreading by new pustules over ball of thumb, ack of hand and wrist, also to back of r. hand.—Burning, smarting soreness, ith deep, angry, ragged cracks of hands; < cold weather.—Hands as cold though handling ice.—Burning of palms.—On putting hands together they veat until it drops from them.—Knuckles of fingers crack and leak.—(Hang-ails.)

23. **Lower Limbs.**—Rheumatic pains in l. hip-joint; < from motion ad cold, yet not > by rest.—Reddish pimples on inside of thighs with itch-g, particularly the l.; < on undressing at night.—Sore, bruised sensation in ont of r. thigh, < from light pressure.—Tingling sensation in one or the her lower limb, like an electric current, ending with a twitch, < on first oing to bed.—Sore pain whole length of lower limbs; esp. in upper portion. -Tired, dull, heavy feeling in lower limbs, with inclination to change posi-on, no position is comfortable.—Child's legs emaciated.—Child cannot walk stand alone at sixteen months of age.—After walking pain begins under oupart's ligament on r. side, extends along course of anterior crural nerve to e inside of joint, then to front, causing limping; > from rest.—Bruised ain in l. ischium.—Rheumatic pains in knee-joints.—Sharp pains in l. knee-int come on suddenly, causing him to cry out.—Tiredness of knees.—Sore, ruised feeling on inside of both knees; < from light pressure.—Severe pain hollow of r. foot; foot swollen, causing restless wakefulness.—Sore, rained feeling in l. foot; < from bending.—Burning of feet, esp. soles, ants to put them in cool place, in water, or uncover them.—Cold, clammy et.—Cramp in feet in bed at night, they are so cold.—Sweat on soles as ough he had stepped in cold water.—Stockings feel sticky.—Sweat between es, making them sore, with foul odour.

24. **Generalities.**—Dread of usual work on account of weakness an exhaustion, with irresistible desire to lie down.—Restlessness ; hard to remai long in one position ; > from motion.—No rest day or night ; always < fro 9 p.m. till after midnight.—Child kicks off clothing even in coldest weather.- Wants to lie on something hard.—Great soreness.—Stiffness and lameness o parts.—(Child looks old, dirty, greasy, and brownish.)—Progressive emaci tion.

25. **Skin.**—Skin dry and flabby.—Itching < by scratching.—Pimples o face.—Boils on wrist.—Eczema exuding sticky fluid : behind ears ; on wrist fingers, toes.—Cracks on fingers.—Skin covered with fine rash all over.—Bod attended with severe itching at night.—(Copper-coloured syphilitic sores).

26. **Sleep.**—Awakes at night with arms under head.—Frequent wakin at night.—Restless, uneasy sleep ; awakens at 3.30 a.m.—Awakes soon afte going to sleep with a start and twitch.—Child is restless during sleep an awakes cross and crying.—She awakens her companion to search for a tram in her room, gets up and looks under the bed for him.—On waking child rub eyes and nose with its fist.—Cannot bear any one to lie close to or touch hin —Lascivious dreams.—Dreams of robbers and cannot sleep till the whol house is searched.—Dreams of murder and remorse.

27. **Fever.**—Chilliness all day ; < in warm room.—The cold air chill him.—Sensation that chills are coming on.—Chill every day at same time.- Chill begins in lower extremities.—Chill every night lasting an hour, begin ning between shoulders, thence extending to arms, fingers, and whole body (intermittent, three weeks after labour.)—Thirst during chill, none durin heat or sweat.—(Chill at 8.30 a.m.—Chill at 5 p.m.—Chill postponing tw hours.—Chill every other day ; fever lasting all night.—Drinks before chill —Whole body feels too hot at night.—Sweat most where limbs cross eac other or touch the bed.—Begins to sweat as soon as covered.—Sweats on firs falling asleep, mostly about neck, wetting clothing through.—Cold, clamm sweat on occiput and neck, those parts feel like a wet stone.—Sweat fron above downward over whole body.—High fever every night with sleepless ness.—Whole body feels too hot at night.—(Wants to move to a cool part o bed.)—Sweats on side lain on.—Hungry during sweat ; water tastes bitter.

Santalum.

Santalum album (India) ; and S. Freycinetianum and S. paniculatun (Sandwich Islands). Sandal Wood. *N. O.* Santalaceæ. Th oil distilled from the wood. Dilutions with alcohol.

Clinical.—Gonorrhœa. Kidney-ache.

Characteristics.—The word *Santalum* is of Persian origin Sandal-wood oil is obtained from several species of *Santalum*, *S. albun* being the chief. Its chief use in old-school practice is in gonorrhœa Shirtliff (*H. W.*, xxxi. 456) observed in a man taking the oil for gonor rhœa, soon after each dose, an acute aching pain felt in the kidne region, so severe that if he was standing he was obliged to sit, which gave some >. On this hint Shirtliff gave it in this case : An elderly man, looking worn and haggard, complained of pain in region of left kidney from ribs to crista ilii, brought on by walking, > leaning forward, completely > by lying down. > Pressing clenched fist into back. The pain had lasted six months, and was very acute when on. *Sul.*, *Berb.*, and *Bry.* gave no relief. *Santal.* (oil), one drop every four hours, soon gave great relief, and entirely removed the pain in two months.

Santoninum.

Santonine. A neutral active principle obtained from Cina (so-called "Semen Cinæ"). $C_{15}H_{18}O_3$. (Colourless, lustrous, right rhombic prisms, odourless, and of a bitter taste. Become yellow by exposure to sunlight. Almost insoluble in cold, somewhat soluble in boiling water ; fairly soluble in chloroform, boiling rectified spirit, and in strong acetic acid, volatile oils, warm olive oil.) Trituration.

Clinical.—*Amblyopia.* Cataract. Convulsions. Cough. Cystitis, chronic. Diarrhœa. Dysuria. Eyes, paralysis of. Enteralgia. Enteritis. Enuresis. Epilepsy. Epistaxis. Gastro-enteritis. Giant urticaria. Hæmoglobinuria. Hemiplegia (l.). Infantile remittents. Strangury. Tetanus. Urination, frequent. Urticaria. Vision, yellow. Vomiting. Worms.

Characteristics.—*Santonin.* is the favourite anthelmintic of the old school, and it is chiefly against lumbrici that it has been given. From 2 to 5 grains are the ordinary doses, but these have caused severe and, in one or two instances, fatal poisoning—convulsions, left-side paralysis, delirium, vomiting, and purging have resulted. A case recorded by Demme was quoted in *Brit. Med. J.*, March 26, 1892 : A boy, 3, was given by his mother during three days fifteen tablets, each containing gr. $\frac{1}{3}$ of *Santonin.* The symptoms produced were : Vomiting, dilatation of the pupils, collapse, cyanosis, dyspnœa, and finally convulsions. After a warm bath with cold affusions to head and spine, consciousness returned. The temperature was 103·5°, epistaxis and hæmoglobinuria occurred, and a scarlatina-like eruption was noticed. The child ultimately recovered. After a dose of 7 centigrammes, a child, 2, was seized with prostation, convulsions, cramps, and icterus, followed on the third day by salivation and ulceration of the gum (*Bull. Ther.* Jan. 30, 1872). Less serious but very characteristic are the effects on the senses, especially the sense of sight. Visions of figures have been produced, and *coloured* vision is a frequent phenomenon, even when the lower triturations have been used. Yellow is the predominant colour, but green and violet vision are also marked. The urine also is yellow coloured and stains yellow, and is passed with much urging and painful burning. A kind of giant urticaria occurred in one case. Hale records that *Sant.* has cured cases of "nervous blindness." It was given to an old man, quite blind, for worms, and his sight partially returned. This led to further trials. It was given in nine cases of cataract, and, according to Hale, four were cured, the rest not benefited. Hale mentions enuresis, strangury, chronic cystitis, as having been cured by it. It has made some "brilliant cures" of chronic catarrh of the bladder. Infantile remittents, with or without worms, have been cured by it. In one prover there was "sensitiveness of the abdomen," which may be a keynote.

Relations.—*Compare :* Cina. Coloured vision, Cycl. Amaurosis, Benz. dinit., Carb. sul.

SYMPTOMS.

1. **Mind.**—Delirium.—Excited, laughs and sings.—Hysterical.—Restless, irritable; wants everything, satisfied with nothing.—Profound and unusual depression, with irresolution and want of confidence, unfitting him for work of any kind; melancholia like that produced by jaundice.—Coma.

2. **Head.**—Vertigo.—Giddiness and intense headaches, every object looks bright green.—Head turning and twisting, restless.—Dulness of head.—Pain in forehead.

3. **Eyes.**—Blue rings round eyes.—Eyes: rolled convulsively; distorted; staring.—Pressure in supra-orbital region.—Pressure in eyes.—Pupils enormously dilated; and insensible.—Photophobia and lachrymation.—Flickering before eyes.—Objects seem to totter and dance; visions of figures, cherries, animals, &c.—Coloured vision: yellow soup looks red; blue evening sky looks green; objects look green; white looks yellow; objects as if in yellow haze or yellow light; violet.

5. **Nose.**—Hallucinations of smell.—Things smell peculiar.—Epistaxis.

6. **Face.**—Convulsive movements of muscles of face, esp. lips and lids.—Face pinched, drawing in of lips over teeth with pinched expression of mouth and nose.—Red, hot face, staring eyes.—Face pale.—Pale round mouth, < afternoon.—One cheek white, the other (l.) red (remains red several days).—Swelling beginning under chin, spreads each way, esp. towards l. parotid gland.—Lips swollen to enormous size, glistening with the distension.

7. **Teeth.**—Grating teeth during sleep.—Teeth clenched.

8. **Mouth.**—Tongue: deep red; dry.—Frothing from mouth.—Burning pains apparently torment her, as she forces everything into her mouth.—Hallucinations of taste.

9. **Throat.**—The glands of neck, parotid and submaxillary, commenced swelling in about five days, and continued to increase till the throat was so filled as nearly to prevent swallowing (fatal effect of gr. vi. in a child of three).

11. **Stomach.**—Deficient appetite.—Thirst: intense; continual for ice-cold water, which she swallowed greedily.—Frequent eructations.—Nausea; and vomiting.—Vomiting: and purging with severe abdominal pains; yellowish, slimy mucus from 11 p.m. till next forenoon.—One night, after eating a teaspoonful of nourishment, he choked and threw up a teacupful of blood and pus and died without a struggle.—Dull pain in pit of stomach.

12. **Abdomen.**—Abdomen: bruised but soft; hot, full; rumbling in;

very sensitive.—Severe abdominal pains with vomiting and purging.—Every night pain in bowels before stool.

13. **Stool and Anus.**—Well-marked tenesmus.—Purging of watery, flaky, foul-smelling stools, followed by vomiting in a few hours.—Stools copious, greyish, putrid-smelling.

14. **Urinary Organs.**—Frequent efforts to urinate; only passes a few drops at a time.—Micturition painful from burning in urethra, constant desire, evacuation of only a few drops that colour linen yellow.—Urine : deep saffron yellow ; thick, sulphur yellow ; greenish.—Hæmoglobinuria.

17. **Respiratory Organs.**—Coughed incessantly all night from tickling in larynx and trachea.—Breath : rapid, sighing ; quick and catchy ; rattling.

18. **Chest.**—Paralysis of lungs; artificial respiration had to be resorted to.

19. **Heart.**—Pulse : quick and full ; rapid ; lowered ; l. absent, r. soft and steady.

21. **Limbs.**—Spasms of limbs.—Twitching of hands and feet.

22. **Upper Limbs.**—Convulsive jerking of upper limbs.

23. **Lower Limbs.**—Gait unsteady and tottering ; staggered.

24. **Generalities.**—Most violent convulsions, unconscious, head hot, face flushed, purplish.—Spasm begins in face and spreads to extremities.—Partial paralysis of one (l.) side.—Great restlessness ; prostration.

25. **Skin.**—Urticaria ; with œdema of nose, lips, and eyelids ; over almost entire lids, with vomiting.

26. **Sleep.**—Sleepy, tired.—Sleep restless.—Sleep disturbed, woke unrefreshed with sickness, frontal headache, and deficient appetite.

27. **Fever.**—Whole body icy cold ; lips and ears blue, face white as snow.—Limbs cold, very clammy coldness crept upward in spite of wraps.—Violent fever, very rapid pulse, burning heat of skin, face puffy, eyes brilliant, fixed.—Heat about head, < every afternoon and evening.—Cold sweats.—Hot sweat in occiput, more clammy in front.

Saponinum.

Saponin. (A glucoside obtained from Saponaria officinalis, Gypsophila, Struthium, Senega, Quillaja, &c.) $C_{32}H_{54}O_{18}$. Trituration. Solution. (Watery solutions speedily decompose.)

Clinical.—Boils. Constipation. Diarrhœa. Dysmenia. Enuresis, when walking. Exophthalmos. Fever. Headache. Leucorrhœa. Rheumatism. Sleeplessness. Spleen, pains in. Strabismus. Temperature lowered. Tongue, strawberry.

Characteristics.—*Saponin.* has had a somewhat extensive proving (in potencies ranging from 1 x to 30th), conducted by A. J. Hills. One prover, who took the 30th, for many years a sufferer from articular rheumatism, had none of his usual pains during the proving, and a great enlargement of the left knee was entirely removed. Two female provers had marked disturbance of the menstrual functions, especially pain and sufferings *before* the flow. A miliary eruption, and colic and leucorrhœa before the menses, pain better but not removed when the flow was established. Severe sore throat, < right side, was experienced by several provers, and Hills had so much swelling of the tonsils that he was obliged to abandon the proving. Nausea and vomiting, colic and diarrhœa, were among the symptoms, and a particular one was "nausea more in œsophagus and throat, < in a warm room." This < by warmth was met with in relation to many symptoms, and is probably a keynote. At the same time there was much chilliness, and lowered temperature is a characteristic feature. One of the provers who took the 12th had had his temperature reduced to 96° on the second day. Allen (*Appendix*) records an experiment which bears on this: 0·1 gramme of *Saponin.* was injected into the left thigh of a man. The immediate effect was to produce intense local inflammation resembling erysipelas, but much more painful; the pain extended to knee and hip, and the glands of the groin swelled. For the first three hours there was rapid increase of temperature, which fell to normal in twenty-four hours. The next two days there was a little fever, evidently kept up by the local irritation, but by the fifth day the temperature had fallen to 93° and the pulse to 65. (The intense local irritation bears on the skin symptoms of the proving, large numbers of boils being produced.) The other symptoms of this experiment were marked bodily and mental depression; and exophthalmos and strabismus of the left eye (the side injected). Among the *Peculiar Symptoms* of *Sap.* are: Involuntary emission of urine when walking. Roughness of mucous membrane of mouth, with raised papillæ on palate and tongue. Strawberry tongue. The symptoms were markedly < by moving; even motion of the eyes < mental labour. < By warmth. > By cold; by cold bathing; while sitting. < Swallowing. Desire to vomit and defecate, < when quiet. > By stool; by onset of menses.

Relations.—*Compare:* Tough mucus, K. bi. > Onset of menses, Lach. Spleen pain, Cean. Kidney pain, Santal. < By movement; moving eyes, Bry. Sleepy but cannot sleep, Bell. Early waking, Bels., Nux. < In warm room, Puls. As if damp stockings on, Calc., Sanic. Strawberry tongue, Frag., Bac. Involuntary emission of urine when walking, Fer., Caust. Compare also, *Seneg.*

SYMPTOMS.

1. **Mind.**—Marked bodily and mental depression.—Irritable; cross wants to be let alone.—Disinclined to study.—Inability to fix mind; to recal names.

2. **Head.**—Dizziness and nausea on stooping.—Dizziness followed th vomiting.—Dull, heavy headache, with depression; < 4–6 p.m.—Afte moving about in morning, dull, heavy sensation in head, mostly forehead esp. over l. orbit, < stooping; eyeball sore and aches; later pain spreads t occiput; heat in forehead > pressure and cold, much < bending over.—Headache < by least mental labour or motion.—Severe pain in head, wit throbbing carotids; < l. side.—Head exceedingly irritable, cannot turn it o

n move eyes without causing nausea.—Headache in temples; sensation as oth temples were pressed out.—Sharp pain in l. temple.

3. **Eyes.**—Could not turn eyes up or around they felt so sore; moving m = pain to dart back to occiput.—Sensation of fulness in eyes, evening. 'onjunctiva yellow and a little congested.—Vision dull.—Pain, exophlmos and strabismus of l. eye (from a subcutaneous injection into l. thigh).

5. **Nose.**—Dry coryza and frequent sneezing.—R. nostril plugged in rning, with headache.—Dull pain at root of nose and in temples.—Nose d and pale.

6. **Face.**—Miliary eruption on face, neck, and head before menses.— e pale.—Lips dry and burning.

8. **Mouth.**—Tongue coated yellowish white on back; red on tip and ges; raised papillæ (strawberry tongue), esp. on tip.—Tongue brown in itre, deep yellow on edges.—Hard palate rough.—Salivation.—Taste: eet, sickish; flat; acrid.

9. **Throat.**—Tough, tenacious mucus on posterior nares, extending to ynx.—Throat sore, < r. side, feeling of constriction, hardly able to swallow. 'hroat: smarting, scraping, raw, rough.—Irritation as from dust.—Tonsils ch swollen, bright red.

11. **Stomach.**—No appetite.—Loathing of food for two days till nausea in.—Thirst not > by drinking.—Nausea, retching, vomiting of greenishlow fluid; with agonising pain in both temples, which disappeared as sire to vomit was >.—On returning home one cold night from place of usement nausea in œsophagus and throat as soon as she got comfortably rm; as nausea increased cold feeling began at tips of fingers and toes and wly spread to abdomen, where they met, giving an electric-like shock; n followed griping pain and diarrhœa and vomiting.—Sinking at pit of mach without appetite; with fulness and heat in forehead.

12. **Abdomen.**—Dull pain in l. hypochondrium, changing to epigasım, very severe, then shooting up under l. scapula, < motion, > sitting.— inful stitches in l. hypochondrium.—Dull pain in umbilical region after ch stool.—Colic 3 a.m. on waking.—For twenty-four hours preceding nses, colic, cramps, and profuse watery leucorrhœa, > when menses ablished.—Sudden colic, > immediately by stool.—Pain in l. inguinal gion.

13. **Stool and Anus.**—Intense itching in rectum, afternoon and night. Burning in rectum.—Smarting in anus, with constipation.—Constant ging, stool insufficient, rather white.—Desire for stool in evening as well as orning.—Diarrhœa with tenesmus.—Stool: profuse diarrhœic, painless but gent; with colic; first hard, then liquid, becomes involuntary; brownish, my; desire to defecate or vomit as soon as there is a little ease, both < by armth.

14. **Urinary Organs.**—Kidneys torpid; sharp pain in region of r. dney.—Burning during micturition.—Waked early to pass water, which ft brickdust sediment.—Involuntary emission of water on walking.—Urine ore profuse and high-coloured.

16. **Female Sexual Organs.**—Menses delayed and diminished.— enses: a week early; profuse, < on motion; blood dark red; paralysed aring down all through period (unusual); before menses, shuddering all

over body, intolerable aching in back and lower limbs ; wants to be let alon —Colic with menses.—For twenty-four hours preceding menses, colic, cramp and profuse watery leucorrhœa ; when menses established pain was less, b persisted through the four days of the period, leaving her weak and depresse —Fine miliary eruption on face, neck, and head before menses.

17. **Respiratory Organs.**—At 4 p.m. peculiar cough, which is excit at every forced inspiration through nose, only one cough at a time.

18. **Chest.**—Formication deep in tissue of lung.—Repeated sharp sta bing in r. lung; middle lobe; dull aching in l. lung.—Dull pains throug thorax.—At time of chill constriction in l. chest.

19. **Heart.**—Dull pain in region of heart.—Pulse: accelerated; wea hardly perceptible.

20. **Back.**—Back and limbs tired walking, boots feel extremely heavy. Dull throbbing in l. scapula, running up.—Severe dull pain in small of bac and sense of weight as if all clothes hanging from back; this sense of suppo ing a heavy weight extended to hips and knees, < from jar of riding in hor cars.—Dull aching in lumbo-sacral region, extending down thighs, wi increased tingling in soles.—Lancinating pains in loins, < walking.

21. **Limbs.**—Exhausted, weary feeling in limbs, with slight inclinati to nausea.—Weakness in hands and feet.

22. **Upper Limbs.**—Sudden pain in l. arm, apparently muscular, region of insertion of deltoid ; arms weak, muscles exhausted, as after lifti heavy weights.—Pain in bones of l. forearm.—Numbness and tingling in third and little fingers (ulnar nerve).

23. **Lower Limbs.**—Dull aching in lower limbs ; and l. loin; muscul pains.—Dull pain in l. lower limb.—Aching in calves.—Soles sore, swolle tender, numb, and tingling.

24. **Generalities.**—Restlessness.—Muscular weakness.—Exhaustion. Faintness : and prostration ; with the chill.

25. **Skin.**—Miliary eruption before menses.—Angry-looking pustules chest.—Boils, single or in crops.—Itching and crawling tingling in vario parts.

26. **Sleep.**—Sleepy.—Sleepy but cannot sleep.—Cannot sleep well aft 4 or 5 a.m.—Waking early, 5.30 a.m. (a very unusual symptom with t prover).—Sleep disturbed by dreams ; dreamed of urinating.

27. **Fever.**—Slight chill accompanied by faintness.—Severe chill ov back on going into warm room.—As nausea increased an icy feeling crept extremities, commencing at very tip of fingers and toes, gradual in ascent a descent, when the two currents met in abdomen it was as if electricity h been applied to them, giving a shock which almost made me jump.—Duri day great coldness of limbs, hands and feet feel as if damp stockings on. Temperature lowered.—Temperature rose steadily for three hours (after su cutaneous injection of 0·1 grm. into inner l. thigh), then gradually fell normal, which it reached in twenty-four hours ; for the next two days the was some fever, but on the fifth day the temperature was far below t normal, reaching the collapse point of 93° ; the pulse, which was somewh elevated at first, fell to 65 on the fifth day.—Feverish and weak.—Head h skin dry.—A sensation of spreading heat, commencing in chest and spreadi both ways, esp. to head.

Sarracenia.

Sarracenia purpurea. Pitcher Plant. (Grows in boggy places from Canada southwards.) *N. O.* Sarraceniaceæ. Tincture of fresh plant. Tincture of root.

Clinical.—Back, pains in. Bones, pains in. Borborygmus. Constipation. Coxalgia. Diarrhœa. Eruptions, scrofulous. Femur, pains in. Herpes. Influenza. Lumbago. Psoriasis. Small-pox Vision, disordered.

Characteristics.—The use of the Pitcher Plant in small-pox is a discovery of the Indians of North America, the spotted appearance of the plant probably suggesting a resemblance to the disease. Hale has collected much confirmatory evidence of its power to antidote the small-pox poison. A proving by T. C. Duncan, Thomas, and others brought out symptoms of fever, backache, headache, and gastric disturbance. Hering quotes these instances of its action: (1) A woman far advanced in pregnancy was cured of small-pox with *Sarr.* 3, 6, and 9, delivery being happily accomplished during her convalescence, the infant bearing on its body numerous red blotches, indicating that it had been affected with the disease. (2) An infant a few months old was attacked with a grave form of small-pox, with variolous angina so severe that it was with difficulty it could take the breast; the mother took *Sarr.* 3, 6, and 9, and continued to nurse the infant, which promptly recovered, the mother not taking the disease. (3) In an epidemic occurring in the environs of Wavre, *Sarr.* was given to two thousand persons living in the very middle of the disease and coming in constant intercourse with it, but all who took *Sarr.* escaped; during the same epidemic two hundred cases were treated with *Sarr.* without a death. Bilden, who used the 1 x tincture in an epidemic with success, concludes that *Sarr.* is to small-pox what *Gels.* is to bilious fever. Hale quotes Surgeon-Major C. G. Logie's (allopath) account of his experience with *Sarr.* (decoction probaby) in small-pox: "Four of the cases in my hospital have been severe confluent cases. They have throughout the disease all been perfectly sensible, have had excellent appetites, been free from pain, and have never felt weak. The effects of this medicine, which I have carefully watched, seemed to arrest the development of the pustules, killing, as it were, the virus from within, thereby changing the character of the disease and doing away with pitting." A number of eye symptoms appeared in the provings, and *Sarr.* has cured disordered vision. A case of "phlyctenoid herpes" has also been reported cured by it. Extreme lassitude and pains in the bones were prominent in the provings. The right side was more affected than the left. *Sensations* were: Light feeling in head. As if he received a knock on the head. As if head were split. Left eye as if congested. Heat in face as if on fire. Swelling in womb as if from a tumour or dropsy. Uterus swollen as if full of cysts. As if bones of leg were too thick. *Sarr.* has the empty, hungry, sinking sensation of the antipsorics. Dryness of mouth and throat. Weak feeling in the arms. Very sensitive to cold air. Faint after stool. There is vesical and rectal tenesmus. Stool smells of musk. The symptoms were < about midnight and at 3 p.m. < Morning. < Rising from lying. < Trying to walk. < In stormy weather. Open air = chilliness, hands and feet cold; = head to be hot and sore, and feel full. Cold air = to feel chilly and < bone pains. Symptoms generally > in fresh air; and > out of bed.

Relations.—*Antidoted by:* Podoph. *Compare:* In small-pox, Ant. t., Merc., Vaccin., Variol., Maland. In bone pains, Eup. perf.

SYMPTOMS.

1. **Mind.**—Melancholia, anxious about everything.—Great depression of spirits with frontal headache.—Brain clearer, buoyant spirits.—Dulness of head, loss of memory, insensibility of r. side; paralysis of hearing and smell.—Want of memory with the headache.—Difficult to concentrate attention, forgetful; feels dull and heavy; sweats freely.—Alternate apathy and intellectual activity.

2. **Head.**—Head feels dull and heavy.—Feels light-headed.—Vertigo: with cramps in neck, spreading to forehead; < night; sensation as if he had received a knock on the head, stupor and staggering gait; obliged to support himself or lie down; with drowsiness in head and contractions in spinal column.—Frontal headache, low-spirited.—Headache: dull at cranial region; severe in afternoon; with chills, nausea, vomiting, dim sight, surring in ears.—Pulsations and burning heat of head, with sensation as if it would split.—Head hot and aches.—Head and body warm.—Frontal bone sore.—Pruritus and heat of scalp.

3. **Eyes.**—Eyes weak.—Dim sight, headache.—Gas flame seems a brilliant yellow ring; sees black objects moving with the eye.—Great photophobia.—Soreness of r. optic nerve, just behind eyeball.—Pain in l. eye as if congested, on waking.—Eyes feel swollen and sore.—Eyes and lids inflamed.—Increased mucous secretion.—Cutting, penetrating pains in orbits.

4. **Ears.**—Surring in ears.—Sticking pains deep in r. ear; transient but recurring often; same in l. ear.—Intense earache; fears he will lose his senses.—Swelling of parotids.

5. **Nose.**—Fetid smell.—Epistaxis nearly producing fainting.—Fluent coryza with cold chills and loss of smell.—Foul-smelling, green, yellowish, or bloody discharges.—Nose swollen, red, with pressure and pulsation at root.

6. **Face.**—Face flushed.—Heat and redness of face.—Face pale, with heat and chill alternating.—Erysipelatous swelling of face.—Miliary eruption on face, with heat as if it were on fire.—Scaly herpes on face and forehead.—Intense neuralgic pains from temples to jaws.

8. **Mouth.**—Tongue: dry; coated brownish white.—Mouth dry; lips and mouth parched.—Toothache at night in bed; from least contact, and cold air.

9. **Throat.**—Throat dry, not > by tea or water; borborygmi.

10. **Appetite.**—Hungry all the time, even after a meal.—Appetite unusually active, but there was a sense of pain about the stomach like that after inflammation or of overtaxed muscle.—Little appetite, but what is eaten agrees.—Great desire to sleep during eating.

11. **Stomach.**—Empty, hungry feeling; for he can keep nothing in his stomach.—Burning pains in stomach with palpitations and contraction.—Pinching pain in stomach, it feels distended and torn.

12. **Abdomen.**—After going to bed whole abdominal region was in commotion, extending along ascending, and descending colon, all in a kind of rolling motion; epigastrium sensitive to pressure.—Transient pains in bowels.—Bloated about navel.—Borborygmi and some pain in bowels with constipation; dry throat.

13. **Stool and Anus.**—Much flatus.—First part of stool natural, last diarrhœic.—Much tenesmus; dysenteric diarrhœa.—Stool at first costive, thin, dark, offensive, soluble.—Costive; stools very hard, covered with mucus, and dark.—Stool copious, dark, fetid, evacuated with great straining, morning.—Rectum and anus swollen and inflamed.—Morning diarrhœa; faint after stool, which is dark, often mixed with blood, foul smelling, or smelling of musk; bloatedness with colic.

14. **Urinary Organs.**—Awoke 3 a.m. with urging to urinate; bladder so full it overcame resistance of sphincter and dribbled away.—Voided 27 ounces of urine of sp. gr. 1024; vesical tenesmus.—Urine phosphatic.—Urine scanty, limpid.

16. **Female Sexual Organs.**—Watery or milky leucorrhœa, foul-smelling, with spasmodic pains in uterus; pulsative pains in womb with swelling as if from a tumour or dropsy; uterus swollen as if full of cysts, esp. r. side; cervix swollen, hot; miliary eruption and heat in vulva; bloody discharge at other times than menstrual period, as during climaxis.

17. **Respiratory Organs.**—Phthisis pulmonalis and bronchial affections, joined to or depending on a psoric state; hæmoptysis, thick cough; continual tickling in larynx and bronchi; cough with desire to vomit, and vomiting, paroxysms of suffocation and epistaxis; hard cough, shaking chest and bowels, and stopping only after expectorating a quantity of compact mucus, tenacious, filamentary, with a bitter, putrid, oily taste.

18. **Chest.**—Pains in third and fourth ribs, with great apprehension of heart disease.—Pain in angle of ribs.—Soreness of pectoralis major.

19. **Heart.**—Feeling of congestion about head, with irregularity of heart's action.—Congestion to chest, heavy feeling about heart.—Slight palpitation in morning.—Pulse: full and strong; 68, general malaise; small; quick.

20. **Neck and Back.**—A pain up r. trapezius muscle with wave-like motion.—Warm sensation passed up back into head.—Weak between and below shoulders.—Back weak, wants to lean on something.—Arms and back tired and sore all over.—Deep-seated pain in back.—Fixed pains in small of back.—Heat in whole r. lumbar region.—Pain in cervical and lumbar vertebræ.—Pain and soreness in sacrum.

21. **Limbs.**—Limbs cold when still, as from deficient circulation.—Limbs easily benumbed.—Weakness of limbs with paralytic debility.—Pains and soreness in diaphyses of all long bones; < humerus, esp. l.—Pain in l. carpus and tarsus.

22. **Upper Limbs.**—Paroxysms of pain in r. shoulder-joint, pain in l. carpus and tarsus; face flushed.—Arms feel weak.—Bruised feeling from shoulders to hands.—Aching, sore pain in l. humerus.—Bones in both arms pain.

23. **Lower Limbs.**—Pain in hip-joints < rising to feet from a lying posture.—Paroxysms of weakness in coxo-femoral joint, with pains of luxation and fear of falling when beginning to walk.—Strange lameness in femur, lower third, < in inner condyle.—Pain in condyles of femur.—Wave-like motion in muscles of femur.—Sensation of fatigue in bones of leg as if they were too thick.—Bruised and luxated feeling in joints.—Pain in r. patella and metatarsal bones.—Knees feel weak.—Bruised pain in knees as after a fall; he falls easily on his knees.—Bone pains in tibia and fibula; intermittent, but bones continually sore.—Bones of feet inflamed; nodes as in gout.

24. **Generalities.**—Debility; heavy, languid.—Dull, heavy, sore feeling in all bones.—Phlegmonous swelling, with a rosy tint on various parts.—Unrefreshed though slept soundly.

25. **Skin.**—Phlyctenoid herpes.—Psoriasis.—Scrofulous eruptions.—Variola; (the decoction taken when eruption is out and beginning to pustulate aborts secondary fever and prevents pitting).—Eruption out, pustules dissipate, first on face, fever lessens, urine though scanty and dark becomes abundant and pale, strength returns.—Eruptions similar to crusta lactea; on forehead and hands papular eruptions, changing to vesicular, with the depression as in small-pox lasting from seven to eight days.

26. **Sleep.**—Sleepy in daytime; sleep disturbed by strange and frightful dreams.—Awakes early: 3, 4, or 5; in a fright; with urging to urinate.

27. **Fever.**—Feverish and shaking chills, < morning.—General chills between shoulder-blades.—Chills, heat, and sweat, 5 p.m.—At 2 p.m. very chilly in open air.—Skin hot and dry.—Hands hot, warm all over.—Head and body warm.—Perspires freely (5th, 8th, 9th d.); although weather still warm, and actively employed, sweat not as free as while taking the drug (11th d.).

Sarsaparilla.

Wild Liquorice. The rhizome of several species of Smilax. (The Officinal Sarsæ radix is imported from Jamaica.) *N. O.* Smilaceæ (by some classed as a sub-order of the Liliaceæ). Triturations and tincture of the dried rhizome.

Clinical.—Asthma. Bladder, affections of. Bones, affections of. Breast, scirrhus of. Bright's disease. Calculi. Climaxis. Constipation. Dysmenia. Dyspepsia. Dysuria. Enuresis. Eruptions. Eyes, affections of. Faintness. Glands, enlarged. Gonorrhœa. Gout. *Gravel.* Hands, chapped. Headache. Hernia. *Herpes*; of prepuce. Hiccough. Intermittents. Marasmus. Masturbation, effects of. Melancholia. Mercury, abuse of. Mycosis. Nipples, retracted. Plica polonica. Renal colic. Rhagades. *Rheumatism*; gonorrhœal. Seborrhœa. Spermatic cords, swelling of. Spermatorrhœa. Strangury. Syphilis. Ulcers. Warts.

Characteristics.—The dried root or rhizome of *Sarsaparilla*, as imported, is of the thickness of a goose quill, many feet in length, reddish brown, scentless, mucilaginous in taste, feebly bitterish, faintly acrid. According to Milne it is "diaphoretic, tonic, alterative. . . . It is given in scrofula and secondary syphilis; and the concomitants of these diseases, such as ulcers, cutaneous eruptions, nodes, indurated glands, caries, necroses, articular swellings, and rheumatism, often improve under a protracted course of it." Some, he adds, "think it a kind of restorative after an exhausting course of *Mercury*." This well summarises the ancient reputation of *Sars.* as a "blood purifier," which Hahnemann's proving has amplified and put on a fixed scientific basis. *Sars.* meets the sycotic as well as the psoric (scrofulous) and syphilitic constitution; and it is "restorative" after over-dosing with *Merc.* because it is a homœopathic antidote to *Merc.* The chief localities of the action of *Sars.* are: The urinary organs; genitals; rectum; skin and bones; right lower extremity; right lower side; inner semilateral head. In the urinary sphere there are symptoms which are very severe and also peculiar: There is great pain at end of micturition, *just as the urine ceases to flow;* inability to pass water freely except in the standing position, when sitting it only dribbles; excessive pain in urethra which may run back into abdomen; passage of gravel which looks like grey sand. Many cases of renal colic and dysuria in infants with passage of sand have been cured with *Sars.* Gonorrhœa and the effect of suppressed gonorrhœa have also been cured with it; herpes preputialis; spermatorrhœa, with swollen cords. In the female generative sphere it has many symptoms of painful and disordered menstruation. A peculiar symptom is "moist eruption in right groin before menses." There are moist eruptions also on scrotum and thighs of the male, and offensive odours about genitals in both sexes. The semen may be bloody. In all cases if the other symptoms are associated with the peculiar urinary symptoms of *Sars.*, this will be a strong corroborative indication. The skin is severely affected by *Sars.* One of its popular uses is for "clearing the complexion." When it succeeds it is by virtue of its homœopathicity, for I have seen a very extensive crop of blotches produced by it in a young lady. *Sars.* produces herpetic eruptions in all parts, and tettery eruptions, moist and dry. Rhagades. Itch-like eruptions prone to appear in spring. Itching eruption on forehead during menses. It causes great emaciation, causing the skin to be shrivelled and lie in folds. It is *suited to* children with faces like old people and enlarged abdomens; to dark-haired persons of lithic or sycotic diathesis. Farrington gives these indications: (1) *Sycotic eruption*, little spots scarcely raised above the skin, often scaling a little, but looking like the roseola of syphilis and itching intolerably, < in spring. (2) Moist eruption on scalp, the pus from which causes inflammation of any part it touches. (3) *Sycotic headache*, beginning at back of head, coming forward and settling at root of nose, with swelling of nose. (4) Moist eruption about genitals or between scrotum and thighs.—*Sars.* has many symptoms relative to the female breast, and scirrhus of the breast has been cured with it. The nipples are soft, unexcitable; they are retracted and cannot be made to come out. Retraction of the nipples is a suspicious sign even when there is no appearance of tumour; and *Sars.* should be helpful in patients of cancerous history when this condition is present. This shrivelling of the nipples is part of the shrivelling, withering, wrinkling, and hanging in folds which characterises the skin generally. Burnett (*H. W.*,

xv. 62) records the case of Miss X., 32, whom he found ill in bed an in great pain. There was vomiting of bitter matter, diarrhœa, an fainting, the initial stage of a painful period. Conjunctivæ yellov and apparently a sharp upset of the liver. *Card. m.* φ removed th pains and vomiting; *Chel.* 1 relieved tenderness of the liver whic remained. The patient had had painful menses for twenty years, tha is, continuously from the commencement, except one year when a school at Tunbridge Wells. She used to begin, generally early in th morning, with bitter vomiting; diarrhœa and fainting fits, wit exceedingly cold perspiration; the pain in back, thighs, and hypo gastrium she described as dreadful. She had to lie down the firs day, the second day the pain continued still very bad, and went off o the third. The *left nipple was considerably retracted*, arising from a fa when patient was a little child, and in addition to the above-name symptoms she had severe pain in left breast extending down left arm and the breast was so tender that she would often hold her hand i front of it to ward off any contact. Twenty-four powders, each con taining *Sars.* 30 gtt. i., were ordered, one at bedtime. The next flov was *painless;* but the breast was as painful as ever. Twelve dose of *Sul.* 30 were given in as many days, and then *Sars.* 30 again. Th painful menstruation remained cured, but the breast was unchange Twenty-four powders were now ordered, the first, twelfth, an eighteenth containing each ten globules of *Sars.* 100, the rest unmed cated. Patient reported: The first two or three weeks she though she had taken a severe cold, as she had such a peculiar pain betwee the shoulders as if the flesh were taken hold of and twisted roun After a few days it got better, and "there has been scarcely any pai in the part since." The retraction of the nipple seemed to Burnett little less. With the same remedy Skinner (*ibid.*) cured many case of retraction or flattening of the nipple in nursing women. On tw occasions with high potencies of *Sars.* he enabled a lady to nurse he child when it was utterly hopeless without the simillimum. *Peculia Sensations* are: As if in a dream. As of a great weight in hea Buzzing as if a large bell had been struck in head. As if he had bee hit with a hammer on top of head. As if something pressing on hea As if gauze spread over left eye. As if a grain of sand in eye. As of needle pricking point of nose. Face as if bruised. Jaw as if bein broken. As if he had eaten nothing. [*Sars.* has the "sinking" se sation of the great antipsorics.] As if diarrhœa would come on. A if bowels were pressed out. As if bound down to bed by a sort c suction. As if breath were stopped by a spasm. Breast-bone as bruised. As if chest were too short. As if tips of fingers ulcerate or as if salt were put on a wound. Limbs as if paralysed. There general sensitiveness. Pains shoot in different directions. Anxie accompanies the pains of *Sars.;* and the pains = depression. Th symptoms are < by touch, pressure, tight clothes, scratching. Scratc ing = itching to begin in another place; = eruption on forehead t become humid. Rest >, motion <. Lying down < asthmati breathing. Sitting <. Standing > (difficult micturition). Stoopin = pains from occiput to forehead. Walking <. < Going up (c down) stairs. Many symptoms are < on moving. < In sprin

Warmth >. Warm diet <. Cold diet >. Warm room < vertigo. Entering cold air from warm room = rash. Cold air > pain in molars. Cold, wet weather <. Washing <. Chilliness <. Seminal emission < dim sight. Bread <. Yawning <.

Relations.—*Antidoted by:* Bell., Merc. *It antidotes:* Merc. *Compatible:* Cep., Hep., Pho., Rhus, Sep., Sul. *Complementary:* Merc., Sep. *Compare:* In sycosis ; warts, Thuj., Nit. ac. Herpes, Nat. m., Petr. "Gone" feeling, Sep. Emaciation, Abrot., Iod., Nat., Sanic. Dry, flabby skin, Bar. c., Op. Pain at end of urination, Berb., Equis., Med., Thuj. Urine passed without sensation (unknown to patient), Caust. Sand on diaper ; child screams before and whilst urinating, Brx., Lyc. Excruciating pains from right kidney downwards, Lyc., Ocim. Nipples withered, unexcitable, Sil. Itching eruption on forehead during menses, Eug. j., Sang., Pso. Bloody emissions, Led., Merc.. < Going up or down stairs ; > on level, Can. s. (Brx. < going down stairs). Faintness during or connected with stool, Ap., Nx. m., Pul., Spi., Ver. (with *scanty* stool, Crot. t., Dulc., Ox. ac., Pet., Sul.). Swelling of spermatic cords from unrequited sexual excitement, Mag. mur. Antidotes to Merc., Bell., Camph., Carb. v., Chi., Dulc., Electric., Hep., Hyo. (loss of voice), Lach., Lyc., Op., Mez., Nit. ac., Sep., Sil., Sul. Stench on genitals, Merc., Sanic. (Sanic. of fish brine). Plica polonica ; right side ; distension after eating a little, Lyc. > Cold diet, Pho. > Loosening cravat, Lach. Flickering before eyes with headache, Ir. v., K. bi.

SYMPTOMS.

1. **Mind.**—Anxiety, with trembling of the feet.—The mental depression is caused by the pains ; anxiety also occurs after seminal emissions.—Thinking about the food he has eaten = nausea.—Despondency, gloominess, amounting to despair.—Moroseness and ill-humour, with inclination to work, but unfitness for exertion.—Irascibility and susceptibility.—Fickleness (changeable disposition).—Impatient ; thinks she cannot bear the headache ; child cannot bear the itching.

2. **Head.**—Vertigo after gazing fixedly on an object for some time.—Vertigo, with nausea and sour risings.—Heaviness in head.—Dull, stupid feeling, cannot keep mind fixed on study.—Staggers, falls forward in open air.—Headache with nausea and sour vomiting.—Lancinating or pressive headache, or else pressive and lancinating at same time.—Pressing and stitching pains in l. side of head.—Semilateral spasmodic pains in head, as if head were squeezed in a vice, with cloudiness of eyes or flickering, necessity to lie down, and vibration in brain at every word that is uttered.—Inner semilateral head, either side ; old neuralgic headaches.—Neuralgic headache, r. side, throbbing, stitching, starting from occiput.—(Headache which = jerking of head to one side and screaming.—Griggs.)—Sensation as of tight band around head and forehead, which is very painful ; as if the hat were too tight, has to remove it often and involuntarily, but without relief.—Sound in the head as if a bell were striking, when talking.—Throbbing pains in head.—Noise and buzzing in head.—Pressive and incisive, or pressive, lancinating

drawing and tearing pains in exterior of head, < by touch and by walking.—Seborrhœa cured by decoction (R. T. C.).—Sensibility of scalp.—Falling off of hair.—Plica polonica.

3. **Eyes.**—Pains in eyes, caused by daylight.—Aching in eyes, esp. in evening when reading by candle-light.—Shootings in eyes.—Burning sensation in eyes and lids.—Stinging in eyes on closing lids, violent pain when closed eyes are pressed on.—Quivering of r. upper lid.—Itch-like eruption on lids.—Agglutination of lids in morning.—Red stripe from cornea to outer canthus.—Internal canthi blue and swollen.—Cloudiness before eyes, like a fog; < after emissions.—A red colour is reflected from white paper in evening.—Flickering before eyes with headache.—Halo round candle.

4. **Ears.**—Shootings in ears.—Shooting pains from l. ear to root of nose.—Contraction and pressure in ears.—Burning, itching scabs on lobes of ear.—Tinkling and ringing in ears.

5. **Nose.**—Epistaxis.—Scabious eruption upon, under, and in nose.—Dry coryza and obstruction of nose.—Very thick mucus in nose.—Base of nose and eyes swollen.—R. nostril stopped up and scabby.—Pain in nose, inflamed spots on septum.

6. **Face.**—Face yellow, wrinkled, old-looking.—Pimples.—Facial eruption.—Itching eruption on forehead, with burning sensation, and oozing after having scratched.—Rough, pale-red spots on forehead.—Thick scabs on the face (like milk crust).—Rigidity and tension in masseters and maxillary joints.—Herpes on upper lip.—Purulent and itching vesicles on chin.

7. **Teeth.**—Toothache, with drawing tearings, from a cold current of air or from cold drinks.—Upper teeth sensitive, set on edge.—Tearing in gums.—Gums swollen, with pain as from excoriation.

8. **Mouth.**—Dryness of mouth.—Aphthæ on tongue and palate.—Offensive breath.

9. **Throat.**—Sore throat (r. side), with shooting pain during deglutition.—Spasmodic pressure at throat, like strangulation, with obstructed respiration; must loosen cravat.—Dryness and roughness in throat, esp. in morning.—Accumulation of viscid mucus in throat.—Trichotomous ulcers after suppression of plica polonica.

10. **Appetite.**—Want of appetite.—Bitter, or acid and clammy, or else sweetish, metallic, and herbaceous taste.—Bread has a bitter taste.—Insipidity of food.—After a meal sensation of emptiness in stomach, as while fasting, or else disgust when merely thinking of what has been eaten.—After eating stomach has no sensation, feels as if he had eaten nothing.—After eating a little, distended as if he had eaten much.—< From warm diet, > from cold.—Drinking water = vomiting.—Thirst, esp. for water, also in morning.

11. **Stomach.**—Risings and regurgitations, esp. during and after a meal, generally bitter or sour.—Belching; with diarrhœa.—Hiccough 6 p.m.—Frequent or continued nausea, with fruitless inclination to vomit.—Sour vomitings.—Constrictive pains in stomach.—Aching at pit of stomach.—Heat and burning sensation in stomach, esp. after eating bread.

12. **Abdomen.**—Contusive pain in the l. hypochondrium.—Shootings in the l. hypochondrium.—Great sensibility of the abdomen to external pressure.—Constrictive and spasmodic pains in the intestines.—Cutting pains, esp. in the umbilical region.—Shootings in sides of abdomen, esp. in l. side.—Severe

ension in r. groin.—Pinching in l. groin.—Hernia.—Soreness in bend of r. groin on appearance of menses.—Sensation of coldness, or heat and burning ensation in abdomen.—Sensation of emptiness and borborygmi in abdomen. —Rumbling and fermenting in abdomen; expulsion of much fetid flatus.—nertia of intestines.

13. **Stool and Anus.**—Hard, retarded, and scanty fæces, often with rgent want to evacuate.—Painful, difficult evacuations, with contractive pains n the abdomen and violent downward pressure.—Obstinate constipation, with equent want to urinate.—Pitchy, sticky, adhesive stools.—Blood with stool. —Loose, acrid, corrosive evacuations, with pains in abdomen.—Fainting uring an evacuation.—Pain as from excoriation, and burning itching in anus. —Wakened in night with sore pain in anus, which changes into a (burning) ching which lasts all day.

14. **Urinary Organs.**—Diminished secretion of urine.—Frequent discharge of pale, copious urine.—Tenesmus, with pressure on bladder, and ischarge of a white and turbid matter, mixed with mucus.—Frequent and neffectual want to urinate, or with scanty emission.—Frequent urination ith hard stool.—Burning while urine passes with discharge of elongated akes.—Frequent and profuse emission of pale urine, day and night, often ithout any sensation in urinary organs.—Turbid urine, like clay water.—iery, scanty, red urine.—Thread-like flakes in urine.—Blood in urine wards the end of an emission (after which the pain, when urinating, abates). —Urine charged with gravel or small pebbles.—(Nephritic calculi.)—Where e patient has gravel, and there is considerable deposit in the urine which oks like grey sand; also pus in urine.—Great pain just as the urine ceases to ow; excessive pain in urethra which may run back into abdomen.—The fant cries before and during micturition, passes large quantities of sand.—an pass urine only when standing; when he sits it dribbles.—Burning sensaon in urethra during every urination.—(Burning in urethra with incontinence urine, < in daytime, < when urine is high-coloured, and < after drinking er.—Much scalding up urethra while urinating, urine high-coloured with hates, enuresis day and night.—R. T. C.)—Cramps in bladder, with ntractive pain.—Stones in the bladder.—Discharge of pus from the urethra, in gonorrhœa.—Jerking sensation along male urethra.—Pain at meatus inarius with women.

15. **Male Sexual Organs.**—Fetid exhalation from genital organs.—flammation and redness of glans.—(Blennorrhœa).—Herpes on the prepuce. Desire for coition, with frequent and painful pollutions.—Bloody pollutions; ermatic cords swollen, sexual excitement makes them ache and sensitive.—velling of cords from unrequited sexual excitement.—Bad effects from norrhœa suppressed by *Mercury*.—Old dry sycotic warts remaining after ercurial treatment for gouty pains.

16. **Female Sexual Organs.**—Catamenia retarded, scanty, and acrid; ry copious, even to hæmorrhage (in an old maid).—During menses, want to inate, excoriation between thighs, pinchings in abdomen, and squeezing, as by a claw, in loins and pit of stomach.—Dysmenorrhœa, began in morning, th bitter vomiting, diarrhœa, and fainting fits, with exceedingly cold sweats; breast so tender held her hand in front of it to avoid contact.—Mucous ucorrhœa.—Leucorrhœa: on walking; pain at meatus urinarius after

urinating.—Climaxis: asthma < lying down; back pains < by pressure —Suppuration of breasts.—Nipples retracted; shrivelled, insensitive, no irritable.

17. **Respiratory Organs.**—Violent cough from a tickling sensation o ulceration in gullet, or from a roughness in throat.—Short and obstructe respiration.—Violent dyspnœa and choking from a sensation of constrictio in throat, and which forces the removal of all clothing from throat and chest

18. **Chest.**—Spasmodic oppression of chest.—Frequent recurrence o deep respiration.—Sensation as if a foreign body had stopped in the back o taking a full inspiration.—Pressure on chest, often with shortness of breath.— Pressive pain on sternum, < by touching it.—Shooting in sides of chest which often forces patient to bend double.—Tensive pain in exterior of chest as from contraction, on rising up.

19. **Heart.**—Palpitation of the heart.

20. **Neck and Back.**—Painful pressure and tension in back and nap of neck, with lancinations on least movement of trunk or head.—Lancination between shoulder-blades and in muscles of neck.—Stitches in back throug into chest on least motion.—Swelling on one side of neck, painful to touch.— Contusive pain in loins, esp. while stooping, and afterwards.—Pains fron small of back down spermatic cords; < at night and from motion; afte emissions.—Tingling in loins.—Tensive pain from loins to hips on leas movement.

21. **Limbs.**—Paralytic tearing in all joints and limbs, often accompanie by trembling of hands and feet, painful tearings in head, and pinchings i abdomen.—Rigidity and immobility of limbs.—Lassitude in the hands an feet.

22. **Upper Limbs.**—Tearings and pressive shootings in arms, forearm and joints of hands and fingers (principally on motion).—Sweating of hand —Herpes on hands.—Numbness of fingers.—Pain in tips of fingers (bruise and sore), as from subcutaneous ulceration.—Purulent vesicles on fingers.— Deep rhagades in skin of fingers (with burning pains).

23. **Lower Limbs.**—Affections of any kind in general, appearing in lower extremity; r. lower side (H. N. G.).—Pressive tearing and shooting i thighs, knees, and legs.—Lassitude in thighs and knee-joints.—Swelling an stiffness of knees, with shootings.—Red, herpetic spots on calves.—Rigidit of legs, as from contraction.—Cramps in legs and calves of the legs.—Draw ing tearing in r. big toe.—Painful pressive throbbing and throbbing-shootin inner side r. sole, later on whole sole when sitting.—Painful sensibility o soles.—Tension and swelling of feet, with heat and redness.—Coldness of fee esp. before going to bed.

24. **Generalities.**—Shooting, tearing, pressive pains.—Darting, prickin sensation in bones.—Paralytic tearing in all joints and limbs, often accon panied by trembling of hands and feet, painful tearings in head and pinching in abdomen.—Arthritic pains (after taking cold in the water; from suppresse gonorrhœa), with diminished secretion of urine.—Rigidity and immobility o the limbs.—Hot and dense swellings.—Great lassitude, esp. in lower limbs.— Lassitude in the hands and feet.—Emaciation.—The pains cause depressic of spirits.

25. **Skin.**—Itching, sometimes over whole body, esp. in evening, in be

ɪnd in morning when rising.—Red and dry pimples, which itch only when ody is warm.—Miliary eruption on going into fresh air from a warm room. -Nettle-rash.—Fine rash on skin of forehead.—Exanthema like milk crust.— ʼurulent vesicles.—Ulcers after abuse of *Mercury*.—Skin slow to heal.— Ierpes on almost all parts of body (esp. on prepuce).—Warts.—Many little varts.—(Horses lose hair with eruptions.)—Shrivelled skin.—Great emaciation, he skin becomes shrivelled or it lies in folds.—Deep, burning, painful rhagades on fingers).

26. **Sleep.**—Complaints concomitant to yawning.—< When yawning.— leep early in evening.—Nocturnal sleeplessness and frequent waking.— 'rightful dreams with frequent starts.

27. **Fever.**—Shiverings night and day.—Chilliness predominating, day nd night).—Coldness, even near the fire, over whole body, except face and hest, but principally in feet.—Rigor, mostly in forenoon, running from feet ɪpwards.—Heat in the evening, with ebullition of blood, palpitation of heart, nd perspiration (only) on forehead.

Scammonium.

Convolvulus scammonia. Scammony. *N. O.* Convolvulaceæ. Triturations of the dried milky juice of the root.

Clinical.—Diarrhœa. Gastro-enteritis.

Characteristics.—*Scam.* is a drastic cathartic, producing copious watery evacuations, and griping a good deal. Sprengel records a case of fatal poisoning in an infant whose mother took a large quantity of *Scam.*, and herself suffered no effects. *Scam.* must be compared with *Jalap.*, another purging convolvulus.

SYMPTOMS.

11, 12. **Stomach and Abdomen.**—Sudden vomiting and copious green stools, distension and sensitiveness of abdomen and death (in an infant whose nursing mother took a large dose of *Scam.* and herself experienced no symptoms).—Slight pain in stomach with evacuation of fæces.—Violent pain and rapid succession of stools, leaving inactivity of lower intestines for several days.—Inflammation of mucous membrane attended with loss of appetite and headache.

13. **Stool.**—Loose evacuation of fæces with slight pain in stomach.— Green stools.—Rapid succession of stools.

Schinus.

Schinus molle. *N. O.* Anacardiaceæ. Tincture of the berries. Tincture of leaves and berries.

Clinical.—Diarrhœa. Liver, griping pain in. Œsophagus, dryness of. Spinal cord, drawing in. Vomiting.

Characteristics.—Allen says *Schinus* is an evergreen shrub, native of Mexico and South America, and frequently cultivated in Southern California under the names "Pepper tree" and "Chili pepper." The symptoms were observed by Dr. P. W. Poulson on a young lady who ate a few berries after dinner, and on himself. Poulson ate leaves as well as berries, and he had heartburn, griping in liver, and "a kind of drawing sensation as in the spinal cord and cerebellum."

Relations.—*Compare:* Anac., Rhus, Comoc.

SYMPTOMS.

11. **Stomach.**—Long-continued vomiting, "as if all the bowels would be emptied out"; vomiting very painful, as the vomiting subsided diarrhœa came on, the diarrhœa being painless.—Heartburn, dryness of œsophagus.

12. **Abdomen.**—Rolling and flatulence in the bowels, and a griping sensation in the liver.

13. **Stool.**—Painless diarrhœa following painful vomiting.—Profuse diarrhœa continuing all night.

20. **Back.**—Drawing sensation as in the spinal cord and cerebellum.

Scilla Maritima.

Scilla maritima. Squill. Sea Onion. (Red variety.) *N. O.* Liliaceæ. Tincture of fresh bulb. Acetum.

Clinical.—Angina pectoris. Asthma; dry; splenic. Bright's disease. Bronchitis. Conjunctivitis, phlyctenular. Coryza. *Cough, catarrhal. Diabetes;* insipidus. *Dropsy;* splenic. Eyes, affections of; watering of. Fidgets. Heart, palpitation of. Hydrothorax. Measles. Pleurisy. Pneumonia. Spleen, affections of. Spleen-cough. Toothache. *Urine, excessive.* Whooping-cough. Worms.

Characteristics.—The genus *Scilla* is distinguished from *Allium* by having the flowers inserted one above the other on the scape, and from *Ornithogalum* by having the petals deciduous. *Scilla maritima* grows on the shores of the Mediterranean Sea, and has had a place in medicine from the most ancient times. If much handled it irritates the skin; and in large doses excites nausea, strangury, bloody urine and hæmorrhoids; fatal inflammation, gangrene of stomach and bowels; in small doses, promotes expectoration and urine; in large doses, vomiting and purging (Meyrick in Green's *lerbal*). "Its cardiac action is exactly the same as that of *Digitalis*" Mitchell Bruce). An old rule runs: "Put squills in every cough-ıixture." The continuous use of squills seems to cause teeth and ums to ache (R. T. C.). "Diuretic, expectorant, emetic, cathartic, nd a narcotico-acrid poison; in large doses it produces inflamma-.on of the alimentary and urinary canals, and a dose of gr. xxiv as proved fatal" (Milne). According to Hamilton (*Flora Hom.*) .ricenna employed *Scil.* "in complaints of the gums, in inveterate oughs, in *diseases of the spleen*, in dropsy and jaundice, and forbids s use in ulceration of the viscera," the last caution also being men-oned by Celsus. The reputation of *Scil.* as a splenic was revived y Rademacher, whom Burnett quotes (*Dis. of Spleen*, p. 89): "I have ound it quickly and surely helpful in painful spleen diseases—affec-ons painful and beyond any doubt in and of the spleen. In those ull pains on the border of the left hypochondriac and epigastric ːgions, there being no signs of any liver affection, I have used *Scil.* s a remedy with advantage." Rademacher also mentions as cured y *Scil.*—(*a*) those so-called "stomach pains" that are made much etter by lying on the left side, and probably in reality splenic; (*b*) ne case of continuous asthma from a splenic affection, with nocturnal xacerbation; (*c*) (possibly) splenic dropsy. Burnett has improved n Rademacher's teachings, and applied *Scil.* successfully in cases of pleen-cough. Hahnemann's proving brought out many symptoms, pparently arising from the spleen, notably stitches under the free bs of the left side. Burnett used the *Acetum scillæ*; and I gave this ive drops of φ in water three times a day) with excellent effect the case of an elderly lady, very gouty, who had a distressing aroxysmal cough, with a pain extending from splenic region into the roat. The cough caused the eyes to pour with tears. Besides lieving the cough, *Scil.* made the motions, which had been very ght, darker and more natural in colour. The gushing of tears with e cough is another *Scil.* indication: The cough causes sneezing, ow of tears, spurting of urine, and even involuntary stools. The dneys are powerfully acted on by *Scil.*, and many of the traditional ses of the drug have been with the idea of eliminating dropsical fusions by producing a great flow of urine. Hahnemann pointed it that the excessive flow of urine accompanying dropsy and other mplaints was one of the best indications for its use. Boger (*H. R.*, . 33) adds the heart to the organs primarily affected by *Scil.* e gives these cases: (1) Mr. B. suffered from angina pectoris; rcible cardiac contractions, *profuse urine*, much loose mucus in roat and trachea, heart pain indefinite but very severe. *Scil.* 30 lieved in a few hours, and kept him free from an attack for three onths. (2) Miss L., pleuro-pneumonia, pulse 132, temperature 103°, spiration 30; must sit erect in bed; *stitching pains in left chest; nstant hacking cough; frequent, hot, scanty urine;* great weakness d anorexia. *Scil.* cm cured. (3) Boy, 7, hay-fever for third year succession. *Teeth show black marks; constantly rubs eyes and sneezes*, oated about eyes and face, loose cough. Under *Scil.* there was mplete relief in two days, and no further trouble that season. The licised symptoms in this case are very characteristic. Boger mentions that Lippe notes " Black teeth " as a symptom of *Scil.* Boger adds that the nails become brittle and split, and that veterinarians use *Scil.* for cracked hoof in horses. The use of *Scil.* as an " expectorant " depends on its power of producing free secretion from the respiratory mucous membranes : in homœopathy this free secretion is one of the leading indications. Hering says *Scil.* is suited to the pleurisy and pneumonia that follow blood-letting. H. P. Holmes (*A. H.*, xxi. 176) has an excellent article on *Scil.*, to which I am indebted for many comparisons in the RELATIONS section. Sherbino (*M. A.*, xxii. 398) gives this verification of a *Scilla* symptom : Miss H., 15, fleshy, light complexioned, blue eyed, large for her age. *Her left eye was much smaller, and lids not so wide open as those of right eye.* *Scil.* 1m (Jen.) was given in May, and repeated each month for three months. Improvement began in the first month. On December 28th *Scil.* 45m (Fincke) was given, and soon after that the restoration was complete the eyes were a perfect match. *Peculiar Sensations* are : Eyes as in swimming in cold water. Nostrils as if sore. As if diarrhœa would set in. As if chest too tight. Tickling creeping in chest. As if intestines would burst through abdomen. Stitches are very prominent : in teeth ; in chest ; in head. The symptoms are : < In morning ; by inspiration ; by motion ; by uncovering. > By rest lying down in bed ; wrapping warmly. Drinking cold water = cough. < Exertion ; ascending ; cold air. > Sitting up. > Expectorating even a small quantity. < Coughing.

Relations.—*Antidoted by :* Camph. *Compatible after :* Bry. *Compare :* Headache ; < motion ; chest symptoms, Bry. (Bry. cough is < change to warm, Scil. cough < change to cold air). Stitches swollen upper eyelids, K. ca. Cold drink = or < cough, Lyc., Sil (> cough, Caust.). Expectoration sweetish and offensive, Calc. Stan. Spurting of urine when coughing, Caust., Alm., Con., Nat. m. Puls. Involuntary stool when coughing, Pho. ; when sneezing, Sul. when urinating, Ail., Alo., Mur. ac., Sul. Convulsive twitching of limbs, " fidgets," Meny., Pso., Rhus, Caust., Zn. Icy-cold feet, rest of body warm, Meny. Sweat only on toes, Scil.—under toes, Tarax Averse to uncover in fever, Nux. Furious, exhausting cough, Coral. Cup., Stan. Cough < in cold air, Carb. v., Pho., Rx. c., Ver. Tickling in chest, Ver. Sensation of cold water in eyes, Lach. (cold tears) Berb., Euphr., Alm., Con., Lyc., Plat., and Med. (cold feeling), Thuj (as if cold air blowing out through eyes). Bloated round eyes in morning, Elaps. Coryza, Agrap. n., Cep., Ars., Phos., Chlor., Ar. t. Anxiety and fear of death, Aco., Ars. Irritable, angry about trifles Cham. Rubs face and eyes, Scil.—Con. rubs and picks nose ; Ar. t. picks nose, lips, and fingers till they bleed ; Sanic. rubs eyes and nose on waking. Splenics, Cean., Querc. Sweetish taste of food Lyc., Merc., Pul.

Causation.—Blood-letting.

SYMPTOMS.

1. **Mind.**—Great anxiety of the mind, with fear of death.—Angry over trifles.—Aversion to mental and bodily labour.

2. **Head.**—Vertigo; in morning; with nausea; as if he would fall eways on rising from bed.—Cloudy dizziness.—Headache in morning on king, with pressing pains.—Some slow stitches extending into r. side of ehead.—Painful sensitiveness of vertex every morning.—Pulsation in head en raising it.—Stinging headache.—Quickly passing pain in occiput, l. to r. Affections of brain: child rubs face and eyes much, esp. eyes, as if to ieve itching; profuse or scanty urination.

3. **Eyes.**—Staring look, with eyes wide open.—L. eye looks smaller than l. upper lid swollen.—Contraction of pupils.—Eyes feel as if swimming in d water.—Phlyctenular conjunctivitis.—Lachrymation and sneezing.

4. **Ears.**—Tearing behind l. ear.—(Tearing pains in both ears.)

5. **Nose.**—Violent, constant sneezing and fluent coryza.—Sneezes ring cough; eyes water, rubs eyes and nose.—Acrid, corrosive, fluent ryza in morning; a regular general snizzle; mucous cough with spurting urine and even of watery stools.—Coryza with ulcerated nostrils.—Nostrils inful as if sore, with violent coryza (in morning).—Humid eruptions under se, with stinging itching.

6. **Face.**—Changeable expression and colour of face.—During the heat lness of face, followed by paleness, without coldness.—Distorted counte- nce, with red cheeks, and without thirst.—Humid, spreading eruption on per lip.—Black, cracked lips and black teeth.—Lips twitch and are covered th yellow crusts.

8. **Mouth.**—Stitches darting upward in both upper canine teeth as if a arp, cold air penetrated the teeth, when eating cold or warm things.—Teeth ow black marks.—Open, dry mouth.—Accumulation of much viscid mucus in outh.—Increased saliva.—Scraping, burning on palate.—Vesicles on tongue.

9. **Throat.**—Burning in mouth and throat.—Irritation in throat with at and tickling, causing constant cough.—Dryness in throat.—Pain in sub- axillary glands.

10. **Appetite.**—Insatiable appetite.—Longing for acids.—Thirst for cold ter, but the dyspnœa compels her to take but a sip at a time.—The food tes bitter, esp. bread; or it tastes sweet, esp. soup and meat.—Tastelessness tobacco when smoked.

11. **Stomach.**—Constant nausea in pit of stomach, alternating with in, as for diarrhœa in abdomen.—Pressure in stomach as from a stone.— usea during the morning cough.—"Stomach pains" > lying on l. side ademacher).

12. **Abdomen.**—Cutting pain in abdomen.—Pain in side of abdomen as intestines forcing through when coughing and walking.—Pressive stinging in in abdominal muscles of l. side.—Bubbling sensation in muscles of r. le.—Pain in spleen.—Cough seeming to originate in spleen.—Splenic hma.—Dull pains on border of l. hypochondriac and epigastric regions.— inful sensitiveness of abdomen and region of bladder.—Frequent discharge very fetid flatulence.—Increased warmth of abdomen.—Griping and incar- ration of flatus in hypogastrium.—Rumbling and gurgling in paroxysms ove pubic region, > by eating.

13. **Stool and Anus.**—Painless constipation.—Diarrhœa; stool very fensive; watery (during the measles) or looking black.—Passes threadworms d white fibres with tenesmus.—Stitches in anus when walking.—Itching in us.

14. **Urinary Organs.**—Sticking in orifice of urethra and somewh further back.—Frequent urging to urinate, with profuse discharge of pa urine (these may occur separately or together).—Continuous, painful pressu on bladder.—Involuntary micturition ; esp. when coughing.—Enuresis no turna.—When urinating fæces escape.— Cannot retain the urine because t quantity is so great.—Dropsy : dropsy of outer parts, dropsy of chest, all wi profuse urination.

15. **Male Sexual Organs.**—Dull stitches in glans causing anxiety.- Compressive pain in testicles.

16. **Female Sexual Organs.**—Atony of cervix uteri.—Hæmorrhag from uterus.

17. **Respiratory Organs.**—Moaning breathing, with the mouth ope —Wheezing breathing.—Frequently obliged to take a deep breath, which : cough.—Shortness of breath from every exertion, esp. when ascending.- Whooping-cough, when accompanied with sneezing, watering of eyes an nose, and the child rubs eyes with the hands ; in all catarrhal affections an coughs, also troubles of the lungs with the above symptoms ; profuse nas secretion.—Cough with expectoration in the morning and none in the evenin —Difficulty of breathing, with stitches in chest when breathing and coughin —Cough in the morning, with copious expectoration of thin, frequent reddish-coloured mucus.—Dry cough morning and night.—Violent dry coug which = shattering pain in abdomen and dryness in the throat.—Intern tickling in region of thyroid cartilage that provokes cough, which, howeve < the tickling.—Short, dry cough in four or five shocks, from tickling beneat thyroid cartilage.—Fits of spasmodic cough with pains in splenic region.- Cough, with a stagnant watery condition of the blood, and enlarged splee (Burnett).—Sputa : white or reddish mucus ; sweetish or empyreumatic o offensive in odour ; in small round balls, very difficult to expectorate.- Rattling precedes the cough, disappears after.—Cough caused by tickling creeping sensation in chest ; from drinking something cold ; from ever exertion.—Cough with stitches in sides of chest ; pain in abdomen ; sensatio of internal heat ; dyspnœa ; headache ; pressure in the bladder and in voluntary spurting of urine.—The loose morning cough is much more sever and causes more suffering than the dry evening cough.

18. **Chest.**—Stitches : in chest, esp. when inhaling and coughing ; shar in scapular end of clavicle during inspiration and expiration ; severe nea sternum, extending downward ; in middle of ensiform cartilage ; recurrent i side ; broad, pressive beneath ribs of both sides ; jerking in r. and l. side o chest near sternum ; broad, blunt in last rib of l. side, in morning in bed waking him.—Contracting stitch in l. side, just beneath last ribs, caused by rapid walking.

19. **Heart.**—Palpitation of heart.—Pulse : small and slow ; slightly hard

20. **Neck and Back.**—Stiffness : of nape of neck ; of l. cervical muscles —Painful jerking above l. scapula.—Painless drawing in l. scapula.—Bubbling sensation beneath scapulæ, in back of l. upper arm.—Perspiration in armpit.

21. **Limbs.**—Convulsive twitchings and motions of the limbs ; convul- sions.—Frequent falling asleep of hands when resting head upon them, and in lower limbs when crossing the legs, during the day.—(Nails become brittle and split.—Cracked hoof in horses.—Boger.)

22. **Upper Limbs.**—Convulsive twitching of arms ; cold hands.—

tretching of upper limbs, with yawning without sleepiness.—Acute stitches ı joints of both hands even when not moving them.—Jerking pain through rists.

23. **Lower Limbs.**—Convulsive twitching of legs.—Soreness between mbs.—Burning pain in ball of r. foot, as after freezing it.—Icy-cold feet.—old foot-sweat.—Perspiration only on toes.

24. **Generalities.**—Weariness.—Spasmodic movements.—Pains over hole body.—Dull rheumatic pains ; < when exercising, > when at rest.—eficiency of blood.—Heat, with aversion to undress or uncover.—Respiration nxious.—Sweetish taste.—Symptoms generally appearing in l. upper ex-emity ; on l. side generally ; in lower belly ; lower part of chest.—< In orning ; during inspiration ; from undressing.—> While lying in bed ; fter lying down ; from wrapping up warmly.

25. **Skin.**—Soreness in the bends of the joints.—Skin of neck painfully ensitive to slightest rubbing of neckband, with red, almost denuded spots.—Iandling the fresh squills caused blisters.—Eruptions like itch, with burning-ching.—Gangrene.—Hard swellings.

26. **Sleep.**—Frequent yawning without sleepiness.—Restless sleep, with uch tossing about.—Dreamed that his body was excessively swollen ; dream vivid, on waking felt himself to see if it was so.

27. **Fever.**—Pulse small and slow, slightly hard.—Chill internally at ight, with external heat.—Chilliness towards evening when walking, not hile sitting.—Heat, dry, burning, internally predominates.—Great sensation f heat in body, afternoon and evening, generally with cold feet.—Whenever e uncovers himself during the heat he suffers from chilliness and pain.—erspiration wanting, even during the violent burning heat.

Scirrhinum.

Carcinominum. The nosode of Scirrhous Cancer. Trituration.

Clinical.—Breast, cancer of. Cancer. Cancerous diathesis. Glands, enlarged æmorrhages. Varicosis. *Worms.*

Characteristics.—Burnett is my authority for this nosode. He roved it on himself, and produced "a tremendous sinking at the avel," which he regarded as a keynote for its use. *Scirrh.* has aided e cure of many cases of breast tumour in Burnett's hands. With he cured a man of hard glands which appeared on the left side the neck after other glands had been removed by the patient's rother, a surgeon. Hæmorrhages and varicosis of legs and feet, ith purple points, have also been cured by Burnett with *Scirrh.* A atient to whom Burnett had given *Scirrh.* mentioned to him that it ad caused the passage of an enormous number of threadworms. On is hint Burnett gave it with great success in many cases of this oublesome complaint ; and I have verified this experience. In veterate cases where *Cina* and *Teucr.* have given little relief, *Scirrh.* as wrought a great change for the better. The time of < of *Scirrh.* from 5 to 6 p.m., and irregularly on through the night.

Relations.—*Compare:* Other nosodes. In helminthiasis, Cin Teuc., Sul., Saba. Sinking sensation, Sul., Sep., Helleb., Hydras Cancer, Con., Hydrast., Phyt., Sang., Cund., Ars.

Scolopendra.

Scolopendra morsitans (and other species). Centipede. *N. O.* Chilc poda (sub-ord. Scolopendridæ). Tincture of living animals.

Clinical.—Angina pectoris. Convulsions. Malignant pustule.

Characteristics.—The effects of Centipede bites have bee observed on several persons. Swelling, pain, inflammation, an gangrene of the bitten part, with appearance like malignant pustul in one case, were constant symptoms. Vomiting and præcordia anxiety occurred, and in one fatal case the paroxysms of vomitin increased in intensity till the child in a convulsive struggle ceased t breathe. A symptom worth noting is "No perspiration of the righ arm for three months."

SYMPTOMS.

2. **Head.**—Vertigo.—Headache.

11. **Stomach.**—Nausea.—Vomiting of a pale yellow, glairy matte continued at short intervals with increasing violence, till the child in a con vulsive struggle ceased to breathe.

19. **Heart.**—Præcordial anxiety.

22. **Upper Limbs.**—Arm greatly swollen; erysipelatous blush extend ing half over arm; black dotted impression in two rows three-quarters of a inch apart, raised in dark lines extending from dot to dot, $5\frac{1}{2}$ inches long thus showing the entrance of every foot; pain deep and dull; no perspira tion on r. (bitten ?) arm for three months.

24. **Generalities.**—Instant complaint which grew rapidly worse, whic was described by the child as being all over (from *S. heros.*—The child, a gi of four, died in 8 h.).

25. **Skin.**—A large red spot, becoming black, in the middle of which a eschar forms as large as a five-franc piece.—The whole affection resembled malignant pustule, and was associated with swelling of lymphatic glands.— Violent itching, followed by violent pain in bitten part.

27. **Fever.**—No perspiration of r. arm for three months.

Scorpio.

Scorpio (several species). Scorpion. *N. O.* Scorpionida. (Class, Arachnida.) Tincture of living animals.

Clinical.—Salivation. Strabismus. Tetanus.

Characteristics.—Scorpion stings are attended with a certai amount of danger, especially to children. The symptoms of th

Schema are from effects of stings. *Scorp.* has not been proved in the attenuations. Pain and swelling of the injured part are first experienced, and constitutional symptoms follow. These include sleepiness, prostration, and possibly tetanus. Strabismus has been observed in some cases; and the pupils are dilated.

Relations.—*Compare:* Vespa., Scol., Tarent., Apis.

SYMPTOMS.

3. **Eyes.**—Pupils dilated.—Slight strabismus.
5. **Nose.**—Frequent sneezing.
6. **Face.**—Trismus.
8. **Mouth.**—Saliva abundant.
12. **Abdomen.**—Meteorism.
24. **Generalities.**—Bitten part much swollen, with violent pains lasting from one to three days.—Heat and pain at bitten spot, sleepiness, sneezing, restlessness; later, abundant saliva, meteorism; later, trismus or tetanus.—Complete prostration.—Always acute pains in and diminished temperature of the part bitten.

Scrophularia.

Scrophularia nodosa (and S. Marilandica, the American variety introduced from Europe and Asia). Fig-wort. *N. O.* Scrophulariaceæ. Tincture of whole fresh plant.

Clinical.—Appendicitis. Breast, tumours of. Colic. Deafness. Dyspepsia. Enuresis. Eyes, scrofulous affections of. Glands, enlarged. Liver, pains in. Palms, cramp in. Pemphigus. Rheumatism. Sigmoid flexure, pain in. Sleepiness. Stiff-neck. Ureter, pain in.

Characteristics.—The plants of the genus *Scrophularia* "have generally an unpleasant smell. The generic name is derived from the property which the roots were supposed to have of curing scrofula. A decoction of one of the common British species, *S. nodosa*, is sometimes used by farmers to cure the scab in swine" (*Treas. of Bot.*). *Scrph.* was proved by Franz, and later in America by W. H. Blakeley, who took from 10 to 60 drops of the tincture several times a day. Pareira gives the analysis of the drug, which shows it to be very complex. It contains much oxalate and carbonate of lime, as well as Magnesia and Silica. The most remarkable of Franz's symptoms were: Excessive drowsiness; in forenoon, in afternoon, and before and after eating; vertigo when in upright position; accumulation of sweetish water in several parts of the tongue; sensation of a soft body in the gullet; constriction of chest; oppression of chest with trembling as after much weeping. Most of these symptoms were confirmed by Blakeley. The chief clinical authority for *Scrph* is Cooper, who has used it on some old indications. Gerarde mentions "hard kernels" and painful and swollen piles as indicating

Cooper gave it to a patient who had been poisoned by an Indian arrow-poison which produced inflammation and suppuration of the glands; *Scrph.* relieved a most painful condition of the rectum and purulent discharge that had kept up years afterwards. Cooper has reduced strumous glands with it; and cured deafness in a "bull-necked" patient; and also cured a case of sycosis menti, using *Scrph.* externally as well as giving it internally. "Nodosities in the breast" is another indication of Cooper's. It has produced, according to Cooper, a sickly, giddy feeling, with a sense of weakness and sinking at pit of chest, too weak to speak; along with pain from forehead to back of head. The provings brought out several symptoms in the lower abdomen. Cooper has seen *Scrph.* in the form of a poultice relieve peritonitis affecting the lower abdomen. Colic from slight vexation occurred in Franz's proving. Blakeley had pain in sigmoid flexure. Both had pains in the liver. The symptoms are: < In morning; by study; in cold air; breathing cold air; deep breathing; lying on right side; by rest; after food; by pressure. > In warm room.

Relations.—*Antidoted by:* Bry. (chest symptoms). *Followed well by:* Dig. (in enlarged glands.—R. T. C.). *Compare:* Botan., Dig., Euphr., Grat. Pains in joints < by rest, > in warm room, Rhus. Sleepiness, Nux m., Op., Lup.

Causation.—Vexation.

SYMPTOMS.

1. **Mind.**—Despondency, much troubled about the past, and very apprehensive about the future; passed off in a few days, leaving intellect clear.—Miserable and sluggish feeling in mind when moving about.

2. **Head.**—Vertigo: in top of head when standing; even with severe aching in supra-orbital region.—Dizziness, fulness, and pressure in vertex.—Heaviness and distress in head, as after eating too much.—On rising the second morning an indescribable pain and fulness in whole head, followed by epistaxis, esp. occiput and vertex, causing congestion of conjunctiva with puffiness.—Darting pain at exit of r. facial nerve from hylo-mastoid foramen, darting to r. eye.—Headache above eyebrows while walking.—Severe headache through temples, appearing every morning, extending to vertex and occiput.—Severe lancinating pain in vertex, forehead, and temples; dull and throbbing, returning periodically; < resting; < in open air; < leaning forward; < by study.

3. **Eyes.**—Severe cutting pains in eyes, unable to move them, passed off with profuse sweat.—Pulsating stitches in r. eyebrow.—Soreness of eyeballs.—Black spots or film before eyes.—On closing eyes visions of objects.—(Scrofulous photophobia; rivals *Con.* in this.—Blepharospasm.—Scrofulous keratitis.—Tinea ciliaris with minute pustulation.—R. T. C.)

4. **Ears.**—Ringing in ears and sudden loss of hearing.—(Deafness in bull-necked boys.—Deafness before and after menses, improving during the flow.—Eczema behind r. ear and round navel.—R. T. C.)

5. **Nose.**—Dry coryza with sternutation.

6. **Face.**—Pleasant warmth in cheeks.—(Recurrent periostitis of lower jaw in a syphilitic.—R. T. C.)

8. **Mouth.**—Teeth feel as if loose, pain in carious teeth, < upper jaw. —Gums bleed very freely.—First great increase of saliva, then mouth dry.—Accumulation of sweetish water in several parts of tongue.—Qualmish, sticking taste just above pit of throat, frequently lasting an hour, with sensation as if a soft substance (a plug of mucus) were lodged there.—Bitter taste in mouth.

9. **Throat.**—Thick, tenacious, offensive mucus in throat, in forenoon.—Rancid taste in throat, with great weakness and stiffness in hollows of knees. —Irritation of œsophagus.

11. **Stomach.**—Appetite greatly increased at first; later nausea with weakness and oppression at epigastrium.—Feeling as if he had missed his regular meal.—(Dyspepsia removed by the proving.)

12. **Abdomen.**—Pain in r. hypochondrium, < deep inspiration or lying r. side.—Cutting in liver on pressure.—Twisting-pinching pain in umbilicus (l. side).—Colic just below navel and some griping in the side in afternoon.—Griping below navel, 7 a.m. (after a slight vexation).—Pain in sigmoid flexure. —Dull, heavy, periodic pain < when abdomen compressed, legs extended.—(Appendicitis as a local remedy.—R.T.C.)

13. **Stool and Anus.**—Several stools daily with tenesmus.—Protruding piles which bleed and pain (R. T. C.).

14. **Urinary Organs.**—Pinching and tearing as if in ureter, extending from anterior superior spine of ilium down to pubis.—Increased secretion of urine with burning in urethra.—Frequent scanty emission of urine in afternoon.—Enuresis somni (R. T. C.).

16. **Female Sexual Organs.**—Recurring metritis with painful piles: irritation, soreness and burning in vagina and anus went away, as well as headache, that prevented her standing up (from local application.—R. T. C.).

17. **Respiratory Organs.**—On turning on either side, violent dyspnœa < on r. than l., with cutting in liver on pressure.

18. **Chest.**—Oppression of chest with tremulous movement as from much weeping.—Pain in whole r. lung, on taking a deep inspiration, which = cough without expectoration.—Cutting in upper l. lung, < breathing cold air.—Constricted feeling in chest, which = uneasiness.—Cramp-like pain transversely across lower chest, as after much weeping.—Pain about bifurcation of trachea.—Stitches in r. chest, about 6th rib, with shivering.—Violent pinching stitches near r. last true ribs, while walking, during rest, seeming to be in liver.

19. **Heart.**—Anguish in præcordia, < after food.—Indescribable sensation in heart, with severe audible palpitation.—Pulse full, regular.

20. **Neck and Back.**—Stiff neck with pain and contraction of r. sterno-mastoid muscle.—Pain in whole spinal column, with slight opisthotonos.

21. **Limbs.**—Drawing rheumatic pain in all flexors of arms and legs.—Tingling in extremities as from a blow on a nerve.

22. **Upper Limbs.**—Deep-seated cutting pain in all muscles of arms.—Tingling or buzzing in arms and hands.—Sticking and drawing in r. palm, from joints of fingers to middle of hand as far as carpal bones (muscular cramp of palms).

24. Generalities.—Weakness; languor; wants to lie down.—Cutting pains in articulations, like those of *Rhus*, but more intense and longer-lasting, < by rest and in open air, > in warm room; darting from knee to ankle-joints, which feel stiff.—(Threatened abscesses that show no sign of disappearing.—R. T. C.)

25. Skin.—Sallow skin.—Burning of surface when rubbed.—Prickling itching all over, < back of hand, inside wrists and between fingers.—Falling off of hair stopped by lotion of *Scroph.* (R. T. C.).—Pemphigus gangrenosus and its allies.—Irritating vesicles on inside of lip, loaded with spindle-celled epithelium (goes from local application.—R. T. C.).

26. Sleep.—Strong disposition to sleep: in morning with weariness and fulness in whole body; irresistible before and after a meal, with prolonged afternoon sleep.

27. Fever.—Chilliness: on moving about in cool air; after rising in morning, for several hours, passing off with profuse sweat, which was followed by stupor and absence of all the symptoms.—Whole body after first day feels very dry and hot, with burning sensation, followed by profuse sweat.

Scutellaria.

Scutellaria laterifolia. Mad-dog Skull-cap. *N. O.* Labiatæ.
Tincture of fresh plant.

Clinical.—Ardor urinæ. Brain, irritation of. Chorea. Delirium tremens. Dentition. Exophthalmos. Flatulence. Headache, nervous. Hiccough. Hydrophobia. Hysteria. Night-terrors. Sleeplessness. Tobacco-heart.

Characteristics.—*Scutel.*, says Hale, who introduced it into homœopathy, is in the domestic practice of North America what *Valerian* is in that of Europe. "Its calming effects on the nervous system have been known ever since the settlement of New England." Provings by G. W. Gordon (*Allen*) and G. H. Royal (*New, Old, and Forgotten Remedies*) give the homœopathic data. Royal (*A. H.*, xxiii. 269) had this indication for *Scut.* given him by a friend: "Nervo-bilious headache with the nervous symptoms uppermost, and *nothing the matter with her.*" He relates this case: Miss M., 32, head of a large school, complained of being used up; unable to sleep or think. Pain in head almost constant, sometimes frontal, mostly at base of brain. Whenever called upon to overdo herself cannot sleep that night, and then there is either a nervous explosion the following day or a nervous sick headache, either being followed by complete collapse. This was in May. *Pic. ac.*, and later *Phos. ac.*, gave relief, and in September patient resumed work. Late in December there was another breakdown, and *Stych. pho.* was given. A week later, after a very long and fatiguing day's work, Royal was summoned at 2 a.m. He found the patient screaming. Every few minutes she had to urinate, and passed only a few drops. Stools frequent, loose, watery. Pulse irregular. *Scut.* φ was given, ten drops every half-hour. Patient was better after the second dose, slept after the fourth.

Since then she has kept the medicine by her, has only taken it when overworked, and has never had a nerve explosion or a headache since. In this case there was "nothing the matter with her"—*i.e.*, no organic defect to which the sufferings could be attributed. Royal's provers took 3x and 30x. Gordon took repeated doses of 10 to 50 drops of ϕ. Hale quotes many eclectic writers who give these indications: (1) Depression of nervous and vital powers after long sickness, over-exercise, over-study, long-continued and exhausting labours. It controls nervous agitation (King). [It was Burnett's chief remedy in the nervous debility after influenza.] (2) Scudder mentions chorea; delirium tremens; and *hydrophobia* (as its popular name suggests). Rafinesque cites cases of *prevention* of hydrophobia; and Hale observed it produce in a patient taking 1x, after each dose —"Spasmodic or constrictive closing of jaws, and a tightness of the muscles of the face." [A writer, quoted *N. Y. Med. Times*, xxiv. 318, says *Scut.* in delirium tremens has the remarkable effect of *calming fear*.] (3) Paine adds these indications: Subsultus tendinum following fevers, in delirium tremens, epilepsy, catalepsy, hysteria. (4) Coe (who uses *Scutellarin*, the concentrated preparation) mentions sunstroke; tenesmus; tetanus; cramps. Hale has used it with success in sleeplessness, night-terrors, hysteria, nervous agitation from pain or exciting emotions, cerebral irritation of children from dentition or intestinal irritation. Like its relation, *Lycopus.*, it caused weak and irregular action of the heart and protrusion of the eyes. It has been found useful in weak heart resulting from cigarette smoking (*M. Cent.*, iii. 463). Churton (*B. M. J.*, quoted *H. R.*, i. 78) gave 60 drops of the tincture every two hours in a case of "severe and rapid hiccough" which *Chloroform*, *Morphia*, and *Pilocarpine* had failed to relieve permanently. After the eighth dose the patient slept, and the spasms gradually diminished, and stopped for good by the fourth day. The hemicrania is > moving about in open air. (But there is also headache < from motion.) All symptoms are > by sleep. < By overwork or over-exertion.

Relations.—*Compare:* Heart, Grave's disease, and botan., Lcpus. Nervous exhaustion, Cypr. (Cypr., according to Hale, acts more on brain, Scut. on spinal cord). Trismus, Nux. Hydrophobia, Agar., Fagus, Lach., Bell., Hdfb. "Overworked women," Mag. c.

Causation.—Excitement. Influenza. Overwork (mental or physical). Tobacco (heart). Pain (causes nervous agitation).

SYMPTOMS.

1. **Mind.**—Mind confused on attempting to study; cannot concentrate attention.—Feeling of stupor on rising.—Apathy.—Irritability.—(Fear.)

2. **Head.**—Vertigo: soon after breakfast; with photophobia.—Dull, oppressive headache; on rising; < by study.—Full, throbbing sensation in head.—Sensation as if cranial contents were confined in too small a space.—Before rising, hemicrania, most severe over r. eye; > moving about in open air.—Pain in occiput.—Headache < by eating; > by motion.

3. **Eyes.**—Eyes feel as if protruding; as if pressed from within outwards.—Aching in eyeballs.—Eyeballs painful to touch.

6. **Face.**—Face flushed towards evening.—Spasmodic, constrictive closing of jaws and tightness of muscles of face (Hale, from 1 x).

8. **Mouth.**—Taste: bad; sour; bitter.

9. **Throat.**—Sensation of lump in throat which could not be swallowed

11. **Stomach.**—Poor appetite.—Sour eructation.—Nausea.—Vomiting of sour ingesta, hiccoughs, pain and distress in stomach.

12. **Abdomen.**—Gas in bowels; fulness and distension.—Colic.—Uneasiness.

13. **Stool.**—Bowels regular with white stools.—Diarrhœa, light-coloured; stools preceded by colic.

14. **Urinary Organs.**—On attempting to urinate, slight difficulty, as if muscles of urethra partially paralysed.—Urine rather scanty.—Bile in urine. —Frequent micturition but quantity small.

18. **Chest.**—Oppression; sticking in heart region.—Dull pain vertically beneath sternum.

19. **Heart.**—Sticking in heart region.—Sensation of throbbing about heart, evening.—Pulse: very variable in force; intermitting.

20. **Back.**—Sharp pains occasionally felt in lumbar region, proceeding mostly from l. kidney region.

21. **Limbs.**—Occasional twitchings in muscles of arms and legs.

24. **Generalities.**—Languor on rising in morning.—Tremulousness and twitching of muscles.—Restless uneasiness; must move about.—Sticking in various parts.

26. **Sleep.**—Frightful dreams.—Sudden wakefulness.—Sleeps late in morning and wakes with severe headache.—Frequent sudden starting from sleep.

27. **Fever.**—Slight chilliness, esp. on getting up.

Secale Cornutum.

Secale cornutum. Spurred Rye. Ergot of Rye. [The black, horn-like spur into which the grains of Rye (Secale cereale, *N. O.* Gramineæ) are changed by the fungus Claviceps purpurea.] *N. O.* Fungi. Tincture of the fresh spurs collected just before harvest.

Clinical.—Abortion, threatened. After-pains. Albuminuria. Anus, incontinence of; open. Asthenopia. *Bladder, paralysis of.* Boils. Carbuncles. Cataract. Chilblains. Cholera; infantum. Chorea. Convulsions. Cramps. Diabetes. Diaphragm, cramp in. Diarrhœa. Distortions. Dysphagia. Epilepsy. Epistaxis. *Feet, cramps in; burning of; coldness of. Fibroma. Gangrene.* Gastritis. Glands, swelling of; suppuration of. Goître. Hæmaturia. Hæmorrhages. Hæmorrhagic diathesis. Heart, palpitation of. Hiccough. Hysteria. Impotence. Liver, enlargement of. Lochia, fetid. Lumbago. *Menstruation, excessive.* Metrorrhagia. Milk, suppressed. *Miscarriage.* Morvan's disease. Myelitis; diffusa. *Nails, degeneration of.* Neuralgia. Night-sweats. *Numbness.* Œsophagitis. *Ovaries, tumours of. Paralysis*; post-diphtheritic; spastic.

Placenta, retained. Post-partum hæmorrhage. *Pregnancy, false pains of.* Purpura. Raynaud's disease. Small-pox, hæmorrhagic. *Spinal irritation.* Stammering. Stomach, cancer of. Strabismus. Stricture, spasmodic. Thrombosis. Tongue, biting of. Typhoid. Ulcers. Uterus, inertia of; neuralgia of; prolapse.

Characteristics.—Rye and grasses are apt to be affected with the Ergot disease in damp seasons, and when grown on damp, ill-drained lands. If breeding cows are turned on pastures where infected grasses grow they are very liable to drop their calves. Ergot has been known as a hastener of parturition from remote times. Its other actions have been for the most part learned from the terrible epidemics of "Ergotism" which have occasionally devastated districts in which Rye infected with Ergot has been ground into flour and eaten by the population. Death takes place in convulsions; or else from gangrene and consequent exhaustion; or from exhausting hæmorrhages or discharges, as diarrhœa. Many who escape immediate death are reduced to a cachectic state, from which they never recover; are paralysed, have limbs distorted and senses impaired. In general the sufferer retains a clear intellect and a good, even abnormally good, appetite to the last. The nervous symptoms of *Sec.* are convulsive. The body is at times rigid; at times rigidity alternates with relaxation. This is especially seen in the hands, which are either clenched or *have the fingers spread widely apart* (a keynote symptom). The muscles of the face and abdomen twitch. There is incontinence or retention of urine. Spasmodic retching, the stomach is violently contracted. Through the like action on the vaso-motor nerves there is first contraction and then dilatation of blood-vessels; the fingers turn bluish black. This stagnation leads to dry gangrene of the parts. *Sec.* shrivels up the skin, makes it dry and harsh; sallow complexion. It is therefore *suited to*—thin, scrawny women, feeble and of cachectic appearance; women of irritable, nervous temperament; of pale, sunken countenance. To very old, decrepit persons. On the other hand, it is also *suited to:* Irritable, plethoric subjects. Women of very lax muscular fibre; everything seems loose and open; no action, vessels flabby: passive hæmorrhages, copious flow of thin, black, watery blood. For *Sec.* lessens the coagulating power of the blood, and produces a hæmorrhagic diathesis; persistent, offensive bleeding. Small wounds bleed persistently. Purpura comes within this category. One grand characteristic of *Sec.*, which will determine its selection in many cases, is: "< By external heat." This applies to cholera, purpura, gangrene, and any condition which may present symptoms of *Sec.* In cholera cases calling for *Sec.* the patient is cold, almost pulseless; there are spasmodic twitchings of muscles in various parts (especially spreading of fingers), eyes sunk, features pinched; surface harsh, shrivelled, dry, as though no moisture were left in the body. *Though cold to the touch, cannot bear to be covered.* In spite of this coldness, *Sec.* has *burning* among its characteristic sensations: burning in all parts of the body as if sparks were falling on the patient. Another characteristic sensation is numbness; tingling as if ants crawling all over, > from rubbing. This may accompany hæmorrhages. loss of other fluids, debility, or skin affections. In the later stages of ergotism there is anæsthesia. The discharges are exhausting and offensive. Diarrhœa is peculiar, involuntary; with wide-open anus. The boils in which *Sec.* is indicated are small and painful, with green contents, mature very slowly, heal slowly, and are very weakening. The eyes are affected in various ways: Pustulous conjunctivitis; suppuration of cornea; dilated pupils, distortion, and strabismus; ptosis; suppressed tears. Catarrh has been caused in many instances. "< From warmth" will be the leading indication in many eye cases requiring *Sec.* Exophthalmic goître has been cured with it; the heart being acted on by *Sec.* as other hollow viscera, and violent palpitation induced. *Sec.* has a great affinity for the uterus, whether gravid or not. Though its use in ordinary doses in obstetric practice is attended with danger, it may be used on its homœopathic indications with perfect safety. It is indicated: (1) In threatened abortion, especially at the third month; prolonged, bearing-down, forcing pains. (2) During labour when the pains are irregular, too weak, feeble, or ceasing; everything seems loose and open, but there is no expulsive action; fainting. (3) For after-pains when too long, too excessive; or when there is hour-glass contraction of the uterus. (4) For suppression or non-appearance of the milk. The menses of *Sec.* are irregular; copious, dark, fluid; accompanied by labour-like pains in abdomen; there may be a continuous watery discharge of blood during the whole time between the periods. Teste records this case: A lady, 50, fat, very soft flesh, had flooding which nothing could stop. After several useless attempts, Teste gave large doses of *Sec.* with scarcely any effect. The patient asked for infinitesimal doses. At that time Teste had no faith at all in infinitesimals, but he yielded to the patient's request, and gave one drop of the 6th. The flooding ceased *immediately* and permanently. *Peculiar Sensations* of *Sec.* are: As if intoxicated while undressing. As if eyes were spasmodically rotated. As of a solid plug in nose. As if tongue paralysed. As if there were some resistance to be overcome in speech. As of a heavy weight in stomach. Region of stomach as if contracted. Anus as if locked up. As if testes being drawn up to inguinal ring. Uterus as if burnt. As if contents of uterus would fall forward. As if soft air were creeping through back. As if sacrum would be forced out. As if something alive creeping under skin. As if fingers asleep. As if limbs had been a long time in hot water. As if sparks of fire falling on different parts. As if mice creeping under skin. Fuzzy feeling in limbs. *Sec.* is indicated in *Suppressions:* tears; lochia; milk; sweat. Thirst with dry mouth or burning. Desires lemonade and sour things. Averse to fat and meat. The symptoms are: < By touch. > Lying doubled up in bed. Motion and any exertion <. Walking = giddiness. Many symptoms (cramps, twitchings) < night. Sinking spells 3 a.m. Open air >. Wants to be fanned. Warm applications <. Warm drink <. Wet bandages > labour pains. Cold applications >. < After eating. All symptoms < just before menses. The right side is predominantly affected.

Relations.—*Antidoted by:* Camph., Op. *Compatible:* Chi. (Teste classes Sec. with Chi. in his Ferrum group), Ars., Aco., Bell., Merc., Pul. *Compare:* In labour, Cinnamon ("In post-partum hæmorrhage,

namon increases labour-pains, controls profuse or dangerous
ding, is always safe, while Ergot is always dangerous."—H. C.
n). Labour-like pains, Pul., Sul., Bell., Calc., Caul., Gossyp., Lil. t.,
., Vib. o. Cold skin, cannot bear to be covered, Camph. >
covering, Aco., Calc., Camph., Fer., Iod., Lyc., Pul., Sul., Ver.
morrhages, Bovist. (flow between periods ; menses flow mostly or
y at night or early morning ; puffy condition of body ; parts feel
rmously large), Mitchella (less passive, blood brighter, dysuria
h the hæmorrhage), Trill. p. (bright red and profuse, faint feeling,
id, feeble pulse), Ham. (with hammering headache), Erig. (flow in
and starts ; with dysuria), Ust. (flow bright red, partly clotted).
. ph., Chi. Hæmorrhagic diathesis, Lach., Phos. Cholera,
ivelled up, gangrene, burning sensation, Ars. (but Ars. is > by
t). Cholera collapse, Camph. (sudden), Ver. (cold sweat on fore-
d). Follicular pharyngitis, K. bi. Cold surface, sunken, pale face,
e lips, tingling in limbs, speech stuttering, Lach. Action on blood-
sels, Bar. c. Diarrhœa discharged with great force, Samb., Crot. t.
us wide open, Apis, Phos. Threatened abortion at third month,
i. Cholera morbus, Colch. Diabetes, Plb. Burning feet, cramp
calves, Sul. Eyes < from warm applications (Asar. > cold wash-
). Exophthalmic goître, Lpus., Scut., Thyr. Spastic paralysis,
th. Old persons, Con. Twitching, coldness, chilblains, cholera,
o botan., Agar. *Compare also :* Ergotinum, which sometimes acts
en Sec. is indicated and fails (see case under *Ergotinum*).

Causation.—Lifting (= abortion). Injury (= gangrene). Sexual
cess.

SYMPTOMS.

1. **Mind.**—Discouragement and timidity.—Great anxiety.—Sadness and
lancholy.—Great anguish.—Furor, with desire to jump into the water.—
dness and inclination to bite.—Fear of death.—Mania.—Weakness of the
ellectual faculties (stupid, half-sleepy condition ; moaning).—Mental aliena-
n.—Delirium.—Loss of consciousness.—Consciousness seems to continue
the last breath ; and just before death it seems as though the patient would
prove.

2. **Head.**—Head confused and stupefied (unconsciousness with heavy
ep, preceded by tingling in head and limbs ; in hæmorrhages from the
rus).—Sensation as from intoxication while undressing.—Vertigo as from
oxication.—Stupefaction, with tingling in head and pain in limbs, which
< from motion.—Diminution and loss of senses, sight, hearing, &c.—
culiar feeling of lightness of head, esp. in occiput.—Attacks of vertigo of
ferent kinds, also chronic.—Headache with dull and painful confusion, esp.
occiput.—Semilateral headache (l.).—Hair falls out.—Scalp sore.—Twisting
head to and fro.

3. **Eyes.**—Eyeballs sunk deep in the sockets ; and surrounded by blue
rgins.—Pupils spasmodically contracted or else dilated.—Convulsed eyes.
Squinting.—Pain in eyes, with feeling as if spasmodically rotated.—Fixed,
ld look.—Cataract, hard or soft ; with headache, vertigo, and roaring in
rs.—Suppuration of cornea ; < from warm applications.—Suppressed

secretion of tears.—Eyes yellow.—Complete blindness.—Double or tri vision.—Mist, spots and a veil before the sight.—Weakness of sight.—Spa ling before the eyes and cloudiness of sight.—Exophthalmic goître.

4. **Ears.**—Humming and roaring in ears; and hardness of hearing Undue sensitiveness of hearing, even slightest sound re-echoed in head made her shudder.—Transient deafness.

5. **Nose.**—Sneezing.—Nose feels stopped yet watery discharge r from it.—Nose stopped l. side as with a solid plug.—Nose-bleed: blood da runs continuously, with great prostration, small, thread-like pulse; in people or drunkards; in young women; from debility.

6. **Face.**—Face discoloured, pale, yellow, wan, with eyes hollow a surrounded by a blue circle.—Distorted features.—Livid spots on face.—F of a deep red.—Swelling of face.—Tingling in face.—Forehead hot.—M cular twitchings, usually begin in face and then spread all over bo sometimes increasing to dancing and jumping.—Lips bluish or deat pale.—Lips and mouth painfully contracted (spasmodic distortion; ri sardonicus).

7. **Teeth.**—Lockjaw.—Grinding of teeth.—Loosening and falling of teeth.—Bleeding from gums.—Difficult dentition.

8. **Mouth.**—Very offensive breath.—Increased secretion of saliva. Dryness of mouth, with thirst.—Hæmoptysis.—Sanguineous or yellowi green foam before mouth.—Tongue discoloured, brown or black; or e loaded with a thick coating (of mucus).—Painful tingling in tongue and thro —Swelling of tongue.—Stammering, embarrassed, indistinct, weak speech; if the tongue were paralysed; or there were resistance to be overcome. Twitching of tongue.—Frequently bites tongue.

9. **Throat.**—Dryness of throat.—Burning sensation or troubleson tingling or crawling in throat.—Follicular pharyngitis; hawks up litt follicular exudation.—Paralysis of muscles of swallowing and speaking; danger of choking.—Inflammation of the œsophagus.

10. **Appetite.**—Dulness of the taste.—Burning, insatiable thirst.—U natural appetite, even when dying from exhausting discharges from bowe —Insatiable hunger, esp. for acid things.

11. **Stomach.**—Frequent risings.—Disgust, esp. for meat and fat things, and nausea.—Continuous nausea; < after eating.—Nausea and inclin tion to vomit.—Hiccough.—Retching and vomiting of bilious, crude matte —Easy vomiting.—Vomiting of food, with great debility.—Vomiting of lur brici.—Vomiting of mucus.—Vomiting of black bile.—Vomiting of dark brow coffee-grounds fluid; of all food and drink.—Hæmorrhage from stomach.- Stomachache.—Cramp in stomach.—Excessively painful sensibility, distres ing oppression (as from a weight), and anguish in pit of stomach, wi ineffectual want to vomit.—Burning sensation in scrobiculus and epigastriur —Great anxiety and pressure in pit of stomach, with great sensibility to touc —Inflammation and gangrene of stomach.—Inflammation and cancer i stomach.

12. **Abdomen.**—Abdomen excessively inflated and tight.—Cuttings an tearing pains in abdomen.—Inflammation and gangrene of the liver.—Liv enlarged.—Burning (or coldness) in abdomen.—Fixed, burning pains i splenic and lumbar regions.—Pains in the loins as from false labour pains.-

c, with pains in sacrum and thighs, frequent risings, and vomitings.—
ıful colic, with convulsions.—Sensation of excessive coldness in abdomen
back.—Burning sensation in abdomen.—Strong pulsation in umbilical
on.—Borborygmi.—Pains in hypogastric region.

3. **Stool and Anus.**—Constipation, with continued and ineffectual
t to evacuate.—Loose, frequent evacuations, with serous, slimy, or else
oloured or brownish fæces.—Diarrhœa of a putrid smell.—Diarrhœa, with
len prostration of strength.—Involuntary (very watery) evacuations.—
nsive, watery diarrhœa (in child-bed).—Cholera; diarrhœa after the
era.—Diarrhœa: frequent brown discharges, dark-coloured; very offen-
; thin, olive green; very exhausting; pernicious.—Hæmorrhage from
bowels.—Expulsion of worms.—Paralysis of rectum and anus.—Anus
open.

4. **Urinary Organs.**—Suppressed secretion of urine.—Scanty, hot,
ing urine.—Emission of urine, drop by drop, difficult, scanty, with con-
d want to urinate.—White urine, clear like water.—Increased secretion
rine.—Urine retained.—Bladder paralysed.—Enuresis: of old people;
watery, or bloody urine.—Hæmaturia; bloody, albuminous urine; thick
blood.—Urinary deposit like white cheese.

. **Male Sexual Organs.**—Numerous erections, even after coition.—
lightness in occiput, strong dragging in spermatic cord, so that testes
ed drawn up to inguinal ring.—After sexual excess palpitation of heart.
ak memory after exhausting coition; impotence.—Chronic spasmodic
ure of urethra.

. **Female Sexual Organs.**—Catamenia too profuse and of too long
ion, sometimes with violent spasms.—Metrorrhagia of a black, liquid
, flowing esp. during a slight movement, sometimes with tingling in legs
reat debility.—Discharge of blood during pregnancy.—Labour ceases,
nstead twitchings and convulsions.—Too long and too painful after-
—Suppression of milk.—Miscarriage (esp. in third month).—Defective
action of uterus after miscarriage.—Swelling and warts on the cervix
which is partially open.—Gangrene of vaginal mucous membrane, with
, slate colour.—Vagina hot or cool.—Sanguineous congestion in uterus.
ensive discharge from uterus causing her to vomit (Ussher).—Lochia
y and fetid, or of too long duration and sanguineous (followed by fever
flammation of uterus).—Puerperal convulsions.—[Female genital organs
eral; pains like labour pains, which are protracted for a long time, skin
nd no wish to be covered, &c.; labour pains ceasing; labour pains too
; abortion in the characteristic patients.—H. N. G.]—Cancer and gan-
of uterus.—Prolapse of uterus.

. **Respiratory Organs.**—Heavy, anxious breathing, with moaning.—
ng of blood, with or without cough.—Feeble voice, inaudible, stammer-
Expectoration of blood during violent efforts to breathe.—Voice hoarse
ollow.—Painless aphonia in morning, as the day goes on he gets hoarse
ced.—R. T. C.).—Anxious and obstructed respiration, with sighs
obs.

Chest.—Dyspnœa and oppression of chest.—Suffocating oppression
st, with cramp in diaphragm.

Heart.—Præcordial tenderness.—Painful sensation over heart.—

Præcordial anxiety.—Violent spasmodic palpitation of heart.—Pulse sm
very rapid, contracted ; frequently intermittent ; fluttering, slow, depresse

20. **Neck and Back.**—Stiffness of nape of the neck.—Profuse mili
eruption on nape of neck and chest.—Sensation of coldness in back.—F
in back and small of back.—Tingling and insensibility in back (extending
tips of fingers and toes).—[Severe pain in (lower) back < when walking m
or sitting long in same position.—R. T. C.].—(Lumbago.)

21. **Limbs.**—Drawing, crawling, tearing, and tingling in limbs
joints.—Distortion of limbs.—Jerks and convulsive movements in lin
which manifest themselves esp. at night, often also periodically, and wh
are > by stretching the parts violently.—Contraction of hands, feet, fing
and toes.—Limbs become cold, pale, and wrinkled, as after being a long t
in hot water.—Disagreeable sensation of sleep and formication in limb
Cramps in legs, calves, arms, hands, and toes.—Burning of hands and fee
Fuzzy feeling in limbs.—Cold gangrene of the limbs ; the dead part separ
at the joints and drops off.—Trembling of limbs.—Weakness, heaviness,
torpor of limbs.—Numbness, insensibility, and coldness of limbs, esp. tip
fingers and toes.

22. **Upper Limbs.**—Spasmodic curvature of the arm, with drawing
the part.—Burning sensation in the hands.—Swelling of the hands, with b
pustules.—Œdematous swelling in the wrist.—Distortion of the hand
Tingling, crawling, with numbness and insensibility in finger-tips.—Cont
tion, distortion, and turning back of the fingers.—Spasms with fingers sp
apart.—Peculiar prickling in tips of fingers that are very sensitive to c
after awhile they began to suppurate, and later the nails separated from t
matrix and fell off one after another, leaving an unhealthy granulating surf
—Degeneration of pulp of nails, the nails are raised.

23. **Lower Limbs.**—Lassitude and soreness in the legs.—Contrac
of the legs and toes.—Distressing cramps in calves and soles, esp. at nigh
Burning sensation in (swollen) feet.—Distortion of feet.—Swelling of
with black pustules.—Feet seem asleep and stiff.—Mortification of to
Gangrena senilis.—Tingling in toes.

24. **Generalities.**—For female complaints chiefly, and esp. when oc
ring in thin, scrawny, wrinkled females or children.—Skin is cold, but
patient does not wish to be covered up.—Copious vomiting of a mixtur
thick, black, pitchy, bilious, and slimy matter.—Dry gangrene, particular
r. side, beginning in toes and running up the limb.—Amaurosis occurrin
patients characteristic of this drug ; hard hearing ; blue colour around
—< From drawing up limbs ; esp. in troubles of childbed.—> From str
ing out the limbs.—Drawing, tearing, and tingling in the limbs and join
Violent and wandering spasmodic pains.—Cramps in legs, arms, and che
Burning sensation in all parts of the body, as if caused by sparks.—T
spasms ; of all extensors.—Tetanus.—Epileptiform convulsions.—Ge
atrophy and emaciation.—Rapid emaciation of paralysed parts.—Unst
gait ; unsteadiness of the whole body ; trembling ; rapid sinking of stre
—Collapse when the patient cannot bear covering.—Syncope.—(
lassitude and indolence.—Paralysis.—Complete mortification of some
by sphacelus.—Affections in general of r. side ; crooked limbs ; sensati
deadness in any part.—Loss of sensation throughout the body.

25. Skin.—Skin sallow, lead-coloured, flaccid, and shrivelled.—Skin rough and dry.—Torpor and insensibility of the skin.—Miliary eruption, esp. on chest and nape of neck.—Petechiæ.—Purpura hæmorrhagica.—Ecchymosis.—Furunculi.—Swelling and pain without inflammation; coldness, blue colour, gangrene.—Black, gangrenous pustules.—Blackness of outer parts; crawling on the skin as of insects.—Subcutaneous tingling.—General desquamation of epidermis.—Ulcers that turn black; skin withered and gangrenous.—Heat, with thirst and want of perspiration.—Sanguineous vesicles, which turn to gangrene, in the limbs.—Anthrax becoming gangrenous.

26. Sleep.—Strong inclination to sleep and coma.—Deep, lethargic sleep.—Sleeplessness, with agitation and dry heat.—Coma with delirium, starts, and fright.

27. Fever.—Violent shivering, followed by violent internal burning heat, with violent thirst.—Excessive coldness in back, abdomen, and limbs.—Coldness of surface of body; esp. of extremities and face; dryness.—Dry heat, with quick pulse, agitation, and sleeplessness.—Small, suppressed pulse (generally slow and contracted, sometimes intermittent, only slightly accelerated during the heat).—Pulse unchanged, even with the most violent attacks.—Cold perspiration.—Cold, clammy sweat all over, esp. above waist-line.

Selenium.

Selenium. An Element. Se. (A.W. 79.5). Trituration.

Clinical.—Alcoholism. Ankle, itching eruption about. *Comedo.* Constipation. Debility. Enuresis. Hair, falling out. Headache. Hoarseness. *Impotence* Laryngitis, scrofulous; tubercular. Liver, affections of; rash over region of. Priapism. Prostatitis. Prostatorrhœa. Psoriasis palmaris. Reveries. Scabies. Scalp, eczema of. *Skin, unhealthy. Spermatorrhœa.* Stammering. Sun, effects of. Syphilis.

Characteristics.—*Selenium* was discovered in 1818 by Berzelius, and was named by him after the moon (σελήνη) because it is found associated with *Tellurium* (Tellus, the earth). It is also found associated with *Sulphur.* All three belong to the same group of elements. "When precipitated it appears as a red powder, which melts when heated, and on cooling forms a brittle mass, nearly black, but transmitting red light when in thin plates. When heated in air it takes fire, burns with a blue flame, giving a gaseous *Oxide of Selenium*, which has a most penetrating and characteristic odour of putrid horse-radish. *Sel.* undergoes a remarkable change in electrical resistance under the action of light: hence the use of Selenium cells" (*Cent. Dict.*). *Sel.* was introduced and proved by Hering. A leading feature of it is the weakness it causes, a weakness involving all parts of the body; easy fatigue from any labour, night-watching, mental exertion, and especially from hot weather. The hotter his body the weaker he is: strength rises as the sun sinks. This debility causes sluggishness: wants to sleep from sheer exhaustion, and is < after. Cannot bear any nervous drain, hence < after coitus or seminal emissions. Impotence. Debility after fevers. When the patient begins to walk after typhoid and feels great weakness in the spine and fears paralysis *Sel.* is indicated. Irritability, headaches, and other troubles following or < by seminal emissions. The headaches are accompanied by profound melancholy, and may be caused by indulgence in alcoholics or in tea, by hot weather, by over-study, and they are < by strong odours, as of musk, roses, &c. The headaches may be periodical, and are frequently located above the left eye. Many chronic liver affections are met with *Sel.*, the guiding symptoms in such cases being : Enlargement of liver with loss of appetite in the morning ; sharp stitching pain < on any movement or pressure, sensitiveness of liver ; and, especially, "fine rash over liver region." There is constipation from atony, with impacted fæces : and dribbling of semen after stool, and also after micturition. Sufferings after seminal emissions—mental confusion, headache, almost paralytic weakness of spine, involuntary escape of prostatic fluid. I have cured with *Sel.* many cases of hoarseness, the special indications being—hoarseness of singers, appearing as soon as they begin to sing ; or after long use of the voice ; with frequent necessity to clear the throat from accumulation of clear, starchy mucus. Scrofulous and incipient tubercular laryngitis have been cured with *Sel.* The parallelism with *Sulph.* is seen all through the pathogenesis of *Sel.*, and perhaps more especially in the skin. *Sel.* causes itching in folds of skin, as between fingers and about joints, especially the ankle-joint. The itching may occur in small spots, and be accompanied by tingling (showing involvement of the nervous system). The scalp is affected with an eczematous eruption which oozes thin fluid after scratching. Hair falls off scalp and all parts of body. I have frequently relieved "psoriasis palmaris" with *Sel.*, which shows that it has a relation to syphilis. Among the *Peculiar Symptoms* of *Sel.* are : Very forgetful in business, but during sleep dreams of what he had forgotten. Coryza ending in diarrhœa. Hungry at night ; longing for spirituous liquors, an almost irresistible maniacal desire. Sensation as if a biting drop were forcing its way out of the urethra. Irresistible desire to lie down and sleep ; strength leaves him suddenly, especially in hot weather. Very great aversion to a draught of air, either warm, cold, or damp. Aversion to salted food. Pulsation in whole body, especially in abdomen after eating [which I have verified]. Great emaciation of face, hands, legs, feet, affected parts, and single parts. *Sel.* is *Suited to* blondes and persons of light complexion. The symptoms are < by touch and pressure. < By motion. > By rest. < After sleep. < By mental exertion. < After seminal losses. < From draught of air, even if warm. < In open air. < From tea ; sugar ; salt ; lemonade ; wine. < In hot weather. < By sun, and with the sun's increase (< towards noon, > as sun declines). > Taking cold air or cold water into mouth. < Every afternoon (headaches).

Relations.—*Antidoted by :* Ign., Puls. (Mur. ac. in a case of mine). *Incompatible :* Chi., Wine. *Compatible after :* Calad., Nat. c., Staph., Pho. ac. (in sexual weakness) Itch checked by Merc. or Sul. often requires Sel. *Compare :* Hunger at night, Cin., Pso., Ign., Lyc. Impacted stool, Alo., Calc., Sanic., Sep., Sel. Impotence (Chlor. sudden). Priapism, glans drawn up, Berb. ; (glans drawn down, Canth.). Aphonia of singers, Caust., Arg. m., Stan., Ar. t., Graph. Prostatitis and urethritis, Lith. c., Dig., Cyc., Caust., Lyc., Cop. Hot weather fatigue, Lach., Camph., Nat. c., Nat. m. Bad effects of mental exertion and loss of sleep, Sul. Impotence, Sul. (Sul. has more coldness and shrivelling of the organs ; Sel. more total relaxation, so that semen escapes involuntarily and dribbles). Exhaustion consequent on protracted diseases, Sul. (Sul. has flushes of heat on least motion ; and gone feeling in forenoon). Periodical headaches, Sul. (Sel. every afternoon, < from tea ; Sul. once a week, < from coffee). Headaches of drunkards or debauchees, Sul. (Sul. < from all forms of alcohol ; Sel. headaches are sometimes > from brandy ; also its gastric symptoms). "Cat-naps," Sul. (Sel. wakes precisely at same hour, before rising time, at which all symptoms < ; Sul. has not the periodic hour for waking, and does not fall asleep again). Itching in folds of skin, Sul. (Sel. has also "tingling in spots"). Chronic enlargement of liver, Sul. Loss of appetite in morning, Sul. (Sul. has increase of thirst ; Sel. has not. Sel. has white tongue ; Sul. has not). Emaciation, Nat. m., Chi. Debility from loss of fluids, Chi. Twitching of face, Tell. Bores fingers in nose, Cin., Ar. t. Throbbing after meals, Nat. c. < From tea, Thuj., Fer. Pain in back with emissions, Cob. Fatigue, Pic. ac. Sun effects, Sol. Larynx, Nat. sel.

Causation.—Alcohol. Tea. Sugar. Salt. Lemonade. Debauchery. Walking. Exertion. Masturbation. Loss of fluids.

SYMPTOMS.

1. **Mind.**—Reveries of a religious and melancholy character.—Great loquacity ; fond of conversing ; esp. in evening.—Excessive forgetfulness, esp. in matters of business.—Great forgetfulness when awake, with distinct recollection during half sleep.—A kind of stammering ; he uses syllables of words in wrong connections, therefore pronounces some words incorrectly.—Difficult comprehension.—Absolute incapacity to execute any business whatever.—Mental labour fatigues him.—Dread of society.

2. **Head.**—The head becomes affected by intellectual labour.—Vertigo : on lifting head, rising from a seat ; raising himself in bed ; moving about ; with nausea, vomiting, faintness ; < (an hour) after breakfast and dinner.—Headache every afternoon.—Headache after drinking lemonade, wine, or tea.—Violent attacks of lancinating pains in head above (l.) eye, with desire to lie down, sensibility in exterior of head, copious emission of urine, anorexia, and melancholy, excited by walking (in the sun) and by strong smells.—Headache of drunkards ; headache after debauchery.—Falling off of the hair when combing it ; also of eyebrows, whiskers, and genitals, with tingling-itching on scalp in evening, oozing after scratching, and with tension and sensation of contraction of scalp, with emaciation of face and hands.—Pain in scalp, as if hair were pulled out.

3. **Eyes.**—Pains deep in orbits.—Spasmodic twitching of l. eyeball.—Itching vesicles on eyebrows and margins of lids.—Falling off of eyebrows.

4. **Ears.**—Ear stopped.—Hardening of wax in (l.) deaf ear.

5. **Nose.**—Itching in nose, in nostrils, and on margins of alæ nasi.—Tendency to bore fingers into nose.—Complete obstruction of nose (chronic).

—Coryza ending in diarrhœa.—Fluent coryza in evening.—Yellow, thick, gelatinous mucus in nose.

6. **Face.**—Greasy, shining skin of face.—Twitching in muscles of face. —Great emaciation of face and hands.—Upper lip cracked.—Comedones.

7. **Teeth.**—Toothache which compels use of toothpick till the blood comes.—Boring in molars.—Teeth covered with mucus.—Toothache from tea.—The teeth become free of mucus, hard, and smooth, and crack when rubbed.—Toothache with feeling of coldness, > taking cold water and cold air into mouth.

8. **Mouth.**—Pain under root of tongue.—Tongue loaded with a thick white coating in morning.—Stammering speech; articulates with great difficulty.

9. **Throat.**—Dryness in throat.—Hawking of lumps of transparent mucus every morning.

10. **Appetite.**—Sweetish, disagreeable taste after smoking.—Anorexia in morning (with white-coated tongue).—Hunger at night.—Dislike to salt things. —Frequent desire for brandy.—Bad effects from: sugar; salt food; tea; lemonade.

11. **Stomach.**—Hiccough and risings after smoking before eating.—Inclination to vomit.—Feels very sick after sleep.—Cramp in stomach.—Pressure in stomach as if cramp would occur.

12. **Abdomen.**—Throbbing of the arteries in the whole body, esp. in abdomen after a meal.—Pain in the liver, esp. on taking an inspiration, extending to the renal region, with sensibility to external pressure.—Red itching, miliary eruption in the hepatic region.—Pains in r. side, around under last ribs, esp. on inspiration, extending to region of kidneys.—Violent shootings in spleen when walking.

13. **Stool and Anus.**—Constipation.—Hard evacuations, followed by a discharge of mucus or of blood when passing the last portion of it; stool so hard and impacted that it has to be removed by mechanical aid.—Stools exceedingly difficult and threaten to tear anus from their immense size; hours spent in effort; stool can be seen through distended anus as an immense, dark, hard ball; sufferings great, patient becomes wonderfully agitated.—Somewhat liquid fæces, with tenesmus.—Filaments, like hairs, in fæces.

14. **Urinary Organs.**—Urine: scanty and red in evening; red sediment, like coarse sand.—Involuntary dribbling of urine when walking.—Dribbling of urine after micturition and after stool.—Sensation in tip of urethra, as if a biting drop were forcing its way out.

15. **Male Sexual Organs.**—Tickling and itching in genitals, esp. in scrotum.—Impotence; with lascivious ideas.—Pollutions, with flaccidity of penis.—Discharge of semen, drop by drop, during sleep.—Lascivious dreams with emissions which waken him, followed by lameness and weakness in small of back.—Flow of prostatic fluid during evacuation and at other times. —Thin and scentless semen.—During coition, feeble erection, too prompt emission, and long-continued voluptuous thrill.—Priapism, glans drawn up. —Gonorrhœa (secondary); gleet.—Debility (weakness in loins) and peevishness after coition.

16. **Female Sexual Organs.**—Menses copious and dark.—Menses delayed about eight days.

17. **Respiratory Organs.**—Hoarseness on beginning to sing (or from singing; talking or long reading; voice hoarse and husky).—Hawking up of mucus and of small clots of blood.—Cough in morning, which fatigues whole chest, with expectoration of blood and small globules of mucus.—Difficulty of breathing when walking in open air.—Frequent efforts to breathe deeply, like sighing.—Respiration obstructed at night, when lying down, by pains in chest, side, and loins.

20. **Neck and Back.**—Cramp in neck.—Pain through l. side of neck and down back of l. leg.—Pain in glands l. side of neck.—Rigidity of muscles of neck and nape, which hinders head being turned.—Hard swelling on back.—Paralytic pain in small of back, > lying on abdomen.—Sensation of paralysis in loins.—Pain as from lameness in small of back in morning.

21. **Limbs.**—Pains in all the limbs, as if caused by a chill.

22. **Upper Limbs.**—Miliaria in forearm.—Tearing in hands at night, with cracking in wrists.—Itching at wrist, in palms; itching vesicles on and between fingers.—Dry, scaly eruption on palms, with itching, having syphilitic base.—Painful hang-nails.—Scabious pimples on hand.—Emaciation of hands.

23. **Lower Limbs.**—Itching pimples on buttocks and thighs, near the scrotum.—Emaciation of legs.—Cramps in calves and soles.—Legs feel weak, with fear of paralysis after typhus.—The knees crack when they are bent (at night).—Flat ulcers on (lower) legs.—Itching in feet, esp. round ankles, in evening.—Blisters on toes.

24. **Generalities.**—[Escape of seminal fluids, particularly when straining at stool, which condition may be accompanied with headache, sleeplessness, weakness, and troubles in general; complaints after stool; impotence of the male; spermatorrhœa; weakness of the sexual powers; nocturnal pollutions.—Deep respiration.—Itch where the pustule comes between the fingers; foul exanthema.—Perspires too easily; on single parts; on forepart of body.—< While drinking tea; after stool; while, or after talking; can't bear to have the hair touched; walking in the open air.—H. N. G.].—< After sleep, esp. on hot days, from lemonade, wine; from very salt food; in the sun.—Excessive emaciation, esp. of face, hands, and legs (thighs).—*Cinchona* produces extraordinary sufferings, and < those which are already in existence to an insupportable degree.—Throbbing in vessels of whole body, esp. felt in abdomen.—Strong inclination to lie down and to sleep, esp. during heat of day.—Symptoms < after sleep.—Inability to bear a draught of air.—Every draught of air, even warm, = pain in limbs, head, &c.

25. **Skin.**—Frequent tingling in circumscribed parts of skin, with great provocation to scratch.—Miliary eruption.—Red rash on region of liver.—Prolonged oozing from parts which have been scratched.—Flat ulcers.—Itching in folds of skin, between fingers and about joints, esp. ankle joint.—Hair falls off head, whiskers, and other parts.

26. **Sleep.**—Disposition to sleep early in evening, with imperfect sleep and frequent waking during night.—Retarded sleep in evening.—Jerks in body when going to sleep.—Light sleep at night, and waking with least noise.—Waking early in morning, and always at same hour.—Sleepless before midnight.—Symptoms < after a siesta; on hot days.—Dreams of quarrels and unnatural cruelty.

27. **Fever.**—Pulse very little accelerated.—Burning heat, extending over

considerable portions of the skin (chest, abdomen, loins, and ribs).—Constant alternation of heat and cold.—Perspiration from least exertion.—Perspiration as soon as he sleeps, day or night.—Tendency to profuse perspiration when walking, or during an afternoon sleep.—Perspiration (on chest, genitals, and under axillæ) which leaves yellow or white spots on linen and stiffens it.—External heat, with burning in skin, and only in single spots.

Sempervivum Tectorum.

Sempervivum tectorum. Houseleek. *N. O.* Crassulaceæ. Tincture of fresh leaves.

Clinical.—Climaxis. Menses, suppressed. Tongue, indurations of.

Characteristics.—Kallenbach (*H. R.*, x. 473) gives some experience with *Semp. t.* In *Hufeland's Journal*, says Kallenbach, "the fresh juice is recommended in chronic aphthæ in grown persons in causal relation to hæmorrhoids, as well as in scirrhous indurations of the tongue." In many countries *Semp.* has a popular reputation for indurations and sores on the tongue. Reichel, of Staben, considers it curative in spasms of the uterus and in menstrual disturbances of all kinds, as well as in cases of too exalted vascular activity in the sexual sphere; also in aural troubles consequent on hardened ear-wax and in inflammatory exudations of the ear. Kallenbach was consulted—(1) By Mrs. S., 44, childless, of sickly looks, for an affection of the tongue. For the previous six months menses had appeared only every eight to ten weeks, and were accompanied with pains darting from small of back to uterus and vulva. During the six months she had stitching pain on right rim of tongue about $\frac{3}{4}$ inch from the point, at which place, after a few weeks, a swelling formed, the size of a small bean, which bled at times, and at night caused a burning sensation as of a small coal, disturbing sleep. Sour food = pain. The swelling is not hard on the surface, but contains two hard nodules, of size of lentils, one of which is denuded and bleeds on touch. Three enlarged veins cross the swelling and enter the tongue muscle behind it. After over a month of treatment with *Aur.*, *Ars.*, *Carb. v.*, in vain, Kallenbach moistened the swelling with the fresh juice of *Semp.* thrice a day. Within three days it was smaller and folds appeared, the enlarged veins were contracted, formed thin, tense vessels crossing the swelling and seemingly tying it. During the next three days the patient applied the juice too energetically, and Kallenbach found the surroundings in inflammatory irritation and very sensitive. The application was stopped, and *Semp.* 2x given internally. After a week's use the swelling had shrivelled to one-third, and ten days later *the menses, which had ceased altogether, reappeared, and continued very profusely for five days.* The swelling shrivelled to the size of a small pea, was firmer, harder, devoid of sensation, and gave no further trouble. The menses continued regular. (2) Mrs. X., 27, mother of a six months' old healthy boy, formerly frequently afflicted with swelling of the glands, very sensitive to homœopathic remedies, complained of a pain under her tongue of ten days' duration, interfering with eating and speaking. There was a bluish red elevation on under side of tongue of size of split bean, hard, and along both sides there were enlarged veins. On one side a denuded spot exuded a whitish albuminous matter which could easily be wiped off: *Semp.* 6, one powder every forty-eight hours. On the second day the swelling was less sensitive, and in a week much smaller. Then *the menses reappeared* (first time since confinement), and in three weeks the whole swelling was gone, leaving only in its place a somewhat engorged vein. Kallenbach treated with applications of 1 x a General v. B. who had nodules on left rim of his tongue with swollen veins, the nodules disappeared, and the sensitiveness was removed, and the patient was so well that he refused to stay for the completion of the cure, and failed to report. My own experience with *Semp.* was in domestic practice. For some childish affection of the eyes in my own case, rags moistened with "Houseleek and cream" (about equal parts of the juice and fresh cream) were applied, and my recollection of it is that the application was exceedingly pleasant.

Senecio Aureus.

Senecio aureus (Variety, Gracilis). Golden Ragwort. Squaw-weed. (United States, North and West; found in swamps.) *N. O.* Compositæ. Tincture of fresh plant in flower.

Clinical.—Amenorrhœa. Ascites. Coryza. Cough. Dropsy. Dysmenorrhœa. Dysuria. Epistaxis. Fainting. Gleet. Gonorrhœa. Hæmorrhages. Home-sickness. Hysteria. Kidneys, inflammation of. Lumbago. Mania. Menorrhagia. *Menstruation, delayed*; early, and profuse; obstructed; vicarious. Nails, brittle. Nervousness. Neurasthenia. Phthisis. Prostatitis. Puerperal mania. Renal colic. Sciatica. Spermatic cord, pain in. Wounds.

Characteristics.—The Golden Ragwort had a reputation in domestic and eclectic practice as a regulator of menstrual functions when Hale introduced it into homœopathic practice. A. E. Small and others proved it, and clinical additions have filled out the picture. Like many other Compositæ, the Ragworts, or Groundsels, have power over hæmorrhagic conditions, whether arising from disease or from wounds. The hæmorrhagic function of menstruation comes particularly under the influence of *Senec.* A very definite relation has been traced between the nose and the female sexual organs, and *Senec.* is indicated when epistaxis or nasal catarrh takes the place of menses when suppressed from any cause. The menses may be profuse and early, or they may be retarded or absent. *Senec.* may be required in a great variety of conditions traceable to non-appearing menses. C. M. Foss (*A. H.*, xxii. 12) reports the case of Miss L., 18, who had seen no period for fifteen months. She was chlorotic, had a dry, hacking cough, with frequent pulse, made still more frequent by any excitement; headache, poor sleep, constipation. The abdomen had been gradually enlarging for six months, and tapping had been decided upon when *Senec.* 1 x was given. All symptoms rapidly cleared up, and the menses returned within a short time. *Senec.* 1 x also cured a girl, 21, who had suppression of urine in addition to chlorosis, ascites, and suppressed menses (*M. A.*, xxiii. 77). S. H. Talcott (quoted *A. M.*, xxiv. 188) reports an important case bearing on the same point. Mrs. X., 26, mother of two children. Before confinement the patient was haunted with the idea that her child would be stillborn. Nine days after its birth, strong and healthy, she was admitted to hospital in a state of violent acute mania, which continued, with high temperature, for three months. With great physical activity, the mental state was that of a wild, violent, and almost uncontrollable person. There was severe pain in the head, great nervous irritability and sleeplessness and hysterical erethism. These symptoms, coupled with the fact (now first ascertained) that the lochia had ceased suddenly after confinement, and the menses had not come on, led to the choice of *Senec.*, which was given in drop doses of the 3x every two hours. Steady improvement resulted, and after a few weeks the patient was allowed out on parole. A relapse followed, and *Bell.* did no good. *Senec.* was again given with good effect, and complete recovery took place. Talcott regards *Senec.* as midway between the pugilistic state of *Bell.* and the tearful state of *Puls.* He remarks that recovery from puerperal mania seldom occurs unless menstruation is re-established. Hale notes that the country people call *Senec.* "Wild Valerian," and use it for nervousness, hysteria, low spirits, sleeplessness, especially in women; and he refers to this "globus" symptom of the pathogenesis: "About the middle of the afternoon, sensation as if a ball was in the stomach, rising up into the throat, lasting for about an hour; sensation of tightness in the throat, with a disposition to attempt to relieve it by swallowing. Talcott's case becomes more significant in the light of Cooper's observation of the brain action of *Sen. jacobæa*. Small, who proved *Senec.*, records this case: Woman, 30, had been ill six weeks, the symptoms steadily increasing till the following picture was presented: Face bloated, abdomen enlarged, feet œdematous; urine alternately profuse and watery, or dark and scanty; frequent desire to urinate day and night. *Senec.* φ, gtt. x, three times a day, cured quickly. Small remarks that he has found *Senec.* useful in the dysuria of women and children when evidently of catarrhal origin; and in dysuria with uterine displacement. Mucous sediment in the urine is an indication. But the benefits of *Senec.* are not confined to the female sex. Small relates this case: Man, 50, nervo-sanguine, subject of renal inflammation affecting right kidney generally, causing intense pain, febrile disturbance, prostration. On one occasion the pain was particularly intense, and the bladder seemed implicated. Every time he passed water he cried out in agony. Urine reddish; very hot and acrid. Bowels constipated. Dull headache; mouth and throat dry; chilly, fever, and perspiration. *Senec.* φ, gtt. xx, in half a tumbler of water; a dessertspoonful every hour. There was relief from the first dose, and the pain soon subsided entirely, leaving the patient freed from recurrence of the attacks. *Senec.* has caused: "Dull, heavy pain in left spermatic cord, moving along cord to testicle. Prostatic gland enlarged, feels hard and swelled to touch. Lascivious dreams, with pollutions." Hale says he has found *Senec.* useful in advanced stages of gonorrhœa, and in prostatic disorders. Hale reports the following case of dysmenorrhœa : Mrs. X., mother of one child, had had an abortion three years before, and another (at the second month of pregnancy) four months before Hale saw her. Since the last abortion she had suffered from painful menstruation, which had not been the case previously. Menses every three weeks, profuse, lasting eight or nine days, accompanied by much cutting pain in sacrum, hypogastrium, and groins. Pale, weak, nervous ; slight cough, generally at night. *Senec.* φ, gtt. v, was given three times a day till the next period, which came on at the twenty-ninth day, and was perfectly normal in quantity and without pain. *Senec.* has a place in coughs and even in phthisis. "It is especially serviceable in mucous coughs," says Hale. "In chronic coughs, catarrhal affections, hæmoptysis, incipient phthisis attended with troublesome cough, *the result of obstructed menstruation*," it has a well-established reputation. *Peculiar Sensations* of *Senec.* are : As of a wave from occiput to sinciput. As if he would pitch forward. As of a ball rising from stomach to throat. Respiration as if greatly fatigued. Pains are radiating, shifting, lancinating. Symptoms alternate. *Senec.* is specially *Suited to :* women and little girls of nervous temperament. Lyman Watkins (quoted *H. W.*, xxxiv. 300) says, "Females taking *Senec.* generally improve in health and strength, accumulate flesh, become light-hearted and cheerful. This may be due to some tonic influence." The symptoms are < at night (cough ; sweat ; sleeplessness ; frequent micturition). < In afternoon (general). < In open air. Very sensitive to open air ; tendency to catarrhs. Colic is > bending forward ; and > by stool. > At onset of menses. < Sitting ; must keep moving about (mind).

Relations.—*Compare :* Botanical, Sen. jac., Arn., Calend., Bels. Uterine, chest, and bladder symptoms, Puls., Helon. Vicarious menstruation, Bry. (Senec. especially bloody expectoration). Homesickness, Caps., Ph. ac. < 4 p.m., Lyc. Prostatitis and gonorrhœa, Sabal ser., Solidag., Puls., Pip. n., Cop., Thuj. Nervousness, Coff., Cham., Val., Ambr. Fidgety feet, Caust., Zn.

Causation.—Venesection. Suppressed menstruation. Wounds.

SYMPTOMS.

1. **Mind.**—Very irritable, worried, undecided ; dissatisfied ; depressed, nervous ; < sitting still ; must move about.—Low spirits alternating with cheerful mood ; sleepless ; sensation of a ball rising from stomach to throat.—Inability to fix mind on one subject for any length of time.—A feeling like homesickness.—(Puerperal mania, wild, violent ; with high temperature, nervousness, sleeplessness, suddenly suppressed lochia, non-appearance of menses.)

2. **Head.**—Dizzy feeling while walking in open air, like a wave from occiput to sinciput ; he feels as if he would pitch forward ; nausea.—Dull,

stupefying headache, with fulness of head, as from catarrh.—Sharp lancinating in l. temple, upper part of l. eye and inside of l. lower jaw.—Dull occipital pain in morning.—Dull frontal pain extending to occiput.—Sharp shooting pains from within outward in forehead ; sharp shooting pains over and in eyes ; catarrh ; suppressed secretion.—Headache preceding leucorrhœa and irritation of bladder.—Forehead hot ; sweaty in evening.

3. **Eyes.**—Dark rings round eyes.—Sharp pains from within outward, l. eye ; lachrymation in open air.—Catarrhal ophthalmia from suppressed secretions.—Eyes and lids burn.—Yellow streak from inner canthus to iris.

5. **Nose.**—Coryza, at first dull headache, dryness of nose and sneezing, burning and fulness in nostrils, later secretion of copious mucus.—Coryza with nose-bleed.

6. **Face.**—Face pale, depressed appearance ; weary, wants to lie down. —Lancinating pain r. side of face, r. shoulder, l. breast.—Lips pale ; dry, feverish.

7. **Teeth.**—Teeth tender and sensitive ; gums pale, dry, feverish.

8. **Mouth.**—Tongue slightly coated ; catarrhal fever.—Mouth and fauces dry, hot.

9. **Throat.**—Throat and nose feel very dry ; later, tightness in throat, wants to swallow.—Fauces dry ; later, mucus fills throat.

10. **Appetite.**—Aversion to all food, esp. sweets and coffee (she is usually very fond of both).—Faint before meals (not hunger).—Full after eating very little.

11. **Stomach.**—Eructations of sour gas and ingesta.—Nausea on rising ; morning sickness of pregnancy.—Nausea from renal derangements.—Stitches in epigastrium.

12. **Abdomen.**—Stitches in hypochondria ; sharp cutting in diaphragm. —Pains about navel, spreading thence in all directions ; > by stool ; griping pains > bending forward.—Rumbling of wind.—Catarrh of bowels, rumbling and watery stools.—Abdomen much enlarged and very tense ; lower limbs œdematous ; urine scanty, high-coloured, not more than eight ounces a day ; pain in lumbar region and in ovaries ; constipation ; cervix uteri congested ; albuminous leucorrhœa ; sense of weight in uterine region (ascites).—About noon, before dinner, stitches running from one part to another in both inguinal regions, lower jaw, shoulders, &c.—Smarting pain in l. groin.

13. **Stool and Rectum.**—Stool thin, watery, bloody ; with tenesmus and colic ; catarrhal dysentery ; evening.—Stool copious with great debility and prostration ; flatulence ; morning.—Stool in hard lumps mixed with yellow mucus.

14. **Urinary Organs.**—Slight pain in region of kidneys.—Attacks of renal inflammation, attacking particularly r. kidney, causing intense pain, fever, and great prostration.—Severe renal inflammation with fever, chilliness, and pain in lumbar region, particularly in l. kidney ; quantity of urine below normal ; urine red, depositing a brickdust sediment ; considerable arterial excitement ; skin hot and dry ; motion caused him to cry out with pain ; constipation.—Intense pain over r. kidney, severe pain during urination, urine red, hot, acrid ; bowels constipated.—Renal dropsy.—Inflammation of kidneys and ureters after passage of gravel.—Tenesmus of bladder ; smarting in urethra, dropsy.—Hæmaturia ; renal pain with nausea.—Tenesmus of

adder, with heat and urging.—Irritation of bladder in children, preceded ' heat and headache.—Renal colic with or without nausea.—Chronic flammation of neck of bladder with bloody urine and tenesmus of bladder. Chronic inflammation of kidneys.—Dysuria: of women and children, idently of catarrhal origin; mucous sediment in urine; with uterine splacement.—Smarting in fossa navicularis before urination.

15. **Male Sexual Organs.**—Lascivious dreams, emissions.—Prostate and enlarged, feels hard and swollen to touch.—Dull, heavy pain in sper-atic cord, moving along cord to testicle.—Gonorrhœa, gleet.—Chronic ostatitis.

16. **Female Sexual Organs.**—Awakened early by great sexual irrita-on, vagina full of mucus, labia swollen; itching and burning exasperates.—rgasm in afternoon after feeling of irritation, and again after sleep.—Aching both ovarian regions, knees, and ankles, and down front of thighs.—Profuse ow of mucus from vagina.—Menses two days early, very scant, less pain an usual, followed by excessive thirst and thin leucorrhœa streaked with ood, and with dull pelvic pains.—Menses every three weeks, very profuse, sting eight or nine days, accompanied by severe cutting pains in region of crum, hypogastrium, and groins; she was pale, weak, and nervous, and had slight cough, generally at night; after an abortion.—Menses premature and ofuse or retarded and scanty.—Dysmenorrhœa with urinary symptoms; itting in sacral and hypogastric regions; flow scanty or profuse or irregular; ile, weak, anæmic; strumous; hacking cough at night.—Amenorrhœa: om a cold; nervous irritability; lassitude, dropsy; wandering pains in back id shoulders; sensation of a ball rising from stomach into throat; costive; young girls with dropsical conditions.—Symptoms as if menses would pear, but they fail; nervous, excitable, sleepless; loss of appetite.—Sup-ession of menses from a cold; after venesection.—Menstrual irregularities consumptive patients.—Itching of vulva, feels sore and chafed; begins hen sitting still, > when mind employed.—Leucorrhœa: preceded by adache, sleeplessness and irritable bladder; in little girls; preceded by adache and sleeplessness.—Chlorosis in scrofulous girls, with dropsy.

17. **Respiratory Organs.**—Hawking of tough white mucus.—Respira-on as if greatly fatigued.—Laboured breathing from mucous accumulation. -Hacking night cough.—Mucous rattling with suppressed cough.—Palliated ough and bloody sputa in a woman far gone with consumption, and brought ack menses, which were absent four months.—Cough with bloody expec-ration.

18. **Chest.**—Catarrh of lungs; loose cough and copious mucous expec-ration.—Hæmoptysis; great emaciation; dry, hacking cough; hectic flush; eeplessness.—Hæmoptysis after venesection or suppressed menstruation.—hthisis with obstructed menstruation; bloody or copious mucous sputa.—harp pain through either lung.—Hot flashes of pain through lungs in orning.—Compression about chest.

20. **Back.**—Pain in back and loins; when sitting long or when lying own.—Sharp, lancinating pains in lumbar region.—Severe pain in small of ack in morning.—Cutting pains in region of sacrum, hypogastrium, and oins, with too early or too profuse menses; she is pale, weak, and nervous, id has a slight cough at night.—Wandering pains in back and shoulders; ain in joints.

21. **Limbs.**—Sharp stitches here and there ; rheumatic pains in joints. Skin dry and nails very brittle.

22. **Upper Limbs.**—Occasionally during the day sharp, lancinati pain in r. shoulder, l. heel, and in r. side of face. -Sharp, sticking pain in shoulder.—Hot pains through arms.—Hands cold and clammy; trembli from nervousness.

23. **Lower Limbs.**—Lower limbs weary.—About 4 p.m. sharp pain neighbourhood of sciatic nerve, shooting down thigh.—Constant desire keep feet in motion.—Feet cold.

24. **Generalities.**—Nervousness, sleeplessness, and hysterical mood.- Lassitude and nervousness.—Tired all morning.—Hysteria.—Wants to down ; pale.—Slight exertion = fainting.—Stitches in different parts of bod

25. **Skin.**—Skin dry, nails brittle.

26. **Sleep.**—Great sleeplessness, with vivid, unpleasant dreams.—Slee lessness of women suffering from uterine irritation, prolapsus, and its atten ant nervousness (it is the *Coffea* of women) ; during climacteric period.— night sleepless, nervous, hysterical ; by day drowsy, languid.—Dreams most of an intellectual character ; memory very active.—Sleep unrefreshing.

27. **Fever.**—Chilly forenoon as after taking cold ; followed by heat an sweat in evening with moderate thirst.—Chilliness followed by urging urinate.—Copious warm sweat towards morning ; catarrh.—Hectic fever.- Heat of forehead.—Hot flushes day and night.—Sweat of forehead.—Dispos tion to perspire.

Senecio Jacobœa.

Senecio jacobœa. St. James' Wort. Staggerwort. Ragwort. *N. C* Compositæ. Tincture of fresh plant.

Clinical.—Brain, affections of. Cerebro-spinal irritation. Depression. Enuresi Headache. Twitchings.

Characteristics.—Cooper has published (*H. W.*, xxxv. 154 observations with *Sen. jac.*, the common Ragwort, which, with it yellow flowers, is such a conspicuous feature of English roadsides and commons throughout the summer months. Cooper (1) gave a lady 57 (who had slight otorrhœa of left ear with deafness on that side), single dose of *Sen. jac.* φ. Immediately after, she began to fee depressed in mind and body ; it seemed as if her brain woul not work, for she talked incoherently. The bowels began acting in gushes, and a bladder weakness was aggravated, so that there wa enuresis night and day for three days. (2) Another woman from a single dose of the same had "exhaustion in the back of the head." (3) A lady, 51, had had depression all her life, coming in fits "Memory and everything goes," cannot talk coherently to herself and dislikes conversation in others. On July 1, 1900, she wrote "Have suffered agony from awful feeling of torpor of brain, which has made it an effort to put words together, memory seemed to go, felt altogether insensible ; bowels have been confined." One dose of

Sen. jac. ϕ was given, and removed the depression and relieved all the other symptoms ; it also produced this : Constant rigidity of muscles, chiefly of neck and shoulders, < at night ; it seems like a habit, "and I try to relax them but find it most difficult ; it seems to run back involuntarily, so that the weight of the head is somehow held in this way, and though touching the pillow does not rest on it. Sometimes in the day the upper part of the legs gets a sort of ague fit of shaking." On this Cooper remarks : " The exhaustion felt after a dose of *Sen. jac.* in the back of the head in case 2, and the cropping up as a new symptom of this strange-looking rigidity of the muscles of the neck, at night chiefly, together with the shaking of the legs in the daytime, points to inco-ordinate muscular action due to deranged cerebral control." Cooper adds this case : A man, 68, many years apoplectically inclined, had constant twitchings at night with vascular deafness of right ear, loss of memory, pressure and heat of head : after a dose of *Sen. jac.* ϕ he remained comfortable for three months and hearing improved. *Sen. jac.* has been used like *Sen. aur.* in cases of menstrual irregularity. Gerarde mentions " green wounds and old filthy ulcers " as benefited by it, also " old aches and pains in the arms, hips, and legs."

SYMPTOMS.

1. **Mind.**—Depressed in body and mind ; it seemed as if her brain would not work, for she talks incoherently.

2. **Head.**—Exhaustion felt in back of head ; after this felt lighter and better.

13. **Stool.**—Bowels (before fairly regular) began acting in gushes, large stools occasionally, but in no way regular.

14. **Urinary Organs.**—The bladder, which had been rather weak, became more so, the enuresis continuing day and night for several days.

20. **Back.**—Constant rigidity of muscles, chiefly of neck and shoulders, esp. at night ; seems like a habit, but finds it most difficult to relax them ; it seems to return involuntarily, so that the weight of the head is somehow held in this way, and though touching the pillow does not rest on it.

23. **Lower Limbs.**—Sometimes in the day the upper part of the legs gets a sort of ague fit of shaking.

Senega.

Polygala senega. Seneca Snake-root. *N. O.* Polygalaceæ. Tincture of powdered dried root.

Clinical.—Amblyopia. Ascites. Asthma. *Bladder, irritable;* catarrh of. Blepharitis ciliaris. *Bronchitis.* Constipation. Cornea, opacity of. *Cough.* Enuresis. Facial paralysis. Hay-fever. Hydrothorax. Hypopion. Influenza. Iritis. Œsophagus, stricture of ; catarrh of. Phthisis mucosa. Pleurisy. Pneumonia. Snake-bites. Sneezing : fits of ; at end of cough. Styes. Throat, sore. Whooping-cough.

Characteristics.—*Senega* was introduced to medical practice by Dr. Tennant, of Virginia, who was led to test its properties through hearing that the Indians used it as an antidote to snake-bites. As it relieved the symptoms of snake venom, Tennant concluded that it might also relieve dyspnœa, cough, and hæmoptysis arising from other causes, and gave it with success in cases of pneumonia, pleurisy, and hydrothorax (Teste). Other old-school practitioners used it as an expectorant in chronic respiratory catarrh, acute phthisis, rheumatic fever, dropsies, incipient cataract, croup. It is at present regarded as "a stimulant, diaphoretic, and expectorant, especially in chronic bronchitis." It is in affections of the chest, eyes, and bladder that homœopaths have found it of most service, and the extensive provings have supplied excellent data for prescribing. Teste (who includes *Seneg.* with *Phos. ac.*, *Cham.* and *Canth.* in his *Conium* group) considers it specially suited to "females of slender and tall make, thin, but having retained a good deal of sprightliness and moral power." He cites this case in which it gave great relief: Lady, 45, had contusion, pressive, sometimes cramping, very old pains in chest, anterior wall of which was sensitive to contact (on both sides); pains at times <, at times > in open air; respiratory mucus at apices feeble, without rhoncus; dyspnœa when walking, and especially when going up stairs; paroxysms of vesicular agitation in chest as if she would faint; catarrhal cough, not very frequent, with ropy, not very profuse expectoration; spitting of red blood now and then; paroxysms of palpitations, during which the rhythm of the heart changed to an almost imperceptible tremor, and which, in some instances, lasted all night, and even longer; menses regular; the palpitation generally took place after the period or in consequence of some moral emotion. This patient was apparently of the type Teste mentions, and the case shows that the correspondence of type must not be too closely considered, for other observers, including myself, have found *Seneg.* more *suited to* plethoric, phlegmatic persons; persons tending to obesity; fat persons of lax fibre; fat, chubby children; and old persons. *Senega* is one of the sources of *Saponin*. It has a nauseous taste, and leaves a scraping sensation in the throat. Guernsey outlines its action thus: "Where there is a great burning in the chest, either before or after coughing; profuse secretion of mucus. Dryness of inner parts which are usually moist; dry skin. General affections of the windpipe; left side of chest particularly; right eye; lower eyelids." Nash (who has only obtained success with low attenuations of *Seneg.*) has cured many cases of "cough with great accumulation of mucus, which seems to fill the chest, with much rattling, wheezing, and difficult breathing." It is especially valuable, he says, with old people, but works well with others. I have used *Seneg.* only in the 30th, and have found it answer to its indications exceedingly well. In the case of a very stout elderly lady, of phthisical family history, who had pneumonia of both bases, especially right, very violent paroxysmal cough, with ropy, difficult expectoration tinged with blood, *Seneg.* 30 quickly relieved a very dangerous condition when other remedies had failed. Leading indications for *Seneg.* in chest cases are: (1) Great accumulation of clear albuminous mucus, which is difficult to expel. (2) Great soreness of walls of chest. (3) Pressure on chest as though lungs were forced back to spine. Whooping-cough in fat, chubby children, clear mucus like white of egg, difficult to raise, cough < towards evening. The soreness of the chest walls makes *Seneg.* appropriate to cases of pleurodynia. There is hoarseness, and the throat is so dry and sensitive it hurts the patient to talk. Cough often ends in sneezing. Clinton Enos (quoted *A. H.*, xxiv. 253) relates this case : A very fat girl, æt. 10, with cold, damp feet and hands and sweating about the head, had spells of sneezing for two years, ever since whooping-cough. Several spells a day lasting about half an hour. Sharp pains in chest and temples during the attacks. In nose a large quantity of mucus with stuffed-up feeling. One dose of *Seneg.* 200 removed the whole trouble in a week. A. R. Macmichael (*N. A. J. H.*, xl. 824) cured Mrs. B., 40, of acute catarrhal laryngitis which had lasted ten days with *Seneg.* 1. There was hoarseness ; hawking of thick, tenacious mucus (profuse, a quart in twenty-four hours) from larynx, especially in morning, with burning sensation. Relief set in within three hours from first dose. *Seneg.* acts on the eyes even more powerfully than on the nose, producing pains, inflammation both of the exterior and interior of the eye and lids, and much disorder of vision. The eye troubles are < when looking intently at an object ; and another modality brought out in the proving has taken the rank of a keynote : > Bending head backwards. The symptom in which it was first noticed was this : "When walking towards the setting sun he seemed to see another smaller sun hover below the other, assuming a somewhat oval shape when looking down, *disappearing on bending the head backwards*, and on closing the eyes." The prover took from 40 to 60 drops of the tincture. "< Bending head forward" and "< stooping" are scarcely less characteristic. Eye symptoms as an accompaniment of head symptoms indicate *Seneg.* : "Violent rush of blood to head when stooping, especially to eyeballs, where a painful pressure is experienced." Extreme tenderness is another note of *Seneg.* : "A sort of aching pain in head, in sinciput, and occiput, not < by pressure ; < sitting in warm room ; accompanied with pressure in eyes, *which did not bear touch.*" Pressure ; dulness ; heaviness are the leading head sensations. There is painful sensitiveness of hearing. The digestive organs are disordered. *Seneg.* has been used as an emetic. The urinary organs are very prominently affected, irritability and catarrh being the leading effects. There is frequent urging, scalding in urethra before or after micturition, and the urine is loaded with mucous threads. *Peculiar Sensations* of *Seneg.* are : Eyes, as if they were pressed out ; as if eyeballs were being expanded ; as if soap in eyes. As if red pepper throughout nostrils and air passages. As if chest too narrow. Dyspnœa as from stagnation in lungs. As if lungs pushed back to spine. As if chest would burst. Wrist as if sprained. Joints as if lame. *Seneg.* has the gnawing hunger and empty feeling well marked. It is predominantly left-sided in its action. The symptoms are < by touch and pressure (but pressure on left side >). < Rubbing. Most symptoms < rest ; > walking in open air. Rest > dry cough. Lying down = tickling in larynx ; fear of suffocation. Lying on right side = pain in chest. Motion = pain under sternum. Motion of arms = soreness of walls of chest. < Going up stairs.

Stepping hard, walking fast, or running = pain through mediastinum; piercing pain between scapulæ. > Bending head back. < Stooping; bending forward. < Morning; and night. Whooping cough < towards evening. < In warm air; in warm room. Lachrymation, sore chest. Cough and chilliness < in open or cold air. Sweat >. < Looking intently at an object.

Relations.—*Antidoted by:* Bry.; also Arn., Bell., Camph. *Followed well by:* Calc., Pho., Lyc., Sul. *Compare:* Saponin (a derivative of Senega root). In bronchial affections, Ammon. Fat, plethoric people disposed to catarrhs, Calc. Muscular asthenopia, loss of voice, paralysis (facial, &c.), Caust. Laryngeal and pulmonary catarrh, Pho. Bronchial catarrh, Spo. Whooping-cough, Coc. c., K. bi. (Seneg. clear phlegm, cough < towards evening; Coc. c. clear phlegm < morning; K. bi. yellow phlegm < morning). Pleurodynia, pleurisy, Bry. Mucous phthisis, Stn.

Causation.—Bites, poisonous. Sprains.

SYMPTOMS.

1. **Mind.**—Hypochondriacal melancholy, with great readiness to take offence.—Excessive anguish, often with accelerated and hasty respiration.—Liveliness, with irritability, and disposition to give way to paroxysms of rage and fury.

2. **Head.**—Head bewildered, with dizziness.—Feeling of confusion and emptiness in head, with aching of eyes (or pressure in them < by touch), and obscuration of sight.—Vertigo, with noise in ears.—Headache which also affects the eyes, is < by heat of a room, and > in open air, or in a cold temperature.—Pressive pain in forehead and orbits after dinner, esp. l. side of head, > in open air.—Drawing in sinciput and temples, extending to face.—Sanguineous congestion in head and eyes when stooping.—Pulsative cephalalgia, with aching of the eyes.—Shuddering and itching in scalp.—Eruption on head.

3. **Eyes.**—Pain in eyes as if dilated and pushed out of orbits.—Aching of eyes in evening, esp. by candle-light and when stooping.—Congestion of blood in eyes when stooping.—Burning sensation in eyes when reading and writing (in evening).—Swelling of lids, with burning pressure and tingling.—Vesicles on tarsal edges.—Styes.—Dryness of eyes.—Lachrymation in open air, and when gazing intently at an object.—Accumulation of hardened dry humour on lids and lashes in morning.—Jerking and spasmodic drawing in lids; in r. outer canthus.—Convulsive contraction of lower lids.—Fixedness of look.—Oculo-motor paralysis.—Opacity of cornea.—Double vision > by bending head backward.—When walking towards the setting sun he seemed to see another smaller sun hover below the other, assuming a somewhat oval shape when looking down, disappearing on bending the head backwards and on closing the eyes.—Sensitiveness of eyes to light.—Confusion of the letters and dazzling of sight when reading.—Weakness of sight and flickering before the eyes when reading; must wipe them often.—All objects appear as if in the shade.—Obscuration of sight, with glistening before eyes, < from rubbing them.—Brilliant spots before sight.—Photophobia.

4. **Ears.**—Aching in ears during mastication.—A cooling sensation equently extends through l. ear.—Painful acuteness of hearing.

5. **Nose.**—Itching in the interior of the nose.—Smell of pus, or as of a ıalignant ulcer, in nose.—Sneezing so often and so violently head grows izzy; followed by thin coryza; with pain as of excoriation in chest.—roublesome dryness of Schneiderian membrane.

6. **Face.**—Sensation as if muscles of (l. half of) face were paralysed.—Ieat in face.—Burning vesicles in commissures of lips, on upper lip (and in orners of mouth).

7. **Teeth.**—The teeth are set on edge.—Digging in the teeth during ıspiration (of damp and cold air).

8. **Mouth.**—Dryness of the mouth, esp. in the morning.—Copious ecretion of saliva.—Putrid breath.—Tongue: yellowish white or slimy in ıorning, with slimy, unpleasant taste; loaded with a white coating.—Burning ensation in throat, mouth, tongue and palate.

9. **Throat.**—Sore throat, as if it were excoriated and raw.—Scraping, urning sensation and dryness in throat, with irritation, which provokes oughing and embarrassed speech.—Accumulation of tough mucus in throat, hich it is difficult to hawk up.—Sensation of constriction in the gullet.—ritation and roughness in œsophagus; burning sensation as if abraded; ·llowed by copious discharge of mucus.—Inflammatory swelling of palate, roat, and uvula.—Copious accumulation of viscid mucus in throat and ılate, which is detached in small clots.

10. **Appetite.**—Impaired taste.—Metallic taste in mouth, or taste of ine.—Clammy taste in mouth.—Anorexia, esp. in morning.—Gnawing ınger, with sensation of emptiness in stomach.—Violent, burning thirst.

11. **Stomach.**—Risings.—Eructations; which > the mucus and hawk-g of mucus from the stomach.—Loathing and nausea, with inclination to ›mit, which seems to proceed from the stomach, with retching.—Vomiting, ith diarrhœa and great anguish.—Spasms (colic) in stomach, with pressive ıin, also at night.—Pressure below pit of stomach.—Burning sensation in omach.—Sensation of emptiness in stomach.

12. **Abdomen.**—Boring and digging pains in abdomen, esp. in epigas-ium and hypochondria.—Gnawing in (upper) abdomen.—Burning and ueezing (oppression) in epigastrium during an inspiration.—Drawing etween the integuments of the abdomen, as by a foreign body.—Flatulent fections, with a sensation of a general bearing down towards hypogastrium.

13. **Stool and Anus.**—Slow, hard, and scanty evacuation, with effort, ıd followed by pressure in anus and rectum.—Frequent, loose evacuations consistence of pap.—Diarrhœa, with vomiting and great anxiety.—Watery ools spirting from anus.

14. **Urinary Organs.**—Diminished secretion of urine.—Increased ·cretion of urine.—Wetting the bed at night.—Urine frothy, or mixed with ımy filaments, and becoming turbid and cloudy when it cools (or deposits a ick sediment, yellowish red, with upper stratum yellow and flocculent).—eddish sediment, with flakes of mucus in urine.—Sensation of an obstruction urethra when urinating.—Shootings and burning sensation in urethra after d during the emission of urine.—Urging and scalding before and after icturition.—Irritability of bladder; subacute and chronic catarrh.

15. Male Sexual Organs.—Increased sexual desire, with painful erc tions.—Slight burning in glans when urinating.—Paroxysmal cramp-like pa in region of glans.—Tickling of prepuce and glans.

16. Female Sexual Organs.—Menses too soon ; has to press her side at tenth rib to relieve gnawing pain.—Slimy leucorrhœa.

17. Respiratory Organs.—Great dryness of the larynx, esp. in mor ing and forenoon.—Sudden hoarseness when reading aloud.—Hoarseness a roughness in throat.—Hacking cough from irritation in larynx.—Tickling a burning sensation in larynx, esp. when lying down, with danger of suffocatic —Abundant accumulation of mucus in larynx and trachea, with short respi tion.—Tearing and stinging in larynx and trachea.—Dry and shaking coug excited by a tickling in larynx, < in open air (and from walking fast). Expectoration of transparent and yellow mucus when coughing.—Coug with profuse expectoration of viscid mucus.—Shaking cough, like whoopin cough, from burning and tickling in larynx in morning, with copious expe toration of tough, white mucus (like white of egg).—The cough is < evening and at night, during rest, in warm room, when sitting, when lying the (l.) side.

18. Chest.—Dyspnœa, with sensation of stagnation in lungs.—Shortn of breath when walking quickly and going up stairs.—Troublesome oppr sion of chest, esp. in open air and on stooping, as if thorax too narrow. Pressure in chest, esp. during repose, and in morning, or at night, on wakin —Great sensibility in interior coats of chest when touched.—Squeezing a spasmodic pains in chest, with agitation and anxiety, esp. when lying on si —Certain movements cause pain, as if chest were too tight ; disposed expand the chest ; this leaves soreness.—Burning, sore pain under sternu esp. during motion and on deep inspiration.—Orgasms of blood ; oppressi with flushes of heat ; oppression, esp. during rest.—Shootings in chest, es when coughing and taking an inspiration.—Burning, aching, and stitches l. half of chest ; < lying on r. side.—Pleurisy r. side of chest with thickenin —Pain as from excoriation in chest, < by external pressure, moveme coughing, and sneezing.—Soreness of walls of chest on moving arms, esp. —Great soreness in walls of chest and great accumulation of clear albumino mucus which is difficult to expectorate ; pressure on chest as if lungs we pushed back to spine.—Accumulation of mucus in chest, larynx, and trach —Phthisis mucosa : hydrothorax.—Profuse secretion of mucus in lungs old people.—Drawing and burning sensation in the chest.—Tingling in t chest.—Violent congestion of blood in chest, with pulsation and ebullitic leading even to syncope.—The majority of symptoms are most viole during repose, but do not obstruct respiration.

19. Heart.—Aching, burning pain in chest becomes seated in region heart, whence it radiates to l. axilla.—Aching and pressure in heart regio during deep inspiration.—Violent shaking palpitation of heart.

20. Back.—Aching and drawing in back and shoulder-blades, as well between and under shoulder-blades.—Pain under r. shoulder-blade, as chest should burst, when coughing or drawing a long breath.—Burni sensation and subcutaneous itching over whole back.

22. Upper Limbs.—Paralytic drawing in forearms as far as fingers. Anxious starting and jerking in upper arm during siesta.—Pain as if sprain in wrists.—Sticking, crawling, prickling in palms.

23. **Lower Limbs.**—Sensation of excessive lassitude in legs, and of paralysis in joints.—Wrenching pain in hip-joint.—Trembling in legs.—Great weakness of feet, esp. in forenoon.

24. **Generalities.**—Where there is great burning in chest, either before or after coughing; profuse secretion of mucus.—Dryness of inner parts which are usually moist: dry skin.—Diseases of mucous membranes.—Dropsy of internal organs (esp. after inflammation).—Inflammation of internal organs.—General affections of windpipe; l. side of chest particularly; r. eye; lower eyelids; < from looking fixedly at any object for a long time.—Sensation of great general lassitude, with trembling, esp. in lower limbs.—Great moral and physical depression, with stretching of limbs, heaviness, emptiness, and throbbing in head.—Great weakness, which seems to proceed from the chest.—Fainting, when walking in open air.—Several symptoms, esp. those of chest, are < by repose, and > by walking in open air.

25. **Skin.**—Bites of poisonous animals or animals when in a state of rage.

26. **Sleep.**—Great disposition to sleep in evening, and deep, lethargic sleep soon after going to bed.—Sleep, towards morning, disturbed by affections of chest, or else by cramps in stomach.—In the morning one frequently wakens from dyspnœa.

27. **Fever.**—Pulse hard and frequent.—Frequent shivering, proceeding from lassitude in limbs.—Shuddering in back, with heat in face, burning sensation in the eyes, dyspnœa, shootings in the chest, and throbbings in the head.—Chilliness and chill almost only in the open air, with weakness in legs and dyspnœa.—Shudders over the back, with heat in face and chest symptoms.—Sudden flushes of heat.—Skin becomes warmer and moister.—Feeling of warmth in l. half of face.—Profuse perspiration commenced and the disagreeable symptoms were quite removed.—Profuse diaphoresis.—Perspiration wanting.

Senna.

The leaflets of several species of Cassia: C. obovata, Alexandrian Senna, is the principal. *N. O.* Leguminosæ. Trituration or tincture of the dried leaves.

Clinical.—Colic; flatulent, of infants. Exhaustion. Nitrogenous waste. Sleeplessness. Sneezing, with heat.

Characteristics.—Used as a laxative in ordinary practice, *Senna* has proved an excellent remedy in the colic of infants, with incarcerated flatulence and sleeplessness. Infantile colic when the patient seems full of wind. The symptoms of the Schema are mostly derived from overdosings. A peculiar symptom is: "Repeated sneezing, which caused heat (especially of hands), exhaustion, and panting breathing." Exhaustion is typical of *Senna*. Farrington says it is one of the best remedies in the materia medica for "simple exhaustion with excess of nitrogenous waste." The exhaustion is exemplified in the sinking immediately after meals. The pods caused a nasty unclean smell from the body of a woman taking them for constipation (R. T. C.).

Relations.—*Compare:* Infantile colic and sleeplessness, Jal. Exhaustion, K. ca. Sinking after meals, Ars., Cin., Lyc., Sil., Stp., Ur. nit., Calc., Iod., Sep., Tab.

SYMPTOMS.

2. **Head.**—Heaviness of the head when stooping, as if it were pressed down.

5. **Nose.**—Repeated sneezing, which caused heat (esp. of hands), exhaustion, and panting breathing.

6. **Face.**—Livid lips.—Commissuræ of lips covered with small burning vesicles.

11. **Stomach.**—Anorexia.—Thirst.—Empty, or watery and fetid, risings. —Loathing and nausea, with inclination to vomit.—Sinking immediately after meals.

12. **Abdomen.**—Colic, esp. in little children.—Painful colic from incarcerated flatulence (particularly in young children).—Sensation of coldness in the abdomen, with emptiness and uneasiness in the stomach.—Accumulation of flatus, with grumbling and fermentation in the abdomen, and discharge of fetid flatus.

13. **Stool and Anus.**—Two liquid stools with griping pains.—Loose evacuation, with tenesmus, and followed by a burning sensation in the anus. —Diarrhœa with straining and prolapsed rectum and sore anus (cured in children.—R. T. C.).

24. **Generalities.**—Universal swelling.—Exhaustion.—Unclean body swell.

26. **Sleep.**—Ebullition of blood, esp. at night, disturbing the sleep.—Sleeplessness, with cries and tossing, esp. in the case of infants.

27. **Fever.**—Heat (esp. of hands).

Sepia.

Sepia officinalis. Cuttle Fish. *N. O.* Cephalopoda. Trituration of dried liquid contained in the ink-bag. [I have found a preparation made from the *fresh* ink-bag, given to me by Dr. Swallow, of Ningpo, in every way superior to the official preparation, which I now rarely use. The provings and recorded cures were, however, made with the dried ink preparations.]

Clinical.—Alcohol, effects of. Amenorrhœa. Anus, pressure of. Apoplexy. *Appetite, depraved.* Ascarides. Baldness. Bladder, irritable. *Cancer. Change of life.* Chloasma. Chorea. Condylomata. Cystitis. *Dandriff.* Dysmenorrhœa. Dyspepsia. *Eczema.* Epistaxis. *Eyes, affections of. Face, yellow. Freckles.* Gleet. Gonorrhœa. Gravel. Herpes; circinatus. Hysteria. *Irritation.* Jaundice. *Leucorrhœa. Liver-spots. Liver, torpid. Menstruation, disordered. Mind, affections of. Nails, pains under.* Neuralgia. Nose, inflamed; swollen. Ozæna. Phimosis. *Pityriasis versicolor.* Pleurisy. *Pregnancy, disorders of;* vomiting of.

Pruritus. Psoriasis. Ptosis. Pylorus, induration of. Quinsy. Rectum, cancer of; fissure of. Ringworm. Sacrum, pain in. Sciatica. Seborrhœa. Smell, sense of, too acute; disordered. Spermatorrhœa. Stye. *Toothache. Urine, incontinence of. Uterus, bearing down in.* Varicose veins. Warts. Whooping-cough.

Characteristics.—The present use of *Sepia* in medicine is due to Hahnemann. Some among the ancient physicians (Dioscorides, Plinius, and Marcellus, says Teste) used either the flesh, the eggs, or even the only bone which constitutes the skeleton of this animal, for "leucorrhœa, gonorrhœa, catarrh of the bladder, gravel, spasms of the bladder, baldness, freckles and certain kinds of tetters"—which is sufficiently remarkable in the light of the provings. *Sep.* is one of the remedies of the *Chronic Diseases*, and was proved by Goullon, von Gersdorff, Gross, Hartlaub, and Wahle. *Sep.* is predominantly, but by no means exclusively, a woman's remedy. It affects the generative organs of both sexes, and a large number of the symptoms occurring in other organs have some relation thereto. Teste describes the *type* to where *Sep.* is *suited* as follows: Young people of both sexes, or, rather, persons between pubescence and the critical period of life; of delicate constitutions, with pure white skins, or skins having a rosy tinge; blonde or red hair; nervous or lymphatico-nervous temperaments; exceedingly excitable and anxious for emotions; and, lastly, particularly such as are disposed to sexual excitement, or have been exhausted by sexual excesses. Hering gives these *types:* (1) Persons of dark hair, rigid fibre, but mild and easy disposition. (2) Women during pregnancy, in child-bed and while nursing. (3) Children who take cold readily when the weather changes. (4) Scrofulous persons. (5) Men who have been addicted to drinking and sexual excesses. (6) Pot-bellied mothers, yellow saddle across nose, irritable, faint from least exertion, leuco-phlegmatic constitutions. Bähr gives: "Sanguine, excitable temperaments inclined to congestions." Farrington adds that the *Sep.* patient is sensitive to all impressions, and that the dark hair is not by any means a necessity. He gives a more complete description: Puffed, flabby persons (less frequently emaciated) with yellow or dirty yellow brown blotched skin; inclined to sweat, especially about genitals, axillæ, and back; hot flushes; headache in morning; awaken stiff and tired; subject to disease of sexual organs; the general attitude is never one of strength and healthful ease, but of lax connective tissue, languor, easily produced paresis. *Sep.* acts on the vital forces as well as on organic tissues. The sphincters are weakened and all non-striated muscles. *Sep.* disturbs the circulation, causing flushes and other irregularities—throbbings all over; hands hot and feet cold, or *vice versâ.* The flushes run upward and end in sweat with faint, weak feeling. Epistaxis may occur either from a blow, from being in a warm room, or from suppressed menses. The upward direction of the *Sep.* symptoms is one of its keynotes. The pains of the head shoot upward; and so do the pains in anus, rectum, and vagina. Also coldness as well as the flushes travels from below up. On the other hand night-sweat proceeds from above downward. The head pains proceed from within out. *Sep.* is one of the remedies which have the "ball" sensation in inner parts. There is vertigo with sensation of something "rolling round" in the head. There is sensation of a ball in inner parts generally; but the most notable one is sensation of a ball in rectum. It may be described as an apple or a potato, and it is not relieved by stool. I have cured both constipation and diarrhœa when that symptom was present. The upward stitches in rectum and vagina, when present, are equally good indications for *Sep.* in cases of hæmorrhoids, prolapse of rectum, and for prolapse or induration of uterus and cervix. As with *Murex* the chief incidence of *Sep.* is on the female sexual organs, though with *Sep.* the menses are generally scanty, as with *Murex* they are the reverse. *Sep.* causes engorgement of the uterus going on to induration. There is either prolapse or retroversion. Yellowish green leucorrhœa somewhat offensive. The bearing-down pains of *Sep.* are of great intensity. They are felt in abdomen and back; and sometimes even seem to interfere with breathing. The bearing down is < standing or walking. The bearing down extends into thighs. There is a constant sense of pressing into vagina, which compels the patient to cross the limbs to prevent prolapse. Connected with the uterine symptoms are: hysteria, erethism, palpitation, orgasm of blood, faintness. The sensation of "goneness" and emptiness, which is one of the characteristics of *Sep.*, is sometimes connected with the pelvic bearing down. The empty sensation is felt in the epigastrium and throughout the abdomen. It is analogous to the great relaxing effect of *Sep.* on connective tissues. This sinking is common in pregnancy; and *Sep.* corresponds to many of the troublesome affections of the pregnant state, as—"morning sickness, vomiting of food and bile in morning; of milky fluid; strains so that blood comes up." "The thought of food sickens her; with sense of great weight in anus." Tendency to abortion is met by *Sep.*; Hering is reported to have said: "All women prone to abortion should take *Sep.* and *Zinc.*" But *Sep.* meets many cases of dyspepsia not originating in uterine disorders. It has cured dyspepsia from injury by overlifting. Portal stasis is part of the *Sep.* action. There is fulness, soreness, and stitches in liver region; as well as stitches in left hypochondrium. The whole urinary tract is irritated, and catarrh of bladder and urethra may be set up. There is frequent strong urging to urinate. Stitches along the urethra. The relaxed sphincters of *Sep.* favour enuresis, and the type which it cures is well defined: "The bed is wet almost as soon as the child goes to sleep, always during the first sleep." It meets the enuresis of light-complexioned boys and onanists. In cases of irritable bladder, although the desire is urgent, the discharge of urine may be difficult, and the patient may have to wait a long time. Gonorrhœa after the acute stage has subsided. Gleet and gonorrhœal warts have been cured with it. Hering gives, "condylomata completely surrounding head of penis." I have cured a crop of small velvety warts completely encircling the mouth of the prepuce. *Thuja* had failed in the case. In reference to warts, I cured with *Sep.* 3x trit. a large horn-like wart on the abdomen of a woman. It was as large as a crown-piece but shaped like a bean, and raised a quarter of an inch from the surface. The skin symptoms of *Sep.* are among its most characteristic features. The skin is delicate, the least injury tends to ulceration. Itching which often changes to burning when scratched. Soreness of skin, humid places on bends of knees. Chloasma. Painful eruption on tip of nose. Herpetic eruption on lips and about mouth. Ringworm-like eruptions every spring on different parts of body. Ringworm on face. Herpes circinatus. Roundness and yellowness of the spots. The nettle-rash of *Sep.* appears on going into open air. It is > in warm room. The itching of *Sep.* may be desperate, especially when it affects the genitals and anus. The action of *Sep.* on connective tissues is again exemplified in the selection of the finger-joints as a seat of ulceration. The sweat is pungent in odour, offensive in axillæ and soles of feet, causing soreness. The skin and the eyes are near akin, and *Sep.* causes all kinds of inflammation of eyes and lids, with impaired vision, black spots, green halo, fiery redness. The eye-symptoms are < by rubbing; < pressing lids together; < morning and evening; > bathing in cold water. *Sep.* is a chilly remedy from lack of vital heat, "chills so easily"; this is especially the case in chronic diseases. *Sep.* is often required in chronic nasal catarrh. Nash had a case in which the discharge was thick, bland, and copious. *Puls.* relieved the catarrh but increased the menstrual flow too much. *Sep.* cured both. *Sep.* is also useful where colds inflame the tonsils and tend to cause suppuration. The characteristic sensations in the throat are: Dryness; pressure as if neck-cloth too tight; plug sensation; stinging; stitching pains on swallowing; contraction of throat without swallowing; sensation of plug when swallowing with feeling of constriction. There are some peculiarities about the mental state of *Sep.* which must be borne in mind: (1) Anxiety: with fear, flushes of heat over face and head; about real or imaginary evils; towards evening. (2) Great sadness and weeping; dread of being alone, of men, of meeting friends; with uterine troubles. (3) Indifferent: even to one's family; one's occupation; to one's nearest and dearest. (4) Greedy, miserly. (5) Indolent. The *Sep.* patient weeps when asked about her symptoms. She is very sensitive, and must not be found fault with. "Faints easily" is a note of the *Sep.* weakness: after getting wet; from extremes of heat and cold; riding in a carriage; kneeling at church. Lorbacher (quoted *H. M.*, xxxi. 142) refers to three important indications for *Sep.* not generally known: (1) Prodromal symptoms of apoplexy; (2) whooping-cough that drags on interminably; (3) hypostatic pleuritis. The symptoms of *Sep.* corresponding to the first are: Stiffness of back of neck; staggering vertigo (< exercising in open air); anxiousness and a feeling of fear of severe sickness; intermitting heart beats; torpor and sleepiness. Lorbacher gives this case: A thick-set farmer, 50, inclined to hypochondriasis, troubled from time to time with piles, without being an habitual drinker was addicted to "nips," Gradually abdominal prominence developed; stiffness of neck; vertigo; occasional throbbing headache; slight transient loss of consciousness; anxiety; fear of apoplexy; *piles less pronounced and less frequently* troublesome than usual. Venesection, performed several times, only partially relieved. Abstinence from alcohol had no decided influence. *Sep.* 12x was given, four drops twice daily at first, then every other day, and later at increasing intervals. In two months the symptoms were reduced, and gradually passed away. The man lived eight years after this, and had no apoplexy, though he did not give up his "nips." *Sep.* is indicated in whooping-cough when it has lasted eight weeks or longer, and the paroxysms, though reduced in number and virulence, do not disappear, and occur especially before midnight. The patients are reduced in strength, dyspeptic, irritable, tearful, easily angered or apathetic. Kunkel reports (quoted *H. M.*, xxix. 670) this case of pulmonary affection : A boy, 14, had been under treatment five weeks for cough and hoarseness. Hoarseness < evening ; during the day cough with purulent sputa. Slept well but dreamed when he lay on left side. Emaciated. *Phos.* 10x produced little change. It was now ascertained that there was remarkable tightness of the chest on breathing, with inclination to take a deep breath ; this was > in open air, on motion, while at work ; < while in the house and at rest. Though the weather was bad he had constant desire to be out of doors. *Sep.* 10x made a rapid cure. Bœnninghausen recommended *Sep.* in cases of cough, either with or without expectoration, with bloody, blood-streaked, purulent, yellow greenish or stinking sputa, and especially in consumption. Nash mentions a case of cholera infantum which he cured with *Sep.* on the indication "always < after taking milk." In moisture oozing from the anus he compares it with *Ant. c.*, which has the first place. *Sep.*, says Bähr (i. 359), "affords considerable help in a certain condition of the system which we have so far only noticed in females. After the exacerbation of a chronic gastric catarrh has lasted a few days with intolerable burning pains, the renal region, more particularly the left side, becomes painful, a violent burning pain is felt in this region, and a quantity of saturated, highly-coloured urine is discharged, which deposits copious quantities of urates, or else a clear urine with copious sandy sediment, coated with uric acid. After the discharge the pains generally abate, and only return if the stomach has not been restored to its normal condition." *Peculiar Sensations* of *Sep.* are : As if every object were in motion. As if suspended in air. Vertigo as if intoxicated. As if brain crushed. As if head would burst. As if waves of pain rolling up and beating against frontal bone. As if something rolling around in head, with vertigo. Stitches as from needles in head. As if roots of hair were sore ; as if cut short near roots. As if eyes would fall out. As of a weight over eyes. As if eyes were gone and a cool wind blew out of sockets. Eyes as if bruised. As if a grain of sand in eye. As if lids too heavy to open. Eyes as if balls of fire. As if lids too tight and did not cover eyeballs. Hollow molar tooth as if swollen and elongated. Gums, as if burned ; as if beginning to suppurate. Tongue and cavity of mouth as if scalded. As of plug in throat. Throat as if raw. As if something twisting in stomach and rising to throat. As if viscera turning inside out. As if stomach sore internally. As if something remained lodged in stomach. As if stomach were being scraped. As if a strap as wide as her hand drawn tightly round her waist. Liver as if bursting. As if everything in abdomen turning around. As of a load in abdomen. As if intestines were drawn into a lump. As of something adherent in abdomen. As of something alive in abdomen. Weight or ball in anus. As if bladder full and contents would fall out over pubes. As if drops came out of bladder. As if bladder and urinary organs would be pressed out. As of everything would issue through vulva. As if everything would fall out of uterus. Uterus as if clutched. As if vulva enlarged. As if something heavy would force itself from vagina. As from a weight in sides. As if ribs were broken and sharp points were sticking in flesh. As if cough came from stomach and abdomen. Chest as if hollow; as if sore. Throat as if filled with phlegm. As if breasts were enlarged. As if heart stood still. Back as if she could not turn or raise herself, or as if she had been in a wrong position, almost as if parts had gone to sleep. Sudden pain in back as if struck by a hammer. Pain in back as from subcutaneous ulceration. As if something were going to break in back. As if limbs would refuse to act. As if shoulder dislocated. Feet as if asleep. Right hip-joint as if bruised. Lower limbs as if beaten. As of a mouse running in lower limbs. As if bones of legs were decaying. As if she could feel every muscle and fibre of her right side from shoulder to feet. As of a ball in inner parts. As of an icy hand between scapulæ. As if she would suffocate. As if feet stood in cold water up to ankles. As of hot water poured over one. "Stiffness" is a prominent feature of *Sep.*: stiffness of limbs < after sleep; stiffness of uterine region. A peculiar symptom of *Sep.* is: "Involuntary jerking of head backward and forward, especially forenoons when sitting." This may occur in hysteria. Open fontanelles in children is an indication for *Sep.* The symptoms are < by touch (except pain in back, which is > by touch). Pressure >. (Pressing eyelids together <.) Binding head tightly >. Loosening clothes >. Rubbing; and scratching <. < Jar; mis-step; slightest blow; overlifting. Many symptoms are both < and > by rest and motion. < Moving arms. Lying on side, and on right side >. Lying on left side <. Lying on back <. Sitting < many symptoms. Faint sitting erect or kneeling. (< Kneeling is characteristic.) Sitting with legs crossed >. Stooping <. Standing <. Hard motion > headache. A short walk fatigues much. Going upstairs <. Dancing and running = no shortness of breath. < Mental labour. < From sexual excesses. < Afternoon and evening. ("Dyspnœa in evening" is characteristic.) < From cold air or during east wind. < In sultry, moist weather. < Before a thunderstorm. < By laundry work. (*Sep.* is the "washerwoman's remedy."—H. C. Allen.) Stormy weather = suffocating feeling. < After sleep (stiffness of legs). < On falling to sleep or in first sleep. > In open air. (Also—warmth of natural bodily heat; very sensitive to cold air.) Cold water > eyes and teeth. > Warmth of bed or hot applications. Cough < in church. < During and immediately after eating. Milk, fat food, acids <. While eating pulsation in pit of stomach, the more he eats the < it becomes. Empty feeling ceases at supper. < From coitus. I have confirmed the experience of Dr. Swallow, who found the fresh preparation of *Sep.* (which I prescribe as *Sep. fr.*) to possess a wider range than the ordinary preparation and to act as an "organ remedy" in a great variety of uterine affections not definitely indicated by the pathogenesis. I have used it in attenuations from the 5th to 30th.]

Relations.—*Antidoted by*. Smelling Nit. sp. d., by Vegetable acids, Aco., Ant. c., Ant. t., Rhus. *It antidotes:* Calc., Chi., Merc., Nat. m., Nat. ph., Pho., Sars., Sul. *Incompatible:* Lach. (but in one case in which *Lach.* in very high potency had caused intensely distressing rectal tenesmus with alternate inversion and eversion of the anus, *Sep.* high proved to be the antidote). *Complementary:* Nat. m. (the cuttle-fish is a *salt-water* animal), Nat. c., and other *Natrum* salts ; Sul. *Followed well by:* Nit. ac. *Compare:* Vesicular eruptions and ulcers about joints, Brx., Mez. Psoriasis, Ars., Ars. i. Chloasma, Lyc., Nux, Sul., Curar. Ringworm, Bac., Calc., Tell. Sadness, Caust., Puls. Mild, easy disposition, Puls. Weeps when asked about her symptoms (Puls., weeps when telling her symptoms). Diseases with sudden prostration and sinking faintness, Murex, Nux m. Washerwoman's remedy, Pho. (Pho., headache after washing). Pains extend from other parts to back (Sabi. the reverse). Pains with shuddering (Puls., with chilliness). Lack of vital heat, especially in chronic diseases (*Led.* in acute diseases). Coldness of vertex with headache, Ver. (heat of vertex, Calc., Graph., Sul.). Indifferent to his occupation, Fl. ac., Ph. ac. Greedy, miserly, Lyc. Must loosen neckband, Lach. Sensation of ball in inner parts, Lach. Herpes circinatus in isolated spots (Tell. in intersecting rings). Empty feeling > eating, Chel., Pho. Constipation during pregnancy, Alm. Pain in rectum long after stool, Nit. ac., Sul. Urine so offensive must be removed from room (Indium, horribly offensive after standing). Bed wet almost as soon as child goes to sleep, Kre. Old-standing gleet, K. iod. Bearing down as if everything would protrude from pelvis, Agar., Bell., Lil. t., Murex, Sanic. Sight or thought of food sickens, Nux. Smell of cooking food nauseates, Ars., Colch. Itching turns to burning by scratching, Sul. Spine pain < sitting than walking, Cob., Zn., Puls., Can. i. Indurated uterus ; vaginismus, Plat. Bearing down, Bell. (Bell. < lying down, Sep. > ; Bell. > standing, Sep. <). Cannot expectorate, Caust., Dros., K. ca., Arn. Spurting of urine with cough, Caust., Nat. m., Fer. Eczema of backs of hands, Nat. c. Prolapsus uteri, Nux. (Sep. follows when Nux ceases to act). Ptosis, Gels. (Gels., sluggish mind ; suffused red face). Urticaria < in open air, Rx. c. Urticaria, Ast. fl., Nat. m., Apis, Chloral., Urtica. Eye affections of tea-drinkers, Thuj. Dyspepsia with thick urine, Lyc. Indurated uterus, melancholy, Aur. Bearing down, sadness, K. fcy. Bearing down, congestion, aching distress, prolapse, Ust., Sec., Vib. o., Vib. t., Inula., Hedeo, Ziz. Uncontrollable fits of laughter, Croc., Ign. Terrible sadness during menses, Lyc., Nat. m, Nit. ac. (Nat. m. is < or > 10 a.m.) Irritable during menses (Nux, Cham., Mg. m. before and during ; *Lyc.* before). < Kneeling, Coccul., Mg. c. Anxious about health, Calc., Pho. Ozæna, clinkers, Pul., Syph., Pso. *Fetid* urine, Calc. (Benz. ac. and Nit. ac., *strong*). Burning, shooting, stitching pains in cervix, Murex. Hot, burning eructations, Pet., K. ca., Hep. Delay in passing water, Ars. (ineffectual desire, Nux). Fear of ghosts, Pho., Pul. Phimosis, Can. s., Merc., Sul., Nit. ac., Thuj. With exhausted feeling in bowels after stool, Plat. Movements of head, Lyc. < From

›itus ; remedy for women, relaxation of tissue, K. ca. As if struck › a hammer in the back (Naj. in nape). Tongue and mouth as if alded, Sang. Turning round in abdomen, Nit. ac. (as if machinery orking in abdomen). Pain as of subcutaneous ulceration, Puls., an. b. Badly healing skin, Hep. Eyes > bathing in cold water, sar. Sensitiveness, Asar. Apoplexy, Ast. r. (a sea animal). < From ilk, Homar. (a sea animal). Chest, Pho.

Causation.—Anger and vexation. Blows. Falls. Jar. Injury. verlifting (dyspepsia). Snowy air. Tobacco (neuralgia). Laundry ork. Wetting. Alcohol. Milk, boiled (diarrhœa). Fat Pork.

SYMPTOMS.

1. **Mind.**—Sadness and dejection, with tears.—Melancholy and morose- ss.—Anguish and inquietude, sometimes with flushes of heat, generally in ening (when walking in open air), and sometimes in bed.—Restlessness, lgety.—Dread of being alone.—Excessively nervous ; sensitive to least ise.—Great uneasiness respecting the health ; and about her domestic affairs. Pensiveness.—Timorous disposition.—Discouragement, often to such an tent as to be disgusted with life.—Indifference to everything (to all sur- undings), even to relations.—Repugnance to customary business.—Great sturbance caused by vexation.—Great excitability in company.—Suscep- oility and peevishness, with great irascibility.—Quarrelsome and caustic sposition.—Weakness of memory.—Distraction.—Aptness to make mistakes speaking and writing.—Unfitness for intellectual labour.—Slowness of con- ption.—Comprehension difficult ; heavy flow of ideas.—Language coming owly.

2. **Head.**—Confusion of the head, which disables him from performing y mental labour.—Fits of vertigo, esp. when walking in open air, or when riting, or even on least movement of arms.—Vertigo, during which all jects appear to be in motion, or with sensation as of something rolling round head.—Vertigo in morning, on rising, or in afternoon.—Sensation of cold- ss on vertex ; < from moving head and stooping, > when at rest and in the en air.—Fits of headache, with nausea, vomiting, and shooting or boring ins, which extort cries.—Headache every morning.—Headache, which does t permit the eyes to be opened.—Headache, with excessive desire for ition.—Headache, on shaking or moving head, and also at every step, as if ain were shaken about.—Semilateral headache, sometimes in the evening, ter lying down, preceded by heaviness of head.—Paroxysms of hemicrania, nging pain as from within to without, in one side of head (mostly l.) with usea (and vomiting) and contraction of eye ; < in room and when walking st, > in open air and when lying on painful side.—Boring headache from thin to without, from forenoon till evening, < from motion and stooping, by rest, when closing the eyes, from external pressure, and sleep.—Heavi- ss of head.—Pressive cephalalgia above eyes, in the clear daylight ; as if the ad should burst and the eyes fall out, with nausea.—Expansive pressure in ad, sometimes when stooping, as if it were about to burst.—Contraction in ad.—Drawing and tearing in and on head, sometimes semilateral.—Lancin- ing cephalalgia, often semilateral or frontal.—Shooting pains, esp. over l.

eye, extorting cries.—Headache at menstrual nisus ; with scanty flow.—Hea
ache in terrific shocks.—Involuntary jerking of head backward and forwar
esp. in forenoon and when sitting.—Fontanelles remain open, with jerkin
of the head, pale, bloated face ; stomacace, green diarrhœic stools.—Perspir
tion on the head, smelling sour, with faintish weakness ; < in evening befo
going to sleep.—Rush of blood to the head.—Throbbing cephalalgia, esp. i
occiput (beginning in the morning, < in evening, from least motion, whe
turning eyes, when lying on back, < when closing eyes and when at rest).-
Violent congestion of blood in head, with heat, esp. when stooping.—Coldne
of exterior of head.—Disposition to take cold on head from dry, cold win
and if head gets wet.—Involuntary trembling, and shocks in head.—Mobili
of scalp.—Scalp and roots of hair very sensitive to touch.—Itching on hea
(nose and eyes).—Eruptions on vertex and back part of head, dry, offensiv
stinging, itching and tingling, with cracks, extending behind ears, feelir
sore when scratching them.—Swelling on one side of head above the templ
with itching ; sensation of coldness and tearing in it ; < when touching i
> when lying on it, or after rising from bed.—Humid scabs on the head.-
(Bald spots on scalp, porrigo decalvans.—R. T. C.)—Falling off of the hair.-
Small red pimples on forehead ; rough forehead. — Swelling of head, es
forehead.

3. **Eyes.**—Heaviness and depression of upper lids.—Pressure on ey
balls.—Itching and smarting in eyes and lids.—Pricking in eyes, by candl
light in evening.—Burning sensation in eyes, esp. in morning on waking.-
Inflammation of eyes, with redness of sclerotica, and shooting pains.—I
flammation, redness, and swelling of eyelids, with styes.—Pustules in tl
cornea.—Scabs in eyebrows.—Glassy, watery eyes, in evening.—Fung
hæmatodes in cornea.—Dry scabs on lids, esp. on waking in morning.-
Yellow colour of sclerotica.—Eyelids pain in morning when awaking as
too heavy, and as if he could not keep them open.—Eyelids red, swolle
styes on them.—Lachrymation, esp. in the morning or nocturnal agglutinati
of lids.—Quivering and jerking of lids.—Paralysis of the lids, and i
ability to open them, esp. at night (and evening).—Confused sight, wh
reading and writing.—Presbyopia.—Weakness of sight, as from amauros
with contracted pupils.—Appearances of a veil, black spots, points, spark
and streaks of lights, before eyes.—Intolerance of reflected light fro
bright objects.—Green reflection round candle in evening.—Great sensitiv
ness of eyes to daylight.—Sight vanishes during the menses, > on lyi
down.

4. **Ears.**—Otalgia.—Shootings in ears.—Stinging in the l. ear.—Pain
ear, as from excoriation.—Swelling, and purulent eruption, in external ear.-
Herpes on lobe of ear, behind the ear and on nape of neck.—Discharge
liquid pus from ear, with itching.—Hearing extremely sensitive, esp. to musi
—Hardness of hearing.—Sudden deafness, as if caused by a plug in ears.-
Buzzing and roaring before ears.

5. **Nose.**—Swelling and inflammation of nose, esp. at tip.—Scabs on t
of nose.—Scabby and ulcerated nostrils.—Hardened mucus in nose.-
Epistaxis, and discharge of blood, frequently, on blowing nose, after being
the slightest degree overheated, or when the nose has been struck by a
thing, even lightly.—Violent bleeding of nose, esp. during menses.—Anosmi

-Smelling too sensitive ; too feeble, yellow saddle across the bridge of nose. –Fetid smell in nose.—Ozæna ; blowing of large lumps of yellow green nucus or yellow green membranes, with blood, from the nose.—Dry coryza.— Dry coryza, esp. of l. nostril.—Dry mucus, which causes an obstruction in nose.—Violent fluent coryza, with sneezing, pain in occiput, and drawing in imbs.

6. **Face.**—Paleness and puffiness of face, with blue circles round the yes, which are red and dull.—Yellowness of face (and of the whites of eyes). —Face emaciated.—Yellow streak on nose, and cheeks, in form of a saddle.— Violent heat in face.—Pale bloatedness of face.—Erysipelatous inflammation, and swelling of one side of face (arising from a carious tooth).—Inflammatory swelling of face, with yellow scurfy pimples, thickly grouped.—Herpes, scurf on face.—Warts on face.—Black pores on face.—Acne < before menses.— tching, and eruption on face and on forehead ; sometimes merely like redness and roughness of skin.—Skin swollen on forehead.—Tumours on the forehead.—Drawing facial pains.—Spasmodic pain and tearing in bones of face.—Neuralgic pains (l. side, from abuse of tobacco).—Dryness and exfoliation of lips.—Tension of lower lip.—Swelling of under lip.—Yellow colour and herpetic eruption round mouth.—Moist and scabious eruptions on the red part of lips, and on chin.—Painful ulcer on internal surface of lips.—Engorgement. and painful sensitiveness of submaxillary glands.

7. **Teeth.**—Toothache, on compressing or touching teeth, and on speaking, also from slightest current of cold air.—Nocturnal toothache, with extreme excitement.—Pulsative shooting, or drawing toothache, extending sometimes into ear (esp. after eating, drinking, or taking anything cold into mouth) or into arms and fingers.—Toothache during the menses.—Toothache ; stinging, pulsating, extending into ear during pregnancy, with shortness of breath, with swelled face and swelling of submaxillary glands, < from every cold draught of air, when touching teeth and when talking.—Toothache with violent ebullition of blood, and pulsation in whole body.—Tearing shocks in teeth.—Bluntness, looseness, easy bleeding, and caries of teeth.—Gums dark red.—Swelling, excoriation, ulceration, and easy bleeding of gums.

8. **Mouth.**—Fetid breath.—Swelling of interior of mouth.—Dryness of the mouth, lips and tongue.—Saline salivation.—Taste bitter, sour, slimy, foul, mostly in morning.—Pain in tongue and palate, as if they had been burnt.— Tip of tongue feels as if scalded.—Excoriation of tongue.—Vesicles on tongue. —Tongue loaded with a white coating.—Soreness of tip of tongue.

9. **Throat.**—Sore throat, with swelling of glands of neck.—Pressure, as from a plug in throat, or pain as from excoriation, and shootings during deglutition.—Pressure in throat in region of tonsils, as if neck-cloth were too tight.—Jerking in throat.—Swelling and inflammation of the gullet.—Inflammation, swelling, and suppuration of tonsils.—Dryness in throat, with tension and scraping.—Clammy sensation in throat.—Accumulation of mucus in throat, and on velum palati.—Roughness and burning in fauces ; < by hawking.—Hawking up of mucus, esp. in morning.—Expulsion of sanguineous mucus on hawking.

10. **Appetite.**—Putrid or sour taste.—Too salt taste of food.—Adipsia or excessive thirst, esp. in morning and in evening, sometimes with anorexia.— Great voracity.—Bulimy, with sensation of emptiness in stomach.—Eager

desire for wine; for vinegar.—Creates aversion to beer.—Repugnance and dislike to food, esp. to meat, and milk, which produces diarrhœa.—Tobacco smoke disagrees.—Disagreeable risings, with nausea, after eating fat food.—Weak digestion.—After a meal: acidity in mouth, frequent risings, scraping and burning sensation in throat, pulsation in scrobiculus, hiccough, inflation of abdomen, sweat, feverish heat, palpitation of heart, cephalalgia, nausea vomiting, pains in stomach, &c.

11. **Stomach.**—Sensation of emptiness in pit of stomach, just below ensiform cartilage; this is a very weak, "gone" feeling, which nothing can satisfy; this symptom may appear in any complication of troubles, in disordered menstruation, &c.—Frequent risings, generally sour or bitter, or else like rotten eggs, or with taste of food.—Painful risings, during which blood comes into mouth.—Acidity, with disgust to life.—Nausea, sometimes when fasting in morning, > by eating a little.—Nausea, with bitter taste and risings—Nausea from motion of a carriage.—Nausea and vomiting after a meal.—Vomiting of bile and of food (in morning, with headache).—Vomiting of bile and food during pregnancy; straining so hard that blood comes up.—Pains in stomach after a meal, sometimes in evening.—Violent pain in cardia, when food passes into stomach.—Pain in the scrobiculus while walking.—Pressure in stomach, as from a stone, esp. during or after a meal, or else at night.—Contractive spasm in stomach.—Waterbrash, esp. after drinking or eating, or preceded by a whirling sensation in stomach.—Vomiting of milky serum (in pregnant women).—Noctural vomiting, with headache.—Cramps in stomach and chest.—Tearing boring in cardiac region, extending to loins.—Cutting boring from stomach towards spine.—Pressive shootings in scrobiculus, and in region of the stomach.—Burning sensation in pit of stomach and scrobiculus.—Throbbing in pit of stomach.—Painful sensation of emptiness in stomach.

12. **Abdomen.**—Pains in the liver, when riding in a carriage.—Aching throbbing, and shooting in hepatic region.—Boring or tensive shootings in hypochondria, esp. during movement.—Shootings in l. hypochondrium.—Attacks of contractive pain in r. hypochrondrium.—Pain across hypochondrium at night on lying down, > from micturition.—Pain in abdomen, in bed in morning.—Pressure and heaviness in abdomen, with sensation of expansion as if it were about to burst.—Excessive distension of abdomen.—Heaviness and hardness in abdomen.—Hardness in pyloric region.—Soreness of abdomen in pregnant women.—Enlargement of abdomen (in women who have had children).—Dropsical swelling of abdomen.—Abdominal spasms, with a clawing pain, as if intestines were twisted.—Incisive colic, esp. after corporeal exercise, or at night, with desire to evacuate.—Digging, cuttings, and aching in the abdomen.—Pain, as from a bruise in intestines.—Coldness in abdomen—Burning sensation and shootings in abdomen, esp. in l. side, and sometimes extending into thigh.—Sensation of emptiness in abdomen.—Lancinations in groins.—Brownish spots on abdomen.—Movements and borborygmi in abdomen, esp. after a meal.—Excessive production and incarceration of flatus.

13. **Stool and Anus.**—Constipation during pregnancy.—Ineffectual want to evacuate, or only with emission of slime and flatus.—Slow, inefficient evacuations, like sheep dung.—Scanty evacuations, with straining and tenesmus.—Fæces too soft.—Difficult discharge even of soft stool.—Great

ifficulty in discharging stool, which seems to stick in anus or rectum as if a all or potato was there.—Difficult stool with sensation of weight in abdomen. -Gelatinous evacuations (small), with gripings (and tenesmus).—Debilitating iarrhœa.—Greenish diarrhœa, often of a putrid or sour smell, esp. in children. -Diarrhœa after boiled milk.—Whitish or brownish colour of stools.—Discharge of blood during the evacuation.—Contractive pain and tension, itching, ngling, burning, and shooting in anus and rectum.—Oozing from rectum.—limy discharge from rectum, with shooting and tearing pains.—Affections of nus and rectum where there are sharp, shooting, lancinating pains running up ito abdomen.—Prolapsus recti, esp. during an evacuation.—Weak feeling in ectum in bed.—Congestion of blood in anus.—Inactivity of the bowels.—rotrusion of hæmorrhoids from rectum (when walking; bleeding when alking).—Bleeding hæmorrhoids.—Excoriation between the buttocks.—ontractive pain in perinæum.—Ring of condylomata round anus.

14. **Urinary Organs.**—Frequent (and ineffectual) want to urinate (from ressure on bladder and tension in hypogastrium).—Aching in bladder.—eeling as if bladder were greatly distended.—Emission of urine at night (has rise frequently).—Involuntary discharge of urine at night, esp. in first sleep.—eep-coloured urine, red like blood.—Turbid urine, with red, sandy, or brick-loured sediment.—With white sediment and a cuticle on surface.—Profuse tid urine, with white sediment.—Urine with a sanguineous deposit.—ediment to the urine like clay, as if clay were burnt on the bottom of the ssel.—Urine very offensive; cannot be endured in room.—Cramp in adder, burning sensation in bladder and urethra.—Smarting in urethra, esp. hen urinating.—Incisive pains and shootings in urethra.—Discharge of ucus from the urethra, as in chronic gonorrhœa.

15. **Male Sexual Organs.**—Profuse perspiration of genitals, and esp. scrotum.—Itching round the genital organs.—Itching eruption on the glans id prepuce.—(Crop of small, velvety gonorrhœal warts round margin of epuce).—Pseudo-gonorrhœa of an acid salt smell.—Ulcers on glans and epuce.—Pains in the testes.—Cutting in testes.—Swelling of scrotum.—eakness of genital organs.—Increased sexual desire, with frequent erections ontinued erections at night).—Frequent pollutions.—Discharge of prostatic iid, after urinating, and during a difficult evacuation.—Intellectual, moral, d physical fatigue after coition, and pollutions.—In either sex, complaints om coition.

16. **Female Sexual Organs.**—Excoriation in vulva, and between ighs, sometimes before menses (soreness and redness of labia and perinæum) Great dryness of vulva and vagina, esp. after menses; painful to touch.—ternal and external heat in genitals.—Contractive pain in vagina.—Swelling, dness, and moist itching eruption on labia minora.—Bearing down in erus, which obstructs respiration.—Pressure as if everything would pro-ude through the vulva (with oppression of breathing).—Pains in both groins d bearing down, with constipation but no leucorrhœa; sleep heavy and non-freshing, coldness all over, tongue flabby (cured in stout woman, 35.—R. T. C.). olapsus of the vagina.—Violent stitches in the vagina upwards.—Prolapsus eri, with congestion, with yellow leucorrhœa.—Prolapsus, with inclination fundus to l., causing numbness in l. lower half of body, with pain, > when ng, esp. on r. side, tenderness of os uteri.—Induration of cervix; burning,

shooting, sticking pains.—Metrorrhagia ; during climaxis or during pregnanc —Menses too profuse.—Menses suppressed, or too feeble, or else too earl (appearing only in morning). —When menses fail to appear in mothers wh do not nurse, with inflation of abdomen.—Colic before menses.—Durin menses : irritability, melancholy, toothache, headache, nose-bleed, and painf weariness in limbs, or spasmodic colic and pressure towards the parts.—Mu cross her limbs to prevent protrusion of the parts.—Dull, heavy pain i ovaries ; esp. l.—Sterility.—Leucorrhœa, or a yellow or greenish red wate or purulent and fetid, sometimes with inflation of abdomen, or shootings i vagina. — Leucorrhœa in place of menses. — Leucorrhœa like milk, wi soreness of pudenda.—Itching, corrosive leucorrhœa.—Inclination to mi carriages. — Abortion after the fifth month. — Tendency to abort fifth seventh month.—Shootings in mammæ.—Excoriation of nipples (which blee and seem about to ulcerate).—Nipples cracked across the crown.—Indur tion of breasts ; scirrhus, stitches, tender, burning pains.—Excoriation children.—Sudden hot flushes of climaxis, with momentary sweat, weakne and great tendency to faint.—Retained placenta after miscarriage.—Soreness abdomen, feels motions of child too sensitively.—During pregnancy yello brown spots on face.—Terrible itching of vulva causing abortion.—Offensi excoriating lochia, very long lasting.

17. **Respiratory Organs.**—Roughness and soreness of larynx a throat.—Sensation of dryness in larynx.—Hoarseness with coryza.—Sensati of dryness in trachea.—Cough, excited by a tickling in larynx or chest.—D cough, which seems to arise from stomach, esp. when in bed in evening (t midnight), and often with nausea and bitter vomiting.—Moist cough, after chill.—Cough only during day, or which wakens one at night.—Expectorati profuse and whitish.—Cough, with copious expectoration of mucus, genera putrid, or of a salt taste, often only in morning or evening, and frequen accompanied by noise, weakness, and pains as from excoriation in chest (as it were raw).—Cough with expectoration in morning, no expectoration evening, or with expectoration at night, none in day ; very severe cough morning on rising, and expectoration of a great quantity of badly tasti substance.—Nocturnal cough, with cries, suffocation, and retching.—Cou like whooping-cough.—Attacks of spasmodic cough, like whooping-cou caused by tickling in chest or from tickling extending from larynx to abdom with expectoration only in morning, evening and at night of greenish-gr pus, or of milk-white, tough mucus, sometimes disagreeably sweet, which l to be swallowed again.—Cough < when lying on l. side ; from acids.—Cou excited by a tickling sensation, and accompanied by constipation.—Diffic expectoration (or being obliged to swallow again what had been raised) Yellow-greenish purulent expectoration during the cough.—Expectoration blood while lying down.—Sanguineous expectoration, when coughing, mo ing and evening, with expectoration of mucus by day.—Lancinations in ch or back during cough.

18. **Chest.**—Dyspnœa, oppression of chest, and shortness of brea when walking and ascending, as well as when lying down in bed, in eveni and at night.—Pain in sides of chest, when inspiring or coughing.—Stitch l. side of chest and scapula when breathing and coughing.—Oppression chest produced by an accumulation of mucus, or by too profuse expectorati

-Pain in chest from movement.—Pressure in chest, esp. when in bed in ·ening.—Heaviness, fulness, and tension in chest.—(Hepatisation of middle ıd lower lobes of r. lung.—Skinner).—Pain in chest, as from excoriation.— ramps in chest.—Itching and tickling in chest.—Sensation of emptiness chest.—Shootings and prickings in chest, and sides of chest, sometimes ıring an inspiration, and when coughing, as well as from intellectual exertion. -Brown spots on chest.—The chest symptoms cease, or are > by pressure hand on thorax.

19. **Heart.**—Ebullition (congestion) of blood in chest, and violent palpita- on of heart.—Intermittent palpitation of heart.—Palpitation : in evening in ·d with beating in all arteries ; during digestion ; with stitches in l. side of ıest.—Heart gives an occasional hard thump.—Wakes up with violent beating heart.—Nervous palpitation > by walking fast.

20. **Neck and Back.**—Tetters on nape, and behind ears.—Claret- loured spots on neck, and under chin.—Furunculus on neck.—Perspiration ı back, and under axillæ.—Swelling and suppuration of axillary glands.— umid tetters under axillæ.—Pressure and stitches in r. shoulder-blade.— tiffness in small of back and neck.—Pains in loins and back, with burning aring.—Throbbing in loins.—Weakness in loins when walking.—Incisive ains, pressure, digging and spasmodic tearings in back.—Rigidity of back nd nape.—Pain in the back, and small of back particularly with stiffness ; by walking.—Tearing in back during menses, with chills, heat, thirst and ontraction of chest.—Aching and dull pain in lumbar and sacral regions, xtending to thighs and legs.—Sprained pain over hips, in evening in bed, nd in afternoon.—Shivering in back.—Brownish spots on back.—Reddish erpetic spots above hip, and both sides of neck.—Stitches posteriorly above hip ; she could not lie on r. side, and when touched it felt sore.—Stitches back when coughing.—Itching eruption on back.

21. **Limbs.**—Drawing in all the limbs.—Drawing and tearing (paralytic ains) in limbs and joints (with weakness).—Heaviness of the limbs.—Arthritic ains in joints.—Tension in limbs as if they were too short.—Easy going to eep of limbs, esp. after manual labour.—Stiffness and want of flexibility in ints.—Easy dislocation and spraining of limbs.—Commotions and jerks in mbs night and day.—Restlessness and throbbing in all the limbs, which dmits of no rest in any place.—Frequent stretchings.—Want of stability in mbs.—Coldness of hands and feet ; but moist.

22. **Upper Limbs.**—Wrenching pain (as from dislocation) in shoulder- int, esp. on lifting or holding anything.—Lassitude in arms.—Sensation of tiffness or coldness in arms, as if paralysed.—Drawing, paralytic pain in arm nd shoulder-joint, extending to fingers.—Swelling and suppuration of axillary lands.—Shootings in arms, wrist, and fingers on fatiguing or moving them.— 'ainful tension in arms, and joints of elbow and fingers, as if caused by con- raction.—Inflammatory, deep red, hard, marbled swelling in middle of arms. –Pustules on arms, with violent itching.—Stiffness of joints of elbow and ands.—Brownish spots, herpetic skin, and itching scabs on elbow (scaling ff).—Itching vesicles on back of hand, and tips of fingers.—Itch and scabs on ands (soldiers' itch).—Herpes on backs of hands.—Swelling of hand, with ruption of vesicles, like pemphigus.—Shootings in wrist on moving the hand. —Burning heat in palms.—Cold sweat on hands.—Malignant scabies, and

scabs on hands.—Arthritic drawing and shootings in joints of fingers.—D tortion of fingers.—Painless ulcers on joints, and on tips of fingers.—(Tingli in tips of fingers, which wakes her up on going to sleep, after which slee well all night.—R. T. C.).—Warts on hands and fingers ; on sides of finger horny.—Flaws on fingers.—Deformed nails.—Panaritium, with throbbing a shooting pains.

23. **Lower Limbs.**—Pain as if bruised in r. hip-joint.—Pain in hi with tearing shootings.—Pain in buttocks and thighs, after having been seat for some time.—Spasms in buttocks at night, in bed, when stretching out t limb.—Paralytic weakness of legs, esp. after a paroxysm of passion.—Stiffn of legs, as far as hip-joint, after having been seated a short time.—Coldness legs and feet (esp. in evening in bed).—Swelling of legs and feet (< wh sitting or standing, > when walking).—Cramp in thighs when walking. Tearing lancinations, or shocks in thighs and tibia, so as to extort cries. Furunculi on thigh and in hams.—Drawing and tearing shootings in kne hams, and heels.—Painful swelling of knees.—Synovitis of knee-joints housemaids (R. T. C.).—Stiffness in joints of knee and ankle.—Cramps calves, sometimes at night.—Restlessness of legs every evening (with forn cation in them).—Itching pimples on legs and instep.—Drawing pain in le and great toes. — Shootings in tibia and instep. — Sensation in legs, as i mouse were running over them.—Jerking in feet when sleeping.—Ulcers instep.—Stiffness in heels and joints of feet, as from contraction.—Pricki and burning sensation of feet.—Tingling and numbness in soles of feet. Profuse, or else suppressed (offensive) perspiration of feet (causing soren between toes).—Stinging in the heels.—Tension in tendo-Achillis.—Ulcers heel, arising from corrosive vesicles.—Indolent ulcers on joints and tips toes.—Corns on feet, with shooting pain.—Deformity of toenails.

24. **Generalities.**—[Affections in general appearing in l. side ; r. upp and r. lower extremities ; eyelids ; internal ear ; hearing very sensitiv region of liver ; inner lower belly ; l. shoulder-blade ; back and small back ; axilla ; axillary glands, esp. where there are darting pains throu them ; upper and lower extremities and joints ; r. lumbar region, with violent pressing or bearing-down pain ; nails turn yellow.—Dark hair ; p face ; exanthema on face, lips, nose, forehead.—Bleeding from inner parts. Spasms : clonic ; tonic ; cataleptic ; great restlessness of the body ; gr aversion to washing.—Debility in general or of particular parts.—Sensation of a ball in inner parts ; pain as if part would burst, were pressed or push asunder ; cramping or drawing pains in inner or outer parts ; sensations emptiness or hollowness in any part, esp. when accompanied by a faint sensation ; jerking in the muscles or elsewhere, as they may be felt in t head when talking, &c. ; knocking, throbbing, or pulsation in inner part pressing as of a heavy load ; vibration like dull tingling or buzzing the body.—< In early morning ; forenoon ; evening, particularly bef falling asleep ; on waking ; stooping ; during inspiration ; while in compan while coughing ; after coitus ; after eating ; from exertion of the min during fever ; female complaints generally ; from loss of fluids ; mastur tion ; music ; milk ; fat pork ; during and after perspiration ; duri pregnancy ; riding in a car ; from riding on horseback, in a swing, & from sexual excesses ; during first hours of sleep ; in snow air ; from stret

ıg the affected part ; while nursing a child ; from water and washing ; from etting wet ; females having leucorrhœa ; during confinement esp.—> From rawing up the limb ; moving ; exertion of body ; drinking cold water ; in olitude ; when walking quickly.—H. N. G.].—Shooting and pricking pains ı the limbs, and other parts of the body.—Burning pains in different parts f the body.—Pains, which are > by external heat.—Pains, by fits, with ıuddering.—Wrenching pain, esp. on exerting the parts affected, and also at ight, in heat of bed.—Rheumatic pains, with swelling of the parts affected, erspiration easily excited, chilliness or shivering, alternately with heat.—reat disturbance, caused by vexation.—Easy benumbing of the limbs (arms nd legs) esp. after manual labour.—Stiffness and want of flexibility in the oints.—Easy dislocation and spraining of the limbs.—Tendency to strain the ack.—Commotions and jerks in the limbs night and day.—Jerking in the ıuscles.—Fits of uneasiness, and of hysterical spasms.—Swelling and supıration of the glands.—Renewal or < of several sufferings, during and nmediately after a meal.—The symptoms disappear during violent exercise, xcept when taken on horseback, and are < during repose, also in the even-g, at night, in the heat of the bed (and in the forenoon).—Painful sensibility the whole body.—Violent ebullition of blood, even at night, with pulsation ıroughout the body.—Great swelling of body, with shortness of breath, with-ıt thirst.—Heaviness, and physical indolence.—Paroxysms of weakness, and ysterical or other forms of syncope.—Fainting fits.—Lassitude, with tremb-ıg.—Want of energy, sometimes only on waking.—The patient is soon tigued, when walking in the open air.—Great tendency to take cold, and nsibility to cold air, esp. in a north wind.—Feverish shivering, syncope, and terwards coryza, after getting wet.

25. **Skin.**—Skin yellow, like jaundice ; chapping of the skin, or cracks ay extend deeply into the tissues, and this is < by washing in water ; xanthema in general, particularly when it is disposed to crack.—Ulceration the exanthema ; bed sores ; brown sphacelus.—Tetters in general.—Ulcers ppurating ; pus too copious ; swollen ; with proud flesh.—Salt rheum.—xcessive sensibility of the skin.—Soreness of skin and humid places in bends joints.—Itching in different parts (face, arms, hands, back, hips, abdomen ıd genitals) which changes to a burning sensation.—Itching and eruption of mples in the joints.—Excoriation, esp. in the joints.—Dry and itching erup-ons, like scabies.—Dry itch ; bad effects where itch has been suppressed by *erc.* or *Sul.*—Brown, or vinous, or else reddish, and herpetic spots on skin. Annular desquamation (annular herpes).—Moist, scabious herpes, with ching and burning sensation.—Boils and blood-boils.—Engorged glands.—cirrhous indurations.—Eruptions of vesicles, like pemphigus.—Itching, nging, lancinating, burning, or sometimes indolent ulcers (knuckles, finger-ints, tips of fingers, joints and tip of toes).—Corns, with shooting pain.—eformity of nails.—Hepatic spots.—Warts : on neck with horny excres-nces in centre ; small, itching, flat on hands and face ; large hard seed arts ; dark colour and painless ; (large horny wart on abdomen).

26. **Sleep.**—Strong disposition to sleep during day, and early in evening. Attacks of coma, returning in a tertian type.—Falling asleep late ; com-ıints preventing sleep ; sleeping late in the morning ; waking frequently ring the night ; very sleepy in the morning ; sleeplessness before midnight ;

sleepiness without sleep.—Awakens at 3 a.m. and cannot go to sleep again.—Sleeplessness from over-excitement.—Early waking, and lying awake for long time.—Frequent waking, without apparent cause.—Agitated sleep, wit violent ebullition of blood, continued tossing, fantastic, anxious, frightfu dreams, and frequent starts (screaming), with fright.—The sleeper fancie himself called by name.—Unrefreshing sleep; sensation in morning, as fror insufficient sleep.—Lascivious dreams.—Talking, cries, and jerking of limb during sleep.—Nightly delirium.—Wanderings, anguish, feverish heat, an agitation in the body, toothache, colic, cough, and many other sufferings a night.

27. **Fever.**—Pulse full and quick during night and then intermitting during day slow.—Pulse accelerated by motion and being angry.—Pulsatio in all the blood-vessels.—Shuddering (chilliness) during pains.—Coldness single parts.—Want of vital heat.—Frequent shivering, esp. when out of doo in evening, and from every movement.—Flushes of heat at intervals durir day, esp. afternoon and evening, while sitting or in open air, generally wi thirst or redness of face.—Paroxysm of heat (transient), esp. when seated, ar walking in open air, also when angry, or engaged in important conversation.-Paroxysm of heat (and of shivering) with thirst.—During chill more thir than during heat.—Continued heat, with redness of face and violent thirst.-Fever, with thirst, during shivering, pains in the limbs, icy coldness of t hands and feet, and deadness of the fingers.—Perspiration in general; pe spires too easily; single parts perspire too easily; perspiration with anxiet with restlessness; sour-smelling or offensive.—Internal chilliness with extern heat.—Perspiration while seated.—Profuse perspiration on the slightest mov ment (more after than during exercise).—Perspiration only on upper part body.—Noctural perspiration, sometimes cold (on breast, back, and thighs). Perspiration in morning, sometimes of an acid smell.—Intermittent fev followed by violent heat and inability to collect one's senses; this is follow by profuse perspiration.

Sepsinum, *see* Pyrogenium.

Septicæminum.

Nosode of Septicæmia (Swan). Attenuations made from contents a septic abscess.

Clinical.—Camp diarrhœa. Dysentery. Typhoid fever.

Characteristics.—Skinner (*H. W.*, xxxv. 246) gave a supply *Septic.* 10m (F.C.) to a volunteer going to South Africa, with instru tions to take a globule every four hours if attacked with anything li sinking or typhoid fever. The young man wrote home that "*Septicæn* is like magic in diarrhœa and dysentery in camp life," and asked more, as his supply was largely drawn on by his friends.

Relations.—*Compare:* Pyro., Malar., Bapt.

Shucks, *see* Zea Mays.

Silica.

Silicea terra. Pure Flint. Silex. Silicic anhydride. Silicon dioxide. SiO_2. Trituration of pure, precipitated Silica.

Clinical.—*Abdomen, distended. Abscess.* Acne. *Anæmia. Ankles, weak.* Anus, fissure of; fistula of. *Appetite, depraved. Back, weakness of. Boils. Bones, necrosis of.* Brain, concussion of. *Brain-fag. Breast, sinuses in. Bunion. Cancer. Carbuncle. Cataract. Cellulitis. Cheloid.* Chin, eruptions on. *Cicatrix. Circulation, feeble. Coccygodynia.* Conjunctivitis, phlyctenular. Constipation. Coryza. *Cough. Debility. Dentition. Diabetes.* Ear, affections of. Elephantiasis. *Enchrodroma.* Enuresis. *Epilepsy.* Eruptions. *Excrescences. Eyes, affections of. Feet, burning; perspiring. Fester. Fibroma. Fistula.* Foot-sweat; suppressed. Foreign bodies, expulsion of. *Fractures.* Ganglion. Gastric catarrh. *Glandular swellings. Headache. Hernia.* Hip-joint disease. Homesickness. Housemaid's knee. *Hydrocele.* Hypopion. *Irritation. Jaw, caries of. Joints, synovitis of.* Lachrymal fistula. *Lactation.* Locomotor ataxy. Mania. *Meningitis.* Metrorrhagia. *Miscarriage. Molluscum contagiosum. Molluscum fibrosum. Morphœa. Morvan's disease. Nails, diseased.* Necrosis. Neuralgia. *Nodes. Nose, tip, redness of.* Panaritium. *Parametritis. Perspiration, offensive.* Phimosis. *Pleurisy.* Prepuce, eruption on. Psoas abscess. *Pylorus, suppuration of.* Rheumatism; chronic; hereditary. *Rickets.* Sinuses. Somnambulism. *Spermatorrhœa. Spinal irritation.* Strains. Strangury. *Suppuration. Teeth, caries of. Tenesmus. Trachea.* Tumours. *Ulcers. Urethra, stricture of.* Urine, incontinence of. *Vaccination. Vagina, spasms of.* Vertigo. *Walking, delay in.* Whitlow. Worms. Writer's cramp.

Characteristics.—Outside homœopathy Flint as an internal remedy is practically unknown. Hahnemann introduced it into medicine, and it was his method of attenuating insoluble substances that enabled him to discover its powers. *Silica* forms one of the most important remedies of the *Chronic Diseases.* A large proportion of the earth's crust is composed of *Silica.* Sea sand (*Silica marina*) is mainly composed of it. The spicules of many sponges are made up of *Silica.* Silicates are taken up by plants and from them *Silica* is often deposited on the surface or in the interior of their stems. The strength of straw is due to *Silica. Equisetum* generally contains as much as 18 per cent. of *Silica* to the fresh plant. Flint supplies the "grit" of the earth's crust, of plant life, and to a large extent of animal life also. "Want of grit, moral or physical," is a leading indication for *Sil.* in homœopathic practice. Teste puts *Sil.* in his *Pulsatilla* group of remedies, the other members of it being *Calc.*, *Hep.*, *Graph.*, *Pho.* According to Teste, *Sil.* is the "chronic" of *Puls.*,—it corresponds to the chronic form of such diseases as *Puls.* cures when acute: Rush of blood to the head, especially to the right temple and vertex; headache every day; photophobia; lachrymation; loss of taste; aversion to fat food with rancid or oily taste in mouth, &c. The symptoms of *Sil.* differ from those of *Puls.* in being more constant, more deep-seated, and lasting longer; for instance, the mucous secretions of *Puls.* become easily purulent under the action of *Sil.* Teste points out that *Puls.* flourishes best on sandy soils (as *Bell.*

does on calcareous soils). Schüssler, who was a homœopathist before he was a Biochemist, describes the sphere of *Sil.* from the Tissue-Remedy point of view as follows: "*Silicic Acid* is a constituent of the cells of the connective tissue, of the epidermis, the hair and the nails.—If a suppurative centre is formed either in the connective tissue or in a portion of the skin, *Sil.* may be used.—After the functional ability of the cells of the connective tissue, which had been impaired by the pressure of the pus, has been restored to its integrity through a supply of molecules of *Sil.*, these cells are thereby enabled to throw off inimical substances (the pus). In consequence, the pus is either absorbed by the lymphatics or it is cast out. In the latter case there is a so-called spontaneous breaking open of the suppurative centre.—*Sil.* may also cause the absorption through the lymphatics of an effusion of blood in any tissue. If the reabsorption of a sero-albuminous exudation in a serous sac cannot be effected through *Calc. phos.*, then *Sil.* may be used; for the delay in the absorption may also be caused by a deficiency of *Sil.* in the subserous connective tissue.—*Sil.* will also cure chronic arthritic-rheumatic affections, as it forms a soluble combination (*Sodium silicate*) with the soda of the urate of soda; this combination is then absorbed and removed through the lymphatics. For the same reason it may also be used in renal gravel.—*Sil.* can also restore the perspiration of the feet when this has been suppressed, and is thus an indirect remedy in diseases arising in consequence of such suppression (*e.g.*, amblyopia, cataract, paralysis, &c.).—When a number of cells in the connective tissue are gradually deprived of *Sil.*, they become atrophied. Such a disease is by no means rare in the external meatus auditorious with old people. The meatus in such a case is dry and enlarged." (Schüssler adds that he generally gives the 12x trituration.) The indications of Schüssler correspond so exactly with those already pointed out by Hahnemann that we are left in doubt as to how much he was indebted to Hahnemann for his facts and how much to his own theories. Be that as it may, the relation of *Sil.* to the connective tissues is a very real one. *Sil.* is a great *evacuant*. *Sil.* produced in the provings sensation of "splinter in the finger," of "a pin in the throat," and whenever foreign bodies have became embeded in the tissues; or whenever portions of the tissues have become necrosed and quasi-foreign, *Sil.* will set up suppuration in the vicinity and bring about their expulsion. (It is this property which makes it necessary sometimes to use *Sil.* with caution; if there are deposits which have became encysted and so far rendered harmless, the administration of *Sil.* might set up suppurative action, to the risk of the patient's life.) *Sil.* both matures abscesses and reduces excessive suppuration. It will also resolve indurations left after suppuration; this has been particularly noted in the case of tonsils which refuse to heal after the pus has been evacuated, and in abscesses which leave sinuses and fistulæ. *Sil.* affects the nails, cripples them, and produces inflammation around and under them. "Sensation as if the finger-tips were suppurating" is one of the symptoms which led to its use in such cases. *Sil.* causes inflammation, swelling and suppuration of all the lymphatic glands and also the glands of the skin. The skin is unhealthy and every little injury ulcerates. Hands and feet are sweaty, and the sweat is generally offensive. The feet may give off an intolerable odour without any sweat. The head sweats, and this may be offensive. *Sil.* corresponds perfectly to many cases of rickets: children with large heads; open fontanelles and sutures; much sweating about the head, which must be kept warm; distended abdomen; weak ankles; slow in learning to walk. This constitutes type No. 1, to which *Sil.* is *particularly suited.* It is also *suited to:* (2) Nervous, irritable persons, with dry skin, profuse saliva, diarrhœa, night-sweats. (3) Weakly persons, fine skin, pale face, light complexion; lax muscles. (4) Constitutions which suffer from deficient nutrition due to lack of assimilating power; over-sensitive physically and mentally. (5) Scrofulous children who have worm diseases during dentition. (6) Stonecutters' ailments (chest affections and total loss of strength.—The action of *Sil.* on the connective tissues may end in new growth as well as in suppuration and ulceration. It has a specific relation to scarred tissue; and I have cured with it a case of recurrent cheloid: Eleanor W., 14, had a growth on left temple. Five months before she had been an inmate in St. Bartholomew's Hospital and had had a tumour removed from the spot, the tumour having existed for two years. A month after the operation a new growth appeared on the scar. Two months later this was removed. But it rapidly recurred, and when I saw her there was a linear elevation an inch long, three lines wide, and raised about two lines. It was red, shiny, and slightly nodulated; was *tender to touch* and the seat of *shooting pain.* Before the first operation there had been no pain and no discoloration of the skin. Hahnemann gives this symptom in the proving of *Sil.* "Stitching, aching pain in the spot where an ulcer had been formerly on the leg." *Sil.* 3 gr. iii., night and morning, was prescribed. There was no further increase in the size of the growth, though it was still painful, the pain being apparently somewhat increased. In three months there was evident diminution in size, and from that time the pain began to diminish. In seven months the growth had entirely disappeared.—The sensitiveness of *Sil.* is one of its key-notes, and an over-susceptibility to nervous stimuli is a frequent accompaniment of conditions requiring *Sil.* The surface is tender and the least touch is painful. The senses are morbidly keen. Brain and spine cannot bear even ordinary vibrations. This condition may be caused by losses of fluids as in spermatorrhœa; by over-worked brain. *Sil.* causes tendency to paralysis and paralytic weakness from defective nutrition of nerves of brain and spinal cord. Constipation is often an accompaniment of these conditions. There may be epileptic convulsions. These have a well-marked course, starting from the solar plexus; are < at full and new moon; and < from any overstrain of mind or emotions. *Sil.* is indicated in locomotor ataxy when the fingers feel stiff with loss of power in them. There is spinal irritation. The neck is stiff causing headache. The small of the back aches as if beaten. The part of the body lain on goes to sleep. The headaches of *Sil.* present one of the grand characteristics of the remedy. They are of the chronic kind, and may owe their origin to some severe disease of youth. They ascend trom the nape of the neck to the vertex, as if coming from the spine, and locate in one eye, especially the right ; < from draught of air or uncovering head ; > pressure and *wrapping head up warmly ;* > profuse urination. The vertigo of *Sil.* in the same way ascends from the back of the neck ; as if one would fall forward (sometimes backward) ; < looking up ; closing eyes ; lying on left side. The sensitiveness of *Sil.* comes out in the mental symptoms : "Sensitive to noise ; and anxiety therefrom." "Sensitive, weeping mood." "Yielding, faint-hearted." "Children become obstinate, headstrong ; cry when kindly spoken to." A curious symptom and one of great value is this : "Fixed ideas : the patients thinks only of pins, fears them, searches for them, and counts them carefully." This symptom enabled me to make a rapid cure of post-influenzal insanity in the case of a man of bad family history, one of whose sisters had become insane and had drowned herself, another sister being affected with lupus. The patient's wife told me one morning that he had "*been looking everywhere for pins.*" *Sil.* 30 rapidly put an end to the search and restored the patient to his senses. *Sil.* has another link with insanity in its aggravation at the moon's phases : epilepsy and sleep-walking are < at the new and full moon. The *Sil.* patient likes to be magnetised, and is > by it. This is related to the persistent want of vital heat which characterises the *Sil.* condition; even exercise will not get up any warmth. Another curious symptom of *Sil.* is : "discharge of blood from the vagina every time the child takes the breast." Another symptom in this relation is important in connection with cancer cases : "nipple is drawn in like a funnel." Always before and during menses there is constipation. The constipation of *Sil.* is characteristic. The stool is difficult as from inactivity of rectum ; with great straining as if rectum was paralysed ; *when partly expelled recedes again.* Fæces remain a long time in rectum. Rushmore (*H. P.*, xii. 530) verified a peculiar symptom of *Sil.* in a lady suffering from scirrhus of left breast. She had a feeling of dryness in her *finger-tips, as if made of paper ; at night.* *Ant. t.* and *Sil.* have this symptom, but only *Sil.* in afternoon. *Sil.* removed this and took away sharp, stinging pains in the tumour as well. *Peculiar Sensations* of *Sil.* are : Susceptibility to nervous stimuli, to magnetism. As if she would die. As if gradually losing senses. As if feeling for pins. Sensation as if she were divided into halves and that the left side does not belong to her. As if one would fall forward. Vertigo as if drunk. As if head were teeming with live things whirling around in it. Headache as if beaten. As if everything would press out and burst skull. As if brain and eyes were forced forward. As if head would burst with throbbing in it, internal and external at same time. As if forehead would be torn asunder ; as from a heavy weight over eyes. As if head were forced asunder. As of water-pipes bursting in head. As if tremendous weight were falling on vertex. Head as if in a cushion and some one were pressing two fingers into it at occiput. As if brain collided with skull. Head as if bruised. As if waves of water from occiput over vertex to forehead.

ck-headaches as if coming from spine and locating over one eye. ead as if too large. As if head were falling off ; as if it were anging by a piece of skin at nape. As if right side of head paralysed. s if looking through a grey cover. As if cornea were a mass of ypertrophied tissue. Eyes as if too dry and full of sand. As of a plinter in upper lid. As if both eyes were dragged back into head y strings. Objects as if in a fog. As if something alive were in ears. s if nasal bone has been beaten. As if a hair were on tip of tongue xtending into trachea. As of a lump on right side of throat. As of a in in throat. Throat as if filled up. As if he could not swallow. s if he swallowed over a sore spot. As of a load in epigastrium. As knives were running into stomach. As if there were no power in ectum to expel stool. As if rectum paralysed. As if anus con-ricted. As of a heavy lump in anus. As if vulva were enlarged. s if tied round chest with a tape. As if sternum were grasped. As of stone under sternum. As if mould were forming over whole body. s if a hand had grasped her breastbone. Cords of neck as if pulled. mall of back as if beaten ; as if dead. Arms and hands as if filled vith lead. As of a splinter in finger. As if a panaritium would form n index finger. As if tips of fingers were suppurating. As if finger vere thick and bone enlarged. As if joints of fingers were being ulled out of sockets. Limbs and feet as if paralysed. Femur as if eaten. Knees as if too tightly bound. Calves as if too short. As if pasms in ankles. As if toe-joints being pulled out of sockets. Nails s if decayed. As if beaten all over. As if he had lain in an un-comfortable position. The direction of the *Sil.* action is upward and *utward :* there are shootings out through eyes and out of ears. The symptoms are : < By touch ; contact ; combing hair. Binding ightly > headache ; but pressure of hat = pain. Pressure <. Rest >. Motion <. Lying down < asthma ; = headache. Lying ight side < pains in liver. Lying left side = vertigo. Sitting <. Gaping or swallowing > stoppage of ear. Opening eyes < pressive pain. Writing = tonic spasm of hand. Walking < ; every step is painfully felt (incarcerated flatus). Open-air < headache ; = lachry-mation ; burning in back. Cold air (especially on head, eyes, back of neck, back) ; cold draught ; changing linen ; uncovering <. < Washing. Change of weather < pain in ears ; < pain in limbs. < Before and during a storm. > Summer. < Approach of winter. < At new moon ; increasing moon (hysteria) ; and full moon. > In warm room ; by warm wraps. < Mental exertion ; talking. Pain in head > while eating. < after eating. Milk < ; = diarrhœa. Aversion to mother's milk and vomiting whenever taking it. Drinking cold water = dry cough. Warm drinks > cough. Averse to warm food. > From magnetism and electricity.

Relations.—*Antidoted by :* Camph., Hep., Fl. ac. *It antidotes :* Merc. cor., Sul. *Incompatible :* Merc. *Follows well :* Bell., Bry., Calc., Calc. p. (in rickets when Calc. p. fails), Cin., Graph., Hep., Ign., Nit. ac., Pho. *Followed well by :* Hep., Fl. ac., Lach., Lyc., Sep. (If improvement ceases under Sil. a dose or two of Sul. will set up reaction, and Sil. will then complete the cure). *Complementary :* Thuj., Sanic., Puls. (Sil. is the "chronic" of Puls.). *Compare :* Head-sweat and open fontanelles, Calc. (Sil. lower than Calc. and offensive) Head must be kept warm, Sanic., Mg. m. Ailments from suppresse foot-sweat, Cup., Graph., Pso. Want of vital heat, Led., Sep. Vertig as if one would fall forward from looking up, Puls. (from looking down K. ca., Spi.). Chronic sick-headaches since some severe disease of youth Pso. Headache > pressure and wrapping up warmly, Mg. m., Stron Constipation before and during menses (diarrhœa before and durin menses, Am. c., Bov). Partly expelled stool recedes, Thu. Fistula i ano alternates with chest complaints, Berb., Calc. p. Somnambulism Luna, K. bro. Vaccination : erysipelas, convulsions, diarrhœa, Thu (Thu. when the fever is high), Apis, Sul., Malan., Vacc., Var. Cicatrix fissure of anus, Graph. Offensive sweat (head, feet, axillæ), Petr Aversion to touch, Cin., Hep., Thu., Lach., Asaf. (Asaf., offensive discharge from tissues, "intolerable soreness round the ulcer, canno bear even the dressing"). Caries, Plat. mur., Ang. (long bones) Stron. c. (femur, with watery diarrhœa), Gettys. (caries with ulcers about joints, discharge excoriating), Calc. (scrofulous subjects ; sweat sour rather than offensive ; foot-sweat does not excoriate ; not sensitive like Sil.). Sweat of head, body dry (Rhus, sweat of body, head dry). Last stage of phthisis, Phell. Perforating ulcers, Nit. ac., K. bi. Headache ascending from nape, Meny. (bursting ; > pressure ; not > warmth), Paris (head feels unusually large), Stron. c., Sang. (to right eye), Spi. (to left eye). Clouded sight after headache, Sil. (*before* headache, K. bi.). < Damp change, Bar. c. Foot-sweat, scrofula, rickets, and headache > wrapping warmly, Mg. m. Catarrhal phthisis, Stn. Abscess of breast, fistulæ, necrosis (of jaw), Pho. (Pho. has more erythematous blush and radiating streaks round opening). Hay-fever, itching at Eustachian orifices, Ars., Rosa, Ran. b. Nervous exhaustion, Pic. ac. Chronic suppuration of middle ear, Caps. Catarrhal diarrhœa, Puls. Tetanus impending, wound suddenly ceases to discharge, Nux. Weakness of ankles, Caust., Sul. ac. < Thunderstorms, Na. c., Pho., Rho., Pet. < From cold or draught (Fl. ac., > cold applications). Nausea when fasting, Pul., Lyc. Calc. Impatient, Cham., Sul. Motes, persistent speck before right eye (Sul., before left ; Macrot., right in morning). "Washed out," but *won't* give in (Pic. ac., *must* give in). Affections of one side of tongue, Calc., Thu. (ulcer right border, Sil., Thu. ; left, Apis ; left side swollen with loss of speech, Lauro.). Hungry but cannot get the food down, Sil., Lyc. Hair sensation on tongue, Nat. m., K. bi. (on back part). Children are obstinate, headstrong, cry when spoken kindly to, Iod. Nipple drawn in like a funnel, Sars. Unhealthy skin, every little injury suppurates, Graph., Hep., Petr., Merc. Crippled nails, Ant. c. Ingrowing toenails, Mgt. aust. Takes cold from exposure of feet, Con., Cup. Takes cold by uncovering head (Bell., by hair-cutting). Difficulty in holding up head, Ant. t. Callosities in feet, Ant. c. < After coitus, K. ca. Evacuant of foreign bodies, Lobel. i. Drinking cold water = dry cough (Caust., >). Ganglion, Benz. ac., Sul. Chronic and hereditary rheumatism, Led. (but Led. has < by warmth, and symptoms extend from below upward, whilst Sil. affects particularly the shoulders and joints). Fibroma, Nat. sf. Cheloid and scars,

Thios. Homesickness, Caps., Ph. ac. Brachial neuralgia, Calc. (*see case under* CALC.).

Causation.—Vaccination. Stone-cutting. Loss of fluids. Injury. Strains. Splinters. Foreign bodies.

SYMPTOMS.

1. **Mind.**—Despondency, melancholy, and disposition to weep.—Nostalgia.—Anxiety and agitation ; yielding, anxious mood.—Taciturnity ; concentration in self.—Inquietude and ill-humour on the least provocation, arising from excessive nervous debility.—Scruples of conscience (about trifles).—Restless and fidgety ; great liability to be frightened, esp. by least noise.—Discouragement.—Moroseness, ill-humour, and despair, with intense weariness of life.—Wishes to drown herself.—Disposition to fly into a rage, obstinacy, and great irritability.—The child becomes obstinate and head-strong ; cries when kindly spoken to.—Excitement with easy orgasm of blood.—Repugnance to labour.—Apathy and indifference.—Weakness of memory.—Incapacity for reflection.—Great distraction.—Tendency to misapply words in speaking.—Fixed ideas ; the patient thinks only of pins, fears them, searches for them, and counts them carefully.

2. **Head.**—Cloudiness.—The head is fatigued by intellectual labour (reading, writing, or reflecting).—Difficulty in holding head up.—Dizziness, esp. in the evening, as from intoxication.—Vertigo of different kinds, esp. in the morning, and principally on lifting up the eyes, or when riding in a carriage, and also when stooping, or after moral emotions.—Vertigo, with nausea and retching, or proceeding from the back to the nape and head.—Vertigo : as if one would fall forward ; is obliged to walk to r. side ; is obliged to sit down ; when closing eyes ; from lying on l. side.—Vertigo, which causes to fall backwards.—Pain which ascends from the nape into vertex, sometimes hindering sleep, at night.—Headache when over-heated.—Headache, with shivering, lassitude, and necessity to lie down.—Headache every morning.—Aching in head, with ill-humour and heaviness in all the limbs, sometimes in morning.—Heaviness of head ; pressing out in the forehead, which seems ready to split, sometimes every day, from morning till evening (< from evening till night, from stepping hard, from uncovering head, or if head becomes cold in open air).—Tension and pressure in the head, as if it were about to burst (ascending from the neck to the forehead).—Drawings in the head, which seem to pass out at the forehead.—Tearing pains in the head, often semilateral, with shootings which seem to pass out through the eyes, and into the bones of the face and the teeth, or which manifest themselves every morning, with heat in the head, principally in the forehead (and great restlessness ; < from a draught of air and motion).—Lancinations (stitches) in head, esp. in temples (principally in the r. from within to without ; < at night, from moving eyes, from talking and writing).—Throbbing headache, generally from congestion of blood in head (pulsating and beating, most violent in forehead and vertex, with chilliness).—Congestion to head, with redness in face.—Painful shocks in head.—Movements and whirling in head, as if everything in it were alive.—Shaking and vibration in brain at every step (roaring and shattering sensation when stepping hard

or knocking foot against anything).—The headaches are < principally by intellectual labour, talking, stooping, noise, jarring, light, and cold air, and are > in warm room ; from wrapping head up warmly ; from binding head tightly.—After the pains in the head, clouded sight.—Painful sensitiveness of exterior of head to least touch.—Profuse perspiration on head in evening, on going to sleep (this looks like *Calc. carb.*, but in *Sil.* the perspiration extends lower down on the neck, and is apt to have an offensive smell).—Burning in head with pulsation and perspiration of head ; < at night, from mental exertion and talking ; > wrapping the head up warm.—Burning and itching, mostly on back part of head ; < from scratching, which causes burning and soreness ; < when undressing in evening and on getting warm in bed.—Tearing pain in scalp < at night and from pressure.—Profuse, sour-smelling perspiration on head only (in evening), with great sensitiveness of scalp, with pale face and emaciation.—Tendency to take cold in head, which cannot possibly be uncovered.—Tuberous elevations on scalp.—Eruption on back part of head and behind ears dry, offensive-smelling, scabby, burning-itching ; when scratching it, burning feeling, more sore, and discharging pus.—Itching pustules and bulbous swellings on hairy scalp and on neck ; very sensitive to pressure, touch, and when lying on it ; > when wrapping it up warm.—Sensitiveness of scalp to pressure (of hat) and to contact ; < in evening and when lying on painful side ; burning after scratching.—Open fontanelles ; head too large and rest of body emaciated, with pale wax-colour of face ; hot, swollen abdomen and fetid stools.—Violent itching in scalp.—Moist scald-head, which itches.—Falling off of the hair.

3. **Eyes.**—Pain in eyes in morning, as if arising from the great dryness, or from the presence of sand.—Pressure and smarting in eyes and lids.—Tearing shooting pains in eyes on pressing them together.—Shootings, which seem to pass out through eyes.—Itching, smarting, and burning in the eyes.—Redness of eyes, with smarting pain in canthi.—Inflammation of eyes.—Affections appearing in angles of eyes, in region of tear-ducts.—Swelling of lachrymal gland.—Lachrymal fistula.—Lachrymation, esp. in open air.—Agglutination of lids, at night.—Fungus hæmatodes and ulcers in cornea.—Cornea thick, rough, warty, as if it were a mass of hypertrophied tissue, scaled off leaving cornea clear.—Specks and scars in cornea.—Weakness ; heat ; quivering of eyes.—Spasmodic closing of lids.—Presbyopia.—The letters appear confused, when reading.—Objects seem to be pale, when reading.—Confused sight, as if directed through a greyish veil.—Blackness before eyes after headache.—Momentary attacks of sudden blindness.—Cloudiness of crystalline lens.—Cloudiness of the sight, as from amaurosis.—Sparks, and black spots before sight.—Photophobia, and dazzling in broad daylight.—Encysted tumours of lids go away after *Sil.* 200 (Bradshaw).

4. **Ears.**—Otalgia, with drawing pain.—Boring and throbbing in the ears.—Shootings in the ears, from within outwards.—Itching in ears (esp. when swallowing).—Inflammation and running from edges of ears.—Scab behind ears.—Swelling of exterior of ear, with discharge (of pus) from the ear, accompanied by a sort of whistling.—Copious accumulation of moist (very thin) cerumen.—Otorrhœa with great sensitiveness to cold air.—Excessive sensitiveness to noise.—Obstruction of ears, which sometimes disappears on blowing the nose, or else with a loud report.—Hard

of hearing, sometimes without noise in ears, or else exclusively for .an voice.—Hardness of hearing, < when the moon is at the full.— ılysed auditory nerves.—Tinkling, clucking, and noise, like the fluttering bird, in ears.—Roaring and singing in ears.—Caries of the mastoid cess.—Swelling and induration of parotids.

5. **Nose.**—Nasal bone painful when touched.—Soreness as if beaten, in l bones.—Gnawing pains (and ulcers) in upper part of nose, with heaviness n stooping, and excessive sensibility to contact and pressure.—Pulsative , as from ulceration in the nose, and extending into the head.—Drawing oot of nose and r. malar bone.—Inflammation in nostrils.—Itching in nose. oluptuous itching about nose, in evening.—Itching and redness of nose the extremity), which is covered with scabious vesicles.—Sore, painful ts below septum of nose, with sticking on touch.—Furunculi on nose.— bs, pimples, and ulcers in nose.—Nose inwardly dry, painful, excoriated, ered with crusts.—Epistaxis.—Anosmia.—Frequent, violent, abortive, rrupted sneezing.—Too frequent, immoderate, sneezing.—Obstinate truction of nose, sometimes arising from (hardened) mucus.—Troublesome inful) dryness of nose, sometimes at night.—Dry coryza.—Continued yza.—Frequent fluent coryza ; or which removes an obstinate obstruction nose.—Alternate fluent and dry coryza.—Acrid and corrosive mucus nose.

6. **Face.**—Pale and earthy complexion.—White spots on cheeks, from e to time.—Red, burning spots on cheeks and nose, esp. after a meal.— at in face.—Shootings in bones of face.—Itching in whiskers.—Furunculus cheek.—Cracks and rhagades in skin of face.—Scirrhous induration in face l upper lip.—Swelling of lips.—Ulceration of commissures of lips.— ıbious eruption on lips, with smarting pain.—Ulcers on red part of lower —Furunculi on chin.—Herpes on chin.—Cramp in maxillary joint.—The iculation of the jaw is spasmodically closed (lockjaw).—Nocturnal shoot- s and drawings in lower jaw.—Swelling and caries in bones of lower jaw. welling of submaxillary glands, with pain when touched, or also with luration.

7. **Teeth.**—Toothache from hot food, or introduction of cold air into outh.—Drawing, jerking, and tearings in teeth, and cheeks, < at night, or e only when eating.—Toothache at night, commonly lancinating, which turbs sleep, < by cold or hot things.—Toothache, with swelling of bone periosteum of jaw, and universal heat at night, which hinders sleep.— gging and boring in teeth.—Bluntness of teeth.—Teeth become loose and l elongated.—Painful inflammation, swelling, excoriation, and easy bleeding the gums.—Gumboils.—Gums painfully sensitive on taking cold water into outh.

8. **Mouth.**—Dryness of mouth.—Fetid breath, esp. in morning.— omacace.—Mucus constantly in mouth.—Sensation, as of a hair on (forepart tongue.—Excoriation of tongue.—One-sided swelling of tongue.—Ulcer r. border of tongue eating into it and discharging much pus (carcinoma).— lcer on the palate.—Tongue coated with a brownish mucus.

9. **Throat.**—Sore throat, with an accumulation of mucus in throat.— vere tonsillitis ("*Sil.* 12x trit. is specific."—Bayes).—Pain as from excoria- on and pricking as from pins (stitches) in throat, during deglutition (quinsy).—

Swelling of the uvula.—Swelling of the palate.—Difficult deglutition, as fr paralysis of the gullet.—Paralysis of velum palati.—Tendency of food to asce into nasal fossæ during deglutition.—Food is ejected through nose.

10. Appetite.—Great appetite ; desire for beer and warm food ; imme ately after eating, appetite and thirst returned.—Ravenous hunger so tha was difficult to fall asleep.—Ravenous hunger before supper, with compl loss of appetite and trembling of all the limbs, followed by chilliness a coldness over whole body, with heat on chest.—Ravenous hunger : mornin evening ; with collection of water in mouth.—Is very hungry ; eats as us and then complains that everything seems to be up in the throat.—Loss taste.—Bitter taste in mouth, also in morning.—Taste sour after eating Sour, putrid taste, or as if blood or mucus were in the mouth.—Violent thi sometimes with anorexia.—Repugnance to all food, esp. to cooked and things, with desire for cold, raw things only.—Aversion to boiled food Loathing of animal food, which proves indigestible.—Aversion of a child its mother's milk, with vomiting after sucking.—After a meal, strong dispo tion to sleep, pyrosis, acidity in mouth, sour risings, fulness in stomach abdomen, or else (often consecutively) aching of stomach, water-bra vomiting, febrile shiverings, congestion in head, heat in cheeks.

11. Stomach.—Risings, with taste of food, sometimes after every meal Sour risings.—Warm uprisings from stomach to throat.—Pyrosis.—Hiccoug before and after eating ; sometimes in evening, in bed.—Nausea, eve morning, with pain in head and eyes, on turning eyes, or else followed vomiting of bitter water.—Continuous nausea and vomiting ; < in morning Constant nausea and vomiting, even at night.—Water-brash, sometimes w shuddering.—Water tastes bad ; vomiting, whenever drink is taken.—Vomiti of food, even at night.—Pressure in stomach, sometimes after every meal, on drinking quickly.—Painful sensibility of scrobiculus, when it is pressed Heaviness in stomach.—Squeezing in scrobiculus, as by claws, sometin after a meal.—Burning sensation in pit of stomach.

12. Abdomen.—Swelling and induration of hepatic region.—Infla mation and induration of liver.—Pain, as from ulceration, in hepatic regi with throbbing ; pains are < by touch, by walking (or when lying on r. si or when breathing).—Shootings in hypochondria, esp. on the l. side.—Pain abdomen ; colic in children from worms.—Colic, during which hands t yellow, and the nails blue.—Aching (pressing) of abdomen, esp. after a me —Abdomen, hard, tight, hot (also in children) and sometimes painful on bei touched.—Enlargement of abdomen.—Colic, from constipation.—Cuttings pinching in abdomen, with or without diarrhœa.—Burning sensation abdomen.—The pains in the abdomen are > by application of hot linen Painful inguinal hernia.—Inflammation and swelling of inguinal glands (lar as peas, painful to touch).—Incarceration of flatus.—Gurgling and borboryg in abdomen, esp. on moving the body.—Difficult expulsion of flatus.—Ve offensive flatulence.

13. Stool and Anus.—Constipation, and slow, hard, difficult, kno fæces (composed of light-coloured lumps).—Hard fæces, with freque tenesmus.—Constipation where the stool comes down with great difficul comes a little way through the anus, and then slips back before it can voided ; obstructed evacuation of bowels ; fetid flatus.—Even the soft st xpelled with much difficulty.—Stool remains long in rectum.—Stool like ; with maw-worms; with tapeworms.—Fæces of consistence of pap, ral times a day.—Diarrhœa (stools horribly offensive) with colic.— dish fæces, or with sanguineous slime.—Frequent discharge of fetid m, of a corpse-like smell.—Cutting and stinging in rectum.—Burning or ging in rectum during stool.—Shootings and itching in anus, and in um, also during the evacuation.—Burning in anus, esp. after a dry, hard l.—Constriction in anus during stool.—Constant but ineffectual desire for l.—Painful hæmorrhoids protrude during stool.

4. **Urinary Organs.**—Urinary tenesmus.—Continued want to urinate, scanty emission (also at night).—Strangury.—Frequent (involuntary) ssion of urine, also at night (with distress from irritable sphincter).— ting the bed (at night).—Reddish sand, or yellow, gritty sediment in the e.—Stricture of urethra.

5. **Male Sexual Organs.**—Itching, and red spots on glans.—Exco- on, itching, and redness of prepuce.—Swelling of prepuce, which is red with itching and moist pimples.—Dropsical swelling of scrotum.— piration and itching in scrotum.—Itching, and moist spots on scrotum.— nce of sexual desire, with weakness in genital functions; or else oderate excitement of sexual desire, with numerous wanton ideas, and g and frequent erections.—Flow of prostatic fluid during urination; and ng of (hard) stool.—After coition, pain in limbs, as from fatigue, or tion of paralysis on one side of head.

. **Female Sexual Organs.**—Menses too early and too feeble, or else profuse.—Increased menses, with paroxysms of icy coldness over whole .—Suppression of the menses.—Discharge of blood before proper d; menses too late; protracted; blood acrid. — Metrorrhagia. — hœa, before the menses.—During the menses, pains in the abdomen, appearance of objects, or burning sensation and excoriation in vulva.— ng in the vulva.—Pressing-down feeling in vagina.—Itching, burning, soreness in pudenda; during menses.—Discharge of blood from the s, while suckling.—Abortion.—Leucorrhœa, which flows when urinating, ter the menses.—Leucorrhœa, like milk, flowing at intervals, and pre- l by gripings in umbilical region.—Acrid, corrosive leucorrhœa.—Inflam- n of nipples.—Darting burning pain in l. nipple.—Sticking pain in l. t.—Painful stitches behind l. breast, with chilliness, all night.—Sup- ion of the mammæ.—Abscess in breast, also with fistulous ulcers; nipple ates.—Indurations in breast.—R. breast hard, painful, and swollen at e, feeling as if "gathering."

. **Respiratory Organs.**—Hoarseness, with roughness and excoriation ynx.—Cough, from cold drinks, or from speaking even for a moment.— ng cough, excited by a suffocating tickling in pit of throat.—Cough and throat, with expectoration of little granules like shot, which, when n open, smell offensively (like *Phosphor.*, excepting the latter remedy hot feeling in throat.—H. N. G.).—Fatiguing cough, day and night, movement, with scanty expectoration of mucus.—Nocturnal, suffocating .—Spasmodic cough.—Hollow, spasmodic, suffocative cough from g in throat-pit, with expectoration only during day of profuse yellowish- pus, or of tough, milky, acrid mucus, at times of pale, frothy blood, generally tasting greasy and offensive-smelling.—Bruised pain in chest v coughing.—Dry cough, with pain in chest, as from excoriation.—Cough, vomiting of mucus.—Profuse expectoration of transparent mucus v coughing.—Cough with expectoration in the day, without expectoratic night.—Expectoration of pus, when coughing.—Expectoration of (frothy) blood, with deep, hollow cough.—Obstructed respiration, when on the back, or else when stooping, running, or coughing.—Deep, sig respiration.—Shortness of breath, during light manual labour, or else v walking quickly, sometimes with dyspnœa during repose.—Panting, r ration, on walking quickly.

18. **Chest.**—Oppression of chest, as from constriction of throat.—A in chest, sometimes only when coughing or sneezing.—Shooting and pri in chest and side, sometimes across back.—Throbbing in sternum.—Ph pulmonalis.—Contusive pain in chest, when drawing breath, or coughing

19. **Heart and Pulse.**—Palpitation and throbbing over whole while sitting.—Violent palpitation on every movement.—Imperceptible p

20. **Neck and Back.**—Purulent ulcer in nape.—Stiffness of nape ; headache.—Swelling of glands of nape, in the neck, and under the (with suppuration), sometimes with induration.—Pimples and furunc nape.—Suppuration of axillary glands.—Caries of clavicle.—Stitches bet the hips.—Coccyx painful, as after a long carriage ride.—Stinging coccygis on rising ; painful to pressure.—Scabby elevation on coccyx, fissure of nates.—Pain in the loins, whether the parts be touched or Spasmodic drawing in loins, which prevents rising up, and forces pati remain lying down.—Inflammatory abscess in lumbar region (on the muscle).—Weakness and paralytic stiffness in back, loins, and nape.— ings and shootings in the back.—Shootings in the loins, when seated or down.—Burning in back when walking in open air and becoming wa Aching, shooting, burning, and throbbing in lumbo-sacral region.—Sw and distortion of spine (curvature of the vertebræ).—Contusive pain be the shoulder-blades.

21. **Limbs.**—Drawing, tearing, and shooting in limbs (arms and le Nocturnal shooting in all joints.—Liability of limbs to become numbed to sleep easily).—Pain in limbs, as though they had been broken, and pa weakness, esp. in evening.—Cramps in arms and legs.—Icy-cold leg feet.—Jerks in limbs, day and night.—Weakness of joints (they giv when walking).—Lassitude and trembling in limbs, esp. in morning.— ness and lameness in limbs.—Nails dirty yellow, crippled and brittle.— about nails.

22. **Upper Limbs.**—Drawings and tearings in arms, hands and fi —Heaviness and paralytic weakness of arms, which tremble on least ex —Numbness of the (fore-) arms when patient is lying upon them or l the elbows on a table.—Throbbing and jerking of muscles of arm.—R ness and trembling in r. arm.—Skin cracked, on arms and hands.—Fur and warts on arms.—Paralytic weakness of the forearm ; everyth dropped from the hands.—Induration of the cellular tissue of the fore Nocturnal shootings in wrist, extending to the top of arm.—Tearing p wrists and ball of hand.—Spasmodic pain in the hands and fingers.— ness of hands at night.—Paralytic weakness of hands.—Tonic spasm o

when writing.—Cramp-like pain and lameness of hand after slight exertion.—Profuse sweat of the hands.—Ganglion on back of hand.—Ulcer on back of hand.—Tingling in fingers.—Burning sensation in ends of fingers.—Pain in joints of fingers, when pressed.—Weakness, rigidity, and want of flexibility in fingers.—Contraction of flexor tendons ; very painful when moving fingers.—Ganglion.—(Ganglion on wrist.—R. T. C.).—Gnawing, purulent vesicles, with burning in fingers.—Tearing, drawing, sticking pain and numbness in fingers, as if suppurating, or as if a panaritium would form.—Numb feeling of a finger, as though it were enlarged and the bone swollen.—Pain as from a splinter in flexor surface of one finger.—Panaritium, esp. with vegetations, cries and insupportable pains day and night.—Finger-nails rough and yellow.—Nails dirty grey as if decayed ; powder when cut and split into layers.—White spots on nails.—Dryness in tips of fingers ; afternoon.

23. **Lower Limbs.**—Tearing, stitching pains in hips and thighs.—Suppurating pains in hip-joint.—Drawing, tearing, and tension in the legs (extending from the hips to the feet).—Easy numbing of the limbs, esp. when seated.—Paralytic weakness of legs.—Pressure, tearing, and shootings in muscles of thighs.—Itching ulcers in thighs and ankles.—Furunculi on thighs and calves of legs.—Softening and ulceration of femur.—Tearings in knee (when sitting, > from motion).—Knee is painful, as if too tightly bound.—Inflammatory swelling of knee.—Fungus in knee.—Drawing pain in legs.—Coldness of legs.—Swelling of legs as far as the feet.—Ulcer on leg, with sticking, burning pains.—Ulcers in the legs, often with sickly complexion.—Red, smarting spot on the tibia.—Caries of the tibia.—Ulcers on lower leg, on tibia.—Tension of calves of legs, as from contraction.—Cramps in calves, esp. in evening, after corporeal labour.—Torpor of calves of legs.—Itching miliary eruption on calves.—Tearing and shootings in calves, heels, and toes.—Lancination in ankle, when treading, or resting on foot.—Numbness of feet in evening.—Coldness of feet, sometimes after suppressed perspiration of feet.—Burning sensation in feet and soles, esp. in evening and at night.—Swelling of feet, generally in morning.—Offensive smell from feet (intolerable carrion-like ; without sweat, every evening).—Profuse, offensive perspiration on feet, with excoriation (and blisters) between the toes.—Suppressed perspiration on feet.—Hard and painful callosities on soles.—Voluptuous tickling in soles, which, when the part has been scratched a little, is almost maddening.—Cramp in the soles of feet.—Gnawing vesicles in heel.—Corrosive ulcer on heel, with itching.—Stiffness of toes.—Constant, violent boring or tearing in great toes.—Ulceration of great toe, with shooting pain.—Bunion.—Itching, suppurating scabs on toes.—Ingrowing toenail ; offensive discharge.—Corns in the feet, with shooting pains ; also under toenails.

24. **Generalities.**—[Affections in general of any kind appearing chiefly in light-haired people ; in r. side ; l. side ; back ; l. lower extremity ; scalp ; external head behind the ears ; external surface of inguinal ring ; inguinal ring and hernia of long standing ; finger-nails, esp. if there are white spots on the nails.—Griping pains with a tearing away feeling, of twisting or of writhing ; or as if something were being torn away.—Sensation of heaviness in inner parts.—Jerking pains.—Debility ; weakness of joints, esp. of ankle-joints.—< In night, chiefly in latter part ; in open air ; in children of *Silica* temperament where they are sickly, have worms, &c. ; when single parts are

cold; from taking cold in the feet; with profuse salivation; on uncovering; from a draught of air; after eating; after drinking; lying on painful side; looking fixedly at an object; from wine; from outward pressure; from reading; stepping heavily on ground or floor; in stonecutters; when the weather changes; from getting feet wet; from worm troubles of any kind; when writing; from uncovering head.—> From wrapping head up; in the room.—H. N. G.].—Tendency to strain back.—Swelling and induration of glands, generally without pain, only sometimes with troublesome itching.—Acid, corrosive discharges.—Trembling when writing.—Epileptic fits; starting, distortion of eyes, twitching of lips, lolling of tongue, stretching and distortion of head and limbs.—Several affections and pains are <, and manifest themselves, at night, and in evening, also during movement.—Symptoms < at new or full moon.—Pains on change of weather.—Feeling as if knives were running into her.—Uneasiness in whole hody, after having been long seated.—Ebullition of blood, and thirst, after drinking wine.—Excessive emaciation.—Children are slow in learning to walk.—Careless, slovenly gait.—General inertia and great nervous debility.—Syncope, when lying on side.—Great fatigue, lassitude, and drowsiness, on approach of a storm.—Strong tendency to suffer from chills, even from the mere uncovering of the feet.—Want of vital warmth even when taking exercise.

25. **Skin.**—Painful sensibility of skin.—Itching over whole body, which is of a crawling or shooting kind (< at night).—Eruption like varicella over whole body.—Tuberous spots on skin, of a light red colour.—Lymphatic swellings and abscesses, even with fistulous ulcers.—Engorgement, induration, and suppuration of the glands.—Painless swelling of the glands; they only cause very unpleasant itching.—Bones very sensitive and tender to touch; bending and caries of bones.—Abscesses which do not break, but burrow under the skin; exanthemata in general which corrode and spread; old and difficult to heal; which itch; fungus articularis; hæmatodes; spongy excrescences.—Tetters in general; corroding and spreading.—Ulcers in general, wherever pus is discharged from any part of the body, or when appearing in the urine; ulcers burning, scabby; indolent; when circumscribed with redness; very high, hard ulcers; with proud flesh; with corroding pus.—Ulcers of all kinds, also after the abuse of *Mercury*.—Ulcers smell very offensive.—Cancerous ulcers.—Inflammation, softening (swelling), and ulceration of bones.—Scirrhous indurations.—Ulcers, which are fistulous, putrid, phagedenic, fungous, &c., with vegetation, or fetid and corroding sanies.—Fistulous openings; parts around hard, swollen, bluish-red.—Mild and malignant suppurations, esp. in membranous parts.—Unhealthy skin; every injury tends to ulceration.—Small wounds heal with difficulty, and suppurate profusely.—Painful pustular eruptions; at last forming suppurating ulcers; on forehead, occiput, sternum, and spine.—Aching, itching, smarting, and boring shootings in the ulcers.—Furunculi.—Carbuncles of a malignant kind.—Ganglions.—Warts.—Panaritium.

26. **Sleep.**—Great sleepiness after eating.—Sleepiness all day.—Excessive sleepiness, without being able to go to sleep.—Frequent yawnings.—Sleep early in the evening.—Retarded sleep.—Sleep too light at night, like dozing.—Not being able to sleep again after waking.—Sleeplessness in general, esp. after midnight.—Talking in sleep.—Sleepless after 2 a.m., with rush of thoughts —

Sleeplessness, caused esp. by ebullition of blood, heat in head, and great flow of ideas.—Frightful visions at night, and many anxious and fantastic dreams, with tears, talking, cries, and frequent waking with a start.—Awakens with erections and desire to urinate.—Jerking of body during sleep.—Lascivious dreams (with emissions).—Snoring while sleeping.—Nightmare.—Somnambulism (gets up while asleep, walks about, and lies down again).—Dreams of robbers, assassins, dogs, voyages, spectres, &c.—At night, congestion of blood in head, with pulsative pains, and throbbing in brain, pain in stomach, nausea and vomiting, or shootings in all the joints, dryness of nose and many other sufferings.

27. **Fever.**—Pulse : small, hard and rapid, frequently irregular and then slow.—The circulation is easily agitated.—Violent chill, evening, in bed, < from uncovering oneself.—Continuous internal chill, with want of animal heat.—Chill in evening with sensation as if cold air were blowing around waist ; not > by wrapping up ; followed by severe fever and perspiration.—Constant chilliness, even when exercising or in a warm room.—Excessively chilly disposition, and shuddering, with frequent shiverings, also on the least movement.—Heat predominates.—Frequently during day short flushes of heat, principally in face.—Violent general heat, with violent thirst in afternoon, evening, and all night.—Periodically returning heat during day, without any previous chill, and followed by slight perspiration.—Perspiration from slight exercise ; most profuse on head and face.—Perspiration only on the head.—Fever, with violent heat in head ; afternoons ; at night, with thirst and catching inspiration.—The perspiration comes periodically ; is < 11 p.m., 6 a.m., or 3 to 5 p.m.—Intermittent fever, heat predominating.—Frequent heat, sometimes transient.—Fever, with excessive heat, generally without shivering, and with little perspiration, commonly from 10 a.m. till 8 p.m.—Perspiration during a moderate walk.—Profuse perspiration at night, sometimes of an (offensive or) acid smell.—Debilitating perspiration in morning.

Silica Marina.

Silica maritima. Sea sand. Trituration. [My preparation was taken from the beach, just as it was left by the tide, on a part of the coast many miles distant from a river estuary or a drained town.]

Clinical.—Constipation. Glands, enlargement of ; suppuration of. Gonorrhœa. Tartar.

Characteristics.—Having seen a statement that *Sil. mar.* had a pronounced action on inflamed glands, I had a specimen triturated and run up to the 30th attenuation. I had not long to wait for an opportunity of testing it. A tall, fair young man of 24, a violinist, presented himself with a mass of scrofulous glands on the right side of the neck softening at one point. I gave him *Sil. mar.* 3, gr. v., three or four times a day, and warned him not to poultice. The mass of glands soon began to diminish. The abscess matured and discharged itself through a minute opening, and eventually healed without leaving a perceptible scar. The rest of the glands in the meantime disappeared. *Sil. mar.* 3, gr. v., three times a day, rapidly cured a case of gonorrhœa in a patient who had had many previous attacks, as well as stricture which had been treated with cauterisations and strong *Arg. nit.* It was this history which partly led me to give the remedy on account of the *Nat. mur.* element contained in it. The discharge was creamy, and there was tenderness in the middle of the urethra. For three days after commencing the *Sil. mar.* there was a sharp aggravation, the discharge became very profuse, was < at night and accompanied by painful erections. In a general way I use this preparation where *Nat. mur.* symptoms are present in a *Sil.* case. Burnett told me an interesting experience of his. He was consulted about a boy who persisted, in spite of punishment, in eating sand when playing on the beach. Burnett advised the parents to let the boy eat as much as he liked. He kept it up for a fortnight, at the end of which time he was vastly improved in health, and he neither wanted nor ate any more sand from that day. W. B. Clarke, of Indianopolis (*A. H.*, xxvi. 237) tells of the use of *Sil. mar.* as a remedy for constipation. He has used it in patients of all ages with excellent results, giving it crude. He prefers the rather coarse sand taken from a river sand-bar. This is thoroughly washed and baked in an oven. He thinks a finer variety may be better for younger patients. The sand is taken plain, or enclosed in capsules, or made into pills. In either case it is washed down with water, and water is to be drunk freely during the treatment. W. B. Clarke mentions this case as the hardest he had encountered: A man, 60, had suffered for thirty years with severe constipation, often sitting at stool for an hour and nearly fainting. He took a teaspoonful after dinner daily for a week, without particular effect. Then he took it three times a day for a week. After this he was able to return to the one dose a day, and soon required it but once a week. "The peculiarity of this treatment is the ease with which evacuation is accomplished after the first impression is made, the discharges being soft, mushy, and yellow, and the regular habit then seems established, for the treatment can then be discontinued." If there is any return of the trouble, a dose or two more will be sufficient to put it right. This experience is of great value and interest as *Sil.* in the potencies (as well as *Nat. m.*) is a great constipation remedy. W. B. Clarke has never observed any ill effects of the treatment. In the case of a child, æt. 4, to whom Cooper gave *Sil. mar.* 6x (my preparation) "a thick mass of tartar which had accumulated behind the front teeth came away in flakes."

Silphium.

Silphium laciniatum. Compass-plant. Pilot-weed. Polar-plant. Rosin-wood. Turpentine-weed. *N. O.* Compositæ. Tincture of fresh plant.

Clinical.—Asthma. Bladder, catarrh of. Bronchitis. Cancer.

Characteristics.—The leaves of this plant, when they first come up, present their faces uniformly north and south; later on, when the leaves become heavy, the winds carry them in different directions and the polarity is not to be observed. The stem of the plant exudes an abundance of resin, as some of its names indicate. Hale mentions that it has been used in all forms of asthma; and in chronic bronchitis with large quantities of stringy, frothy, light-coloured mucus, and in catarrh of the bladder. Hale made a proving of it, and his symptoms comprise the Schema. He gives this case: Mr. H., 55, had phthisis twenty years. On the slightest exposure or cold he would have congestion of mucous surfaces, followed with copious expectoration of stringy, frothy, light-coloured mucus (from one to three pints in twenty-four hours), causing rapid exhaustion and at times keeping him in bed for weeks. *Silph.* 2x trit. was used, gr. 2 every two hours. During the next night less than a teacupful of mucus was raised, and its sudden decrease alarmed the patient so much that he left off the remedy until his doctor assured him that he was very much better, and that the remedy had been more successful than he himself had expected. Cooper has used *Silph.* (in single doses of ϕ) with notable effect in cases of cancer of the throat and mouth. The great "goneness" of the proving shows a relation to the cancer cachexia.

SYMPTOMS.

5. **Nose.**—Irritation extends from throat up posterior nares to nose causing sneezing, followed by discharge of limpid, acrid mucus, attended with constriction and pressure in supraorbital region.

8. **Mouth.**—Tongue: whitish slimy coat, with dry sensation as if burned with hot soup.

9. **Throat.**—Scraping, tickling, and irritation of fauces and throat.—Desire to hawk and scrape throat and throw off a thin viscid mucus.—Engorgement and thickening of mucous membrane of throat extending down.

11. **Stomach.**—Nausea, sick, faint feeling, and a sense of *goneness* in epigastrium.

13. **Stool.**—Stool natural, but covered with slimy mucus.

14. **Urinary Organs.**—Urine: high-coloured, scanty. — Frequent micturition, with sense of heat or burning at meatus during micturition.

17. **Respiratory Organs.**—Rough cough, attended with expectoration of yellow mucus.

18. **Chest.**—Constriction and tightness of lungs, with constant disposition to raise; hacking, spasmodic cough.

Sinapis Alba.

Brassica alba. White Mustard. Senf-Kohl. *N. O.* Cruciferæ. Trituration and tincture of the seeds.

Clinical.—Anus, itching of; affections of. Flatulence. Gastric ulcer. Gastritis. Headache. Heartburn. Lactation, dyspepsia of; sore mouth of. Mouth, inflammation of; ulceration of. Œsophagus. Pregnancy, dyspepsia of; sore mouth of. Salivation. Threadworms. Vomiting. Worms.

Characteristics.—*Sin. alb.*, like *Sin. nig.*, is indigenous in Great Britain. "Its seeds are larger than those of Black Mustard, and of a yellow colour externally. Chemically they differ in containing a crystalline substance known as sulpho-sinapisin. Moreover, its myrosine yields with water a pungent oil of a different character from the Volatile Oil of Mustard" obtained from *Sin. nig.* (*Treas. of Bot.*). The seed-leaves or cotyledons of *Sin. alb.* furnish the "mustard" of "mustard and cress"—the "cress" being *Lepidium sativum*. Bojanus proved *Sin. alb.*, taking substantial doses of the triturated seeds and of a tincture made therefrom. The well-known emetic effects of mustard were produced by it, and also its "burning" sensations in many parts, notably anus, stomach, and œsophagus. Flatulence, headache, (> walking in open air; < in warm room) and salivation were among the observed effects. Under *Sin. alb.* the prover, who had had no sign of threadworms since his thirteenth year, passed many both living and dead; and had all the usual rectal symptoms which accompany their presence. The urine, too, was turbid, as is often the case in helminthiasis. A. L. Fisher (*Med. Vis.*, xiii. 316) says that for twenty years *Sin. alb.* has had a prominent place in his armamentarium. He has used it on the indications of the proving, and he found that the conditions of pregnancy and lactation seem to favour the development of the conditions calling for it. He has verified these: "Excessive accumulation of watery saliva or mucus." "Acute bruised pain, even on slight pressure, just beneath ensiform cartilage." "Vomiting, ejecta consisting of flakes of mucus with blackish veins like clots of blood." "Crawling and burning in anus, with griping in abdomen." "Spasmodic griping in anus, appearing at intervals, and especially noticed after swallowing anything." He has cured with *Sin. alb.* "Sore mouth with intensely red mucous membrane, dotted with minute white ulcers, the least food, even of blandest character, increasing the burning that is present all the time, and also in the throat." *Sin. alb.* has a number of *Peculiar Sensations:* As if head hollow. As of a plug in throat; of hard substance high up in œsophagus under manubrium sterni; something hard lying in stomach, after a moderate meal; hard substance in rectum not > by stool. Bojanus noticed an alternation between the symptoms of the anus and those of the pharynx. I have cured with *Sin. alb.*: "Sharp, shooting pain in right frontal eminence, < in warm room, > moving about and in open air." The symptoms are < by touch. < Pressure. < Motion. > Rest. < Swallowing (crawling in anus). < After eating (sensation of hard substance in stomach). < Warm room. > Rest. > Open air.

Relations.—[An overdose of table Mustard, which contains both Sin. alb. and Sin. nig., with starch, &c., is immediately antidoted by smelling bread.] *Compare:* Sin. n. Plug sensation, Anac. Ball in anus, Sep. Lump in stomach, Bry., Ab. n., Nux, Pul. Helminthiasis, Teucr., Sant., Cin., Naphth., Scirrh.

SYMPTOMS.

1. **Mind.**—Distracted in mind, while reading must make great efforts to keep thoughts from wandering.

2. **Head.**—Dulness, with obscured vision, esp. of forehead over eyes;

< walking.—Sensation as if head hollow.—Rush of blood to head.—Headache > in open air < in warm room.—Heaviness in forehead, as from intoxication, or too great warmth of room.—Pain in l. frontal eminence, paroxysmal, pressive, in the evening.—Pressive pain in r. frontal eminence < moving head back and forth.

3. **Eyes.**—Sudden sensation of warmth with stitching in l. eye compelling winking; eye fills with tears, after which the sensation disappears.

8. **Mouth.**—Root of tongue thickly coated yellow on rising in morning; later extends along sides, esp. l.—Profuse salivation; with nausea; nausea > at rest, < walking about.—Saliva frothy, salt.

9. **Throat.**—Scraping in fauces, provoking frequent hawking.—Sensation as if a large morsel of food had been swallowed.—Burning: in pharnyx; in œsophagus rising up from stomach like heartburn; and pressure in œsophagus.—Sensation of hard body high up in œsophagus; < swallowing hard food and on empty swallowing; in afternoon seems as if a plug sticking in pharynx (this sensation alternated with biting and crawling in anus).—Sensation of constriction on swallowing hard food.

11. **Stomach.**—Thirst with heartburn.—Thirst without heartburn; drinking water = sensation of heaviness and fulness in abdomen as after eating.—Eructations: frequent, tasteless and odourless; of acid liquid with griping scalding in pharynx; aggravating the heartburn; tasting of food.—Heartburn: violent; with eructations.—Nausea; qualmishness; inclination to vomit; salivation.—Nausea > at rest, < by movement.—Retching and vomiting of water, with violent retching and burning in stomach and abdomen, extending to both sides under false ribs and whole chest with extreme discomfort and anxiety in stomach-pit.—Vomits: Flakes of mucus with blackish streaks; yellow, odourless, tasteless matter, with much tenacious, jelly-like mucus.—After vomiting, scraping in throat and burning rising from stomach.—Burning; pressure; fulness and distension in pit of stomach.—Pit of stomach painful to pressure.—Very acute bruised pain, even on slight pressure, in pit of stomach, just beneath ensiform cartilage; pressure on it took away the breath.

12. **Abdomen.**—Rumbling and gurgling, with emission of odourless flatus.—Emission of offensive flatus.—Griping colic.—Movements in abdomen.—Heaviness as of a weight, fulness and distension in abdomen.

13. **Stool and Anus.**—Sensation as though a hard substance were lying in anus and could not be evacuated; not > by stool.—Burning in anus, obliging to scratch.—Violent, sudden stitch in anus, obliging him to cry out.—Burning; burning itching in anus.—Spasmodic griping in anus, appearing at intervals, < after swallowing anything.—Immediately after a stool, sprained sensation, as though anus were drawn up into rectum, with sticking, itching, burning and biting in anus.—Sensation as if something hard were lying just by anus, soon followed by a stool, which, however, was evacuated only with great pressure and was unsatisfactory; first part hard, crumbling, dark brownish green, covered with mucus and containing threadworms, followed by the same sensation as before the stool.—Crawling biting in anus.—Stool: blackish, hard, covered with mucus, followed by prickling burning in anus; small, thin, soft, greenish, with dead threadworms; copious, pasty, partly hard partly soft, sour, fermented; yellowish grey.

14. Urinary Organs.—Urine: dark yellow, soon forming transparent cloud; bright golden yellow; dark-brown like beer.—The urine has a cloud of mucus, and contains numerous small granules looking like frog-spawn; on the surface of the urine, at the bottom and on the sides of the glass, a number of small red granules.—Many grains of red sand deposited, and iridescent film on surface.—Thick, fatty pellicle.—Cloud remains suspended in urine.—Sediment: white; flocculent; like chalk, and containing grains of white sand.

15. Male Sexual Organs.—Emissions, without lascivious dreams.

18. Chest.—Oppression of chest compelling frequent deep breathing.—Burning beneath sternum.

20. Back.—Pains in small of back and coccyx, as if sprained and bruised, with urging to stool.

23. Lower Limbs.—Heaviness in lower limbs.

26. Sleep.—Sleep: in afternoon with vivid dreams; after eating.—Vivid dreams of dead people and of death.—Dreams: confused and unremembered; of foreign countries and dangerous expeditions.

27. Fever.—Pulse full and hard.—Creeping chills on moving about; over whole body after vomiting, with coldness of hands and feet and frequent eructations of gas.—Inclined to perspire.

Sinapis Nigra.

Brassica nigra. Black Mustard. *N. O.* Cruciferæ. Trituration and tincture of seeds.

Clinical.—Amenorrhœa. Apoplexy. Asthma, pituitous. Catarrh. Chlorosis. Chordee. Chorea. Constipation. Coryza. Cough. Diarrhœa. Hæmorrhoids. Hay-fever. Headache, dull, heavy. Heartburn. Hiccough. Intermittents. Menses, premature. Mucous fever. Post-nasal catarrh. Priapism. Scurvy. Variola.

Characteristics.—"*Sin. nig.* yields the greater part of the condiment so generally used in this country. The plant is indigenous, but is nevertheless largely cultivated in Yorkshire and Durham. The seeds are of a reddish-brown colour. Mixed with those of *Sin. a.* they are crushed between rollers, and subsequently powdered and sifted twice or oftener. From the residue left on the sieve a fixed oil is obtained by pressure. The powdered mustard is usually mixed with a considerably quantity of wheaten flour and a small quantity of turmeric powder. The term 'flour of mustard' is not quite accurate, as the mustard seeds themselves contain little or no starchy material. The chemical ingredients are somewat complex. Among them are a peculiar acid called *Myronic acid*, noticeable as containing a large proportion of *Sulphur*, and which, when mixed with water and a peculiar substance called *Myrosine* (analogous to albumen), also found in mustard seeds, yields a volatile Oil of Mustard, which has no separate existence in the seeds, but is formed artificially in the manner just stated. This oil is very acrid, and has been used as a rubefacient. The fixed oil before mentioned as existing in the seed itself has little or no acridity, and has been used as a purgative and vermifuge" (*Treas. of Bot.*). *Thiosinamine*, which is extracted from Oil of Mustard, belongs to the same group os Urea. It has been used in cheloid, and for removing scar tissue, and so in tinnitus aurium (Spencer, *H.M.*, Jan., 1899). As the chemical constituents of the two mustards (see *Sin. alb.*) are not identical, and as they have been proved independently, I have kept them separate. The yellow colour of mustard suggests *Sulphur*, a large amount of which is contained in the seeds. Like many other Crucifers *Sin. n.* has antiscorbutic properties; and it has cured cases of ague; mucous fever; catarrh of bladder, of stomach, and of air passages. It is in the treatment of hay-fever that it has been most used. The special indications are: Mucous membrane dry and hot; no discharge; < afternoon and evening; either nostril may be affected alone, or they may be affected alternately. Hansen adds these: "Acute coryza with thin, watery, excoriating discharge, lachrymation, sneezing. hacking cough, > lying down. Acute pharyngitis, throat feels scalded, hot, inflamed. Loud coughing spells with barking expiration, heard at a great distance. Cooper (*H. W.*, xxxvi. 16) suggests the use of *Sin. n.* as an aperient. He considers that the chief agent in effecting dislodgement of fæces in constipated states is flatus. His method of producing this is as follows: A tumblerful of hot water is to be taken in sips in the early morning; the same at breakfast time with some plain brown bread or with no solid food at all, and at 11 a.m. one or two capsules of pure mustard (*Sin n.*), each containing about five grains of the powder, to be taken, followed by half a tumbler of hot water. "This last is most important, as the water drives on the capsule and prevents its lodgement about the cardiac orifice of the stomach and consequent distress to the patient; and it also causes contraction of the walls of the stomach and consequent expulsion of flatus into the duodenum." *Peculiar Sensations* of *Sin. n.* are: Vertex as if empty. As if she had taken cold. As if scalp was adherent to bones. As of pins sticking in eyeballs. Eyeballs as if pressed on from above. As if nostrils stopped up. As if movements impeded all round the chest. As if something heavy oppressed her on all sides from neck to diaphragm. As if cheeks were bulged out by a bubble of air below malar bone. Skin of lips as if stiff. As if blisters on tip of tongue. As if a load on stomach. Pain as if heart were on right side. As of hot water in blood-vessels.—"Sweat on upper lip and forehead" is a symptom worth noting; also these: mucus hawked or coughed from posterior nares felt *cold*. The symptoms are < by touch and pressure. > Lying down at night. < Leaning forward; stooping motion <. Damp weather <. > Sitting erect. < In warm room. < Thinking of symptoms; > by study or mental diversion. > Shutting eyes. > Hearty meal. Laughing = cough. < Evening, 4–6 p.m. and 7 to 9 p.m. < July and August.

Relations.—*Antidoted by:* Smelling bread (immediate effects of taking excess of condiment). Nux, Rhus; when blistering has been produced by a mustard poultice, soap is the remedy. *Compare:*

Sin. a., Thios., Armor. Scalded sensation on tongue, Sang. Cough < laughing, Arg. n., Pho. Cough > lying down, Fer., Mang. < From 4 to 6 p.m., Lyc. Amenorrhœa, Sul., Pul. As if hot water in blood-vessels (Rhus as if blood running cold).

Causation.—Damp weather. Summer season.

SYMPTOMS.

1. **Mind.**—Irritable ; difficult to think and study.—Unreasonably cross. —Mind worked rapidly.

2. **Head.**—Vertigo : of old people ; violent attacks, with hard hearing after eating heavy food ; esp. fat.—Head dull, heavy, > when mind occupied by study ; > shutting eyes ; > in open air ; < in warm room ; < when thinking of it.—Dull feeling in vertex as if empty.—Frontal headache, most over bridge of nose and round edge of orbits, > when eating, < after eating ; > by rest.—Headache over r. eye < stooping.—Heavy, drawing feeling in r. temple towards night.—Sensation as if scalp were adherent to bones. —Forehead hot and dry.

3. **Eyes.**—Eyes feel weak ; pressure = pricking in them.—Pressing feeling in eyes as from above, difficult to keep lids open ; > shutting eyes ; > by hearty meal.

5. **Nose.**—Symptoms of a severe cold.—Immediately on touching the tongue pungent odour went into nostrils causing sneezing.—Dryness in both nostrils, < l., tender to pressure ; discharged some mucus.—L. nostril stopped up : in afternoon and evening ; all day, scanty discharges, acrid, making skin smart.—Scurvy with copious and frequent nose-bleed.

6. **Face.**—Shrunken features.—Burning prickling in face.—Red round mouth with smarting of lips.—Sensation as if cheek were bulged outward by a bubble of air, just below malar bone, in afternoon.—Lips dry and feel as if integuments were stiff.

8. **Mouth.**—Teeth sensitive to warm drinks and cold air, esp. stopped teeth.—Swollen bleeding gums.—Tongue : fissure in middle line ; dirty white coat in middle ; sore, raw, also gums, could not bear to eat anything hard ; dry and sticky ; burning scalding feeling ; fore part feels blistered.—Black tongue.—Breath offensive, as after eating onions.—Mouth : dry ; burning, extending to stomach.—Profuse saliva.—During proving, mustard (of which he was usually very fond) had a very unpleasant taste, and nearly caused nausea.—Taste : of garlic, causing nausea ; of horseradish.

9. **Throat.**—Dry sensation back of nose and throat > by swallowing or by efforts to cough, which brings up with difficulty a little white, tenacious mucus, in lumps.—Throat sore, left side, on swallowing saliva, less on swallowing food or drink, whole throat behind uvula injected light red.—Sore throat r. side extending to l.

11. **Stomach.**—Appetite good.—Aversion to sweets.—Eructations : of gas ; constantly accompanying other symptoms ; all food tasting of horseradish, later tasteless.—Hiccough.—Heartburn and belching.—Stomach : load in ; burning in.—Ulceration of stomach and intestines.—Pain in region

stomach with sensation of faintness compelling to bend forward, which ,—Dull pain running directly across epigastric region < leaning forward sitting erect.—Pressure in epigastric region.

12. **Abdomen.**—Dull pain in l. hypochondriac region.—Heavy, dull in as from weight below umbilical region.—Severe twisting in umbilical gion.—Pain from l. of umbilical region to l. iliac region ; later to r. side, cending colon.—Accumulation of flatus with twinges of pain about ıbilicus.—Rumbling.—L. inguinal gland swollen and painful.—Sharp pain r. inguinal gland.—Dull pain in r. inguinal region > by pressure.

13. **Stool and Anus.**—Smarting, cutting pain low down in anus, after stool.—Desire for a stool without passage.—Diarrhœa.—Stools offensive.—rst stool normal, second loose.—Before stool uneasy feeling in rectum; ter stool, smarting cutting low down in rectum and anus.—Constipated; ools hard, like balls.—(Constipation and piles cured in the proving.)

14. **Urinary Organs.**—Pain in bladder, in morning, before urina-g.—Desire frequent ; flow increased.—Urine, pale, straw-coloured, without diment.

15. **Male Sexual Organs.**—Violent erections during day and night; stinate, painful, and continued.—Awakening him at night ; with lascivious oughts ; lascivious dreams and emissions at night.

16. **Female Sexual Organs.**—Menses appear in a few hours long fore the proper time (several cases).—Amenorrhœa and chlorosis.—ssation of catamenia.

17. **Respiratory Organs.**—Hoarseness, evening from 4 p.m.—Cough, ort, hacking ; all evening ; 7 to 8 p.m. ; seldom during day.—Cough mostly y or with expectoration of lumps of mucus < in cold air ; > lying down d (temporarily) by eating; excited by laughing.—Expectoration: from sterior nares much mucus, which felt cold ; white, in tenacious masses.—phyxia.—Pituitous asthma.

18. **Chest.**—Wandering pains in chest.—Pain in l. side of chest in gion of heart.—Respiration at base of l. lung roughened.—Sensation in chest as if heart were on r. side.

19. **Heart.**—Dull, continual pain in heart toward apex, in evening; emingly in heart substance.—Heart pains return daily 10 a.m. and 4 to 6 n.—Sensation as if heart were on r. side.—Pulse : accelerated ; full.

20. **Back.**—Severe, dull, pulsating pain under inferior angle of l. scapula. Slight bachache, becoming intolerable towards bedtime ; restless all night om pain in back and hips ; > motion.

21. **Limbs.**—Weariness in limbs with cramps in calves.

22. **Upper Limbs.**—Occasional dull pain in left shoulder-joint.

23. **Lower Limbs.**—Weakness in calf-muscles.—Dull, heavy ache in gs.—Pain constant in ankles and calves.

24. **Generalities.**—It seemed to double him up ; could hardly stand ; ırs ran from eyes ; intense pain across epigastric region.—Rose late, feeling re and stiff all over.—Weakness in all muscles.—Symptoms < 7 to 9 p.m. ; lying down at night, except dreams.

25. **Skin.**—Skin turns red.—Burning heat and stitches in skin.—Frightful ppuration and gangrenous inflammation reaching down to sternum (fatal ects of mustard applied to swollen glands of neck).—General ecchymosis.—

Chronic eczema.—Small-pox; ("to be given until sulphocyanides appe in the saliva").—Ulcers on legs.

26. **Sleep.**—Sleepiness; during day, sleepless at night.—Sleeps little night, but does not feel loss of sleep.—Dreams: vivid; or lascivious.

27. **Fever.**—Severe chills, chattering of teeth, sensation of gene coldness, with shrunken feeling (from mustard bath).—Heat through who body, esp. down spine.—Quartan ague and inflammatory fever.—Sweat a feeling of hot water in all blood-vessels, > when menses came on.—Sw general; esp. on forehead and upper lip.—Sweat free on exertion (mental physical), and from external heat.

Sium.

Sium latifolium. Water-parsnip. *N. O.* Umbelliferæ. Tincture of root.

Clinical.—Convulsions. Tetanus.

Characteristics.—Our knowledge of Water-parsnip is deriv from cases of poisoning through eating the root. The symptoms be a strong resemblance to those of the other poisonous Umbellifer The most pronounced features of the convulsions of *Sium* were t drawing of the arms to the middle of the body, flexure of the finge and the preponderance of the contractions on the left side. T lack of mental energy recalls the action of *Æthusa*.

SYMPTOMS.

1. **Mind.**—Much excited.—Fear of death.—Lack of mental activity.

2. **Head.**—Dizziness; headache.

3. **Eyes.**—Pupils dilated, responded steadily to bright light.

9. **Throat.**—Burning along alimentary tract, esp. œsophagus.

11. **Stomach.**—Nausea and vomiting, at end of which he fell int convulsion.

12. **Abdomen.**—Sense of swelling and flatulence about bowels.

17. **Respiratory Organs.**—Breathing slow and stertorous.

24. **Generalities.**—Muscles in a state of tonic contraction; arms dra to middle of body; fingers flexed; opisthotonos; greater contraction of musc of l. side than of r.—Every few minutes spasms, at first violently clo diminishing with each succeeding convulsion till they became little m than tremors; by degrees the character changed until the last one (in wh circulation and respiration ceased), which was a pure tonic spasm.—Loss voluntary motion.—Prostration.

27. **Fever.**—Skin cold and clammy.—Head hot, rest of body colc Wet with perspiration.

Skookum Chuck.

Skookum Limechen Chuck ("Strong Medicine Water"). Medical Lake. A lake in Western U.S. containing in grains per gallon: Sodic carbonate 63·54, Sodic chloride 16·37, Sodic silicate 10·63, Potassic chloride 9·24, Ferrous carbonate ·526, Magnesia carbonate ·237, Calcic carbonate ·186, Aluminic oxide ·175, with traces of Lithic carbonate, Borax, and Potassic sulphate. Trituration of the dried salt.

Clinical.—Breast, tumour of. Catarrh. Eczema; vaccinal. Hay-fever. Lithæmia. Ozæna. Rheumatism. Urticaria. Vaccination.

Characteristics.—The information respecting the remedy known by the Indian name, *Skookum chuck* (which I will shorten into *Skoo.*), is collected in *New, Old, and Forgotten Remedies*. Gentry introduced it to homœopathy in an article in *U.S. Med. Month.*, 1889. He commenced to prove it, but the severity of the catarrhal symptoms led to its discontinuance. Gentry has himself cured with *Skoo.* many cases of catarrh, and he considers it a remedy in hay-fever. The cure of many cases of inveterate skin disease is on record; the external use of *Skoo.* soap or ointment has been employed as well as the internal administration. D. de F. Cole gave *Skoo.* 3x in water to a girl, æt. 12, who had severe urticaria which did not yield to *Apis* or *Urt. ur.* It cured the urticaria and improved the patient's health. W. D. Ingalls reports (1) the case of Mrs. D., 48, who had eczema plantaris, fissured, exuding an acrid secretion, and so excessively sore that the patient had not been able to wear shoes or walk any distance for two years. *Skoo.* 2x was given internally; an ointment of a drachm to the ounce of vaseline applied, and Skookum soap used for washing. In two months the patient was able to wear shoes, and in three months the feet were well. (2) Mrs. H., 23, had a benign growth in left breast, noticed eight months. No history of phthisis or cancer in family. *Skoo.* was given thus: for the first week, one grain of 1x every four hours; for the second week, two grains of 2x every four hours; for the next seven weeks, five-grain powders of 3x, when the patient was cured. (3) Mr. J., chronic nasal catarrh; discharge greenish yellow having odour of ozæna, was greatly relieved and apparently on the way to cure.—B. F. Bailey reports (1) the cure of Mrs. X., 40, of lithæmic diathesis; never free from eczematic trouble for years. At times much rheumatism. Not unfrequently the rheumatism disappears and is immediatety followed by styes on the eyelids. Former treatment allopathic and also homœopathic. *Skoo.* 3x every four hours. Improvement soon showed itself, and the patient was well in three months and remained so. (2) Mrs. Y., 26, lithæmic, with flushed face and yellowish background. Urine, 1030, and with marked uric acid deposits. Much difficulty of digestion. Great dryness of skin, especially of scalp. Hair falling out to such an extent that baldness was feared. *Skoo.* 3x every four hours. Hair ceased to fall out. The heated, congested feeling of head and face disappeared, and the patient became well. *Skoo.* has also cured vaccinal eczema.

Relations.—*Antidoted by* Tabac. *Compare:* In general, Nat. c
Nat. m. Skin, Graph., Medor., Melit., Maland., Vacc.

Causation.—Vaccination.

SYMPTOMS.

5. **Nose.**—Profuse coryza with constant sneezing as in hay-feve symptoms so severe had to discontinue the remedy; (symptoms continu until antidoted by tobacco).

11. **Stomach.**—Appetite increased.

20. **Back.**—Heaviness in sacrum.

21. **Limbs.**—Severe rheumatic pains in limbs.

Slag.

Silico-sulpho-calcite of Alumina. Slag of blast furnaces in which irc is smelted. Trituration.

Clinical.—Anus, itching of; soreness of. Constipation. Diarrhœa. Flatulenc Hæmorrhoids. Housemaid's-knee. Lumbago. Phthisis. Spleen, affections of.

Characteristics.—*Pulverised Slag*, or blast-iron-furnace cinder, now recognised as one of the best fertilisers of our fields and garden It was introduced into medicine by J. Meredith (*H. W.*, xxiv. 92) wh gave the 6x trit. to a patient suffering from housemaid's-knee, and i addition to relieving this it took away "a dreadful anal itching, pile and constipation as if by magic." Meredith confirmed the rectal pow of *Slag* by experiments on his own person. The specimen of *Slag* use by Meredith was analysed and found to contain in 100 parts th following: *Silica* 36·6, *Alumina* 15·, *Calcium* 36, *Sulphur* 3—part these occur as *Calc. sulph.*,—*Ferrum* 1·, *Phosphorus* 0·5 (Meredith queri if the blue tint of *Slag* is due to *Fer.* and *Pho.*), *Magnesium* 6· *Manganum* 1·0. Loss 0·5. Turner, of Mason College, gives th formula of *Slag* as $2Al_2O_3\ 3SiO_2$, $6(2CaO, SiO_2)$. Acting on Meredith suggestion, George Herring instituted a proving with the 3x o himself and others (*ibid.* p. 358) Herring's only symptom was creeping irritation of the skin or under the skin, in the umbilic region, sufficiently severe to keep him awake. On prover No. 2 *Sla* produced no symptoms, but did something better: it cured him flatulent distension in the evening, and an oppressive feeling over th heart. No. 3 had constipation relieved; but *Slag* produced "sorene of anus." His general health was much improved. No. 4, a delicat lady, of phthisical history, had *Slag* 3x gr. i. twice a day. It set up diarrhœa, debility, quick pulse, lumbago, with pain in back, distensic of stomach, so that she had to loosen her dress [the very symptom cured in one of the men], profuse night-sweat; cough and expector tion. *Pho.*, *Ph. ac.*, *Carb. v.* were given to this patient in successic and all did good. Another proving of *Slag* was made by F. C. I (*ibid.* 453). The prover, whose symptoms are marked (B) in th Schema, was 33, rather dark, nervo-bilious; had chronically enlarge nsils, and tendency to colds in the head. He took *Slag* by way of :periment, hoping to cure his tonsils. It had no better effect than medies previously taken, but it produced a number of symptoms, ominent among them being: drowsiness in evening; dull, stupefying ontal headache, and stiffness at back of head and neck, and pain :tween shoulders; spleen pain and stitches in heart. A pain (dull, :avy sensation) alternated between inter-scapular region and spleen.

Relations.—*Effects were relieved by:* Pho., Pho. ac., Carb. v. *ompare:* Constipation, flatulence, Lyc., Carb. v., Sul. Anal mptoms, Graph., Nit. ac. Intolerance of tight clothing, Lach. ousemaid's-knee, Stict. p., Ap.

SYMPTOMS.

2. **Head.** — On waking, dull, stupefying, frontal headache, want of ergy, pains in limbs (B).—Frontal headache extended to r. temple with nsation of stiffness at back of head (B); (this headache was constant roughout the proving; at a later stage of the proving, it was slightly > oving about).

5. **Nose.**—Cold in head (B).

8. **Mouth.**—Thickly coated, greyish tongue, with terra-cotta streak wn middle (B).—Awoke with slimy tongue (B).

9. **Throat.**—Throbbing in l. tonsil (B).

11. **Stomach.**—Very little appetite (B). Distended stomach, must osen her dress.

12. **Abdomen.**—Creeping irritation of the skin or under the skin in abilical region; kept him awake some time (3x).—In a gouty prover 3x noved distension of abdomen necessitating unbuttoning top button of ousers in evening.—(Flatulent distension.)—Aching in region of spleen ernating with pain between shoulders, in l. elbow (B) — Pain in leen (B).

13. **Stool and Anus.**—Took away a dreadful anal itching, piles and nstipation as if by magic (6x).—Constipation relieved (3x).—Soreness of us produced (3x).—Diarrhœa, great debility, quick pulse: pain in back, lated stomach, had to loosen dress; profuse night-sweat; cough with pectoration (3x. gr. 1 twice a day; in a delicate lady).

14. **Urinary Organs.**—Very frequent urination.—Urine darker than ual (B).

17. **Respiratory Organs.**—Cough with expectoration; profuse ght-sweats.

19. **Heart.**—Stitches in region of heart (B).—(Oppressed feeling over the art.)—Pulse quick.

20. **Neck and Back.**—Stiffness at back of neck.—Lumbago; with tulence.—Aching, dull pain over small of back (B).

21. **Limbs.**—Pain in limbs.—Aching between shoulders, and in l. elbow ernating with aching in region of spleen.

22. **Upper Limbs.**—Pain in l. elbow.—Shifting pains in l. elbow, anging to r., and then back again.

23. **Lower Limbs.**—Pains in both knee-caps, sometimes dull, some-

times aching.—(Housemaid's knee.)—Occasional shooting aching throu knees; < going up stairs.

24. **Generalities.**—Want of energy.

26. **Sleep.**—Unusually drowsy in evening.—Sleep disturbed by creepi sensation about navel.

27. **Fever.**—Quick pulse.—Profuse night-sweat.

Sol.

Sun-light. Saccharum lactis is exposed to concentrated sun's rays a stirred with a glass rod till saturated. Attenuations by Fincke.

Clinical.—Cancer. Freckles. Headache. Lupus. Menses, premat Paralysis. Sunburn. Sunstroke.

Characteristics.—Thanks to Finsen, of Copenhagen, the pl of Light in therapeutics is on the way to be defined so far as *direct* properties are concerned, though Finsen is reviving and c firming, rather than originating, light-therapy. O. V. Tha (*H. R.*, viii. 463) published in 1893 a series of cases in which he h used concentrated rays of sun-light (solar cautery), including ca of epithelial cancer, rodent ulcer, parasitic diseases, moles, sn wens, birth-marks, &c. H. T. Webster (*H. R.*, xv. 126) gives det of a case of epithelioma in which the growth was removed by sol cautery and a scarcely perceptible scar left. Swan and his coadjut investigated sun-light from another point of view. In 1880 (O iii. 275) Swan published a pathogenesis of *Sol*, which I have embod in my Schema. Swan's data were obtained from four provers, fr experiences obtained from sensitives by Reichenbach (*Der Sensi Mench*), from an observation by "Highwood" quoted by Fincke fr *American Observer*, ix. 210. Reichenbach's observations I have tinguished by "(R)," Highwood's by "(H)." The remaining syn toms are those who took principally the 1m attenuations of Finc The 15m was taken by one. Two of Reichenbach's symptoms w observed on two of the provers also, and the letters "(F)" and "(refer to these. Cured symptoms will be found in brackets. common effects of strong sun-light, as sneezing, freckling, and s stroke, may be added to the list.

Relations.—*Antidoted by:* Aco., Bell., Glon., Gels., and ot sunstroke remedies. *Compare:* Luna, Elec., Mgt. Dislike of s Lach., Nat. c.

SYMPTOMS.

1. **Mind.**—Excitement and anxiousness in all her nerves, at first trembling at heart, finally it remained in stomach-pit; all that night and day very sensitive and easily frightened; it was as if all the nerves v trembling inside of them; the anxiousness in stomach-pit passes off second evening.—Anxiousness if somebody comes towards her, b frightened thereat (F and R).

2. **Head.**—Violent headache from vertex down to forehead, pressing, th sensation of heat in face; this headache was repeated the second day ·ee times; it seems to be in connection with the excitement and anxious- ss at stomach-pit (first night).—All the sensitives are very sensitive to the mediate action of sunshine on the vertex (R).—Extreme painfulness if the nshine strike the bare-head (R).—Most violent stitches in brain (R)—Dis- reeable feelings, such as from retrograde passes, go into brain, cause tches and headache, and if she does not gain the shade, stomach-ache and usea follow (R)—Violent headache (R).—L.-sided headache (R).—Head- he from sunshine on bare head, > by laying a glass of water on stomach- : (R)—In morning, severe pain in crown, and then in neck, passing off er breakfast (L and R).—(Heavy pressive pain in vertex.)—Intense entire phalalgia.—Pain in forehead; it seems as if forehead would crush itself wn upon the eyes.—(Sensation of undulating or floating in head after ental excitement, such as attending to business or writing a letter.)— stantaneous shock to brain, followed by prostration, and a scalding nsation on top of head (remedied by orange-coloured cloth in stove-pipe t) (H)—Excessive perspiration of head and neck.

3. **Eyes.**—Sun-light diminished the sensitivity of eyes; od.-blindness).—Suffusion of veins of sclerotica.—Sensation of swelling, as if eyes would rce themselves out of sockets.—Light offends eyes.

4. **Ears.**—Sharp shooting pain from l. ear to nose, continued at intervals r some time.—Partial deafness.

5. **Nose.**—Sneezing, with a little sore throat, as if she had taken cold.

6. **Face.**—Jaws rigidly set as in trismus.

7. **Teeth.**—Grinding of teeth as in helminthic spasms.

8. **Mouth.**—Tastes like something she cannot tell.—She puts anything e is going to eat in the sunshine, because then it is more palatable to her).—Two glasses of water of equal temperature, the one put in the shade, e other in the sunshine for a quarter of an hour, the latter tastes agreeably ol to sensitives, and stale and disagreeable to non-sensitives, whilst the her tastes quite the reverse (R).—Stupid; cannot articulate a word.— rticulates with difficulty.

11. **Stomach.**—Slight inclination to or actual vomiting.—Heat in pit of omach.—Empty feeling in stomach, as if she had not eaten anything bstantial yesterday and to-day.—Sensation of faintness and vacuity in omach-pit.

12. **Abdomen.**—In abdomen, distension and hardness, as large as a ild's head, as if it were in womb, and running throughout from it into ammæ, as if milk would rush in as when a child nurses; this lasted the hole first night till morning; before the distension and hardness came on sensation as after childbirth or at conception (with great excitement).—A ass of water exposed to the sun for six to eight minutes propagates coolness, ot only in stomach, but round about in the viscera (R).

13. **Stool.**—Constipation.

14. **Urinary Organs.**—Had to urinate five times in night.—Urine and ool invariably suspended.

16. **Female Sexual Organs.**—Menses six to seven days too soon.

18. **Chest.**—Weakness about heart.

20. Back.—Pain in back.—Backache.

21. Limbs.—After riding about on horseback in his woods in the su shine all forenoon, and lying down about noon on his bed to rest, he sudde gets peculiar attacks drawing through all his limbs; after rising and maki a few steps up and down, they disappear; this repeats itself several tin (R).—(The r. side, arm, and foot, which had been weak as from part paralysis, became equally strong as l.)—Hands and feet cold.

22. Upper Limbs.—The back of hand exposed to sunshine feels war while at same time a coolness appears in palm, and runs up whole arm i temple (R).—Cool, refreshed hands from holding a stick partially exposed the sun (R).

24. Generalities.—> Of bad effects of the sun by every cloudy v drawing over the sun (R).—If beds and wearing apparel have lain too lo in the sunshine, the agreeable feeling after using them turns suddenly i the most disagreeable, so that she cannot bear it, and falls into headache a spasm (R.)—Spasm coming with sunrise and ceasing with sunset (R.)—So spasms appearing at sunset (R).—Faintness.—Prostration.—(General stiff ing up of the system; the bodily strength seems more equalised.)

25. Skin.—Dermatitis, which often, with cold extremities, degenera into megrim (R.).

26. Sleep.—She could not sleep the first night, except from 3 to 4 a.n otherwise no idea of sleep the whole night long.—Head very much excite could not sleep for hours.—Great sleepiness all through the head, and merely in the eyes; heavy, sound sleep all through night.

27. Fever.—An agreeable coolness extends over whole body, thou the surface of the body perceives the physical heat of the sun's ra simultaneously a kind of coldness interiorly pervades whole body, so t the sun makes warm and cold at the same time, but the feeling of c supersedes that of warmth to such a degree that the latter is overlooked (—Running chills of increasing sensation of cold in all limbs from holdi wires partially exposed to the sun (R).—Felt cold in night; drew up m cover and perspired.—Congestive chill from exposure to sun after drinki cold water freely.—Perspiration streaming out of stomach-pit over wh body (from the crude saturated sacch. lact., in one of Fincke's provers).

Solaninum.

SOLANINUM. An alkaloid obtained from various Solanums, especia S. dulcamara and S. nigrum; also from the Potato pla S. tuberosum. $C_{43}H_{69}O_{16}$. Trituration. Also

SOLANINUM ACETICUM. $C_{43}H_{69}O_{16}C_2H_4O_2$. Trituration. Solution.

Clinical.—Lungs, paralysis of. Tetanus. Ticklishness.

Characteristics.—My first practical acquaintance with *Sol* was through seeing the excellent effect of *Solan. acet.* 2 in soluti given by Dr. Hughes to a diabetic and semi-paralytic man of 60, w had frequent threatenings of respiratory paralysis with accumulations of mucus which he was unable to expel. *Solan. acet.* more than any other remedy rescued him from danger and prolonged his life. From that time I have frequently had occasion to use it in similar conditions. *Solan.* is obtained from many of the Solanaceæ, and especially from *Dulcamara.* It exists in potatoes, and under certain conditions of germination potatoes may contain a poisonous amount. An accident of the kind occurred to soldiers at Pfuhl who were supplied with potatoes containing about 24 per cent. of *Solan.* (*Med. Press*, June 5, 1901). Sixty-six soldiers had marked poisoning symptoms: Shivering, fever, vomiting, syncope, and in one case convulsions. Skin and conjunctivæ were tinged yellow. *Solan.* was proved by Clarus and Schroff and others. Experiments were also made on animals. Slowed and oppressed respiration was a marked feature. Respiration was slowed in inverse proportion to the increase in the pulse rate. There was cerebro-spinal irritation; hyperæsthesia and convulsions < by touch. Skin more easily tickled than usual. In animals the hind limbs were rigid and paralysed; and in the provers the lower limbs were weakened.

Relations.—*Compare:* Dulc., Bell., S. car., S. nig., S. tub., S. t. ægrot. (Botan). In respiratory paralysis, Dulc., Bell. Sleepy but cannot sleep, Bell. Hyperæsthesia, Nux, Tetanin.

SYMPTOMS.

1. **Mind.**—Stupefaction without previous excitement.

2. **Head.**—Vertigo.—Head: hot, heavy, dull, painful.—Pain in occiput.—[(In rabbits:) Injection of cerebro-spinal passages, esp. of medulla oblongata; spasms < by touch; pendulum-like swinging of head and snapping with the mouth.]

3. **Eyes.**—Pupils slightly contracted.

8. **Mouth.**—Salivation.—The pure alkaloid has a cooling, acid, and salt taste, and when chewed causes a glutinous sensation in pharynx and throat, with scraping which extends to stomach, where it becomes a peculiar sticking pain.—Bitter taste.

9. **Throat.**—Scraping in throat.

11. **Stomach.**—Constant eructations.—Nausea, and diarrhœa; and vomiting.—Nausea, violent, ineffectual efforts to vomit.—About 5 p.m., vomiting three times without previous nausea, or pain, or any intestinal symptoms.

12. **Abdomen.**—Rumbling in abdomen.

14. **Urinary Organs.**—Albumen in urine.

17. **Respiratory Organs.**—Hoarseness.—Respiration: slow; superficial; difficult; oppressed; distressed, esp. on inspiration.—[Decreased frequency of respiration in inverse proportion to increase of pulse.—Moist rattle during inspiration.—Frequent violent outcry (from action on medulla oblongata).—Masses of mucus in larger air-passages (post mortem).—Paralysis of respiration. (Rabbits poisoned with *S.*)]

18. **Chest.**—[Convulsions of muscles of thorax, with which were soon

associated tonic spasms of extremities, at first gentle, gradually increasing, and a short time before death suddenly attaining an enormous height; < by touch. (Rabbits.)]

19. **Heart.**—Pulse: increased in rapidity; weak; thready.—Pulse and respiration slowed.—[Increased pulse rate; respiration slowed.—Post-mortem, rigidity of heart muscle, all its cavities full of dark, cherry-red coagulated blood. (Rabbits.)]

20. **Neck and Back.**—[Cerebro-spinal meningitis. (Rabbits.)]

23. **Lower Limbs.**—Slight tonic spasms of lower limbs.—Weakness of lower limbs.—[Incapable of moving hinder feet forward.—Hind legs quite stiff, toes stretched out; then great dejection, retching, and signs of pain. (Rabbits, from the *sulphate*.)]

24. **Generalities.**—Weakness.—Sensitiveness to light, noise, and touch.—Convulsions.—Fainting.—[Sudden rapidity and convulsive embarrassment of respiration, general convulsions, tetanic spasms, and strong dilatation of pupil. (Dog.)]

25. **Skin.**—Skin dry.—Hyperæsthesia; creeping along spine when touching the skin; more easily tickled than natural.—Itching.—Yellow discolouration of skin.

26. **Sleep.**—Frequent yawning.—Great sleepiness with inability to sleep.—Sleep restless, frequently disturbed by frightful dreams.—Sleep frequently interrupted without dreams.

27. **Fever.**—Extremities cold.—Shivering, fever, vomiting, and syncope.—Profuse perspiration without weakness.

Solanum Arrebenta.

Solanum rebenta. Arrebenta cevallos (Brazilian name). Trituration of the leaves. Tincture of the leaves.

Clinical.—Apoplexy. Boils. Breasts, swelling of. Glands, swelling of. Urticaria. Vertigo.

Characteristics.—Mure, who proved *Sol. arr.*, says of it: "The bush grows spontaneously in the provinces of Rio Janeiro, along roads and in cultivated places. It is from ten to sixteen inches high." Among the symptoms "Redness of face and rush of blood to brain" recalls *Bell.*, as do the swelling and pains in breasts.

SYMPTOMS.

1. **Mind.**—Impatient and irritated by trifling causes.

2. **Head.**—Vertigo after bathing.—Headache.

6. **Face.**—Redness of face, and rush of blood to brain.

8. **Mouth.**—Doughy mouth in morning.

10. **Appetite.**—Loss of appetite.—Constant thirst.

11. **Stomach**—Swelling of stomach.—Difficult digestion.

18. **Chest.**—Superficial ulceration below l. nipple.—Pain at pectoralis major.—Glandular swelling in r. breast.—Lancinations in breasts.

22. **Upper Limbs.**—Painful boil below r. axilla.—Swelling of axillary glands.

25. **Skin.**—Suppuration of boils.—Urticaria.—Paleness and greenish colour of the skin after a few days of proving.

26. **Sleep.**—Waking with a start.—Dreams about quarrels and murders.

27. **Fever.**—Slight fever.—Flash of heat all over.

Solanum Carolinense.

Solanum Carolinense. Horse-nettle. *N. O.* Solanaceæ. Tincture of fresh ripe berries.

Clinical.—Convulsions. Epilepsy. Tetanus.

Characteristics.—*Solan. car.* is a domestic remedy in the Southern States for "convulsions," and it has been tested by several old-school authorities (*H. R.*, xi. 20) in cases of epilepsy with some success. Doses of from 30 to 60 drops were given three times a day, the only unpleasant effects being a "mild diarrhœa" in some cases. Grahn (*H. R.*, xii. 462) relates a case of hysterical tetanus in a young negro woman. She had laughed whilst holding a pin in her mouth, and the pin had lodged in her throat. She had managed to get rid of it by coughing, but had hurt the throat, and the tetanic spasms followed. *Passiflor.* did good, but the supply gave out, and *Sol. car.* was given instead. By error of an attendant, maximum doses (two drachms every forty minutes) were given, and a state of dangerous stupor followed. However, all muscles were relaxed, and remained so the rest of that day. Next day a slight return of the spasms was remedied with half-drachm doses of *Sol. car.* It was several days before the disease was entirely overcome.

Solanum Mammosum.

Apple of Sodom. *N. O.* Solanaceæ. Tincture of fresh ripe fruit.

Clinical.—Coxalgia. Hæmoptysis. Irritability. Sleep, abnormal. Thought, difficult. Tobacco, effects of.

Characteristics.—Hering is the authority for *Sol. mam.* The chief symptoms were: Irritability and inability to think; sleepiness, without being able to sleep; a kind of stupor < at time of flood tide, at the full moon, > with ebb tide; hawking of blood-streaked mucus; sensitiveness to tobacco.

SYMPTOMS.

1. **Mind.**—Becomes exasperated at what he thinks may happen.—Inability for continuous thought, though with perfect comprehension of his subject; he could, when writing, only express himself in short, broken sentences.

13. **Stool.**—No stool (2nd d.); stool occurred later than usual, and after much pressure (3rd d.).

17. **Respiratory Organs.**—The mucus hawked from the larynx contains streaks of bright blood.

20. **Back.**—Twitching of large muscle below r. scapula; as if the flesh were pinched up by the hand and shaken back and forth.

23. **Lower Limbs.**—Sticking pain in l. hip-joint that made him quite lame, frequently during and after walking, disappearing after standing and sitting down.

24. **Generalities.**—Uneasiness; inability to keep quiet.—Everything is seen as in a fever with a hard pulse.—Sensitiveness to tobacco.

25. **Skin.**—Causes blotches over whole body (from poisoning).

26. **Sleep.**—Great weariness and desire to sleep without ability to sleep, followed by slumbering without real sleep, and afterwards deep sleep for several hours, from which he awoke and could not collect his senses for a long time, and remained long in an irresolute condition (this condition occurred at time of flood-tide at full moon; with the ebb tide, a general refreshing as after a crisis).—Even after a long sleep during the day he was sleepy in evening, and slept well all night.—Dreams of death with violent weeping.

Solanum Nigrum.

Solanum nigrum. Black nightshade. *N. O.* Solanaceæ. Tincture of fresh plant.

Clinical.—Amaurosis. Chorea. Headache. Heartburn. Hydrocephalus. Mania. Meningitis. Night-terrors. Parotitis. Peritonitis. Puerperal convulsions. Scarlatina. Small-pox. Stammering. Tetanus. Trismus. Tympanites. Typhoid fever. Varicosis. Vertigo. Ulcers.

Characteristics.—*Sol. n.* is a common weed found in waste places. It has white flowers and black berries. "The leaves applied externally ease pain and abate inflammation. Too large a quantity occasions violent sickness and headache, giddiness, drowsiness, and other dangerous symptoms. The Arabians apply the leaves to burns and ulcers, skin diseases, and scrofulous and cancerous affections; they are diaphoretic, diuretic, and purgative" (Green's *Herbal*). Hale says some country practitioners used it with much success under the impression that it was "an indigenous Belladonna," having been misled by the name "nightshade." Hale verified its use in meningitis and headache; in scarlatina when the eruption is *blotchy*. Hale justly points out the close affinity of *Sol. n.* with *Bell.*:—Delirium, headache, flushed face, sparkling eyes, pains coming and going suddenly, fiery rashes, burning skin and sweat. The Schema is made up of provings and symptoms of poisoning cases—all are unusually distinctive. A curious feature of the skin effects of the Black nightshade is that they have a tendency to *blackness*: "The swelling is very painful, it enlarges, becomes shiny, hard, and deep red; and in several places, quite black." "The black hue of the swollen parts grows deeper, the fingers are stiffened," &c. "The tip of the nose, the hands, from the finger-tips to the knuckles, and the toes to the tarsal joints become quite black as if regularly dyed." Corresponding to the black appearance is a bruised feeling all over the body.—The headaches of *Sol. n.* are described as "frightful." They are splitting, throbbing, bursting, piercing, and are < by least movement of head, light, noise, stooping; by least movement after sitting; < in a close room, and rather > in open air. The day after taking a single dose of φ a patient of Cooper's had this: "Head feels full across forehead, eyes heavy, and forehead burns; could not apply himself to work." The vertigo is < on moving the head. Sensation as if the bed was being rapidly turned in a circle. Inclines to left on walking. The delirium is characterised by the cephalic cry, efforts to escape, and by stammering speech. Dilatation of the pupils is as marked as with *Bell.*, and there is the same dryness of mouth and throat. Spasms, convulsions, and tetanic rigidity of the whole body have been induced. The most peculiar feature of the convulsions is this: "In the midst of these convulsions the children frequently stretch out their little hands, then carry them eagerly to their mouths, and go through the motions of mastication and swallowing." The skin symptoms are very marked. After one dose of φ this condition disappeared in a patient of Cooper's: patches of psoriasis, knees, elbows, and forehead, scaly, with red irritating spots at roots of hair. *Peculiar Sensations are:* Brain as if swimming. As if things moving in a circle, when stooping. As if bed turning rapidly in a circle. As if brain shaking about in skull, on moving head. As if head would split. As from a blow on forehead. As if sand in eyes. As if splinter in right tonsil. Tongue as if scalded. Pains come and go suddenly. Symptoms extend upward. Right upper, left lower. Alternate coldness and heat. The symptoms are < by touch. < Motion. < Moving head. < Moving. < Beginning to move after sitting. < Walking (inclines to left). < Mis-step. < Swallowing. < Light. < Bright sunshine (eyes). > Closing eyes (headache = him to close eyes). There is very great sensitiveness to cold air, but headache is < in warm room and > in open air. Many symptoms are < morning on waking. Headache at 10 a.m.

Relations.—*Compare:* In general Bell, and other Solanaceæ. Cerebral cry, Apis. Stammering, Stram. Headache 10 a.m., Nat. m. Splinter sensation, Nit. ac., Hep. Tongue as if scalded, Sang. Pain in back of neck, Hell. Sensation of a blow, Naj. (Naj. on occiput, Sol. n. on forehead).

SYMPTOMS.

1. **Mind.**—Delirium : with stammering speech, efforts to get out of bed ; with piercing cries and convulsions.—Complete cessation of mental faculties.—Apoplectic stupor, muscles relaxed, face flushed, pulse full and irregular.—Coma with twitching.

2. **Head.**—Vertigo : on rising and moving about, with dizziness before eyes ; with nausea and colic ; on stooping ; on rising in morning ; > in open air.—Brain seems to swim, < on moving head. — Sensation as if bed was turning rapidly in a circle (ten minutes after going to bed).—On stooping sensation as if everything moving in a circle.—While walking, body inclines to l.—Headache : dull, heavy throbbing ; followed by dilatation of pupils.—Lightness in head.—Frightful headache.—Headache < beginning to move after sitting ; > walking in open air.—Very severe pain in head immediately over eyes, makes him partially close eyes ; < by light ; by stooping ; 10 a.m.—Headache < in close room.—Feeling as if head would split.—Feeling on least motion after sitting as if brain would burst from forehead.—In forehead : dull, heavy pressure ; sensation as from a blow ; throbbing during whole afternoon.—Severe pain through temples as if head would split.—Severe throbbing pain in l. temple < slightest mis-step, and < stooping at 1 p.m.—Sharp gnawing pain in r. temple 9 a.m., causing him to grasp his hand and shut his eyes.—Throbbing of temporal and carotid arteries, 11 a.m.—Pain in small circumscribed spot on vertex.—Pressure on vertex and forehead.—Eruption on forehead of small red pimples, sore to touch and very hard ; when one went another came.—Scalp sore on moving hand through hair.—Scalp sore as if hair had been severely pulled.

3. **Eyes.**—Wrinkles round eyes.—Eyes wide open, moist, and sparkling.—Eyes : red ; full and tense ; dull and heavy ; burning ; very sensitive to light ; sensation as if sand in them.—Pain : over l. eye ; severe in supraorbital region on waking in morning ; < motion and stooping ; heavy, bruised sensation.—Sharp shooting over r. eye.—Burning in lids.—Burning in lid-margins.—Lids swollen and itching.—Lids agglutinated.—Pain in l. inner canthus.—Lachrymation.—Pupils dilated : enormously and insensible ; alternating with contraction.—Vision weak, < by bright sunlight.—Erethritic amaurosis.—Muscæ ; flickering black points and streaks ; darkness before eyes ; everything seemed too bright.—Sparks before eyes (with nausea).

4. **Ears.**—Most violent parotitis.—Stitches in ear.—Sounds seem distant.—Buzzing before ears.

5. **Nose.**—Nose deep red.—Considerable sneezing.—Discharge of thin, watery substance ; from r. nostril, l. being closed.—Burning in nose.—Nose swollen, painful, and black.—Tip of nose black.

6. **Face.**—Wrinkles round eyes, on upper lip and on fingers.—Face highly congested, wild anxious.—Face ; red, swollen ; bloated ; itching.—Expression : fatigued ; of fright and terror ; as if intoxicated.—Face pale.—Sloughs detached from face.—Sharp, neuralgic-like pains shooting from lower jaw up into l. ear, coming and going suddenly (10 a.m.).—Lips dry and blistered ; as if scalded.—Trismus.

8. **Mouth.**—Lips and tongue dry as if scalded.—Tongue sore as if burnt.—Dryness : of back of tongue and arch of palate ; of mouth.—Insipid

taste (with pain over eyes) on waking in morning.—Utterance becomes uneasy.

9. **Throat.**—Throat sore as if burnt.—Stitches in r. side of throat.—Raw sensation in throat, painful on swallowing, solids or liquids.—Tickling in throat causing cough.—Fauces: dry; sticking in, < on swallowing, at times stitches shooting to drum of r. ear.—L. tonsil swollen.—Feeling as if splinter in r. tonsil.—Cramp in œsophagus —Violent beating of carotids.

11. **Stomach.**—Appetite lost.—Great thirst, for large quantities, often.—Empty eructations with burning in stomach.—Heartburn.—Nausea with sparks before the eyes, continuing till he went to sleep.—Nausea and retchings.—Nausea and efforts to vomit, followed by profuse vomiting, at first of mucus, afterwards of bluish or greyish-black fluid.—Vomit: ingesta; blackish-green liquid, thick.—Severe pain in region of stomach, extending into heart region and l. shoulder (5 p.m.).—Pressure in stomach; constant or in paroxysms.—Cramps; cutting; burning in pit of stomach.—Burning in stomach extending up into œsophagus.

12. **Abdomen.**—Violent cutting in umbilical region.—Abdomen excessively distended and tense.—Colic; and ineffectual urging.—Pain 5 p.m., as if intestines were cut with knives.—Pains in abdomen and desire to lie down.

13. **Stool and Anus.**—Tenesmus in anus.—Stools: natural but more frequent; semi-fluid; yellow, watery.—Stools followed by burning pain in stomach, extending up, with nausea.—Constipation, small, dry, hard stools.

14. **Urinary Organs.**—If a sweat did not break out an extraordinary discharge of urine occurred, frequently followed by purging.

17. **Respiratory Organs.**—Respiration: rapid; difficult; quick but easy; stertorous.

18. **Chest.**—Chest: oppression of; constriction of.—Pressure on sternum and at tenth dorsal vertebra.—Cutting pains in l. side.—On upper part of sternum a large round blotch, deep red.

19. **Heart.**—Anxious feeling in region of heart.—Pulse: rapid, scarcely perceptible; irregular; slow, small, soft.

20. **Neck and Back.**—Neck sore, stiff, as if bruised; < moving head.—Severe pains in muscles of neck.—Great pains in back of neck and shoulders, and in lower limbs.—Pains in back of neck and between shoulders.—Bruised feeling in back and limbs.

21. **Limbs.**—Restlessness in limbs and carphologia.—Wandering pains, first in shoulders, then down arm, then in lower limbs.—Severe pains in all the limbs, 8 p.m.—Painful drawing in arms and feet.

22. **Upper Limbs.**—Arms heavy, prostrated, < r.—Dull, heavy pain in r. arm extending to finger-tips (10 a.m. to 3 p.m.).—Lancinating pains down l. arm.—Pain shooting through l. arm and wrist.—Pain in l. shoulder and r. wrist.—Palms greenish blue.—Tips of fingers black as if dyed.—Vesicles appear on back of hands, break and discharge an acrid fluid.—Eruption like small-pox; sloughs form on fingers.

23. **Lower Limbs.**—Gait unsteady, heavy, insecure.—Trembling of lower limbs, esp. of muscles of thighs, like small successive jerks.—Lower limbs prostrated, < l.—Thighs weak.—Pain in r. knee extending up to hip.—Legs feel sore on walking as if bruised.—In l. calf: compression, crawling.—Swelling of feet.—Tearing on back of l. foot.—Chronic ulcers on feet.

24. **Generalities.**—Coma, convulsive agitation, plaintive cries.—In midst of convulsion the children stretch out their hands, as if to grasp something, carry them eagerly to their mouths, and go through the motions of mastication and swallowing.—Most violent, convulsive agitation.—Convulsions, tetanic rigidity and death.—Lies on back in entire prostration, disturbed at intervals by spasmodic movements.—Increased distension and prominence of varicose veins.—All muscles sore to touch.—Bruised feeling of whole body.—Great sensitiveness to cold air.

25. **Skin.**—Red blotches like scarlatina; irregularly dispersed over whole surface.—Great swelling and intolerable itching of face, eyelids, lips, hands, and feet.—Hands, feet, and nose painful, swollen, and black.—Black hue of swollen parts; shiny, painful.—The swelling and black discoloration diminish together, and are followed by desquamation.—Itching burning of extremities.—Vesicles on back of hands; sloughing on fingers; blisters discharge acrid fluid over arms.—Sloughs are detached from face, but r. hand swells up again.—Face cleans off, but hands are again covered with hard and very painful crusts, which fall off and are soon replaced by new ones.—Swelling of feet, arms, abdomen, scrotum, and penis.

26. **Sleep.**—Sleepiness; during forenoon; all day.—Deep sleep.—Night very restless, sleepless, with hallucinations and carphologia.—In middle of night he wakes up uttering groans, which are wrung from him by violent headache.—Feeling on waking as if he had lost several nights' sleep.—Dreams: waking him in terror, with sensation of falling from a great height; of snakes.

27. **Fever.**—Alternation of coldness and heat.—Flushes across face, 3 p.m.—High fever followed by profuse sweat.—High fever, 12 p.m., with great pain in back of neck, shoulders, and lower limbs.—Heat, redness of face.—Fever, painfulness in præcordia, distension of abdomen with at times screaming and grasping at abdomen, and constipation.—Burning dry heat.—Skin burning, sweating.—Heat in face, hands, and along back.—Flashes of heat run up and down back.—Frequent sweats.—Whole body bathed in profuse sweat.

Solanum Oleraceum.

Solanum oleraceum. Juquerioba. *N. O.* Solanaceæ. Tincture of flowers.

Clinical.—Breasts, swelling of. Catarrh. Glands, swelling of. Herpes Lactation, profuse. Leucorrhœa. Pustules. Sleep excessive. Stye. Urticaria.

Characteristics.—This plant, says Mure, is herbaceous, stem somewhat woody, the upper branches being covered with short and crooked thorns. It grows on the shores round Rio Janeiro in damp and shady places. The most remarkable symptom of the proving was "Swelling of the mammary gland with profuse effusion of milk" occurring in a negro woman of 60. Other symptoms were: "Pain and swelling of face and throat with inflammation." "Cold feeling n left chest after drinking." There was drowsiness with headache, and the generally deranged sleep of the other Solanaceæ.

SYMPTOMS.

1. **Mind.**—Sad.—Irritable.

2. **Head.**—Drowsy with headache.

3. **Eyes.**—Stye on r. lower eyelid.—Pain at internal canthi of eyes.—nflammation of l. upper lid.

5. **Nose.**—Discharge of fetid, yellow mucus from l. nostril.—Acute atarrh.

6. **Face.**—Pain in face.—Pain and swelling of face and throat with nflammation.—Continual redness of face.—Violent pain in l. cheek, spreading ver whole face.

7. **Teeth.**—Toothache.—Toothache at night.

8. **Mouth.**—Tongue coated white.—Ptyalism.

9. **Throat.**—Sore throat.

10. **Appetite.**—No appetite.

11. **Stomach.**—Difficult digestion.—Lancinating pain in stomach not asting long.

14. **Urinary Organs.**—Scanty urine.

16. **Female Sexual Organs.**—Short-lasting menses.—Discharge of vhite mucus from vagina.—Swelling of mammary glands with profuse ffusion of milk, on the second day.—Shortly after taking the drug the reasts of a negro woman of 60 began to swell and discharged a quantity of milk.

17. **Respiratory Organs.**—Suffocating cough.

18. **Chest.**—Sense of chilliness in l. side of chest, after drinking.

20. **Neck.**—Swelling of cervical glands.

23. **Lower Limbs.**—Tickling at the lower limbs.—Herpetic eruption on ankle.

25. **Skin.**—Pustules all over, first white, then red, with an intolerable itching now and then.—Nettle-rash with fever.—Itching.

26. **Sleep.**—No sleep for two nights.—Drowsy for four hours in the middle of the day.—Drowsy all day.—Drowsy with headache.

Solanum Pseudo-Capsicum.

Solanum pseudo-capsicum. Jerusalem Cherry. *N. O.* Solanaceæ.
Trituration or tincture of fruit.

Clinical.—Pupils, dilated. Somnolence.

Characteristics.—The few symptoms of this medicine were observed on a child who ate three or four ot the berries.

SYMPTOMS.

3. **Eyes.**—Dilatation of the pupils.
11. **Stomach.**—Nausea.
12. **Abdomen.**—Very acute pains in lower abdomen.
26. **Sleep.**—Somnolence.

Solanum Tuberosum.

Solanum tuberosum. Potato. *N. O.* Solanaceæ. Tincture of th berries. Tincture of green potatoes. Tincture of fresh plant.

Clinical.—Amaurosis. Cramps. Iritis, rheumatic. Stammering. Trismu Tumours.

Characteristics.—The poisonous properties of the berries an leaves of the potato plant are well known, and the tubers are popularl believed to have anti-scorbutic properties when eaten as food. Unde some conditions the tubers have been known to contain poisonou quantities of *Solanin*. The symptoms of the Schema are the result o eating new potatoes, green potatoes, an extract, and the berries The last proved fatal in a number of instances. Sickness an diarrhœa with tenesmus, giddiness, dilated pupils and indistinc vision, a paralytic condition of the tongue, cramps, and tetani spasms are the main features of the poisonings. Cooper relieve with a single dose of *Sol. t.* φ a case of rheumatic iritis. Burnet cured a case of tumours feeling like masses of potatoes in th abdomen with *Sol. t.*; and it assisted him in the cure of a case o tumours all round the cervix uteri. *Url. ur.* finished this cure.

Relations.—*Compare:* Solanin. In paralysis of tongue, Dulc Iritis, Bell. Stammering, Stram.

SYMPTOMS.

1. **Mind.**—Almost lost consciousness.

2. **Head.**—Vertigo; headache; stupor.

3. **Eyes.**—Eyes deep in sockets.—Staring look.—Eyes for most par open.—Pupils dilated.—Vision indistinct.

6. **Face.**—Hippocratic face.—Expression anxious.

8. **Mouth.**—Constantly spitting through the closed teeth viscid, frothy phlegm.—Tongue covered with brown, moist fur.—Tongue heavy, difficult t move; hardly able to articulate.—Speech thick.—Speechless.

11. **Stomach.**—Violent retching followed by vomiting and diarrhœa.—Felt sick, a darkness over her eyes, skin cold, cramped all over.—Epigastri region sensitive to pressure.

12. **Abdomen.**—Violent colic and vomiting.—Pain in bowels.—Tumours.

13. **Stool and Anus.**—Diarrhœa with tenesmus.—Tends to rela bowels.

16. **Female Sexual Organs.**—(Tumours round cervix uteri.)

17. **Respiratory Organs.**—Respiration: hurried; irregular; at times ıppressed; usually short and incomplete, only seldom slow and sighing; ifficult.

19. **Heart.**—Pulse small, rapid, scarcely perceptible.

21. **Limbs.**—Cramps, esp. in calves, with spasmodic contractions of ngers and thumbs.

24. **Generalities.**—Tossing to and fro in bed.—General rigidity.—atient exceedingly weak.—Faintness.

25. **Skin.**—Skin livid.

27. **Fever.**—Skin cold.—Face, chest, and extremities cold.—Skin bedewed ith cold, clammy sweat.

Solanum Tuberosum Ægrotans.

Diseased potato. Tincture of the affected tubers.

Clinical.—Anus, prolapse of; patulous. Breasts, painful. Breath, offensive, onstipation. Epistaxis. Headache. Ileus. Irritability. Menses, interrupted. oma. Odour of body, offensive. Pruritus vulvæ. Rectum, prolapse of. Scalp, ainful. Sciatica. Scurvy. Skin, darkness of. Tenesmus. Tongue, cracked. ertebræ, pain in; pulsation in.

Characteristics.—The "Potato murrain" is characterised by the rapid putrescence of the leaves and haulm, which is first inicated by the presence of a little mould, *Peronospora infestans*, which reys upon the tissues, spreading rapidly in every direction. The ıbers also exhibit brown spots on their surface and within their ssues, and according to circumstances decay with greater or less ıpidity" (*Treas. of Bot.*). In 1846 the sudden inroad of this disease d to the fearful famine in Ireland, which resulted in the death of ıousands. Mure made the first proving of *S. t. æ.*, using a potato in an entire state of decomposition, without, however, being comletely rotten." Effects of eating diseased potatoes, some of them ıtal, have been observed, and these have been added to Mure's. he symptoms of the proving were pretty severe, and one of the ıost important—prolapse of the rectum—has been confirmed by the oisoning cases. A man and three children ate boiled diseased potatoes, ıd among their symptoms were these: "Pain of an acute character as referred to the region of the anus, which on examination was ound perfectly patulous and exquisitely tender to the touch. Two f the four patients had prolapsus ani, which was probably caused y the violent and ineffectual efforts to discharge the contents of the ectum. There had not been an evacuation of the bowels, nor had ıey passed water, except in drops and with extreme suffering, for x days. On introducing the finger into the rectum, which caused cute pain, it was found that the intestine was completely filled, to ithin an inch of the orifice, with a solid substance." The foul dour of the diseased potato is reproduced in the breath and body-odour of the patients. Lips cracked and raw ; gums bleeding ; tong coated, thick, cracked ; throat inflamed and ulcerated with sensatic of something sticking in it or a fleshy growth. In one poisoni case a condition of noma of left cheek was induced. *Peculi Sensations are :* Of water splashing on head ; as if brain were leapir in skull (on stooping). As of something sticking in throat. As there were a fleshy growth in throat. As if a spring unrolled in le hypochondrium. As if a hollow body were turning rapidly in ches Of stoppage in trachea. Of something becoming detached fro sacrum. The urine has an oily pellicle. Excruciating muscul pains. The symptoms are < by touch and pressure. Headache < on waking ; by smell of alcohol ; walking at 5 p.m. ; sleepin working (headache). Cold water = shock.

Relations.—Mure gives the following as the closest analogues S. t. æ.—the order indicates their relative importance : Bry., Ars., Pl Nux, Sep., Stron., V. tric., Scil., Puls., Graph., Alm., Merc., Na. n Ign., Calc. *Compare:* Sensation of machinery inside, Nit. ac. Co stipation, black balls, Op. Prolapsus ani, Pod., Ruta. Patulous anu Ap., Pho.

SYMPTOMS.

1. **Mind.**—Quarrelsome, irritable mood.—Bad temper.—An uninte ligible expression irritates her so that she would like to break everything ar bite her hands.—Dread of work.—Hypochondriac mood.—She wants to enj a change of scenery, &c.—She fancies she is miserable, and dwells much the future.—Rises in the night imagining that there are thieves behind t curtain, but dares not look, asks others to do it.—Crowd of ideas.—H attention is easily disturbed by other things.

2. **Head.**—Confusion.—Heat in head, evening.—Heaviness of the hea in the vertex ; on stooping and then raising head again.—Catarrhal dulness head ; esp. forehead.—Sensation on stooping as if brain leaping in skull. Lancinations as if brain would burst open.—Sensation of water splashing head.—Headache at noon, < by the smell of spirits.—Head feels too heav she has to make an effort to support it.—Pressure above eyes, on waking.— the forehead : violent pain, all day ; stitching pain ; with dulness of head, ar disposition to fall forwards.—Slight beating in temples.—Sensation as if t hair would be torn out on vertex.—Painful sensitivenes of scalp and roots hair ; cannot bear combing ; > after stirring about and talking.

3. **Eyes.**—Prickling about the lids, the surface of which is red. Spasmodic contraction and twitching of l. upper lid.—Burning in lids. Prickling and burning in eyes.—Congestion of the conjunctiva.—Profu lachrymation ; on waking.

4. **Ears.**—Ringing in the l. ear.

5. **Nose.**—Repeated sneezing, followed by feeble cough.—Nose-blee —Pressure at root of nose.—Smell of blood.

6. **Face.**—Face hot and red.—Mounting of heat to face, now and the —Red pimples on cheeks.—Desquamation of face.—Face pale, bloodle much swollen, esp. about eyelids, nearly closing them.—Bluish-black, fet ulcer of l. cheek.—Upper lip bleeding, cracked.

7. **Teeth.**—Swelling of mucous membrane of the inner margin of the vo incisors.—Teeth loose and very painful.—Gums, esp. lower, spongy, ozing blood.—Teeth covered with white mucus.

8. **Mouth.**—Dry mouth.—The mucous membrane of the velum palati eems to become detached here and there.—Tongue pale.—Thick tongue, a.m.—Tongue swollen, cracked, early in the morning; coated white or ellowish white; or coated white, with red tip, or yellowish along the median ne.—Prickling in r. half of tongue.—Breath horribly fetid.

9. **Throat.**—Mucus accumulates in throat and seems to cover whole nterior part.—Feeling as of a fleshy growth in throat.—Feeling as if someing sticking in throat which she cannot bring up, followed by expectoration a small, hard, yellowish-grey lump.—Fauces and mouth inflamed; ulcerated patches.—Inflamed fauces, unable to swallow saliva.

10. **Appetite.**—Canine hunger.—Salt taste.—Taste of raw potatoes.—ood tastes as bitter as gall.—Great desire for spirits and oranges.—Burning irst.

11. **Stomach.**—Eructations followed by rumbling in stomach.—Sour uctations causing a cough.—Acidity, bitterness, and gulping-up, after eating. -Cardialgia after, breakfast, dinner, and supper.—Pain in stomach, with red ce, after breakfast.—Spasmodic pains, griping-tearing at night.

12. **Abdomen.**—Sensation as if a spring were unrolled in l. hypochonium.—Pains and working in the bowels, early in the morning.—Painfulness abdomen to contact along the median line.—Belly hard, swollen, dropsical. -In abdomen: pain after eating; spasmodic pains, as though the bowels ecame twisted together; dull pains in the hypogastric region, at night; ain with chilliness; rumbling; the clothes cause a feeling of tightness.—mission of flatulence, also with colic.—Pain, as if sprained, in r. groin.—itch in r. groin near inguinal ring.

13. **Stool and Anus.**—Frequent urging to stool.—Stool scanty, with aining, passing off in small, black lumps (balls).—Has to strain until tears me.—Hard, large, lumpy stool; with violent burning in anus and rectum. Stool hard and large, followed by two liquid stools.—Copious greenishllow diarrhœic stool.—Constipation for five days.—Violent colic previous stool.—Alternate protrusion and retraction of rectum during stool, with eling of chilliness of body.—Prolapsus recti.—After stool rectum alternately lls and returns again.—Contraction of sphincter ani.—Strong pulsations in rinæum and r. ring finger.—Acute pain in anus, which was found perfectly tulous and exquisitely tender.—Great heat in anus.

14. **Urinary Organs.**—Region of bladder distended.—Difficult micrition.—Heat (and pain) in urethra after urinating.—Constant micturition aile at stool.—Urine reddish, mingled with mucus.—Urine: very thick, coming covered with white mucus after standing; soapy; turbid, of a ngy yellow, with copious white sediment; turbid, dingy yellow, covered th an oily pellicle.—Pain in urethra, after urinating.

15. **Male Sexual Organs.**—Weight in r. testicle all day.

16. **Female Sexual Organs.**—Twisting pains through uterus.—Feeling dislocation in hip-joint with pain in womb after a slight exertion.—Flatuice presses on uterus.—Menstrual blood rose-coloured.—Suppression of the enses.—Menses smelling of foul fish, mixed with black coagula.—Small

pimples and intolerable itching of labia.—Spasmodic pains striking throug uterus.—Burning and itching in vagina.

17. **Respiratory Organs.**—Constriction and difficulty of breathin caused by dryness of mouth.—Hoarseness on walking.—In trachea: tearin prickling, with cough; tearing, with phlegm; sensation as of an obstacl followed by cough and expectoration of a lump of hard, yellowish-gre mucus.—Cough with expectoration of yellow mucus, at night.—Dry coug day and night.—Cough as from stoppage in pharynx.—Expectoration lumps of black blood, early in the morning.—Constant involuntary sighin —After eating choking and difficult breathing caused by dryness of mouth.- Suffocation owing to previous day's dinner not digesting well; has to ri 3 a.m.

18. **Chest.**—Oppression in chest after supper.—Tearing in chest, al with dryness of mouth.—Sensation on making the least motion, as though hollow body were turning rapidly round in chest quickly and with a nois after which she fancies she will faint, early in morning.—Prickling as from thousand pins on the inner surface of sternum.—Violent stitching pain abo r. breast.—Congestions to chest.—Acute pain in l. side, like a stitch.—Painf stitches in r. side.—Mammæ painful, esp. when raising arm.

19. **Heart.**—Weight and pain in heart region.—Lancinations in hea —Palpitation of heart: for moments; at night; when lying; when raisi oneself; as though the heart would turn; with fainting feeling; with o pression of chest (less when lying); irregular (after eating).—Pulse: irregula sometimes weak; hard and tense.

20. **Neck and Back.**—Swelling of muscles of neck, shoulders, a arms with pain so acute he winces on slightest pressure.—Sense of weig in the back part of the neck.—Violent beating in spine, early, when lying.- Prickling sensation in spine, during sleep, waking her.—Stinging pain in t large dorsal muscle, r. side, when drawing breath.—Burning and painf sensation on the fifth dorsal vertebra, caused by friction of the clothes.- Sensation of weariness in whole back.—Stiffness in muscles of back.—Sens tion as if something on the os-sacrum became detached.—Pain in sacru when walking or touching the part.—Tingling in sacrum.—Beating in shoulder.—Prickling in psoas muscles.—Violent beating in loins.—Pain lumbar vertebræ, impeding walking.—Intolerable pain in lumbar regio obliging her to walk bent.

21. **Limbs.**—Joints swollen and very painful.—Sense of weariness in the limbs on waking.—Inclination to stretch the limbs.

22. **Upper Limbs.**—Feeling of weariness in muscles posteriorly.—Pa as if sprained in r. upper arm, after leaning on elbow.—Beating in midd portion of triceps brachealis.—(Cannot clench hands.)—Heat in hands. Stinging in l. little finger.—Beating in r. ring finger.

23. **Lower Limbs.**—Acute pains in hip-joint caused by least motion. Painful pressure on hip-joint, as with an iron bar, compelling her to lie dow —In l. gluteus muscle: beating; pain, accompanied by loathing.—Lancir tions in posterior part of r. thigh.—Weary feeling in muscles of r. side, aft walking.—Feeling of dislocation in hip-joint, with pain in womb, after a slig exertion.—Shooting pain in posterior and inferior femoral muscles, wh bending knee.—Beating in internal femoral muscles.—Alternate beating a

robbing above patella in both limbs.—Pain as if sprained in whole vertebral lumn, striking through posterior parts of thigh, and extending down to eels.—Drawing pain in posterior part of r. lower limb, from gluteus muscle own to heel.—Legs œdematous.—Shuddering of r. leg.

24. **Generalities.**—A peculiar and most offensive odour immediately erceived on approaching the bed.—Cannot walk erect.—General and artial debility.—Debility, she is about to faint.—Weariness in all the limbs, waking.—Pain as if bruised, in bed, preventing her from stirring.—Muslar pains excruciating.—Cold water (whether drinking it or washing with causes a sense of oppression and shock.

25. **Skin.**—Skin over whole body tender, tumefied, and preternaturally rk.—Rose-coloured patches appear and as suddenly vanish.—Small pimples the back; causing a violent itching.—Small red pimples on cheeks.—The in in the face peels off a little.—Small pimples on back = violent itching.

26. **Sleep.**—Irresistible drowsiness.—Very sleepy in evening.—Restless eep.—Starting from sleep, as in affright.—Sleepless.—Confused dreams, about es, revolution, corpses, thieves, &c.—Amorous dream.—He dreams that he to dress or draw the body of a drowned person, but is prevented in conquence of the body falling all the time on the clothes or paper.—Dreams out men who become transformed to talking animals; that his hands are t to pieces; that he is falling from a steeple.—She dreams that she is eating man flesh; that she is swimming in a river, and cannot get out of it.

27. **Fever.**—Pulse irritated; irregular; hard and tense.—Chilliness and nsation of internal coldness.—Repeated chilly creepings through whole dy, in evening.—Feeling of coldness all over, unable to get warm, her eeks being very red, in afternoon.—Heat all over, with sweat.—Pyrexia, d afterwards dropsical appearance.—Violent paroxysms of heat, suddenly ssing through the whole body, and proceeding from the vertex.—Alternate rning heat and chilliness, at night, in bed.—Exhalations from the skin, when rforming the least work.—Sweat all over, early in morning, in bed, cold ght-sweat.—The sweat smells of potatoes, in bed.

Solidago.

lidago virgaurea. Golden-rod. *N. O.* Compositæ (Tribe, Corymbiferæ). Tincture of whole fresh plant. Tincture of flowers. (Infusion of dry leaves and flowers.)

Clinical.—Albuminuria. Calculus. Croup. Deafness. Dysuria. Eruptions. ut. Leucorrhœa. Ophthalmia, scrofulous. Phosphaturia. *Prostate, enlarged.* eumatism. Sciatica. Scrofula. Urine, scanty; suppressed.

Characteristics.—The common Golden Rod is the only British ecies of *Solidago*. It is common in woods and heathy thickets. "This b," says Rademacher, "is a very old and good kidney medicine. is a specific for kidneys, and brings the patients back to the rmal condition." I quote from a paper by M. Gucken in *H. R.*, 205. Gucken confirms Rademacher's observations and quotes

further confirmations and cures by Dr. Buck of Würtembur[g]
According to Buck *Solid. v.* is *Specially Suited* to scrofulous subject[s]
but not exclusively to them. The grand keynote of this remedy li[es]
in *the condition and the action of the kidneys and the quality of the*
secretions. Diseases arising from or complicated with defective actio[n]
of the kidneys are very likely to be benefited by *Solid.* Pain an[d]
tenderness in kidney region; pains extending from kidneys t[o]
abdomen, bladder, and down limbs; urine dark, red-brown, scant[y],
thick, voided with difficulty; albuminous, mucous, and pho[s]-
phatic urine—these are the leading symptoms. Affections of an[y]
other parts or organs complicated with these symptoms will pr[o]-
bably find their remedy in *Solid.* Buck mentions scrofulous inflammation of the eyes. I have seen very sharp attack of conjunctivit[is]
produced in a patient who was taking *Solid.* for prostatic trouble[.]
The following are Buck's cases: (1) A boy, æt. 8, had severe membranous diphtheria with scarlet rash, which was removed by *Merc. c*[.]
and *Bell.;* but fever of typhoid type remained. The urine was alb[u]-
minous and scanty, pulse weak and intermittent, feet swollen. *K*[*ali*]
ars. 4 was given, but the symptoms grew worse. A thorough examin[a]-
tion of the patient showed great *sensitiveness of the kidneys to pressu*[*re*]
in spite of the otherwise apathetic condition. *Solid.* 3x was give[n],
and in one day the urine became more profuse with correspondi[ng]
improvement in the general condition. The boy peeled and r[e]-
covered completely. (2) Clerk, 45, had sleeplessness and pain [in]
the back. He casually mentioned that it took him a long tim[e]
to urinate for want of the necessary pressure. This he attribut[ed]
to gonorrhœa, which he had had years before. No sleep till 3 a.m[.],
when he got some sleep, which was not refreshing. On rising, tire[d],
especially upper part of thighs; then would begin the pain in t[he]
back, which extended to the loins and lasted till bedtime. *Nux* d[id]
not relieve. The urine was found dark, slimy, reddish, slightly ac[id],
not albuminous. *Kidneys sensitive to pressure.* *Solid.* 3x, taken stead[ily]
for three months, cured. A year afterwards there was a relapse, b[ut]
this time it took the form of sciatica, and *Solid.* again proved to [be]
the remedy. (3) Mrs. F., 53, wife of a farmer, stout, fresh-looki[ng],
had had her present trouble twenty-six years. After her confi[ne]-
ment, which was difficult, and followed by prolapsus uteri—s[till]
existing—her legs began to swell and an itching rash broke out [by]
degrees. Menstruation had always come on at the proper time, b[ut]
suddenly stopped six months before Buck saw her. Since then t[he]
itching had been almost intolerable, the legs more swollen, and alwa[ys]
cold. Appetite very poor; constant bitter taste in mouth, tong[ue]
thickly coated; at the same time a rising from the stomach as [if]
she would suffocate, and at the least exertion she lost her brea[th].
Urinated very little, and mostly at night. No pains in the back, b[ut]
the *kidneys were sensitive to pressure.* "The appearance of the low[er]
limbs of this patient," says Buck, "frightened me. From knee [to]
heel they formed a bluish-red mass in the shape of a stove-pipe, a[nd]
were covered with little blotches and crusts." The prolonged [use]
of *Solid.* 3x, though it did not effect a cure, produced a mitigation [of]
the whole body, so that the lady induced her eldest son to cons[ult]

the doctor. (4) This man had also trouble in his lower limbs not unlike his mother's. A year before he had had some severe throat trouble, after which his lower limbs began to swell and itch. They were also tinted blue-red and covered with vesicles, his *urine was scanty, and his kidneys sensitive to pressure. Solid.* 3x cured him in a few months. Gallavardin (*Alcoholism.*, p. 131) tells of a lady who cured her husband, who had been compelled to use the catheter for more than a year, by administering an infusion of the dried leaves and flowers of *Solid.* morning and evening. He mentions the case of seven patients, of ages varying from 42 to 74, who had been obliged to catheterise themselves for weeks, months, and years, and who were all cured with *Solid.* 1 x. "Clear, stinking urine" is an indication of Cooper's.

Relations.—*Compare:* In prostatic and urinary affections, Sabal., Santal., Hydrang., Triticum. Kidney-ache, Santal. Gonorrhœa and its effects; sciatica, Medor.

SYMPTOMS.

2. **Head.**—Headache.

3. **Eyes.**—Scrofulous, herpetic inflammation.—(Given in a case of prostatic enlargement it caused inflammatory redness of eyeballs.)

4. **Ears.**—Sudden deafness, with ringing in ears and albuminous urine.

5. **Nose.**—Nose dry; inner surface covered with blood-crust; scalding and very scanty brown urine.

8. **Mouth.**—Flat ulcers in mouth and throat.—Continuous bitter taste, disturbing rest, esp. at night.—Tongue heavily coated, does not become clean till urine becomes normal.

12. **Abdomen.**—Chronic catarrh of bowels.—Sensation of pain in abdomen on both sides of the navel, on deep pressure.—Flatulent distension.—Severe pricking in both hypochondria to region of kidneys, reaching to lower limbs, with bitter taste, brown urine, &c.

13. **Stool.**—Diarrhœa with scanty dark urine.—Dysentery.—Costiveness.

14. **Urinary Organs.**—"A very old and good kidney medicine" (Rademacher).—Pains in kidneys.—Region of kidneys painful on pressure.—Pains in kidneys which extend forward to abdomen and bladder.—Dysuria; scanty and difficult.—Urine: dark, red-brown, with thick sediment; dark with sediment of phosphates; slightly sour, neutral, or alkaline; with numerous epithelial cells or small mucous particles; epithelial cells with gravel of triple phosphates or phosphate of lime.—Bright's disease.—Clear, stinking urine.

15. **Male Sexual Organs.**—(Enlarged prostate; obstructing flow of urine.)

16. **Female Sexual Organs.**—Hæmorrhage.—Chronic leucorrhœa in connection with copious watery urine and sediments of mucous particles and uriniferous tubules; epithelium.

17. **Respiratory Organs.**—Heavy expectoration on coughing.—Croup, with little blotches on hands and diminished urine.—Chronic catarrh of lungs.—Continuous dyspnœa.—Periodical asthma with nightly dysuria.

18. **Chest.**—Rheumatism of intercostal muscles.

20. **Back.**—Chronic pains in loins.

23. **Lower Limbs.**—Limping, dragging gait.—Rheumatic pains in legs.—Pains in thigh.—The legs can be moved horizontally, but when moved perpendicularly they feel lame.

25. **Skin.**—Scrofulous rash.—Little blotches on hands and feet, itching very much.—Very obstinate itching exanthemas.—Exanthema of lower limbs without swelling of inguinal glands, but with disturbance in urinating (catarrh of kidneys).

26. **Sleep.**—Insomnia.

27. **Fever.**—Rheumatic fever.—Very frequent pulse.—High fever.

Sperminum, *see* Orchitinum.

Sphingurus.

Spiggurus Martini (Mure). Histrix subspinosum. Histrix prehensilis. Tree Porcupine. *N. O.* Sphingurinæ. Trituration of prickles taken from one of the sides.

Clinical.—Hair falling out (head ; beard). Jaw-joint, pains in. Stammering. Zygoma, pain in.

Characteristics.—The Old World porcupines have the name Histricinæ, those of the New World Sphingurinæ. Mure proved the 3x trituration of the prickles. The most noteworthy symptoms were—falling out of the hair, of whiskers especially ; pain in the jaw-joint and right zygoma. Itching of the pubes after taking tea. Embarrassed speech. Nausea at sight of food. The symptoms are : < Lying down. < After tea. > Walking in open air. > After dinner.

SYMPTOMS.

1. **Mind.**—Capricious mood.—Everything is disagreeable to him.

2. **Head.**—Dizziness behind the head.—Prickings on vertex.—Darting through l. skull-bones.—Hemicrania.—Boring pain in skull after breakfast.—The hair falls off.

3. **Eyes.**—Lachrymation.

4. **Ears.**—Deafness in l. ear.—Whizzing and buzzing in ears.

6. **Face.**—Pain in articulation of jaw.—Pain in right zygoma.—Desquamation of whiskers.

8. **Mouth.**—Bleeding of gums.—Bitter mouth, with salt taste.—Embarrassed speech.

11. **Stomach.**—Nausea, with piercing pain in back.—Desire to vomit at sight of food.—Drowsy after dinner.—Constrictive pain in stomach.—Dry and full feeling in stomach at night.—Shootings in epigastrium.

12. **Abdomen.**—Sense of fulness in abdomen.—Painful swelling of abdomen before dinner.—Pain around navel.

14. **Urinary Organs.**—Violent pains in l. kidney.—Pain in urethra after urinating, < stooping.—Itching of pubes after taking tea.

17. **Respiratory Organs.**—Cough with pain in chest.

18. **Chest.**—Pain in intercostal muscles.—Pain in r. side as from a plug.

19. **Heart.**—Stitch in heart.

20. **Neck.**—Constriction from neck to diaphragm.

22. **Upper Limbs.**—Pain in r. arm, as if broken.—Pain at lower end of r. forearm.—Pain in r. arm as if extension were prevented by a string.

23. **Lower Limbs.**—Knees give way.—Heat and numbness of feet.—Cracks between toes.—Lancing pain in r. big toe.

24. **Generalities.**—Passing pains in toes, r. temple, and one canine tooth.—Weakness.—Numbness.—Symptoms < lying down ; > walking in open air ; > after dinner.

25. **Skin.**—Itching all over with bleeding after scratching.

26. **Sleep.**—Yawning.—Morning dream about a serpent.—Merry dreams.

27. **Fever.**—Shuddering.—Shuddering with chattering of teeth.

Spigelia.

Spigelia anthelmia. Demerara Pink-root. *N. O.* Loganiaceæ.
Tincture of dried herb.

Clinical.—Adenoids. Amaurosis. *Angina pectoris.* Ciliary neuralgia. Cold. *Constipation. Depression of spirits.* Diaphragm, stitches in. Exophthalmic goître. *Eyes, pains in.* Gastric catarrh. *Glaucoma. Headache. Heart, affections of.* Hernia, inguinal. Iritis. Jaw-joint, pain in. *Neuralgia.* Otalgia. Post-nasal catarrh. Prostatorrhœa. Pterygium. Rectum, cancer of. Rheumatism. *Scarlatina.* Sigmoid flexure, cancer of. Stammering. Strabismus. Tinnitus. *Tobacco habit. Toothache. Worms.*

Characteristics.—*Spigelia anthelmia* is a common weed in South America. : *S. Marylandica*, "Pink-root" or "Worm-grass," is a native of the Southern States of North America. *Spigel. anth.* is an acro-narcotic. It was known in Europe in Hahnemann's time as an anthelmintic, this property of the drug having been learned from the negroes of the Antilles. Hahnemann's proving (*M. M. P.*) revealed many other virtues. He says of the plant that it has this peculiarity : the primary action of a single unrepeated dose usually increases somewhat daily during the first seven to ten days, so that pure experiments with it should be conducted with caution, seeing that 60, 80, to 100 drops of the tincture produce violent effects even in robust persons. *Violence* is a note of the *Spigelia* action. The pains are intense, and it produces pains in all parts. It is a neuralgia remedy *par excellence.* I was once written to by a patient in the country, and the only definite points that I could make out of the case were that there was neuralgia and that it affected the left side. I ordered *Spi.*, and it speedily cured.

Spi. is more left-sided than right, but by no means exclusively left-sided. The pains are burning, jerking, tearing, pressing and stitching; they radiate and extend to other parts; are < by noise, jar, movement; change of weather—especially stormy weather. Head, eyes, face, teeth, and heart are the principal seats of *Spi.* action. Hochecker (*H. R.*, x. 147) relates the case of Miss O., 27, blonde, tall, robust, who had neuralgia for several weeks, without traceable cause. Pains came suddenly, twitching and tearing of left side of face, now in ear, then in lower jaw, and were particularly < by mastication. A peculiarity was that whenever the pains were about to commence a diarrhœa set in. A single powder of *Spi.* 6 cured. Hochecker also cured with *Spi.* 3, 6, 10, and 20 a case of tic-douloureux of *right* side of fifteen months' duration. In this case each lower attenuation after first relieving caused an aggravation. That was why the attenuations were successively raised. *Spi.* 20 completed the cure. This patient had dark hair and dark complexion. She attributed her trouble to taking cold in a draught when heated by dancing. Sensitiveness to cold, to wet and stormy weather, is one of the notes of *Spi.* The left-sidedness of *Spi.* is shown in its affinity for the heart. Sometimes the heart, eyes, and head are affected together. A case is quoted in *A. H.* (xxii. 417) in which there were darting and aching pains in head, nose, and eyes, and similar pains about the heart with slow, irregular action, but no murmur. Vertigo on stooping and heat of head. Sudden pains at bottom of back. The pains were < night and morning and in damp weather. In one prover the accustomed evening smoke caused violent toothache. I cured with *Spi.* a case of cardiac neuralgia caused by tobacco. I have frequently seen cardiac murmurs appearing in acute rheumatism disappear under *Spi.* In the eye, neuralgias, inflammation, amaurotic conditions, glaucoma presenting the symptoms of *Spi.* have been cured with it. The pains of *Spi.* are largely *out*-pressing, and proceed from within outward and below upward. A migraine comes from occiput and settles in or over left eye. In the eyes themselves there are intolerable pressive pains < on motion; but there are also stabbing pains through eye *backwards* into brain. The combination of heart and eye symptoms marks *Spi.* as the remedy in many cases of exophthalmic goître. The anthelmintic properties of *Spi.* must not be lost sight of by homeopaths. It has the cardiac symptoms of helminthiasis: itching of anus and nose, colic, and borborygmus. Hering gives this case: "Helminthiasis: dilated pupils; strabismus; putrid smell from mouth, itching of nose, griping pain in belly; throat inflamed, swallows often, pale redness in throat and swelling of mucous membrane; palpitation." Masses of lumbrici have been expelled and also threadworms. Fetid breath and fetid flatus are marked features of *Spi.* There is both constipation and diarrhœa. I have found it especially useful in heart cases where constipation has been a troublesome complication. The bodily sensitiveness of *Spi.* is paralleled by the mental irritability. But the most peculiar mental symptom is "fear of pointed things as pins, &c." Meninger (*A. H.*, xx. 282) had a severe case of nausea of pregnancy which he cured with *Spi.* The only leading symptom in the case was this: She was afraid of pointed things and asked her husband to take away a fork, crochet-needle, &c. (*Sil.* has a somewhat similar symptom, but the *Sil.* patient hunts for pins although afraid of them.) *Spi.* corresponds to rheumatism as well as to heart affections the consequence of rheumatism. A patient whom I successfully treated for a serious heart affection with *Spi.* 3 told me that under the treatment he had lost a pain in the right knee which he had had for eighteen months, and which he had not mentioned to me at first. The pain was as if dislocated ; unable to rise from kneeling ; cannot find an easy position, often for hours at night. *Peculiar Sensations* of *Spi.* are : As if he would fall. As if intoxicated. As if head would burst. As of a band around head. As if head tightly bound. As if electric sparks in temples. Brain as if loose. As if nerves being cut with a fine instrument in forehead and temple. As if eye would be pushed out of head. As if hairs or feathers on lashes. Upper lids as if paralysed. Eyeballs as if too large. As if sand in eyes. As if needles thrust into eyeball. As if eye would be pressed out of socket. As if eye would fly into pieces. As if eye were being pulled forward and backward. Pain in eye as if it would drive him crazy. As if ear loosely stopped or a thick mist before it. As if back of nose were lightly touched by hair, or as if a gentle wind were blowing across it. Face feels as if it had been scorched. As if all muscles of left side of face from head to neck and left axilla were pierced with red-hot needles. Teeth as if too long. As if left side of lower jaw would be torn out of its joint. Sensation resembling purring of cat. As of a worm rising in throat. As of a half fluid body ascending in throat. As of a hard lump in throat. As if abdomen would burst. As if all intestines would be constricted. Suffocating as if from a quantity of water poured into windpipe. Pulse as if a thread pulled through arteries. As if heart compressed or squeezed with a hand. As if heart being crushed. As if everything in chest were too short, loose, and wabbling about. As if something tearing in chest. In left scapula sensation as though blood dripping through a valve. *Spi.* is *Suited to :* Anæmic, debilitated subjects, of rheumatic diathesis ; to scrofulous children afflicted with ascarides and lumbrici ; to persons with light hair ; pale, thin, bloated, weak ; with wrinkled, yellow, earthy skin. The body is painfully sensitive to touch, the part touched feels chilly ; touch sends a shudder through the whole frame. *Spi.* is a *sun* remedy : headache beginning at sunrise, at its height at noon, declining to sunset. In chest affections there are stitching pains synchronous with the pulse. Stammering : repeats first syllable three or four times ; with abdominal ailments ; with helminthiasis. The symptoms are < by touch. Contact and pressure of clothes is unbearable. (Pressure > neuralgia.) < Jarring ; hard step. Rest >. Motion <. Moving, shaking head <. Moving eyes <. Moves very carefully. Lying with head high ; or on right side >. < Rising ; stooping ; bending forward. > Whilst eating, < immediately after. Warmth > ; (< headache). Open air = pain in eyes ; > headache. < Slightest draught ; cold, damp, rainy, stormy weather ; cold air ; cold washing ; (cold application > neuralgia temporarily). < Morning on waking. Pain increases and declines with sun. < (Also sometimes >) from tobacco. Opening mouth < headache.

Relations.—*Antidoted by:* Camph., Aur. (restlessness in limbs); Cocul., Puls. *Antidote to:* Merc., Colch. (heart). *Compatible:* Aco. (endocarditis); Ars., Dig., K. ca., Zn. (heart); Iris (prosopalgia); Arn. (carbuncle). *Compare:* Botan. Nux, Ign., Curar. Pains; left eye, Aco. Neuralgia in left eye, Ther. Headaches, coming and going with sun, Na. m., Sang., Tab. Neuralgia, Act. r. (Act. r. < right). Catarrhs, Puls. Eye pains, Bell. (Bell. more right-sided; more congestion). Heart pains; white stools, Dig. Ciliary neuralgia, Ced., Mez. (mercurial), Thuj. (pains go up and backwards). Stitches in heart, Hep., Na. m., K. ca., Ars., Caust. Headache begins occiput and goes to left eye (Sang. to right; Sil. to both). Tic-douloureux, Thu., Coccin. Aversion to be washed, Ant. c., Clem., Hep., Rhus, Sep., Sul. Faintness connected with stool, Ap., Nux m., Pul., Ver. (with *scanty* stool, Crot. t., Dulc., Ox. ac., Pet., Sars., Sul.). Neuralgia with pallor (with redness, Bell.). Nausea at sight of food, Colch., Lyc., Mosch., Ph. ac., Saba. Worms, Saba., Cin., Teuc., Scirrh., Stn. < Moving head, Sol. n. Coughing, loud speech = head pains, Bry., Caps., Nat. m., Sul. Illusions of vision, Cycl. (Cycl. when with any trouble, headache, sick stomach, &c., one always sees countless stars). < Tight clothing, Lach. Contraction of fingers, Gels., Guaiac. Sensitiveness to touch, K. ca. As if eyes too large, Act. r., Comoc. Sensation of band round heart, Cact., Carbl. ac., Sul. Post-nasal catarrh, offensive, causing choking at night, Hdrast. Scirrhus of sigmoid flexure or rectum, atrocious, unbearable pain, Alumen. Dyspnœa, must lie on right side with head high, Cact., Spo. Toothache from tobacco, Plant. Teste puts Spi. in his Arn. group; he considered it a "chronic" of Arn.

Causation.—Chill. Tobacco.

SYMPTOMS.

1. **Mind.**—Sadness and discouragement.—Agitation and anxiety, with restless care concerning the future.—Timidity.—Afraid of pointed things, pins, &c.—Sits as if lost in thought, stares at a single point.—Moroseness, to the extent of suicidal mania.—Great dejection in evening; he could have killed himself (with chilliness of body).—Weakness of memory.—Absence of ideas.—Difficulty of thinking.—Unfitness for intellectual labour.

2. **Head.**—Head confused, as from intoxication or dizziness.—Giddiness when looking downwards.—Vertigo, to such an extent as to fall down when walking, standing, or looking down.—Vertigo, with nausea.—Headache, on shaking head, with vertigo, and sensation of heaviness.—Neuralgic pains flying from one part to another.—Headache beginning in cerebellum, morning, spreading over l. side of head, causing violent and pulsating pain in l. temple and over l. eye, with stitches in left eye; returning periodically. Painfulness of cerebellum with stiffness of neck.—Stitches in l. side of head and out of l. eye.—Headache like a heaviness; on drawing the facial muscles it seems as though the skull would burst upward and asunder.—Fine burrowing-tearing pains in brain, esp. violent in l. parietal bone; < on false step.—Sharp shaking just behind and above r. frontal eminence.—Pressive pain in r. side of head involving r. eye, morning in bed, < after rising; pain

deeply seated, unaffected by pressure, very acute on motion; on suddenly turning head brain seemed loose; < every jar, step, even straining at stool. —Stitches like electric sparks in head.—Pains in head < by slightest movement, by least noise, and by opening mouth.—Headaches are < from least noise; > when lying with head high, and from washing head with cold water.—Painful tenderness of the occiput, with sensation of numbness and stiffness in nape of neck.—Periodical headaches.—Pressing asunder in head, esp. in r. temple; < from motion and opening mouth; > while at rest.—Pressure in head, compressive or expansive, < by stooping.—Sensation of a tight band around head.—Pain, as if head about to burst, when coughing and speaking loud.—Tearing, digging, or boring headache from within to without, in forehead, vertex, or cerebellum, < during movement.—Sensation of soreness in forehead and vertex.—Tearing in forehead in paroxysms, with fixed eyes.—Pulsative lancinations in forehead, with noise as of hammering before the ears.—Commotions and blows in head, while walking in open air. —Shaking in brain at every step, and at every movement of head.—Burning pain in exterior of forehead and temples as far as eyes.—Tension in scalp.—Painful tenderness of scalp when touched; < when moving the scalp.—Head feels too large.

3. **Eyes.**—Neuralgia of eyes, esp. where there is great soreness, and can scarcely bear a touch; affections of the eyeball; eyelids; optic nerve; dilated pupils; ocular illusions—sees strange things, fiery, luminous rays, sparks, &c. —On shutting eyes a sea of fire appears.—Illusion as if hairs or feathers on lashes; < on moving them.—Impending amaurosis.—Pains in eyes, deeply seated in sockets.—Aching (pressure) in the eyeballs, esp. when turning them. —Pains in the eyes during movement, as if eyeballs were too large.—Digging, boring, and shootings in eyes, penetrating into head, sometimes with pain, which drives to despair.—Pains as if needles thrust into r. eyeball.—Movement of eyes and muscles of face < the pains.—Tingling in eyes.—Itching in r. eyeball, returning after rubbing.—Dry heat and burning sensation in eyes, which forces them to close.—Redness of sclerotica, with injection of blood-vessels.—Inflammation of eyes and of cornea.—Inflammation and ulceration of lids, with smarting pain as from excoriation.—Eyes confused and dull.—Profuse lachrymation.—Acrid, smarting tears.—Great sensitiveness of eyes to light.—Hanging down of lids as from paralysis.—Sensation as of a hard substance under r. upper lid, > by rubbing.—Violent burrowing stitch in middle of eye and in inner canthus that does not prevent vision, but presses upper lid down.—Upper lids feel hard and immovable.—Pain as if l. orbit were pressed from above downward.—Tendency to wink.—Weakness of eyes; in whatever direction they are turned they remain.—Difficulty in raising the eyelids, with painful sensation of stiffness.—Contraction and involuntary movement of eyes.—Squint; convergent.—"A dose of *Spigel.* always produced squint in us when children" (American lady's testimony.—R. T. C.).—Strabismus whether from worms or not (Macfarlan).—Pupils dilated.—Loss (momentary suspension) of sight.—Presbyopia.

4. **Ears.**—Earache with an ichorous, scalding discharge; hearing very sensitive; noise in the ear as of something fluttering.—Pain in margin of l. concha.—Drawing in l. antitragus.—Itching in r. concha.—Pressive pains in r. ear.—Otalgia, with pressive, troublesome pain, as if there were a plug in

ear.—Jerking tearing in ears.—Squeezing, itching, and burning sensation in external ear.—Itching in r. vesicle.—Stoppage of ears, with or without dysecoia.—Periodical deafness.—Sensation of distant ringing in ears, with sensation as if the ear were loosely stopped or a thick mist were in front of it.—Roaring, buzzing, and pulsation in ears.—Noise of hammering before ears.

5. **Nose.**—Itching in nose, with tickling.—Tickling on back of nose, as if lightly touched by hairs, or as if a gentle wind were blowing across it.—Tingling, shooting, boring, smarting and itching in nose.—Herpetic eruption on nose with pain, as from excoriation.—Stoppage and dryness of anterior nose, with copious discharge of whitish and yellowish mucus from posterior nares.—Frequent sneezing; discharge of bloody mucus.—Mucus at one time white, at another time yellow, is discharged from nose; at same time much mucus is discharged from mouth.—Fluent coryza, which recurs frequently, esp. after slightest chill.

6. **Face.**—Face pale and wan, with yellow circles round eyes.—Redness of face; perspiration on face.—Cheeks and lips at one time a deep red, at another time pale.—Burning in r. side of upper lip.—Bloatedness of face, esp. after sleeping.—Facial muscles seem distorted and swollen, morning on rising.—Prosopalgia (mostly l.-sided).—Jerking tearings, burning sensation, and aching in region of zygomatic process; or violent pains, which cannot bear the slightest touch or least movement, with shining swelling of side affected.—Periodical neuralgia; from morning until sunset; < at noon; < from motion or noise.—Semilateral pains in face, with præcordial anxiety and great agitation.—Exostosis of the temporal part of the orbit.—Lips tense and burning.—Small blackish pimples on upper lip.—Pressive pain in angle of lower jaw, as if in the jaw or in the teeth, proceeding from the ear.—Tearing in lower jaw, radiating to ear and about it as far as nape; could not move head without pain.—Pain as if r. side of lower jaw would be torn out of its joint, only when chewing.

7. **Teeth.**—Toothache (in evening) after customary smoke in evening.—Toothache > by tobacco smoke.—Pain, like pressing asunder, in the teeth, immediately after a meal, or at night, which does not permit continued lying down.—Toothache so that he was unable to sleep at night; it drove him out of bed; not during day, except just *after* eating, not *while* eating.—Toothache > by warmth of bed.—Toothache like a pressure outward; < lying on r. side.—Jerking toothache, or with pulsative tearings, esp. in carious teeth, < by cold water after eating or by contact with the open air; > whilst eating and when lying down.—Toothache with prosopalgia, paleness and bloatedness of face, yellowish circles round eyes, palpitation of heart, shivering and agitation.

8. **Mouth.**—Offensive exhalation from the mouth, noticed only by others.—(Stinging) lancinating dryness in mouth on waking in morning.—Much white, frothy saliva in mouth.—White or yellow mucus in mouth and palate.—Tongue cracked.—Vesicles, with burning pain, on tongue and palate.—Took away the pain of cancer of tongue (Bayes, *H. W.*, xviii. 3).

9. **Throat.**—Sore throat, with lancinations and swelling in palate.—Discharge of mucus from fauces all day, most from posterior nares.—Cervical glands swollen.

10. **Appetite.**—Putrid, fetid taste.—Anorexia, with violent thirst.—epugnance to tobacco-smoke and snuff.—Dislike to coffee.—Bulimy, some-mes with nausea and thirst.

11. **Stomach.**—Risings after every meal.—Sour risings.—Nausea (in the orning) when fasting, with a sensation as if something were ascending from omach into throat.—Accumulation of mucus in the stomach.—Pressure in omach and scrobiculus as from a heavy body (as from a hard lump).—Lan-inations in pit of stomach and diaphragm, sometimes with obstructed espiration.—Dull stitches in pit of stomach, < from inspiration, with ppression of the chest.—Inability to bear tight clothing round scrobiculus; e least contact causes anguish, with redness and heat of face, and sensation s if something were torn away in chest.

12. **Abdomen.**—Griping in abdomen, as if intestines constricted, with nxiety and difficult breathing.—Abdomen hard, and painfully tight.—Stitches region of diaphragm, l. side, arresting breathing.—Pressure in umbilical egion, as by a hard body.—Colic, with pinching pains, cuttings (from worms) the umbilical region, with shivering, diarrhœa, and copious secretion of rine.—Lancinations (stitches) in the abdomen.—Tensive pain in the groins hen touched.—Grumbling and borborygmi in the abdomen.—Painful pres-ure in lower abdomen, as if it would burst, esp. in evening before a soft ool; sometimes > after.—Expulsion of fetid flatus.

13. **Stool and Anus.**—Frequent, urgent, and ineffectual want to vacuate.—Soft, liquid fæces.—White stools daily.—Nodular stool with iolent pressure.—Faints during stool.—Hard, difficult evacuations, with uch mucus.—Discharge (of large lumps) of mucus from anus, without vacuation.—Liquid diarrhœa of fæcal matter and of mucus.—Diarrhœa, ith pinchings in abdomen and coldness in body.—Discharge of fæces with orms.—Ejection of lumbrici and ascarides from rectum.—Itching and sen-ation as if something were creeping in rectum and anus.—Boring stitches in erinæum.—(Scirrhus of sigmoid or rectum, atrocious, unbearable pains.—I. C. Allen).

14. **Urinary Organs.**—Urine, with whitish sediment.—Frequent want urinate, with profuse emission, even at night.—Sudden and involuntary ibbling of urine, with burning sensation in anterior part of urethra.—ischarge of prostatic fluid from the urethra.

15. **Male Sexual Organs.**—Tingling round glans penis.—Semilateral welling of glans.—Erections, with lascivious ideas, without voluptuous excite-ent.—(Discharge of prostatic fluid.)—Itching stitch in r. testicle and penis, om behind forward.

17. **Respiratory Organs.**—Catarrh, with hoarseness, continual dis-harge of mucus from nose, dry heat without thirst, prominent eyes, istressing headache, and disposition to weep.—Nocturnal catarrh, with ough.—Cough in open air, with pain in chest as from excoriation.—Dry ough, violent and hollow, caused by irritation low down in trachea, with espiration obstructed, even to suffocation.—Short, dry cough causing sore-ess of chest.—Shortness of breath, esp. when talking, with anxiety and edness of cheeks and lips.—Dyspnœa when moving in bed; can only lie n r. side; or with the head very high.—Danger of suffocation on least ovement, and esp. on raising arms.

18. Chest.—Aching at the chest, with painful oppression.—Contractio of chest, with anguish and obstructed respiration.—Stitches in diaphragn with dyspnœa.—Noise in the chest like that made by a spinning-wheel, esp in region of heart.—Pressure, burning or incisive sensation, pain, as fron ulceration and tearing in chest, esp. on lifting arms.—Cutting tearing beneatl l. nipple, extending to region of scapulæ and upper arm, < during inspira tion and deep breathing.—Sensation of trembling in thorax, < by movin arms.—Spasmodic sensation in chest, proceeding from pit of stomach an causing choking.—Tensive lancinations in chest, esp. when drawing breath.

19. Heart.—Violent palpitation of heart, perceptible to sight and hearing often with anxious oppression of chest, < by curving chest forwards and b sitting down.—Noise in chest, like that made by a spinning-wheel, esp. i region of heart.—Sudden attack of suffocation, with palpitation of heart an anguish.—Heavy aching in region of apex, with feeling as if a dull-pointe knife were slowly driven through it.—(Organic diseases of the heart; rubbing bellows sounds.)—Sensation in heart as if squeezed with hand; as if crushed —Lancinations in region of heart.—Stitches in heart, sometimes synchronou with the pulse.—Sensation of trembling in heart.—The beatings of the hear do not correspond with those of the pulse.—Pulse weak, irregular, trembling —Undulating movement of the heart.—In affections of the heart, particularl if the whole l. side is sore from the affection, and possibly the eyes als from sympathy; purring of heart as of a cat; palpitation of the heart wit anguish; trembling pulsation of the heart; sympathy of the chest with hear troubles.—(Visible pulsation of heart.—Violent, oppressive action of heart ex tending to top of head.—Tumultuous action of heart in acute rheumatism an other acute disorders.—R. T. C.)

20. Neck and Back.—Needle-like stitches in upper dorsal vertebræ in r. scapula.—Sensation in l. scapula as though blood were dripping througl a valve, a kind of bubbling.—Red pimples on neck, with pain as from excoria tion when touched.—Hard and painful swelling of glands of the neek.—Pain in nape, < when still, > by motion.—Intermittent drawing in posterior cervica muscles and up to occiput.—Sticking pain in r. side of neck; on swallowing pain in parotid gland.—Itching of anus and coccyx.—Pain in back as fron a fracture, also during movement.—Bruised feeling in spine, even durin rest.—Lancinations (stitches) in back, sometimes on drawing breath.

21. Limbs.—Fatigue.—Drawing, tearing, twitching pains in limbs an joints.—The limbs are affected mostly when walking.

22. Upper Limbs.—Heaviness and trembling of arms.—Easy numbin of arms and hands.—Jerking of muscles of arms and forearms.—Violent lan cinations and shocks in bend of elbow and joints of hands and fingers.— Spasmodic drawings and tearings in bones of hands. Hard nodosities in th palms, with burning itching.—Hands of a pale yellow colour.—Contractio of fingers.—Purulent pimples on fingers.

23. Lower Limbs.—Pain, as of a fracture, tension and shootings i thighs, almost exclusively, when walking, or during rapid movements.— Stitches in the joints of the legs and feet and in the thigh.—Violent lancina tions in knee on bending it.—Painful stiffness in knee-joint.—Lancinating shocks in joints of feet.—Excrescences, like warts, on toes.

24. Generalities.—[Very violent neuralgia, followed by an extreme sores; boring pains; pains as if parts were pushed or pressed asunder, or as if y would burst; sensation of extension in size; feeling as of a lump in the er parts; darting pains in inner and outer parts; darting pain from within ward; in the joints; pains of a dragging or rooting character.—Affections general of r. side of face and nose; stool with maw-worms (oxyuris ver-ularis); discharge of urine too copious, sensitiveness of outer parts; rsion to washing; trembling pulse that can scarcely be counted.—< On oping; when blowing nose; during expiration; after rising from a seat; m touching the parts affected; when walking in open air; from having rms.—> While taking an inspiration.—H. N. G.].—Arthritic, shooting, or ring pains in the limbs.—Stinging pain in the limbs and principally in the ıts.—Tearing in the vicinity of the joints, as if the bone were scraped.—aviness and soreness in the body when rising from a seat.—Sensitiveness body to touch, with chilliness of the parts touched; or it sends a shudder ough whole body.—Great weakness, esp. mornings.—Heaviness and sen-ion in limbs as if fractured.—Convulsions.—Lassitude, esp. after slight rcise, and in open air.—Syncope, esp. when making an effort to evacuate, in a warm room.—Great sensitiveness to cold air, with sufferings from lking in open air.—Great liability to suffer from a chill.

25. **Skin.**—Pale, wrinkled skin of body.—Painful sensibility of entire n when touched.—Painful glandular swellings.—Red pimples, with pain, from excoriation, when touched.

26. **Sleep.**—Strong disposition to sleep by day, and also in morning or ning; but without sleeping until long after lying down.—Sleep at night, efreshing, agitated, with uneasiness in limbs.—Heavy, stupefying sleep.—ıfused dreams, which cause him to awake wearied, and which he cannot ıember.

27. **Fever.**—Pulse irregular, generally strong, but slow.—Trembling se.—Frequent shiverings, esp. in morning or during slight exercise.—ll, frequently returning at the same hour in the morning.—Chill, alter-ing with heat or perspiration.—Chilliness on some part of the body, on ers heat.—The chill extends from the chest.—Frequent heat, sometimes ısient.—Heat, esp. in back.—Heat in face and on hands, with chill in k.—Thirst for beer during the heat (with flushes of heat at night).—At ht putrid perspiration with heat at same time.—Clammy perspiration.—d perspiration.

Spigelia Marilandica.

gelia Marilandica. Pink-root. Worm-grass. *N. O.* Loganiaceæ. Tincture of root.

Clinical.—Mania. Strabismus (r.).

Characteristics.—The symptoms of *Spi. m.* are mainly from rdosing. A state of mania was induced in a boy from large and quent doses of a decoction of the root. Strabismus of right eye was ted in one case.

SYMPTOMS.

1. **Mind.**—Suddenly affected with complete mental derangeme exactly like that of *Stram.*, countenance distorted, running and skippi fits of laughing and crying, pupils greatly dilated, talk wild and incohere (lasted 24h.).

2. **Head.**—Vertigo.

3. **Eyes.**—Wild, staring, ludicrous expression.—Irregular movement adductors and abductors of eyes.—Strabismus of r. eye.—Pain in and about t eyes.—Sensation of stiffness of eyelids.—Pupils dilated.

6. **Face.**—Much swelling of face and about eyes.—Face flushed.

8. **Mouth.**—Tongue pointed and tremulous.

19. **Heart.**—Pulse : accelerated ; irregular.

24. **Generalities.**—On attempting to assume erect position, seiz with general tremor lasting a few seconds and leaving her exhausted.

26. **Sleep.**—Drowsiness.

27. **Fever.**—Skin hot and dry.

Spiræa Ulmaria.

Spiræa Ulmaria. Queen of the Meadows. Meadow-sweet. *N.* Rosaceæ. Tincture of fresh root.

Clinical. — Conscientiousness, morbid. Convulsions. Epilepsy. Eyelic affections of. Hydrophobia. Œsophagus, stricture of. Ptosis. Urine, deposits i

Characteristics.—Bojanus proved *Spiræa*, taking substanti doses. A leading symptom was the production of *heat*, general an local. Heat in throat ; in œsophagus ; under manubrium sterni; und ensiform cartilage. Bojanus was seized with remorse, a kind of morbi conscientiousness. Fulness and heaviness of head. Washing wi cold water was very unpleasant, and caused a feeling as if the hea were too large. A scurfy condition of eyelids and heaviness of li after siesta were noted. The urine was turbid as if mixed wi clay, and deposited red sand ; had an oily film on the surfac Hansen mentions *Spir.* as having been recommended in hydrophobi epilepsy, and eclampsia. The burning in œsophagus was > by eatin and drinking but not by empty swallowing. Symptoms were < indoors ; > in open air. < Moving head. < Sneezing. > Movin about.

SYMPTOMS.

1. **Mind.**—At 1 a.m. was attacked with remorse over a long-past slig indiscretion, with most fearful qualms of conscience and loathing of himsel could not rest on account of it, obliged to rise and walk about.

2. **Head.**—Vertigo with heat in cheeks.—Headache : < shaking head with increased warmth of body, as if blood flowing more rapidly throug vessels ; > towards evening. Dulness and heaviness in head with pressi

adache.—On lying down at 11 p.m. sensation like vertigo, as if all senses aished and all blood left the head, with a prickling in face.—Pain over ole head as if a ring were tightened about head with heaviness ; on shaking ad, brain seemed to wabble to and fro.—After washing, head felt large.—essive headache and fulness in forehead, < in house, > in open air.

3. **Eyes.**—Eyes full of mucus, dried to crusts on waking.—Lachrymation l. eye, increased warmth in it ; sclerotic bright red.—On waking lids so vy cannot open them for a long time.—Sensation as if something hot unted to eyes, causing biting and burning and sensation as if tears would v, but they did not.

6. **Face.**—Face red.—Sensation as if blood mounted to face with reased heat.

8. **Mouth.**—Slight drawing toothache in l. back teeth.

9. **Throat.**—Increased warmth in pharynx, extending down to stomach ; ning pressure in œsophagus, generally > at night; > eating and drinking, on empty swallowing.—Sensation as if œsophagus too small, constricted.—d sensation in œsophagus extending to both sides of chest.—Warmth in ophagus opposite the manubrium sterni.

11. **Stomach.**—No relish for smoking.—Frequent eructations.—Burning small spot beneath ensiform cartilage as if something hot or acrid had n taken.

12. **Abdomen.**—Frequent emission of very offensive flatus.—Movings gripings in hypogastrium during stool.—After eating moving in navel.

13. **Stool and Anus.**—Prickling, crawling, sticking in rectum and anus.—kling, constrictive sensation long after stool.—Frequent desire for stool, that denly disappeared.—Stool delayed, evacuated with pressure and straining, l, scanty, like sheep's dung.—About 10 p.m. somewhat hard stool, accomied and followed by burning and soreness in the anus, and a sensation as e anus were drawn up into rectum and something hard were still remain-there.

14. **Urinary Organs.**—Burning at orifice of urethra while urinating ing stool.—Urine bright yellow when passed, becomes cloudy, forming posit like clay with red, gritty sand.

15. **Male Sexual Organs.**—In morning in bed, violent erections with t sexual desire.

17. **Respiratory Organs.**—At 7 p.m. cough, at first dry, afterwards e, with tickling and scraping in throat, that continued long after the gh.—On inspiration air of room seemed very cold as if he had been wing peppermint.

18. **Chest.**—Pressure beneath manubrium sterni as if he had swallowed large a morsel ; or a large piece of hard-boiled egg.

19. **Heart.**—Pulse : hard and tense ; weak, soft ; small, contracted, hard, wards full and large.

22. **Upper Limbs.**—Cramp in muscle of forearm on lifting anything.—s in hands distended.

23. **Lower Limbs.**—Heaviness in lower limbs as if full, esp. on ascend-steps.

24. **Generalities.**—In afternoon, exhaustion with stretching and yawn-—Discomfort after siesta.

26. **Sleep.**—Overpowering sleepiness, heaviness in limbs and dulness head.—Difficult falling asleep in evening; restlessness, frequent waking Dreams: vivid during midday nap; in evening lascivious and emission.

27. **Fever.**—Great heat over whole body.—Heat like rush of blood head and face.—While eating, and after, heat over whole body and rush blood to head, with slight outbreak of sweat on chest, face, and hands.

Spiranthes.

Spiranthes autumnalis. Lady's Tresses. *N. O.* Orchidaceæ. Tinct of the root.

Clinical.— Breasts, painful. Breath, putrid. Burns. Coryza. Dyspar Eczema. Hysteria. Kidneys, pain in. Lumbago. Milk, excessive. Skin, affec of. Vision, dimness of.

Characteristics.— The genus to which this orchid belo received its name from the spiral arrangement of the flowers. tuberous roots of *Spir. autum.* were "formerly esteemed as an ap disiac" (*Treas. of Bot.*). The tincture of the root was proved Dr. Patti Chagon, Duc de Sorentino, who says of it: "The actio this drug begins with decided symptoms of inflammation of the e chin, chest, which become red and hot; the whole skin is dry hot; the hands are burning, the extremities of the feet are cold n of the time; there is a sensation of oppression and heat, with pal tion and a desire to uncover." This condition lasted two hours gave place to others, including desire to meditate and comp vertigo, pains in shoulders, *ennui*, loss of appetite. The symptoms to appear are: pains in scalp, on vertex, distres kidneys and intestinal troubles after eating. The secretions of urine milk were first diminished, afterwards increased. The aphrodi property of *Spiran.* was shown in some of the symptoms of the prov and this bears on the increased secretion of milk. A numbe symptoms appear in the lower abdomen, and the globus hyster rises from thence to œsophagus. Heat in lower abdomen; prece eructations; caused by laughing. Among the *Peculiar Symp* are: cerebral troubles on bending or raising the arm. Sensatio a band tied round head. Sensation of a foreign body in th Coldness of teeth. Pulsation in arteries over whole body. Cold of the affected part. Preference for lying on left side; or els back. Pain followed by numbness. The symptoms are < by to < Bending or raising arm. < Raising breast. Laughing = hea lower abdomen. Least emotion = palpitation. < Mental ef > Lying on left side. > Lying on back. < Bending over (rheuma of shoulders). < Stooping.

Relations.—*Compare:* Botan., Cypr. Skin and mucous m branes, Ar. t. Desire for tight clothing; dryness of vagina, Na Pain followed by numbness, Gnaph.

SYMPTOMS.

1. **Mind.**—Melancholy.—Complaining and sobbing.—Ill-humour.—Con-
usion of ideas.—Indolence and *ennui.*

2. **Head.**—Vertigo : obliged to lean head against wall ; on rising
·om bed ; < sitting or lying.—Heaviness and heat in brain.—Brain troubles
< bending or raising arm.—Sensation of band tied about head.—Weight on
›rehead.—Pain in forehead and nasal bone.—Pain in roots of hair.—Hair
ılls out.

3. **Eyes.**—Eyes brilliant ; fixed.—Pain in eyes on looking up.—Burning
ı eyes and lachrymation.—Heaviness of brows.—Lids swollen.—Eyes hot,
ıflamed.—Vision: dim; obscured, with sleepiness; instantaneously lost; objects
t a distance seem to move ; on closing lids, sees wheels of fire.

4. **Ears.**—Pain in l. auditory canal.—Itching in ear, externally and
ıternally.

5. **Nose.**—Dry coryza.—Epistaxis : in clots.—Dripping of water from
ose.—Pain in (r.) nasal bones.—Burning itching at root of nose.—Itching of
ala.—Smell very acute.

6. **Face.**—Face : swollen ; red and hot ; blackish ; pale.—Fixed, medi-
.tive expression.—Burning in upper lip.—Chin : red ; pain in.

8. **Mouth.**—Pain and elongation of teeth.—Toothache only at night.—
ensation of coldness in teeth.—Gums red and burning.—Numerous small
xcrescences on palate, which was bloody.—Putrid odour from mouth.—
rritation of sublingual glands.—Taste : acid ; sweetish, like nitre ; bitter in
ıorning.—Salivation with dryness of mouth.

9. **Throat.**—Globus rising from lower abdomen to œsophagus.—Sensa-
on of foreign body in throat.—Incessant desire to clear throat, caused by a
ıick mucus.—Tickling in throat, provoking cough.—Burning in pit of throat.
-Irritation of tonsils.—Sensation of acidity and burning in œsophagus.—
ıcarceration of air in œsophagus.—Pain on swallowing.

11. **Stomach.**—Desire for acid food.—Loss of appetite.—Constant
ıirst.—Regurgitations.—Eructations : preceded by heat in lower abdomen
ıd lancinations in colon ; acid ; bitter ; difficult ; empty.—Nausea : after
ıting.—Vomiting ; of food after eating.—Epigastrium : distended, intolerant
f touch ; painful after a meal, the pain corresponding to the pain in loins.—
leat rising from stomach to head.

12. **Abdomen.**—Pain : in liver ; and spleen ; on pressure.—Inter-
ıittent pressure in umbilical region.—Pain ; weakness ; tympanites ; after a
ıeal.—Borborygmi.—Desire to tighten clothes.—Piercing, lancinating, in-
ıpportable pain in colon ; on becoming erect.—Laughing = heat in lower
›domen.—Eruption in groin.

13. **Stool and Anus.**—Burning and itching in anus < during evacua-
on.—Stool preceded and followed by prickling and itching in anus.—
·iarrhœa or constipation ; stools sour in children.

14. **Urinary Organs.**—In kidneys : cramp-like pain at night, obliging
ıange of position ; burning ; pain preventing stooping ; < going up stairs,
· lying on back ; coldness and heat.—In bladder : pain on urinating ; pain
ıd burning after waking.—Urine : abundant ; scanty ; decomposes rapidly ;
eposits a gelatinous red sediment.

15. **Male Sexual Organs.**—Erections, on waking; constant.—Pricking pain in cords.—Great desire for, or repugnance to, coition.

16. **Female Sexual Organs.**—Redness of vulva with pruritus.—Pressing pain in uterus.—Bloody discharge from vagina.—Yellowis leucorrhœa.—Burning in vagina.—Burning pain in vagina during coition.—Dryness of vagina.

17. **Respiratory Organs.**—Burning in larynx.—Hacking cough, cause by tickling in larynx.—Dry cough at night, with burning in throat.—Dı cough.—Respiration: difficult; short; panting on walking.

18. **Chest.**—Sensation of dilatation of l. lung.—Sensation of weakness lungs.—Pleuritic and intercostal pains, < l. side.—Milk, abundant: more i l. breast.—Pain in breast on raising it.—Burning on tips of breasts, esp. l.

19. **Heart.**—Pain in heart.—Palpitation: with difficult respiration from least emotional excitement.—Pulse full and hard at beginning of provin afterwards small and quiet.

20. **Neck and Back.**—Cramp-like pain in neck at night compelli change of position.—Lumbago preventing walking.—Pain in centre scapula.—Pain in scapula, when standing, < walking.

21. **Limbs.**—Trembling in limbs; weakness.

22. **Upper Limbs.**—Shoulders: heavy pain in; boring in r., extendi to r. breast and preventing breathing; pressure on and in chest; lancin tions < bending over.—Arms: trembling; weakness; numb and hea (esp. r.); desire to stretch.—Pain in forearms by the pulse; in r. puls —Rigidity of muscles of forearm.—Sudden pain in forearm followed by num ness.—Hands: swollen, esp. r.; veins swollen; blackish; yellowish; red a perspiring; burning, numb.—At night numbness of hand on which he rest cheek.—Pressing pain in extremities.

23. **Lower Limbs.**—Eruptions on nates; in groins; on thighs.—Sciat pain in limbs, esp. r.—Drawing pain in r. limb.—Knees: weak; pain i pain in r.—Pain in r. malleolus.—Feet (esp. r.) swollen.—Pain in heels.

24. **Generalities.**—One appears intoxicated.—Pulsations in arteries ov whole body.—Lies on l. side rather than r.

25. **Skin.**—Dryness of skin.—Whole skin red; red in spots.—Jaundic —Yellow spots.—Miliary rash.—Eruption of red points on nates with itchi and heat.—Vesications as from a burn, with purulent secretion from the gro and in folds of skin about neck.—Pricking over whole body.—Burning itchi in l. cheek near mouth.—Itching: in axillæ; in pubes; scrotum; forear at night; backs of hands; tip of l. thumb.

26. **Sleep.**—Incomplete, yawning.—Sleeping during day.—Starting during sleep.—Late falling asleep, evening.—Sleeplessness in infants.—Lascivious dreams with emissions.

27. **Fever.**—Coldness, evening, esp. of hands.—Alternations of cold a heat.—Affected part colder than rest of body.—Coldness of feet; and toes.—Fever, followed by thirst.—Fever at night, sweat in morning.—Heat of wh skin; flushes of heat in head, followed by sensation of cold.—Heat of he on waking.—Heat and itching over head.—Heat and redness; external e —Heat of face, esp. r. side.—Hands very hot.—Sweat of palms.

Spongia Tosta.

Common Sponge, roasted. *N. O.* Cœlenterata. Tincture (20 grains in 400 drops of alcohol).

Clinical.—Aneurism. Angina pectoris. Asthma. Catalepsy. Chin, affections of. Clumsiness. Constipation. *Cough. Croup.* Diplopia. Exophthalmos, Fainting. *Goître;* exophthalmic. Heart, hypertrophy of. Hernia. Jaw-joint, pain in. Laryngismus. *Laryngitis.* Myopia. Rheumatic fever. Rheumatism. *Testicles, inflammation of.* Tuberculosis. Varicosis. Whooping-cough. Worms.

Characteristics.—According to Hahnemann, Toasted Sponge was first mentioned as a specific for goître by Arnald von Villanova in the thirteenth century; but it was generally given mixed with other substances, and had fallen into disuse when Hahnemann proved it. The virtues of *Spongia* have been attributed to the *Iodine* contained in it, and partially liberated by the presence of roasting. But *Spongia* contains many other elements besides *Iodine*, and it has a distinctive action of its own. It is antipodal to *Iod.* in this respect, that it is best *Suited to* blue-eyed, fair-haired patients, whereas *Iod.* acts best on brunettes. *Spo.* is suited to scrofulous affections, and is often indicated with women of lax fibre, and children. One of the keynotes of *Spo.* is *Dryness of mucous membrane*—of tongue, pharynx, larynx, trachea. Cough is caused by dryness. The cough itself is dry, intensely hacking, crowing, "dry as a bone," or sounding like a saw being driven through a pine board. Dry asthma. In laryngismus, croup, and asthma the patient rouses up generally after midnight with fear of suffocation and death. The sputa cannot be raised, must be swallowed, swallowing >. In laryngismus there is contraction of larynx as if suddenly grasped. With the dyspnœa there is terrible sinking; he seems to be sinking down in a pit. The larynx is sensitive, but has not the hyperæsthesia of *Lach.* Like *Lach. Spo.* has < after sleep. Rouses up in sleep as if in a great fright. Cough is excited by talking; by dry, cold winds; > by eating or drinking; by swallowing; especially > by warm food. Sweets <. *Spo* meets some cases of true tuberculosis; of larynx; of apices, with commencing solidification; tubercles spreading downwards. Congestion of chest coming on when the patient is moving about with sudden weakness as if he would fall. *Rawness* in the chest is another note of *Spo.* The action of *Spo.* on the respiratory organs is closely connected with its action on the glandular system, the lymphatics, the thyroid, and testes are indurated. The blood, heart, and veins are also involved, and with the protruding eyes a perfect picture of exophthalmic goître is produced. Hypertrophy of the heart is frequently met by *Spo.*, and it is especially indicated when the right heart is affected and when asthmatic symptoms are associated with it. *Spo.* meets some cases of croupous deposit on the valves of the heart as it does croup of the larynx. The *Spo.* patient in phthisical and other conditions is subject to frequent flashes of heat. The chill commences usually across the back. He shakes near a warm stove. The heat which follows extends over the whole body except the thighs, which remain numb and chilly. In the heart affections the patient is aroused from sleep as if smothering ; sits up in bed with an anxious look, flushed face, and hard, rapid breathing. Kent (*M.A.*, xxv. 17) gives this indication : " Rheumatic fever after having been over-heated, with arising heart complications." Nash gives this keynote of *Spo.* in valvular diseases : " Awakes out of sleep from a sense of suffocation, with violent, loud cough, great alarm, agitation, anxiety, and difficult respiration." He says it is better than *Lach.* here ; and relieves the " dry, chronic, sympathetic cough of organic heart disease " more frequently and more permanently than *Naja.* *Spo* meets also thickening of joints after rheumatic fever. In orchitis, with heaviness and screw-like squeezing pain in cord and testicle, *Spo* is the chief remedy, though others are generally needed before that stage is reached. Timidity, fear, and terror are leading mental symptoms. Any excitement and thinking of symptoms <. *Peculiar Sensations* are : As if head would fall to one side. As if tipsy. As if all her blood were mounting to head. As if skull would burst. As if hair were standing on end. Eyes as if twisted around. As if a battery of guns were discharged in ears. Stitches as if passing through tympanum. Nodule in concha as if it would gather and break. Jaw as if dislocated. As if eruption were to appear near chin. Left side of chin as if ulcerated. As if something had got jammed between teeth in chewing. As if gums and teeth were swollen, the latter being lifted. Outside of throat as if something were being pressed out. As of a plug in throat. As if he had drunk a great deal of luke-warm water, relaxation of stomach, and œsophagus. Pit of stomach as if growing together. Stomach as if standing open. Of obstruction in abdomen (and in trachea). As if something alive moving in abdomen. As if something alive beneath skin of abdomen. As if diarrhœa would ensue. As of a plug in larynx. As if a stopper or valve were in larynx. As of a nail pressing in larynx. As if larynx and trachea were removed. As if she would suffocate. As if child could not get breath. As if breathing through a sponge. As if chest would burst. Chest as if sore and bloody. As of a large accumulation and weight at chest. As if a broad body armed with points were pressing upward. As if a weight were dragging down on chest. As if she had something hot inside chest. As if blood would burst out of chest. As if cervical glands were swelling. As if skin of neck were compressed between fingers. As if air were passing up and down thyroid and cervical glands. Thyroid gland as if hardened. As if everything were shaking and moving about in goître. As if goître were alive. As if a pointed instrument were thrust into scapulæ. As if bones of forearm were being pressed together. As if parts in and between wrists were weakened by decay. As if a muscle were too short in upper end of thigh. As if knees would give way. As if weight hanging on lower end of tibia As of pins in heels. As if she were going to faint. As if everything were in flames. As if sweat would break out. There is excitement of the nerves ; tendency to start ; twitching of muscles, with fever. Stiff without ability to move. " Conscious but unable to act on her limbs " (as in a cataleptic state). Clumsiness of body. Faint when losing her breath. Feeling of numbness of lower half of body.

< When thinking of her symptoms. Complaints extend downwards; from within out; from right to left. There are cramp-like pains. Bitter taste in *throat.* Aversion to tobacco. Desire for dainties (but sweets <). The symptoms are < by touch and pressure. Scratching does not > biting itching. < Motion; walking; stooping; rising; raising arms (becomes faint); talking; singing. Bending forward > dyspnœa; < symptoms of circulation. > Descending. > Resting in horizontal position. Lying with head low <. Lying right side <. < At night. Before midnight: croup <; dry sound of breathing and cough; sleepless until midnight. After midnight: wakes with palpitation; with suffocation. < Warm room. > Warm food or drink. Frosty weather > cough. Dry, cold weather > headache. Cold weather = coryza. Cold air < cough. < Sudden changes of atmosphere. < At full moon. < Periodically; every night. Eating and drinking > cough; drinking = cough. < Sweets. < After sleep.

Relations.—*Antidoted by:* Camph. *Follows well:* Aco., Hep. *Followed well by:* Bro., Carb. v., Hep. [Bœnninghausen's croup powders consisted of a sequence of Aco., Spo., Hep., given in that order. Spo. is dry; Hep. rattling; Spo. < before midnight; Hep. < after.] *Compare:* In general affections, Chlo., Bro., Iod. (Iod. dark, Spo. fair subjects), Thyroidin, Badiaga. Laryngitis, Samb. (with Samb. the spasms occur frequently); Lach. (sensitive to touch; Lach. from hyperæsthesia; Spo. from inflammation of cartilages). Cough > by eating, Anac. Dry tongue, Nux m. (with *Spo.* the dryness extends downwards; not with Nux m.). > Warm drinks, Ars., Alm., Lyc., Nux, Rhus (> cold drinks, Ver.). Heart, Naj., Sep., Kalm., Abro., Lach. Orchitis, Gels., Pul., Ham. (intense soreness), Merc. (with a little yellowish-green gonorrhœa)—Spo. comes after these when there is induration. Bitter taste in throat (Ruta, nausea in throat). Jaw-joint as if dislocated, Rhus. < Thinking of symptoms, Ox. ac., Pip. m. Tubercular diathesis, Bac., Tub. Voice fails, Alm., Dro.

SYMPTOMS.

1. **Mind.**—Disconsolate and lachrymose humour.—Timidity and tendency to be frightened.—Combative and boastful humour.—Immoderate and mischievous gaiety.—Great inclination to sing.—Mental obtuseness, with complete disinclination and incapacity for attending to intellectual labour.—Distraction of mind.—Pert, witty humour.—Alternately gay, lachrymose, and cross.—Conscious but unable to act on her limbs.—Fancies appear on shutting eyes.—Fretful and anxious about her condition, fears she will die of suffocation.—Anxious sweat and faintness—She is very timid, and is esp. pursued and incessantly tormented by a frightful scene of some mournful event of the past.—Anxious as from presentiment.—Fright awakens.—Satiety of life, with the heat.—Obstinacy.—Every exertion < the cough.

2. **Head.**—Vertigo, with giddiness, to such an extent as to fall, sometimes in evening, or else with a sensation as if head were about to fall on one side.—Vertigo, with nausea, on waking at night.—Heaviness and fulness of head.—Dull semilateral headache on entering a warm room from the open

air.—Headache, with lachrymation, when looking fixedly at an object.—Pressive headache, sometimes with compression.—Pressing headache in (r.) frontal eminence, from within to without, < when sitting, when entering a warm room, after walking in the open air, when looking intensely at anything; > when lying on back in a horizontal position.—Sharp stitches in l. temple extending to forehead.—Pains in head as if it were about to split, esp. in forehead.—Throbbing and pulsation in head.—Congestion of blood in head, with pressing, beating, and pulsation in forehead, with redness of face, anxious look, restless sleep, > in a horizontal position.—Disagreeable tenderness of exterior of head.—Sensation as if hair were standing on end (on vertex).—Troublesome (violent) itching in scalp.

3. **Eyes.**—Eyes dull and clouded, with puffing in lids.—Eyes deeply sunk; or protruding, staring.—Maculæ of cornea.—On looking intensely at one spot lachrymation and headache.—Pressure and shootings in eyes.—Eyes burning, red, and weeping.—Agglutination of lids.—Eruption of yellow scabies in eyebrows (painful to touch on l. eyebrow).—Pressive heaviness of lids.—Contraction of lids in morning.—Myopia.—Sees visions on closing eyes.—Double vision > lying down.

4. **Ears.**—Otalgia, with contractive pain.—Pressure in ears.—Ulceration of external ear.—Pain in cartilages as from soreness, not affected by touch.—Boils on l. ear painful to touch.—Inflamed nodule in l. concha.—Red swelling of l. helix.—Heat in ears.—Hard hearing.—Dull ringing in ears; in r.

5. **Nose.**—Epistaxis, esp. after blowing nose (at dinner).—Fluent coryza, with much sneezing.—Dry coryza; nose stuffed up.—Eruption on point of nose.

6. **Face.**—Paleness of face, with dulness of eyes (with sunken eyes).—Face bloated, red, or bluish, with anxious expression; heat on one side of face, renewed when thinking of it.—Cold sweat on face.—Swelling of cheeks.—Itching and shootings in cheeks.—Eruption on lips.—Spasmodic pain in maxillary joints.—Tension in articulation of l. jaw (when walking in the open air).—Stitches transversely through l. upper jaw.—Cramp-like pain from l. jaw-joint to cheek in evening when eating.—Swelling of the submaxillary glands with tensive pain; painful to touch.—Numbness in chin.—Heat in chin.

7. **Teeth.**—Sensation of bluntness and looseness in teeth while masticating.—Itching and shootings in teeth.—Heat in teeth.—Swelling of gums, with pain during mastication.

8. **Mouth.**—Mouth and tongue covered with vesicles, with burning and shooting pain (on that account cannot eat any solid food).—Salivation.—Speech difficult.—Tongue dry and brownish.—Vesicles on edge of tongue.

9. **Throat.**—Burning sensation and stinging in throat.—Rawness, swelling, and scraping in throat.—Penetrating tickling in throat, toward ear.—Sore throat < after eating sweet things.—Throat symptoms > lying down.—Constantly recurring needle-like stitches above pit of throat, externally, in lower part of goître.—Sticking internally in throat, esp. after eating.—Thyroid gland swollen and hard, with suffocative attacks at night; stitching pains and pressure.—Bitter taste in throat.—In œsophagus: heat; relaxed sensation.—Swelling in fauces projecting from r. to l.—Swallowing difficult.—On

swallowing : stitches in neck pass off ; violent straining pain ; pain in goître ; moving sensation in goître.—(Goître painful, pain synchronous with cardiac pain.—R. T. C.)

10. **Appetite.**—Diminished taste.—Bitter taste, sometimes only in throat. —Sweetish taste in mouth—Moderate appetite and speedy satiety.—Increased appetite.—Excessive, insatiable hunger.—Desire for dainties.—Thirst, sometimes insatiable.—Thirstlessness ; rarely thirst with chill.—Violent thirst after smoking.—Tobacco smoke is disagreeable.—After a meal, fulness and pains in abdomen, as from difficult digestion.—Eating and drinking > cough.— Drinking milk, ale, spirits, cold or hot tea, cold water = cough.

11. **Stomach.**—Risings, sometimes with cuttings and tearings in stomach. —Bitter risings.—Sour regurgitations.—Frequent hiccough.—Nausea, with acidity in mouth.—Craves dainties ; after eating has dyspeptic distress and fulness of stomach ; > from warm drinks, esp. colicky pains in abdomen.— Vomiting after having partaken of milk.—Relaxation of stomach, with sensation as if it were open.—Aching in stomach and scrobiculus.—Pressure of (tight) clothing on stomach is unbearable.—Contractive pains in stomach.— Stitches in region of stomach from least pressure.—Chill in pit of stomach.— Craving at stomach before menses.

12. **Abdomen.**—Abdomen hard and tight.—Spasms in abdomen.— Violent action of abdominal muscles during inspiration. — Viscera drawn up against diaphragm.—Pain in l. side of abdomen ; digging and choking ; > after discharge of wind ; at times as if something alive were moving there.—Pain in abdomen instead of menses.—Fine stitch externally in abdomen.—Heat in abdomen.—Digging and obstruction in abdomen.— Gripings in abdomen, after a meal.—Rumbling in the abdomen, esp. in evening and morning when lying down.—Pain as from a hernia in inguinal ring.—Swelling and inflammation of l. inguinal ring.—Swelling of inguinal glands.

13. **Stool and Anus.**—Hard (insufficient) and retarded evacuations.— Loose, whitish evacuations.—Before the evacuation shootings in the anus and gurgling and rumbling in the abdomen.—During the evacuation tenesmus in the anus.—Itching, smarting, and pain as from excoriation in anus.—Passage of ascarides from rectum and tingling in rectum.—Diurnal dirrrhœa with a large number of ascarides, after which she always feels great relief.

14. **Urinary Organs.**—Increased secretion of urine.—Frequent want to urinate, with scanty emission.—Incontinence of urine (in whooping-cough). —Small stream of urine.—Frothy urine.—Thick, whitish, greyish, or yellow sediment in the urine.

15. **Male Sexual Organs.**—Spasmodic contraction in the testes.—Hard swelling of the testes, and of the spermatic cord, with pressive pain.— Drawing, painful stitches extending from body through glans.—Voluptuous itching at point of glans for several hours, urging him to rub it.—Pinching, bruised, squeezing pain in testicles.—Stitches from testicles into spermatic cord.—(Gouty pains in testicles in old men.—R. T. C.)—Heat in genitals, penis, scrotum, testes, and cords.—Sexual desire very moderate.—Absence of erections.

16. **Female Sexual Organs.**—Catamenia too early and profuse.— Before the catamenia, palpitation of the heart, following pain in back.—

During the catamenia, drawing in the thighs.—Enlargement and induration of ovaries.

17. Respiratory Organs.—[Affections in general of larynx and trachea, particularly in all such affections as croup, asthma, &c., where everything is perfectly tight and dry, no loose rattling sound appearing in the breathing or cough.—Burning sensation is felt in throat after coughing, suffocative attacks of breathing (as in asthma), without any mucous rattle; respiration loud; very hollow voice, all without any rattling sound, or any looseness.—H. N. G.]—Hoarseness (voice cracked); sometimes with cough and coryza.—Weak, husky voice, which fails in singing and conversation.—Pain in larynx on touching it, and on turning head.—Pressure in larynx when singing.—Sensation of obstruction (as from a plug) in larynx, with impeded respiration.—Dyspnœa > by bending the body forward.—Roughness and dryness in throat.—Burning pain in larynx and trachea.—Cough, proceeding from bottom of chest with pain as from excoriation and burning sensation.—Cough, with yellowish expectoration and hoarseness.—Great dryness of larynx, < from hawking.—Sensation in region of thyroid and cervical glands on breathing, as if forced in and out.—Hollow, dry, barking or whistling cough, day and night, < towards evening, and sometimes with pain in larynx.—Laryngeal cough, croupy-sounding, always goes away with a dose of *Spo.* (woman, 65.—R. T. C.).—Cough, with expectoration of viscid mucus.—Expectoration: scanty, of saltish mucus; tenacious, yellow, indurated, sour; loosened mornings but must be swallowed again; smelling like milk; of yellow mucus in little lumps; of cutaneous masses.—Dry cough, excited by a burning tickling in the larynx.—Slow and deep respiration, as from weakness.—Wheezing respiration.—Wheezing, whistling, sawing, anxious breathing; < during inspiration and when lying down (with violent labouring of abdominal muscles).—Mucous râle in trachea by fits.

18. Chest.—Respiration, quick, anxious, and difficult, sometimes with fits of suffocation, and mucous rattling in chest.—Short, panting respiration, surging from heart into chest, as if it would force out upward.—Awakens from sleep with suffocative sensation.—Fixed, lancinating, and pressive pain in region of bronchia.—Spasmodic, constrictive pains in whole chest (and larynx).—Pain in chest, with dyspnœa.—Fulness and obstruction in chest.—Shootings in chest.—Burning sensation, which ascends into chest.—Burning; rawness, soreness in chest.—Ebullition of blood (congestions) in chest after slightest effort and least movement, with obstructed respiration, anguish, nausea, and weakness, which induces syncope.

19. Heart.—Pains and anxiety in region of heart.—Constricting, stinging, pressing pain in cardiac region.—Palpitation of heart (before menstruation), with suffocation, violent gasping respiration, pain in heart.—Rheumatic affections of valves of heart (fibrous deposit on valves).—Violent palpitation of heart, beats rapid (each beat was accompanied by a loud blowing as of a bellows), awakens him after midnight, with a sense of suffocation, loud cough, great alarm, agitation, anxiety, and difficult respiration.—Pulse full, hard, and frequent.

20. Neck and Back.—Painful tension and rigidity in muscles of neck, nape, and throat; on l. side when turning head to r.—Neck cold in evening.—Back of neck snaps on stooping.—Goître large and hard, with pressure, tingling, and shootings.—Cramps in the muscles of neck.—Coldness in back, not > by warmth of stove.—Sacrum sore before menses.—Sensation of numbness in loins and buttocks.—Drawing, tearing, and pressive pain in loins.

21. **Limbs.**—Painful weariness in arms and legs.

22. **Upper Limbs.**—Jerking of muscles about l. shoulder-joint.—Heaviness and trembling of forearms and hands.—Drawings in forearms and joints of hands.—Large blisters in the forearm.—Swelling of hands, with stiffness of fingers.—Redness and swelling in joints of fingers, with tension when they are bent.—Numbness in points of fingers.—Cramp-like pain in ball of (r.) thumb; on moving hand it extends to thumb.

23. **Lower Limbs.**—Nates and thighs numb and cold.—Jerking of muscles of buttocks.—The thighs are spasmodically drawn forward or backward.—Irritation and restlessness of both legs.—Tearing in tibia all afternoon.—Rigidity of legs.—Drawing and tearing in legs and feet, sometimes at night only.

24. **Generalities.**—Uncomfortable feeling of the clothes, they being an oppression and annoyance to the wearer; growing pains; darting pains from within outward; itching, no better from scratching.—Troubles in general of any kind appearing in the sexual organs, esp. r. side; testicles and spermatic cord; anterior surface of thigh.—Phthisis pulmonalis, cough, breathing, &c., being very tight and dry.—< From turning head; on ascending (going up stairs, up a hill, rising from a chair, &c.); from tobacco; wind; from the west wind.—> On descending.—Stinging pain in limbs, esp. joints.—Painful sensitiveness of body to touch, with chilliness on the parts touched, or with tingling running through whole body.—Sensation of torpor in lower part of body.—Heaviness when walking in open air, must sit down.—Heaviness (and soreness) of the body (when rising from a seat).—Excessive moral and physical dejection.—Extreme exhaustion and heaviness of the body after slight exertion, with orgasm of blood in chest, heat of face, vessels hard and distended, great anxiety, and difficult breathing.—More relief is experienced from lying down quietly than from any other position.—Fits of anguish, with pain in region of heart.

25. **Skin.**—Swelling and induration of the glands.—Itching shootings in the skin, esp. on becoming warm in bed.—Sensation of something creeping over the skin, with redness and heat of the part when it has been scratched.—Red, itching spot (blotches) on the skin.—Itching eruptions.—Miliary eruptions.—Tetters.

26. **Sleep.**—Sleepy, yawning, no activity, afternoons.—Sleeplessness, with fantastic dreams and delirium on going to sleep.—Sad, anxious, frightful dreams.—Awakens towards morning from a jerk upwards from the larynx, as if she would suffocate, must sit up, and raises sour, salty mucus.

27. **Fever.**—Pulse full, hard, and quick.—Frequent shiverings over the whole body, esp. the back (even near a warm stove).—Violent heat, soon after the chill, with dry, burning heat all over the body with the exception of the thighs; they remain numb and chilly.—Anxious heat, with red face and weeping, inconsolable mood.—Cool perspiration on the face in evening.—Morning, sweat over the whole body.—Flushes of heat.—Feverish heat, with skin dry and hot, continued thirst, headache, and delirium.—Nocturnal perspiration.

Stachys Betonica.

Stachys betonica. Wood Betony. *N. O.* Labiatæ. Tincture of whole fresh plant.

Clinical.—Cold. Diaphragm, paralysis of. Headache. Vertigo.

Characteristics.—Berridge published the proving of *Stach.* made by Croker and himself with some others. Dizziness, fulness in head and eyes with disposition to take cold were the most prominent symptoms. A feeling of oppressed breathing as from paralysis of diaphragm is a peculiar symptom. *Stach.* has been used in eye-waters, and as a remedy for headaches.

Relations.—Compare Lycopus and the Labiatæ.

SYMPTOMS.

2. **Head.**—Dizziness > open air ; < closing eyes, or moving head.—Fulness over and in eyes as if they would burst.—Dull, heavy action in frontal region > walking about in room.

3. **Eyes.**—Heavy, sleepy feeling in eyes.—Pain in eyeballs as if too tense ; < looking at light, reading, thinking, bending head down.

4. **Ears.**—Slight earache.

5. **Nose.**—Frequent sneezing ; on going indoors from open air ; increased nasal mucus.

11. **Stomach.**—Eructations ; tasting of drug.—Warmth in stomach ; increasing to sharp cutting pain.—Weight in stomach with feeling of sickness.

14. **Urinary Organs.**—Woke with desire to urinate in night.—Urine : high-coloured ; ammoniacal.

17. **Respiratory Organs.**—Breathing oppressed as from paralysis of diaphragm ; constriction just behind ensiform cartilage, on walking up hill must keep mouth open.

24. **Generalities.**—Tired, esp. in legs.—Great sensitiveness to take cold.

27. **Fever.**—Free diaphoresis.—In night profuse sweat, limited to head, neck, and chest.

Stannum.

Stannum. Tin. Sn. (A. W., 118·8) Trituration of the pure metal.

Clinical.—Anæmia. Asthma. Bronchitis. Chilblains. *Colic. Consumption.* Convulsions. Cramps. Debility. Dentition. *Diaphragm, pains in.* Dyspepsia. Ears, ring-holes, ulceration of. Epilepsy. Epistaxis. Gastralgia. Hæmatemesis. Hæmoptysis. Headache. Hectic fever. Hemiplegia. *Hypochondriasis.* Hysteria. Lachrymal fistula. Lachrymal sac, suppuration of. Milk, altered, Nails, splitting. *Neuralgia.* Neurasthenia. Opisthotonos. Paralysis. Phthisis pituitosa. Ptosis. Sleeplessness. Styes. Tapeworm. Trachea, affections of. Uterus, prolapse of. Vagina, prolapse of. Worms.

Characteristics.—*Stannum* is the Jupiter of the alchymists. "The ancients have recorded wonderful cures of the most serious diseases with Tin," says Hahnemann, but in his day, until he proved it, its only use was as a vermifuge. Alston obtained indirectly from "a woman of Leith in Scotland" this prescription, of which he has witnessed the efficacy in a case of tapeworm : "Take an ounce and a half of Tin (pewter metal) and grind it small to powder, mix it with sugar syrup, and take, on a Friday before the change of the moon, one-half of it, the following day the half of the remainder, and the Sunday following the rest, but on the Monday a purgative." Alston also says, in his *Materia Medica*, that he has seen hæmatemesis cured by this as if by magic. Hahnemann's proving appears both in his *Materia Medica Pura* and in his *Chronic Diseases*. A number of worm symptoms appear in the pathogenesis : Sinking, empty, all-gone feeling, diaphragmatic and abdominal pains ; tendency to excessive mucous secretions ; pale, sunken, sickly countenance, with dark rings round eyes ; convulsions. Many of these symptoms occur in conditions not due to helminthiasis, and *Stan.* will be the remedy. Pains in the hypochondria, associated with the hypochondriac or hysterical mental state. Diaphragmatic neuralgia. Colic > by hard pressure, as by laying the child with its abdomen across the knee or on the point of the shoulder. This is one of the keynotes of *Stan.*; but the most important one is in the type of the *Stan.* pains : they begin lightly, increase gradually to the highest point and then as gradually decline. Other remedies have pains of this type but not to the same characteristic degree. This feature applies to the headaches, facial and dental neuralgias, abdominal and other pains. Another cardinal feature of *Stan.* is *weakness :* exhaustion of mind and body. The chest is so weak as to make talking impossible. The patient is so weak, she *drops into* a chair instead of sitting down. While dressing in the morning has to sit down several times to rest. There is weakness and aching of the deltoid and arm, and this has the curious modality that it is felt *when singing or otherwise using the voice. Stan.* is an important remedy for singers and public speakers. The weakness of *Stan.* makes it an appropriate remedy for many states of neurasthenia, nervous exhaustion. A peculiarity of the weakness is that it is felt much more on going down stairs than on going up. The relaxation of tissue is probably responsible for the weak, empty, sinking sensation felt at the epigastrium ; and also for the uterine prolapse. In the dyspepsias of *Stan.* there is nausea and vomiting from the smell of cooking ; and the gastralgia compels the patient to walk about for relief, yet the *weakness* is so great that he is soon compelled to rest. The weak, empty feeling in the chest is one of the notes of *Stan.* in phthisical conditions, and the stitches are another ; hectic fever ; deep, hollow, shattering cough ; expectoration, profuse like white of egg, sweetish, salty ; sour, putrid, musty ; yellow-green pus ; deep, husky, hollow voice, > for the time by hawking or expectorating mucus make up the rest of the picture. *Stan.* is a low-spirited remedy, and when phthisical patients are despondent and without hope (they are usually the reverse) *Stan.* will most likely be needed. (The *yellowness* of the *Stan.* secretions is worth noting : The tongue is yellow ; sputa and leucorrhœa are also yellow.) Palpitation and anxiety occur from ever so slight exertion, as giving directions about the household. Trembling of arms and legs; limbs as heavy as lead. The pains of *Stan.* are frequently compressive and cramp-like; and cramps and spasms are a marked feature of the *Stan.* effects. The convulsions are opisthotonic; the thumbs are drawn in. They are such as are met with in teething children; or in children who masturbate; or who have worms. A typical case of *Stan.* neuralgia is quoted in *Clinique* (xxi. 62): Man, 30, suffered for eight years off and on, and for some months continuously, with neuralgic headache. Pain centres over one or other eye (usually right) and extends over whole or part of head and is at times unbearable. It begins in early morning (4 to 5 a.m.), increases gradually to noon, when it gradually declines to sunset, reappearing again the following morning. Two doses of *Stan.* cured in a fortnight. There is sexual excitement in both sexes. Emissions with excessive prostration. In the female the menses are early and profuse. Orgasm is easily produced: "Scratching arm produces an intolerable sensation of pleasure in genital organs which extends to uterus and produces orgasm." The uterine and vaginal prolapse of *Stan.* has this distinguishing feature: it is < during stool; especially during pressure. Labour pains are spasmodic and put the patient out of breath. The milk of nursing woman is changed, and the child rejects it. Hering gives as cured by *Stan.* "Monday constipation"—that is, constipation occurring on days following rest-days. *Stan.* has marked periodicity. T. H. Urquhart (quoted *H. R.*, iv. 147) cured in two months an affection of the nails characterised by breaking and splitting, a sequel of scurvy, by applying to them *Stannum oleate* on a narrow flannel bandage. *Peculiar Sensations are:* As if all objects were too far off. As if forehead were shattered. As if forehead would be pressed inward. Pain as if from an ulcer in hypogastrium. As if there were a hole in his side. As if there were no sensation in bladder. Chest, as if eviscerated; as if internally constricted. Epigastric region as if beaten. Tickling as from soreness in trachea. Inclination to hawk as if mucus were in chest. As if she would faint. As if limbs beaten. As of a heavy load in affected arm and side of chest. As if sweat would break out. The "girdle" sensation of *Stan.* accompanies yawning. The secretions of *Stan.* are bland. The symptoms are < by touch. > By pressure. > Lying across something hard. < Rest. < Lying; (but must lie down from weakness of chest). < Lying on r. side. Sitting bent over > (cough). Bending double >. Walking > pains, but must soon rest. Motion > pains in head, but < other symptoms. < Using voice (laughing, talking, singing). < Going down stairs (faintness). Blowing nose = shrieking noise in ear. Warm drink = cough. Open air >; (< vertigo). < During stool.

Relations.—*Antidoted by:* Puls. *Complementary:* Puls. *Follows well:* Caust., Cina. *Is followed well by:* Calc., Phos., Sel., Sul., Bac. *Compare:* Sour sensation in stomach, Chel., Pho., Sep. Weeps all the time, but crying < (Nat. m. < by consolation), Pul. (menses scanty, delayed), Sep. < Descending; can go up well enough, Brx. (Calc. opp.). Pain increases and decreases gradually, Plat., Stro. c. (Arg. m. has headache increasing gradually and leaving off suddenly). Weakness seems to proceed from chest; (from abdomen, pelvis, Pho., Sep.). Nausea from smell of cooking food, Ars., Colch. < Laughing, Arg.

< Warm drinks ; (< cold drinks, Spo.). Weak from talking, occul., Ver., Sul., Calc. Prolapsus uteri < during stool, Pod. (Pod. ith diarrhœa, stool green and coming with a rush). Catarrhal thisis, Sil. (more induration ; old people), Pho. (more blood in uta), Seneg. (lungs feel pushed back to spine ; fat persons of lax ore), Colch., Bals. peruv., Eriodict., Teuc. scorod., Illic., Pix., Myos. aralysis by emotions, Stph., Nat. m. > Hard pressure, Coloc., Pb. ain like subcutaneous ulceration ; bland discharges, Puls. Claw nsation, Bell. Nausea in throat, Cycl., Ph. ac., Val.

Causation.—Emotions. Fright. Masturbation. Dentition. Using oice.

SYMPTOMS.

1. **Mind.**—Sad, hypochondriacal humour.—Great agitation and anguish, elancholy and disposition to weep.—Sad, despondent, feels like crying all e time, but crying <.—Quiet fretfulness; answers unwillingly and abruptly. Continued restlessness with anxiety.—Her distress of mind ceases as soon menses begin to flow.—Uneasy, does not know what to do with himself ; ains > by walking, but so weak he soon must rest.—Earnest application to siness, with inability to complete anything undertaken.—Discouragement. Ill-humour, with taciturnity and dislike to society and conversation ; hope- ssness.—Sudden fits of passion.—Nervous excitement.

2. **Head.**—Vertigo, during which all objects seem too far off.—Vertigo sitting down, with loss of ideas.—Headache, usually neuralgic, which mes on gradually and grows steadily < till it reaches its height or severest int, when it begins to grow > and goes away just as gradually as it came —*e.g.*, if it was twelve hours in coming on, it will be twelve hours in going f.—Headache, with nausea and retching, sometimes with burning sensation the sinciput, eyes and nose, or else in the morning, with ill-humour.— eaviness in head in evening.—Heaviness and stunning pressure in head, p. traversing forehead.—Shooting pains in head, esp. in forehead, and < ter a fit of coughing.—Spasmodic pains in head, as from tension or squeez- g (as from a band in whole upper part of head, and in forehead, slowly creasing and decreasing).—Intermittent tearing pain in r. half of forehead, on stooping.—Crushing pain in forehead.—Sharp jerking in r. anterior be of brain, above orbit.—Pressive drawing and tearing in the head.— oring pains in head.—Throbbing pains in temples.—Painful jerks through temple, forehead and cerebellum, < during rest, > from motion.—Burning forehead with nausea, > in open air.—Painful shocks across head.—Pain from suppuration in head externally.—Burning tension on scalp just above forehead.

3. **Eyes.**—Eyes sore, and, as it were, excoriated by rubbing.—Pressure lids and canthi.—Burning lancinations in lids.—Itching, smarting, and urning sensation in eyes.—Nocturnal agglutination of lids.—Pressive pain in inner canthus, as from a stye.—Styes.—Ulcer in the internal canthi (pustular welling of l. inner canthus) like a lachrymal fistula.—Eyes dull (sunken), and ouded.—Jerking and quivering of eyes.—Convulsed or prominent eyes.— ariegated areola round candle.

4. **Ears.**—Earache, with drawing tearings.—Ulceration of holes pierce for earrings.—Tinkling in ears.—Ringing in l. ear.—Cries (screeching) in ear on blowing nose.

5. **Nose.**—Heaviness, and sensation of obstruction, in upper part c nose.—Inflammation of interior of nose.—Burning sensation in nose.—Epi taxis : on moving, on rising from bed ; immediately on waking.—Dry coryz on one side only, with soreness, swelling, and redness of nostrils.—Ove sensitiveness of smell.

6. **Face.**—Pale and wan countenance, with (deep, sunken) eyes ; sickl expression ; features elongated.—Pains in the face, with pressive drawin esp. in zygomatic process, and orbits.—Burning, lancinating pain in muscle of face.—Swelling of cheeks and upper jaw.—Spasm in jaw.—Painful swellin of submaxillary glands.

7. **Teeth.**—Toothache after a meal, with jerking pain and heat in th face.—Sensation of elongation and looseness in teeth.—Ulcer on gums, wit swelling of cheeks.—Epileptiform convulsions from teething ; child > lyin with abdomen across something hard ; clenching of thumbs.

8. **Mouth.**—Fetid exhalation from mouth.—Flow of acid saliva.—Diff cult, weak speech, occasioned by weakness, esp. on chest.—Tongue coate with a yellowish mucus.—Tongue yellow.—Tongue red.

9. **Throat.**—Sore-throat, as from an internal swelling, with drawin and tension.—Sensation in velum pendulum as if a foreign body were there or some mucus which could neither be hawked up nor swallowed ; sam sensation in posterior nares.—Sensation of stinging dryness in throat, wit lancinations (< when swallowing).—Cutting in pharynx and œsophagus o swallowing.—Ulcerated sensation in r. side of throat.—Roughness and scrapin in throat, esp. in evening.—Accumulation of thick, viscid, greyish, blood mucus in throat and mouth, with necessity to hawk, followed by a sensatio of excoriation (efforts to expel it excite vomiting).—After hawking mucus th voice for singing is higher.—Tobacco has a sharp, dry taste in the fauces.— Permanent rawness and dryness in throat : during swallowing a painful feelin as of being denuded.—Rawness and dryness in throat, without thirst.—Nause in fauces and pharynx.

10. **Appetite.**—Bitter and sour taste.—Bitter taste of all food (excep water).—Bitter, herbaceous taste of beer.—Increased hunger, which canno be satisfied.—Increased thirst.—Nausea and vomiting after a meal.—Excessiv weakness of digestion.

11. **Stomach.**—Bitter risings ; or with a taste of rotten eggs.—Sou risings, with scraping in throat.—Frequent hiccough.—Nausea and vomiting in the morning ; from odour of cooking food.—Nausea, esp. after a meal, fol lowed by bitter and watery vomiting.—Vomiting : of bile ; of blood.—Violen retching, followed by vomiting of (undigested) food.—Aching in stomach sometimes very violent.—Tensive pressure at scrobiculus, which is painfu when touched, as from subcutaneous ulceration.—Cramps in stomach, some times with bitter risings, sensation of hunger and diarrhœa, or else wit nausea, and pale and sickly complexion.—Squeezing, as from a claw i stomach, and umbilical region, with nausea.—Sinking, gone feeling i epigastrium.

12. **Abdomen.**—Dull blows across hypochondria.—Cramps in region o

aphragm.—Pressure and burning sensation in hepatic region.—Pressure, asmodic pain, and shootings in the l. hypochondrium.—Abdomen painfully stended, and sensitive to touch.—Spasms (colic) in abdomen, with pains ove and below navel.—Hysterical spasms in abdomen.—Digging, pinching, d griping in abdomen; before every stool.—Burning sensation, and shoot-gs in abdomen.—Feeling of excoriation in abdomen, < by touch.—Severe in causing the patient to lie over the sharp corner of a table or sofa, or mething hard, and to press the abdomen firmly against it, as in this way > afforded.—Griping as of something being torn away.—Sensation as if retched in (r.) abdominal muscles.—Squeezing, as from a claw, in umbilical gion, followed by nausea.—Sensation of emptiness (hollowness) in abdomen; en after eating.—Incarceration of flatus.—Stitches from both sides through ps.

13. **Stool and Anus.**—Hæmorrhoidal pimple on l. side of anus, with inful soreness when touched.—Violent shooting, like needle pricks at base rectum extending to anus.—Soreness and smarting at anus, with fine itches, immediately after a stool.—Itching stitch in rectum.—A corroding in about anus, while walking and sitting.—Burning in anus; constant hing.—Constipation.—Frequent, ineffectual want to evacuate.—Hard, dry, otty fæces, or else scanty and greenish.—Stools: green, curdy, with colic; sufficient with renewed desire afterwards.—Slimy evacuations.—Violent sentery, urging and tormina, stools bloody, mucous with intolerable tenesmus. Violent diarrhœa.—Passes worms; lumbrici; tænia.

14. **Urinary Organs.**—Dull stitches inward in kidney region.—Sensitive essure in neck of bladder and urethra after urinating; seems as though ore would follow; some drops pass when the pressure is <.—Blister on argin of meatus.—Retention of urine.—Scanty emission of urine.—Frequent ant to urinate, sometimes with scanty emission.—Absence of want to urinate, from insensibility of bladder (only a sensation of fulness indicates the cessity to urinate).

15. **Male Sexual Organs.**—Increase of sexual desire.—Violent and luptuous excitement during emission.—Frequent pollutions; with excessive ostration.

16. **Female Sexual Organs.**—Increased sexual desire; early orgasm. Catamenia too profuse.—Before catamenia, anxiety and melancholy.—ıring the catamenia, colic.—Cramps in uterus.—Prolapsus of the vagina, th hard stool.—Bearing down in uterine region; prolapsus uteri et vaginæ. Prolapsus strangulated tends to gangrene.—Leucorrhœa of transparent or llowish mucus, with considerable prostration of strength.—Itching in vulva, evening (*Stan. mur.*).—Spasmodic labour pains; they exhaust her, she is out breath.—A child leaves the breast of its mother, and will not suck.

17. **Respiratory Organs.**—Hoarseness and roughness in larynx, with kling, which excites a cough.—Catarrh, with hoarse voice, sensation of igue in chest, obstructed respiration, and cough with expectoration.—eat accumulation of mucus in trachea, which is easily detached.—The voice louder in singing, after having hawked up the mucus.—Cough excited by ghter, talking, and singing, or by a tickling in chest; or by warm drinks.—chest affections, when talking, reading aloud, singing, &c.; they cause a very ak feeling in throat and chest, an exhausted, "given-out" sensation, and

produce hoarseness; using the voice produces weakness in the arms betwe the elbow and shoulder, then the weakness extends all over the body. T above symptoms are very often found in operatic singers, actors, auctionee —all who use the voice a great deal.—Dry, violent, shaking cough, in bed, evening, until midnight, or more violent in morning.—Shattering, deep coug —Fatiguing, paroxysmal cough, so that epigastric region was painful, as beaten.—Short cough from weakness of chest, having a hoarse, weak soun —Cough concussive, with paroxysms of these coughs.—Cough excited lying on the r. side.—Cough, with retching and vomiting of food.—Coug with frequent expectoration of mucus.—(Cough coming after whoopin cough in girl, 9; very profuse, white, thick expectoration, hoarse, tong coated, sleepless, no appetite, rapid emaciation and debility, with contract chest and pleuritic adhesions.—R. T. C.)—Expectoration when coughi (during the day, in morning expectoration is most profuse and) is greeni sweetish, or yellow; saltish; or else viscid, and in lumps; or serous, a composed of liquid mucus, or of a putrid smell (after coughing and expec rating the patient feels hollow and empty).—During and after the cough, p as of excoriation, and shootings in the chest.—Phthisis pituitosa.

18. **Chest.**—Obstructed respiration at night, esp. when lying down; by day, on least movement.—Dyspnœa, esp. in evening, with sensation emptiness in scrobiculus, and anguish, which causes the patient (to loosen tear his clothes.—Oppression at chest when walking or ascending.—Asth when attacks gradually come on, culminate, and gradually decline.—Rattli of mucus and wheezing in chest.—Agreeable sensation of lightness on taki a full inspiration.—Contusive pain in chest.—Heavy pressure in chest as b weight.—Tension in chest (hydrothorax).—Constriction of chest, sometim in evening, with anguish.—Lancinations in the l. side of the chest, duri inspiration, or when lying on the r. side.—Sharp, cutting stitches in l. side chest, < from stooping.—Burning stitches on l. chest, < on expectoration. Suddenly, a long stitch in l. side of chest beneath axillæ, causing fright Pain, as from excoriation, in chest.—Sensation of weakness in chest, as if were empty, esp. after speaking or expectorating.—Itching-tickling in ches

19. **Heart.**—Pain in præcordial region and hiccough.—Pulse: freque small; indistinct, fluttering.

20. **Neck and Back.**—Lancinations in the shoulder-blades, and na of the neck.—Weakness of the muscles of the nape of the neck, and cra ing of the vertebræ of the neck when shaking the head.—Opisthotonos Stitches in back, in small of back, and into limbs.—Violent tearing in lum vertebræ, from both sides into region of kidneys, < on every motion of tru —Dull thrusts in lumbar region with a sensation of external coldness agai him.

21. **Limbs.**—Great heaviness and paralytic weakness in arms and le —Swelling of hands and feet in evening.—The pains in limbs < gradua and > in the same manner.—Insupportable restlessness in all the limbs.

22. **Upper Limbs.**—Paralytic pain in the shoulder-joint.—Paraly heaviness in the arms; if he holds a light weight even a short time.—Press tearings in muscles of joints of the arms, hands, and fingers.—Weakness a trembling of hands.—Swelling of hands, esp. in evening.—Jerking of han —Violent burning sensation in hands.—Small red spots on backs of hands

hilblains on hands.—Contraction of fingers.—Retraction of thumbs.—Shoot-gs in joints of fingers.—Stitches in finger-tips.—Painful flaws in nails.

23. **Lower Limbs.**—Drawing and pressive tearings in hips, extending sacrum, and also to legs and knees.—Paralytic lassitude and heaviness of gs.—Bending of knees when walking.—Stiffness and tension in ham.—ensation of heat, and burning sensation in feet.—Swelling of ankles in vening.—Swollen ankles in delicate girls (R. T. C.)—Tearing shocks in nkles, extending as far as toes.—Swelling of feet, esp. in evening.—Red welling of feet.

24. **Generalities.**—Pressive and drawing pains, esp. in limbs, gradually ecoming very violent, and decreasing in the same way.—Affections in general f l. chest; l. side; trachea and inner chest; upper part of chest; inner rface of thighs.—Consumption.—< After moving; lying on side; using the oice; from motion; when descending.—> When lying on back; from osening garments; from walking (except weakness).—Attacks of epilepsy n children during dentition), with retraction of thumbs, and tossing about f body; or else with throwing back of head, paleness of face, convulsive ovements of hands and eyes, and loss of consciousness; the attacks come n sometimes in evening.—Excessive emaciation.—Pain as if paralysed in xtremities.—Paralysis (of arms and legs).—Great heaviness and indolence.—xcessive dejection (weakness), and physical and moral depression, with embling, esp. during gentle exercise (or when talking), and with disposition perspire easily.—Profuse debilitating sweat, night and morning; hot, even n slight movement; with mouldy, putrid smell.—Nervous excitement.—ysterical spasms, with pain in abdomen and in diaphragm.—Insupportable neasiness in body.—Excessive fatigue after conversation.—The sufferings em to disappear during a walk, with the exception of the depression, which then excessive; they reappear as soon as the patient is at rest.—Extreme rostration; must sit or lie down continually.—Faintness in going down airs; can go up without difficulty.—Pains commence lightly, increase radually to a very high degree, and decrease again as slowly.

25. **Skin.**—Itching (burning) shootings over skin of whole body (or l. de).—Itching pimples; on face, sore to touch or on washing.—Chilblains.—laws in nails.—Painful hang-nails.

26. **Sleep.**—Tendency to sleep during day.—Frequent yawning, with ppression of chest, as if it were encircled by a belt.—Sleep retarded.—eeling, in morning, as after insufficient sleep.—Deep sleep.—Nocturnal gitation and many vivid dreams, anxious or lascivious.—Moaning, weeping imid supplications), and plaintive lamentations, while sleeping.

27. **Fever.**—Shivering and shuddering in morning, with coldness in hands, nd numbness of points of fingers.—Chill every forenoon (10 a.m.).—Slight hilliness with violent chattering of teeth.—Shivering in evening, which runs ver back (preceded by heat with perspiration); or only in head, with thirst. -Burning heat in limbs, esp. in hands.—Sensation of anxious heat, on least novement.—Heat every afternoon (4 to 5), with perspiration at the same me.—Perspiration smells mouldy.—Small, quick pulse.—Debilitating per-piration from least exertion.—Very debilitating perspiration at night.—'rofuse perspiration in morning.

Stannum Iodatum.

Iodide of Tin. Sn I_2. Trituration.

Clinical.—Phthisis.

Characteristics.—*Stan. iod.* has been used in preference to th metal in some phthisical cases in which the general features of *Stan* were present. O. S. Haines (*Clinique*, vii. 11) considers it especiall indicated where the patient "has a clear complexion and long eye lashes, and where the progress of the disease is rapid." He uses th 2x trituration. M. D. Youngman (*H. M.*, Jan. 1895) finds it a deepl acting drug, chiefly of value in chronic chest diseases characterise by plastic tissue changes. It is indicated in cases that "hang fire and need an "alterative." He gives this keynote: "A persisten inclination to cough, excited by a tickling dry spot in the throa sometimes in one place, sometimes in another, often apparently a root of tongue." This cough, which begins as a weak-sounding cough accompanied by shortness of breath, soon gathers strength an sound and induces raising of a free, copious, pale yellowish expecto ration, which at first >, but is soon followed by a feeling of dryness weakness in throat and chest, and increased oppression. An in veterate smoker, who had a cough of this kind, said it came from hi throat, and ascribed it to his smoking. Youngman found consoli dation areas in middle of right lung. There was weak feeling i chest after coughing. *Stan. i.* 3x trit. greatly relieved. The ma was sent to a high altitude, where he enjoyed perfect health an was freed from his smoking habit.

Staphisagria.

Delphinium staphisagria. Stavesacre. *N. O.* Ranunculaceæ
Tincture of the seeds.

Clinical.—Adenoids. *Anger, fits of.* Anus, itching of. Backache. Bashfu ness. Blepharitis. Bones, diseases of. Cauliflower excrescences. Chalazion Condylomata. Cough. Cysts. Dentition. Dysentery. Dysparunia; in newl married women. Eczema. *Eyes, tumours on.* Fistula dentalis. Gastralgi Glands, affections of. Hip-joint disease. Hypochondriasis. Impotency. Iritis syphilitic. Jaw-joint, easy dislocation of. Lumbar abscess. Mania. Masturba tion, effects of. *Neuralgia.* Night-sweats. Nymphomania. Ovaries, affections o *Pediculosis. Perspiration, offensive.* Pregnancy, nausea of. *Prostate, affections o* Psoas abscess. Ranula. Rheumatism. Sciatica. Scurvy. Sea-sickness. Seborrhœ *Self-abuse.* Spermatic cords, affections of. *Spermatorrhœa.* Steatoma. Stif neck. *Styes.* Swallowing, constant while talking. *Teeth, caries of.* Testicle affections of. Tibiæ, pains in. Tobacco, effect of. Toenail, ingrowing. Tonsilliti *Toothache.* Tumours; tarsal. Voice, nasal; hoarse. Warts.

Characteristics. — The seed of Stavesacre was known t Dioscorides as an agent for producing vomiting and salivation, an for the cure of toothache; "the origin of which application," say

Hahnemann (*M. M. P.*), "was evidently domestic practice. J. H. Schultze, when suffering from toothache, took some of the seed in his mouth, but it gave him such a violent exacerbation that he thought he should go mad. . . . As an exterminator of vermin this seed was called by the Greeks φθειροκοκκον, and as such it still enters into the composition of an officinal ointment (*unguentum pediculosum*)." This last is the only use of *Staph.* now known to orthodox medicine (Brunton). Teste (who groups *Staph.* with *Caust.*) remarks that *Staph.*, which shares this property with *Coccul.*, is, like *Coccul.*, used in some countries for the purpose of stupefying fish. Again, Teste found *Staph.* (he gave it in 6th dil.), like *Coccul.*, a remedy for sea-sickness. To be successful, *Staph.* had to be taken at the moment when dizziness and nausea commenced, *before* vomiting set in ; and it always helped "nervous persons, not over fat, and disposed to sadness." *Staph.* produced in Teste himself these symptoms : "Long-lasting vertigo, accompanied by continued nausea as in sea-sickness," and this : "Vertigo, which ceases on rapidly turning round on one's heel." This corresponds with one of Hahnemann's symptoms : "Wheeling vertigo, especially while sitting, > by walking about (in a circle)." It is noteworthy that *Staph.* and *Coccul.* are both head-remedies and both effective against head lice. Both also affect the genitals, *Staph.* more especially, and both are remedies for crab lice. An application of a dilution of the tincture of the strength of one part to four of water will destroy the parasites, though the state which favours their presence needs internal treatment (probably with a dilution of the same remedy) at the same time. In Teste's experience, *Staph.* was no less effective in the nausea of pregnancy than in the nausea of sea-sickness. *Tabac.* is another remedy for sickness, and Teste cured with *Staph.* effects of tobacco smoking (excoriated tongue ; gastralgia) ; and he also cured with it the habit of "swallowing the tobacco smoke." The use of *Staph.* in the sickness of pregnancy arises out of its power over the genital functions. It produces both physical and moral sexual disturbances, provokes excesses and irregular sexual appetites, a tendency to masturbation, and a physical state corresponding to the effects of that habit. It is one of Gallavardin's chief remedies (*Passion Génitale*) for removing the habit of masturbation in children, and for removing improper appetites in adults. *Staph.* is one of the remedies which has "< from coition" (in men), dyspnœa occurring during or after the act ; dyspnœa and prostration also follow an emission. In women coition is painful because the external parts are excessively sensitive. This property (which is also allied to the vulnerary power of *Staph.*) makes *Staph.* a remedy of extreme value to women in the early days of married life. Some women suffer very acutely (in mind as well as body) during and for some time after the first coitus. I have seen *Staph.* 30 give unspeakable relief in such cases. "Constant urging to urinate in young married women" is the characteristic. Another urinary peculiarity is burning in the urethra when *not* urinating. Urinary difficulties after severe labours. Prolapse of bladder. I have seen cystocele relieved by *Staph.* Sensitiveness ; stinging, stitching, shooting pains < by touch ; itching—are the chief notes of *Staph.* in affections of the genital organs of both sexes. It has cured prostatitis in the man, with pain running from anus along urethra ; inflamed testicles with shooting and drawing in the cords ; stitching towards groin and testicles. In one female prover *Staph.* brought on the menses a year after they had ceased, at the new moon. The symptom did not recur the following month, which led Hahnemann to conclude that this "was only the primary action of the drug." *Staph.* is not only a remedy for ovarian and other affections, it also meets the conditions following operations on ovaries. Effects of "wounds made by clean-cutting instruments" is the keynote. P. C. Majumdar (*Ind. H. Rev.*, v. 134) gives two cases in which *loss of memory* following masturbation and seminal emissions was cured with *Staph.* 30 : (1) A student, naturally robust and intelligent, lost his memory when he contracted the habit of masturbation. His symptoms were : Vacant countenance ; no aptitude or inclination for mental work ; despair of the future ; great languor and weakness ; occasional nocturnal emission ; constipation. When he read anything he forgot it the next moment. Heaviness, headache, and vertigo after the least mental exertion. *Staph.* 30 was given morning and evening. Improvement began at once and the cure was complete in a month. (2) Another student had constant involuntary emissions, weak memory, languor ; headache every morning on rising ; no appetite ; constipation. *Staph.* 30, once a day, cured. "Hypochondriasis, apathy ; weak memory ; caused by sexual excesses or constantly dwelling on sexual subjects," is how the symptom is given. But the mental state of *Staph.* need not necessarily have a sexual origin. *Staph.* is a remedy for anger and for the effects of anger, especially if *the indignation cannot have its natural expression.* "Was insulted ; being too dignified to fight, swallowed his wrath, and went home sick, trembling and exhausted." The mental state of *Staph.*, like its physical, shows great sensitiveness to the least impression, "the least word that seems wrong, hurts her very much." The touchiness may take the form of sudden, violent outbreaks provoked by mere trivial causes. I have known *Staph.* 30 remedy this state when the impulse to throw things at persons who had caused a trifling or imaginary irritation, had almost passed into a mania. This irritability may be manifested in sensitiveness to criticism. Irritated by trifles. Want of self-control. Fear : afraid of his shadow. Among the consequences of anger which are met by *Staph.* is colic : "Colic of screaming, ugly, pot-bellied children, especially if they suffer much from their teeth, which turn black, with tender, spongy gums, sensitive and painful." The irritability of *Staph.* is shown in the intestinal tract in "< from least food or drink." This applies to vomiting, colic, or dysentery. When colic follows operations on the ovaries or intestines, *Staph.* is as useful as in colic from anger. The action of *Staph.* on the teeth is only one of many points in which it touches *Merc.*, and which makes it one of the best antidotes to *Merc.* The characteristic of *Staph.* is : "Teeth turn black, and have dark streaks through them ; cannot be kept clean ; crumble ; *decay on edges ;* scorbutic cachexia." The toothache of *Staph.* occurs during the menses ; affects sound as well as decayed teeth ; < from touch of food or drink; but not from biting or chewing; is < drawing cold air into mouth; < from cold drinks and after eating. *Staph.* has the "sinking" sensation to an extreme degree. The stomach and abdomen feel as if hanging down relaxed. There is extreme hunger even when the stomach is full. There is ravenous hunger for days before an attack of fever; craving for tobacco; and a cough excited by tobacco smoke is an indication for it. "Inability to perspire" is one of the notes of *Staph.;* as also is sweat smelling of rotten eggs. Bibby (quoted *A. H.*, xxiii. 405) has used with much success *Staph.* φ (three drops in two ounces of water; a teaspoonful every two hours) in cases of night-sweat "in patients bordering on consumption." Eruptions, like the sweat, when moist are foul-smelling. There are dry, scaly eruptions over the ends of bones. Pressing, stinging, tearing pains in periosteum. Exostoses and gouty nodes on fingers and toes. Sycotic and syphilitic condylomata. Seed warts. The ulcers of *Staph.* are generally very painful and sensitive. *Peculiar Sensations* are: As if legs would go under him. As if stupefied. As of a round ball in forehead. As if head would burst. As if brain were compressed. As if bones would be pressed out. Brain, as if torn to pieces. As if occiput hollow. As if back of brain were made of wood and couldn't think. As if occiput compressed externally and internally. As if hard substance were pressing on skull. As if eyes were very dry. As if a hard substance were lying beneath left upper lid. As if wind blew into ears. As if cheek swollen. As if glands beneath chin were swollen. As if teeth were hollow. As if stomach were hanging down. As of a heavy weight lying on stomach. As if abdomen would drop. As if bladder were not yet empty. Testicle feels as if compressed. As if something were loose in pit of stomach. As if chest were bruised. As if small of back were broken to pieces. As if a hard skin were drawn over tips of fingers of left hand. As if toes would be drawn down. Whole body as if bruised. As if done up after much hard work. Compressive pains are marked with *Staph.* Sensation of squeezing between stones or in a vice, in intestines, testes, head. The symptoms are: < By touch. < By pressure (as of hat). But pressure > toothache. Motion <. Rest >; (but < pain in back). Sitting <. Swallowing < pressure in throat-pit. Eating and drinking <. < From drinking cold water. < Anger; emotions; excitement. Heat; cold; washing; open air; change of air; winter < (but warmth > pain in kidney and neuralgia of scalp; and cold water > pain in stye). < Evening to morning; night; early morning. Periodicity is marked. Croupy cough alternates with sciatica. Nightly twitching. < New moon; every month before full moon. More symptoms appear on left side than on right. < By coitus. < *After* urinating; when *not* urinating.

Relations.—*Antidoted by:* Camph. *Antidote to:* Merc., Thuj., *Complementary:* Coloc. *Compatible:* Caust. (Caust., Coloc., Staph., follow well in this order). *Inimical:* Ran. b., before and after. *Compare:* Effects of sexual abuse, Plat. (spasms, emaciation), Calad. (glans flabby), K. bro. (depression; weakness of legs), Gels., Dros., Nux, Sul., Calc., Lyc., Nat. m. Colic from mental causes, Cham.

(hot face, red cheeks, hot sweat), Coloc. (bends double). Teeth, Kre. (premature decay of milk teeth; first become yellow, then dark, then decay; Stp., turn black and decay), Ant. c., Cham., Coff. Styes and tarsal tumours, Graph. (cystic tumours midway between inner and outer surface), Calc. Figwarts and condylomata, Thu. (Thu. sessile; Stp., on pedicles). Bone affections, Stillin., Merc., Ka. iod., Stront., Aur. mur., Plat. mur., Gettys. Arthritic ophthalmias, Coloc. (gout of eyes). Stomach hanging down, Ipec., Tab. Diarrhœa, with flatus smelling like rotten eggs, Cham. (Stp. is < on any attempt to take food or drink). Clean-cut wounds and operations, Arn. Crusta lactea, Vinc. m. Lumbar pains compel early rising, Rhe. Paralysis with tingling in affected parts, Aco. Paralysed by emotions, Stan., Nat. m. Throwing things from him, Kre. Irritated by trifles, Sul., Ig. Cauliflower excrescences, Pho., Thu. Stitches from throat into left ear on swallowing, Lach. Perspiration impossible, Lach. Diarrhœa immediately after eating, Alo., Ars., Chi., Lyc., Pod., Tbd. (Fer., *while* eating). Ravenous hunger, Ars., Calc., Cin., Iod., Sil. Sinking immediately after meals, Ars., Cin., Lyc., Sil., Ur. n. Dyspnœa towards end of coitus, K. bi. < After coitus, K. ca. Relaxed Stomach, insufficient gastric juice, Selen. Cross, puny, sickly children, Syph. Nodosities on eyelids after styes, Con., Calc., Mag. Teeth decay on edges (Mez., Thu. at roots). Urging to urinate after difficult labour, Op. Painful sensitiveness of sexual organs, can hardly wear a napkin, Plat. Cough excited by tobacco smoke, Spo. Nodosities on fingers, Caul., Colch., Lyc. Pain in small spot, K. bi. Wind blowing into ears; eruptions; Mercury antidote, Mez. Urinating with cough, Caust. < After stool, Nit. ac. Involuntary stool when passing flatus, Alo. Black marks on teeth, Scill.

Causation.—Anger. Anger suppressed or reserved. Injury; falls; clean-cut wounds; operations. Coitus. Masturbation. Sexual abuse. Sexual craving. Emissions. Dentition. Tobacco. Mercury.

SYMPTOMS.

1. **Mind.**—Hypochondriacal humour, with indifference to everything (after onanism).—Apathetic; gloomy.—Sadness, with fear for the future.—Weeping, and grief respecting the state of health.—Susceptibility.—Patient is so sensitive that the least action or word troubles or annoys his feelings. —Amorous dreams.—Desire for death.—Anxiety and agitation, which allow no rest.—Ill-humour, irascibility, spitefulness, inducing patient to fling violently whatever is at hand; in the morning.—Justifiable ill-humour over what has happened or has been done by oneself; weeping and dejected over the supposed ill consequences of it.—Hypochondria and hysteria after unmerited insults (or sexual excesses), with complaints of flatulence.—Dislike to conversation, meditation, and all intellectual and serious labour.—Weakness of memory; a few minutes after reading anything can recollect it only dimly, and whenever he thinks of anything the sense escapes him; can scarcely recall it after long reflection.—Instability of ideas. Excessively dull intellect, with inability to attend to any occupation.—Delusions with

respect to past events.—Illusion, as if all surrounding objects were lower, and the patient himself much taller than in reality.

2. **Head.**—Head confused and embarrassed; dull feeling of head with inability to perform any mental labour.—Whirling vertigo, sometimes in evening, in bed, or during day, when sitting or lying; > by walking; or by turning rapidly round on the heel.—Fine, burning, needle-like stitches, externally on vertex.—Hard, pressive pain in vertex.—Headache in the morning on waking, as if brain were bruised.—Stupefying, pressing headache, as if brain were compressed.—(Stupefying headache that she had had for three days goes away at once.—R. T. C.)—Pain in l. side of head with inability to keep eyelids open (produced.—R. T. C.).—Stunning pain in the head, sometimes alternately with boring.—Heaviness in head, esp. forehead, above root of nose (> by resting head upon hand).—Pressing in forehead as from a very heavy lump (wedge of wood or plug) which will not be shaken off; < in morning, from motion and from stooping; > when at rest, and when leaning head against something.—Dulness in small spot in middle of forehead.—Violent pressing boring stitches in l. half of forehead, from within outward, in morning.—Drawing, tearing, or lancinating pressure in the head.—Headache, as if forehead were about to split, on moving it, or on stooping.—Burning in l. temple; internally and externally, as if bones would be pressed out, < from touch.—Compressive or expansive pains in head.—Semilateral headache, as if a nail were driven into brain.—Lancinating headache.—Sensation as if brain were loose.—Feeling as if occiput were hollow or empty, or as if brain were not large enough for the space.—Feeling as if all back part of brain was wood and couldn't think.—Feeling as if the occiput were compressed, internally and externally.—Head becomes more pulled down (agg. in an old rheumatic.—R. T. C.).—Neuralgia of scalp.—Rheumatic and drawing pains in exterior of head.—Tingling itching, sometimes also gnawing, in scalp, with pain as of excoriation; the skin peels off, with itching and biting; < in evening and from getting warm.—Much itching dandriff on scalp.—Moist, fetid scald-head, with violent itching.—Humid, scalding-itching, fetid eruption on back part of head, sides of head, and behind ears; when scratching, the itching changes place, but makes it more humid.—(Eczema of scalp and other parts.—Scald-head; hair matted together, very stinking.—R. T. C.)—Falling off of hair.

3. **Eyes.**—Eyes sunken, with blue raised rings around them.—R. eye much larger than usual (lids wider open).—Pupils dilated.—Eyes sleepy.—Aching in the eyes, lids, and canthi.—Itching in margins of lids.—Itching and biting smarting in internal canthi.—Smarting and burning sensation in eyes when writing.—On looking at sun, hot water runs out of l. eye, scalding cheek and making eye smart.—Violent lancinations in eyes on fatiguing them.—Inflammation of eyes, which are surrounded by pimples.—Inflammation in margins of the lids.—Styes.—Steatoma of eyelids (Koch).—Nodosities in margins of lids.—Great dryness of the eyeballs and lids.—Syphilitic iritis with bursting pain in eyeball, temple, and side of face, < from evening to morning, and on using eyes by any light.—Laceration of cornea with prolapse of iris (after *Aco.*).—(After operations for cataract.)—Much purulent dry mucus in canthi.—Obstinate catarrh with swollen eyelids (Baehr).—Nocturnal agglutination of eyes.—Spasmodic closing of lids.—Pain in upper lid,

< on closing eye.—Pain as if a hard substance were beneath l. upper lid.—Diminished power of sight.—Confused sight, as if water were in the eyes.—Black flashes and luminous sparks before eyes.—Sparkling before eyes in the dark.—Areola round candle in evening.

4. **Ears.**—Shootings in ears.—Tensive stitches in l. ear.—Eruption behind ears.—Hardness of hearing, as from enlargement of tonsils, < after abuse of *Mercury*.—[Perforated tympana with deafness as in winter.—Deafness in children, < at meals, with stuffy cold, thick voice and snuffles (adenoids).—R. T. C.].—Tinkling in ears.—Ringing in ears on moving head; reports in ears; sensation as if wind blew into them.—Noises in ears like sawing of wood, with swollen tonsils and vertigo; and shooting pains from temple to temple (much relieved.—R. T. C.).

5. **Nose.**—Nose ulcerated, with scabs, deep in interior.—Violent fluent coryza, with obstruction on one side of nose, frequent sneezing, and lachrymation.—Sneezing without coryza.—Coryza, with ulcerated nostrils.—Coryza; at first discharge of only thick mucus, after of thin water.—Obstruction of nasal fossæ, with nasal voice.

6. **Face.**—Face wan and sharp (countenance sunken, nose peaked), with eyes hollow, and surrounded by a blue circle.—Bashful look.—Bluish and brownish colour of face, when excited by passion.—Distressing pressive and throbbing pain in face, from teeth into eye.—Sharp, burning stitches in l. cheek, which provoke scratching.—Prosopalgia in an old lady; on touching lips with spoon or fork inexpressible pains shot from lips over face; fluid food had to be eaten with fingers, could take no solid food: mastication impossible.—Inflammation of bones of face, with burning shootings, or incisive drawings and pressive tearings.—Facial eruption, with itchings and shootings.—Lips scurfy, covered with ulcers and scabs, with burning pain.—(Neuralgia that affects l. upper lip, with shootings up side of face.—R. T. C.)—Neuralgia of *Staph.* is < by holding cold water in mouth (R. T. C.)—Swelling of lips.—Easy dislocation of maxillary joint.—Painful swelling and induration of submaxillary glands.—Painfulness of submaxillary glands, with (or without) swelling.—Sensitive induration, like a cartilage, beneath chin, pain on swallowing and on touch.—Caries of lower jaw, following osteitis after tooth extraction.

7. **Teeth.**—Toothache, with swelling of cheeks and submaxillary glands.—Toothache, immediately after a meal, and after mastication, and also after cold drinks, and the introduction of cold air into mouth (but not when biting on them), < at night or in morning.—Tearings and pressive drawings in carious teeth, or in the roots of those which are sound (in open air), and also in gums.—Teeth sensitive to touch, esp. at night and in the morning.—(Front teeth get loose from alveolar periostitis going on to caries of jaw.—R. T. C.)—Gnawing pain in carious teeth.—Blackness, brittleness, and caries of teeth (which exfoliate).—Dentition: child very sensitive; teeth decay as soon as they are cut.—Toothache so sensitive that one can't bear to move the tongue (hard pressure frequently > the toothache); black streaks running through teeth.—Affections of teeth on r. side chiefly; decayed teeth very often excessively tender on being filled; can't bear the operation.—Painful sensitiveness, swelling, and easy bleeding of gums.—Painful nodosities and excrescences on the gums.—Tearing in gums of lower incisors, and their roots while eating.—Gums pale, white, ulcerated (spongy).

8. **Mouth.**—Mouth and tongue covered with vesicles; stomacace.—Conditions of mouth and throat like scurvy and mercurial poisoning.—Painful excrescences on interior of cheek.—Ulcers in mouth.—Salivation.—Sanguineous saliva.—Constant accumulation of mucus in mouth.—Swelling of glands under tongue.—(Cysts in connection with salivary ducts.—R. T. C.)—Ranula.—Tongue: white-coated; dry, with tough mucus stopping posterior nares; stitches in tip; sore pain in anterior part; sticking in margins.—Shootings in tongue, as from splinters.—Low voice, from weakness of the organs of speech (after anger).—Nasal voice from stoppage of posterior nares.—While talking she swallows continually.—(Chronic winter throats with enlarged tonsils.—R. T. C.)

9. **Throat.**—Roughness (dryness) and scraping in throat, with feeling of excoriation, when swallowing and speaking.—Constant deglutition when speaking.—Dryness and shootings in palate and throat.—Sticking in throat on swallowing.—Tonsillitis, on swallowing a stitch runs up from throat into ear.—Swelling of tonsils (also after the misuse of *Mercury*).—Painful drawing from hyoidal arch into throat, < touching side of neck.—Tonsillitis: both tonsils inflamed and swollen; l. sends stitches into ear on swallowing.

10. **Appetite.**—Mawkish and watery taste, with normal taste of food.—Bitter taste of all food.—Sour taste of bread.—Appetite, with want of taste.—Voracity.—Bulimy, even after a meal, sometimes with waterbrash.—Child cries as soon as it eats.—After eating: cutting in abdomen; dysenteric stool; after meat, cough <. After drinking: cutting in abdomen; dysenteric stool.—Great desire for milk.—Tobacco has an acrid taste, and produces pyrosis.—Appetite for liquid food only (soup).—Craving for wine, brandy, and tobacco.—Thirstlessness.

11. **Stomach.**—Eructations, generally empty or scraping.—Bitter risings after acid food.—Salt and bitter risings after eating meat.—Frequent hiccough.—Sobbing risings.—Waterbrash.—Nausea, with inclination to vomit every morning.—Frequent nausea.—Pressure at the stomach, as from a weight, in morning in bed.—Sensation as if stomach were hanging down relaxed.—Tension and pressure in stomach, < or > by eating, esp. bread.—Fulness, pressure, and shootings in scrobiculus.—Digging pain in stomach.—Anxious tension across hypochondria, in morning, with obstructed respiration.

12. **Abdomen.**—Biliary colic, after domestic disturbance.—Tensive pressure in abdomen.—Hard pressure in r. side beneath umbilicus.—Pinching stitch in l. viscera.—Enlargement of the abdomen in children.—Drawing pains across abdomen.—Sensation of weakness and bearing down in abdomen, as if it would drop; wants to hold it up.—Gripings after all kinds of food and drink.—Colic with urging to urinate.—Spasmodic cuttings, with want to evacuate.—Frequent production and incarceration of flatus (smelling like rotten eggs).—Eruption of pimples as large as peas on whole abdomen and thighs, itch; when scratched off are moist and then burn.—Frequent discharge of hot or fetid flatus.—Painful swelling of inguinal glands.—Inguinal hernia.

13. **Stool and Anus.**—Constipation.—Hard evacuations.—Frequent want to evacuate, with scanty evacuations, hard or soft.—Evacuation tardy, without being hard.—Difficult evacuation.—Obstinate constipation sets in

two weeks after a single dose of φ (R. T. C.).—Loose evacuations, preceded, accompanied, and followed by tenesmus and gripings.—Diarrhœa : < after drinking cold water ; < after eating ; in children.—Loose evacuations, with frequent expulsion of fetid wind.—Involuntary evacuation of liquid stools.—A thin stool passes unconsciously, as if flatus would pass.—Dysenteric stools ; with pressing and cutting in abdomen before, during, and after stool.—Smarting, sore pain in rectum for long after stool.—Itching in anus, while sitting.—Burning cuttings, pressure, and constriction in anus, during evacuations.—Hæmorrhoids, with enlarged prostate ; intense pain in back and through whole pelvis.—Flatus : hot, smells like rotten eggs.

14. **Urinary Organs.**—Itching, needle-like stitches in region of kidneys.—Pressure on bladder on waking from sleep.—Very frequent want to urinate, with emission drop by drop, or else of a slender stream of deep-coloured urine.—Excessively painful emission of urine.—Frequent (profuse) emission of clear watery urine (with much urging).—Frequent emission of red urine.—Constant micturition at night (produced.—R. T. C).—Bloody urine (produced.—R. T. C.).—Involuntary emission of urine when coughing.—After having urinated, a fresh want is felt, as if bladder were again full.—Burning sensation in urethra, esp. (after and) when urinating (with urging, as if the bladder were not emptied).—Constant urging in young married women.

15. **Male Sexual Organs.**—Soft, moist excrescences, upon and behind the glans (sycosis).—Inflammation of testes, with burning shootings, or pressive drawing and tearings.—Pressing pain in l. testicle when walking ; and after rubbing ; < from touch.—Drawing, tearing, in r. testicle, as if compressed.—Drawing, burning, extending from r. inguinal ring, as if in spermatic cord, into r. testicle.—Chronic prostatitis in old men ; pain extending from anus along urethra.—Sensation of worms crawling in back of scrotum.—A very marked increase of sexual desire, with frequent erections, esp. at night.—Voluptuous itching in the scrotum, which provokes emission.—Frequent pollutions, even during a siesta.—Effects of onanism ; face sunken, abashed look ; melancholy ; nocturnal emissions ; backache, legs weak ; organs relaxed.—Seminal emissions followed by great chagrin and mortification ; great prostration ; dyspnœa.—Dyspnœa (towards the end of, and) after coition.—Discharge of prostatic fluid, during a hard evacuation.

16. **Female Sexual Organs.**—Nymphomania, with extreme sensitiveness to mental and physical impressions ; mind dwells too much on sexual subjects.—Painful sensitiveness of genital organs (esp. when sitting).—Prurigo senilis ; or from pediculi.—Smarting and lancinating itching in vulva.—Sufferings after coitus in newly married women.—Inflammation of the ovaries with burning, stinging, and pressing-drawing.—Very sharp shooting pains in ovary, which is exceedingly sensitive to pressure ; pains extending into crural region and thighs.—Flow of blood from genitals a long time after critical age.—Menses which had ceased for a year, reappeared with cutting colic and violent rumbling, at the new moon.—Spasmodic pains in vulva and vagina.—Menses : irregular, late, and profuse ; sometimes wanting ; first of pale blood, then dark and clotted ; occasionally spasmodic uterine contractions.—Amenorrhœa from chagrin with indignation.—Granular vegetations of vagina.

17. **Respiratory Organs.**—Hoarseness, with accumulation of mucus,

which adheres to larynx and chest.—Sensation of pressure and contraction in pit of throat, after a fit of passion, < by deglutition.—Roughness, rawness, in larynx, after much speaking.—Dry, hollow cough, excited by a tickling in the larynx.—Violent cough, with expectoration of viscid mucus, in evening, after lying down.—Violent spasmodic cough, with (tough) purulent, yellow expectoration, esp. at night.—Croupy cough in winter, alternating with sciatica in summer; cough excited by tobacco smoke.—Expectoration of blood, when coughing.—Dyspnœa: with constriction; after seminal emissions; towards end of coition.—Pain (soreness and rawness) as from ulceration in the chest, during cough.—Dyspnœa with constriction and restlessness in chest.

18. **Chest.**—Aching in chest, with heaviness in that part when sitting, mitigated by walking.—Contractive oppression, and great agitation in chest.—Itching stitches in costal cartilages.—Itching in sternum beneath pit of throat.—Lancinations in chest.—Pain in chest, as from excoriation and ulceration.—Cramp in diaphragm, after a fit of passion.—Miliary eruption on the chest, with redness and itching when heated.—Herpetic eruption on lower ribs, with burning itching.

19. **Heart.**—Tremulous palpitation of heart; on least movement; after least intellectual fatigue; when listening to music; after a siesta.—Stitching pains in heart, or region of heart; stopping breathing.—Heart feels weak (produced.—R. T. C.).

20. **Neck and Back.**—Drawing, rheumatic pressure, and tension in nape, with rigidity.—Stiff-neck, shoulders sore to lie on (produced.—R. T. C.)—Weakness of muscles in nape and neck.—Eruption of itching pimples on nape.—Painful swelling of glands of neck, of nape, and under axillæ.—Lancinations under axillæ.—Pain, as if broken in loins, or sensation as from overlifting, or straining the back, esp. during repose, and principally night and morning.—Pain in loins on rising from a seat, or on turning in bed.—Itching stitches in region of kidneys.—Violent (stitches) lancinations, which pass up back.—(Suppurating swelling in the psoas muscle.)—Lumbar abscess.

21. **Limbs.**—Drawing, tearing, stitching pains in extremities.—Limbs feel beaten and painful, as after a long walk, below shoulders and below hip-joint.

22. **Upper Limbs.**—Aching of shoulders.—Stitches in shoulder-joints, < on touch and motion.—Dislocation pains in r. shoulder-joint, only on moving.—Stiffness of shoulder-joint in morning.—Shoulders sore to lie on, and stiff-neck (produced.—R. T. C.).—Pains in bones of arms, during movement.—Pressive, paralytic, drawing, and lancinating tearings, in arms (< on motion and touch), and forearms, shoulders, hands, and fingers.—Painful pressure in bone of arm.—Paralytic drawing in metacarpal joints, < from motion.—Hands become anæmic from cardiac inertia; gouty pains in little finger, index and thumb of l. hand at night, and loss of power in l. thumb with pain in r. shoulder (produced.—R. T. C.).—Herpes on hands.—Herpes with scabs on elbows.—Numbness in ends of fingers.—Jerking tearing in fingers, esp. in the tips.—Burning itching in l. thumb.—Arthritic nodosities in joints of the fingers.—Osteitis of phalanges of fingers.—Cramps in fingers.—Convulsive movements of fingers.

23. **Lower Limbs.**—Pulsating pain in hip-joint as from beginning suppuration.—Stiffness of coxo-femoral joint in morning.—Nates ache while sitting ; pain extends to small of back, sacrum, and hip-joint.—Daily pains beginning at crest of ilium, r. side, extending backward and downward to thigh, < early morning, on rising or on sitting down, > standing and from warmth.—Exceedingly severe pain in r. leg, extending into genitals, esp. testes ; attacks followed by great prostration.—Painful weakness of thighs and legs, esp. of knee-joint.—Pain as of a fracture in thighs when walking.—Itching tetters on thighs and legs.—Itching on inner side of thighs.—Drawing shootings in the knees and knee-joints (< on motion).—Drawings, and pressive tearings in tibia, and bones of feet.—Boring stitches in r. tibia during rest.—Nocturnal cramps in calves and soles.—Tearing in muscles of legs when sitting and standing.—Stitches in r. calf.—Swelling of instep.—Swelling of metatarsal bones.—Burning itching in toes, as if they had been frost-bitten.—R. toe inflames round nail and forms an abscess (produced.—R. T. C.),

24. **Generalities.**—[Flatulent colic, where the flatus is incarcerated ; gnawing pains ; darting pains ; sensation of trembling in inner parts.—Pains in zygoma ; in cheeks ; in under jaw.—Affections of angles of eye, particularly the inner ; glands about neck and lower jaw ; diseased ovaries, particularly r. one.—Yellow scabs behind ear.—Flat taste ; obstructed evacuation of bowels.—Micturition too frequent ; too sparing.—Polypus ; arthritic nodes ; restlessness of the body ; scurvy.—< From : mental affections ; anger ; grief ; mortification, esp. if caused by offence ; from loss of fluids ; tobacco ; *Mercury ;* sexual excesses ; sleeping in afternoon ; touching the parts (as in toothache, can't bear to have the tongue, drink, or anything touch the teeth) ; from the least touch on affected parts.—> After breakfast ; from breaking wind.—H. N. G.]—Has been used as an application for healing recent wounds.—Paralytic drawing in joints, esp. during movement, or when the parts are in a false position.—Drawing tearing in muscles, esp. when seated. — Twitches at night. — Acute, penetrating, deep lancinations in different parts.—Cramps in limbs.—Painful inflammations of bones ; suppuration of bones and periosteum.—Swelling of bones.—Semilateral paralysis, after a fit of anger.—Syncope.—Painful sensibility of all muscles, when touched, and of joints, when using them.—Mechanical injuries from sharp-cutting instruments.—Painful weariness and excessive lassitude, esp. during movement ; > by sitting or lying down.—Continued disposition to remain lying down.—Great fatigue, early in morning, with stiffness of all joints.—Sore and stiff all over, swollen fingers and sore tibiæ (produced.—R. T. C.).—After a siesta, cloudiness, with heaviness in limbs.—Relieves pains of cancer (R. T. C.).

25. **Skin.**—Tingling, as from insects, over whole body, esp. in morning.—Chronic miliary eruptions, sometimes with convulsive jerks at night.—Eruption of itching, oozing nodosities, with burning pain.—Scald-head with yellow scab, smells badly, itches very much, &c.—Exanthema on cheeks, face, or particularly if it is yellow ; with a creeping itching.—Incised wounds, with great pain.—Herpetic eruptions, with itching in evening, and burning sensation after scratching them.—Arthritic nodosities on the joints.—Dry, crusty tetters on the joints.—Painful engorgement and induration of the glands.—Unhealthy skin, easily suppurating.—Frequent furunculi.—Ulcers,

ith tearing shootings (gnawing pains), or itching smarting.—Jerking and earing round ulcers, esp. morning and evening.—Wens and encysted tumours urst after *Staph.* 200 (R. T. C.).

26. Sleep.—Strong tendency to sleep all day.—Violent yawnings and retchings, which cause tears to come into the eyes.—Sleep retarded by mental activity (crowding of ideas); or in consequence of an itching and urning sensation in the tetters and ulcers, or of violent pains in calves.—leepy all day; awake all night; body aches all over.—Jerking of limbs, when sleeping.—Disturbed sleep, with unquiet dreams, and frequent waking with a start.—Child wakes, pushes everything away and wants everybody to go away; restless at night as from frightful dreams; calls for mother often. –Lascivious dreams, with emissions.

27. Fever.—Pulse very fast but small and trembling.—Frequent shivering and shuddering, also at night.—Fever in evening, manifesting itself only by chilliness.—Chilliness and coldness predominate.—Violent chill in evening with heat in face.—Chilliness 3 p.m.; > when exercising in open air.—Chill scending from back over head.—Chill running down back.—Before and after the paroxysms of intermittent fever, ravenous hunger.—Tertian fever with symptoms of scurvy, such as putrid taste), bitter taste, bleeding gums, anorexia, and constipation.—External burning heat, with ebullition of blood, and thirst (after midnight, followed by chill towards morning).—Burning heat in hands and feet, at night, which renders it needful to uncover them.—Great tendency to perspire by day, even when seated quietly; or else inability to perspire, with paleness of face and headache.—Profuse perspiration at night, sometimes with putrid smell (like rotten eggs).—Cold sweat on orehead and feet.

Stellaria Media.

Stellaria media. Chickweed. *N. O.* Caryophyllaceæ. Tincture of whole fresh plant in bloom.

Clinical.—Gout. Liver, inflammation of. *Rheumatism.* Psoriasis.

Characteristics.—The first mention of *Stel.* appeared in *H. W.*, xxviii, 284 (June, 1893). F. H. Brett gave an experience with the tincture applied externally, in the case of his wife to enlarged, inflamed gouty fingers-joints, and in his own case to painful, aching great toes. In each case a few applications removed the trouble. Brett was led to this use by having heard a rumour that "chickweed poultices" were good for gouty joints. In the same volume, p. 560, F. Kopp published a proving of the tincture on himself. The symptoms of the proving make up my Schema. Kopp took frequently repeated doses of the tincture, and also chewed some of the weed. The pains induced were of a rheumatic character, and were so severe that they had to be antidoted with *Nux* and *Bry.* Kopp confirms Brett's observations in the value of external applications of *Stel.* Internally he gave the 2x. The most prominent symptom, apart from the rheumatic effects, was the pain, swelling, and soreness of th liver. The pains were > by motion, and were accompanied b soreness. Bellairs (*H. W.*, xxi. 24), published this case: "E. B., 18 had had rheumatic fever which had left him in a hopeless state o chronic "shifting" rheumatism: pains now in ankle, now in knee now in arm, wrist or fingers. *Stel.* 2x, taken three times a day, com pletely cured in a month. Bellairs suggests that "shifting-pains" ma be a keynote; and Kopp confirms this. Brett (*H. W.*, xxxiv. 93 cured himself with *Stel.* 1 of a violent attack of sickness, with shar pains in stomach, increasing in violence and culminating in an ex plosive vomit. The liver was much enlarged, hard to the touch The pain began in the region of the gall bladder. Vomiting ceasec after the first dose, and the liver enlargement quickly subsided Cooper gave much relief with a single dose of ϕ in the case of a woman, 55, who had psoriasis, dating from twenty-one years back with irritation in the spots, chiefly on flexures of joints, with much irritation of scalp and soreness of eyeballs.

SYMPTOMS.

2. **Head.**—Rheumatic pains over r. side of head, esp. at back; sore to touch.—Rheumatic pains; darting through whole head < r. side; through l. half of forehead, over eye; sore to touch.

3. **Eyes.**—R. eyeball sore to touch.—Flushes of heat below r. lid.—Darting pain in r. eye.—Vision dim.

5. **Nose.**—Dryness of nostrils.

6. **Face.**—Neuralgic pains r. side of face.—Burning on lower lips.

8. **Mouth.**—Persistent taste of the drug with slight acrid feeling.—Heat and dryness of mouth; numbness of lower gums and tip of tongue.—Sensation as if incisors set on edge.

9. **Throat.**—Numbness and dryness in throat, followed later by sharp stitches in l. tonsil.

11. **Stomach.**—Slight nausea with frequent eructations, tasting of the drug.

12. **Abdomen.**—Stomach and bowels sore, < by touch.—Navel sore to touch.—Soreness and dragging pains in lower bowels.—Wandering pains around navel, settling between navel and liver.—Sensation as if liver too large for body.—Burning pains all over liver.—Liver sore to touch.—Burning pressure in region of liver.—Bilious feeling.—Pains in r. groin.

13. **Stool.**—Stools loose, dark brown, attended with slight pain.

14. **Urinary Organs.**—Kidney region sore to touch.

17. **Respiratory Organs.**—Short cough from tickling on upper chest, < deep inspiration.—Hawking of viscid, saltish mucus.

18. **Chest.**—In chest: tickling, upper part; constricted; oppression; heat.

20. **Back.**—Rheumatic pains across small of back, < bending.—Loins stiff and sore.—Dull pain under r. scapula.

21. **Limbs.**—Joints stiff.

22. Upper Limbs.—Darting, rheumatic pain: down r. arm, and in iddle of index finger of l. hand.

23. Lower Limbs.—Rheumatic pains: in r. hip; l. foot; ankle; l. knee, radually extending along thigh; below r. knee-cap; in calves which are nsitive.

24. Generalities.—Pains < on motion; parts sore to touch.—Symptoms ome on rapidly after taking the drug; next morning on rising bruised feeling l over thighs as from over-exertion.

26. Sleep.—Sleeps well but unrefreshed on waking.

27. Fever.—Pulse slightly raised but temperature normal.

Sticta Pulmonaria.

Sticta pulmonaria. Lung-wort. *N. O.* Lichenes. Tincture.

Clinical.—Angina pectoris. Anus, pain in. Asthma. Bronchitis. Catarrh. lergyman's sore throat. Cold. Cough. Diabetes. *Diaphragm, rheumatism* . Diarrhœa. Glands, swollen. Hay-fever. Headache. *Housemaid's knee.* ysteria. Influenza. Laryngitis. Levitation. Measles, cough of. Migraine. ilk, scanty. Neuralgia. Ozæna. Phthisis. Post-nasal catarrh. Pott's disease. heumatism. Seminal emissions. Sick headache. Sleeplessness. Syphilis.

Characteristics.—There cannot be much doubt whence *Sticta* eceived its name of *Pulmonaria*. The likeness of the plant to lung ssue is self-evident. It was a popular remedy of great repute in atarrhs and coughs when Hale introduced it to homeopathy. S. P. urdock, C. H. Lutes, and S. Lilienthal proved it and elicited some ery remarkable and valuable symptoms. Hering added many no less aluable clinical symptoms. Dewey (*Trans. Paris Int. H. Cong.* 1900, . 317) conducted another proving on several persons which has rther enriched the pathogenesis. His additions are marked (D) in e Schema. "It was first used," says Hale, "for severe, harassing ough," and such good results accrued that provings were made to scertain its full value. It was found to cause severe coryza, with iolent sneezing, intense headache, and conjunctivitis. These attacks ere preceded or followed by rheumatic pains and swelling of the nall joints." The catarrh of *Stic.* is for the most part *obstructive;* nd if there is discharge it dries quickly, and forms crusts or scurf. onstant need to blow the nose, but no discharge comes on account f dryness. In syphilis, or any other disease where this condition is resent, *Stic.* will be the remedy. A grand characteristic both of eadaches and catarrh is a "dull, heavy pressure (or stuffed feeling) root of nose." The cough of *Stic.* is also dry. "Dry night cough" a keynote: cough dry, < evening and night; can neither sleep nor lie own; must sit up. P. C. Majumdar (*Ind. H. R.*, v. 109) cured two cases f whooping-cough with *Stic.* 6x. The cough began just after sunset, nd went on till vomiting occurred, and all the contents of the stomach ere thrown off. *Stic.* will often cure coughs left by measles, hooping-cough, influenza. Hard, dry barking coughs following colds.

In cases of phthisis and hæmoptysis it is of great service. "Oppressio at chest; sensation as if a hard mass on it. Sudden pain from sternur to spine, constant, < on movement," are leading symptoms in such case in addition to those of the cough. Phthisis and rheumatism nc infrequently occur in different members of a phthisical family; an *rheumatism* (as the word implies) is related to catarrh. *Stic.* meets a these conditions; and it has, like *Bacil.*, "a deep-in headache." Elia C. Price (in *Southern J. of H.*) relates this case: Boy, 8, had acut rheumatism with inflammation and redness of one knee, ankle, toe wrist, and fingers; valvular heart disease from a previous attack. *Ac* and *Sul.* failed to relieve. *Stic.* 1 x was given every hour. Next da there was a *considerable quantity of fluid in the knee-joint* [an aggr vation by *Stic.* apparently], but otherwise the boy was better. *Sti* was continued. Next day half the fluid was gone, and the third da it was all gone, and the boy was cured in nine days. Price remark that he had noticed one symptom so frequently present in the cases h cured with *Stic.* that he began to regard it as a characteristic althoug it was not in the provings: A *spot* of inflammation and redness o the affected joint like the hectic flush on the cheeks in phthisis. I housemaid's-knee *Stic.* comes as near being a specific as a remed ever can. M. D. Youngman (*H. M.*, 1893, p. 360) related a numb of cases of catarrhal and pulmonary affections cured with *Stic.* the indications being: Harsh, racking, incessant, "unprofitable cough of spasmodic type. He considers it especially *Suited* neuralgic, rheumatic, gouty individuals. Here is one of his cases Mrs. H., 42, had an attack of bronchitis in January, and when see March 29th, had a harsh, racking cough, with pain all through che on coughing; spongy state of mucous membrane of pharynx, whic bleeds easily; has had several attacks of asthma; has hay-fever eve August; paroxyms of cough often end in convulsive sneezing, whic she dreads because it is followed by asthmatic symptoms. "Sh takes cold in her head, which in a day or so goes down in her throa and thence into her chest." Every cold she gets does this. *Stic.* 1 gave relief in five days. Hale says *Stic.* is indispensable in Februar March, and April in the American climate. L. O. Rogers (*S. J. of H* prescribed *Stic.* for a patient with the cough of the remedy the time she was nursing her seventh child. She had always bee annoyed because of a scantiness of milk; it had been occasional entirely suppressed. Whilst taking *Stic.* the flow became ample, an remained so as long as an occasional dose was being taken. Roge subsequently verified this effect in a number of cases. Another us of *Stic.* is in sleeplessness, which is due to nervousness, or to coug This is part of its action on the nervous system. *Stic.* is one of th remedies which produce the levitation symptom: the legs feel as floating in the air; head as if floating off; as if the body and lim did not touch the bed. Hysterical chorea coming on after pr fuse hæmorrhage has been cured by *Stic.* *Peculiar Sensations are*: if she cannot keep her tongue still. As if stomach full of yeas Throat and mouth burn as if scalded. As if hard mass collected lungs. As if floating in air. The right side is more prominent affected. The symptoms are: < By touch. < Motion (also: must g up and move about for relief from pain of knee). < Turning eyes. Pressure >. Lying down > headache ; < cough. Influenza is > in open air. Many symptoms are < as the day advances, lasting all day. Cough < nights (comparatively free from it during day). Coughing < cough (the more he coughs, the more he wants to).

Relations.—*Compare:* Lung affections ; deep-in headache, Bac. Catarrhs and coughs, Dros., Nux, Rx. c., Samb., Meph. Rheumatism, Act. r., Stellar. Nerve symptoms, Asar, Tarent. Asthma of consumptives associated with splitting headache, Rx. c., Meph. Levitation symptoms, Calc., Sil., Can. i. Sensation of lightness of body, Coccul., Gels. The more he coughs, the more he wants to, Ign. Heaviness from front to back, Naja. Headache as if skull being raised and lowered, Can. i.

Causation.—Fall. Hæmorrhages.

SYMPTOMS.

1. **Mind.**—Confusion of ideas, cannot concentrate them.—Great desire to talk about anything and everything, doesn't care whether any one listens, cannot keep her tongue still.—Lively, wanted to strike out ; lay on the lounge and began to "kick up her heels" ; when reproved said she couldn't help it but felt as if she wanted to fly away.

2. **Head.**—Slight vertigo (D).—Dull sensation in head with sharp darting pains through vertex, side of face, and lower jaw.—Dull, heavy pressure in forehead and root of nose, increasing in intensity during the day.—Pain in r. supraorbital region ; became more acute and extended through brain on r. side ; deep in brain.—Headache extending through brain, almost intolerable. —Headache as if entire skull were being raised up and lowered again, comes on after dose of ϕ in man, 43, with arthritis deformans ; the pain had been felt before but not so severely (R. T. C.).—Darting pains in temples, increasing in intensity the entire day.—Catarrhal headache before catarrh sets in.—Sick-headache, must lie down ; < from light and noise ; nausea and vomiting, nearly to faintness.—Headache with severe pain in eyes felt on closing lids or turning eyeballs.—Scalp feels as if too small, or as if drawn too tight.—[Painful weight on back of head.—Confused, heavy sensation on head.—The head seems as if flying in space.—Frontal migraine > by cold ; < by pressure.—Slight pressive headache deep in.—The head seems full and confused by every dose (D).]

3. **Eyes.**—Eyes feel heavy.—Burning in lids with soreness of the ball on closing lids or turning eyes ; increasing during the entire day.—[Eyes : painful as if inflamed.—Sight dim as if he had read too much.—Pain in l. internal canthus.—Right eye painful as if something were in it (D).]

4. **Ears.**—Acute neuralgic pains in mastoid apophysis, rather deep in.

5. **Nose.**—Fulness at root of nose.—Constant need to blow nose, but no result on account of dryness.—Excessive and painful dryness of mucous membrane ; secretions dry rapidly, forming scabs difficult to dislodge.—Incessant sneezing with fulness in forehead and r. side of nose, tingling in r. side of nose.—Desire to put finger in nose to clear out gluish secretion. –Coryza < afternoon ; > in open air.—Constant desire to blow nose without dis-

charge (tertiary syphilis).—[Slight epistaxis.—Slight liquid coryza.—Sensation of obstruction in nose.—Yellow, thick discharge for several days (D).]

6. **Face.**—Darting pains in side of face ; and in lower jaw.—[Pain in malar bone.—Sensitiveness of lower jaw.—Pain in r. submaxillary gland, < by pressure.—Pain in parotid gland (D).]

8. **Mouth.**—Mouth and throat burn as if scalded.—[Thick yellow coat on posterior half of tongue with a narrow yellow stripe running along centre to tip ; many red papillæ show through.—Patch covered with pearly white coat, rough and hard to dislodge ; saliva abundant and foamy (D).]

9. **Throat.**—Excessive dryness of soft palate, feels like dried leather, causing painful deglutition.—Dropping of mucus from posterior nares, throat feels and looks raw.—Sore throat ; coryza from slightest cold.—[Scraping sensation in throat.—Obstruction in throat (D).]

11. **Stomach.**—Slight pyrosis with acid and bitter regurgitation ; sleepy after dinner and diminished appetite (D).—Dull, oppressive pain in cardia. —Severe pains from sternum to spinal column, and a feeling of rumbling burning in stomach as if full of yeast.

12. **Abdomen.**—Dull pains in r. hypochondrium.—Feeling of fulness in l. hypochondriac region.—Rumbling as if full of yeast.

13. **Stool and Anus**—Mucous diarrhœa and loose cough.—[Thick diarrhœa ; stools profuse, frequent, little colour.—Constant desire for stool with no result.—Profuse stool 1 a.m., driving him hurriedly from bed.—Foamy stool, with flatus.—Stool 3 a.m. with effort.—Constipation with acute tetanic pain in anus, lasting half an hour after stool (D).]

14. **Urinary Organs.**—[Bladder seems distended.—Urine thicker than usual, and increased in quantity.—Sensitiveness or pain in bladder.—Urine much increased.—Frequent necessity to urinate ; must rise several times at night.—Efforts to urinate with emission of a small quantity (D).]

15. **Male Sexual Organs.**—[Pollutions for several nights.—Pollution whilst he slept in afternoon.—Mind drawn to sexual subjects (D).]

16. **Female Sexual Organs.**—[Uneasiness in the pelvis.—Menses more abundant and paler than usual (D).]—Scanty milk became abundant.

17. **Respiratory Organs.**—Tickling in larynx and trachea causing cough.—Tickling in r. side of trachea below larynx.—Clergyman's sore throat, characterised by great dryness of mucous membranes.—Hay-fever, with dryness of membranes.—Cough : dry, < evening and night ; can neither sleep nor lie down ; dry, noisy ; severe, dry, racking with splitting frontal headache. —Cough after influenza ; after measles ; after whooping-cough ; barking ; < night and morning.—[Cough : dry ; spasmodic ; the more he coughs the more he wants to.—Spasmodic cough which he cannot stop.—Dry cough, causing pain in upper part of sternum (D).]—A lady had catarrhal asthma so badly was refused admission to an hotel ; *Sti. p.* 1 x was given, and next day she walked into the hotel without any sign of asthma (R. T. C.).

18. **Chest.**—Slight oppression of lungs.—Feeling of a hard mass in chest. —Sudden pain through chest from sternum to spine ; constant, < on movement ; arms powerless from extreme pain if an attempt was made to move them ; difficult breathing and speaking.—Pulsation from r. side of sternum down to abdomen.—Coryza with expectoration of dark blood brought on by every cold, damp spell.

19. **Heart.**—Dull, oppressive pain in cardiac region.—Attacks of anxiety about heart; awakes with strange sensation about heart and for a few moments feels as if floating in air.—[Pulse uneven, drops every third or fourth beat.—Veins of hands feel distended, also superficial veins of arms and legs (D).]

20. **Neck and Back.**—Cervical glands swollen, l. side, neck sensitive.—[Woke with heavy pain in second and fourth lumbar vertebræ, > sitting upright or bending forward.—Great weakness in the back in afternoon (D).]

21. **Limbs.**—Darting pains in arms, legs, and shoulders, beginning in muscles of arms, then in fingers, joints, thighs, and toes.—Swelling and stiffness of hands and feet.—Rheumatism of joints.—Hands and feet tend to be cold (D).—Red spots of inflammation on affected joints (Price).

22. **Upper Limbs.**—Rheumatism in r. shoulder-joint, deltoid, and biceps, extending at times to forearm; commencing at night; > during day.—Lancinating pain in second joint of middle finger, increasing in intensity all day.—Rheumatism of wrists; wrists and hands swollen, little redness, very painful on moving.—On movement, painful bruised sensation in muscles, esp. of forearm (D).

23. **Lower Limbs.**—L. leg felt as if floating in the air, feels light and airy without any feeling of resting on the bed.—(Fluid in knee-joint.)—Rheumatism of r. ankle, swollen, very painful.—Knee painful from a fall.—Housemaid's-knee.—[Lancination in knees and legs.—Feet cold and sweating (D).]

24. **Generalities.**—Dulness.—Very soon after taking *Sti. p.* prover said, "I feel that medicine all over me."—General feeling of weariness.—Burning, biting, sticking pains all over body during entire day.—Feeling of levitation of different parts.—Hysteria after loss of blood.—Swelling and painfulness of lymphatic glands.

26. **Sleep.**—Sleeplessness: from nervousness; from cough; of children; after surgical operations (*e.g.*, setting broken leg).

27. **Fever.**—Increase of temperature.—Shudder through the whole body, esp. of toes and fingers.

Stigmata Maïdis, *see* Zea.

Stillingia Sylvatica.

Stillingia sylvatica. Queen's Delight. (Pine barrens from Virginia to Florida.) *N. O.* Euphorbiaceæ. Tincture of the root after flowering.

Clinical.—*Bones*, diseases of; nodes on. Clergyman's sore throat. Elephantiasis. Hæmorrhoids. Headaches, syphilitic; mercurial; catarrhal. Hip-joint disease. Influenza. Larynx, affections of. Liver, affections of. Nodes. Periostitis. Psoriasis. *Rheumatism.* Scrofula. *Syphilis.*

Characteristics.—*Still.* has long been a popular remedy for syphilis in the southern states of U. S. T. Y. Symons introduced it into professional medicine, and Hale to homœopathy. H. R. Frost, A. B. Nichols, J. M. Cunningham, and others proved it, chewing the root or taking the tincture. One prover chewed the bark. The proving shows an action closely parallel with that of syphilis, attacking the genito-urinary organs, throat (pharynx, larynx, and trachea), mouth, head, and bones. I have cured with it syphilitic cough of the hoarse, barking type. In one case of secondary syphilis the patient (who was taking *Still.* 1) complained that the medicine made his legs and feet feel tired and his feet feel sore. *Still.* attacks the periosteum and produces pain in the bone. It has removed nodes on the forehead, tibia, and elsewhere, and arrested caries of the nasal bones. Pain in the cranial bones and the headaches of syphilis. It is not confined to syphilitic cases in its action. It has a popular repute in scrofula, skin affections, liver diseases, and rheumatism—all of which the provings confirm. One prover was cured of a pustular eruption during the proving. In chronic rheumatism Hale classes it with *Phyt.* and *K. iod.* *Peculiar Sensations* are: As of a heavy substance pressing on brain. Tongue as if scalded (*Still.* has the irritating properties of the Euphorbians). As if room were too warm. Pains are sharp, shooting, darting. The cartilages of larynx and trachea are sore and feel bruised. *Dryness* is a common feature. Hale quotes a case of secondary syphilis treated by Preston, one of the provers. The patient, a man, suffered extreme torture from bone pains. After receiving *Still.* he slept well. The immense nodes disappeared from head and legs; and "from the most deplorable, down-hearted (sometimes almost raving from derangement), miserable, thin-looking object, he changed into a buoyant, joking, rotund-looking fellow." The symptoms were < by movement. < Walking. Pressure > pain in forearm. < Exposure to cold or to air. Warmth > itching of legs.

Relations.—*Antidote to:* Merc. *Antidoted by:* Ipec. (nausea from the fumes). *Compare:* In syphilis, Syph., Med., Merc., K. iod. Chronic rheumatism, Guaiac., Phyt. Nodes, Mang., Corydalis, Staph. Hip disease, Nat. s. (Still. secondary or inherited syphilis, pains in and through hip < night, < wet weather; Nat. s. hydrogenoid constitution, pains < night rouse patient from sleep, > turning over in bed).

SYMPTOMS.

1. **Mind.**—Depression of spirits; and gloomy forebodings.—Intellect dull and stupid.

2. **Head.**—Dizziness and throbbing in head.—Persistent dull headache in vertex.—Dull, heavy pain in r. side of head.—In frontal region a feeling as of a heavy substance pressing on brain, becoming sharp and darting, almost unendurable.—Pains in head, with inflamed and watery eyes, and general soreness of muscles.—Sharp darting pains in r. occipital protuberance.—Mercurial, spyhilitic, and catarrhal headaches.—Bone swellings in head and forehead, in latter size of hen's eggs.—Mercurial periostitis of skull.

3. **Eyes.**—Eyes inflamed and watery, with severe headache and general nuscular soreness, as if he had taken cold.—Sharp darting pain over l. eye; achrymation of both eyes, esp. after reading; r. eye <.

4. **Ears.**—Burning in l. ear in evening; next morning a vesicular ruption.

5. **Nose.**—Catarrhal discharge, first watery then muco-purulent; ollowed by small abscesses on inside of r. nostril.—Sharp burning sensation n r. nostril, 6 a.m. on waking.—Influenza.—Necrosis of bones of nose.

6. **Face.**—Pains under malar bone, extending transversely through ace.—Stinging darting pains in face; with frontal headache.—Periostitis of acial bones.

8. **Mouth.**—Paroxysms of neuralgic toothache.—Tongue: coated ieavily; yellowish white; white; feels rough and sore.—Scalded sensation on tongue, with soreness in region of larynx.—Heat in mouth and fauces.—Taste: salty; bitter in morning.—Increased flow of saliva.

9. **Throat.**—Smarting, stinging, dryness and rawness of fauces.—Contriction of throat.—Intense burning in fauces and throat extending to tomach; < on any attempt to swallow.

11. **Stomach.**—Appetite: increased; lost.—Regurgitation and vomiting of ingesta.—Pyrosis daily, 3 p.m. to bedtime.—Nausea with constipation.—Sickness and salivation.—Faint, empty sensation in stomach.—Distress; griping; cramps in stomach.

12. **Abdomen.**—Torpidity of liver with jaundice, great depression, constipation.—Severe cramps in both hypochondria.—Sharp darting in l. hypochondrium, followed by passage of flatus. — Borborygmi. — Colic, periodical.—Heavy pain in hypogastric region.

13. **Stool and Anus.**—Severe attack of piles lasting several weeks.—Pain in rectum and sphincter with stool; burning and tenesmus; lasting half an hour after.—Bowels loose and irregular.—Stools: copious, acid, rothy, bilious; papescent; white like curds; dysenteric.—Constipation, tools delayed.

14. **Urinary Organs.**—Dull pain in region of kidneys.—Incontinence of urine.—Violent smarting burning through whole length of urethra < by nicturition, with difficulty in voiding urine.—Urine: increased; flocculent, nucous sediment.

15. **Male Sexual Organs.**—On micturating, sharp pain in glans extending up urethra, so severe as to cause perspiration.—Slight drawing up n r. testis.—Dull tearing pain in l. testis.—Gonorrhœa.

16. **Female Sexual Organs.**—Both ovaries pained very severely.—Copious muco-purulent leucorrhœa, with rheumatic pains.

17. **Respiratory Organs.**—Laryngitis, esp. if syphilitic, with hoarseness and dry spasmodic cough; or cough may be loose.—Hoarseness and chronic aryngeal affections in public speakers.—Croup.—Slight uneasiness and ickling in trachea and bronchi, < on rising in morning.—Tickling ensation in trachea in evening which = dry, spasmodic cough.—Slight lame eeling seemingly in cartilages of larynx.—Hoarse cough.—Bruised feeling n trachea.—Short, hacking cough.—Cough deep and loose.

18. **Chest.**—Oppression of chest.—Darting pain in thorax, with tickling in throat and short, hacking cough.—Sharp darting pains through chest

and shoulders.—Sore aching above l. clavicle.—Raw feeling in chest who length of sternum.—Incipient phthisis in persons of strumous habit.

19. **Heart.**—Boring pains about region of heart, with irregular pulse.- Pulse weak and very irregular.

20. **Back.**—Aching in back and down thighs and legs.—While sittin pain in l. lumbar region, darting forwards.

21. **Limbs.**—In evening pains in r. elbow and leg, aching and pulsatin with soreness.

22. **Upper Limbs.**—Pain in r. scapula runs up neck.—Soreness an aching in humerus.—Sharp shooting pains in both arms, from middle thi of humerus down to fingers.—Very large node on olecranon.—Aggravatir pains in l. elbow, shooting towards shoulder and head; slighter in r. elbo and wrist.

23. **Lower Limbs.**—Aching pain in r. leg.—Pains in l. lower anteri third of leg.—Burning-itching of legs.—Enlargement of tibia to suc a degree as to deprive the child of all power of motion; limbs contract and swollen.—Ulcers on legs, venereal, chronic, and indolent.—Periosti and nodes of tibia.—Syphilitic and gonorrhœal sciatica; l.-sided complain —(Legs and feet feel tired, and feet sore.)

24. **Generalities.**—Soreness of muscles all over; feels as if he ha taken a severe cold.—Weak and emaciated.—Symptoms lasted eight week —Nothing seemed to >; much < by exposing parts to cold or even to ai > from the aggravation only by covering with flannel or getting into bed.

25. **Skin.**—(Pustular eruptions healed rapidly during the proving.)—Itc ing and burning-itching of legs < exposure to air.—Vesicular eruption c ears.—Scrofulous, venereal, and other skin diseases.—Ulcers with unhealt skin.—Elephantiasis.—Lepra.

26. **Sleep.**—Unusual drowsiness all day, with general malaise ar headache.—Very sleepy after eating.

27. **Fever.**—Cold on going to bed; immediately after broke out sweat, with excessive warmth all night.—Feverish heat, evening.—Fev 1 a.m.; gets into heavy sleep.—During day, room felt too warm.—Gre warmth in face like catarrhal fever.

Stramonium.

Datura stramonium. Thorn-apple. Jamestown-weed. Stink-wee (Grows in vicinity of cultivation on rank soil where refu is deposited in all parts of the world.) *N. O.* Solanace Tincture of fresh plant in flower and fruit.

Clinical.—Anasarca (after scarlatina). *Aphasia.* Apoplexy. Burns. Cat lepsy. Chordee. *Chorea. Delirium tremens.* Diaphragmitis. Ecstasy. Enures *Epilepsy. Erotomania. Eyes, affections of.* Headache; from sun. Hiccoug *Hydrophobia.* Hysteria. Lochia, offensive. Locomotor ataxy. *Mania.* Meningit Nymphomania. Œsophagus, spasm of. Scarlatina. *Stammering. Stari* Strabismus. Sunstroke. Tetanus. *Thirst. Tremors.* Trismus. Typhus.

Characteristics.—The first to use *Stram.* in medicine, accordi to Teste, was Stoerck, who was one of Hahnemann's predecesso oerck first tried it in mental alienation, *because* it was supposed to oduce "a marked and persistent disorder of the mental faculties." ahnemann proved it, and introduced it into the homœopathic ateria medica. In his introduction to the remedy he points out that, ough it produces many uncomfortable symptoms, it does not in its imary effects cause actual *pain*. Hahnemann attached a good deal importance to this. "*Stram.*," he says, "allays some spasmodic ovements, and restores suppressed excretions in several cases which absence of pain is a prominent symptom." In addition to e absence of pain there is with *Stram.* (and in many mental cases) extreme muscular mobility. This mobility affects muscles of pression and muscles of locomotion. The movements of *Stram.* e generally gyratory and graceful when they occur in the ms. The forms of mania specially mentioned by Teste as calling r *Stram.* are: Nymphomania of lying-in women. Certain forms of ligious monomania, in exaggerated and ridiculous scruple of con-ience. Fixed notion that some unpardonable sin has been com-itted (which the patient is nevertheless unable to remember); that he possessed of the devil. Hallucinations. The delirium of *Stram.* is r the most part terrifying. It corresponds exactly to many cases of elirium tremens. Visions of animals enter largely into it. In a case severe pleuro-pneumonia of right side, supervening on scarlatina, e patient, a young man, said he saw a large black dog about the om. This led me to give *Stram.*, which rapidly altered the whole se for the better, including the pneumonia, and resolved a situation of o little anxiety. *Stram.* is also called for in congestions without actual flammation, but with high mental exaltation and furious delirium d little or no fever; without pain but with some coma. J. Emmons riggs (*New Eng. M. Gaz.*, xxx. 151) relates this case of poisoning: riggs had an urgent call to see James M., 4, in "convulsions." He und him lying on the bed in a state of wild delirium, requiring the nstant combined efforts of two people to keep him in bed. Face ceedingly flushed; expression becoming in rapid alternation leasant and anxious. Pupils widely dilated; iris scarcely visible, iving the eye a very brilliant appearance. Marked convergent rabismus, skin hot and dry, resembling scarlatina eruption. Abdomen nse. The most alarming symptom was rapidly recurring convulsions ith twitching of the arms and lower limbs. Thirty or forty of ese spasms occurred in rapid succession, followed by a moment uring which the countenance brightened and seemed at rest, only to followed in an instant by a series of clonic contractions. rasping at imaginary objects before the eyes, when expression equently became anxious, as if the patient was trying to ward f imaginary foes. At times the mind was very active, and e patient talked rapidly and incoherently. Between the spasms ughter and crying frequently occurred. The boy, it transpired, d been chewing a Thorn-apple. When he came home he emed rather dazed, and vomited. He then threw himself on the fa and slept very soundly till he awoke in the convulsions. The y recovered under *Kali bro.* in five-grain doses, though it was with eat difficulty that he was made to swallow. This difficulty of swallowing is a marked feature of *Stram.*, and with the intense thirst delirium, and hallucinations completes the picture of many cases o hydrophobia. Another symptom indicating it here is "< by brigh light, mirror or surface of water." S. A. Jones (quoted *A. H.*, xxii. 410 relates the case of a little girl with brain symptoms for whom he ha prescribed a remedy. The report was brought late at night, that th patient was much worse. "She vomits," said the father, "if she eve raises her head from the pillow." The vomit was *green*. Jone found this under *Stram.* by aid of the Cypher Repertory. He gav *Stram.*, and the next morning the case was entirely changed for th better. Acting on this analogue, Jones also cured a "vomiting o green stuff always induced by bright light." On the other hand, th *Stram.* patient is dependent on light and company; cannot walk i the dark (hence it is indicated in locomotor ataxy); and going throug railway tunnels without a light in the carriage may cause fainting Some of the head-movements of *Stram.* are characteristic: Continuall jerks head up from pillow; head bent back; boring head into pillow The twitchings of single muscles and the squint mark *Stram.* as th remedy for many cases of chorea. I find it correspond to about a equal proportion with *Agaricus;* and when there is fright in the causa tion *Stram.* will almost certainly avail. *Stram.* has a relation to th hip-joints, and *Stram.* has cured both coxalgia and morbus coxæ (left) This is accompanied by very severe pain, and is one exception to th "painlessness" of *Stram.* affections. The effect of *Stram.* on the secre tions is to suppress them; and this makes *Stram.* an excellent remed in many cases of illness due to suppressed secretions—menses, lochia sweat, eruptions. *Stram.* causes high fever with rashes, some scarlet like scarlatina; petechiæ; spots on the arms like flea-bites vesications; and it corresponds also to burns and scalds. *Stram.* 3 caused the face of a boy to whom I gave it to swell and come out i blotches soon after commencing the remedy. (I have seen *Dulc.* 3 produce *furfuraceous* rash on the face in the same way.) In a case o mine *Stram.* relieved an extensive eczematous eruption which cam on after a fright. As a result of suppressions convulsions occur. Thes may be general, or they may be partial or choreic. The convulsant spasmodic properties of *Stram.* are shown in the respiratory spher in constriction of the chest, asthmatic symptoms, and cough of th whooping-cough type. The common practice of smoking Stramoniu leaves for asthma is roughly homœopathic. *Peculiar Sensations* o *Stram.* are: As if spinning or weaving. As if objects were smalle than they really are. As if dizzy. As if he had no limbs. As i drunk. Head as if drawn backward. Starts as if a shock o electricity had been passed through her body. As if eyes wer forced out. As of sparks of fire rushing from stomach to eyes Eyelids as if swollen, or as if oppressed with sleep; as of win rushing out of ears. As if sawing cheek-bone; as if a hole wer there and the brain were touched. As if nose were shifted. As i pins and needles were in forehead. As if he was seeking something As if bones were sawed through. As if front teeth would fall out Teeth as if pressed together. Moving fingers as if searching fo something. Cries as if from sight of hideous objects. As if lip would grow together. Inner mouth as if raw. Soft palate as if drawn down. As of boiling water in throat. As if a ball were wedged in throat. As if falling. As if he would vomit. As if navel were to be torn out. Abdomen as if puffed up. As if abdomen were expanded to extremest degree. As if urine could not be passed on account of narrowness of urethra. As if a cylindrical body were being passed through urethra. As if he had not power to close neck of bladder. As if very tall. As if something turned round in chest. Limbs feel as if gone to sleep. As if parts of limbs were completely separated from body. Hands and feet as if loose in joints. As if cold water were poured down back. *Stram.* is an ill-smelling plant, and the discharges and secretions it causes are often foul and even cadaveric in odour. *Stram.* is *Suited to:* Ailments of young, plethoric persons; especially of children (chorea, mania, fever, delirium). The symptoms are: < By touch; by pressure. Motion <; removing head from pillow = vomiting of bile; walking = involuntary micturition; walking in dark = vertigo. < After motion (vomiting of bile; palpitation; pain in back, shoulder, and abdomen). Whilst sitting: involuntary micturition; cough = lower limbs to be jerked up. Lying > pulsating heat of vertex; in evening = prosopalgia in l. cheek; = cutting pain in sternum. Lying on side < vertigo. Warmth >. Wind <. Cold <. < Evening and night. < In dark. > In light. > In company. < Looking at shining objects, water, &c. < Sun. Great desire for acids; citric acid >.

Relations.—*Antidoted by:* Lemon-juice, Vinegar, Tobacco injections; Senna for cerebral symptoms; Bell., Hyos., Nux; and "Particularly Camphor" (Teste). *Antidote to:* Merc., Pb. *Follows well:* Cupr., Bell. *Incompatible:* Coffea. *Compare:* Metrorrhagia, from retained placenta with characteristic delirium, Sec. (Sec. often acts when *Stram.* fails), Pyro. (with fever and septic tendency). Delirium, Bell., Lach., Agar., Cupr., Zn. Illusions of shape, Bapt., Petr., Thuj. Erysipelas, Bell., Rhus. Stuttering; unable to combine consonants with vowels, Bov. Bright light = convulsions, K. bro. > Light, Stro. Hiccough, Ign. (< after eating, smoking, emotions), Ver. (after hot drinks). Hears voices from far off talking to him; behind him, Anac. Body bathed in hot sweat, Op. Gyrating movements (Hyo., angular). Loquacity, Cup., Hyo., Lach., Op., Ver. Hands constantly on genitals, Zn. Laughs and weeps by turns, Aur., Pul., Alm., Lyc., Caps., Graph., Phos., Sep., Sul., Ver. Tetanic convulsions < touch and light, Nux (Stram. with mania; Nux, mind clear). Desire to escape in delirium, Bell., Bry., Op., Rhus. Hydrophobia, Hfb. Painlessness, Op. Sleepy, but cannot sleep, Bell., Cham., Op. < After sleep, Apis, Lach., Op., Spo. Objects appear small, Plat. Night-blindness, Bell., Nux.

Causation.—Shock. Fright. Sun. Childbirth. Suppressions.

SYMPTOMS.

1. **Mind.**—[The principal range of this remedy is found in the mental affections.—In young people who are sometimes hysterical, showing the

following condition : praying and singing devoutly, beseeching, entreating, &c.—Young women with suppressed menses may be affected in this manner. —In some kinds of fevers, where the patients can't bear solitude or darkness, if they are left alone or are in a dark room, the mental affections are very much < ; also in unconscious delirium when the patient will every now and then jerk up the head from the pillow, then let it fall again, this being kept up without intermission for a long time ; women in puerperal fever or convulsions have many absurd notions—that they are double, that some one is in bed with them, and other strange and unmeaning fancies.—Affections of the intellect in general ; madness.—H. N. G.]—Melancholy.—Sadness, with deadly anguish, and copious tears, esp. in evening, in bed.—Anguish of conscience.—Inconsolable disposition, and susceptibility to irritation by trifles.—Great activity and rapidity of movement.—Obstinacy and self-will.—Bursts of laughter, alternating with choleric passion or moaning.—Howling and groans.—Murmurs, or continued cries.—Ungovernable fury, desire to bite, to strike and to kill.—At one time great indifference to matters of business, at another time fear of being found incapable of discharging them properly.—Love of procrastinating and loss of will-power (cured in a man, 75 —R. T. C.).—Desire to run away.—Desire for society, candle-light, sunshine, because darkness and solitude < the moral symptoms.—The moral symptoms are < after the autumnal equinox.—Loss of memory (loses thoughts before she can utter them ; calls things by wrong names).—Dulness of all the senses, insensibility to external influences (insensibility to mental impressions).—Dizziness, with internal agitation.—Mental derangement, esp. in drunkards.—Loquacious delirium and mania.—Mania-à-potu with clonic spasms and desire for light and company.—Deliria, generally characterised by terror, with visions of frightful spectres.—Loss of consciousness, so that the patient forgets his own relations.—Fixed ideas ; the body is supposed to be cut in two.—Carphologia.—Delusions of fancy, in which all surrounding objects appear to be very small, and the sufferer himself very large, and on an elevation.—Deliria, with strange ideas.—Mental alienation, with praying and pious actions (prayers, hymns, devout aspect, &c.).—Mania, generally with endless fictions of imagination, lascivious talking, conversation with spectres, affectation of importance, dancing, laughter, and blows, or ridiculous buffoonery, in constant alternation with sad and serious behaviour.—Hallucinations : a voice near r. mastoid process scolding her ; frightful, of rats, mice, cats, dogs, and animals moving.—Hallucinations that = terror or rage. —Saw people coming out of all corners.—Rush of blood to head with furious loquacious delirium.—Fear : of losing his senses ; that his lips will grow together ; that he will suffocate ; of falling ; of everything falling on her.—Boy seemed to see black objects, spoke of black people, black clouds, and grasped at air.—Awakens with a shrinking look as if afraid of first thing she sees.—Dulness of senses before a rash.—Conversing in different languages. —Talking in Jewish jargon.—Ecstatic.—Mania from shock.—Nervousness and restlessness.

2. Head.—Intoxication and dizziness.—Vertigo ; cannot walk in the dark, falling to l. or backward.—Vertigo, with giddiness and staggering, or with clouded sight, headache (red face, colicky pain and diarrhœa).—Vertigo, head feels drawn backward.—Stupefaction with vanishing of vision l hearing, and convulsive movements of head.—Headache, with clouded at and dysecoia.—Headaches with tendency to speak incoherently (much eved.—R. T. C.).—Anæmia of the brain in old people (relieved.—R. T. C.).)istressing sensation of lightness and weakness in head.—Woke up with rful headache and extreme sickness, got up at noon but could hardly ak to any one all day; this went on for three days and then left (pro-ced in a woman, 60, fourth day after single dose of ϕ.—R. T. C.).—ad feels empty, hollow; sensitive to every sound.—Throbbing pains in tex, with syncope.—Congestion of blood to head, with heat.—Congestion blood to head, pulsation in vertex, loss of sight and hearing, bloated, turgid e, total loss of consciousness, and painlessness.—Inflammation of brain, h heat and pulsation of vertex, attacks of fainting, loss of sight and hear-, convulsive movements of head, frequently raising head up or bending it kward; > while lying still.—Hydrocephalus with convulsive movements head, sensation of lightness of head, and frequently raising head up.—nful dark-red swelling of the highly congested head and turgid face, with avulsive movements, delirium, and desire for light and company.—Retrac-a and convulsive movements of head.—Lifting head frequently from ow when lying down.—Bores head into pillow.—Bends head backward.—side of head numb.—Head perspires more than usual.

3. **Eyes.**—Eyes red (inflamed) and swollen.—Pressure and tension in s and lids.—Inflammation of margins of lids.—Eyelids ulcerated.—oluntary lachrymation.—Nocturnal agglutination of eyes.—Eyes wide n, staring, prominent.—Conjunctiva injected, as if the vessels were filled h dirty liquid.—Eyes fixed, wide open, and sparkling.—Eyes half open in p.—Photomania.—Vague, melancholy look.—Paralysis and spasmodic sing of lids.—Eyes convulsed.—Contortion of eyes and lids.—Marked avergent strabismus.—Pupils dilated and insensible.—Cloudiness of sight. 'ransient blindness.—Blindness (at night), periodical.—Objects appear e.—Myopia.—Diplopia.—Indistinct, confused sight.—(Everything looks abled up.—R. T. C.)—(Used as a lotion to prevent cataract by a well-own oculist.—R. T. C.).—Amblyopia.—Confusion of letters, when reading.—'ors of vision; objects appear oblique or coloured.—Illusions of vision.—llucinations dark; black spots before eyes.—Luminous vibrations; fiery rks.—Sees balls of fire roll over the counterpane.—Sensation as of sparks ire rushing from stomach to eyes.

4. **Ears.**—Wind rushes out of both ears.—Dryness in Eustachian tube. 'ains in ears.—Pain in l. ear pressing down to l. side of cheek.—Tearing n in r. ear with shooting through forehead and vertex.—Hearing very te.—Hallucinations of hearing.—Deafness.—Deafness of r. ear improves nce from 30th (twitching of pomum Adami led me to it.—R. T. C.).

5. **Nose.**—Obstruction of the nose.—Alæ nasi white, face red.—Nasal charge yellow, bad-smelling, quickly liquifies.—Nose feels obstructed and , though she is able to breathe through it.—The cold of *Stram.* is accom-aied by catarrh of nasal passages and shooting pains over r. eye (pro-ced.—R. T. C.).—Spasmodic sneezing.

6. **Face.**—Dull and bewildered air, with timid behaviour.—Stupid, dis-ted countenance.—Anxiety and fear is expressed in the countenance.—donic grin.—Painful distortion of features.—Facial muscles in constant

play during delirium.—Twitching in muscles of face; frowns on forehead L. side of face for moments distorted with painless convulsions; contract of zygomatic muscles draws cheeks and mouth from below up, and from f backward to temples.—Face deeply furrowed and wrinkled.—Face bloat puffed with blood, sometimes with an idiotic expression.—Circumscril redness of cheeks.—Hot cheeks.—Blood rushing to face.—Deep red, or v pale colour of face.—Fainting with paleness of face, dryness in throat, subsequent red face.—Erysipelas on one side of face and nose.—Boils co out on face while taking *Stram.* (R. T. C.)—Lips dry and glued together A yellow streak in red part of lips.—Quivering in lips.—Distortion of mouth.—Crawling sensation on chin.—Chewing motion with mouth.—Mo spasmodically closed.—Lock-jaw.

7. **Teeth.**—Grinding of the teeth.—Pulsative toothache, as if the te were going to fall out.

8. **Mouth.**—Dryness of mouth (dry fauces and dry, sticky lips) Dribbling of glairy saliva from mouth.—Copious salivation.—Saliva decreas —Sanguineous froth before mouth.—Hæmoptysis.—Tongue swollen paralysed.—Tongue felt stiff, dry, and parched to the very root; as if ed rolled up as hard and dry as leather.—Tongue paralysed, trembles when out.—Imperfect speaking and stammering (with distortion of face) Continued murmurs.—Complete loss of speech.—A trembling tongue.

9. **Throat.**—Spasmodic constriction of throat.—Impeded deglutiti with shootings in throat, or pressure in submaxillary glands.—Deglutit obstructed, sometimes by dryness in throat.—Dryness of throat and fau not > by any sort of drink.—Paralysis of pharynx and œsophagus Contracting, tearing in throat; sensation as if a ball were lodged in thro —Twitching of pomum Adami, up and down movement as in swallow (R. T. C.)—Spasm of œsophagus.

10. **Appetite.**—Loss of taste.—Food tastes only of sand, or straw has no taste at all).—Violent thirst (for large quantities, drinking with avidi —Violent thirst, esp. for acid drinks.—Constant bitterness in mouth, with bi taste of food.—Burning thirst, generally with dread of water and all liquids

11. **Stomach.**—Risings, with sour taste.—Nausea.—Watery vomiti with colic and diarrhœa.—Vomiting of mucus, which is greenish, or of a s smell.—Vomiting of green bile after slight exercise.—Convulsive hiccough Pain in stomach, with smarting or pressive sensation.—Anxietas precordi with obstructed respiration.—(Inflammation of stomach.)—Diaphragmit delirium; burning along diaphragm; short-breathed; spasms; strug against the water offered.

12. **Abdomen.**—Abdomen painful when touched.—Abdomen distend not hard.—Abdomen inflated, hard, distended.—Contusive pain in abdom during movement.—Violent pains in abomen, as if navel were being torn —Hysterical spasms in abdomen.—Swelling of inguinal glands.—Borboryg and fermentation in abdomen.—Expulsion of much flatus.

13. **Stool and Anus.**—Constipation (unsuccessful urging to go stool).—Tenesmus.—Fetid fæces (painless) of a corpse-like smell.—Diarrh with pain and borborygmi in the abdomen.—Discharge of coagulated bl from anus.—Suppression of both stool and urine.—(Stools passed unc sciously and very frequently loose, with mental derangement.—R. T. C.)

14. **Urinary Organs.**—Suppression of secretion of urine (in typhus).—Emission of urine, drop by drop, with frequent want to urinate.—Involuntary emission of urine.—Urine : profuse flow ; sudden ; and burning.

15. **Male Sexual Organs.**—Lasciviousness (exalted sexual desire in both sexes).—Constant uncovering of genitals ; indecent talk.—Priapism.—Scrotum œdematous.—Testes retracted, penis erect as in chordee.—Onanism, causing epilepsy.—Impotence.

16. **Female Sexual Organs.**—Nymphomania.—Increased catamenia, with discharge of large masses of coagulated black blood.—(Menses too profuse and attended with headaches.—R. T. C.)—Increased sexual desire. — Metrorrhagia (with characteristic mental symptoms). — Eclampsia. — During catamenia, fetid smell from body, great loquacity, drawing pains in abdomen and thighs.—Sobs and moaning after catamenia.—Too profuse secretion of milk in nursing women.—During pregnancy : mania ; faceache ; is full of strange fancies.—Cadaverous odour of lochia ; she is full of strange fancies and visions.

17. **Respiratory Organs.**—Voice : hoarse and croaking ; high, fine, squeaking ; indistinct.—(Sudden aphonia in hysterical girl just recovering from chorea.—R. T. C.)—Twitching of pomum Adami.—Constrictions of larynx.—Periodically returning attacks of painless, barking, spasmodic cough, in fine, shrieking tone, from constriction of larynx and chest, without expectoration.—Voice loud and bawling.—Want of breath.—Difficult (hurried or) sighing respiration.—Suffocating obstruction of respiration.—Oppression with desire for open air.—(Asthma continually recurring, with some gouty tendency : attacks < at night.—R. T. C.)—Dyspnœa on waking up every morning, cold winds catch her breath, "can cough at any time" (much relief.—R. T. C.)

18. **Chest.**—Constrictive oppression on chest (with dyspnœa).—Pressure on chest, < by speaking.—Sensation, as if something were turning over in chest.—Spasm in pectoral muscles.—Red rash on chest.

19. **Heart and Pulse.**—Pressure about heart.—Angina pectoris.—For a week after single dose of ϕ felt as if heart beat insufficiently, and had a suffocating feeling in throat (R. T. C.).—Palpitation.—Pulse rapid, full, strong ; irregular, hard, slow, small, frequent.

20. **Neck and Back.**—Neck stiff, cannot bend head backward.—Pain in nape, from neck over head.—Sensitiveness along spine.—Pain as of a fracture in back, when moving.—Drawing and tearing in the back and loins.—Spine sensive ; slightest pressure = outcries and ravings.—Drawing pains in middle of spine ; in sacrum.—Opisthotonos (with distorted countenance).

21. **Limbs.**—Twitching of hands and feet ; of the tendons.—Trembling of limbs ; they fall asleep.

22. **Upper Limbs.**—Convulsive movements of arms, above head.—Convulsive movements of arms and hands ; carphologia.—Contractive pain in arm, with acute lancinations in forearm.—Distortion of hands.—Clenched fists.—Cramps in hands.—Trembling of hands.—Numbness of fingers.

23. **Lower Limbs.**—Coxalgia, l. hip ; violent, distracting pain when abscesses form.—Pain in muscle of outer side of r. hip.—Morbus coxæ, l.—Drawing pains in thighs.—Jerking in legs, as from a shock, with retraction.—

Drawing pains in thighs.—Bending of legs when walking (he falls over his own legs).—Trembling of feet.—Contractive cramps in feet.

24. **Generalities.**—Face red and bloated.—Cannot walk or keep on the feet in a darkened room, is sure to fall.—Restlessness of the body; staggering when walking; pithy, numb feeling of outer parts.—Complaints concomitant to morbid sleep.—< During perspiration; after sleep, when first awakens from sleep will shrink away as if in fear; in the dark; in solitude.—> In company.—The *Stram.* patient longs for light; if lying down, longs to sit up, and dislikes having head on pillow.—Spasmodic, drawing, paralytic pains in muscles and joints of limbs.—Contractive cramp in limbs.—Tingling in the limbs.—Sensation as if limbs were separated from body.—Slow contraction and extension of limbs.—Attacks of cramps of different kinds.—Tetanus.—Opisthotonos (the body is bent backwards with distorted countenance).—Cramps, and other hysterical sufferings.—Stiffness and contraction of several of the limbs.—Attacks of cataleptic stiffness in body, with loss of consciousness, preceded by headache with vertigo.—Easy movement, or great heaviness, of limbs.—Involuntary motions; hydrophobia.—Excessive aversion to liquids.—Convulsions, which resemble St. Vitus' dance.—Convulsions (in children) with profuse perspiration followed by sleep.—The movement of the muscles subject to the will is easier and increased.—Convulsive jerking of limbs, with weeping.—Convulsive movements and jerks, esp. on touching, or fixing the eyes on brilliant objects (such as a candle, a mirror, or water), or else appearing periodically.—Convulsions, as in epilepsy, but without loss of consciousness.—Puerperal convulsions.—Syncope, with stertorous breathing.—Unconscious snoring; jaws hang down; hands and feet twitch; pupils dilated.—Trembling of limbs (also in drunkards).—Tottering of limbs, when walking, and when standing upright.—Paralysis, sometimes after an attack of apoplexy.—(General paralysis of insane.—R. T. C.)—Symptoms as from old age, sight becomes dim, has to use glasses, mind gets weak, cannot complete sentences, avoids people and suspects them; wakes with r. arm over his head and cannot get it down again (produced.—R. M. Theobald.)—Weakness, with necessity to lie down.—Suppression of all secretions and excretions.—Painlessness with most all ailments.—Movements hurried.—Restlessness and nervousness beyond description.—Whole body sensitive to touch and every movement <.

25. **Skin.**—Suppressed eruptions and the consequences thereof.—Intense, bright, scarlet-red rash over whole body.

26. **Sleep.**—Strong disposition to sleep by day.—Deep sleep, with snoring, cries, and howling.—Lies on back with open, staring eyes.—Restless sleep, with tossing about, twitching, and screaming.—(Restlessness of old age; she constantly wakes up those about her.—R. T. C.)—Comatose somnolency, with a ridiculously solemn expression of countenance on waking.—(Boy wakes in a great fright from indefinable terrors; stammers and puffs on least excitement.—R. T. C.)—Agitated sleep, with vivid dreams.—Frightful visions during sleep.—Kneeling position in bed, and starting at least touch, with shrieks and wild gestures.

27. **Fever.**—Coldness of whole body, esp. of limbs, with shaking and shivering and general jerking.—Coldness of hands and feet, with redness of face.—General coldness in afternoon after previous heat of head and face,

followed by general heat.—During chill great sensitiveness to being uncovered. —Chill running down back.—Heat over whole body, with red face and perspiration.—Profuse perspiration already during the heat with violent thirst.—Greasy, oily, putrid-smelling perspiration.—Cold perspiration.—Intermittent fever.—Chill over whole body without thirst, followed by heat and anguish; sleep during hot stage, and violent thirst after waking up, which causes a stinging in throat, until he drinks something.—Heat, with anxiety, and redness of cheeks, or else with thirst and vomiting.—At first, heat in head, then general coldness, followed by heat and thirst.—Pulse very irregular, generally full, hard, and quick, or small and rapid, at times slow and scarcely perceptible, occasionally intermitting and trembling.—Frequent profuse sweat. also at night.—Retention of urine in any fever.

Strontium Bromatum.

Bromide of Strontium. $SrBr_2$. Trituration. Solution.

Clinical.—Dyspepsia. Gravel. Legs, swollen. Phlebitis. Varicosis. Urine, offensive.

Characteristics.—Cooper gives me the following experiences with *Str. bro.*: (1) A woman, 40, had tenderness of limbs, and veins of legs show up and incline to inflame (chronic cellulitis), left ankle inclined to swell; vertigo, at times darkness comes over sight; appetite not good, bowels regular, menses every three weeks, cannot keep awake in evening. Great relief came from *Str. bro.* 3x, but after taking it for ten days, severe ardor urinæ, with constant enuresis day and night, set in, which yielded to *Ferr. phos.* 6x., after failure with other remedies. (2) Woman, 60, had left leg and left foot swollen, hard and tender, red and pitting; right also but less in degree; indigestion with pain after food, and sickness after food for seven or eight years; is rheumatic and has had sciatica, off and on, for two years; bowels confined, sleep very restless generally. *Str. bro.* 3x was given, and in two weeks the legs had gone down very much and she felt altogether better, urine had become clear, but though ravenous for food had to stop eating and felt more sick, and the bowels were more confined. After this patient got quite well without further medicine. (3) *Str. bro.* 30 gave great relief to a lady broken down by sorrow who could not digest food. (4) *Stro. bro.* 6x produced in a woman, 70, the following symptoms: Urine thick, and offensive and dark-looking, with grains of red sand.

Strontium Carbonicum.

Strontiana carbonica. Strontianite. $SrCO_3$. Trituration.

Clinical.—Angina pectoris. Ankle, sprain of. Anus, burning in. Apoplexy. Bones, diseases of. Cardialgia. Constipation. Cramp. Diarrhœa. Emaciation. Enuresis. Feet, cold. Femur, caries of. Hæmorrhoids. Headache; congestive;

tensive. Heart, affections of. Hiccough. Hoarseness. Leucorrhœa. Menses, disordered. Phlebitis. Sciatica. Sprain. Sternum, pains in. Sycotic eruptions. Varicosis. Vision, affections of.

Characteristics.—Native Strontium Carbonate, a mineral named Strontianite, was first discovered in the lead-mines of Strontian in Argyllshire, from whence it received its name. It occurs in massive, fibrous, stellated, rarely orthorhombic crystals. The metal *Strontium* is dark yellow. *Stro. c.* varies in colour from white to yellow and pale green. It was proved by Nenning, Schreter, Seidel, Trincks, and Woost. Among the prominent symptoms were flushing in the face and violent pulsation of the arteries ; congestion to heart, lungs, and head. The distinctive feature about these states with *Stro. c.* is that they are > by warmth and wrapping up and < by cold. This also distinguishes the headaches of *Stro. c.* The headaches are boring, pressive, and *tensive.* There are various expressions of the congestive state. One of the tensive pains is peculiar : "Tension from vertex to upper jaw, as if head were expanded from within, and as if scalp were too tight, < in evening when lying with head low, slowly increasing and decreasing, > from heat. The *pressure* appears in the stomach ; it is > by eating ; and < by walking. There is also pressure after eating. There is both diarrhœa and constipation, the stools of both are accompanied and followed by burning in the rectum. A. P. Bowie (*H. R.*, ii. 62) cured this case occurring after a tedious labour : Stools large and hard, expelled with great effort, followed by great pain in anus, burning, lasting a long time and compelling patient to lie down. Anus violently contracted after stool. Complains of coldness in spots on calves of legs. *Stro. c.* 6 entirely relieved. The diarrhœa is < at night, and the stools are yellow. Walking < all complaints : headache ; leucorrhœa ; dyspnœa ; pressure in sternum. The symptoms about the chest and sternum, with the < by walking, suggest angina pectoris, and a similar but less serious state often met with in gouty patients. The *tension* is manifested in the nape, as if the tendons were drawn up ; tensive drawing in dorsal and lumbar muscles. In the arms there is venous tension : "the veins of the arms and hands are injected and tense, with great prostration and ill-humour"—suggesting phlebitis and varicosis. *Stro. c.* has a relation to sprains and bone affections. The femur is especially affected by it. It is particularly suited to bone affections of scrofulous children when associated with diarrhœa. The diarrhœa of *Stro. c.* is < at night ; is very urgent ; can scarcely leave the vessel before having to return ; > after 3 a.m. *Stro. c.* is indicated in chronic sprains of the ankle when œdema exists. C. M. Boger (*H. R.*, xv. 339) cured with *Stro. c.*, after other remedies had failed, a sciatica accompanied by œdema of left ankle. *Sensations* of *Stro. c* are : As if a load on chest. As if head were expanded from within. As if scalp were too tight. As if tendons of neck were drawn up. As if bruised in back and sacrum. As if all power had left right arm. Gnawing as if in marrow of bones. Symptoms as if in marrow of bones. Symptoms like phantoms difficult to locate. External soreness is a note of *Stro. c.* ; also numbness. Emaciation has been caused by it. The symptoms are < by touch ; by rubbing ; by scratching. Lying ith head low < tension in head. Motion <; walking especially . Stooping <. Exertion <. Motion > weakness of right arm. Evening; night, and early morning, 2 or 3 a.m. Warmth, vering >. Heat of sun > tension in head. Least draught <. ain and itching alternate. Right side most affected. Pressure in omach is > by eating; and < after a meal.

Relations.—*Antidoted by:* Camph. *Compare:* Bar. c. (closest ngener; scrofulous, apopletic conditions; chilliness). In headache wrapping up warmly, Sil. (Sil. headache comes up spine and over ead; Farrington says Stron. has the same). > Wrapping; sheeping stools, Mag. m.. Sprains, Arn., Rhus, Ruta. Caries of femur ith watery diarrhœa, Sil. Scrofulous bone affections, Staph. ains increase and decrease gradually, Plat., Stan. > By light; ersion to darkness, Stram., Am. m., Calc. Bar. c., Ars., Carb. a., arb. v., Caust., Lyc., Pho., Puls., Rhus, Val. (Cin., aversion to light). Walking, Æsc. h. Threatened apoplexy, Ast. r.

Causation.—Operation (photopsia). Sprains. Hæmorrhages hronic sequelæ).

SYMPTOMS.

1. **Mind.**—Inquietude and anguish.—(Depression of spirits.—R. T. C.)—pprehension as from a bad conscience.—Peevishness, with tendency to fly o a rage.—Excessive forgetfulness.

2. **Head.**—Headache, with nausea and vertigo.—Troublesome pres-re in forehead.—Threatening apoplexy; violent congestion to head; > apping head up.—(Dizzy when talking to people.—R. T. C.)—Burning forehead.—Tensive headache as if all the skin were being drawn wards the vertex, and the contents of the skull pressed outwards; < in ening when lying with the head low, slowly increasing and decreasing, from heat.—Chilliness over scalp and upper part of back, < in evening, night, and in cold air.—Tension on head (externally and internally), in evening, and from cold, > from warmth, esp. in heat of the sun. Tension from vertex to upper jaw.—Distensive pressure in entire head; l. side of head.—Lancinating headache.—Stitches in head.—Vibration in nples in evening.—Sensation of burning heat in head and face, when walk-g in afternoon, with redness of face, anguish, and sleepiness.—Boring in all spot r. side of occiput.—Dull, pressive pain in occiput.—Sensation of at of head and face, with red face, anxiety, and sleepiness.—(Tendency of ir to fall out with irritation of scalp.—R. T. C.)

3. **Eyes.**—Burning in eyes.—Burning, drawing, and redness in eyes.—essure on upper part of eyeball.—Violent jerking and quivering of eyelids. Red and blue circles before eyes, after rubbing them, with pressure, as by nd.—Sparkling before eyes.—Luminous vibrations before the eyes.—otopsia, remaining after an operation, esp. when objects appear covered th blood.—Green spots before eyes in the dark.

4. **Ears.**—Tearing in front of r. ear as if in the bone.—Sticking in ont of l. ear extending into it.—Boring and tearing in r. ear.—Roaring and ring in r. ear in frequent paroxysms.—Humming in the ears,

5. **Nose.**—Quivering on one side of nose.—Blowing of (dark) guineous scabs from nose.—Twitching of l. side of nose.

6. **Face.**—Redness of face, with burning heat.—Itching of face; cheek, < by scratching.—Jerking, tearing and boring in zygomatic proce —Twitching of l. malar bone extending to frontal eminence.—Violent bo pain in (r.) malar bone.—Stitch in l. side of chin extending into jaw-joint.

7. **Teeth.**—Toothache, with jerking pain.—Sensation in teeth a screwed together.—Tearing at root of teeth.—Grasping pain in te preceded by copious accumulation of saliva.—Gums swollen, painful w touched.

8. **Mouth.**—Bad odour from mouth.—Sensation of numbness of dryness in mouth, in morning (early when waking), without absenc saliva.

9. **Throat.**—Roughness and dryness of throat.—Inflammation palate, with pain during deglutition.—The fauces are inflamed and pai (stinging) during deglutition.—Sticking in throat on swallowing.

10. **Appetite.**—Earthy taste in mouth.—Violent thirst, esp. for bee Appetite only for brown bread.—Hunger after dinner.—(Ravenous, but comfort prevents him eating more than a few mouthfuls.—R. T. C.)

11. **Stomach.**—Nausea, with burning heat in face.—Violent hicco —Sickness after all food, sometimes quickly, sometimes after an hour or (produced.—R. T. C.).—(Heartburn, distension of abdomen, flatus with aching across waist and aching in l. temple.—R. T. C.)—Pressure in stom > by eating; < on walking.—Constriction in stomach with uprisings of c water.—Stitches in stomach now r. now l. side.—Pressure in stomach, sensation of fulness in abdomen, esp. after a meal.

12. **Abdomen.**—Pressive, bruised pains in hypochondria.—Abdo distended and painfully inflated.—Colic in umbilical region.—Gripings, diarrhœa, with chilliness, and shiverings.—Lancination in sides.—Grumb in abdomen, with abundant expulsion of very fetid flatus.

13. **Stool and Anus.**—Hard, knotty fæces (compact and in l lumps), evacuated slowly, with effort and much pain (in anus).—The sto passed in lumps like sheep-dung, and only with great effort so that she tho she would faint, and with most frightful pain followed by boring in anu Diarrhœa, of yellow water, with gripings and pinchings in abdome Diarrhœa < at night, is scarcely off the vessel before he must retur towards morning at 3 or 4 o'clock.—Tenesmus after (the diarrhœa-like) s —Burning sensation in anus, during and after a stool.—Pain, as hæmorrhoids in rectum.

14. **Urinary Organs.**—Diminished secretion of urine.—Incre secretion of a yellow, deep-coloured urine.—Nocturnal emission of urin Pale urine, with a strong smell of ammonia.—Urine has a normal appear with a strong smell of *Iodine*.—(Urine strong-smelling.—R. T. C.)

15. **Male Sexual Organs.**—A very transient, pressive pain i spermatic cord while urinating.

16. **Female Sexual Organs.**—Retarded catamenia, at first se (like meat-water), afterwards in clots.—Menses too early and of too sh duration.—Leucorrhœa while walking.

Respiratory Organs.—Hoarseness and roughness in throat, w excites a cough.—Dry cough, excited by irritation in trachea, < at night.—Dyspnœa, when walking, with heat and redness of face.

18. **Chest.**—Pressure at chest.—Drawing pain in muscles of chest.—Constriction ; pressive pain < walking.—Spasmodic drawing and clawing ; stitches on coughing and inspiring.—Painfulness of sternum to touch.—Slight burning l. side of sternum extending upwards.—Pressure in sternum.—Pressive pain beneath sternum, at night, disappeared in morning on rising.—Slight sticking in ensiform cartilage on walking in open air.—Dull stitches deep internally beneath ensiform cartilage, taking away the breath.—(Pain in l. breast with oppression < after meals.—R. T. C.)

19. **Heart.**—Dull, intermitting pressure in præcordial region.—Violent beating of arteries and of heart.

20. **Neck and Back.**—Tearing tension in nape as if tendons were drawn up.—Sensations as if bruised in back and sacrum, < from stooping and when touched.—Pain, as of a fracture, in loins and back.—Drawing pain in back, and lumbar region.—Slight drawing pain along spine in afternoon, changing to a seated dull tearing in joints of legs, < walking.

21. **Limbs.**—Tearing (rheumatic pains) in the limbs, esp. in the joints, < in the evening, and at night in bed.—One side of the body is generally only affected (r. side).—Immobility of the limbs, on one side only (the r. side of the body), like paralysis, in the evening.—Trembling of the limbs.

22. **Upper Limbs.**—Painful paralytic sensation in l. shoulder and elbow-joint at night.—Constant burning pains in r. shoulder-joint.—Veins of arms and hands injected and large ; prostration ; ill-humour.—Tearings in arms hands, and fingers, esp. in joints.—Numbness, almost paralytic, of the forearms and hands.

23. **Lower Limbs.**—Paralytic drawing in limbs.—Swelling and caries of femur, usually on scrofulous children ; diarrhœa.—Cramp in calves and soles, esp. in people who suffer from cold feet.—Sprains, esp. of ankle.—Jerking of legs.—Jerkings and tearings in legs, feet, and toes, esp. in joints.—Swelling of feet.—Sensation of icy-coldness in outer surface of calf (in spots).—Icy-cold feet, evening.

24. **Generalities.**—Excessive emaciation.—The majority of the pains, the exact situation of which it is difficult to determine, seem to be in the medulla of the bones (?).—The symptoms imperceptibly increase to a certain intensity, and diminish in the same manner.—Predominance of symptoms on one side of the body.—Violent involuntary starts of the body ; tension in inner or outer parts ; heat, with aversion to undress or uncover one's self.—Affections in joints of legs.—< In night ; evening ; from cold in general ; from undressing ; after lying down and rising again ; from rubbing ; in darkness.—> from light ; from a very bright light ; from warmth in general ; from wrapping up warmly.—> In open air, esp. from heat of sun.—Great lassitude and depression, morning and evening.

25. **Skin.**—Tension of skin in different parts, when in bed, in evening.—Skin adherent to scar in forearm becomes looser.—Eruption of small pimples in different parts, with burning itching, esp. after scratching.—Sycotic eruption on face and elsewhere in mouth, itching, burning.

26. **Sleep.**—Retarded sleep.—Jerking in body and starts when sleeping.—Frequent waking at night, principally caused by a dry cough.—Sleep, with many fantastic dreams.

27. **Fever.**—Pulse full and hard, with violent pulsation in the arteries.—Chill in forenoon, descending from sacrum to posterior part of thighs.—Chilliness from head over shoulder-blades.—Shiverings, morning and evening.—Heat seeming to stream from nose and mouth, with thirst.—Dry heat at night (with thirst).—Profuse perspiration at night, and when a limb is uncovered pain is instantaneously felt in the part.—Perspiration of parts affected (during morning hours).

Strontium Nitricum.

Nitrate of Strontium. $SrNO_3$. Solution.

Clinical.—Cravings, morbid. Ears, eczema behind. Headache. Kidneys, congestion of. Menses, scanty.

Characteristics.—C. M. Boger (*H. R.*, xv. 337) records the following cases: (1) Miss D., 18, brunette, had dull pains over eyes < by sunlight, motion, loss of sleep, sewing, reading; > after stool. With the headache, swelling of upper lids, < in morning. Sometimes bad taste in mouth. Menses irregular, profuse, dark. Feels tired and weak. Is addicted to eating cloves. In hot weather sweats profusely and easily about head and chest, staining yellow. Very susceptible to cold. Cough provoked by oppression of breathing and talking. Formerly had catarrh; now has right-sided deafness. Had typhoid fever two years before, and during the fever was allowed unlimited quantities of ice. Preceding the fever she had a post-auricular eczema suppressed by salves; now is anæmic and bloated. The urine contained epithelium, excess of chlorides, calcium oxalate and a trace of albumen (due probably to the clove habit). *Glonoin* helped the case, but for a time only. *Stront. nit.* was chosen because *Stront.* irritates the kidneys, and *Nit. ac.* corresponds to the vaso-motor disturbance, besides having cravings for odd things. *Stront. nit.* 6x was given, and in a few days the headache vanished. At the end of a month the post-auricular eruption had reappeared. Five months later there had been no return of headache or palpebral œdema; the craving for cloves had gone; the patient had taken on good flesh and colour. The eruption had not all gone. (2) A case of passive congestion of the kidneys was completely relieved by *Stront. nit.* in a woman at the climacteric. The menses, which were usually exceedingly scanty, became profuse.

Strophanthus.

Strophanthus hispidus. Inee. Onaye. Onage. Poison of Pahonias. *N. O.* Apocynaceæ. Tincture of the seeds.

Clinical.—*Alcoholism.* Anæmia. Cough. Diplopia. *Dropsy; cardiac.* Hæmoptysis. Heart, affections of. Levitation.

Characteristics.—*Strophanthus* is an ornamental, evergreen climbing shrub, native of Tropical Africa and Asia. It is used as an arrow-poison by natives of Africa. T. R. Fraser experimented with it on animals, and his conclusions are marked (F) in the Schema. Piedvache proved the tincture (*C. D. P.*), but only with reference to the pulse. His symptoms are marked (P). Gisevius (*H. R.*, xii. 502) proved *Strop.* φ, beginning with 5 drops, increasing to 80 drops during the five days of his proving. His symptoms are marked (G). Matthes (*ibid.* 508) proved *Strop.* φ (10 drops), and *Strop.* 2 (10 drops). His symptoms are marked (M). Some well-marked symptoms were produced on two chemists from preparing the tincture (*C. D. P.*). Other effects curative and pathogenetic have been observed on patients taking the drug. *Strop.* disorders the digestion, causes burning in the œsophagus and stomach, nausea, vomiting, and diarrhœa. A. P. Skworzow (*H. W.*, xxix. 534) gave to a dipsomaniac, 63, for weak heart and intermittent pulse, in 7-drop doses three times a day, an infusion of *Strop.* The first dose caused nausea, and a repugnance to alcohol which proved to be permanent. The man entirely discontinued the habit. On this hint *Strop.* was given to two other alcoholics, with the same result of abolishing the taste for alcohol. It caused nausea and profuse sweating, and the sudden withdrawal of alcohol was not attended with delirium. A case of mine illustrates the gastric and cardiac action of the remedy (*Dis. of Heart*, p. 191): W. G., 16, a delicate-looking boy, was admitted to hospital, having had rheumatic pains about him for three months, and an attack of rheumatic fever two years previously. He had been laid up a month before admission, and a week before was taken with cough, shivering, and occasional vomiting. When admitted he had a frequent, short, dry cough, < lying down; had to be propped up in bed; had œdema of feet, especially left. Tongue white; unable to retain any food for three days; no pain after food, but much flatulence, eructations giving much relief. Heart greatly dilated, pulsation diffused; double mitral bruit. Dulness at bases of both lungs, moist râles halfway up right lung. Expectoration of bright blood seven days. *Strop.* φ, one drop every four hours, was given. Improvement in all the symptoms was immediate; sickness, cough, hæmoptysis, and dropsy all disappeared; and the heart sounds had cleared up to a large extent when the boy went home, less than three weeks after admission. Hamer mentions that *Strop.* has cured "functional disturbance of the heart from alcohol, tobacco, and tea." This agrees with the relation of *Strop.* to alcoholism, and to symptoms of indigestion. A writer (*A. H.*, xxiii. 304) gives his experience with *Strop.* (in 5-drop doses of 1x tincture) in urticaria—which again bears out the gastric relations of *Strop.*): A lady had constant outbursts of urticarial rash dating from exposure to an offensive effluvium from a dead whale cast on the sands. The attacks would recur after drinking a glass of table beer. *Strop.* cured. Any accompanying cardiac weakness would be an additional indication. The same writer considers *Strop.* of great service in the anæmia of young girls when palpitation and breathlessness are marked features.—An accidental proving on a girl of five (*H. R.*, iii. 175) was made through the mother giving twenty drops of the tincture by mistake. Some half an hour later this condition was found: Face flushed, lips scarlet, eyes brilliant; temperature raised, skin dry, tongue normal. Pupils quivering, dilating, and contracting every few seconds. Pulse 140, arteries distended. Heart sounds vigorous, slight regurgitant mitral murmur. Intellect clear; precociously loquacious during the five hours the poisonous symptoms lasted. An *Ipec.* emetic was administered. No urine passed for ten hours after the dose.

Relations.—*Compatible:* Fer. (in anæmia). *Compare:* Botan., heart, dropsy, Apocy. c. Heart, Dig. (Dig. is cumulative; Strop. is not), Cretæg., Phas., Cact. Anæmia, Fer. Alcoholism, Chi., Nux, Aven., Querc.

Causation.—Alcohol. Tea. Tobacco.

SYMPTOMS.

1. **Mind.**—Irritative humour (G).—Precociously loquacious (child).

2. **Head.**—Some vertigo (M).—Stitches in l. temple; later in r. (M).—Waving and bubbling in whole head; stitches in l. temple, later r. (M).—Severe headache about junction of skin and hairy scalp, gradually spreading to temples; accompanied by double vision; (from preparing tincture).—Pulsation in head and heart (G).—Undulating sensation in head and whole body (M).—Twitching pain in occiput (M).

3. **Eyes.**—Impaired sight of l. eye; with nausea and faintness; following the headache and double vision (from preparing the tincture).—Eyes brilliant.—Pupils quivering, dilating, and contracting alternately every few seconds.

6. **Face.**—Face flushed, lips scarlet.

9. **Throat.**—Burning in œsophagus.—Burning in throat and œsophagus to stomach, compelling empty swallowing (M).—Dryness of tongue and fauces (M).

11. **Stomach.**—Eructation and hiccough (M).—Twitching in stomach (M).—Burning in œsophagus and stomach with loss of appetite and extreme gastric distress, which not rarely rose to vomiting; sometimes there was diarrhœa.—Nausea without actual vomiting (from preparing tincture).—Loathing of food, followed by choking and vomiting after eating.—Repugnance to alcohol.

12. **Abdomen.**—Pressure in hepatic region (G).—Shooting pains in r. hypochondrium (M).—Stitches in r. renal and hepatic regions (M).—Colic (G).—Rumbling in abdomen and pinching at navel (M).—Stitches in region of sigmoid flexure.

13. **Stool and Anus.**—Diarrhœa.—Frequent diarrhœa with violent colic but good appetite (G).—Stool with burning and tenesmus in anus.

14. **Urinary Organs.**—The kidneys become hyperæmic not only in the cortex and medullary portions but esp. at tips of pyramids.—No urine passed for ten hours after the dose (child).—Quantity of urine decreased about one-third after the first two or three days (P).

17. **Respiratory Organs.**—(Expectoration of bright red blood.—Cough < by lying down.)

18. **Chest.**—Pressive pain middle of r. third rib on anterior half < by pressure (G).

19. **Heart.**—The heart is easily and powerfully affected; systole is increased and the contractions slowed by small doses; the heart is paralysed in rigid contraction by large doses; this action is produced if the influence of the cerebro-spinal system be altogether removed (F).—Pulse slowed at first; increased after drug discontinued (P).—Evidence of the physiological discrotism of the pulse obliterated (P).—(Chronic degeneration of cardiac muscle, pulse small, frequent and irregular; great difficulty of breathing, and œdema.—Nervous palpitation and arrest of breathing.)—Lively perception of action of heart; then pressive sensation of anguish, tending to deep respiration; pressure on hepatic region (G).—Intense palpitation from comparatively slight exertion (G).—Distinct stitching and restlessness towards apex of heart, increased impulse with peculiar pulsation and twitching throughout body (M).—Stitches and twitches at apex beat.—Loud heart sounds, slight regurgitant mitral bruit (child).

21. **Limbs.**—Heaviness and pains in forearm and fingers, then same pains in l. hip-joint, extending into drawing twitches in top of l. shoulder, extending into joints of foot, which is quite painful when moved (M).

23. **Lower Limbs.**—(Swelling of legs.)—Itching and stitching in both feet (G).—Dorsum of foot painful and tense (M).

24. **Generalities.**—Coldness of extremities and faintness (from preparing tincture).—Increases contractile power of all striped muscles, rendering their contractions more complete and prolonged (F).—In lethal doses it causes the rigidity of contraction to pass into rigor mortis (F).—During afternoon nap, sensation as if being lifted from the couch (G).

27. **Fever.**—Coldness of extremities.—Temperature raised; skin dry.—Profuse sweat.

Strychninum.

STRYCHNINUM. Strychnia. Strychnine. An alkaloid obtained from several species of Strychnos. $C_{21}H_{22}N_2O_2$. Trituration. Solution. [The Liquor Strychniæ of B. P. is a solution of the alkaloid in a very weak solution of hydrochloric acid and alcohol, the proportions being: Strychnia gr. iv., diluted hydrochloric acid ♏vi., rectified spirit ʒii., distilled water ʒvi.]

STRYCHNINUM NITRICUM. Nitrate of Strychnine. $C_{21}H_{22}N_2O_2HNO_3$. Solution. Trituration.

STRYCHNINUM PHOSPHORICUM. Acid Phosphate of Strychnine. $C_{21}H_{22}N_2O_2H_3PO_42H_2O$, Solution. Trituration.

STRYCHNINUM SULPHURICUM. Normal Sulphate of Strychnine. $(C_{21}H_{22}N_2O_2)_2H_2SO_47H_2O$. Solution. Trituration.

STRYCH. VALERIANIC. Valerianate of Strychnine. $C_{21}H_{22}N_2O_2C_5H_{10}O_2$. Solution. Trituration.

Clinical.—Amaurosis. Aorta, pain in. Aphonia. Asthma. *Athetosis.* Bladder, paralysis of; pains in. Breasts, pains in. Cough, explosive. Cramps Diaphragm, spasms of. Emphysema. Enuresis. Exophthalmos. *Eyes, optic nerve, sclerosis of* (*n*). Headache. Hemiplegia. Influenza. Joints, stiffness of. Laryngeal crises of locomotor ataxy. Locomotor ataxy. Malar bones, pains in. Neurasthenia (*p*). Night-blindness. Paraplegia. Proctalgia. Rheumatism. Scrotum, abscess of. Spinal irritation (*p*). Tetanus.

Characteristics.—Poisonings innumerable with *Strychnine* are on record, the symptoms being convulsions of a tetanic nature, in the fatal cases ending in asphyxia. The spasms are intermittent, and the least touch or movement is sufficient to induce an attack. Lying on the back is the only tolerable position. Here is a case: "Lying on her back, body rigid, jaws set, arms and hands flexed, the thumbs nearly touching across the chest, and the whole muscular system convulsed, with short, jerky spasms, which would continue for about a minute and then remit, the muscles remaining contracted and as hard as wood during the intervals between the paroxysms." The convulsions generally take the form of opisthotonos; cries, terror, hippocratic countenance, and frothing at the mouth are common occurrences. The *Liquor strychniæ* is responsible for many of the poisonings, the powdered crystals, either pure or mixed in pills or rat-poison, for others. *Strychnia* itself is very sparingly soluble in cold water (1 in 5760). I have not attempted to distinguish between the different salts of *Strych.* An extensive proving of the *Liquor Strych.* was made under the supervision of Henry Robinson on two provers, a man and a woman (*M. H. R.*, xii. 252). The man took 900 drops in twenty-three days; the woman 445 drops in fifty-three days. These have furnished the most distinctive symptoms. Extreme nervous excitability; visions of an ugly face; fits of laughing, with light, swimming sensation in the head and giddiness; involuntary, idiotic-like chuckle; confusion of ideas, stupor and weariness—were some of the mental symptoms. The drowsiness was a well-marked feature and characterised some of the headaches. The headaches were frontal largely, or momentary dartings like electric shocks. A lady to whom I gave *Strych. ph.* 3x in five-drop doses twenty minutes before meals felt at once constriction of the throat, and after each meal violent headache in forehead over the eyes. The choking sensations were a constant feature in provings and poisonings. A patient now under my care suffering from locomotor ataxy has had among other manifestations alarming laryngeal crises with choking attacks. For these Felix Semon had given him subcutaneous injections of *Strychnine*, which was exquisitely homœopathic to the case, and gave marked relief. The direct "tonic" action of *Strych.* was shown in one of Robinson's provers, who had "unusually good appetite, she enjoys her food amazingly." Gamper, of St. Petersburg (*C. D. P.*), experimented with *Strych. nit.* on healthy young hospital assistants and found that it increased the amount of gastric juice secreted, the general acidity, and the quantity of free acid in the secretion. It hastened the absorption from the stomach, and strengthened the mechanical movements. The effects continued some time after the administration was stopped. The action of *Strych.* on the rectum and genito-urinary organs was as pronounced as that of *Ign.* and *Nux*; the male prover had his left testicle and cord swollen, and an abscess of the scrotum developed and discharged. Meyhoffer (*C. D. P.*) experimented with *Strych.* on himself and two other persons, one of whom was a woman of ymphatic temperament. "It always brought on electric shocks, occurring whenever the prover was touched or whenever any one ightly shook the bed on which he or she was lying. This happened o all, only the woman (lymphatic and feeble) needed a stronger dose." This prover also had this curious symptom : Any touch on any part of the body = a voluptuous sensation. Hale mentions the following uses of *Strych.* and its salts as observed by him and others : (1) In the tetanic spasms of cerebro-spinal meningitis. *Strych.* 6. (2) Amaurosis from atony of retina. (3) Diplopia, and night-blindness. Facial neuralgia and neuralgic headache, *Strych. sul.*; (and in one case when all other *Strych.* preparations had failed, *Strych. val.* cured). (4) Spasm of œsophagus in an hysterical woman, *Strych.* (5) Brain exhaustion of women in whom high nervous erethism exists. *Strych. val.* 2x. (6) Chorea, when the convulsions do not cease during sleep. *Strych.* 12, or 30.—A suggestion of Cooper that many cases of persistent cough recurring after influenza are met by *Strych.* I have found to be correct. The influenza cough has in it a strong spasmodic and asthmatic element, whether dry or not, and this seems to give one point of correspondence. C. W. Lawson (quoted *H. W.*, xxxiv. 134) relates the case of a medical man who took continuously for two years *Liq. Strych. Hydrochlor.*, 5 to 10 minims, thrice daily, with a little *Sal volatile.* He was at first benefited, but afterwards experienced a desire to take abnormally deep inspirations, "and he felt that to do so would overcome the inhibitory power over the lung, probably the action of the diaphragm." One morning, after a dose of *Strych.*, he was taking such an inspiration, and from that moment experienced the sensations complained of : inability to take a deep breath ; fixation of chest walls compelling him to stoop ; weakness on exertion, great confusion of thought and memory ; occasional clay-coloured fæces, usually greater in amount than ordinary. After six months the apex beat descended to the 6th interspace, and headache and drowsiness became marked. He travelled for six months without benefit. All attempts to act on the heart with drugs increased the headache. Lawson then found the heart dilated, wide subcostal angle, chest emphysematous, moving *en masse.* After a year of treatment *Hyoscyamus* tincture, ♏xx. at bedtime, was ordered and proved strikingly beneficial, drowsiness ceased entirely and improvement in all other respects followed.—*Peculiar Sensations* of *Strych.* are : Feeling as if head and face were enlarged. [Hence *Nux* and *Strych.* are remedies for the after-affects of debauches.] As if an iron cap were on head. Paralysed feeling in left half of head and face. Scalp sore, as if hair had been pulled. As if nerves suddenly pulled out of teeth. As of a lump in throat. As if water dripped off right elbow ; at intervals ; and off right shoulder. As if chopped in half at waist, at night. The pains and sensations of *Strych.* come *suddenly* and return at *intervals.* Sudden palpitation. Darting, pinching lancinating, fulgurating, electric pains. "Gurgling noise in rectum with electric darts" is a symptom of one prover. Many pains centre about the lips and eyes. Pains and chills occur in the occiput and nape and run down whole length of spine. There is much itching of the whole body and "violent itching in roof of mouth," which should prove a useful symptom. Jerkings, twitchings, and shocks in all parts run throughout the pathogenesis. The sensitiveness is shown in the increased activity of the spinal senses; the dread of touch; shrinking from draughts of air; and in Meyhoffer's prover touch anywhere excited a voluptuous sensation. *Stiffness* is a leading note of *Strych.*, and Cooper gives "rheumatism with stiff joints" as an indication. The symptoms are < in morning. < By touch; noise; motion; exertion; walking. < After meals. > Lying on back.

Relations.—*Antidoted by:* Passiflor. (?) (suggested by Hale); Hyo. (drowsiness, respiratory affection); Tobacco, Chlorof., Camph., Acon. have been advised. See also under Nux. Osterwald (*Med. Press*, January 6, 1901) found inhalation of Oxygen an effective antidote in animals. Black draught (Senna and Epsom Salts) relieved the constipation better than any other aperient. Sul. 30 in globules dry on the tongue brought about a rapid and almost complete relief of all the rectal symptoms of Robinson's male prover. *Compare:* Headache extending from occiput down spine, Pic. ac. Sudden pains, Bell., Lyc. Itching on palate, Glon. Sensation as if cut in two at waist, Ars. Headache with drowsiness, Bruc. Head jerked forwards and backwards, Stram. Spasm of throat, inability to swallow, Stram.

SYMPTOMS.

1. **Mind.**—Delirium: like that of hydrophobia; like delirium tremens; frightened; shrinks from persons; from currents of air.—Shouted out, "They are coming for me!"—Extreme nervous excitability; painful nervousness.—Immoderate fits of laughing, with light, swimming sensation and giddiness.—Moaning; sobbing; screaming.—Exceedingly despondent.—Irritable.—Confusion of ideas.—Loss of memory.—Consciousness perfect till death; though there may be loss of consciousness.

2. **Head.**—Vertigo: inclines to fall forward; with roaring in ears; while lying, with nausea.—Jerking of head forwards; and backwards.—Veins of head, and neck and face turgid; red, protruding eyes.—Violent headache with bursting pains in forehead, esp. l. side.—Stupid headache with extreme drowsiness.—Severe pains over l. eye and behind ears, with a feeling of stupor and drowsiness, 8 p.m.—Sensation as if an iron cap on head.—Violent thumping pains in head, esp. r. half and over l. eye.—Shattered sensation in head with drowsiness.—Sharp, darting pains in l. temple and round to back of l. ear.—Rapid pulsation in l. temple and l. hypochondrium.—Sudden pain and pressure in vertex and l. eye.—Peculiar paralysed feeling in l. half of head and face.—Dull pains in back of head and temples.—Constant pains on back of head and nape of neck.—Boring pain in occiput.—Pains on back of head, extending down whole length of spine.—Sharp pains in occiput, extending to l. eye and back of r. ear.—Sore pains in scalp as if hair had been pulled.—Intense itching of scalp and nape.

3. **Eyes.**—Eyes highly congested and in constant motion, as in great affright.—Eyes red; injected and protruding.—Eyes: sunken; rolling; distorted; turned to one side; turned to r. and fixed, with dilated, insensible pupils and red conjunctiva.—Aching, smarting, dull pains in eyes, with misty

vision.—Burning in eyes, < l.—Feeling as if eyes were suddenly stiffened and drawn back.—Burning; intense, sudden; in eyes and lids.—Feeling as if cold in eyes.—Rolling of eyes as if they were two cold bullets.—Tender, bruised feeling over l. eye.—Rapid pulsation over l. eye; in l. upper lid with weakness, swelling, discharge.—Increased lachrymation.—Needle-like pains in balls.—Pupils dilated, eyes staring.—Pupils contracted.—Vision: dim; confused, misty; persistent amaurosis.—Sparks before eyes, blackish, white, or red.—Increased peripheric sensibility for blue.—Enlargement of field of vision.—Everything seemed to turn green and he fell on the floor.

4. **Ears.**—Creeping, tingling sensation in external ears.—Sudden burning itching in ears, nose, lips, and eyes; in l. ear in afternoon.—Intense aching behind ears and down spine.—Sharp, darting pains behind r. ear; behind ears and back of head and neck.—Digging pain deep in l. ear.—Intense fulness in ears.—Hearing extremely sensitive, hears slightest sounds. —Roaring; burning; noise like wind.

5. **Nose.**—Face swollen and burning hot, eyes half closed as if stung by bees.—Face puffy, pale, distorted.—Muscles stiff.—Risus sardonicus.—Expression of extreme terror.—Face: livid; flushed and bathed with cold, clammy sweat.—Sharp, needle-like pains in cheek-bones; in l. cheek-bone shooting into teeth.—Lips: blue; livid; swollen; retracted.—Trismus.—Stiffening of jaws affecting speech.—Dull pains in jaws generally shooting into temples.—Needle-like pains under jaws.—Pulsation in chin.

7. **Teeth.**—Teeth clenched.—Toothache: at midnight; in l. upper teeth shooting into cheek-bone; as if nerves suddenly pulled out, at night: drawing; shooting.

8. **Mouth.**—Tongue: dry and papillæ erect; dry, with white moisture on edges; gums and lips violet; hot; sore, and roof of mouth.—Frothing at mouth.—Violent itching in roof of mouth.—Taste: bad; feverish; hot and bitter; dry.—Mouth filled with (frothy) saliva.—Articulation difficult.—Speech: indistinct; lost.

9. **Throat.**—Choking sensation in throat; as if something were held tightly round it.—Dry; spasmodic; contracted feeling; intense difficulty in swallowing.—Feeling as of a lump in throat, evening.—Dry, hot feeling; soreness (l. side); scraping.—Every attempt to swallow = violent spasms of muscles of pharynx.—Severe dull pains in muscles and glands of neck and at back of ears.—Sharp pains in glands of neck, behind ears and back of head.

11. **Stomach.**—Unusually good appetite, enjoys her food amazingly.—Thirst: intense; feverish.—Eructations: of bitter wind before vomiting; bitter, greasy; with bad taste.—Nausea.—Almost constant retching.—Violent vomiting.—Vomiting thin, colourless liquid.—Heavy feeling in stomach.—In pit of stomach: intense pain; sharp pain; intense twitching; violent jerks; spasm.—Spasm of pit of stomach, suddenly, while at dinner, lasting an hour with severe pain and feeling of suffocation, compelling to loosen clothes.—Burning along œsophagus and in stomach.—Immediately felt a burning sensation in stomach for about a minute then felt as if the blood ran cold.

12. **Abdomen.**—R. hypochondrium: aching at intervals, with sick, faint feeling; tense pain in r.; sharp, needle-like and cutting pains.—Sharp pains in l. hypochondrium shooting to pit of stomach.—Rapid pulsation in l. hypo-

chondrium and l. temple.—Abdominal muscles rigid in tetanic spasms.—In muscles: sore, contracted, bruised feeling.—Rumbling.—Griping, cutting, gnawing pain in bowels.—Sharp, cutting pain in r. lower and l. upper half of abdomen.—Uneasiness in bowels and constipation.—Deep-seated, sore, contracted, cramp-like feelings in lower abdomen.—Sharp, needle-like pains in l. groin.

13. **Stool and Anus.**—Gurgling sounds in rectum, with spasms of darting pain compelling him to sit on the ground as if shot.—Two agonising darts of pain during the night.—Two darts like shocks from a strong galvanic battery before going to bed.—Spasmodic jumping in anus.—Diarrhœa: copious, watery.—Fæces discharged involuntarily during the spasms.—Stools: lumpy and dry, flatus smelling of fresh putty; lumpy with mucus.—Very obstinate constipation; with griping.

14. **Urinary Organs.**—Contraction of bladder; it expelled urine apparently as fast as it was secreted.—Bladder paralysed.—Painful pressure in bladder and rectum.—Uneasiness about bladder and urethra < walking or sitting on anything hard.—Darting and shooting pains from bladder down thighs; from back of bladder down rectum; from front wall of bladder along urethra; finally the pains left the bladder and settled in glans penis.—Scalding in urethra.—Constant urging.—Urine: copious; scanty; variable, natural, dark like beer, thick, red sediment, albuminous-looking masses floating in it.

15. **Male Sexual Organs.**—L. spermatic cord painful, l. testicle swelled, painful only on standing or walking; hard, swollen, later burning pain on l. side of scrotum where the skin was tense on the testicle, and a large abscess formed in the dartos and cellular tissue; this was opened by a small incision and yielded a very large quantity of semi-transparent fluid, partly mixed with blood, after the discharge of which the size of the testicle became somewhat less; there was no connection between the testicle and the abscess.

16. **Female Sexual Organs.**—While falling asleep, quite suddenly several hysterical jerks as from the womb, with burning, irritating heat and violent pulsation in the passages; also feeling of great pressure and bearing down.—Darting pain and thrilling sensation in vagina with momentary pulsation coming on at intervals.—Violent tearing pains in womb, at intervals.—Menses at proper times, lasted only two days and were scanty.—Any touch on the body, it mattered not where, excited a voluptuous sensation.

17. **Respiratory Organs.**—Spasm of muscles about larynx and of arms; she felt and looked as if strangled; the muscles on each side of larynx became tense like cords.—Spasm of respiratory muscles, breathing irregular, intermittent, difficult.—Voice: weak; low; hoarse.—Aphonia.—Occasionally spasmodic, explosive cough; dry.—Breathing: hurried; difficult; choking; tight; with great pain in præcordia; sobbing; moaning.—Asphyxia.

18. **Chest.**—Walls of chest fixed.—Oppression.—Chest moves *en masse*, is hyper-resonant.—Tightness.—Pain: severe, sharp, contractive, spasmodic, darting, on chest, neck, and back.—Sharp needle-like pains: in upper chest and small of back; in r. (and l.) upper chest; in l. side under the ribs.—Severe stabbing pains in r. breast passing through to back at intervals.—Violent tearing in l. breast, at intervals.—Sharp pains in l. breast.

19. **Heart.**—Tightness about præcordia.—During day, dull pain, shifting

along line of aortic arch.—Fluttering sensation about heart with faintness.—Sudden palpitation.—Tumultuous action of heart.—Feeling as of heart coming into throat.—Heart fluttering like a wounded bird.—Pulse: irregular; accelerated; corded, tense, strong; full, rapid; nearly extinct in the paroyxsms.

20. **Neck and Back.**—Neck swollen; jugular veins distended.—Neck stiff, muscles like rigid cords.—Stiffness: painful; extending down back; momentary in l. half of neck.—Darting, knife-like pains: in muscles of neck and top of shoulders; chest, abdomen; with sick feeling.—Violent pain (stabbing, darting) in nape and down spine.—Back stiff.—Convulsive jerks in the back, and spinal column.—Intense aching or icy-coldness in entire back.—Agonising, gnawing pain in back and neck and muscles of legs.—Cutting in l. half of back.—Sudden stiffness in lower back and hips.—Sharp, needle-like pain in back about waist.—Suddenly violent cutting pain in back about waist, as though she were chopped in half, extending r. and l. to stomach at night.

21. **Limbs.**—Fingers and toes violet-coloured, fingers spasmodically drawn in, toes drawn back.—Limbs outstretched and rigid, at times jerking movements.—Cramps.—Darting pains in muscles.—Rheumatic pains in arms and legs.—Crawling in limbs after spasms.

22. **Upper Limbs.**—On washing his hands, half an hour after touching an abrasion on l. thumb with *Liquor. Strych.*, immediately felt numbness extending from thumb to whole of l. hand and wrist and rapidly to elbow and shoulder; in two hours joints of all fingers swollen and numbness gone; later enormous swelling of whole limb.—Arms stretched out, hands clenched.—Soreness, tenderness of muscles.—Sharp rheumatic pain in socket of r. shoulder.—Sharp pains in back of l. upper arm and fore part of thigh.—Sharp pain r. elbow-joint.—Sensation as though a drop of cold water were dripping off r. elbow at intervals; at times as if cold water dripped off r. shoulder.—Subsultus tendinum.—Trembling of hands.—Violent twitching in veins of r. hand; it seemed as if the blood had stopped and then flowed on.—Hands: partially paralysed; spasmodically clenched.—Momentary stiffness of fingers.—Cramp-like; rheumatic, sharp pains in hands.—Prickling, numbed sensations: in l. hand, at intervals; sudden in fingers.

23. **Lower Limbs.**—Painful convulsions in lower limbs and nape, with lightning-like pains in lumbar region, constantly shooting.—Loss of power of lower limbs.—Stiffness; rheumatic pains; sharp, needle-like pains in joints and limbs.—Trembling of legs.—Sudden jerking of legs; at night.—Hard rigidity of legs.—Stiffness of l. leg and back.—Agonising, gnawing pain in muscles of thighs.—Cramp-like pains in r. foot and leg.—Severe pains in r. ankle-joint < walking.—Cramp-like pains in feet.—Sharp, darting pains in feet, esp. in bottom of heels.—Thrilling from toes up legs.—Stiffened, twisted feeling in toes.—Violent itching-tingling in soles and palms.

24. **Generalities.**—Spasmodic, convulsive twitchings.—Every muscle of the body in a state of constant twitching.—Extremely violent twitching, first in limbs then in whole l. side.—Violent, electric-like starting and shuddering; followed by opisthotonos.—Shocks in muscles so violent that r. thigh is dislocated.—Constant inclination to bend towards r. side.—Convulsions recurring regularly.—Every attempt to move threatened a convulsion.—Convulsive jerks on falling asleep.—In convulsions, skin hot, bathed in perspiration and steaming.—Everything seemed to turn green and he fell on the floor.—Can lie in no

position but on her back ; any other = convulsions.—An attempt to take liquids = violent, spasmodic fit preventing her swallowing it.—Pains cramp-like, made her feel as though she would be stiffened.—< Evening.—< At night. —< From 8 to 10 p.m.

25. **Skin.**—Skin : pale at first ; then livid and bluish.—Burning ; prickling sensation ; formication.—Formication on tips of fingers.—Intense itching of skin of entire body ; esp. of scalp, face, arms, and legs.

26. **Sleep.**—Yawning ; extreme drowsiness.—Sleeplessness : from internal uneasiness and anxiety ; from dread of rectal spasms ; with visions of dead persons.—Extreme restlessness and talking in her sleep with peculiar working in back of brain.—Restless nights with profuse perspirations.—Dreams : disagreeable ; strange wanderings of the imagination.

27. **Fever.**—Extreme chilliness ; and drowsiness.—Peculiar creeping chilliness all over with a tremulous sensation in the jaws.—Extreme chilliness even in a warm room.—Icy coldness : painful ; of entire body ; sudden.—A single cold chill down entire length of spine ; afterwards she felt deathly cold. —Icy coldness down spine.—Extremities cold.—Lower extremities cold and perspiration flowing in a stream from head and chest.—Fever of adynamic intermittent type.—Intolerable sense of heat over whole body though some parts cool to the feel.—Burning heat with hot sweat.—Bathed in warm sweat. —Profuse sweat after the spasm.—Sudden cold sweat and icy coldness of entire body.—Cold sweat with the convulsive shocks, and increased shaking and stiffening.

Succinum.

Electron. Amber. (A mineralised resin not to be confounded with Ambergris, Ambra.) Trituration. Solution of the non-rectified oil (Oleum Succini non rectificatum) prepared by dry distillation of Amber. Solution of Succinic acid. $C_4H_6O_4$.

Clinical.—Asthma. Fear ; of trains and close places. Globus. Hay-fever. Hiccough. Hysteria. Leucocythæmia splenica. Spleen, affections of.

Characteristics.—Dr. Morris Weiner (quoted in *New, Old, and Forgotten Remedies*, tested *Succin. ac.*, which he prepared himself from Amber by dry distillation. The fumes of the crude acid, he says, are inflammable, and produce asthma, cough, sneezing, weeping, dropping of watery mucus from nostrils, pain in chest, and headache. On this indication he treated thirty persons suffering from hay-fever, and cured them all, and saved them the necessity of making an annual exodus. He gave one or two grains of the 3x trit. of *Succinum* itself diluted in twelve teaspoonfuls of water ; a teaspoonful every two hours. Burnett (*Dis. of Spleen*) used the non-rectified oil as an organ remedy in spleen affections, especially when accompanied by nervous and hysterical phenomena. The crude oil is a thick brown liquid having a strong empyreumatic odour. It is a powerful local irritant, and has been used with success as such in lumbago, rheumatism, and sciatica. It enters into the composition of "Roche's Embrocation," and "Haarlem

Oil," and has a popular reputation as a remedy for whooping-cough, the directions being for it to be rubbed into the spine night and morning (Murrell, in *Brit. Med. Jour.*). A tablespoonful dose, says Murrell, has caused persistent vomiting, diarrhœa, and symptoms of collapse; and the patient aborted. These observations are of value in relation to Burnett's experience. He gave the oil thus: To six ounces of Acorn-water are added half a scruple of the oil. They do not mix chemically, but by shaking each time a dose is taken the required division and attenuation is attained. Burnett's keynote is: "Painful spleen affections wherewith there are convulsive attacks such as the hysterical and hypochondriacal often have." Burnett relates in his book a most remarkable case of "chronic enlargement of the spleen, with hemi-hyperæsthesia, cephalalgia, dyspnœa, orthopnœa, convulsions" in a young lady "towards the end of her teens." After years of treatment under others and himself, Burnett concluded from Rademacher's account of *Succ. ol.* that it might provide the remedy. It was given in five-drop doses three times a day. In forty-eight hours the convulsive attacks ceased for good, and all the phenomena slowly disappeared. Burnett has also found *Succ. ol.* curative in splenic leucocythæmia. A keynote of Burnett's is: "Fear of trains and close places." His dose is five drops of the oil three times a day.

Relations.—*Compare*. Splenics, Cean., Nat. m., Querc., Mang. ac., Nat. sul.

SYMPTOMS.

1. **Mind.**—Fear of trains and close places.
2. **Head.**—Headache.
3. **Eyes.**—Lachrymation.
5. **Nose.**—Sneezing; dropping of watery mucus from nostrils.
9. **Throat.**—Globus.
11. **Stomach.**—Persistent hiccough.—Violent vomiting.
13. **Stool and Anus.**—Persistent diarrhœa and vomiting.
16. **Female Sexual Organs.**—Abortion.
17. **Respiratory Organs.**—Asthma.—(Incipient phthisis.—Chronic bronchitis.—Whooping-cough.)
18. **Chest.**—Pain in chest.
24. **Generalities.**—Symptoms of collapse; the patient aborted, but recovered.—Hysterical convulsions in women (from the smell.—Burnett).

Sulfonal.

Diethylsulphone-dimethyl-methane. $(CH_3)_2C(C_2H_5S)_2$.
Trituration.

Clinical.—Albuminuria. Cramps. Cyanosis. Ears, noises in. Epilepsy. Headache, with tinnitus. Hæmatoporphyrinuria. Locomotor ataxy. Paralysis, ascending. Reflexes abolished.

Characteristics.—*Sulfonal* was at first regarded as one of the safest of hypnotics, but many cases of poisoning by medicinal doses have occurred, and my Schema is made up of reported effects produced on patients. The accounts will be found in recent numbers of *H. W.* Prominent symptoms were: Stupor. Headache, with noises in ears. Vomiting and diarrhœa. Urine retained, or secretion arrested; claret-coloured; containing albumen; porphyrin. Ataxic gait and diminished or abolished reflexes point to locomotor ataxy. Ascending paralysis has been observed. The heart is weak; fainting occurs; and death takes place by heart failure. Rashes have been noticed on the skin, purpuric, erythematous, &c. One man (*H. W.*, xxxii. 174) observed uniform skin effects every time he took *Sfo.*, more intense the larger the dose. This occurred from gr. v.: Patches of erythema appeared (1) first on inner side of first phalanx of right little finger; (2) next over proximal ends of metacarpal bones of left thumb and index; (3) on posterior surface of left forearm a little below elbow; (4) fourth on prepuce. The symptoms were > by cold douches.

SYMPTOMS.

1. **Mind.**—Stupidity.—Unconscious, with dilated and fixed pupils and profuse sweat.

2. **Head.**—Headache and tinnitus aurium.

3. **Eyes.**—Pupils dilated and fixed.

4. **Ears.**—Tinnitus.

8. **Mouth.**—Breath smells of onions.

6. **Face.**—Face livid.

11. **Stomach.**—Vomiting, diarrhœa, and violent chills.—Constant retching, vomiting, and soreness over epigastrium.—Great disturbance of digestion with scanty urine.

12. **Abdomen.**—Spleen enlarged; hyperæmic.

13. **Stool and Anus.**—Diarrhœa and vomiting.—Great constipation.

14. **Urinary Organs.**—Dark brown urine.—Urine very scanty albuminous; almost solid when cooled.—Hæmatoporphyrinuria and death urine oscillated between deep claret and light claret colour.—Retention of urine; had to be drawn off; dark-coloured.—Urine cherry-colour, later like dark port wine.

15. **Male Sexual Organs.**—Erythema on prepuce.

18. **Chest.**—Œdema of lungs.—Signs of broncho-pneumonia.

19. **Heart.**—Death from heart failure and œdema of lungs.—Heart's action feeble, occasionally intermittent.

20. **Back.**—Chronic leptomeningitis, circumscribed softening of dorsal portion of cord, with hypostatic pneumonia of r. lung, and cyanosis of liver and kidneys (post mortem of poisoning cases).

23. **Lower Limbs.**—Gait ataxic; reeled about.—Plantar reflex deficient.—Paralysis of lower limbs.—(Cramps of legs and single muscles.)

24. **Generalities.**—The symptoms disappear slowly.—Paralysis of body.—> By cold water; cold douches.—Great prostration.—Progressive paralysis affecting legs first then arms.—Paralysis sometimes progressive sometimes with hyperæsthesia and abnormal sensation.—Twitching of muscles, esp. of face and flexors: < by voluntary movement, but alway

present in sleep.—Reflexes abolished.—(Epilepsy, inveterate cases with over-excitability of the cortical substance.)—Fainted and vomited.—Livid, esp. face.—Cyanosis.—Death by respiratory failure preceded by unconsciousness.

25. Skin.—Discoloured patches like purpura on skin.—Patches of erythema, of intensity proportionate to dose:—(1) On inner side of first phalanx of *r.* little finger; (2) over proximal ends of metacarpal bones of *l.* thumb and index; (3) on posterior surface of l. forearm, a little below elbow; (4) on prepuce.—Erythematous measles-like eruption.

26. Sleep.—Stupor.—Heaviness and drowsiness.—Sleepiness and weariness with unsteady gait.

27. Fever.—Violent chills.

Sulphur.

Brimstone. Sublimed Sulphur. S. (A.W. 31·98). Trituration of "Flowers of Sulphur." A saturated solution of Sulphur in absolute alcohol constitutes the φ tincture. [A trituration of amorphous Sulphur has also been used. Effects of "Milk of Sulphur" or Precipitated Sulphur, *i.e.*, Sulphur prepared by precipitation from a solution of Calc. sulph. with Hydrochloric acid, are included in the pathogenesis.]

Clinical.—*Acne. Adenoids.* Ague. *Alcohol habit.* Amaurosis. *Amenorrhœa.* Anæmia. Anus, prolapse of. *Asthma.* Atelectasis. Bed-sores. *Biliousness. Boils. Brain, congestion of.* Breasts, affections of. Bright's disease. *Bronchitis.* Cataract. *Catarrh.* Chagres fever. Chancre. Cheloid. *Chest, pains in. Chilblains.* Chloasma. Climaxis, sufferings of. *Cold. Constipation. Consumption.* Corns. *Cough.* Crusta serpiginosa. Dental fistula. Diabetes. *Diarrhœa. Dysentery.* Dysmenorrhœa. *Ear, affections of. Eczema.* Emaciation. Enuresis. Epilepsy. *Eructations. Eruptions. Eyes, affections of. Faintness. Feet, burning; perspiring. Fever.* Freckles. Ganglion. Glands, affections of. Gleet. Globus hystericus. Gonorrhœa. *Gout. Hæmorrhoids. Headache.* Head, rush of blood to. Herpes. Hip-joint disease. Hydrocele. *Hydrocephalus. Hydrothorax. Hypochondriasis.* Impotence. *Influenza. Intermittents. Irritation. Itch.* Jaundice. *Laryngitis. Leucorrhœa. Lichen. Liver, derangement of. Lumbago. Lungs, affections of. Lupus.* Mania. *Measles. Memory, weak.* Meningitis. *Menstruation, disorders of. Miscarriage.* Molluscum. *Nettlerash. Neuralgia.* Nipples, sore. *Nose, bleeding of; inflammation of.* Œsophagus, constriction of. Ophthalmia, acute; scrofulous; rheumatic. *Pelvic hæmatocele.* Phimosis. Phlegmasia dolens. *Peritonitis. Pleurisy. Pneumonia. Pregnancy, disorders of.* Prostatorrhœa. *Rectum, affections of. Rheumatic fever. Rheumatism, acute; chronic; gonorrhœal. Ringworm.* Sciatica. *Self-abuse. Sinking. Skin, affections of. Sleep, disordered. Smell, illusions of. Spinal irritation.* Spine, curvature of. Spleen, pain in. *Startings.* Stomatitis. *Taste, illusions of. Tenesmus. Thirst. Throat, mucus in. Tongue, coated.* Tonsillitis. Toothache. *Trachea, irritation in. Ulcers.* Urticaria. Uterus, prolapse of. *Vaccination.* Varicocele. Varicosis. *Vertigo. Warts.* White swelling. *Worms.* Worry. *Yawning.*

Characteristics.—*Sulphur* is an elementary substance, occurring in nature as a brittle crystalline solid, burning in the air with a blue flame, being oxidised to Sulphur dioxide (*Sulphurous acid*). The reputation of *Sulphur* as a remedy is perhaps as old as medicine. "As early as 2,000 years ago," says Hahnemann, "*Sul.* had been used as the most powerful specific against the itch. . . . The itch, with which the workers in wool are so much affected, causes an *intolerably agreeable, tingling, itching*, gnawing as of vermin. Some designate it as an intolerably voluptuous titillating itching, ceasing as soon as the parts are scratched and commencing to burn, which burning continues after the scratching. *Sul.* frequently produces in healthy persons burning-itching pimples and vesicles resembling the itch vesicles, and especially itching in the joints, and in the night." The specific power of *Sul.* to cure itch was abused. It was applied externally as baths and ointments, and the skin affection was not cured but repelled, and a host of secondary affections appeared in its place. Hahnemann found in *Sul.* the homœopathic counterpart of the peculiar constitutional dyscrasia which tends to manifest in itch-like eruptions, and which he named *Psora*. *Sul.* is the chief of the antipsoric remedies. A proving of *Sul.* appears in the *M. M. P.*, and this is amplified in the *Chronic Diseases*. The domestic use of *Sul.* (in the familiar "Brimstone and Treacle") as a "Spring medicine" is based on its antipsoric properties. "It is one of the most popular diaphoretics of the day," says Milne, "few old women failing to use it when any eruption is supposed to be struggling through the skin." It is this property of *Sul.* to divert to the surface constitutional irritants which renders it the chief of Hahnemann's antipsorics. *Sul.* has also an antipsoric action independently of its power of "bringing out" rashes. The psoric poison may be present and active in a case of disease and "apparently well-indicated remedies may fail to act" in consequence. In such cases one or two doses of *Sul.* will frequently antidote, as it were, the psora, and either clear up the case, or open the way for the action of other remedies. In such cases there will almost certainly be some *Sul.* indications present. *Sul.* is a potent antiseptic, and is one of the most certain destroyers of the acarus of itch. The exact relation of acarus itch to psora and other itching eruptions need not be considered; but as *Sul.* has the power of repressing constitutional eruptions when locally applied, as well as the power of destroying the acarus, it is best to use other means (*e.g.*, Oil of Lavender) for the latter purpose, and give *Sul.* or other indicated remedies internally. In my experience the psora of Hahnemann (which is a very real and definite dyscrasia) is generally inherited. The symptoms of latent psora are set forth in detail in Hahnemann's *Chronic Diseases*, and they are for the most part almost exact reproductions of the symptoms of *Sul.* But whilst *Sul.* is the chief of antipsorics, it is only one of many; and *Sul.* is in no way limited in its uses to cases of latent or declared psora. Much more important is it to know the leading features of the drug's action, which are sure guides in any case. (1) A key to many of the *Sul.* conditions is to be found in an *irregular distribution of the circulation*: flushes of heat; rush of blood to head, chest, heart; plethora from suddenly suppressed eruptions, piles, discharges; heat and burning sensation of all parts or coldness, sweating of many parts. These irregularities may go on to actual inflammation with effusions; and to fever of intermittent or other types. Another manifestation of this is found in the *redness* of orifices and parts near orifices: red ears, red nose; red eyelids and red borders round eyelids: brilliant red lips; bright red anus in children; red meatus urinarius ; red vulva. The orifices are not only red and congested, but they are sore and hypersensitive as well ; the passage of all discharges or excretions is painful. (2) The other side of this feeling of fulness is a feeling of *emptiness.* There is no medicine which has this symptom in a more extreme degree than *Sul.*, and there is no single symptom that is of greater value to the homœopathic prescriber than "Faint, sinking, all-gone sensation at 11 a.m." When that symptom is marked I give *Sul.* (generally 30), and get all the good I can out of the remedy before prescribing anything else, and very rarely am I disappointed. There is no need to wait to be told the symptom, or to ask patients directly if they experience it. I generally ask if they get hungry out of their usual mealtimes ; and if they say "Yes" ; I ask "What time ?" The time need not be exactly eleven ; though that is the most characteristic time. People who "must have something between breakfast and dinner-time" are generally benefited by *Sul.* This ravenous hunger at 11 is often associated with other *Sul.* symptoms, as heat at vertex ; dyspepsia ; portal congestion ; constipation with ineffectual urging ; piles ; constipation alternating with diarrhœa. When the dyspeptic gets food and relieves his hunger he begins to feel puffed up, feels heavy and sluggish, and is low-spirited, he scarcely cares to live. The dyspepsia of *Sul.* is often the result of suppressed eruptions. It is well known that drunkenness "runs in families," and the underlying disease of drunkenness is often psora. *Sul.* both causes and cures craving for beer and spirits. Gallavardin cured many apparently hopeless drunkards with *Sul.* 1m. The sinking, empty, all-gone sensation" is a common feature in the dyspepsia of drunkards. Dyspepsia from farinaceous food. Cannot take milk ; vomits it at once ; sour vomit with undigested food. Voracious appetite is a frequent symptom of scrofula, and scrofula and psora are frequently convertible terms. The child clutches at all food offered to it as if starved to death. Defective assimilation ; hungry yet emaciated. Stopped catarrh ; nose obstructed indoors, > out of doors. The child looks dried up, a little old man ; skin hanging in folds, yellowish, wrinkled, flabby. Head large in proportion to body. Lymphatic glands enlarged. Defective assimilation. When scrofula exists without particular symptoms *Sul.* will develop them. Allied to scrofula is tuberculosis ; in connection with which many symptoms of *Sul.* appear : marasmus with hunger at 11 a.m. ; sore, red orifices ; flushes of heat. In tuberculosis of the lungs a keynote is "body feels too hot." The patient must have windows open no matter how cold the weather may be. The caution is usually given to repeat *Sul.* seldom in cases of tuberculosis ; and to give it only in the early stages. (3) "< By heat" is another keynote of *Sul.*, and marks it out as the remedy in a large number of cases ; the < is most noticeable by *warmth of the bed.* Whenever a patient says he is all right till he gets warm in bed, *Sul.* must be examined, it will generally cover the case. (In some cases *stove* heat >.) The cases of rheumatism and sciatica requiring *Sul.* will generally have > morning and < at night in bed. (4) "< At night" is scarcely less characteristic. *Sul.* is related to both the sun and the moon, which makes it one of the most important of periodics. Cooper cured many cases of neuralgia < at noon or at midnight. He regards every twelve hours as the most characteristic periodicity, but it may be multiples or divisions of twelve. Lippe cured with "a single dose of *Sul.* at new moon" a case of menorrhagia, patient had not been well since her last miscarriage. Skinner gave to a man who had paresis of the lower limbs a single dose of *Sul.* cm, with instructions to take it on a certain date (when the moon was full). The man recovered almost suddenly. Cooper has had some important experience with *Sul.* in intermittent fevers. He generally gave two pilules of *Sul.* ϕ every four hours. Correspondents of his found this treatment preserve them from fever in India, and one, an officer, by means of it kept his regiment of sepoys in health when many others were in hospital. One writer treated nine cases with the pilules, and arrested the fever in twenty-four hours. One of the cases was a particularly obstinate one, and had been pronounced by the doctors to be complicated with liver affection. *Quinine* had been tried before the *Sul.* cured. In a case of "Chagres fever" (of West Indies), which had lasted three months, Cooper ordered a Sulphur bath as well as the *Sul.* pilules. That single bath seemed to alter the whole condition; from being an unhealthy, anæmic, bilious-looking man, the patient rapidly became the picture of health. Cooper recalls the fact that workers in Sulphur mines, though in malarial districts, enjoy a complete immunity from intermittent fevers. The power of *Sul.* in acute inflammatory conditions is allied to its action in intermittent fevers. *Sul.* is the chronic of *Acon.* in the effects of chills; and if *Acon.* does not promptly solve the difficulty, *Sul.* will be required. In the acute inflammations of the high South African plateau, where the variations of temperature are extreme, and chills and their consequences are very common, Van den Heuvel tells me that for the pain, fever, and anxiety before physical signs have appeared, *Acon.* is his first remedy. But if the fever does not yield in twenty-four to forty-eight hours, *Sul.* will clear it up. "Chill" is "suppression" in another form. *Sul.* is a remedy of such universal power that it may be misleading to speak of it as more related to one side than to another. Taken altogether there are more symptoms on the left side than the right. It acts strongly on the left side of the chest: "Sharp stitching pains through left lung to back, < lying on back, < by least motion," is characteristic. In a case of left pleuro-pneumonia following a violent hæmoptysis, *Sul.* 30 rescued a patient of mine from a condition which seemed desperate. *Sul.* acts on the whole respiratory tract, from the nose to the lung tissues. It causes a condition often met with in scrofulous patients, nasal catarrh where the nose is stopped indoors and free out of doors. All the features of asthma are produced in the pathogenesis, and *Sul.* has the alternation between skin irritation and asthma often met with in asthmatics. Villers (*H. R.*, xv. 563) relates the case of a girl, 22, afflicted since three years old with eczemas of the most varied form, mostly moist, the chief seat being the region about the pudenda, armpits, fold behind ear; but the whole body was defaced, the only parts which had remained white and normal being the breasts. She had been continuously under treatment for the nineteen years, the worst effects resulting when external applications had been used to dry up the eruption. Then most frightful asthma occurred, which lasted till the corrosive, ill-smelling eruption appeared again. She had recently come under the care of a homœopath, who gave *Ars. iod.* 3. From this there resulted a condition of which the patient said, "I cannot describe it, but I felt as if I was being killed." Her doctor then sent her to Villers, who sent her for three months to a water-cure before he would commence treatment. Her general health was somewhat improved thereby, but the skin remained the same. He then thought of some very high potencies he possessed, and gave a few pellets of *Sul.* cm. Three days later he was sent for in a great hurry late one evening, and on arrival found the patient had torn off all her clothes, was rolling about on the floor of her room, continually trying to rub her back and her legs on the legs of chairs or the edge of the door. Then she jumped up, brought a knife from the kitchen and scraped her whole body; would eat nothing and only drank enormous quantities of cold beverages. This lasted five days, after which she slept for two full days. Then this happened: The eruption dried up completely and scaled as after scarlatina. The girl had always had very weak menses; the next three were increasingly strong and intolerably fetid. There was very disagreeable discharge from the ears, corrosive secretion from the eyelids, and a dreadfully tormenting and burning discharge from the pudenda, strongly exciting to voluptuousness. Under the action of the single dose steady improvement occurred, and in four months she was a youthfully blooming maiden in the full flow of all her functions, and the skin in perfect condition. To test this Villers made the patient wear rough wool; dip her hands in first hot and then cold water; and for two weeks he made her rub her body daily with pretty coarse sea-salt. The only effect of these measures was to make the skin improve in texture.—*Sul.*, when indicated, will cause absorption of effusions, pleuritis (plastic, or hydrothorax), hydrocephalic, or synovial. I have frequently cured ganglion of the wrist with *Sul.* cm and lower, given on general indications. In the rheumatism of *Sul.* the affection begins below and spreads upwards. (This is analogous to the "from without inwards" direction of the psoric complaints which *Sul.* meets and reverses.) *Sul.* acts on the right eye and on all regions of the head—forehead, vertex, and occiput. It is the remedy for a large number of *periodical* headaches; headaches occurring every week; every month. Sick-headache. The headaches are accompanied by red face and hot head; are > in warm room; at rest; < in open air; < from stooping. There is also a headache on coughing. I have cured a severe occipital headache < on coughing with *Sul.* 30. Among the characteristics of *Sul.* are: (1) Aversion to be washed, always < after a bath. (2) Complaints that are always relapsing (menses, leucorrhœa, &c.); patient seems to get almost well when the disease returns again and again. (3) Congestions to single parts: eye; nose; chest; abdomen; ovaries; arms; legs; or any organ of the body, marking the onset of tumours or malignant growths, especially at climacteric. (4) Chronic alcoholism; dropsy and other ailments of drunkards; they reform but are continually relapsing. (5) Sensation of burning: on vertex; and smarting in eyes; of vesicles in mouth; and dryness of throat, first right then left; in stomach; in rectum; in anus, and itching piles, and scalding urine; like fire on nipples; in chest rising to face; of skin of whole body, with hot flushes; in spots below scapulæ; burning soles, must find a cool place for them at night. (6) Hot head with cold feet. Lutze (*N. A. J. H.*, xv. 286) finds that *Sul.* 1m will make feet that have been cold for years comfortably warm. (7) Cramp in calves and soles at night. (8) Hot flushes during day, with weak, faint spells, passing off with a little moisture. (9) Diarrhœa: after midnight; painless; driving out of bed early in morning; as if bowels were too weak to contain their contents. (10) Constipation: Stools hard, dry, knotty, as if burnt; large, painful, child is afraid to have stool on account of pain; or pain compels child to desist on first effort; alternating with diarrhœa. (11) Boils: coming in crops in various parts, or a single boil is succeeded by another as soon as the first is healed. (12) Skin: itching, voluptuous; scratching > ("feels good to scratch"); scratching = burning; < from heat of bed; soreness in folds. (13) Skin affections that have been treated by medicated soaps and washes; hæmorrhoids that have been treated by ointments. (14) Nightly suffocative attacks, wants doors and windows open; becomes suddenly wide awake at night; drowsy in afternoon after sunset, wakefulness the whole night. (15) Happy dreams, wakes up singing. (16) Everything looks pretty which patient takes a fancy to; even rags seem beautiful. (17) Ailments from the abuse of metals generally. (18) Offensive odour of body despite frequent washing. (19) Red nose < by cold: the colder the redder. (20) Cutting, stabbing pain in right eye. (21) Poor breakfast eaters. (22) Worried by trifles. (23) White, frothy expectoration. (24) Empty sensation (head; heart; stomach; abdomen). [*Sul.* aggravates much more in high dilutions than in lower ones; especially where extensive collections of disease-tissue exist, a single globule of 200th will often set up violent disturbance. The domestic use of *Sul.* is interesting. In one form or other *Sul.* is used in various countries for allaying pain; a piece of stick *Sul.* carried in the pocket is much used in England to ward off rheumatism. Natives of South America apply *Sul.* in solid form to parts in pain, and allow it to act for an hour before result is effected; and for lumbago and chronic rheumatic pains a bag filled with Flowers of Sulphur and applied heated to the part, immediately relieves the pain. An experienced sea captain testified to the extreme frequency of rheumatism amongst his sailors; but, he added, when carrying cargoes of *Sul.*, he had never had a case of it (acute rheumatism) on board. In the treatment of croup and diphtheria the local application of *Sul.* to the fauces has been highly spoken of by many practitioners. Dr. Laugardière, of Toulouse, reported recently to the Academy of Medicine that he has discovered a cure for croup—a tablespoonful of Flowers of Sulphur dissolved in a tumbler of water. After three days of this treatment his patients were rescued from imminent death, and fully recovered. Nettlerash is often relieved by a little Flowers of Sulphur and water; and *Sul.* mixed with sea-sand and rubbed over itch vesicles destroys the acarus at once. In the early days of vaccination it was found that the action of *Sul.*

on the frame was decidedly adverse to the receptivity of vaccine. According to Dr. Tierney, Dr. Jenner failed in vaccinating thirty soldiers, all under treatment by *Sul.* (*B. M. J.*, Jan. 6, 1872. George Gascoin, letter on antiseptic treatment of small-pox). Seeing that operatives in sulphur mines enjoy an immunity against ague when prevalent in surrounding districts ; and that, before going on hunting expeditions in malarious districts, men in Ethiopia submit themselves to fumigations with *Sul.*, and find it an efficient prevention of ague, the probability of *Sul.* having a power of destroying the organisms in the blood of ague patients is certainly great, and deserves investigation (Cooper)]. *Sul.* is a great *resorbent*, and is frequently needed after acute illnesses which do not entirely clear up. *Peculiar Sensations* are : As if a band were tied tightly round forehead ; round cranium. Vertigo as if swinging. As if bed were not large enough to hold him. As if one stood on wavering ground. As if hair on vertex stood on end. As from a weight pressing on top of brain and a cord tied around head. As if head soft ; brains bashed in. As if brain were beating against skull. As if eyes were pressed down. As if he had taken too much alcohol. As if hair would be torn out. As if head would burst. As if head were enlarged. As if she would sneeze. As if head had been beaten. As if top of head were being pressed against wall. Occiput as if hollow. As if flesh of scalp were loose. As if scalp had been beaten. As if cornea had lost its transparency. As if eye were gone and a cool wind blew out of socket. As if eyes had been punctured. As if a needle or splinter were sticking in eye. As if a thick veil were before eyes. As if eyeballs were dry. As if balls rubbed against lids. As if eyes were rubbed against spicules of glass ; eyeballs dry ; salt in eyes ; cornea covered with fine dust ; lids would become inflamed. As if sounds did not come through ears but forehead. As of water in ears. As if he smelt perfume. As if nose were swelled. Nostrils as if sore. As if lower jaw would be torn out. As if air just in front of her were hot. Teeth as if too long ; as of a hot iron in teeth. As of a hard ball rising in throat. As if swallowing a piece of meat. As of a lump in throat. As of a hair in throat. As if throat too narrow. Stomach as if puffed up ; as if torn with pincers. Intestines as if strung in knots. As if hernia would form. As if muscles of abdomen and peritonæum had been bruised. As if obliged to urinate, in urethra. As if something in larynx. As of a lump of ice in (r.) chest. As if lungs came in contact with back. As if strained in chest. As if he had fallen upon chest. As if chest would fly to pieces when coughing or drawing a deep breath. Heart as if enlarged. As if muscles of neck and back were too short. As if vertebræ gliding one over the other. Small of back as if beaten. Left shoulder and hip as if luxated Like a weight on shoulder. As if something heavy hanging on upper arm. Arms as if beaten. As of a mouse running up arms and back. Thigh as if broken. As if too short in popliteal space. Skin as if denuded and sore. Sweat may occur on one side of the body only ; or on neck only. *Sul.* is *Suited to :* (1) Lean, stoop-shouldered persons, who walk and sit stooped ; standing is the most uncomfortable position. (2) Persons of nervous temperament, quick-motioned, quick-tempered, plethoric, skin excessively sensitive to atmospheric changes. (3) Dirty, filthy people, with greasy skin, and long, straight, matted hair, prone to skin affections. (4) Children who cannot bear to be washed or bathed; emaciated; big-bellied; restless, hot, kick off clothes at night; have worms. (5) Persons of scrofulous diathesis, subject to various congestions, especially of portal system. (6) Lymphatic temperaments, nervous constitutions disposed to hæmorrhoids, with constipation or morning diarrhœa; diseases caused especially by suppressed eruptions, peevishness, sudden and frequent flushes of heat all over body, followed by perspiration, hot palms, soles, and vertex; faintness in epigastrium in forenoon. (7) Children, emaciated, old-looking faces, big bellies, dry, flabby skin. (8) Full-blooded persons with great irritability, restlessness, and hastiness. (9) Old people. (10) People with hot, sweaty hands. (11) "Ragged philosophers"; dirty-looking persons who are always speculating on religious or philosophical subjects. (12) Freckled people. (13) Light-complexioned people. (14) Red-haired people. (15) Dark-complexioned people; negroes. (16) People who refer all their sufferings to the epigastrium: "everything affects me there." The symptoms are: < By touch. < Pressure (pressure > pain in head when coughing). Rest <. Standing <. Stooping <. Lying on (r.) painful side >. Motion > pains in head, hips, knee, hæmorrhoids; < other symptoms. Moving arms <. Every step <. Rising <. Ascending <. Talking = fatigue of whole body. Vivacious talking = hammering headaches. < 11 a.m.; 12 noon; midnight; morning; evening; night; after midnight. Wants doors and windows open. Susceptible to temperature; warm things feel hot. Indoors = nose stopped up; > emptiness in occiput. Open air <. Draught of air <. Raw air <. Warmth <. Sun < (headache). Washing <. Cold, damp weather <. Cold food and drink < thirst. Cold water > head; left eye; whitlow. < Before a storm. < After sleep. < From milk; sweets; alcohol. > By eating; < after. < Before eating. > By warm food. < Before, during, and after menses (headache; leucorrhœa). < Looking down. < Crossing running water. < Raising arms. Hearing is < eating and blowing nose.

Relations.—[Sul. frequently serves to rouse the reactive powers when carefully selected remedies fail to act (especially in acute diseases; in chronic, Pso.). In this respect it is a close analogue and ally of Medor. and Syph., which should be studied with it.] *Antidoted by:* Aco., Camph., Cham., Chi., Merc., Puls., Rhus, Sep., Thu. *Antidote to:* Aco., Alo., Chi., Iod., Merc., Nit. ac., Olean., Rhus, Sep., Thu.; ailments from abuse of metals generally. *Compatible:* Calc., Calc. ph., Lyc., Sars., Sep., Puls. (Sul., Calc., Lyc.; and Sul., Sars., Sep. frequently follow in this order. It is generally said that Calc. should not be used *before* Sul.). *Follows well:* Merc. *Complementary:* Alo. (Sul. is generally the remedy when Alo. has been abused as a purgative), Aco., Nux, Puls. (Sul. is the "chronic" of the last three. If a patient is sleepless Sul. may be given at night. If the patient sleeps well it is best given in the morning, as it may disturb sleep if given at night; Nux may be given at night and Sul. in the morning when their complementary action is desired). Sul. complements Rhus in paralysis. Follows and complements Ant. t. and Ipec. in lung affections, especially left; atelectasis. An interpolated dose of Sul. helps Sil. in indurations. Pso. complements Sul.; Pso. loves heat, Sul. hates it. Teste includes in the Sul. group: Crot. t., Merc. c., Bov., Æth. c., Kre., Lob. i., Merc. sol., Aster., Cic., Rat. *Compare:* Meningitis, Apis. Injuries to eyes, Aco. (Sul. follows). Early-morning diarrhœa, Bry. (as soon as he moves), Nat. s. (with much flatus), Rx. c., Pod. (stools changeable; go on all day, though < at noon; Sul. raw, sore anus), Diosc. (colic flying to other parts). Defective reaction, Pso., Cup., Lauro., Val., Ambr., Carb. v. Flushes at climaxis, Lach., Sul. ac., Amyl., K. bi. Intermittent fever and neuralgia, Chi., Ars., Bapt. Ravenous hunger with heat at vertex, Calc., Pho. Tuberculosis, Bac., Calc., Pho. Itch, Merc., Sep., Caust. Dyspepsia, Nux, Sep. Excessive venery, masturbation, Nux, Calc. Yellow-brown spots, Sep., Lyc., Curar. Rheumatism, paralysis, Rhus. Sour stools, sore anus, Cham. Pneumonia, restoration imperfect, Sang. Paralysis from cold, Aco., Caust., Rhus. Accumulation of flatus, sour and bitter taste, Lyc. (with Sul. patient refers accumulation to left groin, region of sigmoid flexure). Bad effects of mental exhaustion; of seminal losses, Selen. (Sel. is a cognate element of Sul. and close analogue; Sel. < from tea; Sul. < from coffee; Sel. has "tingling in spots"). Morning aphonia, Carb. v. (Carb. v. also evening). Edges of eyelids, Graph., Bac. Congestion of lumbar spine, Pic. ac. Atrophy of infants, Ars. Sinking < 11 a.m., Na. m., Pho., Indm., Na. c., Zn. (nervous symptoms, Arg. n.). Prophylactic of cholera, Cup. Weak from talking, Stan., Cocc., Ver., Calc. Falls easily, Na. c. Hasty speech and action, Bell., Lach., Dulc., Hep. Weak ankles, Sul. ac., Caust. > Open air; desire to be uncovered, Pul., Lyc. Wetting bed in deep sleep, Bell. (in first sleep, Sep.). Effects of losses of fluids, Ars., Calc., Chi., Fer. Persistent speck before left eye (right Sel.). Vision mostly green, Sang. Rhagades of hands, Na. c. Hard, horny hands, Na. m., Graph. (opp. Calc.). Left to right, Lach. Stitches up vagina, Sep., Pho., Nit. ac. (also down and out), Alm., Berb., Pul. (Sul. stitches go to head). Left ovarian and left inframammary pain, Lil., Lach., Caulo., Vib. o., Pul., Ustil. Bearing-down pains, Bell., Sep., Gossyp., Pul., Sec. < On awaking, Lach., Na. m. Alarmed about soul's salvation, Ver. < Hearing water run, Hfb. Violent movements of fœtus, Op., Croc., Thuj. Dread of losing mind, Calc., Lyc., Nux. Hollow sensation in region of heart (Lil. as if heart empty). Earthy complexion, Na. m. Tall, slender people, Pho. (Sul. with stoop). Aversion to be washed, Ant. c., Clem., Hep., Rhus, Sep., Spi. (Puls. baby likes being washed). Fear of ghosts, Aco., Ars., Bro., Carb. v., Cocc., Lyc., Pho., Pul., Ran. b., Sep., Zn. (I have been frequently asked by patients taking Sul. not to give them "that medicine" again as it made them "see faces," generally described as horrible). < Heat of bed at night, Bry., Merc., Pul., Cham. (toothache), Dros., Led., Sbi., Apis. Laughing alternately with weeping, Aur., Pul., Lyc., Croc., Pho., Ver. Vertigo looking down, Olean. (Calc. turning head, Pul. looking up). Throbbing headache, Glo., Calc., Pul. Drowsiness with headache, Bruc.,

Strych., Gins., Herac., Na. s., Gels., Nux m. Passes almost pure blood from rectum, Merc., Aco. Diabetes with impotence, Mosch. Phimosis, Can. s., Merc., Nit. ac., Sep., Thu., Rhus, Sbi. Hunger at night, Chi. s., Pso., Pho. (with febrile heat, unappeasable), Lyc., Ign. Hot breath, Calc., Rhus. Sharp splinter sensation on slightest touch, Arg. n., Hep., Nit. ac. Throat, right then left, Lyc., Bar. c., left side, Lach., Sul. Freckles, Adren. Weak chest when speaking, Calc. Acid smell from mouth, Nux. Taste of blood, Ham. Sensation of hair in throat, K. bi., Sil. Intolerance of pressure of clothes, Lach. Blackish stools, Lept. Burning between scapulæ, Pho., Lyc. Sinking sensations, worms, Scirrh. and other cancer nosodes. Vividly remembered dreams, Chi. Mistakes time of day, Merc., Lach. Boils, Anthrac. Vaccination effects, Thu., Malan. Red lips, red borders round eyelids, Bac. Offensive body smell; checked eruptions and discharges, Med. Excessively sensitive to atmospheric changes, Hep., K. ca., Pso. (Pso. is generally extremely chilly, Sul. hot). Restless, hot, kicks off clothes at night, Hep., Sanic. Wants to find cool place for feet, Sanic. Relapsing alcoholism, Pso., Bac.

Causation.—Suppressions. Alcohol. Sun. Sprains. Chills. Over-exertion. Reaching high. Falls. Blows. Bed-sores.

SYMPTOMS.

1. **Mind.**—Melancholy and sadness, with grieving ideas; uneasiness respecting the patient's own condition and prospects, and about business affairs, so as to become exceedingly unhappy, disgusted with life, and even to despair of eternal salvation.—Egoistic.—Dwells on religious or philosophical speculations; anxiety about soul's salvation; indifference about lot of others. —Vexatious and morbid ideas of the past arise and cannot be got rid of.—Hypochondriac mood (through the day, in evening he is inclined to be merry). —Strong tendency to weep, and frequent weeping, alternating sometimes with involuntary laughter.—Disconsolate humour, with scruples of conscience, even with respect to the most innocent actions.—Fits of anguish, esp. in evening; timidity and great tendency to be frightened.—Precipitation, restlessness, and impatience.—Peevishness; childish peevishness in grown people.—Ill-humour, moroseness, quarrelsome disposition, disposition to criticise, and dislike to conversation.—Irritability, disposition to anger and passion.—Great indolence and repugnance to all exertion, both mental and bodily.—Too lazy to rouse himself up, and too unhappy to live.—Indecision, awkwardness (at his work), inadvertence, anthropophobia, with feeling of giddiness.—Stupidity and imbecility, with difficulty in understanding and in answering correctly.—In afternoon, stupefied state after a glass of wine.—Great weakness of memory, chiefly for proper names.—Misplaces or cannot find the proper word when he speaks.—Mistakes as to time, thinks it earlier than it is; at vesper bell (7 p.m.) insists it is only 5 p.m., quite angry when one attempts to convince her of her error.—Forgetfulness of that which is about to be uttered.—Great flow of ideas, for the most part sad and unpleasant, but sometimes gay, and interspersed with musical airs.—Strong tendency to religious and philosophical reveries, with fixed ideas.—Incoherent

peech.—Mania, with a settled idea of having all things in abundance, ossessing beautiful things, &c.—Delirium, with carphologia.—Errors re- pecting objects, a hat is mistaken for a bonnet, a rag for a handsome gown, ;c.—Foolish happiness and pride; fantastic illusions of the intellect, esp. if ne turns everything into beauty, as an old rag or stick looks to be a beautiful iece of workmanship; everything looks pretty which the patient takes a ancy to.—Melancholia and epilepsy, with strong impulsive tendency to uicide by drowning or leaping from window; five fits a day with at times wo hours of unconsciousness, always < during menses (*Sul.* 10m cured).

2. **Head.**—Confusion in head, with difficulty in meditating; or weak- ess, dizziness, and stupor, sometimes with necessity to lie down, and esp. in orning or in evening, or when walking in open air, or when going up an scent.—Vertigo and staggering, esp. when seated, or after a meal, or when xercising in open air, when stooping, looking down, walking, going up an scent, rising from a seat, lying on back, passing over running water, and lso in morning, in evening, or at night, and often with nausea, syncope, veakness, and bleeding at nose (with inclination to fall to l. side; with anishing of sight).—Headache as if caused by incarcerated flatus, by bstruction in head, or by a debauch.—Painful sensibility of head, chiefly of ertex, on least movement, with pain at every step, when coughing, blowing ose, or masticating.—Sensitiveness of the vertex, pressing pain when touch- ng it, < from heat of bed, in morning when waking, on scratching it, it bites nd burns.—Fulness, pressure, and heaviness in head, chiefly in forehead (< hen raising head and after sleeping and talking, > when sitting or when ying with head high) and occiput.—Tearing or stitches in forehead or mples, from within to without, < from stooping, > when pressing head gether, or when moving about.—Sensation of emptiness in back part of ead, < in open air and when talking, > in room.—Pulsation in head with eat in brain, pulsation of carotid arteries and of heart, < on waking in orning, when moving about, on stooping, when talking, in open air; > hen at rest and in warm room.—Hammering headache on vivacious talking. -Throbbing all over head with furious pain taking away her sight and pre- enting her from stooping: it affects vertex more and is < by washing her ead (produced.—R. T. C.).—Heat on crown; cold feet; frequent flushings. -Painful tingling on vertex and in temples.—Violent pain in vertex in even- g, as if hair would be torn out; it bristles on the most painful spots.— ain in vertex, r. side, < 5 to 8 p.m., > by warmth.—R. T. C.)—Boring eadache on top, beneath vertex; the spot is painful to touch externally.— evere burning in vertex; went off after getting up; succeeded by cool eling in same place.—Aching; burning; throbbing; pressing in vertex.— ertex very sensitive when touched; and when not.—Tension in forehead d eyes on exercising brain; < when lifting up eyes, after sleeping; > hen sitting in room.—Tension and painful contraction in brain, sometimes ith a sensation as if head were compressed by a band (with the sensation as the flesh were loose around it, followed by inflammation of the bones and ries; < in wet, cold weather and when at rest; > from motion).—Expan- ve pressure, as if head were about to burst, principally in temples.—Sharp d jerking pains, or drawing and shootings in head.—Painful sensation, as brain were wounded or bruised.—Sensation as if the head were soft;

as if the brains had been bashed in.—On moving head brain strikes agains
cranium.—Congestion of blood in head, with pulsative pains, clucking, an
feeling of heat in brain.—Rush of blood to head ; a pressure out at eyes
with roaring in ears and heat of face ; during menses ; during soft stool ; a
night in bed ; arising from chest with throbbing ; < when stooping, talkin
in open air ; > sitting in warm room.—Tinkling, buzzing, roaring, and vibr
tion in head.—The headache is often only semilateral, or confined to verte
or to occiput, or to forehead above eyes, with inclination to frown or to clos
eyes, confusion of sight, unfitness for meditation, humming in ears, and nause
with inclination to vomit.—Quotidian, periodical, and intermittent headache
appearing principally at night, or in evening in bed, or in morning, or after
meal ; (every 3, 4, 6, 12, or 24 hours ; 12 noon or 12 midnight ; < midsumme
or midwinter).—Movement, walking, open air, and meditation often excite o
< the headaches.—Pimples with itching in head, principally in forehead.–
Dry or thick yellowish scabs in scalp, with secretion of a thick and fetid pu
but always with great itching.—Dry (seldom humid), offensive, scabby, easil
bleeding, burning, and sore paining eruption on back part of head and behin
ears, with cracks, > from scratching (tinea capitis).—(Scabby eruption ove
head and on various parts of body ; with hard lumps that discharge and irr
tate and prevent sleep.—R. T. C.)—Coldness in head, sometimes only i
circumscribed places.—Painful sensitiveness of the roots of hair and of scal
when touched.—Mobility of scalp.—Falling off of hair ; with great drynes
of the hair, painfulness of scalp to the touch and violent itching in evenin
when getting warm in bed, with swelling of glands on neck (also in lying-i
women).—Fontanelles remain open too long.—Head bent forward whe
walking.—Itching in head, with impatience.—Exanthema and itching o
forehead.

3. **Eyes.**—Heaviness and aching in eyes and lids, with a sensation o
friction as from sand.—Itching of eyebrows.—Itching, tickling, and burnin
sensation in eyes, canthi, and lids.—Pains as from a bruise or wound, an
smarting in eyes and lids.—The pains in eyes often extend into head, and ar
< by movement of eyes, and also by light of the sun, which sometimes <
them to an insupportable degree.—Pain (cutting) in r. eye, renewable b
touching r. side of tip of nose.—Stinging in eyes, esp. in sunshine and from
light of a candle.—Inflammation, swelling, and redness of sclerotica, conjunc
tiva, and eyelids.—Pain in lid, as if rubbed against spiculæ of glass.—Smartin
pain as from dryness of margins of lids.—Redness of borders of lids.—Ulcera
tion in the margins of the eyelids.—Pustules and ulcers round orbits as far a
cheeks.—Inflammatory redness of iris.—Affections in general of the cornea
eyeball ; sclerotica.—Opacity of cornea, as if covered with dust, or cloudec
with a deposit of greyish lymph between the lamellæ.—Specks, vesicle
(pustules), and ulcers in the cornea (with redness of eye).—Injection o
vessels of conjunctiva.—Pupil unequal, or dilated and immovable ; or con
tracted.—Cloudiness of crystalline lens.—Nodosity, like hordeolum, in lids.–
Eyes water, itch, and feel hot.—Profuse lachrymation, esp. in open air ; o
great dryness of eyes, < in a room.—Pain as from dryness of eyeballs, and a
sensation as if they rubbed against the lids.—Lachrymation in morning, wit
burning.—Retinitis, caused by over-use of eyes, congestion of optic nerve.–
Oily tears.—Copious secretion of mucus in eyes, day and night.—Nocturna

agglutination of lids.—Palpitation and quivering of eyelids.—Contraction of eyelids in morning.—Trembling of eyes.—Confused sight, as if directed through a mist, or as if down or a veil were before eyes.—Dim-sightedness, cataract.—Great dimness of vision, as if cornea had lost transparency, confusion of head and dull aching in forehead.—Objects seem more distant than they are.—Presbyopia.—Myopia.—Clouded sight when reading.—The eyes are dazzled by daylight.—Dazzled by looking long at an object.—Sparks and white spots, or dancing flies, black points, and spots before eyes.—Night-blindness.—Visions of faces appear on closing the eyes.—Objects appear to be yellow.—Great sensitiveness (and aversion) of eyes to light, principally to that of the sun, and during warm and oppressive weather.—Halo around a lamplight; cataract.—Yellowish colour of sclerotica.

4. **Ears.**—Itching in ears (in external ear).—Stitches in l. ear.—Sharp or drawing pains, or shootings in ears, sometimes extending into head or into throat.—Recurring earaches in tubercular meningitis.—R. T. C.)—Burning heat which goes out at ears.—Gurgling in ears as if water were in them.—Discharge of pus from ears.—Otorrhœa, < l. ear.—Discharge from both ears, dirty, very offensive; profuse, of a penetrating odour; at times causing an eruption about auricles; objects strongly to having ears washed.—Bad effects from suppression of otorrhœa; hard hearing, esp. if ears are very dry; noise in ears in general, particularly a humming.—Otitis; in psoric subjects.—Furunculus on tragus.—Great acuteness of hearing; the least noise is insupportable, and playing the piano occasions nausea.—Something seems to come before ears.—Swashing in ears.—Hardness of hearing preceded by hypersensitiveness of hearing.—Dysecoia, esp. for human voice; from disposition to catarrhs; < after eating or blowing nose.—Obstruction and sensation of stoppage (pressure and pain when sneezing, as if ulcerated) in one ear, often when eating or blowing nose.—Tinkling, humming, and roaring in ears (in evening in bed); sometimes with congestion of blood in head.—Cracking in ear, like the breaking of a bladder full of water.—Excoriation behind ears.—Ears very red with children.

5. **Nose.**—Boring in root of nose.—(Itching and) burning in nostrils.—Inflammatory swelling (redness) of nose, chiefly at extremity, or in alæ nasi (< in r.).—Tip of nose red and shiny.—R. ala nasi and entire septum inflamed and painful to touch.—Inflammation, ulceration, and scabies in nostrils.—Cracking in nose, like the bursting of a bladder full of air.—Ephelides and black pores in nose.—Herpes across nose, like a saddle.—Obstruction of nose, sometimes semilateral.—Great dryness of nose.—Dry coryza, or fluent coryza, with copious secretion of mucus.—Burning coryza in open air, obstructions of nose in room.—Discharge of burning mucus, or secretion of a thick, yellowish, and puriform mucus in nostrils.—Blood or sanguineous mucus is blown from nose.—(Discharge of watery fluid from nose tinged with blood, and synchronous with præcordial pain, severe headache and pains in soles of feet, high-coloured urine and confined bowels: symptoms followed on a severe wetting.—R. T. C.)—Bleeding of nose, esp. in morning, and sometimes with vertigo (at 3 p.m., afterwards it feels sore when touched).—Frequent, even spasmodic sneezing, sometimes preceded by nausea.—Smell increased or diminished, and also entirely lost.—Offensive odour of nasal mucus on blowing nose.—Smell of inveterate coryza, of burnt horn or of smoke.—Offensive odour of nasal mucus, as of an old catarrh.

6. **Face.**—Face pale or yellowish, with sickly complexion ; and ey deep sunken, surrounded by a blue circle.—Heat and burning sensation i face, with deep redness of whole face, circumscribed redness of cheeks, o else red spots, also on neck.—Pale or red swelling of face.—Swelling o cheeks, with lancinating pain.—Pain : tearing in r. half of face ; pressure o malar bone and beneath eye ; stabbing below l. zygoma with darting up sid of head.—Pain in all three divisions of fifth nerve (l.) ; from exposure to cold draught of air ; worry ; beginning 5 p.m., lasts with slight intermissions thre or four days ; besides sharp dartings every few moments ; extreme extern sensitiveness.—Drawing, sharp pain, sensation as from a bruise, pressive an burning sensation in cheek-bones.—Erysipelas of face (beginning on r. ea and spreading over face).—Phlegmonous erysipelas in face, chiefly in eyelid nose, and (l.) ear.—Roughness and redness of skin of face.—Eruption o pimples on face and on forehead.—Itching and moist tetters over whole face chiefly above nose, round eyes, and in eyelids ; small white vesicles in group and forming scabs.—Ephelides and black pores in face, chiefly on nose, lip and chin.—Lips dry, rough, and cracked.—Burning sensation and continue heat of lips.—Yellowish hepatic spots on upper lip.—Tinea faciei.—Tremblin and jerking of lips.—Swelling of lips.—Swelling of lower lip with eruption o it.—Scabious ulcer on red of lip.—Cancer of the lips.—Herpetic eruption i corner of mouth.—Painful eruption round chin.—Sharp, lancinating, an drawing pains, and painful swelling in jaws.—Swelling of submaxillary glands with pains and lancinations when touched.

7. **Teeth.**—Great tenderness of teeth.—Great sensitiveness of points o teeth.—Jerking, shocks, sharp or drawing pains ; shootings ; throbbing pains boring and burning sensation, both in carious and in sound teeth.—Tearing toothache on l. side.—Pulsation and boring in teeth, < from heat.—The toothache often extends as far as ears or into head, and is sometimes accom panied by congestion of blood in head, with shiverings and disposition to sleep, or with swelling of cheek.—Appearance or < of toothache, prin cipally in evening ; at night ; or in open air ; also from a current of air ; from cold water ; when masticating, and sometimes when taking anything hot.— Toothache with congestions to head, or stitches in ears.—Brownish mucus on teeth.—Painful loosening, elongation, setting on edge, and easy bleeding o teeth.—Bleeding, sensation of unfixing, and swelling of gums, sometimes with throbbing (heating) pains.—Fistula dentalis.—Hard, round swelling of gums with discharge of pus and of blood.

8. **Mouth.**—Dryness, heat, and burning sensation in mouth, some times in morning with moist tongue.—Great dryness of palate with much thirst ; obliged to drink much.—Mouth dry, insipid, and sticky in morning —Ptyalism from abuse of *Mercury* or during a fever.—Accumulation o saliva in mouth : sanguineous ; salt ; acid ; bitter ; or mixed with blood even after eating.—Fetid, sometimes acid, smell from mouth, esp. in morning or in evening or after a meal.—Vesicles, blisters, and aphthæ in mouth and on tongue, sometimes with burning, or with pain of excoriation when eating.—Exfoliation of membrane of mouth.—Burning sensation and tickling on tongue.—Pain, swelling, and inflammation of tongue for three days.—Tongue dry, rough, and cracked, of colour of cinnabar ; or loaded with a white coating, or covered with brownish, thick, and viscid mucus.—

uttering when speaking.—Accumulation of saltish mucus in mouth.—Taste : tter ; pasty ; offensive ; of blood ; sweetish ; metallic.—Bilious taste in outh when fasting ; though food tastes right.—Bitter taste with dulness head and ill-humour.—Acid taste all day.

9. **Throat.**—Scraping, roughness (rawness), and dryness in throat awking and clearing throat).—Pressure as from a plug or from a tumour in roat, sometimes with difficult deglutition.—Stitches in throat on swallowing. Sensation as if a hard ball were ascending throat, and would close pharynx d take away the breath.—Contraction and painful sensation of constriction throat when swallowing.—(Sensation of contraction in throat.—R. T. C.) Dryness of throat.—Pain as from excoriation, burning sensation and shoot-gs in throat, < during empty deglutition (soreness begins on r. side and goes l. ; redness of tonsils).—Burning in throat as from sour eructations.—nsation during empty deglutition as of swallowing a piece of meat.—Sen-tion as of a plug in throat, with empyreumatic taste.—Sore throat, with elling of glands of neck.—Elongation of palate ; swelling of palate and nsils.—Sensation of a hair in throat.—Angina gangrenosa.

10. **Appetite.**—Bad taste in mouth, mostly acid, bitter, or putrid and eetish or mawkish, < in morning on waking.—Taste bitter or too salt or sipidity of food.—Complete anorexia and dislike to food, principally to eat, rye bread, fat, and milk.—Dislike to sweet and acid things, or craving such things, with anorexia.—Continued thirst, even at night, often with sire for beer.—Craving (in drunkards) for wine and brandy.—Immoderate petite and attacks of bulimy, sometimes with headache, lassitude, and want lie down.—Ravenous hunger which obliges him to eat frequently, gets adache and has to lie down if he does not.—Hungry, but appetite vanishes sight of food, feels full in abdomen ; when he begins to eat is averse to it. Desire for sweets.—Complaints from eating sweets.—Complaints from inaceous food.—Desire for raw food.—Great weakness of digestion, prin-ally for meat, fat, milk, acids, and farinaceous food, all of which some-es cause great suffering.—Food sweetened with sugar < the pains in the mach and abdomen.—Milk produces sour risings, an acid taste in mouth, d even vomiting.—Beer is followed by a prolonged after-taste, and causes ullition of blood.—Disgust for drinking wine.—After a meal oppression chest, nausea, pressure, and cramps in stomach, colic, inflation of abdomen, tulence, vomiting, great fatigue, shivering, confusion and pain in head, heat face, burning sensation in hands, flow of water from mouth, and many er sufferings.

11. **Stomach.**—Continued eructations, principally empty, or with taste food, or acid and burning, bitter, or fetid, with taste of rotten eggs, esp. er a meal or at night.—Loud eructations as soon as he presses on stomach. Heartburn.—Abortive risings.—The food rises into throat.—Regurgitation food and drink, often with acid taste.—Pyrosis, often with burning and gling in chest.—Hiccough.—Qualmishness.—Nausea, which sometimes en induces fainting, with trembling, weakness, and frequent eructations, . after a meal, in morning, at night, or when riding in a carriage.—Water-sh, < in morning or after a meal, sometimes with aching or digging in domen.—Retching and vomiting of food, and of acid or bitter substances, blackish, or sanguineous, &c. ; esp. in morning, in evening, after a meal, or

at night, and sometimes with nausea, pains in stomach, and cold perspiration on face.—After eating but little stomach feels completely full.—(Pains in stomach following a headache, < 10 p.m., causing him to bend forward to ease himself, with flatus and prostration at stool.—Tight crampy feeling in stomach on laughing and sneezing, preventing him rising from his seat.—R. T. C.)—Heaviness and fulness, or pressure and compression, or else contractive and spasmodic pains, or digging and shootings in stomach and præcordial region, < after a meal at night or in morning, often with nausea and vomiting, anxiety, and inflation of abdomen.—Uneasy, unpleasant feeling in stomach as if several hard things were lying in it, and all in different directions (cured.—J. H. C.).—Pressure in pit of stomach during menses.—Sensation of coldness, or heat and burning sensation in the stomach.—Great sensitiveness in the region of the stomach when touched (or pressing upon it—even the bed-cover causes pain).—Swelling of the præcordial region.—Pulsation in the pit of stomach.—Swelling at pit of stomach.—Weak, empty, gone, or faint feeling in stomach, about 11 a.m.; and at other times.

12. **Abdomen.**—Painful sensibility of hypochondria, as if they were wounded; pressure of clothes disagreeable.—Drawing, pressure, tension, and shootings in regions of the liver and spleen, swelling and hardness in both regions.—Stitches in spleen, < when taking a deep inspiration and when walking.—Frequent shoots in splenic region.—Inflammation, swelling, and induration of liver.—Bile increased.—Fulness, heaviness, tension, and pressure, as from a stone in abdomen, chiefly in epigastrium and hypochondria.—Enlargement and hardness of abdomen.—Gripings, or sensation of tearing or contractive and spasmodic pains in abdomen.—Intestines feel as if strung in knots.—Shootings (stitches) in abdomen, < on the l. side when walking (coughing) or taking a deep inspiration (about navel).—After food sensation of weight r. side of navel when he breathes (cured with three doses of *Sul.* 1m in a case of mine).—The pains in the abdomen have generally a tendency to attack the l. side, or to extend into stomach as far as chest and back, with obstructed respiration, nausea, anxiety, and hypochondriacal humour.—Pains in abdomen, chiefly at night, or after eating or drinking, or else periodical; < by food sweetened with sugar; > by bending forwards.—Movement and digging in abdomen, or sensation as if something were pushed outwards.—Movements in abdomen as of the fist of a child.—Pains as from contusion and bruising in integuments of abdomen.—Painful sensibility of abdomen when touched, as if all interior were raw, or formed one large wound.—Inflation of abdomen, with pressive pains from incarcerated flatus, principally in l. side (with constipation).—Pressure: towards anus; downward while lying in bed at night; it woke her.—Borborygmi and rumbling in abdomen.—Frequent escape of very fetid flatus.—Cutting in hypogastrium, with thin stool.—Griping in lower abdomen; pain in small of back (and chilliness over body) during menses.—Between 4 and 5 p.m. boring, shooting pain now in r. groin, now in spermatic cord, extending to testicle, now within inguinal ring in abdominal cavity; followed by sharp, cutting pain in r. great toe.—Painful swelling, and also suppuration of inguinal glands.—Violent protrusion of hernia, with incarceration.—Dropsy.—Portal stasis; hæmorrhoidal congestions; indigestion; constipation, &c.—Symptoms threatening peritonitis, terrible pains extending over entire lower

›domen followed a teaspoonful of *Sul.* taken for constipation ; relief follows
ırgation by castor oil.—(R. T. C.)

13. **Stool and Anus.**—Constipation, and hard, knotty, and insufficient 'acuations.—Frequent and often ineffectual want to evacuate, chiefly at ght, and sometimes with pressure on rectum and bladder and pain in anus. Urgent want to evacuate.—Looseness of bowels ; redness about anus ; ›structed evacuation, particularly if hard stools are retained.—Diarrhœa, ırticularly where there is the red line about the anus, and the patient can't ıit, must go immediately desire is felt ; also waking early in morning with ırrhœa, which drives one out of bed in a great hurry ; tenesmus in the ıme way, drives one in a great hurry ; rumbling and rolling in bowels.—ıolera asiatica ; as prophylactic, a pinch of the powdered milk of Sulphur ›rn in stockings in contact with soles of feet ; diarrhœa commencing tween midnight and morning, vomiting at same time ; numbness of limbs, amp in calves and soles, blue under eyes, cold skin, indifference ; during nvalescence, red spots, furuncles, &c. ; susceptibility to temperature, warm ings feel hot ; nerve symptoms (Hering).—Diarrhœa with frequent evacua-›ns, chiefly at night, and often with colic, tenesmus, inflation of abdomen, spnœa, shivering, and weakness to the extent of fainting.—Evacuations : ıcous, watery, frothy, or acid, or of a putrid smell, or of undigested sub-ınces.—Stools : nearly black, loose, viscid, greasy, with pungent odour of lphuretted hydrogen.—Stool hard, as if burnt.—Stool, with sensation as if ıe remained, and as if the stool had been insufficient.—Discharge of liquid ›m anus, followed by fæces at night during sleep.—Diarrhœa : painless ; in ›rning compelling one to rise from bed (at 5 a.m., one stool an hour till a.m.) ; undigested, involuntary ; diarrhœa in children, green, of bloody ıcus, with crying and weeping.—Dysenteric stools at night, with colic and ›lent tenesmus.—Colic before every loose evacuation.—During stool, dis-ırge of blood ; pain in small of back ; palpitation of heart ; congestion of ıd ; itching, burning, and stinging at anus and in rectum.—After stool ıesmus, constriction at anus.—Whitish, greenish, discoloured, or brownish-l fæces.—Involuntary evacuations (when sneezing or laughing, with emis-n of flatus).—Evacuations mingled with mucus, blood, and purulent matter. Discharge of mucus, even with hard fæces.—Ejection of lumbrici, ascarides, d also of pieces of tænia from rectum.—Prolapsus recti, esp. when evacuat-; (a hard stool).—Sharp and pressive pains, itching, shootings, stitches, and rning in anus and rectum, even when not at stool.—Burning in anus, 'ore, during, and after stool.—Prostration follows stool.—Dull ache just ide coccyx, awful dead ache as if the heart would stop.—All pains seem to to rectum, life-taking pains.—Blind piles with burning as if something re biting at anus, going away when lying down, coming on when standing walking about (produced.—R. T. C.).—Hæmorrhoids which protrude, ooze l bleed.—Anus inflamed, swollen, covered with red veins.—Excoriation l swelling of anus.—Much itching about anus ; itching runs back along inæum and adjacent parts.—Involuntary discharge of moisture from anus, h itching in it.—Suppressed hæmorrhoids, with colic, palpitation, conges-ı to lungs ; back feels stiff as if bruised.—Constant bearing down towards ıs ; forcing down after sitting.

14. **Urinary Organs.**—Violent pain in region of kidneys after stooping

a long time.—Aching in small of back all day, esp. < while urinating.—Sup pressed or very scanty urine.—Frequent and sometimes very urgent want t urinate.—Frequent, profuse, and watery urine, sometimes gushing out witl much force, esp. at night.—Retention of urine.—(Neuralgia of neck o bladder, aching and forcing down with smarting and burning in urethra.— R. T. C.)—Rigor when urinating.—Pressure soon after urinating, as from a ful bladder.—Involuntary emission of urine (and stool), esp. when coughing, o expelling flatus.—Wetting the bed (lie awake for some time, then fall into deep sleep, in which they wet the bed).—Red urine with sediment; or els whitish, turbid, or deep-coloured.—Urine like yeast; muddy, turbid, scanty —Oily pellicle over urine.—Fetid urine.—Urine smelling of chamomile te (produced.—R. T. C.).—Discharge of (white) mucus from urethra.— Secondary gonorrhœa.--Whitish or thick or reddish sediment, like flour, i the urine.—Urine discharged by drops.—Painful emission of some drop of sanguineous urine after much effort.—Discharge of blood and mucu with the urine.—Itching, sharp pains, shootings, and burning sensatio in (orifice of) urethra, chiefly when urinating.—Both flow of urine and dis charge of fæces are painful to parts over which they pass.—Urine excoriatin parts.—Redness and inflammation of orifice of urethra, and pain as at com mencement of gonorrhœa.—Discharge of mucus from urethra.—Hæmorrhag from urethra.—Shootings in bladder.—Dragging in bladder in morning afte urinating.—Small and intermittent stream of urine.—Spasmodic pains in loin and inguina.

15. **Male Sexual Organs.**—Affections of the genitals in general.— Itching about genitals on going to bed at night.—Fetid perspiration in parts —Excoriation between thighs and in groins, chiefly when walking.—Shooting in penis and glans.—Prepuce stiff, hard, like leather, with copious secretion o fetid smegma.—Inflammation, swelling, and phimosis of prepuce (with dis charge of fetid pus), with deep cracks, burning, and redness.—Deep (suppu rating) ulcer with elevated margins in glans and prepuce (with puffed edges) —Aching, tension, and shootings in testes and spermatic cords.—Swelling an thickening of epididymis.—Excoriation and oozing in scrotum.—Increase sexual desire and voluptuous irritation of the parts, often without erection.— Weakness of the genital functions, often with icy coldness, bluish colour o glans, prepuce, and penis, and retraction of prepuce.—Testes relaxed an hanging down.—Hydrocele.—Frequent pollutions, also at noon.—Water semen.—Involuntary discharge of semen, with burning in urethra.—To quick discharge of semen during coition.—Escape of prostatic fluid, chiefl when urinating and while at stool.—Impotence.—(Induration of testes.)

16. **Female Sexual Organs.**—A weak feeling in genitals.—Sor feeling in vagina during an embrace.—Labour-like pain over symphysis.— Uterine pains running from groins to back.—Moroseness and apprehensio with uterine pain.—Pressure on the parts.—(Bearing down with nightl enuresis.—R. T. C.)—Excoriation, troublesome itching and burning sensatio in genitals; with papular eruption around them.—Burning in the vagina is scarcely able to keep still.—Ascarides of vulva.—Inflammation of labia —Menses too late; too short.—Delay of first menses.—(Amenorrhœa, dread ful depression and apprehension, head feels full and heavy, followed b violent headache, numbness of arms and legs, cramp and sick feelin

at molimen.—R. T. C.)—(Imperfect development of the genital organs, menstruation does not appear at the usual age; breasts imperfectly developed; pains about the shoulders, in the stomach after meals, in l. side on inspiration; anorexia and vertigo.—R. T. C.)—Catamenia premature and too profuse; or too feeble or entirely suppressed (particularly in psoric individuals), with colic, abdominal spasms, headache, pains in loins, pressure at stomach, congestion in head, and nasal hæmorrhage, agitation, and even attacks of epilepsy.—Menstrual blood thick, acrid, corroding thighs; scanty, dark; dark, putrid, clotted.—Before menses: headache, itching in the parts; spasmodic colic; inquietude; cough; toothache; pyrosis; epistaxis; leucorrhœa, and asthmatic sufferings.—Bearing down in pelvis; congestion to uterus.—Sterility, with too early and profuse menstruation.—Prolapsus: from reaching high; with pain in hypogastrium, esp. r. side; with metritis; with dropsy of uterus.—Promotes expulsion of moles.—Morning sickness of pregnancy not amounting to vomiting, faint, sickish spells forenoon, profuse salivation, taste of which = nausea; aversion to meat; craves beer or brandy.—Hæmorrhoids during pregnancy and in childbed.—After menses: itching in nose.—Menstrual blood too pale or of an acid smell.—Leucorrhœa sometimes corrosive; gnawing and yellowish, preceded by colic.—Cancer of uterus; offensive, corrosive, ichorous leucorrhœa; sensation of heat in crown of head; coldness of feet; flushes of heat pass off in a perspiration with faintness; weak at pit of stomach 11 a.m. to 12; violent burning in vagina, with painful soreness during coitus.—Hot flushes at climaxis, with hot head, hands, and feet, and great goneness in stomach.—Excoriation and itching in nipples.—Cracks in nipples, with burning sensation, easily bleeding, and ulceration (the nipple smarts and burns very much as soon as the infant lets go of it).—Mammary glands engorged and inflamed.—Erysipelatous inflammation of mammæ; they are hard, with red rays extending from nipple, and stitching pains.—Swelling of mammæ.—Nodosities in mammæ.—Scirrhus of breast.

17. **Respiratory Organs.**—Catarrh, with fluent coryza, cough, pain in chest, as if it were raw, and shivering.—Hoarseness, evening and morning, roughness, and scraping in throat, with accumulation of mucus in chest.—Pain as from excoriation, and tingling or tickling in larynx, with tendency to cough.—Coldness in throat during an inspiration.—Voice hoarse and low, or entirely extinct, generally in cold and damp weather.—Sensation as if larynx were swollen, or as if a foreign body were in it.—Short, dry cough.—Dry cough, sometimes fatiguing and shaking, with retching, vomiting, and spasmodic constriction of chest, esp. in evening, or at night, in a recumbent position, or in morning, or after a meal.—(Constant cough with irritation of throat and wheezing.—R. T. C.)—Moist cough, with profuse expectoration of thick, whitish, or yellowish mucus, like that of a coryza of long standing.—Cough with expectoration during day, without expectoration at night.—Short, dry cough, with stitches in chest, or stitches in l. shoulder-blade.—Spasmodic whooping-cough in successive double attacks, shortly following one another, from tickling in larynx as from dust; only with expectoration during day of either dark blood or yellow-greenish, purulent matter, or of cold, milk-white mucus, generally tasting sour, or putrid, or salty, or like old catarrh.—Fetid expectoration of a greenish-yellow colour, like pus, and of a salt or sweetish taste, while cough-

ing.—Febrile cough, with hæmoptysis.—Cough in general with bloody expectoration; esp. with heat in chest; hæmorrhage with the same sensation. —When coughing, pain as from excoriation, or shattering pains, or shootings in chest, pain as from a bruise, or shootings in head, pain in abdomen, cloudiness before eyes, pains in hips and loins.—Respiration and conversation sometimes excite the cough.—Feels suffocated, wants doors and windows wide open.—Oppressed respiration, particularly from congestion to the lungs; if with a sense of heat all through the chest.

18. **Chest.**—Congestion of blood to chest, with sensation of fulness in it. —Shortness of breath; frequent chokings, obstructed respiration, dyspnœa, and fits of suffocation, esp. when lying down at night, and also during sleep, and sometimes also when speaking or walking in open air.—Dyspnœa; shortness of breath and oppression of breathing on bending arms backwards.—Asthma at night.—Asthma: attacks every eight days; has rough, harsh hair; following swelling of hæmorrhoids; alternating with fits of gout or psoriasis; from suppressed eruptions or discharges.—Inability to take a full inspiration, with sensation as if chest were contracted.—Frequent, short, or wheezing respiration.—Snoring and rattling of mucus in chest.—Shooting pains in back and sacrum during an inspiration.—Painful sensation in chest, as of something falling forwards in it, when turning the body in bed.—Pain as from a bruise in thorax when the part is touched.—Painful obstruction in the l. side of chest, with anguish, and inability to lie on side affected.—Heaviness, fulness, and pressure as from a stone in chest and sternum, < in morning, also when coughing, sneezing, and yawning.—Pain when coughing and sneezing, as if chest were shattered or bursting.—Periodical spasms in chest, with sensation of constriction, spasmodic pains, shortness of breath, bluish colour of face, and inability to speak.—Pulsations in chest and sternum.—Weakness of chest, felt particularly when speaking, with great fatigue in lungs after speaking or sighing.—Shootings in the chest or sternum, or extending to the back, or into the l. side, < when coughing, lying on the back, during least motion, when taking a full inspiration, or when lifting the arms (over the head).—Pain in chest from over-lifting or after inflammation of lungs.—Sensation as if lungs were touching (or scraping) the back.—Exudation after pneumonia.—*Sul.* acts in pneumonia a part analogous to that of *Bell.* in brain affections (Hartlaub, confirmed by Curie).—The pains in the chest chiefly affect the l. side.—Sensation of coldness or burning in chest, sometimes extending to face.—Sensation as of a lump of ice in r. chest.—Red spots all over the chest; also brownish or butternut-coloured spots.—Deep yellow spot began on l. breast and spread all over body (chloasma).—Cheloid on sternum.

19. **Heart and Pulse.**—Stitches and blows in region of heart.—Sharp pain at heart goes through to between shoulders; esp. with dyspeptic symptoms.—Cutting pains about heart, as with knives, which decrease or increase, last a few hours, with redness of face, followed by general coldness; attacks only when waking up.—Great orgasm of blood with violent burning in hands. —Violent congestion of blood towards chest and heart, sometimes with ebullition in chest, uneasiness, faintness, and trembling of arms.—Sensation of emptiness in the cardiac region, or pressure and sensation as if the heart had not room enough.—Affections in general of heart; also external chest.—Sensation as if heart were enlarged.—Frequent palpitation of the heart, some-

times even visible, and with anxiety; at night; in bed; on falling asleep; when going up an ascent.—Heart beats too rapidly and her throat felt as if a string were tied round it; and she did not sleep till 5 a.m. (produced.—R. T. C.).—Pulse hard, full, and accelerated.

20. **Neck and Back.**—Stiffness of neck; in nape, with paralytic, sprained pain.—Child cannot hold head up neck muscles so weak.—Tetters on nape.—Swelling and inflammation of glands of nape and of neck.—Fetid perspiration in axillæ.—Swelling and suppuration of axillary glands.—Cracking in vertebræ of neck, esp. on bending backwards.—Weakness and wrenching pains, or pain as from a bruise in loins, coccyx, and in back, esp. on walking, or rising from a seat.—Gnawing pain in small of back.—Pain in small of back not permitting one to stand erect.—Finds himself at night lying on back.—Cannot lie on back on account of rush of blood to head.—Pain in back after manual labour.—Shootings in loins, back, and shoulder-blades, sometimes with obstructed respiration.—Sharp and rheumatic pains, drawing, tension, and stiffness in loins, back, and nape.—Pinching and burning sensation between the shoulder-blades.—Tension and bruised pain between scapulæ and in nape, which on moving head goes to shoulders.—Stitches beneath scapulæ which take away the breath.—Drawing in r. scapula, evening on going to sleep.—Tearing in l. scapula while sitting.—Needle-shoots at point of l. scapula.—Sprained pains in back.—During whole day aching in small of back, < when urinating.—Distortion (curvature) of spine.—Vertebræ softened.—Cracking of vertebræ on bending head backward.

21. **Limbs.**—Sharp and drawing pains, or shootings in limbs, esp. in joints, and sometimes with want of strength, stiffness, and sensation of torpor in the parts affected.—Wrenching pains, as from contraction of the tendons, cramps, and spasms in several parts.—Cracking in joints, esp. of knee and elbow.—Inflammatory swelling of joints, with heat and redness.—Tingling in limbs, esp. in calves of legs and arms.—Tendency of limbs to go to sleep.—Weakness and trembling of limbs, esp. hands and feet.—Unsteadiness of joints.—Limbs "go to sleep," esp. when lying down.—Bruised feeling, and drawing, tearing pains in limbs (in outer parts, in muscles and joints, from above downward).—Cramp-like pain in muscles of limbs on motion.—Arthritic swelling and heat.

22. **Upper Limbs.**—Pressure on shoulders as from a weight.—Rheumatic pain in shoulders, esp. l.—Stitches extending from shoulder into chest on motion.—Stitching beneath r. axilla.—Sweat on axillæ smelling like garlic.—Jerking of shoulders, hands, and fingers.—Jerking, sharp pains (tearing), and shootings in joints and muscles of arms, hands, and fingers, and also in shoulders, chiefly at night in bed.—Nocturnal cramps in arms.—Tingling in arms and fingers.—Swelling of arms, sometimes with heat, hardness, and lancinating or tensive pains.—Exostosis in arm.—Warts on arms, or itching miliary or red, burning spots, which appear after washing.—Purulent vesicles in bend of elbow.—Sprained pain and stiffness in wrist, < in morning.—Ganglion.—Paralytic weakness of arms and hands.—Swelling of hands and thumbs.—Rigidity and wrenching pain in joints of hands and fingers.—Trembling of hands, esp. when occupied with fine work.—Involuntary contraction of hands, as if about to grasp something.—Coldness in hands and fingers.—Great burning in palms.—Perspiration on hands (in the palms) and

between the fingers.—Eruption of small, red pimples on hands and fingers, with itching.—Warts on fingers.—Desquamation, hardness, dryness, and cracking of skin of hands.—Itching vesicles on backs of hands.—Cracking and chapping on finger-joints.—Burning in balls and tips of fingers.—Cramps and jerks in fingers.—Contraction of tendons of hands and fingers.—Large and shining swelling (erysipelatous) of fingers.—Dead fingers.—Nodosities on fingers.—Ulcers about nails.—Flaws in nails.—Hang-nails.—Panaritium.—Chilblains (thick, red) on fingers, with itching in a warm temperature.—Swelling and inflammation of points of fingers, with subcutaneous ulceration and boring and pulsative pains at night.

23. **Lower Limbs.**—Pain, as from subcutaneous ulceration, in buttocks and in ischiatic tuberosities, esp. when touched, and after having been seated for a long time.—Purulent and painful swellings on buttocks.—Pain as from a wrench, and as from a bruise in hip, on least movement, with shooting pains at every step.—Pain in hip with contraction of leg.—Sharp and drawing pains in legs, esp. at night in bed.—Heaviness of the legs, sometimes with tension in thighs and knees, esp. at night.—Red, oozing, painful spots on the internal surface of thighs.—Middle of thigh as if broken.—Tension in hams, as from contraction of tendons.—Large (white, or) shining swelling of knee, with stiffness and painful weariness.—Phlegmasia alba dolens.—Cracking, drawing, sharp pains, and shootings in knees.—Tetters on hams.—Restlessness in legs and feet.—Torpor and numbness of legs.—Painful fatigue and paralytic weakness of legs, chiefly of knees, which yield frequently.—Sticking in knee and tibia.—Red spots and itching miliary rash on legs.—Transparent swelling of legs.—Erysipelas in leg and foot.—Bluish spots and swollen and varicose veins in legs.—Pain in calves when walking.—Cramps in calves and soles, esp. at night (in the soles at every step).—Tension in hollow of knee, as if contracted on stepping.—Painful sensibility of soles when walking.—Easy dislocation of foot when walking.—Stiffness of knee and ankle-joint.—Stiffness of maleoli.—Sprained pain in l. ankle when standing and walking.—Ankles weak.—Stiffness and wrenching pain in instep.—Tingling in legs and calves.—Burning and inveterate ulcers on legs or feet.—Tetters on ankle.—Shootings in feet.—Coldness in feet, esp. in evening, in bed, or burning sensation, chiefly in soles of feet.—Burning in feet, wants to find a cool place for them; puts them out of bed to cool them off.—Burning in soles; on stepping after sitting a long time; and itching, esp. on walking; wants them uncovered.—Cramp in soles at every step.—Soles cold and sweating.—Sweat on r. foot.—Sharp shooting, as from a blunt nail, in rapid succession at root of nail of great toe.—Swelling of feet, and esp. of the ankles.—Red, shining swelling of the toes.—Itching in the toes that had formerly been frozen.—Chilblains: redness and swelling with tendency to suppurate; thick and red with cracks on joints; itching < warm in bed.—Gnawing vesicles on soles.—Ulcer on instep.—Cramps and contraction of toes.—Coldness and stiffness of toes.—Tingling in ends of toes.—Large and shining swelling of toes.—Ulcerated and gnawing vesicles in toes.—Corns, with pressive or shooting pains.

24. **Generalities.**—[Affections in general of any kind appearing in l. side; hair of head; external front of head; inner belly, esp. l. side; back; small of back; axilla; lumbar region; upper extremities in general; posterior and inner surface of thigh; lower extremity in general; of the nails.—Inflam-

mation of mucous membranes in general; swelling of the glands.—Affections of the brain from suppressed cutaneous eruptions.—Very often when rash in scarlet fever will not come out, cannot bear to be washed.—Face pale, or reddish yellow.—Diminution of saliva.—Back is so stiff that one cannot rise from a stooping posture, and is always < before a storm.—Bleeding from inner parts in general.—Dropsy of inner parts, particularly in psoric persons, or resulting from a suppressed eruption.—Dryness of inner parts which are usually moist.—<: On waking, after eating; from exertion of body, unable to stand much exercise; from leaning against anything; after menstruation; from taking milk; during perspiration; from suppressed perspiration; from wet poultices; from abuse of *Mercury;* on rising; from any quick motion, as running; during sleep; after a long sleep; during stool; in children whose bowels are regular but who suffer great pain at every passage (when bowels are moved causing much pain, stools hard and lumpy, *Nitr. ac.*); on stretching limbs, esp. the affected limb; when swallowing food; from talking; from water and washing; ascarides; worms in general; from suppressed menstruation; from vomiting; on getting warm in bed.—>: From drawing up the affected limb—can't bear to have it extended.—H. N. G.]—Muscular palpitation.—Jerks and shocks in certain parts or throughout body, esp. when sitting or lying down.—Attacks of spasms.—Epileptic convulsions; excited by a fright or by running, and sometimes with cries, rigidity of the limbs, clenching of the teeth, and sensation as if a mouse were running over the back or arms.—Fainting fits; or hysterical or hypochondriacal uneasiness, sometimes with vertigo, vomiting, and perspiration.—Is very nervous, can't bear to be spoken to, could cry at anything (produced.—R. T. C.).—Trembling of limbs, esp. the hands.—Sensation of trembling in interior of body.—Sensations of: heat in chest; of heat anywhere; with any trouble; of sudden and frequent flushes of heat all over the body; of contraction of inner parts, chiefly in abdomen, with feeling as if it should be bandaged up or supported; of a hoop or band around the parts; buzzing or vibration in the body; of knocking or throbbing in outer parts; as of a lump in inner parts; of roughness in inner parts; of tightness or stiffness in outer parts; of sometimes being very small and then again being very large.—Attacks of uneasiness in whole body, which do not permit the continuance of a sitting posture, with desire to stretch and to contract the limbs alternately.—Great nervous agitation; towards night; could not sleep.—Great uneasiness and orgasm of blood.—Violent ebullition of blood, sometimes with burning heat in hands.—Great exhaustion, with great fatigue after the least conversation or the shortest walk, disposition to remain always seated, and profuse perspiration, even when sitting, reading, eating, lying down, or walking.—The sensation of fatigue is sometimes removed by walking.—Muscular weakness, esp. in knees and arms, and also in legs, with unsteadiness of gait.—Stooping gait. —Cannot walk erect; stoop-shouldered.—Standing is the most disagreeable position; every standing position is uncomfortable.—Extraordinary emaciation, sometimes with weakness, fatigue, and burning sensation in hands and feet.—Great sensitiveness to open air and to the wind; with pains in limbs on a change of weather, disposition to take cold, and many sufferings produced by exposure to open air.—The affections of head and stomach are those which are chiefly < in open air.—The majority of the sufferings are <

or appear at night, or in evening, and also during repose, when standing for a long time; and on exposure to cold air; they disappear on walking, on moving the parts affected, and also in warmth of a room; but the heat of the bed renders the nocturnal pains insupportable.—Several symptoms appear periodically.—When carefully selected remedies fail to produce a favourable effect, esp. in acute cases, *Sul.* will frequently excite reaction and clear up the case.—Complaints that are constantly relapsing.

25. **Skin.**—[The greatest general psoric remedy for almost every kind of itch, sore, ulcer, &c.; very colicky babies with pimples, itch, or eruption on skin, or roughness of skin.—Troubles of very long standing resulting from suppressed eruptions—*Sul.* will very often bring these out and cause their cure.—Exanthema in general on any part of the body which is < by any heat, from getting warm at work, in bed, &c.; freckles; cancerous ulcers.—Skin dry; rough; scaly; voluptuous itching—"feels so good to scratch"; ecchymosis; chapping of the skin, esp. when it ulcerates; chapping of the skin after being wet; soreness of the skin in children (soreness in folds of skin); brown sphacelus.—Tetters in general; chapped; scurfy; painful tearing; pulsating, &c.—H. N. G.]—Itching in skin, even of whole body, < at night, or in morning, in bed, and often with pain as of excoriation, heat itching (soreness), or bleeding of the part which has been scratched.—Eruptions, like those which often follow vaccination.—(Eczema rubrum.—Gouty eczema with much oozing.—R. T. C.)—Seborrhœa of scalp (used locally.—R. T. C.).—Scabious eruptions and tetters of a greenish yellow colour, commencing with small itching phlyctenæ, with a red areola.—Herpetic, red irregular, furfuraceous spots, or covered with small phlyctenæ, discharging a serous lymph.—Scabious eruptions.—Ecthyma with itching day and night.—Miliary eruptions, principally on limbs.—Nettle-rash.—Burning itching of the eruptions.—Hepatic spots of a yellow or brownish colour (on the body).—Erysipelatous inflammation, with pulsative and shooting pains.—Weals even from the slightest contusion.—Bright scarlet redness over whole body.—Tingling in the skin throughout the body.—Red, swollen, and ulcerated chilblains, with itching in heat of a room.—Callous warts, esp. round the fingers.—Skin cold, pale, dry.—The skin cracks easily, esp. in open air; cracks, with pain, as from excoriation.—Rhagades after washing.—The nails crumble off.—Skin of hands hard and dry.—Desquamation and excoriation of skin in several places.—Pityriasis of head and chest.—Unhealthy skin; slightest injuries are followed by inflammation and ulceration.—Ulcers with elevated margins, surrounded by itchy pimples, red or bluish areola, sharp, lancinating, and tensive pains; bleeding readily, and secreting a fetid and sanious or yellow and thick pus.—Ulcers with itching in the sore.—Proud flesh in the ulcers.—Fistulous ulcers.—Furunculi.—Encysted swellings, or pale, tense, and hot swellings; inflammatory abscess.—Inflammation, swelling, and induration or suppuration of the glands.—Nodosities on skin of whole body, but principally in the breast, from swelling of the subcutaneous glands.—Dropsical, burning swelling of external parts.—Inflammation, swelling, and painful sensibility of the bones.—On the bones sensation of constriction, or as if a band were around them.—Repugnance to ablutions.

26. **Sleep.**—Unconquerable drowsiness, esp. in afternoon and in evening by candle-light.—Irresistible drowsiness by day, wakefulness by night; i

bed every place appeared hard for his head and he keeps moving it hither and thither.—Goes to sleep late.—Sleeps with his eyes half-open.—Frequent yawning.—Retarded sleep at night, or sleeplessness, sometimes caused by a great flow of ideas or from over-excitement.—Sleep too light; or agitated with frequent waking, often with starts, and in a fright.—Waking too early with inability to go to sleep again.—Morning sleep too much prolonged; sometimes deep and lethargic, with difficulty in rising in morning.—Unrefreshing sleep.—Waking frequently during night when one becomes wide awake suddenly.—Pains, uneasiness, and tingling in limbs, anxiety and heat, colic at night; gastralgia, vertigo, headache, visions and illusions of senses, palpitation of heart, asthmatic sufferings, hunger and thirst.—Inability to sleep otherwise than on back, with head high.—When sleeping, agitation and tossing, shocks in body and jerks in limbs, starts and fright, talking (talks loudly while asleep), cries, murmurs, wanderings, delirium, lamentation, and moaning, snoring, eyes half-open, lying on back with the arms above head, nightmare, and somnambulism.—On waking, illusions of senses, frightful visions, and fear of ghosts.—Frequent, fantastic, anxious, frightful, and horrible, anger-exciting, disgusting, and agitated dreams; dreams of fire, of dogs which bite, of being possessed of fine clothes, of falling, of danger, of death; dreams, with a presentiment concerning the events of the morrow.—Vivid, beautiful, pleasant dreams.—Singing during sleep.—Happy dreams when one wakes up singing; busy all the time; wishing to touch something with inability to do so.—Vivid dreams, remain impressed on the memory.—After waking mind long confused.—Immediately after closing eyes, horrible strange grimaces appeared to her, could not banish them.—Lay in a reverie and talked of whatever vision appeared to him, with open eyes, for three nights in succession.—Voluptuous dreams with seminal emissions.—Vivid dream that she is seated on the chamber, which causes her to wet the bed.

27. **Fever.**—Chilliness from want of natural heat.—Chilliness, coldness, shivering, and shuddering, < in evening or at night in bed (followed by heat and profuse perspiration), as well as in afternoon, and when walking in open air.—Chilliness in forenoon; heat with cold feet in afternoon.—Chilliness externally with internal heat and a red face.—Chilliness, beginning in the toes.—Slight chill, 10 a.m., continues till 3 p.m., followed by heat lasting two hours, mostly in head and hands, with desire for beer.—Partial shiverings, principally in back, chest, and arms, coldness in hands, feet, and nose.—Chill constantly creeps from small of back up back.—Chill and fever; no reaction; constantly sinking.—During the shiverings paleness or heat in face, headache, and sometimes flushes of heat.—Frequent flushes of heat.—Heat, < at night or in evening or in morning, and also in afternoon, and often with (circumscribed) redness of cheeks, ardent thirst, burning sensation in hands and feet; partial shiverings, partial sweats, principally in head, face, and hands; fatigue and painful weariness in limbs, hoarseness and cough, anxiety, &c.—Heat at night without thirst, preceded by chilliness with thirst.—Febrile attacks both in forenoon and afternoon, or in evening, manifesting themselves by heat, which is preceded by shiverings, and followed or attended by perspiration, or else by heat in face, followed by shiverings.—During the fever palpitation of heart, delirium, weakness, obstruction, and scabs in nose, with violent thirst, which last symptom may also occur before the shiverings.—Swollen veins.—

Pulse hard, quick, and full (at times intermitting).—Perspiration in general of single parts ; on back part of the body ; great disposition to perspire ; perspiration, with anxiety ; compound or intermittent fevers.—Thirst.—Want of perspiration.—Frequent and profuse perspiration, day and night, evening and morning, in bed, aptness to perspire during labour, partial perspiration, chiefly on head, nape of neck, hands, &c., acid perspiration.—Perspiration very debilitating, pungent smell, very seldom offensive, at times cold.—Sweat smelling of sulphur.—Perspiration only on one side of body ; < at night and in morning.

Sulphur Hydrogenisatum.

Hydrogenium sulphuratum. Sulphuretted Hydrogen. H_2S. Solution of the gas.

Clinical.—Asphyxia. Asthma. Convulsions. Delirium. Mania. Tetanus. Typhoid fever.

Characteristics.—*Sul. h.* is a colourless, inflammable gas, having a sweetish taste and an exceedingly fetid smell resembling rotten eggs. It is extremely poisonous when inhaled. It is evolved when animal or vegetable tissues containing *Sulphur* decays ; and it also occurs in mineral springs, being liberated by the reduction of gypsum or other sulphates through the action of a microbe (*Cent. Dict.*). *Sul. h.* is one of the agents which give rise to "blood poisoning" when bad smells are encountered. Asphyxia, tetanus, delirium, low continued fever have been observed as resulting from the gas. J. Wiglesworth (*B.M.J.*, July 16, 1892) has recorded two cases of insanity, one certainly, and both probably, due to inhaling the gas : R. H., 32, engineman at chemical works, had been kept at home with an attack of bronchitis for ten days. A few days after his return to work he became "gassed" (*i.e.*, accidentally inhaled *Sul. h.*). This caused headache, stupor, prostration, compelling him to stay at home for a few days, when he became wildly delirious. He passed rapidly into a very excited state, shouting and gesticulating ; said he was Jesus Christ, &c. ; tried to bury his head in the floor and to raise his feet above his head. Three days later he was admitted to Rainhill Asylum, and was there still very violent and excited, gesticulating and talking incoherently, chiefly on religious subjects. At the end of a month there was some improvement, and he was discharged, recovered, five months after admission. In the other case, that of a labourer at chemical works, Wiglesworth is not quite certain that *Sul. h.* was the poison inhaled. This patient was greatly excited ; threw his arms about ; shouted and laughed by turns ; was excited and talkative. He remained permanently insane.

SYMPTOMS.

1. **Mind.**—Loss of consciousness.—Coma ; commencing as natural sleep.—Three days after exposure became delirious ; passed rapidly into a

olent excited state, shouting and gesticulating; said he was Jesus Christ, c., tried to bury his head in the floor and raise his feet above his head.—esticulating and talking incoherently on religious subjects (the mania lasted ıree weeks; complete recovery in five months).

2. **Head.**—Headache; and prostration.

3. **Eyes.**—Eyes sunk with darks rings round them.

6. **Face.**—Face pale.—Lips blue.

11. **Stomach.**—Nausea.—Sickness and debility.—Vomiting and diarrhœa, oth very painful.

12. **Abdomen.**—Diffused pains in abdomen.

17. **Respiratory Organs.**—Respiration: rapid and irregular; laboured; asmodic attempts to get air into lungs.—Immediate asphyxia.

19. **Heart.**—Pulse: rapid; at first weak then hard and rapid; irregular: feeble flutter.

24. **Generalities.**—Blood brownish black.—Muscular system flabby ıd emaciated.—Convulsions.—Spasms.—Tetanic spasms, sometimes preeded by delirium, sometimes by pains in stomach, faintness and difficult eathing, and the mouth fills with white froth, while the pulse sinks.—rembling.—Sudden weakness and loss of motion and sensation.

27. **Fever.**—Skin cold; deathly.—Low fever and delirium.

Sulphur Iodatum.

Iodide of Sulphur. S_2I_2. Trituration.

Clinical.—Acne; punctata. Barber's itch. Coryza. Ears, noises in. Eczema, eeping. Gonorrhœa. Hay asthma. Influenza. Kidneys, pain in. Lichen planus. p, upper, eruption on. Parotid glands, hypertrophy of. Prostate, affections of. alp, soreness of. Spine, weakness of. Stricture, urethral. Tongue, thickening . Tonsils, chronic hypertrophy of.

Characteristics.—*Sul. iod.* was proved by Kelsall on himself and ome others. Hale has used it in "obstinate skin diseases, notably *ırber's itch*, for which it is almost a specific." The provings indicate ıis in "pustular eruption on upper lip" and "erythema on chin." ale used the 3x trit. internally and applied a cerate (of one or two rains of *Sul. iod.* to an ounce of Cosmoline). It is also useful, Hale ıys, in large and painful suppurating acne. Dr. Berlin (quoted *. W.*, xxxi. 216) treated with *Sul. iod.* two cases of "weeping eczema" ssociated with varicose veins of the leg and pronounced itching. Also child with eczema of arms. The keynote in all is: "dark red, vollen, and weeping eczematous surface which itches terribly." The x trit. was given. The symptoms of *Sul. iod.* are < in morning; leanıg forward; stooping; rising; ascending stairs. > By expectoration. *eculiar Symptoms* are: Hair feels as if erect. As if heat in heart. esire for acids. As if a band across forehead. Hansen mentions mong the therapeutic uses of *Sul. iod.* Thickness of tongue remaining fter parenchymatous glossitis. Hypertrophy of parotids after parotitis.

Chronic hypertrophy of tonsils. Lichen planus, chronic and simple Bradford (*H. M.*, quoted *Org.* iii. 111) reports the following cases: (1 Burning at end of penis; dull pain in prostatic region; weaknes across kidneys: frequent desire to urinate with slight flow; eats ver little; does not go out of doors; is much discouraged about himsel *Sul. iod.* 3x cured. (2) Violent attack of pain in renal region, wit shootings down ureters; pain and weakness about kidneys; constar desire to urinate; urine thick and whitish with creamy sediment *Sul. iod.* 3x and 6x cured. (3) Stricture after gonorrhœa; chordee very painful urination, twisted stream. Yellow discharge: *Sul. io* cured.

Relations.—*Compare:* Band across forehead, Manc. Difficu expectoration, K. bi. Heat in heart, Lachn., Rhod. Sleepy by da restless at night, Staph. Acne, Bellis, K. bro., Arct. l.

SYMPTOMS.

1. **Mind.**—Doubtful.—Anxious.—Unsteadiness of ideas.—Apathy ar inaptitude for business.—Dread of exertion.

2. **Head.**—Headache; frontal, tightness.—Shooting and throbbing i temples; when stooping.—Sides of head ached; as if squeezed in a vice.- Scalp sore; on vertex.—Hair feels as if erect.

3. **Eyes.**—Eyes bleared; esp. l.—Inclination to close eyes, as if t press out tears.—Lids heavy.—Eyes: water much; dim.

4. **Ears.**—Itching, tingling, and buzzing in ears.—Singing in ears; wi feeling of tightness above eyes, as if a band was drawn tightly over forehead with sore throat, with heat above pit of stomach.

5. **Nose.**—Coryza.—Thick green mucus in nostrils.—Acrid discharge.- Burning tickling in r. nostril every time handkerchief is used; strong odo of *Iodine* perceived.—All the agonies of "grippe."—Excoriation of nostrils.- Acuteness of smell.

6. **Face.**—Face dry, hot and yellowish.—Erythematous eruption upper lip with yellowish pustules, painful, sore and tender, quickly disa pearing in dry scabs.—Erythema on chin.

8. **Mouth.**—Teeth felt soft to tongue and were coated with dark fur.- Tongue dry and hard, furred at root, red at point.—Taste: bitter; nasty ar fetid breath.

9. **Throat.**—Throat dry and painful to touch, feeling as if swelled.- Sore throat in morning.—Drawing, creeping sensation at back of throat. Uvula and tonsils slightly enlarged and red.—Constant disposition swallow saliva: throat and gullet parched; the saliva did not allay t dryness.

11. **Stomach.**—Anorexia; desire for acids, pickles, lemonade.—Thirs —Sensation of heat about pit of stomach.—Soreness and sinking in epiga trium.

13. **Stool and Anus.**—Itching in rectum.—Bowels constipated.

14. **Urinary Organs.**—Itching in urethra.—Frequent micturitic esp. mornings.—Ardor urinæ.—Urine smells like raspberries.—(Stricture. Pains in kidneys shooting down ureters.—Urine thick, whitish, creamy.)

15. **Male Sexual Organs.**—(Chordee and yellow discharge.)

17. **Respiratory Organs.**—Accumulation of dark, purulent mucous in trachea, continued inclination to swallow saliva, which does not moisten it; mucus removed with difficulty and by violent, hacking, coughing and straining.—Tickling in larynx.—Sensation of dryness in trachea; thick, hard clots of mucus collected about top of windpipe difficult to detach, and which caused tickling and irritation of larynx and cough.—Much troubled with cough during early part of night, accompanied by a nasty taste in mouth and fetid breath.—Inclined to expand chest, and take a deep inspiration; leaving a fluttering sensation.—(Hay asthma, with sneezing, catarrh, &c.—R. T. C.)

18. **Chest.**—Tightness across chest; difficulty of expanding it; with prostration.

19. **Heart.**—Boring pain as if in heart, with some difficulty of respiration.—Sensation of heat in region of heart.—Palpitation.

20. **Back.**—Weakness of spinal column with pain in loins as if bruised, with weakness of spine.

23. **Lower Limbs.**—Weakness of knees and joints.—Legs ache and feel weak.—Tickling in calves and feet.—Trembling and aching of ankle-joints.—Soles of feet ache and burn and are sore when standing.

24. **Generalities.**—Prostration, with difficulty of expanding chest on inspiration.—Weakness as from influenza.—Faint and sick.—Much < on waking in morning; sleepy; leaning forward; rising or ascending stairs.

25. **Skin.**—Pustules on upper lip.—Erythema on skin.—Itching rash, like nettlerash on arms.—Acne punctata (specific in dilution.—R. T. C.).

26. **Sleep.**—Sleepy by day, restless at night.—Sleep unrefreshing; confused dreams; awakened by fright; sleep with mouth open.

27. **Fever.**—Occasional chills.—Febrile excitement.—Dry heat.

Sulphur Terebinthinatum.

Terebinthinated Sulphur. [One part of purified Sulphur is dissolved by heating in one hundred parts of Turpentine.] Dilutions.

Clinical.—Chorea. Chronic rheumatic arthritis.

Characteristics.—*Sul. tereb.* is referred to in the Hon. Robert Boyle's works (Shaw's edition, vol. iii. 584). A 1 x dilution cured a most obstinate case of St. Vitus's dance, and has often relieved pain in chronic rheumatic arthritis (Cooper).

Sulphuricum Acidum.

Sulphuric acid. H_2SO_4. Dilution.

Clinical.—*Acidity.* Alcoholism, chronic. Aphthæ. Back, stiffness of. Bowels, looseness of. Brain, concussion of. Breath, offensive. Cancer. Cancrum oris. Chafing. Chilblains. Climaxis, sufferings of. Constipation. Corns. Diabetes.

Diarrhœa. Diphtheria. Dyspepsia. Erythema nodosum. Flushing. Gangrene. Gastralgia. Glossitis. Hair, grey; falling out. Heartburn. Hernia, inguinal. *Hiccough.* Impotence. Intermittents. *Irritation.* Liver, affections of. Menorrhagia. Metrorrhagia. Myopia. Nightmare. Œsophagitis. *Paralysis, lead.* Perspiration, excessive. Phthisis. Pneumonia. Pregnancy, sickness of. Purpura. Rheumatism. Scurvy. Spleen, affections of. Sterility. Ulcers. Uterus, prolapse of. Vagina, prolapse of. Varicosis. Warts.

Characteristics.—*Sul. ac.*, according to Teste, was a favourite remedy of the Middle Ages, being used extensively in dilution in the treatment of scrofulous, phagedenic, cancerous, and venereal ulcers; as a gargle and mouth-wash for aphthæ, ulceration of the gums, and diphtheria. It was given as "Mineral Lemonade" in cases of lead poisoning. [This use I have verified, giving water acidulated with the 3x.—J. H. C.] The "Acid Soap" of Achard was prescribed as a dissolvent in scirrhus of the breast and calculous nephritis, obstinate intermittent fevers, visceral obstructions, dropsy, jaundice, cachexia, and "certain tumours of the feet." *Elixir of vitriol* (a mixture of the acid, alcohol and water) is a popular remedy for nervous weakness in women at the present day. Dippel, Haller, and others each had an "Elixir," differing only in the proportions of the chief ingredients. The elixirs were used in: Intermittent, putrid, malignant, contagious fevers; comatose and petechial fevers, scarlatina, confluent and malignant variola; dysentery; plague, lepra, itch, and other cutaneous diseases; nocturnal emissions; suppression of menses and piles, calculous nephritis, and gout; pituitous phthisis; chorea. Hahnemann proved *Sul. ac.*, and says that it has cured affections characterised by: "tension in the eyelids in the morning, shortsightedness; hardness of hearing; inguinal hernia; chronic looseness of the bowels; profuse menses; metrorrhagia; roughness in the throat; *asthma*; swelling of the feet; coldness of the feet" (*Chron. Dis.*). Teste gives this experience of his own: "Two or three times I have used this drug with success against round syphilitic spots, of a bright red colour, of the size of a penny, rather itching, running into each other, secreting a humour sometimes, and generally seated at the upper and inner surface of the thighs, between the shoulders, on the face, and at the posterior surface of the forearms and hands. The subjects on whom this acid seemed to act best were lymphatic, ate a good deal, and were disposed to a constant looseness of the bowels, so that their evacuations were rarely in shape." Hahnemann's proving with homeopathic experience has confirmed many of the old uses of *Sul. ac.* and brought out characteristic indications. Weakness is a keynote to *Sul. ac.* The patient is weak and exhausted. *Sul. ac.* is suited to cases where the weakness is out of proportion to the disease. Weakness which seems to come from deep-seated dyscrasia. There is as well a sense of general internal trembling; as if trembling from head to foot, but without visible trembling. It is useful for inebriates who are "on their last legs," long after *Nux* had ceased to help. Hering says the craving for liquor has been subdued by taking for two or four weeks, thrice daily, ten to fifteen drops of a mixture of one part of *Sul. ac.* with three parts of alcohol. The indications are: "Vomiting in morning;

acidity in stomach; burning in œsophagus and stomach; sour, acrid, or foul eructations." *Sul. ac.* has this characteristic: in spite of great thirst, water is not tolerated; unless qualified with alcohol it chills the stomach. This is a common symptom with hydrogenoid patients. *Sul. ac.* has a keynote symptom in the mental sphere. *Hurry*—hasty, quick, sullen, impatient; angry because things move so slowly. Like *Sul.*, *Sul. ac.* is periodic and has an important place in agues and periodic neuralgias. Cooper with reason contends that many ague cases, supposed to have been cured with *Chi. sul.* (Sulphate of Quinine), were really cured by the *Sulphuric acid* used in dissolving it. "Moreover," says Cooper, "in all epidemic diseases—influenza, cholera, small-pox, &c.—*Sul. ac.* is often called for by the concomitant symptoms. In the neuralgia of influenza it has cured very severe pain over the whole left side of the head, face, and neck, coming on from exposure to draught; in the diarrhœas of cholera times it certainly arrests mischief; in the diarrhœas of emaciated children it is often called for. A chemist in Covent Garden used to use a lotion of *Sulphuric acid*, well diluted, for all the cases of itch that came before him, and they were many." There is a keynote of *Sul. ac.* in respect to neuralgias which is of great service; the pains increase gradually and end abruptly; the most characteristic kind of pain is dull pressure—as of a plug thrust in. There is external soreness and sensitiveness. The piles of *Sul. ac.* are external, sensitive to touch and accompanied by itching. *Sul. ac.* is a great hæmorrhagic; there is bleeding from every orifice; bleeding under skin (purpura); the menses are too early, too profuse, and sterility may be a consequence of this; oozing of dark thin blood. Many sufferings of *Sul. ac.* seem to arise from the generative organs, especially of the female. With *Sul. ac.* 30, a dose every night, I gave great help to a delicate woman who had *nightmare, waking in a fright, before each menstrual period.* The local "weakness" of *Sul. ac.* may amount to prolapse of vagina and uterus. *Trauma* is another indication for *Sul. ac.*; it follows *Arn.* in bruises of soft parts, *Con.* in bruises of glands, *Ruta.* in bruises of bones. It also removes long-lasting black and blue spots with soreness and stiffness of the parts. Flushing is another feature (as at climacteric), and with the flushing there is sweating. Easy sweating is a note of *Sul. ac.*, and the sweat affects mostly the upper part of the body. The body odour of *Sul. ac.* is *sour* and cannot be washed off. This is especially observed in children. Heartburn with sour eructations that set the teeth on edge. *Sul. ac.* is *Suited to:* (1) Old people; especially women. (2) Light-haired people. (3) Pains at climacteric. (4) When some deep-seated dyscrasia prevails, the child is weak with no other symptoms. (5) Sour babies. *Sensations* are: As if brain were loose and falling from side to side. As if one side of head filled with smoke. As if a plug were thrust quickly into head. As from subcutaneous ulceration in scalp. As of a foreign body on right outer canthus. As of a leaf lying before ears. As if white of egg had dried on face. As if skin of cheek and chin were pinched. As of want of elasticity of vocal organs. As if there were a lump in throat. As if menses would come on. As if hernia would protrude. As if rectum were torn to pieces during stool. Many symptoms appear on right side, but the left cheek and left parotid are most affected. Pain travels from left to right round hypochondria Other *Peculiar Symptoms* are : Pains felt during sleep and disappearing on waking. Jerkings on falling asleep. Seriousness alternating with buffoonery. Pain in bladder unless call to pass water is immediately attended to. The symptoms are : < By touch ; pressure ; chafing mechanical injuries. Open air <. Warmth >. Cold <. Rest > Lying on affected side > gnawing in face. Motion ; lifting arms rising ; walking ; riding <. < Morning ; (also evening and night) < Drinking cold water. Wine <. Warm food = sweat. The cauterising property of *Sul. ac.* is of the phagedenic order, which makes it suitable to many gangrenous conditions.

Relations.—*Antidoted by:* Puls. *Antidote to:* Lead poisoning *Complementary:* Puls. *Follows well:* In injuries, Arn., Con., Rut *Compare:* Cough followed by belching wind from stomach, Ambr. Ver. Dyspepsia of drunkards, Carb. v. (Carb. v. is a putrid remedy Sul. ac. more sour). Acidity sets teeth on edge, Rob. Weaknes and giving way of ankles, Caust, Sul., Sil. Scarlatina, blue spots diphtheritic membrane, Mur. ac. (Mur. ac. has > uncovering) Sprains, Am. c. (hot and painful). Falls easily, Nat. c., Caust., Sul Pains increase gradually, end suddenly (Bell., Lyc., pains begin and end suddenly ; Stn., pains begin and decline gradually ; Col., begin suddenly and end gradually). Aphthæ, Sul. ac., Borax, Nat. m. K. chl. Piles, Nit. ac. Drinks chill the stomach, Elaps. Flushing a menopause, Lach. (Sul. ac. with sweating). Throbbing headache a menses, Lach. (Sul. ac. with sweating). Inguinal hernia, Lyc. (Lyc right, Sul. ac. left). Sour children, spite of washing, Hep., Mg. c. Rhe. Sensation of brain loose in forehead and falling from side to side, Bell., Bry., Rhe., Spi. Prostration, Acet. ac. Hæmorrhages o black blood from all outlets, Crotal., Mur. ac., Nit. ac., Tereb. Wea and exhausted from deep-seated dyscrasia, no other symptoms, Pso. Sul. Weakness, Pic. ac. Sensation of white of egg on face, Alm Sensation of subcutaneous ulceration, Puls. Alcoholism, Querc Prolapse of vagina, Staph. Larynx sensitive, Lach. Warmth o genitals (Sul. coldness).

Causation.—Lifting arms. Falls. Bruises. Concussion (o brain). Chafing. Surgical operations. Sprains.

SYMPTOMS.

1. **Mind.**—Mental excitability ; and exaltation.—Melancholy dejection —Inclination to weep.—Anxious apprehension and mistrust.—Despondency —Agitation, precipitation, and impatience.—One feels in a very great hurry feels that everything must be done in a hurry (also *Arg. nit.*).—Restlessness —Irritability, nervous fatigue, and tendency to take fright.—Peevish morose ness, and dislike to conversation.—Disgust to life.—Seriousness, alternatin with buffoonery.—Extraordinary absence of mind.—Dulness of intellect.

2. **Head.**—Semilateral confusion of head, as if the part containe smoke.—Vertigo when seated, disappearing in the open air.—Sensation a if brain were loose in forehead, and was falling from one side to the othe

< when sitting quiet in the room.—Headache, which at first increases, then uddenly disappears.—Sensation of weakness in head.—Headache, as if rain were lacerated.—Rush of blood to head.—Throbbing headache during nenses, with sweating.—Pressive headache.—Sensation of heaviness and ulness in brain, as if head would burst.—Sensation of constriction in head.—'ainful shocks in forehead and temples, < in forenoon and evening.—Head-che as if a plug was thrust quickly by increasingly severe blows in head.—hocks and blows in the head.—Violent jerk beneath l. frontal eminence, uddenly disappearing.—Headache, with dull lancinations, or drawings and earings.—Sensation of wavering of the brain.—Sensation in exterior of head s if suppurating, or ulcerated, painful to touch.—Itching and eruption in calp.—Hair turns grey and falls off.—Pimples on forehead and side of nose.

3. **Eyes.**—Burning aching in eyes, in open air, or when fixing eyes on n object in a room.—Tension in lids in morning.—Smarting, burning ensation in eyes, and lachrymation, esp. when reading.—Sensation of a oreign body in r. outer canthus, in morning when walking.—Eyes red, with hotophobia.—Chronic inflammation of eyes.—Difficulty in opening eyelids. -Myopia.

4. **Ears.**—Tearing in ears.—Tearing and shaking in r. ear.—Violent ckling in concha.—Dysecoia, as if there were a band over the ears, or as if leaf were before them.—Rhythmical roaring in ears.—Ringing of bells efore ears.—Humming in ears, in evening.

5. **Nose.**—Epistaxis in evening.—Dry coryza, with loss of smell and iste.—Coryza : thin, lemon-coloured discharge.—Pimples on side of nose.—'low of water from nose, with obstruction of one nostril.

6. **Face.**—Paleness of face.—Contusive pain in zygomatic process.—'earing of bones of face.—Dry shrivelled spots on face.—Sensation as if face vere swollen, and as if it were covered with the white of eggs dried.—Lips re cracked, and exfoliate.—Lips swollen, red, painful to touch.—Pain, as om excoriation, in commissures of lips.—Inflammation and swelling of ubmaxillary glands.

7. **Teeth.**—Toothache, more violent in evening, in bed, < by cold air, > by warmth, generally with tearing digging, or gnawing.—Bluntness of teeth. -Toothache with tenderness and pain along side of head and down spine R. T. C.).—Teeth on edge.—Swelling and easy bleeding of gums.—Ulceration f gums.

8. **Mouth.**—Aphthæ in mouth ; in children.—Sensation of dryness in outh.—Tongue dry.—Tongue ; horribly swollen ; swallowing impossible ; overed with wrinkled white skin ; tip and edges red ; denuded at tip and tensely red.—Ulcers on inflamed tongue.—Talking difficult as from want of lasticity in parts.—Breath very offensive.—Profuse salivation.—Hæmorrhage om mouth.

9. **Throat.**—Sore throat during deglutition, with lancinating pain, sp. in evening (swollen as if a lump were in it ; < on l. side).—Thick ellow membrane on fauces, sticks like glue.—Swelling of uvula and roof of alate.—Swelling and inflammation of submaxillary glands.—Roughness in iroat.—Mucous membrane of palate and pharynx swollen, injected and lcerated.—Stringy, lemon-yellow mucus hangs from posterior nares, in iphtheria.

10. Appetite.—Putrid taste.—Bread has a bitter taste, and is heavy c stomach.—Bulimy, with rumbling and borborygmi in abdomen.—Desire f fresh fruits (plums); brandy.—Loss of appetite and great debility.—Chron alcoholism; vomiting in morning; acidity of stomach; burning in œsophag and stomach; sour, acrid or foul eructations.—After eating; pain in stomac and rising of food by mouthfuls.—After warm food, sweat.—After a me agitation, gripings, and digging in abdomen, or excessive inflation of stomac —Cold perspiration, immediately after hot food.—Lassitude and flatulen after drinking milk.—All drinks chill the stomach, if a little spirit is not add to them.

11. Stomach.—Empty or bitter risings.—Acid, bitter, salt, or el sweetish regurgitations.—Sour eructations, violent heartburn.—Violent hi cough.—Pyrosis.—Nausea in the stomach, with shivering.—Vomiting, first water, then of food.—Vomiting of drunkards.—Very painful sensitiveness region of stomach.—The water (or every drink) causes cold of the stomac if not mixed with some alcoholic liquor.—Fulness and pressure in stomach. A contracting sensation in stomach in evening, as from a chill.—Contracti in stomach and scrobiculus (< from hard food).—Cuttings round stomach. Sensation of coldness or burning in stomach.—Cold, relaxed feeling stomach.

12. Abdomen.—Lancinations in spleen.—Spleen enlarged: hard a painful; hurts when coughing; after intermittent fever.—Stitches in liver a spleen.—Shootings in the hepatic region.—Shooting in loins.—Colic abdomen, like labour pains, extending into hips and loins.—Movemen gripings, and pinchings in abdomen, sometimes at night.—Sensation of he in umbilical region.—Jerking throughout hypogastrium, esp. at surface. Throbbing, tearings, and shootings, in inguina.—Smarting in inguinal regic —Inguinal hernia, much protruded.—Flatulent colic in the hypogastriu with grumbling and borborygmi, and sensation as if a hernia were about descend.—Weak feeling as if menses would appear.

13. Stool and Anus.—Tenesmus.—Ineffectual urging to go to stool. Evacuations retarded, hard, knotty, and black.—Fæces of a very large size. Chronic relaxation of abdomen.—Loose evacuations, of consistence of p (yellowish-white; partly solid, partly liquid), greenish, and watery.—Wate diarrhœa, very offensive.—Diarrhœa, of frothy slime only, with burni sensation in rectum.—Diarrhœa, with great debility.—Soft stool, followed a sensation of emptiness in abdomen.—Evacuations of mucus, streaked wi blood.—The child frequently has a stool as if chopped, saffron yellow, string slimy.—Very fetid stools of a putrid smell.—Discharge of blood duri the evacuation.—Sanguineous congestion in rectum.—Hæmorrhoidal excr cences in anus, with shootings, burning sensation, itching and oozing. Hæmorrhoids feel damp and are painful to touch; itch violently; pain stool as if rectum were torn to pieces; stools like sheep's dung; piles in ha drinkers.—Pressing in anus during and after pasty stool.

14. Urinary Organs.—Diabetes; lassitude; debility; despondency. Diminished secretion of urine, with burning sensation when urinating Emission of urine at night.—Urine watery (brown, diminished secretion and as if it contained earth (or loam).—Slimy sediment in the urine Sediment like blood in the urine, which is covered with a fine pellicle.—P in the bladder, when the want to urinate is not immediately satisfied.

15. **Male Sexual Organs.**—Excessive heat in genital parts and testes.—Emission of semen, without voluptuous sensation.—Itching pain in upper margin of glans.—Scrotum relaxed.—Orchitis (r.).

16. **Female Sexual Organs.**—Strong desire for coition, from irritation of the external genital organs (in females).—Catamenia premature and too profuse.—Catamenia of too long duration.—Metrorrhagia.—Nightmare before menses.—During menses, lancinations in abdomen and vagina.—After menses; great desire for, or else great aversion to, coition.—Sterility, with catamenia premature and too profuse.—Acrid and burning, or milklike leucorrhœa.—Discharge of sanguineous mucus from vagina.—Prolapse of vagina; parts look greenish and smell badly.—Climacteric age with constant hot flushes, and a feeling of tremor all over body, with great debility, and as if everything must be done in a hurry; spitting of blood; constipation; symptoms are < by smelling (not drinking) coffee.—Nausea and vomiting during pregnancy; never vomited food, but could not eat because of increased distress in stomach and vomiting of mucus.

17. **Respiratory Organs.**—Hoarseness, with dryness, and roughness in throat and larynx.—Pain in larynx, with embarrassed speech, as if the parts were not sufficiently elastic.—Larynx excessively sensitive; to pressure.—Cough, excited by open air.—Cough < from walking, riding, cold water, and when smelling coffee.—Dry, short, panting cough, sometimes in the morning, after rising.—Moist cough, with slimy expectoration.—Long-continued hæmoptysis.—Cough, with hæmoptysis.—Cough with expectoration in morning, without expectoration in evening.—Cough from irritation in the chest, with expectoration in morning of dark blood, or of a thin, yellow, blood-streaked mucus, generally of a sourish taste.—After the cough, eructations.—Profuse hæmorrhage from the lungs.—Risings and regurgitation of food after coughing.

18. **Chest.**—Dyspnœa.—Great weakness in the chest, with difficult speech.—Aching in the l. side of chest, and in scrobiculus.—Cutting pain in front of l. axilla.—Pains along sternum; beneath sternum; cutting, burning.—Sternum sore as if beaten.—Dull stitches in l. side of sternum by costal cartilages.—Dull tension in l. side of chest.—Stitches from chest to l. scapula.—Pneumonia l. side of chest and in pit of stomach.—Dulness of base of r. lung, pneumonia, collapse, death.—(Many cases of poisoning by *Sul. ac.* are followed by pneumonia.)—Slight pulsating, twitching beneath l. side.—Lancinations in chest.—Violent sticking in r. breast; frequent and continuous; when pressing on it pain extended deeper.

19. **Heart.**—Palpitation of heart (with or without anxiety).—Lancinations across heart.—Præcordial region very painful.

20. **Neck and Back.**—Neck swollen.—L. neck painful on pressure.—Large suppurating swelling l. side of neck.—Sensation, as from excoriation, and as of a fracture, in the back and loins.—Drawing in the back and loins.—Pain in small of back.—Boring in small of back.—**Furunculi on back.**—Stiffness of back several mornings; on rising.—Painful sensibility and swelling of axillary glands.

21. **Limbs.**—Convulsive movements of arms and legs.—Pains in joints felt during sleep, disappear on waking.—Tearing in all limbs during menses, esp. **in evening.**—Inclination to cramp in hands and feet.—Wrists and other

large joints painful and swollen, but not red.—Limbs livid.—Twitching of tendons.

22. **Upper Limbs.**—Heaviness of the arms.—Spasmodic, paralytic contractions in arms.—Shootings in joint of shoulder, on lifting arm.—Tensive pain in elbow-joint.—Bluish spots on forearm, as from ecchymosis.—Cramps in hands.—Shocks and blows in bones of hand, when writing.—Eruption on hands, and between fingers.—Lancinations in joints of fingers.—Chilblains on fingers.

23. **Lower Limbs.**—Inner surface of thighs red, sore, excoriated after riding.—Heaviness of legs.—Torpor and numbness of legs.—Want to stretch and retract limbs.—Tearing in varices of legs.—Painful weakness of knees, with dull lancinations, shocks, and blows in those parts.—Red, itching spots on tibia.—Stiffness of ankles.—Coldness in feet.—Swelling of feet.—Tearing and lancinations in corns and feet.

24. **Generalities.**—For any affections arising from general debility, as prolapsus uteri, retroversion, any uterine trouble whatever, the patient having a sense of tremulousness all over.—Burning darting pains in muscles ; shocks as from pain ; black and blue spots in body ; in a bruise (esp. if an old person) when the injured part gets black and blue, and seems as if it would mortify.—Hæmorrhages of black blood from all the outlets of the body.—Affections in general occurring in r. abdominal ring ; sexual organs r. side ; r. upper side l. lower side ; inguinal hernia.—< Afternoon and evening ; from surgical injuries in general ; in the open air ; from smelling coffee.—Tearing pains throughout body, also in face.—Stitches in joints.—Cramps in limbs.—Pains felt during sleep.—Icteric sufferings.—Jerking of the tendons.—Appearance or < of symptoms, morning and evening.—The patient feels < in open air.—The l. side seems to be more particularly affected.—Slowly increasing but suddenly ceasing pain, as if a blunt instrument were pressed against the part.—Sensation of soreness as if bruised over the whole body.—Weakness of the whole body with sensation of trembling.—Extreme weakness and exhaustion, with sensation of tremor all over the body, without trembling.—Sour odour of body.—Great weakness and emaciation with backache in young girls (R. T. C.)—General weariness in a plethoric woman and pain in lower back chiefly l.-sided, with weakness in lower abdomen, < at menses, furred tongue and constipation.

25. **Skin.**—Bad effects from mechanical injuries, as from bruises, falling, knocking, pressure of blunt instruments, and contusions (esp. in old women) —Gangrenous tendency after a bruise.—Itching over whole body.—Red itching spots on skin, or small, red, livid, and bluish spots, as from ecchymosis —Excoriation of skin, also with ulceration like gangrene (becomes easily chafed when walking or riding).—Furunculi.—Gnawing (eating pain in the ulcers.—Painful sensitiveness of glands.—Chilblains.—Corns in feet, with tearings and shootings.—Warts.

26. **Sleep.**—Retarded sleep and early waking.—Sleepiness.—Sleeplessness from mental excitement.—Jerkings during sleep.—Anxious dreams.—Jerking of fingers during sleep.—Nightmare before menses.

27. **Fever.**—Chilliness during the day, < in room, > when exercising in open air.—Frequent chills running down body.—Heat in evening and after lying down in bed.—In evening frequent flushes of heat, esp. when exercising

—Flushes of heat with perspiration (in climacteric years).—Heat predominates. —Small, feeble (accelerated) pulse.—Perspiration on least movement (which continues for a long time after sitting down).—Profuse perspiration in morning. —Perspiration at night.—Cold perspiration as soon as one eats warm food.

Sulphurosum Acidum.

Sulphurous acid. H_2SO_3. Sulphurous anhydride. SO_2. Sulphurous acid gas dissolves in water and constitutes 9·2 per cent. by weight of the solution.

Clinical.—*Acne rosacea.* Colds. Constipation, scybalous. Croup. Diphtheria. Eczema marginalis. *Favus. Hands, chapped.* Influenza. Nipples, sore. *Pityriasis versicolor.* Pyrosis. *Stomatitis, ulcerative.*

Characteristics.—Some forty years ago, when the germ theory of disease in its present form was in its infancy, Dewar, of Fife, conceived the idea that *Sulphurous acid* was an innocent and at the same time universal germ destroyer, and consequently universal remedy. His views met with cordial acceptance, and inhalations of *Sulphurous acid* given off from burning *Sulphur* became the fashion. Dewar's method was simple. A few red cinders were put in a kitchen shovel; this was placed in the centre of a room and flowers of sulphur sprinkled thereon. In a very short time every person in the room was sneezing violently, coughing and wheezing, and running at the eyes and nose. Dewar also used the ordinary solution and a spray. Among the special diseases arrested by *Suls. ac.* Dewar named: Chilblains; chapped hands; diphtheria; scarlatina maligna; erysipelas (a local application of equal parts of the B.-P. acid and glycerine); cold in the head, influenza, asthma, bronchitis, croup, clergyman's sore throat, chronic phthisis; typhoid fever. Wounds, sore nipples, bruises were also amenable to its local use. As one who has undergone the "fumigation" process (it was supposed to *prevent* all sorts of maladies, as well as cure, and I suppose it was with that object that I was made to "prove" *Suls. ac.* in my boyhood), I can testify to its homœopathicity in the "cold, coughs, asthma, and influenza" part of Dewar's recommendations. *Suls. ac.* doubtless shares the antiseptic properties of *Sulph.* The symptoms of the Schema are from observations of the effects on workmen in mines, from air contaminated with *Suls. ac.*, with a few additions of my own. Milne sums up its virtues thus: "Antiseptic, disinfectant; a powerful deoxidiser and destroyer of vegetable life." As a gargle it is used in the strength of one to six. In parasitic skin affections the B.-P. solution is used and is effective. Internally, says Milne, it "does good in sarcina" in doses of ℳ xxx. to lx., well diluted with water. Ringer (who endorses most of Dewar's recommendations) says that ten to fifteen minims taken ten minutes before each meal will remedy pyrosis in most instances, and prevents flatulence and fermentations; and that "the solution, either strong or diluted, in varying proportions, speedily removes thrush." This case touches a homœopathic characteristic of *Suls. ac.*—ulcerative inflammation of the mouth. It has cured this in the attenuations. The headache of *Suls. ac.* is > by vomiting. C. Wootton tasted the acid (*H. W.*, xxvi. 204) with this result—it at once stopped the mucous secretion of the bowels, producing scybalous motions. The constipation was so severe that he was in misery for nine months, till he took *Hydrast.*, which cured. The use of *Suls. ac.* as a hair-wash at a later time produced the same result.

Relations.—*Antidoted by:* Hydrast. (constipation). *Compare:* Sul. In ulcerated sore mouth, Nat. m., Caps. The effects on the back recorded by Hahnemann as from the fumes of burning Sulphur were *antidoted by* Electric shock.

SYMPTOMS.

1. **Mind.**—Quite furious.—Disposed to fight.—Extreme terror and efforts to escape; imagine every one wants to lay hands on them.—Listless.—Singing and praying.—As if intoxicated.—Great anxiety.

2. **Head.**—Giddy, lost recollection, as after spirits.—Violent pain and beating in head, with ringing in ears.—Insufferable headache, somewhat > after vomiting.

4. **Ears.**—Ringing in ears with pain in head.

5. **Nose.**—Sneezing and coryza.

8. **Mouth.**—(Ulcerative stomatitis.)

11. **Stomach.**—Many vomited, others had inclination but could not.

13. **Stool and Anus.**—Severe constipation, scybalous motions, lasting nine months; complete dryness of intestinal tract; (*Hydst.* cured at last).—Some evacuated contents of rectum; others had the desire but could not.

17. **Respiratory Organs.**—Persistent choking cough, with copious expectoration of thin mucus.—A difficulty of breathing and frequent involuntary deep inspirations.

18. **Chest.**—Extreme tightness of the chest.

19. **Heart.**—Heart palpitated violently.—Pulse: quiet, feeble; or slow, feeble and irregular.

20. **Back.**—[Stiffness (painful) of spine between scapulæ, during and after movement, with pain as though it were broken.—Painful stiffness in the junction of sacrum with base of pelvis; in morning there occurred very painful jerks. (From the fumes of burning *Sulphur*).]

23. **Lower Limbs.**—Lower limbs weak, very painful immediately above the knees.

Sumbul.

Ferula sumbul. Sumbul. Musk-root. *N. O.* Umbelliferæ. Tincture of the powdered root.

Clinical.—Acne. Asthma. Breasts, pains in. Chorea. Diarrhœa. Epilepsy. Fainting. Heart, palpitation of, nervous; affections of. Pneumonia. Hysteria. Infra-mammary pains. Neuralgia. Porrigo capitis. Spermatorrhœa. Throat, catarrh of; spasm of. Typhoid fever. Worms.

Characteristics.—*Sumbul*, as its name, "Musk-root," implies, has an odour resembling that of musk. The resemblance is so close that *Sumbul* is used to adulterate musk. *Sumb.* was proved by Lembke, Cattell, and others, and the symptoms are as like to those of *Moschus* as the physical resemblance would imply. Hysterical mood; easy fainting; nervous palpitation; are common to both. Hale gives the following indications: (1) Nasal and pharyngeal catarrh, with nervousness, sleeplessness, and tendency to spasms (especially in children); discharge of tenacious, yellow mucus. (2) Ascarides, with bloated, drum-like abdomen and constipation, picking nose (cured with *Sumb.* 15). (3) Oily pellicle in urine. (4) Pain in left uterine region. (5) Asthma: catarrhal, spasmodic, or cardiac. (6) Climacteric flushings. (7) Neuralgia: facial or ovarian, in women of quick and lively nervous constitutions. (8) Neuralgia of left hypochondrium, simulating angina pectoris; with palpitation; in nervous women. (9) Insomnia of chronic alcoholism. *Peculiar Sensations* of *Sumb.* are: Tongue as if scraped. Like a string pulling in right breast. Corkscrew pains in (left) uterus and appendages. Clogged sensation in left chest. As if heart beating in water. The left side was more affected than the right. The symptoms are < by motion. < After sitting. < By inspiration. < By cold. > By warmth. < Thinking of symptoms. < In morning. Music = faintness.

Relations.—*Compare:* General symptoms, Mosch., Asaf. Porrigo, Melit., Medor., Mez. Oily pellicle on urine, Sul., Pul., Petr. Tenacious, yellow mucus, Hydras. Infra-mammary pain, Act. r., Pul., Lil. t. < Thinking of symptoms, Ox. ac., Pip. meth.

SYMPTOMS.

1. **Mind.**—Intellect dull in morning; inability to study; clearer in evening and in warmth.—Happy disposition with continued smiling; expression idiotic; fear of becoming insane (chorea).—Hysterical mood even in men; alternate laughter and tears; easily excited; emotional; irritable, fidgety, at first spirits are exalted, then depressed.

2. **Head.**—Vertigo: on stooping; using warm water; moving about or rising from a seat; feeling a want of security.—Hysteria, with tendency to faint from slightest cause.—Fits with falling forward.—Ebullition of blood in head, lightness and exalted feeling.—Cold in the head, < morning.—Porrigo in infants, l. side of scalp; spots round and dry, slightly raised and reddened at edges with bran-like scales in centre.

3. **Eyes.**—Sensation of foreign body in eyes.—Tight feeling in eyes.—Quivering and swimming before eyes.

4. **Ears.**—Loud surging and hissing in both ears; in r.

5. **Nose.**—Cold in head, < morning.—Coryza: watery; of yellow mucus.—Alæ nasi sore at edges.—Stuffing in nose.—Tenacious yellow mucus in nose; < l. nostril.—Loss of smell.

6. **Face.**—Acne punctata, black pores on face.

8. **Mouth.**—Brown (or white) coating on tongue, morning.—Tongue feels rough as if scraped, with heat in throat.—Increased saliva.

9. **Throat.**—Erosion, burning heat and rawness in throat, with tenacious mucus.—Catarrhs of children with great nervous irritation and spasms.—Choking constriction at top of gullet, constant swallowing.

11. **Stomach.**—Appetite increased.—Eructations; empty.—Nausea and salivation.—Pressure; rumblings; slight shootings in stomach.

12. **Abdomen.**—Tension, pain, and gnawing in r. hypochondrium.—Abdomen feels distended, painful.—Gnawing in r. hypochondrium.—Glands in groins painful.

13. **Stool and Anus.**—Ascarides with bloated, drum-like abdomen and constipation; pricking at nostrils.—Chronic diarrhœa, from inert condition of intestinal canal; discharges cause alarm; diarrhœa in typhoid fever.—Rectum protrudes.—Hæmorrhoids excited.

14. **Urinary Organs.**—Urine: clear; yellowish-red; clouded at bottom, and an oily pellicle on surface.—Frequent desire.—Stitches up urethra.

15. **Male Sexual Organs.**—Absence of erections and all sexual desire.—Itching in genitals with increased desire.—Erythema of scrotum.

16. **Female Sexual Organs.**—Leucorrhœa, white, esp. after sitting.—Menses: premature; of short duration, with deficient quantity; retarded.—Corkscrew pains in l. region of uterus and appendages.—Tensive pain like a string in r. breast.—Tensive pains in l. breast, evening.—Lancinations and biting pains in l. breast, < deep inspirations.—Flushings at climaxis.

17. **Respiratory Organs.**—Hoarseness.—Asthma: catarrhal; but more esp. spasmodic, hysterical.—Hacking cough.

18. **Chest.**—Tightness in chest with diminished secretion.—Paroxysm of dull pressure under sternum.—Tightness, tensive, stretched feeling across chest, between l. breast and sternum and in l. breast, < on inspiration.

19. **Heart.**—Pulse: very irregular, compressible; want of elasticity in vessels.—Nervous affections of heart; rheumatic carditis; heart's impulse strong, jerking, esp. after exertion or during digestion; action of heart full and sharp, strokes at times irregular, rapid, then slow; bellows murmur; flushings of heat in floods from back; sharp pains like a knife in chest; oppression in l. chest, clogged sensation; < on stooping; l. arm numb, heavy, weary, with sharp, wiry shooting in fingers; hysterical mood.—Nervous palpitation in hysterical subjects; or at climaxis.—Heart beats softly, as if in water, with sinking of heart and sickliness and faintness all over.—Palpitation on least excitement, < on paying attention to it.

20. **Neck and Back.**—Cannot keep warm; least draught is felt down spine.—Nape of neck, r. side, swollen.

21. **Limbs.**—L. arm and foot easily chilled.—Fulness of arms and feet.—'remulous tingling, dry, in palms and feet.

22. **Upper Limbs.**—Weakness, beaten sensation, and numbness in rms.—L. arm numb.—Hands red, veins distended.—Fingers swollen.

23. **Lower Limbs.**—Aching, rheumatic pain, weakness of lower limbs. -Pain in knee, with stiffness, impeding walking.—Felt as if her legs were not er own.—Trembling of feet.

24. **Generalities.**—Chorea: constant jerking of head and limbs, with rotusion of tongue; voracious appetite.—Dropsy dependent on impaired ervous vitality.—Clogged sensation in body, esp. in head and stomach.—Iysteria.—Epilepsy; falls forward, foaming at mouth.—Tendency to faint rom slightest cause.

25. **Skin.**—Acne punctata; black pores on face.—Porrigo in infants, l. ide of scalp.—Skin cold, white, shrunken, and dry, as if washed in acrid vater.—Miliary spots on back, r. shoulder-blade, and hip.—Reddish spots on orehead, chin, and cheeks, containing either water or thick, white, curdy natter.—Itching.

26. **Sleep.**—Drowsy in the cold.—Drowsy during day.—Wakefulness at ight.—Sleep interrupted by startings of limbs.—Dreams; of falling; vivid; of coitus, followed by profuse *sudden* emission.

27. **Fever.**—Coldness.—Chilliness, esp. down spine; sensitiveness to east draught.—Too easily chilled; want of elasticity in the vessels.—Numbness and coldness of tips of fingers.—Dry, transient heat all over body. —Typhoid fever with cerebral excitement; low and nervous fevers succeeding typhus.

Symphoricarpus Racemosus.

Symphoricarpus racemosus. Snow-berry. *N. O.* Caprifoliaceæ. Tincture of fresh ripe berries.

Clinical.—Pregnancy, sickness of.

Characteristics.—An account of *Smpho. r.* by E. V. Moffatt is quoted in *New, Old, and Forgotten Remedies.* S. P. Burdick gave the tincture to a lady, who said its effects were "precisely like the morning sickness" she used to have during pregnancy. On other women it produced effects varying from qualmishness to intense vomiting. Moffatt gives these as the leading indications: Qualmishness and indifference to food. Deathly nausea; vomiting continuous, violent retching. One patient was > lying on back. (No particular morning < was observed.) Moffatt gives this case: A young lady, three months advanced in her first pregnancy, had deathly nausea, with vomiting and retching so prolonged and violent as to produce hæmatemesis. The smell or thought of food was repugnant in the extreme. Moffatt gave *Smpho.* 200 (obtained from Dr. Burdick) in the middle of a violent paroxysm. In a few minutes she stopped vomiting, and said she felt soothed and quieted all over. In half an hour nausea began again, but a few pellets checked it promptly and she fell asleep. A few more doses completed the cure. A relapse following over-exertion a month later was speedily remedied by *Smpho*.

Symphytum.

Symphytum officinale. Bone-set. Healing Herb. Comfrey. *N. O.* Boraginaceæ. Tincture of fresh root-stock collected before flowering and in autumn. Tincture of fresh plant.

Clinical.—Abscess. Backache, from sexual excess. Bone, cancer of; injuries of. Breasts, sore. Eyes, pains in; injuries of. *Fractures;* non-union of; nervous. Glands, enlarged. Gunshot wounds. Hernia. Menses, arrested. Periosteum, sensitive, painful. Psoas abscess. Sexual excess, effects of. Sprains. Stump, irritable. Wounds.

Characteristics.—*Symphytum* may be considered the orthopædic specific of herbal medicine. "The roots of Comfrey stamped, and the juice drunk with wine, helpeth those that spit blood and healeth all inward wounds and burstings. The same bruised and laid to in manner of a plaister, doth heal all fresh and green wounds, and are so glutinative, that it will solder and glue together meat that is chopped in pieces, seething in a pot, and make it in one lump" (Gerarde). Peter Squire (*Squire's Companion to B.P.*, 6th ed.) gives as the "medicinal properties" of *Symph.*: "Astringent, mucilaginous, glutinous; useful to form cases for injured limbs. The black rind (of root) is scraped off and the mucilaginous root is then scraped carefully into a nice even pulp; this spread of the thickness of a crown-piece upon cambric or old muslin is wrapped round the limb and bandaged over; it shortly stiffens, and forms a casing superior to starch, giving support and strength to the part." P. Squire knew a bone-setter who practised fifty years ago, and rendered himself famous for setting compound fractures with this root, which he kept secret, and he never removed the bandage after the first dressing until the limb was well (R. T. C.). *Symphytum* has not received its names for nothing. *Consolida* is one of them; and "Comfrey" is derived from *Confirmare.* The glutinous juice of the root seems, according to Gerarde, to have given the key to its action as a vulnerary. H. C. Allen (*Med. Cent.*, quoted *Ind. H. Rev.*, v. 60) refers to the following indications for *Symph.* given by Lippe: (1) When the bone or periosteum has been injured and the soft parts have recovered from the bruised soreness under *Arn.*, the remaining pain and soreness of periosteum may be promptly relieved by *Symp.* (2) In traumatic injuries of bone or periosteum (as from a snowball or anything else on the face), *Symp.* was the only remedy Lippe has seen efficient. He cured many cases after others had used *Arn.* and failed. (3) Here is one of his cures: "More than a year ago fell and struck knee on a stone; wound healed and scarcely left any trace, but there remained an acute stitching pain at point of injury, felt when the part was touched by clothing as when knee was bent." Allen also gives the following cure reported by Fowler: Mrs. J. stepped on the edge of a scantling, which rolled, and she turned her ankle. In a few minutes the ankle began to swell and become painful, pain increasing rapidly, so that in an hour or two patient was in great agony. She declared her leg was broken, she "could feel the rough ends of the broken bones jagging into the flesh"; could not bear any one to approach her for fear of being hurt. No discoloration whatever. *Symp.* promptly relieved, so that she went about her usual duties in forty-eight hours. Allen regards *pricking* pain as a guiding symptom. Next to bone injuries in importance are injuries to the *ball* of the eye, as distinguished from injuries to the *soft parts* around. "I have long since ceased to use *Arn.* in injuries of the globe of the eye, *Symp.* having given such prompt and permanent relief" (H. C. Allen). [I have, however, seen *Arn.* speedily clear up hæmorrhage into the vitreous from a blow of a cork from a soda-water bottle.—J. H. C.] Allen gives these indications: Severe pain in globe of eye after an injury by a blunt instrument (snowball; cane; point of umbrella; infant's fist), the soft parts remaining intact. Croserio (*New, Old, and Forgotten Remedies*) was one of the first to use *Symp.* in the potencies for fractures. P. P. Wells translated Croserio's *Connection of Homœopathy with Surgery*, in which this passage occurs: "Injuries of the bones are healed most promptly with *Symp.* 30, internally, once a day." Wells gives these cases of his own: (1) Boy, 14, broke bone of forearm at junction of middle and lower thirds, two years before. Had twice repeated the fracture by slight falls. Ends now slightly movable on each other, arm of little use. Three doses of *Symp.* made a perfect cure, and the boy became robust and much better in health than he had ever been before. (2) Boy, 8, fractured humerus near junction of condyles and shaft. *Arn.* 30 immediately arrested the spasmodic jerks of muscles of injured arm. *Arn.* was continued three days, by which time all traumatic fever had subsided. *Symp.* 3, one drop in half a tumbler of water; a teaspoonful morning and evening. The splints were removed the ninth day, and the bone found consolidated. The cure was entirely without pain. F. H. Brett (*H. W.*, xxv. 304) cured himself of inguinal rupture by rubbing the part with tincture of the root. On another occasion a blow on the lower part of the back from a fall resulted in a secondary affection of the spine in the mid-dorsal region, a protuberance as if from a slight dislocation appearing at the spot. Again *Symp.* φ was applied. The tenderness at the point subsided after three applications, and in a few days the protuberance disappeared. Brett mentions (*ib.*, 379) a case he had heard of: A diseased arm which had begun to mortify was dressed with a poultice of Comfrey root, and this "drew off the mortified substance, and the arm became sound again." Sir Wm. Thomson, of Dublin (*Lancet*, Nov. 28, 1896) relates a case of malignant tumour of the antrum which had extended to the nose. Microscopical examination proved it to be round-celled sarcoma. The patient, a man, was advised to have the jaw removed. This advice was refused at the time, and was repeated by Felix Semon, who saw the man later. After still further delay Thomson performed the operation in the month of May, 1896. A month later the growth began to show again, increased rapidly, closed the right eye, was blue, tense, firm, lobulated, but did not break. Thomson declined to operate again. Early in October the man walked into Thomson's study well: "The tumour had completely disappeared from the face, and I could not identify any trace of it in the mouth." The man had applied poultices of Comfrey root, and the swelling disappeared. Cooper (*H. W.*, xxxii. 403) gives this experience of a patient of his: Just before her marriage she had a dangerous attack of scarlatina, leaving abscesses on both sides of the neck and great internal swelling, so that she could swallow only liquids, and that with great difficulty. The external swelling extended from ear to chin, and was hard and very painful. Poultices of Comfrey root were applied. The pain was immediately relieved and her abscesses decreased rapidly until they were entirely absorbed, without external opening so far as the patient could remark. Hering (from whom I have taken the main part of my Schema) says *Symp.* has had a fragmentary proving by Macfarlan. Gerarde adds to the uses of *Symp.* quoted from him above that it eases pains in the back from violent motion as wrestling, or from excessive sexual indulgence, even when spermatorrhœa has been induced thereby. *Arn.* has an analogous use. *Peculiar Sensations* are: As if upper lid passed over an elevation on closing eye. As if ears were stopped up. The symptoms are: < By touch. Sitting = pain about navel. Stooping = weight in forehead. Walking = pain opposite spleen.

Relations.—*Follows well:* Arn. (for pricking pains; and after the bruising of the soft parts is healed). *Compare:* Fractures, Calc. ph. Injuries, Arn. (Arn., soft parts, Symp., hard; Arn., painful swelling with discoloration, Symp., without discoloration; Arn., sore, bruised lame; Symp., pricking, stitching, jagging pains), Calen., Fl. ac., Hep., Sil., Stp., Led., Rhus, Hyper. Effects of sexual excess, Arn. *Antidote to* Canthar. (Green's *Herbal*).

Causation.—Fractures. Injuries (to eye; bone; periosteum). Falls. Blows. Sexual excess.

SYMPTOMS.

2. **Head.**—Headache in occiput, in top of head, in forehead, changing places.

3. **Eyes.**—Pain in eyes after a knock or contusion of an opaque body.—After being struck upon eye with a cane by a child, no visible injury, but a sensation on closing eye as if upper lid passed over an elevation on bulb of eye; on waking eye could not be easily opened, seemed spasmodically closed.

4. **Ears.**—Cannot hear well; feels as if ears were stopped up.—Inflamed ears.

5. **Nose**—Pain comes down bone of nose, and sometimes down both sides of nose (produced.—R. T. C.).

6. **Face.**—(Malignant tumour of r. antrum.)—Inflammation of inferior maxillary bone; hard, red swelling.

11. **Stomach.**—Pains across epigastrium from one side to other, < pposite spleen, in walking; when sitting < about navel; griping pain.

13. **Stool and Anus.**—(Dysentery.—Inflamed and bleeding piles.)

14. **Urinary Organs.**—Stricture of urethra (curative in some forms.—R. T. C.).

15. **Male Sexual Organs.**—Testicles become painful and tender and revent walking (produced.—R. T. C.).—(Backache from excessive sexual ndulgence; with spermatorrhœa.—Gerarde.)

16. **Female Sexual Organs.**—Menses stopped; headache, weight in orehead when she stoops; has it almost all time; a good deal of fever every ther hour; cold all day, cramp and diarrhœa; nose sore inside alæ, wants o pick it; wants to rub her eyes; inflamed ears; feels as if something were n them, stopped up, cannot hear well.—(Leucorrhœa.—Sore breasts.)

20. **Neck and Back.**—Pain in back from a fall; from sexual excess.—Pott's disease from fall.—Psoas abscess.—Much used among herbalists in aries of spinal and other bones (R. T. C.).

21. **Limbs.**—Seems to act specially on the joints; a woman, 50, after ingle dose of ϕ complained of loss of power in the large joints, they seemed o get fixed, being particularly painful on turning in bed; and then followed great working in all the joints, esp. in feet, with prickings and shootings in oes of both feet (R. T. C.).

23. **Lower Limbs.**—More than a year ago struck knee upon a stone; wound healed and left scarcely any trace, but there remained an acute titching pain in the place, felt when clothing touched part, or when knee was ent.—Man suffering from a spontaneous luxation of thigh since childhood, ell and received a fracture of affected thigh; after two months fragments were quite movable, and as union was despaired of, an apparatus was made which allowed him to sit on a chair during day; *Symp.* 4, four globules very six hours, brought about complete union in twenty days.

24. **Generalities.**—Bruises, sprains; sore breasts.—Inflammation of bones; diseased spinous processes.—Psoas abscess.—Facilitates union of ractured bones and lessens peculiar pricking pain; favours production of callous.—Pricking, sticking, jagging pains.—"A conserve of the roots cures he whites, and a decoction of them is excellent in coughs and soreness of the breast. Dried and powdered they are good against fluxes of the belly attended with griping pains and bloody stools. [*Symph.*] is also serviceable n defluxions of the lungs, spitting of blood, and other disorders of the chest.—Bruised and applied to foul ulcers it cleanses and disposes them to heal. It removes the inflammation and stops the bleeding of piles; and is of considerable efficacy in ulcerations of the kidneys and urinary passages, particularly if occasioned by the use of *Cantharides*" (Thos. Green's *Herbal*).

Syphilinum.

Luesinum. Lueticum. Syphilitic virus. A nosode. Attenuations

Clinical.—Abscess; succession of abscesses. Alcoholism; hereditary cravin for alcohol. Anus, fissure of. Aphasia. Asthma. Breasts; sensitive. Bubo Constipation. Crying of infants. Deafness. Deltoid rheumatism. Dentition Diplopia. Dysmenorrhœa. Epilepsy. Headache; syphilitic. Hoarseness; befor menses. Iritis. Leucorrhœa; infantile. Mouth, ulcerated. Myopia. Neuralgi Night-sweats. Ophthalmia. Otorrhœa. Ovaries, affections of. *Ozæna.* Pemphigu Psoas abscess. Ptosis. Rectum, stricture of. Rheumatism. Sciatica. Sleepless ness. Spine, caries of. Strabismus. Stricture. Sunstroke. Syphilis. Teeth, carious Throat, ulcerated. Tibia, pains in. Tongue, cracked, ulcerated. Ulcers Whitlow.

Characteristics.—I learnt the value of this nosode from Skinner who has made with it some very brilliant cures. It has been proved by Swan in the potencies, and Hering's Schema, from which mine is taken, comprises also disease symptoms—marked "(n)"— and cured symptoms, which have generally the name and the disease appended. Cured cases of secondary syphilis I have marked "(s.s.)." The widespread distribution of syphilis, acquired and hereditary, and the virulence and persistence of the virus, give this nosode a high degree of importance in homœopathic practice. It has been mainly, almost exclusively, employed by those who are familiar with the use of high attenuations. I have used no potency lower than 200, and rarely repeat the dose oftener than once a week The leading features of the disease are the keynotes for the use of the remedy, and (1) first in importance is the "Night <": "Pains from *darkness to daylight;* begin with twilight and end with daylight." "All symptoms < at night." "Terrible dread of night, on account of mental and physical exhaustion on awaking." This night aggravation will be found in a large proportion of the cases needing *Syph.;* in ophthalmia, the pains are < at night, and during the night the lids grow together. Neuralgia, and headache, asthma, coughs < from sunset to sunrise, whether syphilitic or not, will be benefited by *Syph* Sleeplessness is itself a leading indication for *Syph.*, which vies with *Sul.* as a sleep restorer. (2) Next to the Night <, is Ulceration: this may affect mouth, nose, genitals, or skin, and the ulcers have greyish bases; in the nose they produce the most offensive form of ozæna with discharge of fetid clinkers. In such cases I have found *Syph.* of the greatest service. Fetid discharges from the ear come in the same category. (3) Abscesses with foul secretions. (All pus formations of *Syph.* are fetid.) *Succession of abscesses* is one of the grand keynotes of the materia medica. Eyes, teeth, and skin give other leading indications. In ophthalmia neonatorum the lids adhere during sleep; pains < 2 to 5 a.m.; pus profuse; > cold bathing Iritis, syphilitic or rheumatic, has been cured with *Syph.* Ptosis sleepy look from drooping lids. Diplopia, one image seen below the other. Teeth decay at the edge of the gums and break off; are cupped have serrated edges; dwarfed in size and converge at their tips. The typical eruption of *Syph.* is copper-coloured spots, but it covers many

ther forms, including pemphigus. The glandular system is affected
iroughout and nutrition impaired, leading to extreme emaciation.
Burnett has recorded in his book on *Delicate Children* many
istances of the power of *Syph.* to free stunted children from this
onstitutional blight. Further indications for *Syph.* are : Pains < and
> gradually; are shifting, and require frequent change of position.
eucorrhœa ; profuse, soaking through napkins and running to heels.
Craving for alcohol in any form. Hereditary tendency to alcoholism.
Bacchus and Venus are close allies). The orifices of the body are
ll affected by syphilis, and *Syph.* has a great sphere in rectal pain
nd constipation. "Obstinate constipation for years ; rectum seems
ed up with strictures ; when enema was used the agony of passage
vas like labour." Bones are affected, and especially bones of head
nd tibiæ. Nodes on the head. H. C. Allen says: "Syphilitics, or
atients who have had chancre treated by local means, and as a result
ave suffered from throat and skin troubles for years, are nearly always
enefited by this remedy at commencement of treatment unless some
ther remedy is clearly indicated." Thomas Wildes (*H. P.*, xi. 267)
ives his experience with *Syph.* In chancre he gives *Syph.* 1m (Swan)
–according to Skinner's calculation this is much lower than 1m of the
entesimal scale—one dose every night. The chancre increases for the
rst two weeks and then gradually fades away, not being followed
y secondaries. Where the edges of the chancre assume the appear-
nce of proud flesh in the third or fourth week, and become everted,
agged, and angry dark red, he gives *Lac can.* cm (Swan) every night
or ten to fourteen days, until the sore takes on a more natural appear-
nce, when *Syph.* 1m is again given to finish the case. For any
emaining induration *Nit. ac.* 30, four times a day, is given. Head-
ches in great variety he cured with it ; aphasia ; ptosis ; paralysis of
ongue ; facial paralysis ; hemiplegia ; "persistent pains in any part
f the body ;" catarrhal and nerve deafness ; itching of nostrils ;
ark purple lines between alæ nasi and cheeks. Itching scabby
ruptions on face or breast ; singly or in clusters, looking like herpes.
Pain and pressure behind sternum. Epilepsy. Wildes cured with
yph. 1m a bookkeeper who for many months had had a piercing,
ressing, excruciating headache over right eye extending deep into
rain. It was so severe, he was losing continuity of thought and
nemory. Under *Syph.* every night the headache disappeared entirely in
en days and the mental faculties were fully restored ; but in six
veeks the whole eyebrow on that side broke out into a sickly, yellow,
yphilitic eczema with a red, angry, and oozing base extending under
he arch to the lid from canthus to canthus up into forehead and down
he side of the nose. The cure of this was tedious, because, Wildes
hinks, he did not stick to *Syph.*, but changed the remedy. This man
ad had syphilis a few years before. In 1879 a lady, 26, extremely
right and intelligent, came to Wildes with a dreadful ozæna. She had
lso curvature of the spine and congestion of right ovary. Always
elicate from a child. *Syph.* cured the ozæna and improved the
ealth, but it "drove out a saddle to which the *Sepia* saddle
 but a shadow"—a furious inflammatory mass of syphilitic sores,
cabs, and eczema, red and angry, with a fiery base extending from

one malar prominence to the other, across nose up to eyes and fore
head. This took eighteen months to cure. The ozæna never returne
A boy, 4, had an obstinate rash, a combination of prurigo and herpes, o
chin, lips, cheek-bone, forehead, and hairy scalp; on arms, chest, bac
bends of joints and on the joints, and on fingers and hands, nowhe
profuse. In spite of authorities to the contrary, Wildes maintai
that syphilitic rashes may itch, and that prurigo is infectious and is or
of the initial stages of leprosy. This boy had a spot of eruption c
the left thigh the size of the top-joint of a man's thumb. This wa
distinctly a leper spot. *Syph.* 1m caused the rash to come out strong
all over the body in patches, the face was one-third covered with
thick, yellow, scabby eruption. The remedy was continued and th
boy got well, wonderfully improved in health, no longer nervou
growing well; sleeping well; appetite good. Girl, 16, had measl
a year before which did not come out properly. A year and a ha
prior thereto subject to neuralgic headaches. Ailing about two years
very despondent, wants to die, headaches growing more viole
During the headaches the temple veins stand out, has pains all ov
the body, is very irritable, restless, *walking about much of the tim*
does not wish to be soothed, *violent on being opposed*, has tremo
and *seems on the verge of convulsions*, dazed, *absent-minded*, and almo
insane. Always washing her hands. Was formerly constipated, b
now subject to "a kind of diarrhœa." Menses never have come
properly, and for the past year have been very irregular, much delaye
scanty, and *always extremely painful.* Often feverish. Sleep anxio
distressed, and often *wakeful* and violently *restless.* The italicis
symptoms indicated *Syph.*, and under this she steadily recovered.
young lady contracted "lepra-syphilis" from vaccination. She h
an immense blood-boil on her arm which would not heal. Fa
broken out with a lumpy fiery rash. With *Syph.* 1m at bedtime s
recovered rapidly; the arm healed quickly and her face became fr
from eruption. Boy, 3, had cluster of yellow blotches on fing
and roots of nails, distorting the nails. The boy's father was epilep
The boy was helped with *Fluor. ac.* and cured with *Syph.*, the na
becoming straight. Many persons, says Wildes, after taking *Syph.*
a few days, complained of heavy, crushing, cutting pains across t
base of the cerebellum; others of heavy aching and stiffness fr
base of neck up through muscles and cords of neck and into t
brain; others of a heavy, clouded, dull feeling at base of brain w
physical lethargy, and sometimes with dizziness, sometimes w
confusion of thoughts and often a feeling as if going insane or ab
to be paralysed. Sometimes a far-away feeling, with a feeling
indifference to the future. Accompanying these there may come
heavy, dragging, dull feeling in lumbar region, with stiffness and wa
of elasticity. *Peculiar Sensations are:* A seething feeling as if
water or hot oil running through all veins of the body, all night lo
As if going insane or about to be paralysed. Tongue feels as
paralysed. A far-away feeling with apathy. As if head were pul
back by a weight. As if blood went to right inner canthus a
temples and could get no further. As if sand in eyes. As if ri
eye were wide open and cold air were blowing in it. Fluttering a

something alive in teeth. As if a worm in tooth. As if teeth had got out of place. Distress as if in omentum. As if rectum were tied up with strictures. As if urethra had been stuffed up and clogged. As if sternum was being drawn towards dorsal vertebræ. As if she would suffocate with cough. As if skin were drawn up in centre of chest on drawing back head. Coccyx as if swollen. As if toes on right foot were disjointed. Like growing-pains in limbs. As if bones were sawed. Palms and soles as if pricked by needles. As if throat tearing to pieces. As if top of head were coming off. As if teeth were loose. As of a nervous chill commencing in anus and running down legs. As if bitten by bugs. A number of *linear* pains have been observed in *Syph.* cases. G. H. Carr (*M. A.*, xvii. 162) relates this case : An old man had been troubled two or three winters with an *intense cold pain* in both legs ; it came on every night on lying down ; and lasted all night, the only relief being by getting up and walking. Magnetic leggings had given most relief. *Syph.* mm, one dose daily, was given. He lost the pain for six weeks, when it returned in milder form. *Syph.* cmm was given, and he had no more pains all the winter. This medicine, he said "made his genitals ache so that he couldn't sit still." This lasted over a month. *Syph.* cm cured (*ibid.*) a lady of "asthma" that she had had for twenty-five years, the attack coming on *only at night after lying down*, or *during a thunder-storm.* Swan (*M. A.*, xxviii. 239) says he gave crying infants, when they developed the propensity immediately after birth and did not cease, one dose of *Syph.* cmm, and it was difficult to make them cry after that. Yingling (*M. A.*, xxix. 135) reports this case : Rev. D., 30, dark, free from venereal taint, had a constant dull, heavy ache above inner angle of right eye, very distressing, with an occasional *thrust as of an iron rod from the same spot* through to lower part of occiput. This thrust was excruciating. He was due to preach next day, but the pain quite incapacitated him, hence his appeal for help. Haggard look. *Syph.* cm, one dose, was given. He was free from pain before he reached home, next morning was perfectly well. The symptoms are < by touch (tibia ; os uteri). Pressure = pain in spot middle of thigh ; > throat ; pressing teeth together > toothache. No position suits. Motion <. Raising arms laterally <. Walking > pain in hips and thighs. < At night. Warmth and cold < and >. Warmth > headache ; of stove > pain in swollen wrist and big toe. Hot or cold things < toothache. Cold water > ophthalmia pains. Damp weather ; warm, damp weather ; thunderstorm ; seaside <. > In mountains. < Winter.

Relations.—*Compare :* In bone diseases and syphilitic affections, Aur., Asaf., K. iod., Merc., Nit. ac. < At night, Aur., Merc., Sul. (Med. and Sycotics < early morning). < At sea-shore ; > inland (Med. opp). < At seaside ; averse to consolation, Nat. m. Dysmenorrhœa, Med. Deep-in headache, Bac. Pains increase and decrease slowly, Stn. Ozæna with offensive clinkers. Sep., Pul., Pso., K. bi. Succession of abscesses (Anthrac., succession of boils). Syphilitic stomatitis, Lach., Lac c., Merc. Nodes, K. iod., K. bi., Mang., Merc. Emaciation, Abrot, Iod. Lancinating pains in heart (from base to apex), Med. (from apex to base), Spi. (from base to clavicle or shoulder).

Fears suffering from exhaustion on awaking, Lach. Ptosis, Caust., Graph. Hereditary tendency to alcoholism, Asar., Pso., Tub., Sul., Sul. ac. Constipation with labour-like pains. Lac d., Tub. Fissure in anus, Thuj. Shoulder rheumatism < raising arm laterally, Rhus, Sang. (r. shoulder), Fer. (left), Urt. ur. Dentition troubles < night (Med. < early morning). Hereditary syphilis ; dentition, Kre. Vertigo < looking up (Sul., looking down). As if teeth out of place (Tub. as if jammed together). Thunder, effect of, Pho.

Causation.—Sun. Damp weather. Thunderstorms.

SYMPTOMS.

1. **Mind.**—Loss of memory (n).—Loses remembrances of passing occurrences, names, dates, &c., while all occurrences previous to inception of disease are remembered as distinctly as ever (n).—Very nervous, weeping without cause.—Cross, irritable, peevish.—Irritable, excited, walking much of the time, does not want to be soothed, violent on being opposed, has tremors, seems on the verge of convulsions, dazed, absent-minded, always washing her hands.—Periodical neuralgia in head (neuralgia).—Very despondent, does not think will ever get better (s.s.).—Teribile dread of night ; always < as night approaches ; leaves her about daylight, which she prays for (spring cough).—Feeling as if going insane, or about to be paralysed.—A far-away feeling, with apathy and indifference to future.—Crying infants, who begin immediately after birth.

2. **Head.**—Vertigo on looking up, seems to be caused by heat.—Headache : linear, from or near one eye backward ; lateral ; frontal ; from temple to temple ; deep into brain from vertex ; as from pressure on vertex ; in either temple, extending into or from eye > by warmth ; in bones of head ; < by heat of sun ; after sunstroke.—Sick-headache, pains intolerable, arteries of head full and pulsating violently ; high fever, frequent retching on trying to vomit ; menses regular, but very scanty.—Lancinating pain in occiput, invariably < at night (n).—Neuralgic headache causing sleeplessness or delirium at night, always commencing about 4 p.m. ; < at from 10 to 11 and ceasing at daylight.—Bursting sensation in vertex as from severe cold.—Pain from eyes through to occiput, with sensation of weight in occiput drawing head back ; or as if it were pulled back ; eyes ache and smart.—Constant linear headache, commencing at both angles of forehead and extending in parallel lines backward—a precursor of epileptic attack.—Heavy, crushing, cutting pain across base of cerebellum.—Heavy, clouded, dull feeling in base of brain.—Headache through temples, thence vertically like an inverted letter T.—Coronal headache (s.s.).—Headaches accompanied by great restlessness, sleeplessness and general nervous erethism.—Syphilitic headache for many months, piercing, pressing excruciating over r. eye ; extending deep into brain ; losing continuity of thought and memory ; makes repeated mistakes in figures.—Suffusion and full feeling in face, throat, and head, with innumerable small enlarged cervical glands.—Sore, one and a half inches in diameter, on occipital bone, covered with a thick, yellow-white scab.—Dirty eruption on scalp.—Great loss of hair (n).

3. **Eyes.**—Red papulous eruption round l. inner canthus, with isolated pimples on side of nose, cheek and eyebrow; these pimples were red, with depressed centre, circumscribed areola, became confluent where they were most dense; pimples bleed when scabs come off; agglutination of lids.—Myopia (n).—Sharp, pulsating pain, occasionally at outer end of superior border of r. orbit, apparently in periosteum.—Upper lids swollen.—Ptosis: paralytica; eyes look sleepy from lowering of upper lid.—Diplopia, one image seen lower than the other.—Strabismus paralytica, eye turning inward, and pupil can only be turned outward as far as median line.—Chronic recurrent phlyctenular inflammation of cornea; successive crops of phlyctenules and abrasion of epithelial layer of cornea; intense photophobia; profuse lachrymation; redness and pain well marked; delicate, scrofulous children, esp. if any trace of hereditary syphilis remains.—L. eyeball covered with fungus-like growth, pain intense, < at night.—Acute ophthalmia neonatorum (n).—Redness and swelling of outer half of both lower tarsal edges.—Syphilitic iritis, intense pain steadily increasing night after night; < between 2 and 5 a.m., coming almost at the minute and ceasing same way (s.s.).—Pain in r. inner canthus as if blood went there and could go no farther; also in r. temple (rheumatic iritis).—Both eyes glued in morning; conjunctiva injected; photophobia, constantly wears a shade.—Eyes dull.—Infantile syphilis.—Ophthalmic pains, < at night, > by cold water.—R. eye alone affected congestion of conjunctiva and sclerotica, with some chemosis; lids inflamed, esp. at outer canthus; sensation of sand in eyes; lids agglutinated in morning; great photophobia (hereditary syphilis).—Neuralgia every night, beginning about 8 or 9 p.m., gradually increasing in severity until it reached its height about 3 or 4 a.m., and after continuing thus for two or three hours gradually decreased and finally ceased about 10 a.m. (rheumatic ophthalmia).

4. **Ears.**—Intense earache in r. ear, incisive pains thrusting into ear; purulent watery discharge from ear with pain.—Gathering in l. ear which discharges a great quantity of pus (hereditary syphilis in a child).—Deafness gradually increasing until she could scarcely hear at all.—Complete deafness; nothing abnormal to be seen.—Catarrhal or nerve deafness with marked cachexia.—Calcareous deposit on tympanum.—Small, acrid, watery discharge occasionally from ears, no deafness (ozæna).

5. **Nose.**—L. side of nose, inside ala, itching.—Nose stuffed up and burning.—Attacks of fluent coryza.—Offensive, thick yellow-green nasal discharge; during sleep dry scabs form in both nostrils; following an application of salve for sore eyes; l. submaxillary gland, which had been swollen and indurated, softens, discharges and, after forty-five days, begins to heal slowly.—Ozæna syphilitica; (*Syph.* brought out an eruption of sores with a fiery-red base on nose and over frontal sinuses).—L. side of nose inside and out very sore, likewise lips and chin; sores itching and scabbing over.—Itching in nostrils.

6. **Face.**—Face drawn to one side, difficulty of speaking, masticating, blowing (n).—Spasmodic twitching of many muscles, esp. in face (paralysis agitans), with great melancholy and depression of spirits.—Facial paralysis r. side, thick speech, hemicrania, jactitation of r. eye and lid.—An old gentleman has had for some years cancer on r. malar bone; no rest, his agony excruciating in extreme (relieved).—Face pale.—Itching, scabby, eczematous eruptions

singly or in clusters, looking like herpes.—Nose and cheeks covered with eruptions and scabs in layers rising to a point.—Dark purple lines between alæ nasi and cheeks.—Lips and teeth covered with bloody mucus.—Sores on lips and chin, esp. l. side scabbing over.

7. **Teeth.**—Single small lunæ cleft in upper incisors, permanent set, which incisors are dwarfed in their general dimensions, and converge at their tips; inherited syphilis (n).—Children's teeth are cupped.—Teeth decaying at edge of gum and breaking off (n).—Felt like a worm in tooth, could not tell which tooth.—Singular feeling as if teeth had all got out of place, and on closing jaws teeth do not come well together.

8. **Mouth.**—Tongue red and thick; two deep cracks running lengthwise in it; one on each side of median line.—Aphasia, difficulty of finding words; debility.—Tongue feels as if paralysed.—Fetid breath.—Tongue coated; white, edges indented by teeth.—Putrid taste in mouth before epileptic fit.—Tongue very red and thick; covered with herpetic eruption, two deep cracks running lengthwise on each side of median line, making it difficult to swallow (s.s.).—Tongue thickly coated, dirty, edges indented or serrated by teeth (n.).—Twenty ulcers in mouth, every part involved, top and under side of tongue, lips, buccal cavity, fauces and nose; septum of nose threatened, both alæ nasi very painful, smarting with burning as if on fire; pains and burning prevented sleep; hungry but could eat nothing but fluids as mastication was impossible; tongue heavily coated white, large quantities of stringy, viscid, saliva running from mouth of a sweetish taste; a putrid, sickening odour filled whole house; all symptoms < toward night (s.s.).—Herpetic eruption in mouth, tonsils, hard palate and fauces, completely covering inside of mouth and throat, making it very difficult to swallow even liquids.—Syphilitic destruction of hard and soft palates.

9. **Throat.**—Chronic hypertrophy of tonsils (hereditary syphilis).—Chancrous ulcer extending across velum palati to l. pillar of pharnyx (s.s.).—Acute pharyngitis (s.s.).

10. **Appetite.**—Appetite indifferent and capricious (psoas abscess).—Total loss of appetite for months, little or nothing satisfies him; formerly was generally ravenous.—Thirst.—Tendency to heavy drinking; alcoholism.—Aversion to meat.—Dyspepsia; flatulence, belching of wind; nervous dyspepsia.

11. **Stomach.**—Nausea.—Heartburn with pain and rawness from stomach to throat-pit, often with cough.—Vomiting for weeks or months due to erosion from superficial ulceration of lining of viscus, herpetic, of syphilitic origin.

12. **Abdomen.**—Pain or distress deep in abdomen as if in omentum.—Feeling of heat internally in hypogastric region.—Pain in r. groin followed by swelling of glands.—Large painless bubo in r. groin opened and discharged freely (s.s.).—Slight lancinating pain in one groin, < at night.—Inguinal bubo.

13. **Stool and Anus.**—Bowels torpid for five weeks (periodical neuralgia in head).—Obstinate constipation for many years; rectum seemed tied up with strictures, when injections were given agony of passage was like child-bearing.—Chronic constipation, with fetid breath, earthy complexion, gaunt appearance.—Stools very dark and offensive (infantile syphilis).—Bilious diarrhœa at seashore, painless, driving her out of bed about 5 a.m.; stools

during day, later causing excoriation; face red, suffers from heat; occasional painless, whitish diarrhœa when at home, always > by going to mountains.—Fissures in anus and rectum.—Two indurated ulcers at mouth of anus somewhat sore; slight itching of anus (primary syphilis).

14. **Urinary Organs.**—Itching in orifice of urethra.—A sensation, in morning on going to urinate, as if male urethra were stuffed up or clogged, about an inch from orifice.—Scalding urine.—Urination difficult and very slow; no pain, but a want of power, so that he has to strain.—Urine infrequent, not oftener than once in twenty-four hours, scanty, of a golden-yellow colour.—Profuse urination after chill; passed during night nearly a chamberful.—Rich lemon-yellow scanty urine.—Frequent urging to urinate all night, at least from 7 p.m. until 5 a.m.

15. **Male Sexual Organs.**—Chancre on prepuce.—Buboes.—Burning in chancre size of a split pea, on prepuce above corona glandis; edges raised, bottom covered with lardaceous deposit; glans purple, on l. side covered by an exudation.—Chancre on penis, third in two years, all on same spot (s.s.).—Aching of genitals, could not sit still for over a month.—After suppressed chancre, disease attacked testes and scrotum, which became painful and swollen; this was supposed to be cured, but ever since, every few weeks, if exposed at all to damp weather would be seized with pain as if in kidneys, seemingly traversing ureters, but instead of passing into bladder followed spermatic cord, down groins and into testes; pain agonising, chiefly in cord, in present attack in r.; pricking in chancre.—Chancroid, phagedænic, spreading rapidly; buboes commencing in each groin.—Inflammation and induration of spermatic cord.

16. **Female Sexual Organs.**—Uterus and all surrounding parts loose, soft and flabby; profuse, thick, yellow leucorrhœa; constant pain across small of back.—Yellow offensive leucorrhœa, watery or not, so profuse it daily soaks through napkins and runs to heels of stockings if much on her feet.—Profuse yellow leucorrhœa, < at night; in sickly, nervous children (inherited syphilis).—Soreness of genitals, and muco-purulent discharge, in a child.—Acrid discharge causing violent itching and inflammation of external organs, < at night from warmth of bed, parts very tender; itching and inflammation > during menses.—Nocturnal < of r. ovarian pain, preventing sleep.—Sore on r. labium majus, extending to l. (s.s.).—Menstruation painful, two weeks too soon; pink-red, bright, profuse, running free for some days; napkins wash easily.—Painful menstruation.—Sensitiveness of os uteri, < to intolerable pain at menses, or on introduction of finger or penis; frequently causes abortion (n).—Sharp zigzag shooting pains in region of uterus.—Ovaries congested and inflamed; tendency to ovarian tumours.—Sore aching in l. ovarian region, extending to r. with darting pains.—L. ovary swollen, during coitus, at moment of orgasm, a sharp cutting pain like a knife, and twice there was smarting as of a sore; ovary swelled so much that its size and shape could easily be felt through abdominal walls (caused by *Buboin*).—Uterine and ovarian diseases with pronounced nervous disorders, esp. in married women.—Mammæ sensitive to touch, feeling sore; during menses, and at other times.

17. **Respiratory Organs.**—Hoarse, almost complete aphonia, day before menses.—Diseased cartilages of larynx (tertiary syphilis).—Chronic

asthma, in summer, esp. when weather was warm and damp ; most frequently in evening, passing off at daybreak.—Pain and oppression at bifurcation of bronchia and in larynx, it hurts her to breathe.—Attacks of spasmodic bronchial asthma for twenty-five years ; they come on only at night after lying down or during a thunderstorm, producing most intense nervous insomnia, entirely preventing sleep for days and nights.—Violent attacks of dyspnœa, wheezing and rattling of mucus, from 1 to 4 a.m.—Cough : hard cough < at night, when it is continuous, preventing sleep.—Hard, constant cough, with thick, yellow, tasteless expectoration.—Dry, racking cough, with thick, purulent expectoration, caused by a sensation of rasping or scraping in throat, always at night.—Whooping-cough with terrible vomiting.—Cannot lie on r. side, as it causes a dry cough.—Muco-purulent expectoration, greyish, greenish, greenish-yellow, tasteless.—Expectoration without cough, quite clear, white, feels like a round ball and rushes into mouth.

18. **Chest.**—Rattling in chest and throat.—Soreness of chest, with great anguish and inability to retain a recumbent position ; in winter, severe bronchial cough succeeded asthmatic attacks ; a regular type of chills and fever developed ; suffered from this many years ago.—Pain in centre of chest as if skin were drawn up, on drawing the head back.—Lack of sleep produces a sudden faintness and sinking sensation in chest ; three spells succeeded each other during a single night.—Oppression of chest to such an extent as almost to arrest breathing ; asthma caused by sensation as if sternum were being gradually drawn towards dorsal vertebræ ; expansion of chest difficult ; confusion of mind as if unconsciousness might follow.—Sensation of pressure under upper part of sternum.—Pain and pressure behind sternum.—Angina ; ptosis l. eye ; facial paralysis l. side, slight aphasia ; impotence (relieved).—Eczematous herpetic eruptions on chest.

19. **Heart.**—Lancinating pains in heart at night, from base to apex (*Medor.* has reverse).—Valvular disease of heart.

20. **Neck and Back.**—Heavy aching and stiffness from base of neck up through muscles and cords into brain.—Caries of cervical spine with great curvature in same region, directly forward ; pain in curvature always < at night (no proof of syphilis).—Enlargement of cervical glands and a number of pedunculated pin-head warts on neck ; cured by *Syco-syphilinum* (hereditary syphilis ; girl, 10).—Enlargement of glands in different parts of body, particularly abundant about neck ; indurated and slightly painful, causing a sensation of fulness and suffusion in face, throat and head (n).—Enormous swelling of glands of head and neck (Hodgkin's disease).—Rigidity of muscles.—A heavy, dragging, dull feeling in lumbar region, with want of elasticity.—Great pain in back in region of kidneys, < after urinating (s.s.).—Pains commencing in sacral regions internally, and apparently coming around to uterus.—Pain at coccyx at its junction with sacrum, sometimes in lower sacral vertebræ ; < on sitting, with a sensation as if swollen, though it is not.—Caries of dorsal vertebræ with acute curvature, for five months, every night most intense neuralgic pains, commencing generally from 5 to 7 p.m., and never terminating till about 5 a.m. ; < by least motion, and slightly > by warm poultices.—Psoas abscess first l. then r.—Nocturnal < of pains in back, hips and thighs.

21. **Limbs.**—Aching pains in limbs like growing pains.—Gradual

rigidity of all joints after eruption ; flexors seem contracted.—Rheumatic swelling of l. wrist and big toe, bluish red, with pains as if somebody sawed at his bones with a dull saw ; > by heat of stove ; < from sundown to sunrise ; no appetite ; has lasted two weeks (rheumatism).—Feeling of numbness in palms and soles, at times a prickly sensation as if numb parts were punctured by a great number of needles.—Excruciating arthritis ; swelling, heat, and redness intense.—Rheumatism, muscles are caked in hard knots or lumps.

22. **Upper Limbs.**—Rheumatism of shoulder-joint or at insertion of deltoid, < from raising arm laterally.—Can only raise arms to a right angle with axilla ; trying to force them higher causes muscles to suddenly become paralysed and they drop pendant (n).—Lameness and pain of arm on motion, < on raising arm up in front as if reaching ; pain located about insertion of deltoid in upper third of humerus, not painful to pressure.—Fingers and thumbs have runarounds (infantile syphilis).—Always washing the hands.—Hands badly ulcerated on backs (s.s.).—R. second finger swollen and stiffened (s.s.).

23. **Lower Limbs.**—Swelling of legs from knees down, soles painful when standing on them ; swelling goes down in morning, comes back at night.—Pains in lower extremities, excruciating, completely banish sleep ; < from hot fomentations ; > pouring cold water on them (n).—Cannot sit in a low chair, or squat down, owing to loss of control over knee and hip-joints (n).—Pains in long bones of lower extremities, also in joints (n).—Dull pain over backs of feet to toes, began soon after getting into bed, lasting until 4 or 5 a.m.—For two or three winters intense cold pain in both legs, < in l., came on every night on lying down, lasting all night ; > by getting up and walking, and in warm weather.—Pain in three toes of r. foot as if disjointed.—Slight contraction of tendons beneath r. knee (psoas abscess).—Tearing pains in hip and thighs, < at night, > about daybreak, > by walking, not affected by weather (improved).—Redness and rawness with terrible itching between toes (s.s.).—Bubo with pain in spot on middle of r. thigh in front, only when standing and on deep pressure, which seemed to touch spot, which was apparently on periosteum.—Two ulcers larger than a crown piece, dirty stinking, sloughing, with jagged, elevated edges, one on thigh above patella another on head of tibia ; two large pieces of bone came away from head of tibia (s.s.).—Osteosarcoma in centre of r. tibia the size of half an ostrich egg, pains agonising at night, growth irregular, spongy, partly laminated, very hard (s.s.).—Contracted, painful feeling in soles, as if tendons were too short.

24. **Generalities.** — Utter prostration and debility in morning. — Epilepsy.—Dwarfed, shrivelled-up, old-looking babies and children.—Epileptic convulsions after menses.

25. **Skin.**—Pustular eruption on different parts of body ; in patches on certain places, particularly on wrists and shins, where bones are nearest cuticle, and isolated other large pustules on other parts, these break, discharging an ichorous fluid for one or two days, then heal, leaving characteristic pockmark cicatrices ; patches take longer to heal, discharging same fluid till healing process commences.—After healing of chancre a fresh pustular eruption appears on different parts of body, which, when pustules have

discharged an ichorous liquid and healed up, leaves fresh coppery pockmarks *Medorr.* removed it permanently, causing it to turn yellow-brown, dry at edges and scale off, leaving skin permanently clear and free.—Biting sensation in different parts of body, as if bitten by bugs, at night only.—Syphilitic rash, very prominent on forehead, chin, arms and front of thorax, an abundance of fine scales peeling off ; large prominent spot on centre of forehead, filled with fluid, as also are some smaller patches (s.s.).—Syphilitic bullæ discharging freely on cheeks, under chin, on back of shoulders, on scalp and other parts of body (infantile syphilis).—Maculæ ; copper-coloured (s.s.).—Pemphigus looking like a pock, often confluent and persistently reappears.—Skin bluish.

26. Sleep.—Great restlessness at night, impossible to keep leg in one position.—Absolute sleeplessness (vies with *Sul.* in producing quiet, refreshing sleep).—Wakes soon after midnight and cannot sleep again till 6 a.m.

27. Fever.—Great pains in head, whole body extremely cold, looked blue ; wanted to be covered with blankets or couldn't get warm ; no appetite sleeping almost continually, could not be roused (s.s.).—Nervous chills preceded by pains in head, esp. occiput and scalp of that part ; pains below waist, in pelvis, legs, esp. tibia, which is sensitive to touch ; bowels torpid cross, irritable, peevish ; pains begin every day 4 p.m., culminate at midnight disappear at daylight.—After retiring nerve chill beginning in anus, running down legs ; desire for stool, > by profuse urination and by eructations.—Fever : dry, hot, shortly after going to bed, parted lips, great thirst ; 11 to daily.—Sweat : profuse at night, sleepless and restless ; esp. between scapulæ and down to waist, with excessive general debility.

Syzygium.

Syzygium jambolanum. Jumbul. *N. O.* Myrtaceæ. Trituration of the seeds (fruit-stones). Tincture of the powdered fruit-stones.

Clinical.—Diabetes. Ulcers.

Characteristics.—*Syz. j.* is a native of India. It has an edible fruit, the powdered stones of which have a popular use in India (*B. J. H.*, xli. 275) as a remedy for diabetes. The dose is five grains of the powdered stones three times a day. Dudgeon used *Syz.* in the lower homœopathic attenuations with marked success, which has been repeated by many others. Hansen mentions as having been cured with *Syz.* "old ulcers of skin, probably of a diabetic foundation." Dudgeon (*H. W.*, xxiv. 540) relates this case : A scientific man, 56 complained of "prickly heat" all over upper part of body and arms. The skin was covered with small red papules, which itched so intensely he could get no rest. He felt very weak, which was perhaps due to his having abstained from all animal food, and confined himself to bread, farinaceous food, vegetables, and fruit. There was much thirst and great flow of urine, which he was obliged to pass every tw hours, night and day ; mouth very dry. Urine 1036, very saccharine. He was ordered chiefly animal diet, very little bread, and no sugar. *Syz.* ϕ, mixed with three times the quantity of alcohol, was given ; of this two drops every three hours. The specific gravity of the urine steadily declined, sugar disappeared, and all the symptoms passed off ; and this in spite of the fact that the dietetic rules were relaxed.

Tabacum.

Nicotiana tabacum. Tobacco. *N. O.* Solanaceæ. Tincture of the fresh leaves collected before the flowers are developed.

Clinical.—*Amaurosis.* Anæmia. Angina pectoris. Anus, prolapse of. Apoplexy. Asthma. Backache. Brain, anæmia of. Brain-fag. Catalepsy. Cholera. Cholera infantum. Colour-blindness. Constipation. Diarrhœa. Epilepsy. Freckles. Glands, enlarged. Heart, intermittent. Hernia. Hiccough. Idiocy. Leg, jerking of. Lip, cancer of. Masturbation, effects of. Ménière's disease. Œsophagus, stricture of. Optic neuritis. *Pregnancy*, pruritus of ; *sickness of;* toothache of. Prostatorrhœa. Pruritus. Pyrosis. Rectum, paralysis of ; stricture of. Sea-sickness. Speech, embarrassed. Strabismus. Tetanus. Toothache. Varicocele.

Characteristics.—*Nicotiana tabacum* received its specific name from Jean Nicot, French ambassador to Portugal, who was the means of introducing the tobacco plant into France about 1560. When Columbus and his followers landed in Cuba in 1492 the practice of smoking tobacco was in common use among the natives throughout the island, and also throughout the continent of America. On their return to Spain the practice rapidly spread throughout the Peninsula. Sir Walter Raleigh and his companions introduced the practice into England in 1586. From that time the cultivation, manufacture, and use of tobacco, either by smoking, snuffing, or chewing, rapidly became universal. The symptoms of the pathogenesis are composed partly of provings made by Lembke, Schreter, and others, and partly of poisonings and over-dosings. Several instructive articles on tobacco appeared in the *Homœopathic News* of 1897, from the pen of M. E. Douglass, then practising at Danville, Virginia, in the midst of tobacco plantations. His third article (July, 1897) was devoted to the "medicinal uses" of Tobacco ; and it seems that it is regarded as a perfect panacea by the Virginians for diseases of men and cattle. One use he mentions is as a palliative for bee-stings and mosquito-bites. A portion of a leaf is moistened with vinegar and applied to the part. This is interesting, as *Ipec.*, one of the antidotes of *Tab.*, has a similar reputation. Strong tobacco-juice is the most effectual destroyer of the burrowing-flea, Chigoe. For headache leaves of Tobacco are moistened with vinegar or camphor solution, and applied to the forehead and nape. The pain is allayed and sleep induced. The local application over the pit of the stomach relieves nausea. Douglass made an involuntary proving on himself when about twenty. He was attending an evening writing-class, when a class-mate gave im a bit of tobacco to chew, and he put it in his mouth. In a few ninutes the bell rang and he took his seat, after first removing the obacco. He soon began to feel dizzy, and could not distinguish his copy ; the letters danced all over the page ; a cold perspiration broke out on the forehead, and extended all over the body. He felt a leathly nausea at his stomach ; his hands trembled so that he could not hold pen to paper. He felt so weak and faint he feared he would all out of his seat. His desk-mate helped him out of the house *into he cold air*, and gave him a *sour apple*, bidding him eat it. It did not seem possible, but he finally tried, and was so much relieved that e ate it all. In half an hour he was able to return to the class, but vas so weak and tremulous, he did not attempt to write. The nausea vas the first symptom to disappear, then the cold perspiration. The dizziness, trembling, and excessive weakness did not entirely leave ill next day. Since then Douglass has used small doses of vinegar n acute symptoms of nicotine poisoning, either chewing or smoking, vith excellent results. Nothing, he says, relieves the sensation of constriction of the œsophagus (in his own case the symptom was a very lisagreeable one, "as of a hand clutching the throat") so quickly as vinegar. One of Douglass's patients, a young man in good health, vho was very fond of cigars, was certain, if he smoked two in an evening, to have an emission on the same night, sometimes with, but ftener without, dreams. Next day he was prostrated, hypochondriacal, ongue furred with a thick, fuzzy, yellow coat at base ; and dull, occipital headache. Prostatorrhœa and impotence are also among he effects of *Tab.* The constrictive sensation is not confined to the hroat ; it affects the rectum, bladder, and chest. There is violent ectal tenesmus ; and there is also paralysis and prolapsus ani. The esical sphincter is paralysed, there is debility of urine, and enuresis. Two of Lembke's provers, students accustomed to smoke and drink coffee and beer, had incontinence of urine ; in one the quantity of urine was not increased, but it was "passed more frequently, and dribbled away involuntarily, with slight itching of urethra" ; in the ase of the other the urine was increased, pale, and he "had to pass t several times in the night, almost amounting to incontinence." The power of *Tab.* to paralyse sphincters and also morbid constrictions accounts for its traditional use in cases of strangulated ernia and obstruction of the bowels, which has been confirmed in omœopathic practice. Renal colic comes under the same heading. The same pair of opposites—relaxation and constriction—are seen in he weakness and paralysis on the one hand, and the convulsions on he other. All shades of nervous tremors, faintings, cramps, jerkings, nd restlessness are noted, and it is by its power of antidoting these onditions that *Tab.* holds its place in society. "After an unusually exatious day," says Douglass, "when I am in that unpleasant condition of mind when it seems as though the slightest word would ause an outburst of passion, nothing else does me quite so much good as a smoke." This is a central nervous action, and if too much ndulged leads to degeneration of nerve tissue, as seen in tobacco-blindness. *Tab.* also produces a condition like brain-fag ; inability to oncentrate thoughts ; this may even go on to a state of idiocy.

Silly talking in boys. A curious state was induced in Mr. Harrison (*C. D. P.*), who slept in the cabin of a sloop, the cabin being full of large packages of tobacco. His sleep was harassed by wild and frightful dreams, and he suddenly awakened about midnight, bathed in a cold dew, and totally unable to speak or move. He knew perfectly where he was, and recollected what had occurred the day before ; but could not make any bodily effort whatever, and tried in vain to get up or change his position. "Four bells" was struck on deck, and he heard the sounds (though rather, it seemed, through their vibrating in his body than by the ears) ; and he was conscious of other things that occurred—so he was not dreaming. At length he became totally insensible for a time, till a roll of the ship roused him, and he awakened and got on deck. His memory was totally lost for a quarter of an hour ; he knew he was in a ship, but nothing more. While in this state he saw a man drawing water, and asked him to pour a bucket on his head. This was done, and all his faculties were instantly restored ; and he acquired a most vivid recollection of a vast variety of ideas and events which seemed to have passed through his mind, and that had occupied him during the time of his supposed insensibility.—The nutrition is profoundly influenced by *Tab.* and it probably retards growth in children. It produces a deathly sinking and craving at the stomach, and it is no doubt by virtue of this, acting homœopathically, that *Tab.* enables persons who cannot have proper meals to endure starvation better than they otherwise would. Decaisne (*C. D. P.*) observed the effects of smoking on youths aged from 9 to 15. Among the effects were : Bruit in carotids and diminution of red corpuscles of the blood. Palpitation. Deficient digestive power. Sluggish intellect. Craving for alcoholic stimulants. Epistaxis. Ulcerated mouth. "The younger the boy, the more marked the symptoms ; the better fed suffer least." "Rapid emaciation, especially of back and cheeks" has been noted among the effects. *Tab.* has a number of backaches, and some are peculiar. C. M. Boger (*Hahn. A.*, xxxviii. 41) cured this with *Tab.* cm : Backache persistent ; < lying down, > walking ; history of anginoid attacks. In cases of cholera, sea-sickness, sickness of pregnancy, renal colic, strangulated hernia, &c., the keynote symptoms are : deathly nausea, pallor, coldness ; icy cold surface, covered with cold sweat ; vomiting violent, as soon as he began to move, > on deck and in fresh air. Terrible faint, sinking feeling at pit of stomach. Terry cured a case of sea-sickness with heat along spine from nape down ; cold sweat ; then vomit. He also cured a case of Ménière's disease with a feeling as if sea-sick. A keynote symptom of much importance in many abdominal cases is : > *by uncovering abdomen.* Child wants abdomen uncovered ; it > nausea and vomiting. There may be coldness of the abdomen at the same time. *Tab.* produces a number of skin affections, notably pruritus. Teste cured with it several cases of freckles ; he repeated the remedy and gave it for weeks at a time : "A country girl had her face and hands covered with freckles, two-thirds of which disappeared completely [under *Tab.*] in summer, the season in which they are most frequent and obstinate." Burnett told me that an infusion of tobacco is a popular German remedy for scrofulous glands. Cooper gives as an indication, "intermittent heart in old people." E. T. Blake (*H. R.*, ii. 68) records a case of rheumatism with rigid joints and spinal insomnia in a lady, 40, who had been heavily drugged with narcotics before he saw her. "Whenever she composed herself for sleep, just as she was lapsing into unconsciousness, the knees would attempt to fly up towards the chest with an abrupt jerk, tearing painfully at the acetabular adhesions." Other symptoms were: sweating, impaired memory, hypochondriasis, drumming in the ears, facial as well as crural clonus, white tongue, epigastric sinking, alternating with nausea and flatulence, heart action increased by day, diminished down to severe fainting during the night. *Tab.* 12 gave three hours' refreshing sleep the first night, more the second, and after the third the leg-jerk departed for good. C. W. (*H. W.*, xxvi. 207) was troubled with spasm of lower jaw, < out of doors. No remedy did good till he remained one evening with two friends who were smoking, and got himself well saturated with the smoke. That cured him. Slight subsequent returns were always removed by *Tab.* J. W. Scott (*H. P.*, xvi. 420) observed a case of epileptiform convulsions brought on by tobacco. For five months the patient had two attacks weekly, and they grew worse in spite of treatment till the tobacco was discontinued. *Sensations* are: Sensation of excessive wretchedness. As if struck by a hammer on right side of head. As if a band round head. As if brains were being bored out. As if black dots filled visual field. As if ears were closed. As of a plug in œsophagus. As if throat gripped by a hand. As if sea-sick. As if stomach were relaxed. As if chest too tight. As if a crowbar were twisted round heart. The symptoms are: > Uncovering abdomen. < By pressure. < Motion of vessel. < Lying; > walking. Lying on left side = palpitation. Motion (even least) <. Coughing = hiccough; stitches in pit of stomach. Rising <. < Morning: vomiting; diarrhœa; sickness of pregnancy; cramps in fingers. Thirst < night. Sight < evening. > In open air; (ear symptoms <). > Cold affusion to head. < Indoors. Symptoms come in paroxysms; are periodical. < By stimulants. Weeping >. Vomiting >. Music = pains in ears.

Relations.—*Antidoted by:* Vinegar, Sour Apples, Camph., Coff.; Ipec. (primary effects: vomiting); Ars. (effects of chewing tobacco); Nux (bad taste in mouth in morning, amblyopia); Phos. (palpitation, tobacco heart, amblyopia, sexual weakness); Spig. (heart affections); Ign., Puls. (hiccough); Clem. (toothache); Sep. (neuralgia in face and dyspepsia, chronic nervousness); Lyc. (impotence); Wine (spasms, cold sweat from excessive smoking). Plant. maj. has sometimes caused aversion to tobacco. Gels. (occipital headache and vertigo); Tab. 200, or 1,000 for the craving when discontinuing its use. *Antidote to:* Cic., Stram. *Compare:* Nicotinum. Cold sweat, Ver. (Ver. on forehead; Tab. all over). Coldness in abdomen, Colch., Elps., Lach. Spasmodic pains along l. ureter, Berb. Ménière's disease, Salicin. Incarcerated hernia, Aco., Nux, Op., Sul. Chills or creeps precede headache (Chel., accompany headache). Sinking immediately after meals, Ars., Cin., Lyc., Sel., Stp., Ur. nit. Hair sensation, K. bi., Sil. (Tab., in eye). Blindness, optic atrophy, Carb. s., Benz.-din.,

Filix. m. Emissions, heart, anæmia, Dig. Retracted abdomen, Pb. Jerking of legs in bed, Meny. As if a hand clutching throat (Bell., intestines).

SYMPTOMS.

1. **Mind.**—Gloomy melancholy.—Inclination to weep.—Anguish and inquietude, generally in the afternoon, > by weeping.—Restlessness, which prompts continual change of place.—Dislike to labour and conversation.—Excessive vertigo ; mental faculties much impaired ; cannot read or study ; sufferings from abuse of tobacco.—Difficulty of concentrating mind for any length of time on one subject.—Feels as if some one were coming to arrest him, or murder him; always with singing in ears (produced—R. T. C.).—Suicidal tendency, gloomy forebodings, inclined to hang down head, breath becomes short, appetite goes (produced—R. T. C.).—Feels intoxicated, hands and feet tremble.—Over-excitement and great liveliness, with songs, dancing, and great loquacity.—The Mexican priests incite courage and bravery by means of an ointment of tobacco.—Abject cowardice, thinks he is going to die and is in extreme terror of death (from smoking many cigars.—J. H. C.).—Frequent laughter without cause.—Silly talk, cannot stop ; loss of memory.—(Attacks of silliness; cannot help talking sillily and memory goes, blames himself for things, inclines to suicide and despair.—R. T. C.).—Idiotic ; epileptic idiocy.—Concourse of confused ideas.—Cataleptic state.—Stupor.—Coma.

2. **Head.**—Emptiness and confusion in the head.—Dizziness.—Vertigo, which often produces loss of consciousness, with nausea (< indoors ; > in open air), and pains in head and eyes.—Vertigo < on rising and looking up—brought on by immoderate use of cigars.—Giddiness in occiput.—Headache, with nausea and vertigo.—Excessive heaviness of head.—Pressive headache, esp. above eyes, vertex, and temples.—Shootings in head.—Headache from one temple to the other, involving orbits, or with shooting in l. eye, > from cold.—While passing urine, suddenly attacked with pains in head, so severe he screamed for assistance ; immediately followed by vomiting.—Congestion of blood in head, with internal heat, and throbbing in temples.—Neuralgic headache, sensation as of sudden blows struck by a hammer.—Periodical sick-headache from fatigue or excitement.—Tightness in head as though a band stretched round it, disturbance of vision, tinnitus, and vertigo.—Headache > in the open air.—Burning and tingling sensation in exterior of head.—Trembling of head.—Hair falls out.—Formication above l. temple.

3. **Eyes.**—Pain in eyes, as from much weeping.—Aching in eyes, extending into bottom of orbits.—Sensation, as if there were a hair in eye.—Smarting in eyes.—Heat and burning sensation in eyes, with redness.—Contraction of the lids.—Pupils : dilated and insensible ; irregularly dilated ; contracted.—Amblyopia with intolerance of light.—Loss of sight on looking steadily at anything white.—Confused sight, in evening, as if looking through a veil.—Sees as through a fog, and hears as through cotton wool (produced—R. T. C.).—Squinting when trying to read.—Insufficiency of internal recti.—Sparks and black specks before eyes.—Central colour scotoma.—White or grey atrophia of optic nerve.—Optic neuritis.—Sudden failure of vision.—

Tobacco-blindness commences in one eye, generally r.; sight < evening.—Photophobia.

4. **Ears.**—Shootings in ears, esp. in open air, and when listening to music.—Hyperæsthesia to music and loud talking.—Jerking tearing in r. ear, and in front of it externally.—Burning heat and redness of the ears.—Hard reddish swelling behind (l.) ear, with shootings.—Ringing; roaring; rushing; humming in ears, < by loud noise or going into open air.—Tinnitus and vertigo.—Fluttering in r. ear both heard and felt.

5. **Nose.**—Burning sensation and tingling in the nose.—Diminished power of smell, which, however, is very sensitive to odour of wine; fumes all but intoxicate her.—Frequent sneezing.—Dryness and obstruction of nose.

6. **Face.**—Deadly paleness of face (during the nausea; face collapsed, cold sweat on).—Burning heat in face, with redness, sometimes of one cheek only, and paleness of the other.—Face covered with cold sweat.—R. cheek glowing, the other pale.—Red spots on face.—Tearings in bones of face (and teeth, in evening).—Pimples on cheeks, wings of nose, and corners of mouth.—Violent tearing in r. facial bones and teeth.—Granulated tuberosities on cheeks.—Emaciation of face.—Lips dry, burning, rough, and cracked.—Epithelioma of lip (27 per cent. in men; $1\frac{1}{2}$ in women).—Eruption on commissures of lips.—Lancinating pains in maxillary joint, when laughing.

7. **Teeth.**—Toothache, with drawing and tearing pains.—Lancinations in carious teeth, when masticating.—Violent tearing in r. teeth.—Throbbing or jumping pains in teeth.—Drawing pain in gums.—Gums pale and parched.

8. **Mouth.**—Dryness of the mouth and tongue, with violent thirst.—Tongue feels swollen.—Tongue: trembles; white; red; furred; dry and parched; covered with blackish-brown crust.—Frothing from the mouth.—Profuse salivation.—Accumulation of white, tenacious mucus in mouth and throat, which must be frequently expectorated.—Swelling of glands under tongue.—Weak, interrupted speech.—Drawling, monotonous style of reading.

9. **Throat.**—Roughness, dryness, and scraping in throat, as from a foreign body.—Dry, hot, sulphur feeling in throat, with dry, parched mouth, comes on after dose of ϕ and remains for a week off and on, but generally < in morning after sleep (R. T. C.).—Throat dry, can hardly swallow.—Crawling and tickling in throat.—Swallowing very painful from spasms in throat.—Peculiar sensation of plug in œsophagus, with constant dull pressure.—Redness of fauces.—Burning in pharynx.—Accumulation of viscid mucus in throat.

10. **Appetite.**—Mawkish and clammy, or bitter and sour taste.—Acid taste of all food.—Acidulated taste of water, as if it contained wine.—Adipsia, and dread of water.—Great thirst; < at night.—Absence of hunger and appetite.—Constant hunger, with nausea if nothing is eaten.

11. **Stomach.**—Frequent empty and noisy risings.—Sour, burning risings.—Pyrosis.—Spasmodic hiccough.—Frequent nausea, esp. during movement, often inducing syncope, with deadly paleness of face, disappearing generally in open air.—Deathly nausea, with vertigo, in paroxysms, body covered with cold sweat; sea-sickness.—Nausea, with inclination to vomit, sensation of coldness in stomach, or pinchings in abdomen.—Vomiting of water only, with yellow and greenish reflection before eyes.—Vomiting of

acid serum, often mixed with mucus.—Violent vomiting ; easy, of sour liquid ; watery, insipid, sometimes bitter in morning.—The vomiting is renewed by the slightest movement.—Stomach-ache.—Squeezing, contractive cramps in stomach, sometimes after a meal, often accompanied by nausea, and an accumulation of saliva in mouth.—Shootings in the scrobiculus, which pass through back.—Relaxation, and sensation of coldness or burning in stomach. --Sinking at the pit of stomach.—Dreadful faint feeling in stomach.

12. **Abdomen.**—Hepatic pain, when pressing on the part.—Hepatic and renal regions sensative to pressure.—Pressure in hepatic region, as from a heavy body.—Shooting in hepatic region.—Shootings in the l. hypochondrium. —Great sensitiveness of abdomen to slightest touch.—Uncovering abdomen > nausea and vomiting—Painful distension of abdomen.—Pressive pains in abdomen, esp. in umbilical region, with spasmodic retraction of that part.—Violent burning in abdomen, horrible pains, must shriek.—Nocturnal tearings in abdomen.—Pinchings and borborygmi in abdomen.—Incarcerated hernia.

13. **Stool and Anus.**—Constipation.—Chronic constipation, great pain and tympanitic distension of intestines ; great dyspnœa.—Stools clay-colour or mottled grey and brown.—Habitual constipation ; paralysis of rectum ; spasm of anal sphincter.—Prolapsus ani ; great drowsiness during day when trying to study.—Frequent tenesmus.—Soft fæces of consistence of pap, also at night.—Violent pain in small of back during soft stool.—Shifting of flatulence, formed by sudden, papescent, yellow-green or greenish, slimy stools with tenesmus.—Violent diarrhœa, fetid or yellowish green slime ; also at night, accompanied and followed by violent tenesmus, and burning sensation in anus.—Cholera-like stools ; watery, urgent, painless.

14. **Urinary Organs.**—Renal colic ; violent pains along ureters ; cold sweat ; deathly nausea.—Paralysis of sphincter, constant dribbling.—Enuresis —Urine yellowish-red, with increased secretion.—Inflammation of the orifice of the urethra.

15. **Male Sexual Organs.**—Frequent erections.—Flow of prostatic fluid.—Nocturnal emissions ; until waking.—Genital organs flabby ; no erections or sexual desire.—Varicocele.—(Masturbation and its consequences —R. T. C.)

16. **Female Sexual Organs.**—Retarded and profuse catamenia.—Leucorrhœa, like sanguineous water.—Leucorrhœa of serous liquid after the menses.—In climacteric period, also during menses; subjective coldness epigastric sinking, palpitation, severe diarrhœa, muscular relaxation, excessive sense of wretchedness.—Morning sickness of pregnancy; nausea and vomiting, patient dreads least movement.—During pregnancy, insupportable pruritus over whole body, pyrosis, toothache, and other gastric symptoms.

17. **Respiratory Organs.**—Dry cough, excited by a tickling in throat in morning and towards evening.—Cough = in pit of stomach sensation as of a wound by some sharp instrument.—Cough, with hiccough (at same time) almost suffocating; (or hiccough after every paroxysm of whooping-cough) —Difficult respiration.—Paroxysm of suffocation.

18. **Chest.**—Oppression of the chest, with anguish.—Constriction of the chest.—Pressure on the chest and sternum.—Shootings in chest and sides of chest, sometimes when drawing breath.—Sticking under sternum with inability to take a deep breath.—(A trembling, frightened feeling across pi

f chest with sudden and irregular sinkings.—Nervous indigestion, constant nking in chest.—R. T. C.)—On taking a deep breath it seemed as if chest vere too tight.—Sensation as if a crowbar were pressed tightly from breast to l. till it came and twisted in a knot around heart, which stopped, hen leaped violently; after the attack heart missed every fourth beat.—Pain, s from excoriation, in chest, during a meal.—Itching pimples on chest.

19. **Heart and Pulse.**—Sudden attacks of extreme faintness; feeling f oppression around cardiac region.—Angina pectoris (single doses of φ elieved much; not to be repeated often.—R. T. C.).—Feeble, irregular pulse. —Palpitation of heart, when lying on l. side.

20. **Neck and Back.**—Stiffness of the neck.—Head drawn back in onvulsions.—Neuralgic pains in neck and between shoulders.—Burning nder scapula.—Neuralgia of back with tightness of throat.—Contractive ains in the loins, esp. after a stool.—Violent pain in small of back and loins renal calculi).—Throbbing in sacral region, evening.—Pain in small of back nd loins, esp. after sitting.—Intolerable pain in small of back much < while itting.—Pains in small of back, constriction; esp. after a stool.—Pressive ain in lumbar region on rising from a seat and beginning to walk, goes off n walking.—Emaciation of the back.—Red, itching eruption on the back.

22. **Upper Limbs.**—Painful weakness of hands and arms, which are, s it were, paralysed.—Constant need to stretch arms.—Shootings and drawing n shoulders.—Red spots on shoulder, which burn when they are touched.— Tension in arm, esp. in elbow.—Pain and shootings in l. arm, which disable t and prevent its extension.—(Coldness and trembling of the limbs), trembling f hands.—Cold perspiration on hands.—Cramps in the arms and hands.— Cramps in single fingers, esp. while washing; early morning.—Cramps and ingling in fingers.—Swelling of fingers.—Itching pimples on fingers.

23. **Lower Limbs.**—Burning pain in knee and soles.—Legs icy cold rom knees down.—Shooting in knee and ham.—Flexion of knees, when walking.—Cramp in toes, extending into knees.—Jerking of legs in bed.— Tingling, crawling, from knee to toes.—Tension in leg when walking, from knee to foot.—Trembling and paralytic weakness of feet.

24. **Generalities.**—Pressive pains, with agitation throughout body, and anxious perspiration.—Sudden breaking out of cold, clammy sweat; with much nausea; feeble, irregular pulse; collapse.—Cramps and tingling in limbs. —Restlessness, wants to change place continually.—Gait slow and shuffling, difficulty in ascending stairs.—Excessive emaciation.—Anæmia of boys and girls, particularly with brain symptoms (cured with dilutions.—R. T. C.).— Paralytic and painful weakness of limbs.—Trembling of limbs.—Great general lassitude.—Jerkings throughout body, with pulsation and palpitation of the heart.—Convulsions, head firmly drawn back, with rigidity of muscles at back of neck; constantly recurring rigid uterine spasms, muscles of back being principally affected, till death a week after he chewed the tobacco.— Epileptiform convulsions.—Symptoms < on l. side; from great heat or great cold, and esp. in stormy weather; from walking, riding in a carriage, and jar of a railway train.—> In the open air; from vomiting.

25. **Skin.**—Itching in skin, as from flea-bites.—Itching over the whole body.—Eruption of itching pimples, or vesicles, with yellow serum and red areola.

26. **Sleep.**—Urgent inclination to sleep, esp. after a meal, and toward evening, with frequent yawnings.—Retarded sleep in evening, and difficulty in waking in morning.—Stupefying sleep at night.—Disturbed sleep at night with fright.—Nightmare.

27. **Fever.**—Pulse full, hard, and rapid, or small, imperceptible, intermittent, slow.—Coldness and shivering, sometimes with chattering of teeth.—Coldness of legs from knees to toes; warm body, cold hands.—Chilliness after eating and drinking.—Frequent attacks of shuddering, sometimes with flushes of heat.—Permanent shuddering, from morning till evening.—Perspiration at night.—Viscid cold sweat, with intermitting pulse.—Cold sweat in hands, on forehead and face.

Tamus.

Tamus communis. Black Bryony. Ladies' Seal. *N. O.* Dioscoreaceæ Tincture of fresh root. Tincture of the berries.

Clinical.—Chilblains.

Characteristics.—*Tamus* is the only European representative of the Dioscoreaceæ. There are two species, *T. communis* and *T. cretica*. The Greeks use the young suckers of both like asparagus, which they much resemble. *T. communis* is the Black Bryony of our hedges. "The root is very great and thick, oftentimes as big as a man's leg, blackish without and very clammy or slimy within; which having been scraped with a knife, it seems to be a matter fit to be spread upon cloth or leather in manner of a plaister of sear-cloth" (Gerarde). Dioscorides, according to the same authority, says the fruit or berries take away sun-burns and other blemishes of the skin; and Gerarde adds that these "very quickly waste and consume away black and blue marks that come of bruises and dry beatings: which thing also the roots perform being laid upon them." The fruits steeped in gin are a popular remedy for chilblains, and the only use that *Tamus* has been made of by homœopaths is as a paint for chilblains. Gerarde says of the root-plaister that it removes scars and deformities; breaks hard apostems, draws forth splinters and broken bones, dissolves congealed blood, and if laid on hip or knuckle-bones or any other part where there is great pain, it takes away the pain speedily.

Tanacetum.

Tanacetum vulgare. Tansy. *N. O.* Compositæ. Tincture of the fresh plant in flower. Attenuations of the oil.

Clinical.—Abortion. Amenorrhœa. Chorea. Dysmenorrhœa. Epilepsy. Eyes, sclerotica inflamed. Hydrophobia. Labia, abscess of. Paralysis. Strabismus (right inward). Worms.

Characteristics.—The common Tansy (the word is derived from *ἀθανασια*, immortality), with its deep-yellow button-like flowers, a close companion of the Rag-wort (*Senecio Jacobea*) on our commons and in our hedgerows, takes a not unimportant part in giving colour to the landscape. In olden times puddings were made containing Tansy leaves, and these puddings were called "tansies" also. "In the springtime are made with the leaves hereof newly sprung up, and with eggs, cakes *or tansies*, which be pleasant in taste and good for the stomach. For if any bad humours cleave thereunto, it doth perfectly concoct them and scour them downwards" (Gerarde). Gerarde also says that the seeds kill and expel worms of every sort; the root is good in gout; and being drunk with wine *Tan.* relieves pain in the bladder, and dysuria when a man is only able to urinate by drops. Like *Senec.*, *Tan.* has an action on the female generative organs, and a large proportion of the observations with it have been on women who have taken it to procure abortion. Other effects are from its use as a vermifuge, and in addition to these are provings by Burt and others. In Russia *Tan.* has a reputation as a remedy for hydrophobia. M. Peyraud (*C. D. P.*) has even used *Tan.* as a substitute for Pasteurian "vaccinations," and reports success. Experiments on animals show that *Tan.* induces all the cardinal features of rabies: convulsions, frothy, bloody mucus in the air passages, hallucinations, convulsions without loss of consciousness, opisthotonos, spasms of pharynx, larynx, and thorax, abundant salivation, sensual excitability, tendency to bite, hoarse cry, diminished sensibility and mobility, momentary paralysis, sub-pleural ecchymoses, infarctions of the liver—*rabies tanacetica*, *simili-rabies* being the name suggested by Peyraud for this drug-disease. Whether the convulsions of *Tan.* be rabic or epileptic, they are sufficiently similar to render the drug useful in either condition. W. H. Pierson (*H. W.*, xxx. 488, quoting *N. A. J. H.*) observed a woman who took two drachms of the oil to procure abortion. The attempt failed, but throughout her pregnancy she suffered from mixed tonic and clonic convulsions, frothing at the mouth, clenched hands, thumbs turned in, followed by exhaustion and a short coma. Since then Pierson treated every case of epilepsy which came to him with drop doses of the fluid extract of *Tan.* four times a day, and with marked success. Hale mentions as having been cured with *Tan.*: Amenorrhœa, dysmenorrhœa, menorrhagia, uterine cramps, and metritis. In one instance it caused a large abscess of the labium majus. Hale says a crystallisable acid identical with *Santonin* has been isolated from it. *Suddenness* is a characteristic of a number of the symptoms. *Peculiar Sensations* are: As if something closed the ears very *suddenly*. His own voice sounds strange in his ears. As though arms and legs *suddenly* swollen. Sensation like a thrill all through body. The symptoms were < at night, and at 4 a.m.

Relations.—*Compare:* In uterine symptoms, Sabi., Tereb., Hedeo., Ruta. In convulsions, Stram., Cicut., Cupr. Worm symptoms, convulsions, paralysis, Sant., Cin., Chenop. Abscess on labium majus (Strych., abscess of scrotum).

SYMPTOMS.

1. **Mind.**—Exhilaration.—Nervousness.—Confusion.—Mind fatigued after least mental exertion.—Indifference and incoherence.—Unable to fix attention on anything; it seemed next instant my reason would leave me.—Uttered a shriek and fell senseless to the floor; continued in comatose state over an hour, when she vomited again and recovered consciousness.

2. **Head.**—Dizziness.—Weariness in head.—Strange fulness and pressure in head amounting to pain.—Dull, frontal headache with cutting in temples.—Occipito-frontal headache, backache, and pains in limbs.

3. **Eyes.**—Sclerotic congested, dark purple glassy-looking, swollen so that cornea appeared sunk.—Eyes open, very brilliant, pupils equal, widely dilated, immovable; sclerotics injected.—Pupils contracted.—Slight inward squint; r. eye.—Occasionally slow, lateral, rolling motion of eyeballs.—Lids agglutinated in morning.—Dull aching in eyeballs.

4. **Ears.**—Stitches in internal ear.—Sensation as if something closed ears very suddenly.—Her own voice sounds strange in her ears.—Roaring; ringing in ears.

5. **Nose.**—Profuse secretion of mucus in nose with fluent coryza.—Dryness of nostrils.

6. **Face.**—Features seemed fixed, giving an expression of deep solemnity.—Fulness of head and face.—Face: dusky; flushed, cheeks bright red.—Mouth and nose drawn a little to r.

8. **Mouth.**—Tongue white coated, feels rough.—Mouth, blood-stained; frothy.—Flat, insipid taste.

9. **Throat.**—Roughness of throat.—Feeling in throat as if I would cough all the time, without being able to cough through the whole proving.—Unable to swallow.

11. **Stomach.**—Thirst.—Constant eructations tasting of the oil.—Eructations of sour air at night.—Nausea; and vomiting.—Faint and sick at stomach.—In stomach: slight glow, burning; great heat (immediate), and in bowels; weight.—Drawing cutting pains in epigastrium many times.

12. **Abdomen.**—Dull pains in r. hypochondrium; sharp in l.—Sharp sticking pains in whole umbilical region; esp. 4 a.m.—Bowels feel as if full of fluid from taking a cathartic.—Frequent spells of sharp, cutting, colicky pains < night, esp. after midnight.—L.-side pain extending from ribs to hip.

13. **Stool.**—Stools: soft, papescent, preceded by colic; two loose, with feeling he would have more.—Constipation (secondary).

14. **Urinary Organs.**—Urine caused slight scalding.—Constant desire.—Marked diuresis, must rise in night to urinate.—First suppression, then profuse flow.—Urine: very fetid; high-coloured; increased, smelling of the drug.

16. **Female Sexual Organs.**—Heat and fulness through hips, increasing as the drug is persisted in until a "show" appears.—Inflammation of vaginal walls, of internal and external labia, which resulted in an enormous abscess in one labium.—(Dysmenorrhœa, bearing-down pains, tenderness, drawing in groins.)—Abortion in early months of pregnancy.—Brought back menses after suppression of several days, not naturally but very profusely,

with severe labour-like pains.—At full term a child was born not larger than a cat; the child lived three weeks.

17. **Respiratory Organs.**—Collection of much (frothy) mucus in larynx and fauces impeding respiration.—Tickling in larynx and fauces causing desire to cough, but no coughing.—My voice had a strange sound in my ears.—Breathing laborious.—[Frothy, sanguineous mucus in trachea and bronchi as in rabies; all other symptoms of rabies also (in poisoned animals)].

19. **Heart.**—Feeble heart-action and all signs of impending dissolution. —Pulse: increased in force and frequency; feeble, frequent; extinct.

20. **Back.**—Severe attack of lumbago all one evening.—Constant dull ache in loins.

21. **Limbs.**—Numbness and sensation as though arms and legs were suddenly swelling.—Cold numbness over limbs, going on to paralysis.— Prickling, coming and going, over limbs and along spine; with flashes of heat.

22. **Upper Limbs.**—L. wrist very lame and sore in morning.

23. **Lower Limbs.**—Great weakness of legs with general prostration of strength.—Unsteadiness of step with an indescribable feeling far worse than pain.

24. **Generalities.**—Trembling.—Convulsions.—Clonic spasms; not convulsive, coming instantaneously and lasting a minute; slight tremor of arms, they were thrown forward, and at right angles to the body, forearm supinated, hands bent at right angles, fingers straight, slightly bent on hands, points of fingers nearly in contact; respiratory muscles strongly affected, air forced from chest slowly but steadily making a hissing noise at lips; in the intervals muscles relaxed, except the jaws.—Great irritability, makes extraordinary movements and curious gestures, stretches himself, draws up his legs, stands on his head; when remonstrated with says, "Leave me alone, it does me good; I can't help doing it;" when he draws up his legs and the muscles will not go farther he pulls them up with his hands and then suddenly stretches them out again; all the time has no pain; lasts half an hour and occurs with each repetition of the medicine (boy, 12, took one and a half ounces of extract for worms).—Bites tongue in convulsions.—Sensation like a throb through whole frame.

26. **Sleep.**—Drowsy.

27. **Fever.**—Surface cool and moist.—Feeling of warmth diffused over whole abdomen.—Cold, clammy sweat.

Tanghinia.

Tanghinia venenifera. *N. O.* Apocynaceæ. Trituration of the seed.

Clinical.—Paralysis. Vomiting.

Characteristics.—*Tanghinia* (the Tanghin or Tanquen of Madagascar) is the only representative of its genus of the Apocynaceæ. The fruit of the tree is ellipsoid, between two and three inches long, having a smooth, purplish skin tinged with green, containing a hard stone surrounded by a thick fibrous flesh. The part used as an ordeal is the seed, which is pounded, and a small piece is swallowed by the person to be tried. Those in whom it causes vomiting escape. Those whose stomachs retain it are quickly killed, and their guilt is held proven. General weakness, even complete paralysis is produced, death being preceded by spasmodic movements of fingers and toes. Numbness is a common symptom ; especially numbness of the hands. The vomiting is intense and distressing, and is accompanied by anxiety and weakness. The Schema comprises symptoms observed on persons undergoing the ordeal.

SYMPTOMS.

1. **Mind.**—Conscious to the last, without delirium.—Delirium occasionally occurs.—Stupor.—Lies as if asleep, and when roused answers like a drowsy man and then relapses into former condition.—Anxiety with the vomiting.

2. **Head.**—Giddy ; staggers.

8. **Mouth.**—Numb tingling in mouth and fauces.

11. **Stomach.**—Vomiting, intense, distressing and repeated, first of contents of stomach. then of bile and mucus.

13. **Stool.**—Purging and urination (purging is a bad symptom, and the worse the more urgent it is).

21. **Limbs.**—Death preceded by spasmodic movements of fingers and toes.

22. **Upper Limbs.**—Hands numb.

24. **Generalities.**—Great debility and anxiety with the vomiting.—Numb feeling over whole body, esp. of hands.—Staggers if attempts to walk, is unable to support his own weight, and falls down helpless and paralysed.

Tannin.

Tannic acid. $C_{14}H_{10}O_9,2H_2O$. [There are two forms of tannic acid, Gallo-tannic acid, derived from nut-galls, and Querci-tannic acid, derived from healthy leaves and bark of the oak. The former is the most used.] Trituration. Solution in rectified spirit.

Clinical.—Constipation. Ileus.

Characteristics.—*Tannin* or *Tannic acid*, of which *Gallic acid* ($C_7H_6O_5$) is a derivative, has produced effects on healthy persons, and on several taking it for diarrhœa. The chief effects were the production of a state of leathery dryness of mouth and intestinal canal ; a condition like ileus ; and a very aggravated state of constipation.

Relations.—*Compare :* Querc., Gall. ac., Op., Pb.

SYMPTOMS.

8. **Mouth.**—Tongue white, dry.—Leathery dryness of mucous membrane of mouth and intestinal canal.

11. **Stomach.**—Loss of appetite.—Thirst.—Vomiting.—Obstinate vomiting of bilious substances.—Painful sensation in epigastric region and abdomen.—Violent pains in stomach.

12. **Abdomen.**—The intestines could be felt like cylindrical enlargements through walls of abdomen.—Ileus.—Colic.—Abdomen: distended; sensitive to pressure but not distended.

13. **Stool.**—Painless and bloody discharge from bowels.—Obstinate constipation; lasted eight days; only dissipated on the ninth day by two drops of *Croton oil*.—Foul stools.

14. **Urinary Organs.**—Urine scanty, dark-coloured.

19. **Heart.**—Palpitation.

24. **Generalities.**—Weakness.

Taraxacum.

Leontodum taraxacum. Taraxacum Dens-leonis. *N. O.* Compositæ.
Tincture of whole plant just before the perfection of the flower.

Clinical.—Ague. Bilious attacks. Debility. Diabetes. Gall-stones. Headache, gastric. Jaundice. Liver, affections of. Neuralgia. Night-sweats. Rheumatism. Tongue, mapped. Typhoid fever.

Characteristics.—The young leaves of the *Dandelion* are sometimes eaten in salads. They have a bitter chicory-like taste, as also has the root. Children eat the flowers, although they are supposed by them to cause bed-wetting. This has given rise to one of the popular names of the plant. Its chief traditional uses are as a remedy for jaundice, liver obstruction, in dysentery, involuntary emissions, and in difficulties in passing water. Hahnemann's provings brought out these leading symptoms: "Painless urging to urinate;" and "frequent urging to urinate with copious discharge of urine." Hahnemann points out that this, with the thirst, may indicate *Trx.* in some cases of diabetes. *Trx.* has caused pains in both splenic and liver regions, and has cured jaundice with enlarged indurated liver. Cooper gives me the following case: An old Indian officer, when in India, suffered much from gall-stones, and was advised to take dandelion infusion every day. This he did, and soon the symptoms left him, and he remained free from them for over twenty years. A symptom in connection with disordered digestion, which has proved a good guide for *Trx.* in some cases, is the "mapped tongue." The tongue is coated white, and clears off in patches, leaving dark red very sensitive spots. *Treas. of Bot.* points out that "the bright-yellow flowers of *Trx.* open in the morning between 5 and 6 o'clock and close in the evening between 8 and 9. Hence this was one of the plants selected by

Linnæus to form his floral clock." The symptoms of *Trx.* are < at night. Hands and nose cold at 8 p.m. "Cold finger-tips" is a guiding symptom. *Peculiar Sensations* are: As if brain was constricted. As if teeth were set on edge. As if larynx were compressed. As if bubbles were forming and bursting in abdomen. As of rolling and gurgling in right scapula. As if limbs were bound or powerless. Some leading indications are: Gastric and bilious attacks, especially gastric headaches; the headaches are generally pressive. Pressure in lower occiput after lying down is characteristic. Debility, loss of appetite, profuse night-sweats, especially when convalescing from bilious or typhoid fever. Restlessness of limbs in typhoid. Sweat between toes. The symptoms are: > By touch (jerking in right calf). Rest <. (Almost all symptoms appear when sitting; lying down; resting.) Motion >. > In open air. Burning in throat is > by drinking. Hahnemann's dosage was a single drop of the φ tincture (*M. M. P.*).

Relations.—*Compatible:* Ars. (night-sweats). *Compare:* In gastric and bilious affections, Bry., Chel., Hydr., Nux. Mapped tongue, Ars., Nat. m., Ran. s. Restlessness of limbs with tearing pains, Rhus.

SYMPTOMS.

1. **Mind.**—Irresolution and dislike to labour.—Loquacity and inclination to laugh.

2. **Head.**—Vertigo, with giddiness and staggering when walking in the open air.—Drawing pain in l. temple while sitting, ceasing when walking or standing.—Tearing pain in occiput.—Pressure and heaviness in lower part of occiput, after lying down.—Headache, as from contraction or expansion of brain.—Heaviness and pressure in head.—Lancinations in forehead and temples.—Violent headache, felt only when standing or walking.—Tension of scalp.

3. **Eyes.**—Pain in eyes, as if a grain of sand were in internal canthus.—(Aversion to light) burning sensation, and burning shootings in eyes.—Burnin l. eyeball.—Inflammation of eyes with lachrymation and photophobia.—Nocturnal agglutination of lids.

4. **Ears.**—Shootings in ears.—Drawing pain in external ear.—Dysecoia in evening.

6. **Face.**—Purulent pimples on face, cheeks, alæ nasi, and (r.) commissures of lips.—Sensation of heat and redness in face.—Shootings and pressure in cheeks.—Upper lip cracked.

7. **Teeth.**—Toothache, with drawing pain in carious teeth, extending to eyebrows.—Pressive pains in teeth.—Teeth set on edge as from acids.—Flow of acid blood from carious teeth.—Bluntness of teeth.—Hawking up of sour mucus, causing teeth to feel dull.

8. **Mouth.**—Accumulation of acid saliva in mouth (with sensation as if the larynx were compressed).—Tongue loaded with a white coating, with exfoliation (it cleans off in patches, dark red, and they are very sensitive).—Tongue dry, loaded with a brown coating on waking in morning.

9. **Throat.**—Sore throat, with pressive pain, as from internal swelling.

—Dryness, shootings, and bitter mucus in the throat.—Hawking up of acid mucus.

10. **Appetite.**—Bitter taste in mouth, with natural taste of food.—Salt or acid taste of food, principally of butter and of meat.—Tobacco-smoke is disagreeable, causes pyrosis, and interrupts respiration.—Great chilliness after drinking, or eating.

11. **Stomach.**—Bitter risings (eructations and hiccough).—Empty risings, esp. after drinking.—Nausea (with inclination to vomit or vomiting) from very fat food, with anxiety and pressive headache, > in open air.

12. **Abdomen.**—Pinching in abdomen.—Pressive shootings in abdomen, and sides of abdomen, chiefly in l. side ; in hypogastrium.—Grumbling and movements (sudden sensation) in abdomen, as if bubbles were bursting in it.

13. **Stool and Anus.**—Inefficient urging to go to stool.—Evacuations several times a day, but accomplished with difficulty (even if stool is not hard).—Fæces of the consistence of pap, followed by tenesmus.—Voluptuous itching in perinæum (compelling one to scratch).

14. **Urinary Organs.**—Frequent want to urinate (pressure without pain), with profuse emission.—Enuresis somni (?).

15. **Male Sexual Organs.**—Pain in testes.—Permanent erections.—Frequent pollutions ; on alternate nights.

16. **Female Sexual Organs.**—Suppressed menses.

17. **Respiratory Organs.**—Sensation as if the larynx were pressed together.

18. **Chest.**—Pressure at chest.—Shootings in chest and sides of chest.—Jerkings in muscles of sides.

20. **Neck and Back.**—Pressive jerkings and shootings in muscles of neck, (throat), and nape.—Tearing from ear downward to the neck.—Pressive pains in loins.—Pressive and tensive shootings in back and loins, when lying down, with obstructed respiration.—Pressing-stinging in spine and sacrum with dyspnœa.—Gurgling and swelling in shoulder-blades and shoulders, with shivering over whole body.—Vibration and quivering in r. scapula.

22. **Upper Limbs.**—Pulsative throbbing and jerking in shoulders and arms.—Jerkings of muscles of arms.—Twitching in muscles of l. forearm.—Shootings in arms and elbows.—Drawings and tearings in forearm and wrist.—Eruptions of pimples on hands and fingers.—Icy coldness of ends of fingers.—Pressive pain in three last fingers of r. hand.

23. **Lower Limbs.**—Shootings in thighs, knees, calves, soles, and toes.—Stitching pain in l. thigh.—Pressive pain in l. calf.—Jerking pain in r. calf, ceasing quickly when touched.—Drawing pain in dorsum of r. foot; when standing; stitches when sitting.—Severe or fine stitching pains in r. sole.—Burning sensation in knees, legs and toes.—Profuse perspiration between toes.

24. **Generalities.**—This remedy acts well in all affections of the liver ; sour taste ; darting pains in outer parts.—Affections in l. upper side ; r. lower side ; back of foot ; sole of foot.—< While lying down ; from fat food ; while resting.—> From moving; when walking.—Painful tenderness of all limbs, esp. when touched, and when they are in a false position.—The limbs are movable, but it feels as if the power to move them were impeded.—Sensation of weakness and uneasiness throughout body, with constant necessity to lie

down or to sit.—Almost all symptoms appear while the patient is seated, and are dissipated by walking.

25. **Skin.**—Unhealthy, pimply, sycotic skins.—Stinging on skin.—Eruption over body and limbs itching severely, and appears to be a mixture of lichen and urticaria.—Biting in skin with sweat.

26. **Sleep.**—Sleepiness, and going to sleep while listening to a scientific discourse.—Sleepiness in daytime, and yawning while sitting.—Vivid unremembered dreams; frequent waking and tossing.

27. **Fever.**—Chilliness, esp. after eating and drinking.—Chilliness, shiverings, all over, with pressive headache.—Chill in open air.—Heat at night on waking, esp. on face and hands.—Violent night-sweats, mostly before midnight, when just going to sleep.—Very debilitating perspiration, causing biting on the skin.

Tarentula.

Lycosa tarentula. Tarantula. *N. O.* Araneideæ. Tincture of the living spiders.

Clinical.—Angina pectoris. Callosities. Chorea. Coccygodynia. Cornea, opacity of. Cystitis. *Depression of spirits.* Diphtheria. Dysmenorrhœa. Epistaxis. *Erotomania.* Fibroma. Headache. Hiccough. *Hysteria.* Intermittents. Kleptomania. *Levitation.* Locomotor ataxy. Mania. Ménière's disease. Migraine. Onanism. Ovaries, enlargement of. Paralysis; agitans. Physometra. Proctalgia. Pruritus pudendi. Quinsy. Septic diseases. Spinal irritation. Spinal sclerosis. Tumours. Uterus, cancer of; neuralgia of. Vertebræ, tumours of.

Characteristics.—The name *Tarentula* covers a number of poisonous spiders, but in homœopathy, unless otherwise distinguished, it refers to *Tarentula hispanica, Lycosa tarentula.* Nunez is our chief authority. He instigated the proving and collected much outside information bearing on the action of the poison. "Tarantella" is a dance named from the city of Tarentum. "Tarantism" is a dancing mania, set up in persons bitten by the *Tarentula*, or in those who imagine themselves bitten. The cure is music and dancing. Here are two illustrations from *C. D. P*: (1) Girl, three months old, was bitten by a tarentula. She appeared at first uneasy, then exhibited dyspnœa, and complained, showed signs of suffocation, vomited, was agitated and much convulsed. Music was played; movements of the limbs were set up, whence resulted profuse sweat, followed by sleep and complete recovery. (2) Francis Mustel, a peasant, was bitten by a tarentula on the left hand, about the middle of July, as he was gathering corn. He went home with his companions but on the way fell as if struck by apoplexy. Dyspnœa followed, and face, hands, and feet became dark. Knowing the remedy, his companions fetched musicians. When the patient heard their playing he began to revive, to sigh, to move first his feet, then his hands, and then the whole body; at last getting on his feet he took to dancing violently, with sighing so laboured that the bystanders were almost frightened. At times he rolled himself on the ground and struck it vehemently with his feet. Two hours after the music began the blackness of his face and hands went off, he sweated freely, and regained perfect health. Every succeeding year at the same season the pain and attending symptoms returned, but less violently; and they could always be averted by music. But if the imminent paroxysm was not averted in time, he was found by his friends struck down as at first and was restored in the same way. These cases bring out some of the cardinal features of *Trn.* (1) Dark red or purplish coloration and swelling of skin and tissue. (2) Apparent imminent choking. (3) Choreic movements; restlessness. (4) > By music: music at first excites and subsequently relieves. (5) Periodicity; deep action returning annually on the date of the bite. *Trn.* is a remedy of *synalgias* and concomitants: Neuralgia of inferior maxillary nerve accompanying pain with irritation in pit of stomach. Snapping and pain in ear associated with hiccough. Throat and eye. Heat of face with heat of palms. Faint feeling in stomach with frontal headache. Many symptoms take their rise from the generative sphere, which is profoundly affected. Desire is excited in both sexes to the point of mania. Coitus only < the sufferings of both. In one male prover the semen was bloody and caused a sensation of heat in its passage. The sexual desire was so excited in one woman that when playing or dancing with men she hugged them before everybody; and was angry when reproved, but did it again. The periods were scanty and pale with severe pains in teeth and buttocks; at times she had a desire to take things which did not belong to her; the "Tarantella" played on the violin produced no effect on her, but as soon as she took in her arms a little girl, she began to cry until it was taken away. Cuttings and contractions in uterus; shootings in vagina; swelling and induration of uterus; expulsion of gas from uterus; pains in other parts associated with uterine pains; restlessness, hysteria. The restlessness is particularly noted in the lower extremities, with desire to cry: must keep moving about though walking < all the symptoms. Many of the mental symptoms, which almost exhaust the protean range of hysteria, were in connection with sexual disorders; sighing, yawning; laughing and crying; joking and profound melancholy. The unceasing movements—twitching, jerking, dancing—are the most constant features. There is hysterical hyperæsthesia: the least excitement irritates, followed by languid sadness; great excitability of nerve endings; tips of fingers extremely sensitive; feels sore and bruised all over, < moving about; spinal irritation, slightest touch along spine = spasmodic pain in chest and heart regions. Farrington gives among the mental symptoms: "When there are no observers there is no hysteria; when attention is directed to her she begins to twitch"; and "cunning attempts to feign paroxysms of wild dancing." The chorea of *Trn.* is most marked on right side. The neuralgias of *Trn.* may be anywhere; in the head they are of great intensity: "as if thousands of needles were pricking to the brain. They are < by noise, touch, strong light, > by rubbing head against pillow. ("> By rubbing" is a keynote Condition of *Trn.* "Termini of nerves become so irritated that some kind of friction is necessary in order to obtain relief.") Constrictive headache with pain in uterus. P. C. Majumdar (*Ind. H. R.*, v. 43) reports this case: Girl, 18, had oppression of chest, suffocating sensation, continued jerking and movement of hands, foam at mouth, complete insensibility, profuse and delaying menses; very sleepy. Hystero-epilepsy was diagnosed. *Ign.* 30 did nothing. *Trn.*, high, brought her out of the fit and restored her completely in a few minutes. But *Trn.* is not a hysteric remedy only. C. M. Boger (*Hahn. Ad.*, xxxviii. 40) cured a case of irritative cough with *Trn.* 30: Mr. B., 41, sore all over, throat feels dry, cough lying down at night and in morning after rising; dry with tearing pain in chest; excited by pressure of phlegm in chest; feels short of breath for at least an hour after each coughing attack; *only* > *from smoking.* Bad taste evening. Three doses cured. Diphtheria; tonsillitis of an intensity to threaten suffocation; cystitis; septic and intermittent fevers have been successfully met in *Trn.* on its indications. In *M. A.*, xvii. 568 a case of hyperæsthesia of finger-tips is mentioned. The patient, a lady, 33, could not dress herself without gloves. The irritation caused at once a sensation in the *teeth as if set on edge by a strong acid.* The pain was not in the fingers. *Trn.* gave relief after *Asar.*, *Gels.*, and *Sul. ac.* had failed. Among peculiarities of *Trn.* are: Stools occur immediately the head is washed. Wetting hands in cold water = symptoms. Snapping and cracking in right ear with pain and hiccough. One pupil dilated, the other contracted. Farrington relates a case of typhoid in a child cured by *Trn.* The child rolled its head and bit its nightgown. *Apis.* and *Agn.* improved. *Trn.* slightly aggravated at first, then rapidly improved. *Peculiar Sensations* are: As if head were knocked, in morning. As if thousands of needles were pricking into brain. As if occiput were struck with a hammer (this sensation as if hammered occurs in many parts and may be considered a general indication). As of a hair in eye. Singing like a tea-kettle in left ear. As if lower teeth were going to fall out. As if a living body in stomach rising to throat. As if body were bruised. As if there were not sufficient space in hypogastrium. Painful uneasiness in coccyx. Motion in uterus as of a fœtus. As of something crawling up legs under skin from feet to uterus. As if heart turned and twisted round. Heart as if squeezed and compressed. As of needles sticking into muscle of neck when touched. As of insects creeping and crawling. Tickling, burning, scorching, and numbness are prominent sensations. *Trn.* is *suited to* nervous, hysterical patients subject to choreic affections; to persons of foxy, mischievous, and destructive tendency; to choreic affections when whole body or right arm and left leg are involved. The symptoms are: < By touch. Rubbing >. Pressure >. Music >; = excitement. Rest <. Must walk about but walking < all symptoms. Can run better than walk. Motion > headache, < uterine pains and pains in coçcyx. < At night. < Washing head, < Wetting hands in cold water. Fresh air >. Warm water >. Coitus <. Light <; = to scream. Cough = headache; involuntary urination. < After sleep. > Riding in carriage (pain in spermatic cords). Epistaxis > throbbing in carotids, &c.

Relations.—*Antidote to:* Lach. (Hering). *Partial antidotes:* Puls.,

Mg. c., Mos., Cup., Chel., Gels., Bov., Carb. v. *Compare:* Irritation of periphery of nerves > exercising and rubbing, K. bro. Chorea, Myg., Act. r., Agar., Stram. Desire to jump, Stram., Croc., Nat. m., Sticta., Asar., Agar., Hyo., Cic. Bores head in pillow, Bell. (*Trn.* is more *rubbing*). Hysteria, alternation of moods, sensation of something alive, epistaxis black clots, Croc. As if occiput struck with a hammer, Naj. Deep-in headache, Bac. Extreme joy, Coff. Unfortunate love, Ph. ac. Ménière's disease ; ague, Chi. sul. Sees faces, Sul. Fidgety feet, Caust, Zn. Satyriasis, Pic. ac. Bloody semen, Merc., Led. Angina pectoris, Lat. mac., < after coitus, K. ca., Stph. Physometra, Bro. Crawling under skin, Coca. Callosities, Ant. c. Heart as from fright or bad news, Gels. Septicæmia, Pyro.

Causation.—Fall. Unrequited love. Bad news. Scolding. Punishment. Sepsis.

SYMPTOMS.

1. **Mind.**—Paroxysms of insanity ; presses her head and pulls her hair ; repeated after intermissions, threatening manners and speech ; restlessness of the legs ; mocking laughter and joy expressed in her face ; comes out of the attack with severe headache, eyes staring and wide open, sees small figures hovering before her eyes, and moves her hands.—Great excitement caused by music, one hour after it general and copious sweat.—Hysteria : with bitter belching ; < by moaning, > by sighing, with repeated yawning ; ludicrous and lascivious.—Visions : monsters ; animals ; faces ; insects ; ghosts.—The colours red, yellow, and green, and particularly black, produce heavy mist before the eyes.—Sees strangers in the room.—Great taciturnity and irritability ; desire to strike himself and others.—Excessive gaiety, laughs at slightest cause ; maniacally happy mood.—Joy and strong emotion with trembling when seeing beloved persons.—Sings until hoarse and exhausted.—Fits of nervous laughing ; followed by screams.—Profound grief and anxiety.—Desire to take things which do not belong to her.—Indifference, disgust, and sadness from morning to 3 p.m. were marked, < after midday ; from 3 p.m. to evening the gay disposition returned.—Wants to be without any light and without being spoken to.—Irritability, rage, fury.—Mischievous, destructive.—*Ennui.* —Fear of impending calamity.—Little intelligence and poor memory.

2. **Head.**—Vertigo : on walking ; after breakfast, with bad taste in mouth ; sudden, in air, on coming downstairs ; transient during the night ; preceded by gastric symptoms, < by carrying anything heavy on head ; causing falling without loss of consciousness ; when fixing sight on any object, with headache, severe pain in cerebellum, accompanied by incomplete erection of penis and formication of soft palate.—Contortions and extraordinary movements of head and hands, with rage and nervous agitation. —Must move head from r. to l. and hit it against some object, with crossness. —Head heavy, difficult to open eyes ; tendency to incline head backward.—Headache on waking compels her to lie down again.—Headache with giddiness when fixing the sight on any object.—Pain in head and heart with cough and nausea, morning on waking.—Deep, intense headache, with restlessness, compelling to move from place to place ; the pain flies to forehead and

occiput with photophobia; a strong light compels to complain and swear.—Compression; hammering; lancinating; burning pains in head.—Great burning in head, the hair troubles to the point of wanting to remove it; continually tossing head without finding a place where to rest it; uneasiness, impatience; ill-humour, oppressive breathing and desire to pull out her hair.—Headache < by touch.—Inclining head forward < frontal pain; inclining backward < occipital pain; inclining to either side < pain in that side.—Frontal headache, pain in vertex and parietal bones as if cold water was poured on the head, with great noise internally.—From 3 to 7 p.m. pain in forehead, esp. r. side.—Neuralgia of temples.—Pain in upper and middle part of head extending to cheek-bones, with nausea and desire to vomit.—Headache particularly affecting l. eye.—Lancinating pain l. side of head; with itching of r. ear.—Pains extending to occiput, with necessity of shutting the hands, which >.—Headache on occiput and temples when coughing, as if striking it with a hammer.—Pain in occiput: as if struck with a hammer; burning, scorching; with burning thirst; as if a nail driven in; compression, extending towards neck.

3. **Eyes.**—Blue circles round eyes.—Eyes glassy, red.—R. pupil much dilated, l. contracted.—Feeling of a hair in l. eye, which pricked it; pricking caused her to rub it, < on waking.—Pain in l. eye as if cold water poured into it.—Sensation: of splinter; sand; eye-lash; pin pricking eyes.—Shooting, lancinating, stinging pains in eyes.—Light irritates eyes; company annoys him.—Itching of eyes and very thick tears.—Pain in eyebrows.—Lids agglutinated on waking.—Itching of lids; herpes.—Photophobia.—Vision: weak, obscure; sees ghosts, faces, flashes.

4. **Ears.**—Profuse mucous secretion from r. ear.—Violent pain at external meatus, < by touch, which = sensation as if a nail were driven through head, or a general shaking.—On rising snap in r. ear followed by thick, brownish discharge.—Snapping cracking in r. ear with pain and hiccough.—Deafness with buzzing, whizzing, and vertigo.—Noise in ears: in night < waking; in r. with mucous discharge; in r. of clear bell on waking vanishing on getting up.—When a snapping or cracking is felt the hearing is >.

5. **Nose.**—Sneezing and coryza (r.).—Profuse epistaxis, with a flow of black, quickly coagulating blood.—Great itching in l. nostril and frequent sneezing.—Epistaxis > throbbing carotids and fulness in head.

6. **Face.**—Face: expression of terror; pale, earthy, strongly contrasting with purple neck; flushed with burning heat, also heat and sweat of palms.—Burning and scorching sensating on lips as after a fever.—Pain in angles of lower jaw, so severe he thinks he is going crazy.—Pain in lower jaw as if all teeth going to fall out.—Pain in direction of r. lower maxillary nerve, with a tickling sensation in stomach, dizziness, vanishing of sight, buzzing in ears.

7. **Teeth.**—Toothache: with sense of formication; with hiccough; as if loose, and electric sparks passed through them; throbbing; < coming in contact with the air.—Great dryness of mouth and teeth.—Painful aphthæ on tongue; with fetid breath.—Tongue drawn backward preventing speech.—Patch of suspicious cancerous nature in mouth and on fauces.—Palate feels scalded.

9. **Throat.**—Sore throat: when swallowing, at same time shooting in

l. eye; when coughing; talking; yawning; with painful constriction when smoking.—Sensation when swallowing of constriction in throat.—Throbbing sore throat.—Sensation as if cold water continually dropping down throat.—R. tonsil: painfully swollen; painful constriction, extending to ear, < by swallowing.—Fauces inflamed purplish.—External swelling of neck so great as to cause danger of choking.—Constant throbbing pain in cervical and submaxillary glands, with occasional sharp stinging pains.—Tonsillitis; high fever, delirium, red face, tonsils so swollen, suffocation feared.—(Diphtheria with same symptoms.)

10. **Appetite.**—Loss of appetite, intense thirst; general prostration; vomiting after eating; and getting out of bed; craving for raw food; disgust for meat.—(Disorders of pregnancy.)—Opium habit.—Taste of food: flat; bitter; salty: piquant.—Flat or sweetish taste in mouth.

11. **Stomach.**—Hiccough; with toothache.—Nausea: with dizziness compelling to lie down.—Vomiting: acid; mucous; with intense burning pains in stomach and œsophagus.—Pain in stomach < by drinking water.—Gastric symptoms with slight pains in roots of teeth, esp. when touching each other.—(Many digestive symptoms are peculiar on account of accompanying sympathetic neuralgic pains, in sides of head, face, ears, teeth, malar bones.)

12. **Abdomen.**—Swelling of hypochondria.—Lancinating pain in spleen, with pain in stomach and uterus.—Hepatic region painful to touch.—Sharp pain in umbilical region; violent burning in abdomen and rectum; stools profuse, dark, fetid, with violent urging; constipation.—Bloating.—Borborygmus.—Fibrous tumour in hypogastrium compressing genitals, and causing uterine discharges.—Burning in hypogastrium with great weight, interfering with walking and causing pruritus of vulva.—Pain in hypogastrium, hips and uterus, as if these parts were compressed; at same time unconquerable drowsiness.—Pain in groins; with relaxed sensation; as from rupture, esp. r., < by cold water.

13. **Stool and Anus.**—Pain and burning in anus after stool.—Repeated shooting in anus.—Violent effort to have a passage; hard stool with blood.—Tenesmus.—Constipation; with involuntary passing of urine on coughing or any effort.—Profuse diarrhœa with prostration, nausea, vomiting, fainting.—Stools: three or four times daily, very dark, fetid, partly formed, containing much mucus, expelled with difficulty, and followed by smarting and burning in anus; stools occur immediately on having head washed.—Weakness of sphincter, fæces appear natural but are passed as fast as accumulated.

14. **Urinary Organs.**—Pain in kidneys; with prostration.—Cystitis; with high fever, gastric derangement, excruciating pains and inability to pass a drop of urine; bladder seems swollen and hard; great tenderness and spasmodic action, debilitating patient, who passes only by drops a dark-red brown, fetid urine, with gravel-like sediment.—Pain in region of bladder; urination frequent, very painful; extremely nervous; could get no relief in any position; < night.—Urine: hot, thick, much sediment; difficult micturition; incontinence and pain in kidneys.—Diabetes.—Incontinence when laughing, coughing, &c.

15. **Male Sexual Organs.**—Extreme sexual excitement, lasciviousness almost to insanity.—Onanism followed by prostatic ailments and hypochondriasis.—Painfulness of genitals; testes relaxed, painful to touch; pain in

groins and stricture of urethra.—Erections.—Emissions.—Indolent tumou developed in each testicle.—Heaviness, pain and great swelling of (r.) testicl and cord.—Drawing pulling in left cord.—During emission of semen a sensa tion of heat is felt in its passage, it is rose-coloured containing some blood.— Difficult coitus, followed by fatigue and cough.

16. **Female Sexual Organs.**—Extreme sexual excitement; menses to early and profuse; pains and spasm of uterus; pruritus vulvæ; leucorrhœa —Violent nymphomania; < from coitus.—Nymphomania; reflex chorea hyperæmia and hyperæsthesia of sexual organs.—Sexual desire in a woma who had a shining callosity on l. index finger.—Fibrous tumour of uteru with bearing-down pains.—Discharge of blood alternately with leucorrhœa —Uterine discharge with pain in groins.—Spasmodic pains < when trying t walk.—Expulsion of gas from uterus.—Anguish, malaise in sexual organs impossible to walk; seems as if a living body moving or tingling in stomacl with tendency to rise to throat.—Sensation as if uterus had not room enougl and were pushing away intestines.—Pain in uterus with constrictive headach —Shooting: in vagina; in genitals followed by leucorrhœa.—Cutting in uteru or pain as if a heavy blow struck on it.—Pruritus vulvæ, after menses.—Pro fuse menstruation: with erotic spasms; crossness; ennui, and deep dissati faction; < after sleep.—Menses seven days too early.—(Uterine neuralgia.— Dysmenorrhœa.)—Sensation of motion in uterus, like a fœtus.—Disorders pregnancy.—Swelling of breasts with itching of nipples.

17. **Respiratory Organs.**—Roughness in larynx and trachea wit some dry cough, and smarting in eyelids.—Aphonia with increased difficult of breathing.—Hoarseness.—Cough: painful; dry; gagging; fatiguing; = distensive pains in head, chest, and uterus with sadness and anxiety; but whe walking in open air a sensation of happiness.—Cough when getting out bed, with vomiting and involuntary emissions of urine.—Chronic suffocatin catarrh.—Loose cough followed by tickling in larynx and bronchial tub which renews cough.—Attacks of suffocation, with crying, screaming, an restlessness.

18. **Chest.**—Great oppression in chest; panting respiration.—Sensatic as of a blow at base of l. lung.—In chest, pains; stinging; pressive; cram like; shooting.

19. **Heart and Pulse.**—Diseases of heart < by wetting hands in co water.—Præcordial anxiety, tremulous beating of heart.—Pain in heart as squeezed, also in aorta.—Nervous spells with pain in l. ovary.—Sensation as heart turned or twisted round.—Palpitation, stitches interfering with breathin —Painful throbbing of carotids, with fulness in head, esp. region of medull > by epistaxis.—Trembling and thumping of heart as from fright or bad new —Pulse: hard, infrequent; irregular.

20. **Neck and Back.**—Neck stiff; cannot move it without pain.—Pa l. side of neck when turning head to r.—Mole on neck with sensation as needles sticking into it when touched.—Pain in neck and back followed l general paralysis.—Swelling (or tumour, or rheumatoid prominence) spinal column with laboured breathing.—Tabes dorsalis.—Scapula: pa in; shooting pain under l.—Shooting in l. loin above hip.—Acute convulsi pains in l. lower part of vertebral column on appearance of menses, ceasi with them.—Repeated lancinating, shooting pain in coccyx.—(Coccygodyr

after confinement ; burning, smarting leucorrhœa, painful uneasiness in coccyx > standing, < slightest movement, sitting, lying in bed, or least pressure).

21. **Limbs.**—Rheumatism checked by putting extremities in cold water, panting respiration, anxiety, cramps in heart or twisting pains ; arm feels tense, stretched ; morning and night cold extremities.—Weakness, numbness, and dulness.—Necessity to move legs extends to hands with desire of taking something and throwing it away ; to roll something between fingers ; followed by general fatigue.—Great pain in knuckles and toes, can scarcely bear the weight of lightest linen.

22. **Upper Limbs.**—Heaviness in arms (soon).—Squeezed pain in l. arm and hand (forenoon).—Pain and swelling in wrists.—Restlessness of hands.—Unbearable pains in thumbs, esp. r., > pressure.—Burning and sweating of palms.

23. **Lower Limbs.**—Uneasiness of legs, must keep moving them.—Weakness of legs, cannot plant them firmly ; do not obey will.—Numbness of legs followed by paralysis.—Convulsive shaking and twitching in r. leg.—Pain in r. internal malleolus.—Shooting : in r. tendo Achillis ; r. great toe ; r. little toe.—Painful cramp in r. sole.—Itching in soles of feet.

24. **Generalities.**—A state like apoplexy or asphyxia comes on ; if music is brought the patient revives, sighs, commences to dance vigorously, and so the symptoms pass off with perspiration ; but they are apt to be renewed the following year in the same season.—Trembling of all limbs.—Intense restlessness.

25. **Skin.**—Ecchymosed spots.—Hepatic spots.—Furfuraceous spots.—Miliary eruption.—Indolent pimples.—Vesicular eruption like crusta lactea.—A small callosity, whitish, indolent, in r. palm between middle and index fingers, increased, with heat and pain, extended, broke, leaving an ulcer with callous edges, healed leaving a small scar.—Painful callosity at end of r. thumb fell off.—Callosity in l. index fell out.—Every year intense pain in toes from re-opened wound.—Formication ; pricking ; itching over whole body.

26. **Sleep.**—Yawning.—Sleeplessness.—Dreams : of business ; of drowning ; sad with weeping.—Wakes up cross.

27. **Fever.**—Constant chill and coldness during four days.—Scorching heat on whole body alternating with icy coldness.—Intermittent febrile attacks ; during heat continued coldness of feet.—Chills and fever with choreic convulsions ; shakes almost continuously with involuntary movements in limbs, abdomen, chest, back and face, < l. side ; could not speak (after a severe scolding or punishment).—Toxæmic fevers of a typhoid or intermittent form ; chilliness or burning heat, chilliness predominating.—Scorching heat of skin, which is scarlet.—Debilitating sweats.—Night-sweats.—Cold sweat.

Tarentula Cubensis.

Mygale Cubensis. Araña peluda. Cuban Tarantula. *N. O.* Araneideæ. Tincture of whole spider.

Clinical.—*Carbuncle.* Chorea. Intermittents.

Characteristics.—"The *Mygale Cubensis*, which may be called the *Cuban Tarentula*, also found in South Carolina and Texas, is a larger spider, of a dark brown colour, less poisonous, and covered with more hairs than the *Tarentula Hispanica*" (Hering). The chief uses to which *Trn. c.* has been put are: (1) Carbuncle, even to sloughing; with great prostration and diarrhœa. (2) Intermittent fever, with evening exacerbation. A keynote symptom is "atrocious pains." A case of chorea in a girl of twelve is reported (*H. M.* March, 1901) cured with *Trn. c.* 6. The movements were confined to the left side, and occurred chiefly at night, when *Trn. c.* was prescribed.

Relations.—*Compare:* In intermittents, Aran. d. Carbuncle Anthrac., Lach., Sil.

SYMPTOMS.

1. **Mind.**—Anxiety.—Delirium.
2. **Head.**—Headache.
13. **Stool.**—Diarrhœa.
14. **Urinary Organs.**—Retention of urine.
24. **Generalities.**—Toxæmia.
25. **Skin.**—The bite is painless; the person is not sensible of it till next day, when an inflamed pimple is found surrounded by a scarlet areola; from the pimple to some other part of the body a red erysipelatous line is seen marking the line followed by the spider over the skin after biting.—The pimple swells, the inflamed areola spreads, chills and fever set in with copious sweat and retention of urine; the pimple becomes a hard, large exceedingly painful abscess, ending by mortification of the integument over it, and having several small openings, discharging a thick, sanious matter containing pieces of mortified cellular tissue, fasciæ, and tendons the openings by growing run into one another, forming a large cavity at this period the fever takes the intermittent type with evening exacerbations.—In two cases, in delicate children, the bite proved fatal; but the majority recover in from three to six weeks.
27. **Fever.**—Chills followed by intense burning fever supervene on second or third day; with great thirst, anxiety, restlessness, headache delirium, copious perspiration and retention of urine.—Later the fever takes the intermittent type, with evening paroxysms, accompanied by diarrhœa and great prostration.

Tartaricum Acidum.

Tartaric acid. $C_4H_6O_6$. Trituration. Solution.

Clinical.—Gastritis. Heels, pain in.

Characteristics.—A proving by Nenning and some poisonings have furnished the pathogenesis of *Tart. ac.* One of the most marked symptoms was intense burning in throat and stomach, feeling "as if on fire." Tongue brown and dry. Almost constant vomiting; vomited matter of deep green colour. Fæces coffee-ground colour. Difficult respiration. Paralytic debility: "Weakness in the evening, can scarcely drag himself along." This should prove useful: "Tearing pain on the soles of the feet, near the heel, which prevents him putting his foot on the ground, after luncheon." All the symptoms were > in open air. The pasty taste is > after eating.

SYMPTOMS.

2. **Head.**—Confusion in head; dizziness.

6. **Face.**—Face instantly became red as fire, and having exclaimed that he was poisoned, became speechless; died on tenth day (drank 2 oz. in solution).—Lips turn brown and blackish on their inner edges.—Constant dryness of lips, must moisten them continually.—Burning of lips.

8. **Mouth.**—Teeth set on edge.—Brown and dry tongue.—Taste, pasty, in morning, ceases on eating.

9. **Throat.**—Burning sensation in throat and stomach as if on fire.

11. **Stomach.**—Very urgent thirst.—Eructations.—Nausea.—Vomiting, repeated and almost continuous.—Vomited matter, deep green.

12. **Abdomen.**—Pain in umbilical region.—Pinching below navel with emission of flatulence; cold feeling in abdomen.

13. **Stool.**—Many stools during night.—Stools of colour of coffee grounds.

17. **Respiratory Organs.**—Hoarseness and scraping in larynx.—Respiration: accelerated; then laborious and slow.

19. **Heart.**—Very weak action of heart.—Feeble pulse.

20. **Back.**—Sharp pain in region of loins.

23. **Lower Limbs.**—Paralysis of thighs and legs.—Tearing pains at soles, near the heel, which prevents him setting his foot on the ground, after luncheon.

24. **Generalities.**—Convulsions just before death.—Extreme weakness.—In evening feels very tired, can scarcely drag himself along.—General bruised sensation, esp. of lower limbs.

26. **Sleep.**—Yawning and stretching.—Frequent yawning.

27. **Fever.**—General cold feeling, evening in bed.

Taxus Baccata.

Taxus baccata. Yew. *N. O.* Coniferæ. Tincture of the fresh young shoots. (Tincture of the berries.)

Clinical.—Ciliary neuralgia. Cystitis. Digestion, too rapid. Dysuria. Ear, polypus of. Eruptions. Fainting. Gout. Hair, falling out. Headache, with photopsia. Heart, affections of. Kidneys, affections of. Knees, abscess of. Lachrymation. Nose, eruption on. Rheumatism. Purpura. Spermatorrhœa. Strangury. Vision, dim.

Characteristics.—The poisonous properties of the Yew have been recognised and disputed from ancient times. Gerarde says that in his schooldays he and his companions ate their fill of the berries of the Yew and slept not only under its shade, but on its branches, without any ill effect. But there is plenty of evidence on the other side. Recently (*Med. Press*, May 29, 1901), a patient of Mullingar Asylum died suddenly from eating Yew leaves. Some years ago a correspondence in the *Times* brought to light instances of the lethal effects of Yew leaves on cattle. One correspondent, Mr. James Simmons, of Haslemere, mentions an observation made by himself and others, that Yew leaves are more poisonous some time after they have been cut than when fresh : "Yew cropped green from the tree has no fatal effect," and animals do not eat it fresh, they prefer grass ; but if Yew has been cut and allowed to wither cattle will eat it in large quantities, and in that state it is deadly poison." "My people," says Mr. Simmons, "once buried some Yew cuttings deep in the dung of a farmyard ; a number of large hogs dug it up, ate it and all died."—The symptoms of the pathogenesis are made up o poisonings by leaves and berries, and also of provings by Gastier Fainting is a very prominent feature with *Tax.*, and the fatal cases end in convulsions, collapse, and syncope. Death from Yew poisoning, says Cooper, is remarkably painless. "Empty feeling" in the stomach was prominent ; and it was noted that the digestion was very rapid. "Must eat frequently" is a characteristic. Gastric catarrh is set up with vomiting of tenacious mucus. The saliva is increased and it also is viscid ; and there is viscid sweat. An intense action on the skin was developed, and *Tax.* is indicated in pustular skin affections, the pustules being large, flat, and strongly itching. On the suggestion of Cooper, I once gave a single dose of *Tax.* φ in a case o aural polypus (bright red) with catarrh, in a youth, with the result that the polypus shrivelled up to one-third of its former size. The shooting pains in the toes suggest the use of *Tax.* in gout. The kidneys and bladder were much irritated ; and the heart disturbed *Tax.* has been recommended as a substitute for *Dig.*, being considered superior to the latter in having no cumulative effect. The symptom were < by pressure. Rubbing > itching of eyelids. Coughing = headache. Deep respiration = cough. < Before and after each meal. < By application of liquids. < After coitus.

Relations.—*Antidoted by:* Staph (prostration with oppressio after an embrace). *Compare:* The Coniferæ. Load at stomach, Ab. n. Rapid digestion, Sul. Podagra, Urt. ur.

SYMPTOMS.

1. **Mind.**—Impatience, which unfits the patient for mental application. —Delirium.—Stupor.

2. **Head.**—Reeling sensation when at rest, on being seated, and when standing upright.—Headache above eyebrows, with brilliant and movable lines before the sight.—Pains in forehead, extending to face, with drawing pains in eyes, and lachrymation.—Heavy pain in region of r. temple and eyebrow, with a sensation of lachrymation, and < from slightest cough.—Squeezing in sides of head.—Aching, esp. in temporal bone.—Burning headache.—Lancinating pain in frontal region.—Heat in forehead.

3. **Eyes.**—In the eyes: drawing with lachrymation and pressure, and headache below the eyebrows.—Itching of external angle of l. eye.—Burning itching in eyelids, disappearing after scratching them.—Abundant lachrymation when eyes are used, even but a little, esp. in females.—Lachrymation of l. eye.—Pupils widely dilated.—Vision dim.

4. **Ears.**—(Polypus of the ears.)

5. **Nose.**—Round spot of a reddish-brown colour, on the end of nose, with desquamation of skin.

6. **Face.**—Looks ill.—Face: pale; livid; convulsed.—Lips: purplish; livid; blackish brown, esp. upper.—Frothing at mouth.

8. **Mouth.**—Sensation of coldness in (upper incisor) teeth.—Burning pricking on tongue.—Tongue: excoriated; moist; tremulous.—Mouth dry. —Saliva: increased; extremely viscid; acrid.—Bitter taste, like that of Cinchona.

11. **Stomach.**—Violent hunger, soon after breakfast, with general uneasiness, and weakness in region of stomach.—Frequent want to eat, with activity of digestive functions.—Nausea with accumulation of saliva.—Sensation of emptiness, without hunger, in stomach.—Retching.—Vomiting ending in death.—Vomit: tenacious, containing bile; Yew leaves embedded in mucus.—Pain in pit of stomach, when touched.—Tension in epigastrium, which is painful to touch.—Aching, burning, and pinching in region of stomach.

12. **Abdomen.**—Tension in abdomen, as if the stomach were overloaded. —Squeezing and tension across abdomen.—Aching in umbilical region.—Borborygmi.

13. **Stool.**—Hard, difficult, dry evacuations.—Occasionally a stool which is soft, or of a natural consistence.—Diarrhœa, with insupportable tenesmus, and burning at every evacuation.

14. **Urinary Organs.**—Cutting pain at base of kidneys which allows him neither to sit still nor stand up, and even prevents turning in bed.—Urinary tenesmus.—Frequent want to urinate, with difficult emission in a fine stream.—Strangury, urine red.

15. **Male Sexual Organs.**—Flow of semen without erection or sexual

pleasure for several successive nights.—Great excitement during coition.—After coition, weakness and great oppression.

17. **Respiratory Organs.**—Violent and fatiguing cough.—Short cough, after every meal, excited by full inspirations, with oppression.

18. **Chest.**—Oppression, esp. when stomach is either too full or too empty, or else with pain below xiphoid cartilage.—Lancinating pain in l. side.—Lungs engorged.—Chest full and hot.

19. **Heart.**—Irregular action of heart.—Pulse : rapid ; slow ; feeble ; small, wiry ; almost imperceptible.

20. **Neck and Back.**—Drawing pain in muscles of neck (l.).—Sacral pains, which allow no rest either in a standing or sitting posture, and which compel the patient to remain in bed.—Incisive pain in sacrum.—Constant pain in back.—Pain in shoulder-blade, which subsequently removes to loins.

21. **Limbs.**—Numbness of limbs and paralysis ; esp. after several sweats.—Sharp, transient, wandering pains.

22. **Upper Limbs.**—Aching pain in elbow near humerus, affecting the bone, felt during motion and rest, but < by movement.—Violent itching in forearm, followed by an eruption of red and hard pimples round wrist, which itch chiefly in evening, and at night, and afterwards occasion a tickling sensation.—Lancinations in hand.—Burning dryness of palms of hands.—Dull pain in joints of fingers.—Rheumatic pain in r. forefinger, renewed by least contact with even warm liquid.

23. **Lower Limbs.**—Pain in hip and knee, with tearing pain and coldness in thigh ; > at night.—Pain in l. hip, with internal heat.—In thighs, distressing coldness of skin, esp. of fore-part.—Tingling in l. thigh.—Painful tingling round patella.—Lancinating pain in knee, with weakness of the joint.—Abscess at r. knee.—Contusive and incisive pain, which hinders walking.—Incisive pain, esp. in l. knee, which awakens patient at night.—Violent pinching in l. calf, with itching in a small circumscribed place.—Large suggillation on sole of l. foot.—Tingling crawling sensation in whole l. foot.

24. **Generalities.**—Pains in the knees, elbows, and back.—Trembling.—Slight tremor over whole frame.—Convulsions.—Faintness.—Fainting and collapse.—Relaxation of muscles.

25. **Skin.**—All hairy parts became denuded (after a month).—Black jaundice.—Skin red.—Body covered with pustules.—On waking, body covered with miliary eruption ; disappeared on third day and abscess formed at right knee.—Large suggillation on l. sole followed by dark petechiæ over nearly whole body, great swelling of face and lips, esp. upper lip, exhaustion and death (boy 5, poisoned by berries).—Eruption of large pimples, slightly elevated, like red spots, on the upper part of both arms.—Dry tetter, red at the base ; and causing much itching, at external angle of l. eye.

26. **Sleep.**—Sleeplessness during whole night, yawning without inclination to sleep.

27. **Fever.**—Commencing with general shivering at 2 a.m., followed by dry heat of hands and feet, and general uneasiness, dryness of mouth, without thirst, afterwards profuse perspiration on forehead ; shaking after breakfast, with general uneasiness, and dryness of mouth, without thirst.—Perspiration attends the least exertion, with great prostration of strength. Profuse night-

sweats.—Offensive viscid sweats, with smart itching and redness in the glandular parts at the surface of the body.—Peculiarly offensive sweat with eruption of vesicles.

Tellurium

Tellurium. An element; (generally considered non-metallic). Te. (A.W. 125). Trituration of the precipitated element.

Clinical.—Axilla, offensive sweat of; tumour of. Barber's itch. Cataract. Conjunctivitis. Coryza. Eczema. Entropion. Eyes, inflammation of. Foot-sweat, fetid. Gleet. Herpes. Hoarseness. Levitation. *Pityriasis versicolor.* Post-nasal catarrh. *Ringworm. Sacrum, pain in.* Sciatica. *Spinal irritation.* Worms. Yawning.

Characteristics.—*Tellurium* occurs in the native state and in combination with gold, silver, lead, and antimony. It resembles *Sulphur* and *Selenium* in its chemical reactions. It was proved and introduced into homœopathy by Hering in 1850. The most notable feature of the proving was the irritation of the skin, including skin of eyelids and ears, of spinal column and of some nerves. The most characteristic form of the skin irritation of *Tell.* is herpes circinatus, and it has probably cured more cases of ringworm, especially of the face and body, than any other remedy. (I cured with *Tell.* an Indian officer home on furlough whose body was covered over with a ring-worm-like eruption.) The odour of the body and of the sweat is offensive and garlic-like. The prover had to sit apart from the rest of the class during a whole session on account of this. In parts where the skin forms openings, as the ear, the effect of *Tell.* is intensified. The characteristic odour of the ear discharge is that of fish brine. The discharge is so acrid it vesicates any part of the skin it touches. *Tell.* is one of the most important remedies in otorrhœa. Nash cured several cases of post-scarlatinal otorrhœa, using the 6th, higher attenuations having failed. Eyelids are inflamed, and the vesicating property extends to the eye itself, setting up phlyctenular conjunctivitis. Other parts of the skin affected by *Tell.* are the hair-roots, the breasts, the perinæum, and the anus. There is itching in the rectum after stool. *Tell.* has caused expulsion of threadworms. The offensiveness of *Tell.* appears in the breath and in the flatus; and it is a leading remedy in offensive foot-sweat. In addition to the inflammation of the eyes caused by *Tell.*, it has pains over the eyes. Skin and nerves are closely allied, and *Tell.* is a remedy in many neuralgic conditions, notably sciatica. The right side is most affected, and these are characteristic Conditions: the pain is < coughing, sneezing, or straining at stool; < lying on painful side. Many of the pains and symptoms of *Tell.* come and go suddenly. The ears are suddenly stopped. There are sudden rushes of blood to the head. *Tell.* has great sensitiveness to touch. This is shown in the neuralgic hyperæsthetic state of the spine. It has also a vulnerary action as shown in a case of Kent's (quoted *A. H.*, xxiii. 439). A boy, 4, slid down banisters and struck his head on a tiled floor. He became unconscious and a surgeon was summoned, who found him in that state and with a clear, watery discharge from the ear, which the surgeon pronounced to be cerebro-spinal fluid. This condition lasted three days, and the case had been pronounced hopeless when Kent first saw the boy. Kent noticed that the discharge was acrid, and reddened whatever part it came in contact with. One dose of *Tell.* was given. In two hours the child vomited, a sign of reaction, and in two weeks was well. Shelton (*H. R.*, vii. 103) relates three cases: (1) Widow, 50, had pain and soreness upper part of back for a long time. She shrank from the slightest touch on the part. The sensitiveness was so acute that *when touched the pain extended into the occiput and all over the upper region of the back. Tell.* 6 cured in eighteen days. (2) Miss X., 45, had a fall, striking a severe blow on the sacrum. She suffered for some weeks from concussion, with one point of great soreness in the sacral region, just above the spot where the blow was received. She was kept in bed for some weeks and improved generally, but the painful spot remained and sensitiveness appeared over the back, especially its upper third. *Tell.* 6 cured all completely. (3) Miss Y., 29, who had had severe spinal meningitis ten years before, consulted Shelton for a burning, pressing pain at base of brain. He diagnosed the condition as pachy-meningitis. The patient grew worse, and gradually ptosis, and then right and then left hemiplegia set in. Finally hyperæsthesia of the back became so distressing that it was a question of finding any support that did not intensify the pain. She could not bear the slightest touch, complaining that *it not only hurt her at the point of contact, but she felt it in the head and in remote parts of the body. Tell.* cleared up the case. Skinner (*H. W.*, xviii. 535) cured two sporting dogs of ringworm with *Tell.* 1m F.C. The irritating property of *Tell.* is shown again in the coryza, post-nasal catarrh, tickling in larynx, hoarseness, and cough. There is a good deal of drowsiness with *Tell.*; yawning after retching; drowsy after eating. I once gave *Tell.* to a child for an eruption, and cured it incidentally of constant yawning, with which it had been troubled. The eruption improved at the same time. *Peculiar Sensations* are: Fear of being touched on sensitive places. As if in air on going to sleep. Brain as if beaten. As if lashes were turned in. As if air whistled through left Eustachian tube. As if strapped together in epigastric region. As if fluid wanted to discharge in lobe of right lung. There is periodicity about some of the symptoms. One prover has a return of them every Tuesday for several weeks. More symptoms appear on the left than on the right side. The symptoms are: < By touch; touch = bleeding from ear; spine sensitive to touch. Pressure = lump in axilla to be painful. Rest <. Lying: > vertigo; on left side = throbbing over right ribs and *vice versâ*; on left side = pain in heart. > Lying on back. Lying on affected side < sciatica. While sitting up: vertigo; face red. Stooping, coughing, laughing, straining at stool <. Many symptoms are < in morning, on being wakened, and at night; eating = drowsiness. Eating rice = vomiting. Eating and drinking > sore throat.

Relations.—*Antidoted by:* Nux (epigastric oppression). *Compare:* Tetradymite, which contains Tellur. Restlessness; garlicky odour, Ars. Coryza, Cepa. Otitis, Puls., Bell., Ter. Ringworm, Bac., Sep., Nat. m. Ringworm in clusters Sep., Calc. Threadworms, Teucr. Pains come and go suddenly, Bell., Lyc. < Laughing, Pho. < Straining at stool, Indm. Cough and skin, Osm.

Causation.—Falls. Rice (vomiting).

SYMPTOMS.

1. **Mind.**—Forgetful.—Fear of being touched in sensitive places.—Excitable, disposed to fly into a passion.—Rough, angular disposition.—Mind depressed.

2. **Head.**—Vertigo; when going to sleep; morning after rising; < walking, sitting up, or turning head; > lying perfectly quiet.—Brain feels as if beaten on slightest movement.—Heaviness and fulness of head in morning.—Violent linear pain in small spot over l. eye; pain, short, sharp, and defined.—Congestion to temples and forehead on waking in morning.—Sudden rush of blood to head.—About 10 a.m. pain above l. eye, came and went suddenly.—Sensation of numbness in occiput and nape.—Red spots and fine blisters on occiput, neck, and behind ears, and on posterior surface of ears.

3. **Eyes.**—Deposit of chalky-looking white mass on anterior surface of lens (cataract).—Pterygium.—Herpes conjunctivæ bulbi; phlyctenules near edge of cornea; < from crying.—Pustular conjunctivitis with eczema impetiginodes on lids and much purulent discharge from eyes; offensive discharge from ears.—Scrofulous inflammation; < l. upper lid; lachrymation, itching, and pressure in lid.—Eyelids: thickened, inflamed, covered with pustules; pale red, œdematous, oozing.—Feeling as if lashes of lower lid were turned in.—Palpebral swelling of l. upper lid; ulceration on outer surface of lid, near outer canthus; pain < at night.

4. **Ears.**—L. ear began to itch, burn, and swell; aching and throbbing pain in meatus, followed by a copious, watery, acrid discharge.—Dull, throbbing pain in ears, day and night; thin, watery, excoriating discharge.—Ears suddenly stopped in forenoon; < l.—Sometimes, for an instant, sensation as if air catches itself in, or whistled through l. Eustachian tube; when snuffing or belching air passes through.—Vesicular eruption on membrana tympani; suppurating and perforating.—Itching and swelling, with painful throbbing in external meatus; in three or four days discharge of watery fluid smelling like fish-pickle, which = vesicles wherever it touches; ear bluish red, œdematous; hearing impaired.—Waked during night with dull aching deep in r. ear, continued three days with depression of spirits.—Eczema behind ears, with formation of thick crusts; scrofulous conjunctivitis, blepharitis, and catarrh of middle ear.

5. **Nose.**—Fluent coryza, lachrymation and hoarseness when walking in open air, with short cough and pressure in middle of chest under sternum; > after being in open air some time.—Nose dry, then becomes fluent with relief of headache; r. eye becomes hot with profuse lachrymation.—Nose obstructed, must breathe through mouth.—Hawks from posterior nares dried yellowish-red phlegm tasting salty, mornings.

6. **Face.**—Sudden flushes of redness over face.—While sitting, face red. —Twitching in l. facial muscles, l. corner of mouth drawn up when talking.—Burning in lips.—Ringworms on face; barber's itch.—Pimples on face.

8. **Mouth.**—Gums bleed easily and profusely.—Tongue somewhat swollen, furred white, shows print of teeth.—Breath has odour of garlic.—Coldness of mouth and pharynx on drawing in air.—Copious saliva.—Tenacious mucus runs from mouth (dog).—Taste earthy, metallic.

9. **Throat.**—Painful dryness of fauces.—In morning hawks from back of nose pieces of yellowish-reddish phlegm tasting salt.—Rough, scratching sensation in throat; < towards evening.—Throat feels sore with a prickly, rough sensation evening and morning; throat sore on simply swallowing; > after eating or drinking..—Pain in throat extends into ear.

11. **Stomach.**—Hungry at night; wants an apple in middle of night.—Longs for beer.—After meals, great drowsiness.—After eating rice obliged to vomit.—Belching with taste of food eaten.—Heartburn with warmth in stomach as from alcohol.—Sensation of weakness like faintness in stomach after local congestion of blood to head and nape, also with chest symptoms. —Fulness in pit of stomach, must lie down after dinner.—Constrictive feeling in stomach as if strapped together.

12. **Abdomen.**—Fulness and oppression in hypogastrium, her dress must be loosened.—Pressing first l. then r. side as from wind.—When lying on l. side, throbbing under r. ribs and *vice versâ*.—Pinching in abdomen.—Frequent spasmodic pains in bowels as from incarcerated wind; mostly from 5 to 9 p.m.

13. **Stool and Anus.**—Passes very offensive wind.—Passes a large quantity of threadworms.—Spasmodic pains with urging to stool, copious stool with feeling of flatulence in bowels.—Costive.—Tetter on perinæum, itching.—Itching in rectum after stool.—Itching at anus.

14. **Urinary Organs.**—Pain and soreness in kidneys.—Increased urination.—High-coloured, acid urine.

15. **Male Sexual Organs.**—Erections all night.—Increased desire, followed by long-lasting indifference.—A drop of viscid fluid glues meatus. —Secondary gonorrhœa.—Herpes on scrotum and perinæum.

16. **Female Sexual Organs.**—Painful soreness in region of kidneys, extending downward like a weight, mostly to r. and in sacrum; < morning, making her irritable.—Shooting deep in pelvis across to l.—Menses too early in climacteric years.

17. **Respiratory Organs.**—Hoarseness in morning with fluent coryza; a rough, pressing, tickling sensation in larynx.—Coughing on laughing < aching in small of back.—Cough towards morning; after a few days looser.

18. **Chest.**—Pain in region of clavicle.—Pain in middle of chest; going through to back; from dorsal vertebræ through to sternum; in or behind sternum.—Shooting in l. chest, fifth rib.—Feeling as if some fluid wanted to discharge, pressing downward in middle lobe of r. lung.—Cutting around and in l. nipple, through to scapula.—Eruption about nipple.

19. **Heart.**—Dull pain in region of heart when lying on l. side; > lying on back.—Palpitation of heart, with throbbing through whole body and full pulse, followed by sweat.

20. **Neck and Back.**—With the pain above the eye, sensation along l.

side of neck as if the blood there had suddenly been retained in one of the large veins, or had streamed backwards.—Numbness in nape and occiput.—When lying on l. ear sharp pressing pain from neck into ear.—Pressing ache in r. scapula, later in l.—Painful sensitiveness of spine from last cervical to sixth dorsal vertebræ ; sensitive to pressure and touch.—Weak feeling in back.—Pain in sacrum, passing into r. thigh ; < pressing at stool, coughing, and laughing.

21. **Limbs.**—Sharp, quick pains in elbows, ankles, and other parts.—Aching all over, mostly in limbs, < r. side and in walking.

22. **Upper Limbs.**—Offensive sweat of armpits, smelling of garlic.—Lump in anterior wall of l. axilla, painful from pressure or motion.—near thumb-joint.—Finger-tips feel dead on stretching hand.—Rheumatism of r. little finger, < moving it.

23. **Lower Limbs.**—Sciatica, r. side ; < lying on affected side.—Sciatica with sensitiveness of vertebral column.—Tonic muscular contraction of long standing.—Contraction of tendons of bends of knees.—Bruised pain in hip-joints after walking.—Feet sweaty, mostly on toes.—Fetid sweat of feet.

24. **Generalities.**—Persistent fetid body odour.—Restlessness.—Lassitude.

25. **Skin.**—Ringworm : on face ; barber's itch ; whole body, < lower limbs ; on single parts.—Stinging in skin.—Small red pimples, very bright red and very sharply defined, with minute vesicles upon them, first on lower limbs, then also on upper, most on l. side ; they began first on calves, then on inside of forearms above wrist and spread from that part, caused very severe itching day and night, < night after going to bed.—Little stinging prickings in various parts, compelling him to rest ; circular vesicular spots appeared.—Body thickly covered with elevated rings of herpes circinatus.—Psoriasis.—Skin dry, hot.—Scrofulous eczematous eruption.—Itching < in cool air.

26. **Sleep.**—Yawning and belching.—Drowsy after a meal.—Sleepless ; restless turning from weariness and bruised feeling.—At night pains all over.—On going to sleep feels as if in air, quick drawing towards feet awakens him.

27. **Fever.**—Chilly, with pains.—Skin hot and dry ; sensation as if overstrained, as if bruised, as if he had taken cold after severe exertion.—Heat : in sinciput ; in face.—Sweat : on face ; on spots with increased itching of these places ; often throbbing through whole body ; generally warm, while sitting in a cool breeze.

Teplitz.

The mineral water of Teplitz in Bohemia. [Contains in 16 oz. Nat. c. gr. 2·28, Nat. m. ·43, Nat. fl. sil. ·13, K. sul. ·43, K. mur. ·1, Calc. c. ·32, Sil. ·31, &c.] Dilution.

Clinical.—Amenorrhœa. Bones, affections of. Breast, tumours in. Epistaxis. Eruptions. Erysipelas. Flatulence. Gout. Hæmorrhoids. Leucorrhœa. Metrorrhagia. Paralysis. Rheumatism. Sciatica. Scurvy. Speech, difficult. Spine, pains in. Tongue, paralysis of. Toothache. Ulcers. Vertigo.

Characteristics.—The waters of Teplitz are chiefly in repute for the treatment of gouty patients, especially those suffering from atonic gout. The springs are alkaline and hot, and the temperature forms a leading feature in their action. The symptoms of the Schema are Perutz', who experimented on himself and several healthy individuals, together with symptoms by Hromada. Symptoms of *Nat. c.* and *Nat. m.* appear throughout. Tearfulness, low spirits, and irritability were noted, and giddiness of much intensity. This symptom has been cured: "Giddiness, when she walks all the houses seem to move too." Some *Peculiar Symptoms* are: On moving head it seems as if something fell from one side to the other. Burning in stomach, > drinking cold water. > From hæmorrhoidal bleeding. Burning sensation in many parts. Hæmorrhage; epistaxis; piles; with stool; metrorrhagia. Vesicles in mouth and on tongue. Vesicular erysipelas. Paralysis of tongue; of limbs. Cold feelings: in upper arm; in foot. Increased sensitiveness to cold. The symptoms are < at night (bone pains). < Motion. > By friction. > Drinking cold water.

Relations.—*Compare:* Nat. c., Nat. m., K. sul., Mang., Lith., Sil., Alm.

SYMPTOMS.

1. **Mind.**—Anxiety.—Irritable, tearful.—Loud speech and absence of thought.—Indisposition to work.—Weak memory.

2. **Head.**—Confusion of head with aching over eyes.—Vertigo: with feeling of paraplegia; with faintness; with noise in ears and dim vision; with feeling, when she walks, as if all the houses moved too.—On moving head, sensation as if something fell from one side to the other, with weak memory.—Tearing in head with pain in throat so that he could not breathe freely.—Bursting headache.—Frontal headache with inclination to vomit.—Throbbing headache in r. temple with swollen red face.—Aching in occiput.—Hair falls out.—Large movable lumps on head with erysipelas of face.—Vesicles on scalp.—Soreness of hairy scalp, every hair causing pain when touched.

3. **Eyes.**—Both eyes closed in morning with white viscid mucus.—Dryness in r. eye and dimness of vision.—Aching and burning in eyes.—Erysipelas of lids.—On r. lid two styes, which disappear without suppuration.—Cramp pain in upper lids, cannot be opened except with the hand.—Lachrymation.—Inflammation of conjunctiva of eyelid and eye ball.

4. **Ears.**—Swelling of l. concha with erysipelatous inflammation.—Purulent discharge from ear.—Tearing pain in interior of r. ear as from a red-hot coal.—Tearing, shooting pain first in one ear, then in the other.—Dulness of hearing, with sensation as if sweat stopped ears.—Tinnitus.

5. **Nose.**—Aching over root of nose.—Pricking and dryness in nose.—Frequent and profuse epistaxis.

6. **Face.**—Face: swollen, red; swollen, pale.—Drawing and tearing in face; in r. side from forehead to jaw, with drawing of the jaw awry and difficult speech.

8. **Mouth.**—Raging toothache, r. cheek and lower jaw drawn to l. side, ɜventing proper speech.—Violent toothache as if all teeth suddenly pierced th a hot iron.—Boring in upper molars.—All incisors feel too long.—equent bleeding of gums with loosening of teeth.—Spasmodic protrusion tongue with difficult speech.—Tongue: paralysed; swollen; moist; coated ite or yellow.—Vesicles on back of tongue with burning pain in throat.—side r. cheek several small vesicles which burst and form ulcers.—Dry outh with burning on tip of tongue.

9. **Throat.**—Pain in throat without redness.—Aching on swallowing.—aring-drawing in muscles of throat and stiffness of neck.—Swelling of ula and tonsils with difficulty of swallowing.—Swelling of cervical glands.

11. **Stomach.**—Canine hunger, soon satisfied, and followed by stomach-he.—Anorexia: with sour taste; with white, viscid coating on tongue; with eling of fulness in pit of stomach.—Heartburn with flow of much water tongue.—Nausea, and faint feeling, and vomiting.—Aching in stomach tending through to back.—Pain in stomach, with burning rising up into roat as if a red-hot coal lay there; > drinking cold water.—Sensation as if omach full of water; seems to splash about when walking.—Full feeling stomach with much wind and eructation.

12. **Abdomen.**—Shooting in r. hypochondrium, esp. on drawing a full eath.—Tearing in umbilical region.—Tense, swollen abdomen, with dis-arge of much flatus.—Rumbling.—Weight in abdomen and bearing down genitals.—Cramp of recti muscles.—Swelling of inguinal glands.

13. **Stool and Anus.**—Profuse bleeding of piles with > of symptoms. Passage of whitish, acrid mucus by anus.—Painful piles and violent burning anus.—Burning in rectum with evacuation of viscid, blood-streaked secretion. Itching in perinæum, with production of eruption.—Frequent urging ithout stool.—Discharge of bright red blood by stool, with colic.—Stool: in, frothy, with burning in anus; hard with bright red blood.—Con-ipation: with nausea; with pain in back and heaviness of lower limbs.

14. **Urinary Organs.**—In urethra: flying shooting; burning in anterior rt.—Urine: copious; scanty; retained; slimy; brick-dust sediment.

15. **Male Sexual Organs.**—Vesicles on glans becoming speedily sore. Suppurating eruption on glans and scrotum leaving blue marks.—Painful velling of testes.—Drawing in r. testis and cord.—Increased desire and eams.

16. **Female Sexual Organs.**—Milk-white leucorrhœa like boiled arch.—Violent tearing pain in abdomen.—Menses a fortnight before time. -Often pain in hypogastrium as if everything would be forced out below; enses, which had never appeared, occurred very copiously.—Metrorrhagia ith frightful pains in abdomen; blood black and coagulated.

17. **Respiratory Organs.**—Aching in larynx > when swallowing.—larynx: dryness; roughness; tickling.—In trachea: catarrh, with expec-ration of viscid mucus; rawness.—Hoarseness to aphonia.—Cough: short, ry; suffocative; at night.—Expectoration: viscid, yellow mucus; copious. -Violent cough with enormous expectoration of grey colour, which only isappears when an eruption appears.

18. **Chest.**—Oppression, as from great rush of blood to chest.—Cramp-ke contraction in chest.—Shooting in intercostal muscles.—Tearing in pec-

toralis major to shoulder.—Burning under sternum.—In r. breast two lum
as large as hazel-nuts with dull pain.—Fine pricking as with needle in
breast.

19. **Heart.**—Violent shooting in heart; with palpitation.—Action
heart: irregular, painful; intermitting.—Pulse: quick, hard; full.

20. **Neck and Back.**—Bruised pain in nape and back.—Tearing ar
drawing in nape with stiffness.—Shooting pains along spinal column, fro
nape to lumbar vertebræ, preventing slightest motion.—Tearing drawin
down back to sacrum; in scapulæ.—Shooting and gnawing betwe
scapulæ.—Eruption of pimples on whole back.—In small of back: pa
< by every movement; drawing into pelvis, to calves.—Aching and stitch
in loins, extend to spine, with difficulty of breathing.

21. **Limbs.**—Weariness and heaviness.—Tearing, drawing, shooting
limbs, esp. joints.—Tearing in hands and feet.

22. **Upper Limbs.**—Paralysis: of r. arm; of both arms, with creeping
finger-tips.—Violent pains in both arms with raised spots like syphilis.—Tearir
in whole arm with contraction of elbow-joint.—Stiffness in l. shoulder-joi
with difficulty in raising arm, esp. backwards.—Violent, ever-increasing pa
in r. shoulder-joint.—Dislocation pain in shoulder.—Paralysis of shoulders.-
Burning or shooting in axilla.—In upper arm: shiny red swelling; co
feeling as if cold wind blew on it; sore, bruised feeling; boring, tearin
cramp.—Elbow: swelling and tearing; cracking, and in wrist; shootin
burning; scab-like eruption round.—Tearing down forearm to fingers.—
wrist: redness, swelling; violent pains; stiffness; sprained feeling in r.-
Hands: tremble; swelling of; gouty nodes on fingers.

23. **Lower Limbs.**—Hip-joints: stiff; tearing; shooting; bruise
pains.—Aching in femur with cold feeling.—Numbness; jerking; cram
swelling in thighs and calves.—Knee-joint: swollen, stiff; cracking in
aching in patella.—Swelling and suppuration of bone in middle of l. leg.-
Sprained feeling in ankle.—Tension in tendo Achillis, preventing putting he
to ground.—Burning in heels.—Shooting-jerking in great toe.

24. **Generalities.**—Weariness and heaviness on waking with congesti
of head.—Increased sensitiveness to draughts.

25. **Skin.**—Redness of skin.—Swelling and profuse perspiration.—Ras
like scarlatina; miliary; pustular; erysipelas, vesicular.—Ulceration.—Prickir
as with needles.

26. **Sleep.**—Sleepiness; by day.—Frequent jerks on falling to sleep.-
Dreams: incompleted; lively with increased sexual desire.

27. **Fever.**—Chilliness, shuddering.—Cold feeling in shoulder; in thig
—Prickly heat, followed by moderate sweat.—Copious sweat.—Sour an
mouldy-smelling sweat.

Terebinthina.

eum terebinthinæ. Oil of Turpentine. $C_{10} H_{16}$. The oil distilled from the oleo-resin (turpentine) obtained from various species of Pinus, purified by repeated rectification with water. Solution in rectified spirit. Ozonised Oil of Turpentine (prepared by exposure of the common oil to sun and air in a half-filled bottle and shaking from time to time).

Clinical.—Albuminuria. Amblyopia potatorum. Asthma. *Backache. Bladder, itable.* Brachial neuralgia. Bronchitis. Chordee. Chorea. Ciliary neuralgia. stitis. Dentition. *Dropsy.* Dysentery. Dysmenorrhœa. *Enteric fever.* ilepsy. Erysipelas bullosa. Erythema. Fibroma. Gall-stone colic. Glands, uinal; swelling of. Gleet. Gonorrhœa. *Hæmaturia.* Hæmorrhoids. Hernia; angulated. Herpes labialis pudendi. Hydrophobia. Hypochondriasis. Insanity. estines, ulceration of. Iritis. Jaundice. *Kidneys, congestion of;* neuralgia of. mbago. Neuralgia; supraorbital. Ovaries, pains in; dropsy of. Pityriasis. rpura hæmorrhagica. Scabies. *Scarlatina. Sciatica.* Spermatorrhœa. *angury.* Stricture. Tetanus. *Tympanites.* Uræmia. *Urine, suppression of;* ention of. Worms.

Characteristics.—*Ter.* was introduced to homœopathy by Hartab. A proving of it appeared in Hartlaub and Trinks' *Annalen.* ny symptoms have been added from poisonings and overdosings in l-school practice. According to Taylor, children are particularly isitive to its action. Illness caused by sleeping in newly painted oms is due in great part to the turpentine. "A stimulant and tonic the mucous membranes, especially of the bladder and urethra: proves useful in gleet, leucorrhœa, and cystorrhœa." This is lnes' account of the old-school use of *Ter.* as an internal remedy. unton gives these points: (1) Applied to the skin *Ter.* acts as an itant and rubefacient, causing a sensation of burning, and vesicles applied for any length of time. (2) Inhaled it causes sneezing, htness across eyes, and dyspnœa. (3) Given internally it causes rning in mouth and salivation; in stomach, sensation of heat or d; gastro-enteritis, with vomiting and diarrhœa; ulceration of estines. The pulse is sometimes slowed, sometimes quickened. spiration is quickened and spasmodic; the drug is partly excreted the lungs and acts on the mucous membrane, lessening its retion. The temperature sometimes rises, sometimes falls. luntary movement is diminished; reflex action lowered; blood-ssure lowered, and vessels dilated. Diminishes the quantity of ne; gives the urine an odour of violets; causes lumbar pain, ning in urethra, painful micturition, hæmaturia. Among the uses *Ter.*, Brunton mentions the treatment of biliary colic. For this it is en in ether in the proportion of one part of the Oil of Turpentine three of Ether. Homœopaths have confirmed the value of this. roughout this list of effects *burning* is a constant note, and gives the to many cases calling for *Ter.*—burning in gums, tongue, tip of gue, mouth, throat, stomach, rectum, and anus, kidneys, bladder, urethra, uterus, air passages, chest, and sternum. The last was ticularly noticed after warm drinks, the pain running along the

sternum with the drink and spreading in the chest. Burning exter
from kidneys along ureters. *Ter.* is an irritative, sensitive reme
Cooper has found it indicated in children (especially teeth
children) when they fly into passions. There is irritation of
meninges and often ascarides or other intestinal worms. In
case of maniacal fury in a man it did good. This irritabi
manifests itself in some cases of spasms and convulsions, and Li
observed a case in point (*H. P.*, x. 480). A woman had made
feet sore by walking, and applied turpentine to them. This
followed by a state like hydrophobia ; she had spasms whene
she saw water or heard it poured, or saw a bright object ;
also whenever she attempted to urinate. *Ter.* is a great hæmorrha
and its hæmaturia is particularly characteristic : Smoky, turbid u
depositing a sediment like coffee-grounds. Dull pain, or burn
pain in region of kidneys, burning during micturition are lead
indications. *Ter.* corresponds to many cases of albuminuria
hæmaturia after scarlatina ; and also to the consequent dropsy. T
last may indicate *Ter.* in many affections of the genito-urinary sph
"Burning in uterus" is very characteristic. Peritonitis, metr
metrorrhagia will probably need *Ter.* if the burning is present.
hæmorrhages of *Ter.* are generally passive ; dark, and fetid. Pur
hæmorrhagica calls for it if there are fresh ecchymoses in g
numbers from day to day. The hæmorrhages may occur from
orifice. Additional keynotes of *Ter.*, which will be decisive if c
bined with others, are : (1) Smooth, glossy, red tongue, as if depr
of papillæ. (2) Excessive tympanites. (3) Drowsiness. In capi
bronchitis, the child is drowsy. Stupor and great weakness
found in many *Ter.* conditions, rendering it appropriate in case
typhus, typhoid, and uræmic poisoning. "Drowsy with reten
of urine." With the tympanites there is generally extreme sensi
ness to touch. With cystitis and uro-genital and rectal troubles t
is sensitiveness of hypogastrium and pains in symphysis pubis. P
go from left to right across bowels and then shoot upward. F
being exposed to turpentine odour, a lady, 35, got pain as
pinchings in the throat, with lifeless feeling in the tongue and dry
of the mouth, followed by pains in r. eyeball, which extended ba
same side of occiput (Cooper). S. H. Roberts (*B. M. J.*, Dec. 25,
maintains *Ter.* has a specific effect in tonsillitis when applied exter
Marc Jousset gave *Ter.* 1x with marked benefit in two cases of bron
asthma. He was led to give it in the first case by coincident hæmat
but this was not present in the second (*L'Art Méd.*, April, 1901)
remedy may be known by its antidotes and antidotal prope
Ter. antidotes and is antidoted by *Phos.* A young man who
badly poisoned by a low attenuation of *Phos.* got more relief
Ter. 3x than from any other remedy. Brunton says it is
Ozonised Ter. that is effective here. The preparation I used wa
ordinary one. Hering says the ozonised oil is recommended
prophylactic in malarial and African fevers, a few drops being
daily on a lump of sugar. George Royal (*Med. Cent.*, ix. 70)
three cases illustrating the action of *Ter.* : (1) Typhoid, third we
man 24. Extreme distension, rapid, small, compressible pulse,

sweat in lower limbs. *Ter.* 6x two drops in water every half-hour. *Oil of Ter.* was applied locally to the abdomen mixed with lard, and later in the evening, when there was already slight improvement, an injection containing turpentine was administered. This relieved the patient of a large quantity of flatus, and next morning he was on the high-road to recovery. (2) Pyæmia after abortion at third month, brought on by patient herself. Enormous distension ; lower limbs covered with cold sweat ; lochia thin, scanty, offensive. *Ter.* given in another case brought about slow improvement for three days, when *Chi.* 30 was indicated and finished the cure. (3) Teamster, 36, had severe nephritis after being out in cold rain. Constant desire to urinate, severe pain in back, down ureter, to bladder ; urine scanty, very high-coloured. Temperature 102°. Pulse weak, 130. *Ter.* 6x every half-hour ; and hot fomentations on kidneys greatly relieved. After three days he was able to leave his bed. Royal considers cold sweat of lower limbs, and rapid pulse with the distension, as leading indications. A keynote of Burnett's for *Ter.* is : "Pains in the bowels which = frequent micturition." *Peculiar Sensations* are : As if he would pitch forward on walking As of a band round head. As if sand thrown violently in eye. As of a sea-shell sounding in l. ear. In ear as of striking of a clock. As from hasty swallowing in epigastrium. As if he had swallowed a bullet, which had lodged in pit of stomach. Sense of anxiety and utter prostration about epigastrium. Umbilical region as if covered with a round, cold plate. As if intestines were being drawn towards spine. As if abdomen distended with flatus. As if diarrhœa would set in. As if inguinal hernia would appear. As if symphysis pubis were suddenly forced asunder. As if foreign body had entered windpipe. As from electric shocks. Twitching of limbs. Crawling tingling as if parts were asleep. As if hot water running through a tube in nerve. Sprained pains, contusive pains, and rheumatic pains appear in the pathogenesis, and notably pressure and drawing pains. These show the suitability of *Ter.* to the effects of injury and rheumatic conditions. It is on this property that certain popular embrocations containing turpentine owe their reputation. *Ter.* is specially *Suited to :* Children (dentition, nose-bleed, worms). Bleeders. Nervous women (amenorrhœa ; dysmenorrhœa ; headache). Complaints of old people ; of people of sedentary habits. Chronic rheumatism and gouty complaints. The symptoms are : < By touch. < By pressure (in region of bladder it = convulsions). Effects of falls and injuries. < Lying on left side, > turning to right. Sitting <. Stooping >. Motion >. (Pain in crest of ilium < from motion and least jar.) Walking in open air <. < Night ; 1–3 a.m. Damp dwellings <. Damp cellar = diarrhœa. Damp weather = neuralgia in legs. (*Ter.* is hydrogenoid.) Cold water > burning in anus. > Belching and passing flatus. Loose stool > nausea.

Relations.—*Antidoted by :* Phos. *Antidote to :* Phos., Merc. *Followed well by* . Merc. cor. *Compare :* Botan., Thu., and other Coniferæ. Hæmorrhage in typhus, Alum. Melæna, Arn. Albuminuria, Ars. Smoky urine, dropsy after scarlatina, dry, glossy tongue, Lach. (Ter. has more tympanites). Capillary bronchitis, drowsiness, lungs clogged up, urine scanty, almost dark from blood, Ipec. Dropsy from kidney congestion, Hell. Renal congestion, smoky urine, Colch. Urticaria after eating shell-fish, Aps., Urt. ur. Glazed tongue, K. bi., Lach., Pyrog. Hæmaturia, Pul. Burning tip of tongue, Mur. ac. Burning in anus and rectum, fainting and exhaustion after stool, Ars. Worms, with foul breath, choking, Cin., Spi. Purpura, fresh ecchymoses in great numbers from day to day, Sul. ac. Burning and drawing in kidneys, bladder, and urethra, Berb., Can. s., Canth. Passive hæmorrhages, strangury, Camph. Metritis, peritonitis, bearing down, burning in hypogastrium, cloudy, dark, muddy urine, tongue dry, red, Bell. Catarrh in children, Pix. Umbilicus retracted, Pb. Kidney-ache, Santal. Warmth at heart, Kalm., Rhod., Lachn. Pains = frequent micturition (Thuj., urging to urinate accompanies the symptoms). Rheumatism, Sul. ter.

Causation.—Alcohol. Falls. Strains. Tooth extraction. Damp cellars.

SYMPTOMS.

1. **Mind.**—Stupefaction ; inability to fix attention (uræmia).—Mania.—Intense nervous excitement.—Children fly into tempers.—Intense irritability, with irritation of membranes of brain (esp. in teething children).—Anxiety on going to bed.—Facility of thought.—Fears apoplexy ; fulness and pressure in head.—Weary of life.—Suicide by hanging in two cases following washing of laces in turpentine and alcohol.—(Frightful maniacal temper, wanders about at night meaninglessly.—R. T. C.)—Intoxication.—Coma.

2. **Head.**—Dizziness, with nausea.—Attack of vertigo, which nearly occasions falling, with cloudiness before eyes.—Headache, with pressive pain and disposition to sleep.—Dull headache, with colic.—Sensation of a band round head.—Excessive heaviness, and troublesome pressive fulness in head.—Tearing cephalalgia.—Rending, tickling pain in l. temporal region, coming and going while in bed in evening ; rubbing removes it.—Erysipelas capitis.

3. **Eyes.**—Eyes sunk.—Ciliary neuralgia with acute conjunctivitis.—Amblyopia potatorum.—When walking in open air, muscæ volitantes and transient dizziness.—Photophobia.—Rheumatic iritis.—Contracted pupils.—Half-opened, up-turned or rolling eyes.—Opened eyes only when swallowing.—Spots and black points before eyes.

4. **Ears.**—Voice sounds unnatural, < r. ear.—Sensation in ears as of striking of a clock.—R. ear hot, l. cold.—Otitis.—Otalgia.—(Earache in children < in l. ; and at night.—R. T. C.)—The internal use of *Ter.* prevents otitis after syringing Eustachian tube (Eugene Weber).—Deafness after measles with high vascularity of meatus and membranes (R. T. C.)—Eczema in front of ear.—Sudden stitch in r. mastoid process.—Tinkling in ears.—Cannot tell direction of sounds.—Loud talking is very painful.

5. **Nose.**—Discharge of serum from nose, without coryza.—Violent nose-bleed.—Passive epistaxis in children.

6. **Face.**—Pale, earthy colour of the face.—Herpes on lips.

7. **Teeth.**—Toothache, with drawing pain.—Gums detached, easily bleeding, with pain as from a burning wound, every morning.—Gumboils

form in a child under *Ter.* (R. T. C.).—Dentition: suppressed urine and convulsions.

8. **Mouth.**—Tongue red, smooth, and glossy, as if deprived of papillæ.—Coating of tongue peels off in patches, leaving bright red spots; or entire coating peels off suddenly, leaving tongue dry and red; burning on tip.—Tongue swollen hard and stiff even without fever.—Foul breath.—Burning in mouth.—Ulcers in mouth.—Mercurial ptyalism; stomacace.—The child dribbles (R. T. C.).—In mouth and angles of lips ecchymoses which bleed.—Stomatitis from mouth to anus.

9. **Throat.**—Scraping, scratching in throat, frequently with coughing in evening.—Burning in throat.—An agreeable coolness in throat.—No power over deglutition.

10. **Appetite.**—Hunger and thirst with debility.—Loss of appetite, great thirst.—Desire to eat more; after a satisfying meal.—Diminished appetite.—Aversion to animal food.—After eating: sick at stomach; loud rumbling in bowels, while pain in hypochondrium disappears; pressure in scrobiculus and distension of abdomen.—Warm drinks = burning in chest.

11. **Stomach.**—Eructations: rancid; flatulent, acrid.—(Continual loud eructations and belching up of much flatus.—R. T. C.)—Belching and nausea.—Nausea and vertigo.—Vomiting: of mucus; of yellowish mucus; of food; of blood.—Retching and vomiting of mucus.—Excessive sensitiveness of region of stomach to touch.—Pressure at stomach and in scrobiculus; as from hasty swallowing; as if he had swallowed a bullet, which had lodged there.—(Severe circumscribed flatulent pain below scrobiculus cordis.—R. T. C.)—Pressing in stomach: > by belching; when lying on l. side, > turning on r. and passing wind.—Burning sensation in the stomach.

12. **Abdomen.**—Burning sensation and pressure in hypochondria.—Pressing below diaphragm, extending l. to r.—Colic from calculi; chronic liver complaints.—Pressing and cutting in l. hypochondriac region while sitting, > moving about.—Pressure, burning sensation and drawing in renal region.—Abdomen very sensitive to touch.—Heaviness, fulness, and pressure in abdomen.—Slight pressing pain in small spot in epigastrium; > stooping, lying down, or taking a deep breath.—Distended abdomen; frequent colic.—Meteorism.—Cuttings in epigastrium and hypogastrium, often extending into thighs.—Sensation of excessive coldness in abdomen, esp. in exterior of umbilical region, which is retracted.—Pains shooting across bowels from l. to r. and upward.—Inflammation of intestines.—Noise, gurgling, and borborygmi in abdomen.—Ulceration of bowels; peritonitis; with tympanites.—Great but obscure pains in lower abdomen.—Sensation of pressure outwards in inguina, as if caused by a hernia.—Painful swelling of inguinal glands.

13. **Stool and Anus.**—Constipation, with distension of abdomen.—Ineffectual urging.—Tenesmus, bloody stools.—Constipation; with abdominal distension.—Hard, scanty fæces.—Dry, brown evacuations.—Fæces of the consistency of pap, with pinchings in abdomen, and burning sensation in rectum and anus (after stool).—Stools consisting of mucus and water; < in the morning.—Intestinal catarrh and diarrhœa, with nephritis.—Loose, liquid fæces, of a greenish yellow, with expulsion of tænia and lumbrici.—With a loose stool, immediate cessation of nausea.—Stools: frequent; profuse; fetid; bloody.—Hæmorrhages: from bowels; with ulceration; epithelial degenera-

tion; passive.—Diarrhœa with tetanic spasms.—Piles, internal, bleeding.—Burning and tingling in anus > applying cold water.—Worms: with foul breath and choking sensation; dry, hacking cough; spasms,—Threadworms.—Burning sensation and tingling in anus (with the sensation as if ascarides would crawl out), during evacuations, and at other times.

14. **Urinary Organs.**—Pressure in the kidneys when sitting, going off during motion.—Sensation of heaviness and pain in region of kidneys.—Violent burning drawing pain in region of kidneys.—(Nephritis that follows an irritation of the skin.—R. T. C.)—Frequent desire to urinate.—Transient movement in region of bladder during a stool as if bladder were suddenly distended and bent forward.—Spasms from any attempt to urinate.—Suppressed secretion of urine.—Strangury, followed by soreness.—Diminished secretion of urine.—Secretion of urine considerably augmented.—Urine smelling strongly of violets; deposit of mucus, or thick, muddy deposit.—Thick, slimy, yellowish white sediment in urine.—Hæmaturia.—Much blood with very little urine and constant painful dysuria (produced in a child from poisoning.—R. T. C.).—Burning sensation in urethra, felt also when urinating.—Urethritis, with painful erections.—Stricture of urethra (Burnett, after Rademacher).—Urine scanty and bloody.—Burning sensation, incisive pains, and spasmodic tenesmus of bladder.

15. **Male Sexual Organs.**—Spasmodic and incisive drawings in the testes (esp. l.) and spermatic cords.—Tearing in mons veneris.—Feels as if symphysis pubis were suddenly forced asunder.—Spermatorrhœa in man, 25, no bad habits; urine turbid, and had a yellowish mucous sediment.—Gonorrhœa; chordee; gleet.

16. **Female Sexual Organs.**—Catamenia retarded and scanty.—Drawing in thighs and colic as if menses would set in, a week after she had had them.—Uterus and ovaries very painful.—Ovarian dropsy.—Terrible burning in uterus, with great bearing-down pain; caused great heat all over; craves drink; inward heat.—Uterine diseases after wearing pessaries.—Fibroids; bloody leucorrhœa; burning in uterus; menorrhagia, black blood.—Herpes labialis.—Abortion.—Neuralgia during pregnancy.—Burning and bearing down in uterus during urination.—Metritis, lochia checked, burning in uterus.—Peritonitis after confinement from tight-lacing.

17. **Respiratory Organs.**—Dryness of the mucous membranes of air passages; feel hot and congested.—Breath short, hurried, and anxious.—Choking sensation (worms).—Emphysema.—Cough as if a foreign body had entered larynx, spasmodic inspiration.—Dry, hacking cough.—Voice gone.—Expectoration streaked with blood.—Respiration impeded by congestion of lungs.—(Pulmonary hydatids with gangrene.—W. Begbie.)

18. **Chest.**—Burning in the chest; along the sternum.—After spasmodic cough, soreness of lower chest.—Pressing behind sternum.—Spastic contraction of muscles of chest and neck.—Râles and crepitation through both lungs.—After warm drinks burning in chest along sternum, gradually spreading through whole chest, disappearing with stitches at both nipples.

19. **Heart.**—Frightful oppression in præcordial region.—Warmth in heart while sitting in evening, obliged to yawn a great deal, with collection of water in mouth.—Palpitation.—Pulse: quick, small, thready, almost imperceptible; intermitting; irregular.

20. **Neck and Back.**—Drawing in nape, extending to occiput. —Drawing pain in the back and loins, esp. in evening, when seated.—Pain and increased warmth in lumbar region.—Backache and soreness in kidney affections.—Pressive pain in back extended up between shoulders and there became a throbbing.

21. **Limbs.**—Numbness of limbs.—Heaviness.—Nerves sensitive.—Intense pains along larger nerves.—Dropsy.—Coldness.—Sudden twitching of limbs as from electric shocks.—Drawings in limbs.—Heaviness of limbs.—Sensation of stiffness in all the muscles, with difficult, slow, stooping gait, as in old age.

22. **Upper Limbs.**—Sprained pain in muscles of l. upper arm.—Drawing in bones of upper arms.—No control over hand when attempting to write. —Trembling of hands.—Fingers insensible.—Neuralgia brachialis or subscapularis.

23. **Lower Limbs.**—Insensibility.—Staggering gait.—Infantile paralysis greatly ameliorated (J. Simon).—Drawing and tearing in hips and thighs.—Pain from hip to forehead ; or from kidneys.—Drawing along thigh.—Pains in groins extending to thighs.—Erythema in thighs and body resembling scarlet rash.—Contracting spasms of thigh muscles during remission of neuralgia.—Swelling and stiffness of r. knee with pain in calf and swelling of vastus externus.—Profuse sweat on legs, evenings, in bed.—Intense neuralgia, esp. in damp weather.—Tearing in feet, now here now there ; chiefly in soles and heels.—Dropsy.

24. **Generalities.**—Hæmorrhage from the urethra.—Worms, particularly lumbrical.—Some forms of gonorrhœa.—Great prostration.—Occasional subsultus.—Spasms every time she saw water, or heard it poured, or saw a bright object, or attempted to urinate (from applying turpentine to feet; *Canth.* relieved).—Violent convulsive paroxysms producing the most frightful opisthotonos.—(Chorea.—R. T. C.)—Shooting, lightning-like pains.—Neuralgia with sensation of coldness in nerve, occasionally like hot water running through a tube.—Has no power of balancing body, stands with feet apart.—Dropsy.—Natural heat increased.

25. **Skin.**—Eruption like scarlatina.—(Scarlatina eruption slow in appearing.)—Purpura hæmorrhagica.—Skin warm and moist.—Pale-red elevated blotches becoming vesicles.—Erythema.—Erysipelas bullosa.—Violently itching vesicles.—Chronic jaundice.—Excessive itching, stinging burning of skin.—General increased sensibility.

26. **Sleep.**—Lethargy.—Retarded sleep.—Agitated sleep at night, with tossing, and frequent waking.—Many dreams.—Nightmare.—(Wakes frightened at night, looks ghastly and shrieks, is nervous.—R. T. C.)

27. **Fever.**—Cold, clammy perspiration all over the body.—Fever, with violent thirst.—(The child is cross and irritable, temper changeable, has a dry, short cough and aching in limbs and head with feverishness.—The little girl is feverish and fretful, and bursts out crying and is very restless in sleep.—R. T. C.)—Profuse perspiration on the legs in bed in the evening.

Tetradymite.

"Rare crystals from North Carolina and Georgia, containing about 60 parts of Bismuth, 33 of Tellurium, 6 of Sulphur, and traces of Selenium and Iron." Trituration.

Clinical.—Coccygodynia. Nails, ulceration of; ingrowing. Tendo Achillis, pain in. Urticaria.

Characteristics.—Hering proved *Tetradymite*, taking about five grains of the 1st trituration. The most prominent symptoms were pains occurring in small spots; ulcerative pains about the nails, and a sharp attack of urticaria from eating shell-fish. Pains in ankles, heels, and tendines Achillis were also severe, and these were < rising from a seat.

SYMPTOMS.

1. **Mind.**—After waking in morning, made anxious by street noise.

2. **Head.**—Pains in r. temple; in occiput.

4. **Ears.**—Pains in l. ear, afterwards in r., as if bones sore.

5. **Nose.**—Repeated sneezing on going out; with discharge of thin mucus.

8. **Mouth.**—Toothache r. lower jaw, afterwards l.—Coated tongue became clean.—Bitter taste.

11. **Stomach.**—Great hunger in morning.

12. **Abdomen.**—Disagreeable feeling in abdomen.—Colic and desire for stool.—Burning, pinching-pressive pain in last ribs.

13. **Stool and Anus.**—Pasty, scanty, lumpy stool, light yellow, with biting burning in anus.—No stool second day; third day, in morning, scanty, soft stool with much pressure and discharge of blood; in evening another soft stool with much black blood.

15. **Male Sexual Organs.**—Violent erections in morning.

17. **Respiratory Organs.**—Hoarseness.—Oppression > by sweat.—difficult respiration in back part of throat and larynx.

18. **Chest.**—Griping as with pincers, followed by violent sticking in upper chest, beneath l. shoulder, repeated at intervals; afterwards in l. elbow.

20. **Neck and Back.**—Pain in nape.—Pain in small of back on rising.—Severe pain in coccyx and lower extremity of r. ischium, esp. when sitting (an old symptom revived).

21. **Limbs.**—Pain in l. leg, and l. elbow.—Frequent pains in margins of nails as if an ulcer would develop, painful on pressure, as if burning and sore in small spots, esp. r. middle finger.

22. **Upper Limbs.**—Stiffness in l. arm as if lame < about elbow-joint, at part where ulnar nerve is exposed, constant inclination to stretch, twist, or turn arm.—Violent pain in hands as if in bones or nerves.

23. **Lower Limbs.**—Sharp pain through l. leg.—Tendines Achillis (esp. r.) constantly painful as if sprained; > walking; < rising from seat. —Pain in ankles, violent while sitting, < rising from seat.—Cramp in r. side.

24. **Generalities.**—Pains in small spots.

25. **Skin.**—Nettlerash, esp. in face after eating crabs; whole face stiff even while eating.—Burning pains as from hot needles.—Crawling itching in r. palm.

26. **Sleep.**—Very sleepy, weary and ill-humoured while riding in carriage.—Awoke 3 a.m. from a dream that a steer was following him, and as though he had often had the dream before, which was not so.

27. **Fever.**—Sweat, esp. on occiput and on nape; at night, though the night was cool and windows open.

Teucrium Marum.

Marum verum. Cat Thyme. *N.O.* Labiatæ. Tincture of whole fresh plant.

Clinical.—*Anus, itching of.* Eyelids, tumour of. Fibroma. Hiccough. Ingrowing toenail. Nose, catarrh of. Polypus. Psoriasis. Rheumatism. Urethra, excrescences in. Worms.

Characteristics.—The Germander group of the Labiatæ, to which the Teucriums belong, had an important place in old herbal medicine, and homœopathy has placed *Teuc. m.* on a firm foundation. Stapf and others proved it. Marked symptoms of helminthiasis, irritation of anus and nose, were elicited, and *Teuc.* has well justified the labour of the provers in this respect. No remedy meets more cases of threadworms than *Teucr.* The nasal symptoms have led to the use of *Teuc.* in nasal polypus. Guernsey gives this as guiding: "Polypus with stoppage of nose on side lain on; large red pimples under right nostril near septum, sore and smarting to touch." A snuff of *Teuc.* has been used in some cases in addition to the internal use of the remedy. But *Teuc.* has a relation to new growth in general as well as of the nose. It has removed a fibrous tumour of the eyelid; urethral granulations following gonorrhœa; and also uterine fibroids. Worms and polypi suggest a tubercular taint, and I have used both *Teuc. m.* and *Teuc. scorod.* in phthisical cases. I was led to think of the remedies by reading an article on the latter, and not being able to obtain it I gave *Teuc. m.* ϕ, in five-drop doses three times a day, to a man of 44 who had phthisis affecting the right lung with severe recurrent hæmorrhages. *Teuc.* helped him much, and with other remedies he got quite well, and has now been at his work for some years. But whilst taking *Teuc.* he noticed that he passed a *large quantity of threadworms*, to which he was not at all subject. C. M. Boger (*Hahn. Ad.*, xxxviii. 40) relates this case of cough: Patient had with the cough a *mouldy taste in the throat when hawking* up mucus. Expectoration profuse. Rapid loss of weight and strength. Anorexia. A brother had died of phthisis four years before with very similar symptoms. *Teuc. m.* 3x helped, and 20x finished the cure. The italicised symptom is a keynote. *Teuc.* has the craving hunger of the antipsorics and worm remedies; it prevents sleep at night. Nervous, irritable, sensitive. There are many rheumatic and gouty symptoms and scapular pains, both in the bones and joints. Limbs go to sleep with tingling when sitting. *Peculiar Sensations are:* As if air forced through mucus in ear. As if right nostril were partly stopped. As if nail had grown into flesh of right great toe. Chill as from abdomen. Sensation as from fleabites. *Teuc.* is *Suited to:* Old persons and children. When too much medicine has produced an over-sensitive condition and remedies fail to act. The symptoms are : < By touch. < Sitting. < Stooping. < On side lain on. Moving >. Disinclined for exertion. < Evening and at night. Desires exercise in open air, which does not fatigue. Warmth <. < Warmth of bed. Wet weather <.

Relations.—*Antidoted by:* Camph. *Compatible:* Chi., Puls., Sil. *Compare:* Botan. Teuc. scorod. Sinking immediately after meals, Ars., Cin. Lyc., Sil., Staph. Hiccough, Ign. (Ign., < eating, smoking, emotions; *Teuc.* after nursing, in infants). Loquacity, Lach. Hyo. Singing, Bell, Croc., Hyo., Spo., Stram. Worms, Scirrh., Cin., Spi. Phthisis, Bac. Polypus < damp weather, Lemn. Nervous phenomena, Nux, Val. Nasal catarrh, K. bi. Nasal polypus, Pho., Sang., Sil. Nails growing in, Mgt. aust., Nit. ac.

Causation.—Concussion (brain). Injuries likely to set up tetanus.

SYMPTOMS.

1. **Mind.**—State of irritability, and irascibility, with sensitiveness so great that fatigue is produced by merely hearing the conversation of others.—Irritability < after eating (with pressure in forehead).—Moroseness.—Indolence, and great aversion to exertion, either mental or physical.—Excessive moral excitement and loquacity.—Irresistible inclination to sing.

2. **Head.**—Headache, with dull, spasmodic pain.—Pressive pains in head, principally in eyes, forehead, and temples, < on stooping.—Skin of forehead feels sensitive to touch.—Tearing by paroxysms, in r. side of head (alternating with the same sensation in r. frontal eminence, and in l. temple).

3. **Eyes.**—Pains in eyes with pressure, as if sand were in them.—Biting sensations.—Smarting in eyes, esp. in internal canthi, with redness of conjunctiva.—Eyes red and inflamed.—Fibrous tumour inside lower lid, one-third inch in diameter; preventing closing lids; bedimmed sight; no pain.—Redness and puffiness of upper lids.—Profuse smarting tears in open air.—Eyes watery, with an appearance as after weeping.

4. **Ears.**—Otalgia.—Shootings and tearings in ears.—Whistling in ears, when speaking, or when producing any sound whatever.—A hissing sound in ear when passing hand over it, when talking, or when inhaling air through nose with force.—Eruption of scaly tetters on the lobe of ear.

5. **Nose.**—Sensation of obstruction in nose.—Tingling in nose.—Frequent sneezing, with tingling in nose; with crawling in nose without coryza.—Stinging, lancinating pain in upper part of the nasal cavity.—Violent crawling in r. nostril, with lachrymation of r. eye.—Sensation as if nostrils were stopped; blowing nose or sneezing does not remove the obstruction; nasal polypus.—Obstruction of nose.—Polypus, with stoppage of the nose on

the side he lies on; large red pimple under r. nostril, near septum, sore and smarting to touch.—Fluent coryza in open air.

6. **Face.**—Sickly, pale complexion, with hollow eyes.—Flushes of heat on face, without redness.—On both sides of under lip, two deep furrows with elevated edges.—Pressive tearing in zygomatic process, extending to teeth.

7. **Teeth.**—Toothache, with tearing pain in roots of teeth and gums (of the r. lower incisors).—Pain in teeth and gums during mastication.

8. **Mouth.**—Mouth clammy.—Much mucus in mouth.—Smarting as from pepper, first on l., later also on r. side.—Smarting and scraping in bottom of gullet, and in root of the tongue (esp. l. side).

9. **Throat.**—Sore throat, with shooting pain, and impeded deglutition.—Pressure or drawing and tearing in throat.—Frequent necessity to hawk, and hawking up of much mucus of a mouldy taste.

10. **Appetite.**—Hunger in morning and evening.—Bitter taste in gullet after dinner.—Appetite increased.—Sensation of hunger, as if the food were unsatisfying, and which hinders sleep.—Cuttings or nausea, with inclination to vomit after drinking water.

11. **Stomach.**—Regurgitation of food, with bitter taste.—Troublesome hiccough when eating, with violent blows in scrobiculus.—Little children, emaciated, jerking hiccough after nursing, and belching without bringing anything up.—Vomiting dark green mucus; hiccough with a stitch through stomach to back.—Pain in stomach, as from emptiness, with gurgling.—Faintness in pit of stomach.—Pressure, and anxious oppression in scrobiculus.

12. **Abdomen.**—Colic (cutting pain) after drinking beer or water.—Colic, with tearing drawings, under hypochondria.—Incarceration of flatus, with drawing, pinching, and gurgling in abdomen.—Pressure in abdomen.—Pressure towards inguinal ring.—Frequent emission of silent, hot, hepatic-smelling flatulence.—Expulsion of much flatus, having the smell of rotten eggs.

13. **Stool and Anus.**—Copious fetid evacuations of the consistence of pap.—Crawling in the rectum after stool.—Expulsion of ascarides (with creeping and itching, and nightly restlessness; < from warmth of bed).—Frequent itching and tingling in anus, often after the evacuations.—Crawling and violent sticking in anus in evening, in bed.—Swelling, itching, and creeping at anus as from ascarides.

14. **Urinary Organs.**—Increased secretion of watery (pale) urine.—Distressing sensation, as from excoriation, and smarting in the upper part of the urethra.—Burning sensation, during and after the emission of urine.—Diminished sexual desire.

15. **Male Sexual Organs.**—Sexual desire decreased.—Drawing pain behind l. side of root of penis, extending to l. side of scrotum, became sore to touch.—Pressive, drawing sensation from abdomen into cords and testes.—Burning, pressing, biting in fore part of urethra when not urinating.—Excrescences in urethra following gonorrhœa removed by injections of *Teuc.* φ for a week.

16. **Female Sexual Organs.**—Smooth pedunculate, pear-shaped polypus of vagina, protruding three inches beyond hymen.

17. **Respiratory Organs.**—Dry cough, excited by a tickling in trachea, as if dust had been inspired (which is < by coughing).

18. **Chest.**—Chest loaded, with sensation of dryness in trachea.—Squeez-

ing pressure in lower part of chest, with anxious uneasiness (without affecting the breathing).

19. **Heart.**—Suddenly in evening pulse begins to be felt, beats rapidly, with gout-like pains in fingers.

20. **Back.**—Burning in l. scapula.—Rheumatic drawing and tension in back.

21. **Limbs.**—Rheumatism in the limbs, esp. in bones and joints.—Tearing in the limbs, esp. in the joints.—Jerking of the muscles.—The limbs go to sleep.

22. **Upper Limbs.**—Painful heaviness in arms and forearms.—Jerking of muscles of arms.—Drawing tearing (rheumatic pains) in bones and joints of arms, hands, and fingers.—Burning in the tips of fingers.—The finger-joints bend over easily.—Panaritium.—Painful pulsations and drawing in the fore-finger.

23. **Lower Limbs.**—Jerking of muscles of legs.—Tearings in joints and bones of legs, feet and toes.—Pain in great toe, as if the nail were entering the flesh.—Nail of r. great toe grows in and ulcerates.—Ingrowing of toe-nails with ulceration.

24. **Generalities.**—Great irritability and nervous excitement, with trembling (sensation in whole body), and dizziness.—Staggering when walking; when walking, placing one foot over another.—Numbness and tingling in limbs.—Great desire for exercise in open air.—Itching shootings in different parts.—[One of the strongest characteristics of this remedy is, patients can't sleep at night on account of an intense itching at the anus (which may be produced by ascarides), causing him to toss and roll about all night, the itching lasts all night.—Hiccough; flatus in general.—Very dry skin; entire absence of perspiration.—Affections in general of the finger-tips; joints of the toes.—H. N. G.]

25. **Skin.**—Sensation as from fleabites.—Rash, burning itching.

26. **Sleep.**—Sleep retarded in evening.—Unrefreshing sleep, and difficulty in waking in morning.—Agitated sleep at night, from excessive excitement (sleeplessness, esp. before midnight; goes to sleep late), with vivid dreams and frequent starts.—Very vivid, most agreeable dreams.

27. **Fever.**—Shivering and shaking, often with icy coldness in hands, and frequent yawning.—Chilliness after eating, and when talking about unpleasant things.—Heat < in evening, with exaltation and great loquacity.—Frequent feeling of flushing in face, without external redness.

Teucrium Scorodonia.

Teucrium scorodonia. Wood Germander. Wood Sage. *N. O.* Labiatæ. Tincture of whole fresh plant.

Clinical.—Bronchorrhœa. Phthisis. Testicle, tuberculosis of. Tuberculosis.

Characteristics.—*T. scorodonia* is an extremely bitter plant with the smell and taste of hops, for which it has been substituted. Some have observed an alliaceous smell, and Cazin says that it gives a garlicky taste to the milk of cows, goats, and sheep which eat it. Dr. Criquelion, of Mons (*Rev. Hom. Belge*, June, 1895, quoted *R. H. Française*, Feb., 1896), tells how Dr. Martiny one day, in the Ardennes, had occasion to examine a man of thirty who was apparently in the last stage of consumption and had a cavity in one apex. Martiny gave his opinion that he had not long to live. A year later, being in the same district, he called at the house and inquired of a man whom he saw there, apparently in perfect health, what had become of the invalid. "*I am he*," was the reply. It was the fact, though it took some time to convince Martiny of it. An old woman had recommended him to make a tisane of the Wood Germander which grew abundantly about there. He had taken it daily, and got well. ["A similar case," says Cooper, "was told me by a distinguished scientist. *Teuc. s.* is allied to *Marrubium vulgare* (Common or White Horehound), a well-known cough remedy; and to *Nepeta glechoma* (Ground Ivy), which was formerly much used with snail-jelly for chest affections."] Martiny introduced *Teuc. s.* into his practice and used a tisane of it with much success in bronchorrhœa and consumptive affections with tuberculous elements and muco-purulent expectoration. I have, myself, confirmed this, using the ϕ tincture in five or ten-drop doses two or three times a day. Criquelion points out that *Teucrine* has been used as a subcutaneous injection in tubercular cases as a substitute for Koch's *Tuberculin*. Criquelion had a patient, a farmer of scrofulous habit, high colour, thick neck, who had had for ten years an enlarged testicle the size of a quince, which he diagnosed to be tuberculous. *Teuc. s.* 6 was given, one drop in four spoonfuls of water; a spoonful three-quarters of an hour before each meal. After three months the testicle was softer; in six months it had almost returned to its proper size.

Relations.—*Compare:* Bac., Tub., Teuc. m., Helix.

SYMPTOMS.

15. **Male Sexual Organs.**—Enlarged tuberculous testicle.

17. **Respiratory Organs.**—Bronchorrhœa with muco-purulent expectoration.—Tubercular phthisis.

18. **Chest.**—Cavity in apex.

Thallium.

Thallium. A Rare Metal. Tl. (A. W. 203·7). Trituration. Solution of the Sulphate.

Clinical.—Baldness. Conjunctivitis. Locomotor ataxy. Paraplegia.

Characteristics.—*Thallium* is a rare metal discovered by Crookes in the residuum left from the distillation of *Selenium* and named Thallium (θαλλός, a green shoot) from the green it gives in the spectrum (*H. W.*, xxxiii. 242). It has been experimented with by Lamy and

Marme. Some symptoms of *Thal. sul.*, which is an energetic poison are included (and distinguished) in the Schema. The symptoms observed on animals were from the sulphate, with which Lamy experimented (*H. W.*, xxxiv. 82). Combermale, of Lille, used *Thal.* with success in the night-sweats of phthisis, but this treatment had the effect of causing profuse falling of the hair, so serious as to contraindicate its use. Huchard had patients become quite bald in several days. Hansen says *Thal.* relieves the violent pains of tabes dorsalis..

Relations.—*Thal.* belongs to the Lead group of metals, and approaches Plumb. closest in its symptoms. *Compare:* Baldness, Jabor., Pilo., Petr. Baldness and phthisis, Pho.

SYMPTOMS.

2. **Head.**—Hair falls off with great rapidity.

3. **Eyes.**—Very frequent conjunctivitis with abundant production of mucus.

8. **Mouth.**—Ptyalism.

11. **Stomach.**—Loss of appetite.—Nausea.—Vomiting.—Pain in stomach and bowels, terribly severe lancinations, following each other with the rapidity of electric shocks (*Thal. sul.*).

12. **Abdomen.**—Gall-bladder distended (dog).—Coating of liver white and granular-looking (duck).—Pain in intestinal canal.—Retraction or depression of abdomen (*Thal. sul.*).

13. **Stool.**—Diarrhœa ; bloody stools.—Constipation (*Thal. sul.*)

17. **Respiratory Organs.**—Slow and difficult breathing.

19. **Heart.**—Diminished frequency of pulse.

23. **Lower Limbs.**—Pain of tabes dorsalis.—Trembling and more or less complete paralysis in lower extremities (*Thal. sul.*).—Great lassitude.—Paraplegia (dog).

24. **Generalities.**—Emaciation.—Hyperæmia, swelling, and excessive secretion.—Anomalies of motion, chorea-like movements.

27. **Fever.**—Remedies profuse sweating in some cases of severe illness.—Night-sweats of phthisis.

Thea.

Thea chinensis. Tea. *N. O.* Ternströmiaceæ (Genus, Camellia). Infusion. Tincture. Trituration of Theine.

Clinical.—Delirium ; tremens. Mania ; suicidal ; homicidal. Megrim. Nervousness. Neuralgia. Paralysis. Sleeplessness.

Characteristics.—The use of Tea has spread from the older civilisations of the East to the newer ones of the West. Tea contains an alkaloid, *Thein*, which is by some considered identical with *Coffein*, and both tea and coffee are used to stimulate jaded faculties and nable persons to endure fatigue, and get more enjoyment out of hemselves than they could obtain by mere food. But coffee and tea re different in their effects though they may be alike in their hemistry. The after-effect of all stimulation is reaction; unless it s kept off by a repetition of the stimulant as the effect of the ast dose wears off. The sign that the last dose of Tea is wearing off is a nervous, restless, depressed, ill-tempered state, which is visible in persons who rely on tea, at about 5 p.m. Another symptom is an all-gone, sinking sensation at the epigastrium. Excessive tea-drinking is a fruitful source of neuralgia and insomnia. It is often noticed in persons who have sensitive kidneys that they can never take tea when they are going anywhere, because they are compelled to pass water almost immediately after. The symptoms of the Schema are made up of observed effects of overdosing and some direct provings. In a woman who was addicted to *eating* tea, very pronounced delirium tremens resulted, indistinguishable from that caused by alcohol, though there was no alcoholism in the case. A woman who kept a pot of tea boiling on the stove and drank several bowlfuls every day developed both suicidal and homicidal mania; impulse to jump out of the window; to cut her baby's throat and throw it downstairs (*Thea* cm, Fincke, cured). A friend of mine who had been many years in the East and was used to one-storey houses, on his return to this country had a curious impulse to jump out of the window, which he traced to tea-drinking, and which disappeared when he left it off. The homicidal impulse appeared in the dreams of one prover (Teste), who was so far from being horrified by his dream-murders that he even took pleasure in them after awaking. The talkativeness of *Thea* is one of its chief allurements. Among tea-tasters, who do not drink the tea they taste, but only hold it in the mouth a short time, yet long enough for the mouth to absorb some, there is sometimes developed what is known as tea-tasters' paralysis, affecting mostly the lower limbs, with loss of sensation of both upper and lower. This case has been recorded: A man after drinking tea had pain in epigastrium going through to back, with feeling as if he wanted to be sick and could not, > sitting down and stretching himself out. *Thuja* 30 cured. Guernsey gives these as indications for *Thea*: "Nervous sleeplessness; heart troubles, &c., of old tea-drinkers; palpitation of the heart, can't lie down." *Peculiar Sensations* of *Thea* are: As if a foreign body in throat. As if on the verge of fainting. As if the stomach hung down relaxed in the body like an empty bag. As if the weight of a sheet on the feet would crush the toes. Cold sensations are prominent; cold, damp feeling at back of head; with pain spreading thence to eyes; also dryness; and swelling of mucous membrane. The symptoms are: < At night; on walking in open air; after meals. > Warmth, external (applying hand or warm clothes to occiput). < By cold water. > Warm bath.

Relations.—*Antidoted by:* Thuj., Fer., Beer. Hering says Coffee-drinkers should drink wine, tea-drinkers should drink beer. Beer caused in one tea-drinker relaxation of bowels which was > by Port wine. But Beer relieved in others nausea; irregularity of pulse; weakness; sleeplessness; nervousness and want of confidence.

Compare : Gone, faint feeling ; sick-headache radiating from one poi and pain in left ovary, Sep. Averse to work, especially writin Hydrast. Relaxed feeling in stomach, Ipec. Desire for acids, Ver Sul., Ant. c., Phos., Sbi.

SYMPTOMS.

1. **Mind.**—Delirium ; with ecstasy, laughed incessantly, talked i rhyme.—Delirium tremens (from *eating* tea).—Sensation as if impelled t suicide, to jump out of the window, put her baby in the boiler with th clothes, cut its throat while cutting bread, throw it downstairs (from excessiv tea-drinking, cured with *Thea* cm, Fincke).—Temporary exaltation.—Dis position to quarrel at the most harmless speech.—Great nervous excitabilit with exaltation of intellectual faculties.—Nervousness and want of con fidence.—Peevish ; ill-humoured.—Nocturnal fright, suicidal thoughts.– During the sleepless nights the mind was in a state of most active an persistent thinking in spite of all attempts at forgetfulness (*Thein*, gr. 12).

2. **Head.**—Vertigo ; with darkness before eyes ; sudden in open air.– Rush of blood to head, with sensation of fulness, esp. in forehead over eyes —Excessively disagreeable headache with throbbing of carotids.—Sick headache ; chiefly at menstrual period ; pain seems to begin in l. ovary anc stomach and go to head.—Neuralgic pain in nape like a cold flat-iron betwee skin and skull passing over whole cranium to forehead region, excruciating.— Throbbing, shooting in temples extending to nose ; with great acuteness of smell.—Every heart throb felt at vertex.—In occiput : tearing pain ; feeling of damp coldness ; electric shocks ; pain extends to r. shoulder ; > application of hand or warm cloth.—Scalp tender ; on vertex ; can scarcely comb hair.

3. **Eyes.**—Eyes : unusually bright, with dilated pupils ; glittering ; dry, with neuralgia of eyes.—Sight : dim ; dark before eyes ; fiery lines ; sparks.

4. **Ears.**—Neuralgic pains in cartilages of ears, with icy coldness ; impossible to warm them ; pains extend to malar bones.—Hallucinations of hearing ; for four nights in succession waked thinking he heard the door bell distinctly.—Roaring in ears.

5. **Nose.**—Nose-bleed before menses.—Sensation at root of nose as if epistaxis would occur.—Dryness ; soreness of nose.

6. **Face.**—Wild, distressed expression.—Face : pale ; with congested redness ; flushed.

8. **Mouth.**—Teeth frequently decayed.—Tongue : clean and pale ; red ; blistered ; painful as if scalded.—Whole buccal cavity dry and sensitive.— Much viscid saliva.—Bitter taste in mouth.

9. **Throat.**—Diphtheritic sore throat.—Uneasy feeling in pharynx, as if obstructed by a foreign body.—Painless swelling of mucous membrane.

11. **Stomach.**—Very hungry, but little satisfies.—Empty feeling, and faintness.—Thirst ; but every mouthful of cold water affects the head like a shock.—Craves acids ; lemons.—Nausea ; and vomiting after eating (cured). —Vomits bile, never food, when pain at its height.—Weakness about stomach ;

seems to hang in the body like an empty bag.—Empty, sinking, craving, ›ne feeling ; pressure ; tickling ; sensitiveness, at stomach.

12. **Abdomen.**—After lunch, stitch below ribs, r. to l. side, in ıroxysms.—Intestines relaxed.—Liability to hernia.

13 **Stool and Anus.**—Swelling of lower end of rectum, with slight :hing.—Chronic relaxed bowels < by beer, > by port wine.—Constipation.

14. **Urinary Organs.**—Very marked increase of urine.—Must pass ater immediately after drinking tea.

15. **Male Sexual Organs.**—Erections.—Unnatural excitement.

16. **Female Sexual Organs.**—Soreness and tenderness of r. ovary.—enses delayed, scanty, with severe cramp-like, uterine bearing down from :ginning to end of period.

17. **Respiratory Organs.**—Œdema of respiratory tract.—Scraping in ·ynx.—Hoarseness.—Cough : dry ; severe and bloody expectoration.—:spiration increased in frequency and amplitude.—Breathlessness on least ertion.—Paroxysm of asphyxia.

18. **Chest.**—Chest : oppressed ; constricted ; fluttering in l. side with lness about clavicles, and feeling of suffocation ; tight across upper part mpelling her to sit up in bed.

19. **Heart.**—Anxiety in præcordium.—Anxious oppression, anguish.—asm in region of heart.—As if on the verge of fainting.—Palpitation ; ›lent.—Pulse : full, quick ; feeble, irregular, intermittent.

21. **Limbs.**—Paralysed numbness of extremities.—Joints of hands and :t tender.—Nervous excitability in wrists, hands, and feet.

22. **Upper Limbs.**—Violent pains inside arms under elbow wake her er half an hour.—Hand trembled violently, could not be held still more ın a few seconds ; regular writing impossible (*Thein*, gr. 12).

23. **Lower Limbs.**—Sensation in under side of either or both thighs, if circulation had ceased, causing great uneasiness and desire to kick out to restore sensibility.—Neuralgic pains in outer hamstrings.—Restless-ss of feet.—Sensation as if the weight of a sheet even would crush toes.

24. **Generalities.**—Enormous indolent swellings or tumours appear :cessively on back, thighs, hands, scrotum and penis, each lasting two days :ste).—Trembling.—Epilepsy (in a child from swallowing a concentrated usion).—Convulsions.—Languor.—Faintness.— < Afternoon.

25. **Skin.**—Skin dry as if pores obstructed.—Skin of finger-ends peels m excessive dryness. — Eruption of red, indolent pimples. — Itching, wling, prickling in different parts.

26. **Sleep.**—Sleeplessness.—Awoke suddenly as from a struggle of ubus.—Nightmare (esp. from green tea).—Horrible dreams, of murdering ›ple ; caused me no horror, and even after waking I found pleasure a long time in the hideous remembrance.

27. **Fever.**—Intense coldness passing over whole head.—Lowered tem-ature.—Hands and face cold as marble, and bedewed with clammy per-·ation.—Almost immediate increase of general heat.—Excessive internal t, with flushes of heat on the surface, coming and going quickly.—Dis-ition to perspire.—Bedewed with chilly moisture.

Theridion.

Theridion curassavicum. Orange spider. *N. O.* Arachnida. Tincture of the living spider.

Clinical.—Angina pectoris. Anthrax of sheep. Bone, affections of. Caries. Climaxis. Cough. Dysmenorrhœa. Eye-teeth, pains in. Fainting. Headache Hysteria. Liver, disorder of; abscess of. Ménière's disease. Nausea. Necrosis. Nose, catarrh of. Ozæna. Photophobia. Phthisis florida. Pregnancy, sickness of. Rickets. Scrofulosis. Seasickness. Spinal irritation. Tetanus. Toothache. Vertigo

Characteristics.—*Therid.* was introduced and proved by Hering in 1832. The spider is found in the West Indies, chiefly in the island of Curaçoa. It is about the size of a cherry-stone, is found on orange-trees, velvety black when young, with antero-posterior lines composed of white dots; on posterior of body there are three orange-red spots, and on the belly a large square yellow spot. It is very poisonous. It produces a highly sensitive, nervous condition with weakness, trembling, coldness, anxiety, faintness, and easily excited cold sweat. There are two well-marked keynotes, one or other of which will be found in most cases calling for *Therid.* (1) Extreme sensitiveness to noise; < by least noise; "*sounds penetrate the teeth.*" The sensitiveness extends to vibrations of any kind, jar of a step, riding in a carriage or in a boat The symptom also shows the relation *Therid.* has to bony structures as well as to the nervous organs they enclose: it meets cases of spinal irritation; and also cases of disease of the spinal and other bones. Caries, necrosis, and scrofulous disease of bones have all been cured with it. "In scrofulosis when the best remedies fail to relieve" (H. C. Allen). (2) "< Closing eyes." This applies to vertigo, and symptoms of the head and stomach. This forms the indication in many cases of seasickness, or sickness of pregnancy The headaches are severe and affect the eyes, especially the left. The ears are highly sensitive. There are hallucinations of sight and hearing, luminous vibrations, and rushing sounds. Although there is "< closing eyes," there is also intolerance of light. A species of intoxication is induced, hilarity, talkativeness. "Time passes too slowly" is a well-marked symptom. *Therid.* has a peculiar cough frequent, convulsive, head spasmodically jerked forward, knees jerked up to abdomen. Chackravanti (*H. W.*, xxxvi. 345) relates a case of headache cured with *Therid.*: Mr. B., 35, well built, of bilious temperament, had for three months severe headache with nausea and vomiting, like seasickness, and shaking chills. Dulness and fulness in the head with throbbing beginning in occiput, preceded by flickering before the eyes. Head feels large and heavy. The pains begin in the morning increase during the day, and last till evening. Excessive irritation with loss of sustaining power. < From least overwork and motion > by keeping quiet in horizontal position. Constipation, stools hard small, dry. *Therid.* 3x was given, one drop in water twice daily. The pain was much better next day, and was gone in less than a week Baruch (*H. P.*, viii. 331) says of *Therid.* "In cases of scrofulosis, where the best chosen medicines do nothing, I always interpolate a dose of

Therid., which must act for eight days, and I have seen the most surprising results from it, particularly in caries and necrosis. For phthisis florida *Therid.* is indispensable, and effects a certain cure if given in the beginning of the disease. In cases of rachitis, caries, and necrosis I depend chiefly on *Therid.*, which, although it does not seem to affect the external scrofulous symptoms, apparently goes to the root of the evil and effectually destroys the cause of the disease." *Peculiar Sensations* are: As if her head was another strange head. As if vertex did not belong to her. Like a pressing pain in root of nose and about ears. As of a veil before eyes. As if too much air passed into nose and mouth. Mouth as if furred, benumbed. As if some one tapped her on groin when raising leg. As if a lump were lying in perinæal region. Like labour pains in lower abdomen. As if a child were bounding in body. As if something in œsophagus were slipping towards epigastrium. As if bones were broken and would fall asunder. As if dying. Burning pains and itching are common; and a stitch high up in apex of left chest has proved a guiding symptom for *Therid.* in the cure of cases of phthisis. "Burning in liver region" has led to the cure of abscess and even cancer of that organ. The symptoms are < by touch; pressure; on ship-board; riding in carriage; closing eyes; jar; least noise. Lying = pain deep in brain; > flickering before eyes. < Stooping; rising; motion; exertion, going up or down stairs; walking. After washing clothes, nausea and fainting. < Every night. Warm water > nausea and retching. Warmth >. Cold <; cold water feels *too* cold. < By coitus (groin pains). < After stool (headache). Left side most affected.

Relations.—*Antidoted by*: Acon. (sensitiveness to noises); Mosch. (nausea); Graph. (more chronic effects). *Follows well*: Sul., Calc., Lyc. (scrofula). *Compare:* Aran. d. and Spiders generally. Hemicrania < closing eyes, < noise, Sep. (but Sep. < from noise is less intense). Vertigo and faintness on closing eyes, Lach. Headache, nervousness, hysteria, Trn. Stooping down, violent stitch high up in l. chest, thence to back, Myrt. com. (through to l. scapula), Pix (3rd. costal cartilage where it joins the rib). Illic. (3rd rib, generally r. side). Time passes too quickly (too slowly Can. i., Arg. n., Nux m.). Vertigo on closing eyes, Lach., Thuj. (on opening them, Tab.; on looking up, Puls. Sil.). Headache < lying down, Lach. Nasal catarrh, thick yellow greenish discharge, Puls., Thuj. Spinal irritation, Chi. s. Bites tongue in sleep, Ph. ac. (Ph. ac. sides; Ther. tip). Effect of washing clothes, Pho. Lump in perinæum, Arg. n. (Sep. in anus). Scrofulosis; deep-in headache, Bac., Tub. As if a child bounding in body, Croc., Thuj.

Causation.—Sea-travelling. Riding. Washing clothes.

SYMPTOMS.

1. **Mind.**—Joyous; he sings, though the head is internally hot; oppressed and heavy.—Imaginative excitement in head at night with rushing in ears.—Talkative; after spirituous beverages.—Inclined to be startled.—Time appears

to pass rapidly, although he does little.—Despair, want of self-confidence, he gives himself up.—Tries to occupy himself constantly, but finds pleasure in nothing.—Sluggishness, with disinclination to rising in morning.—Thinking is hard when it is of a comparative nature, but not when it is creative.

2. **Head.**—Vertigo : on turning around ; < stooping ; with blindness caused by pain in eyes ; with nausea increased to vomiting ; in sleep, waking her at 11 p.m. ; with slow pulse ; from every noise ; on board vessel.—Whenever she closes her eyes, nausea and vertigo < by noise and motion.—Headache : at the beginning of every motion ; evening when walking, with depression ; deep in brain, so that she must sit up or walk, it is impossible to lie.—Thick feeling in head : with nausea and vomiting on least motion, < closing eyes ; as if it were another head, or as if she had something else upon it.—Oppression and heaviness hindering his studies.—Painless, indescribable sensation.—Headache like a band in root of nose and around ears.—Violent frontal headache, with heavy, dull pressure behind eyes.—Headache on beginning to move.—Headache deep in sockets of eyes, < l.—Throbbing or pressive headache, sudden, over l. eye.—Aching behind eyes.—Stinging in l. temple.—Pressing together in temples.—Oppression behind ears, with fulness.—Itching on head and nape in evening.—Violent headache, with nausea, cannot bear the least noise ; a feeling as if vertex were separated from rest of head, or as if she would like to lift it off.—Effects of sunstroke, with most intolerant headache, nausea and vomiting.—Itching on scalp ; on head and nape, evening.

3. **Eyes.**—Twitching in r. eye.—Burning pain internally above inner canthus on waking.—Sensitive to light, objects look double ; fluttering, nausea, cold hands.—Hard, heavy, dull pressure behind eyes.—Closing eyes < ; = nausea, vomiting, vertigo.—Nausea while closing eyes ; changed into nausea while opening eyes (which was > by *Mosch.*).—Vision lost, everything seemed very far, as if a veil were before her, with blazing and flickering, when closing eyes, then affection of head and weakness.

4. **Ears.**—Least noise < ; every shrill sound and reverberation penetrates whole body, esp. teeth, < vertigo, = nausea.—Loud noises make too strong an impression (> *Acon.*).—Pressure above ears ; fulness behind ears.—Violent itching behind ears.—Roaring in ears.—Rushing in ears like a waterfall, with impaired hearing.

5. **Nose.**—Nose dry, as if too much air passed in ; itching in nose.—Sneezing: in evening, with running coryza ; all day, with discharge of water from nose, but without coryza ; violent, with frequent necessity to blow nose.—Pressure in root of nose and heaviness.—Chronic, offensive-smelling discharge, thick, yellow, or yellowish green ; (nasal catarrh ; chronic ozæna).

6. **Face.**—Face pale.—Froth before mouth with shaking chill.—Jaw immovable in morning on waking and at other times of the day, then opening involuntarily.

7. **Teeth.**—Teeth feel as if cool water were too cold.—Burning and tensive pain in teeth, gums and palate.—Every shrill sound penetrates the teeth.—Raging pain in all teeth in afternoon and evening, causing weeping, but drawing particularly in roots of sound eye-teeth.

8. **Mouth.**—Gums, mouth and nose dry, and feeling as if too much air passed into mouth.—There is no proper taste, her mouth feels furred, benumbed.—Salty taste, hawking of salty mucus.

9. **Throat.**—Sore throat; chilly; bones sore; difficult swallowing; constipation; urine scanty and high-coloured.—Pressure in lower part of œsophagus towards epigastrium, taking away the breath.

10. **Appetite.**—Constant desire to eat and drink, he knows not what.—Appetite for acidulous fruit.—Craves oranges and bananas.—Increased desire to smoke tobacco.—Thirst: great after midday sleep; for wine and brandy.

11. **Stomach.**—Nausea: in morning; on rising; from vertigo on least motion; on closing eyes; on opening eyes (> *Mosch.*); like seasickness; when looking steadily at an object; on motion; on talking; from fast riding in a carriage.—Sensitiveness in region of stomach and epigastrium.

12. **Abdomen.**—Violent burning pains in hepatic region < from touch; retching, bilious vomit.—Abscess of liver.—Anthrax of sheep.—Emission of more flatus than usual.—Pains in groins: after coition: in region of groin on motion, when she draws up her leg it seems as if some one tapped her hard on the groin.

13. **Stool and Anus.**—Stool: papescent, scanty, urgent, next day thin and scanty, omitted on third day.—Stool difficult towards the end, though not hard.—Bowels open twice with colic and flatulency, after which headache is <.—Anus protrudes and is painful, < sitting.—Spasmodic contraction of rectum and anus.—Heaviness in perinæal region, which he has had for a very long time, is now felt at every step, with feeling of a lump there.

14. **Urinary Organs.**—Urine increased.—Has to rise four or five times in night to micturate; does not pass much during day.

15. **Male Sexual Organs.**—Red spots on glans.—Erections: strong in morning, without desire; weak during coition; absent; desire vanished.—Scrotum shrivelled.—Violent and profuse emission during nap after dinner (had taken *Anise* during the day).

16. **Female Sexual Organs.**—Hysteria, during puberty; at climaxis.—Menses omitted in a woman at climaxis; gave birth to a son the following year.—Bruised, sore pain in both ovarian regions; < motion and pressure; labour-like pain in lower abdomen, with sensation as if child bounding in body; tickling in both sides.—Dysmenorrhœa, intense, in l. ovary, with intense headache, extreme sensitiveness of the cervix, chilliness, &c.

17. **Respiratory Organs.**—Cough at night.—Convulsive cough, with the peculiar vertigo.—Violent cough, with spasmodic jerking of head forward and knees upward.—Increased inclination to take a deep respiration, to sigh.

18. **Chest.**—Violent stitches high in chest beneath l. shoulder, felt even in throat.—Pinching in l. pectoral muscle.—Pressure as if something in œsophagus were slipping towards epigastrium, taking away breath for a few moments.

19. **Heart.**—Anxiety about heart, sharp pains radiate to arm and l. shoulder.—Pulse slow with vertigo.

20 **Neck and Back.**—Itching on nape, at top of shoulder and on back.—Pain between the shoulders.—Spinal irritation; great sensitiveness between vertebræ.—Sits sideways in a chair to avoid pressure against spine.—Could not bear least noise, and jar of foot on floor was so aggravating it made her cry out.—Loins affected after vomiting.

21. **Limbs.**—Heaviness in all limbs after breakfast, necessity to lie down, internal chill so that he trembles.

22. **Upper Limbs.**—Stinging from elbow to shoulder.

23. **Lower Limbs.**—Peculiar drawing in r. hip, passing down thigh in evening when sitting and afterwards, with internal coldness below knee; > external warmth.—Knees trouble her in afternoon.—Feet swollen.—Pain in little toe as if pressed in walking.

24. **Generalities.**—Tetanus with trismus.—Every shrill sound and reverberation penetrates her whole body, < teeth, and increases the vertigo, which then causes nausea.—Pain in all bones, as if every part would fall asunder, feeling as if broken from head to foot, then coldness.—Weakness: in morning, with sleepiness; with tremulousness and perspiration.—The sudden, violent symptoms were > by *Acon.*; later symptoms were > by *Graph.*

25. **Skin.**—Hard pimple beside ball of thumb.—Itching: on back; calf; nape; at edge of shoulder in morning; on nates with knots; burning, on inner and upper part of l. ring-finger, with redness.

26. **Sleep.**—Sleepy in morning.—Sleeps all day.—Deep sleep at night.—He often bites tip of his tongue in sleep, so that it is sore next day.—Sleep long and dreamful at midday, dreams of journeys in distant regions and of riding on horses (in one who scarcely ever sat upon a horse).—Dreams that he broke off a tooth.

27. **Fever.**—Shaking chill: with foam at mouth; with headache and vomiting.—Sweats easily after walking and driving.—Icy sweat covering body, with fainting and vertigo, and vomiting at night.

Thevetia.

Thevetia nereifolia. Cerbera thevetia. Ahovai-baum (of the Antilles). *N. O.* Apocynaceæ. Tincture or trituration of the seeds.

Clinical.—Diarrhœa. Somnolence. Throat, affections of. Vomiting.

Characteristics.—J. Balfour observed the effect of eating the seeds on two boys, 8 and $6\frac{1}{2}$. This peculiar symptom was noted: "A tendency to sleep, disturbed every three to four minutes by irritation in the throat, and the discharge of a mouthful of frothy mucus with a sort of gulp; then the child would lie down and close his eyes until again disturbed."

Relations.—*Compare:* Apocy. Stroph. Upas.

SYMPTOMS.

9. **Throat.**—Tendency to sleep, disturbed every three to four minutes by irritation in the throat and discharge of a mouthful of frothy mucus with a sort of gulp; then the child would lie down and close his eyes again until again disturbed.

11. **Stomach.**—Vomiting.

13. **Stool.**—Bowels moved twice or thrice.

Thiosinaminum.

llyl sulphocarbamide. (Derived from Oil of Mustard-seed.) Trituration of the crystals. Solution in alcohol.

Clinical.—Adhesions. Cicatrices. Lupus. Lymphatic glands, enlarged. ectum, stricture of. Strictures. Tinnitus aurium. Tumours.

Characteristics.—*Thios.* belongs to the same chemical group as *rea.* The colourless bitter crystals are soluble in water, alcohol, and ther. *Thios.* has been used externally and internally in cases of lupus, hronic glandular tumours, and for dissolving scar tissue; and internally or resolving tumours of the uterine appendages. The usual internal ose in old-school practice is 4 to 8 grains once a day given hypoderically in a 15 per cent. solution. C. H. Pennoyer (quoted *Pac. C. . of H.* viii. 199) relates this case: Mrs. C., 69, had been several years l with gastric distress, sciatica, pains in hips down to knees; < by notion. Indigestion, flatulence of stomach and bowels, < after eating. Pain in back. Inability to walk; much perspiration; depression of pirits; and subnormal temperature. Her father had died at 69 of tomach trouble; mother at 58 of stricture of the bowel. Examination showed stricture of rectum two inches above anus, there being a ense fibrous band forming a ring opening, which would not admit the ndex finger. Bougies and mechanical measures failed to relieve. Veakness was so great, patient would faint at stool. Under general reatment nutrition improved, but the local condition was unchanged. year later the stricture was slightly increased. *Thios.* was now iven, gr. ii. twice daily. The following year the patient was found much mproved. Examination showed that the *cicatricial band had gone*, the peculum could be introduced, and the mucous membrane was normal n appearance, though not as distensible as a normal rectum should be. W. Spencer (*H. M.*, xxxiv. 55) has applied this property of resolving icatricial tissues in cases of tinnitus aurium "where the ossicles are bound down, and the function of the tympanic cavity so much mpaired by fibrous bands or adhesions." In such cases he has had ncouraging success. Enlarged lymphatic glands have been reduced n the same way. A few symptoms observed on patients under treatment I have arranged in the Schema with some cured symptoms.

Relations.—*Compare:* Botan., Sinapis and Cruciferæ. Uterine umours, Thlasp. b. p. Diuresis (also chemical) Urea. Lupus, Tub. Cicatrices. Sil., Fl. ac. Affections of rectum, Nit. ac., Graph., Scirrh.

SYMPTOMS.

4. **Ears.**—Tinnitus caused by fibrous bands.

11. **Stomach.**—Appetite increased.

13. **Rectum.**—Stricture of rectum resolved.

14. **Urinary Organs.**—Urine increased in quantity; no albumen or ormed elements.

16. **Female Sexual Organs.**—Tumours of uterine appendages.

17. **Respiratory Organs.**—Accelerated respiration.

24. **Generalities.**—Sensation of heat and burning in affected parts.—Bodily weight increased.—Glandular swellings reduced.

25. **Skin.**—Distinct local reaction in lupus cases after a few hours. Urticaria.—Lupus.—Scar tissues.

Thlaspi Bursa Pastoris.

Capsella bursa pastoris. Shepherd's Purse. *N. O.* Cruciferæ.
Tincture of fresh flowering plant.

Clinical.—Abortion, hæmorrhage after. Dropsy. Dysentery. Dysuria. Fibrom Gall-stones. Gonorrhœa. Hæmaturia. Hæmorrhages. Leucorrhœa. Liv affections of. Metrorrhagia. Ranula. Renal calculi. Strangury. Uric acid diathes Uterus, hæmorrhages from ; affections of ; cancer of. Whitlow.

Characteristics.—"Shepherd's purse," says Gerarde, "staye bleeding in any part of the body, whether the juice or the decoctio thereof be drunk, or whether it be used poultice-wise, or in both, any way else. In a clyster it cureth the bloody flux ; it healeth gree and bleeding wounds ; it is marvellous good for inflammations ne beginning and for all diseases which must be checked back ar cooled." Gerarde adds that the decoction will stop diarrhœa, bloo spitting, hæmaturia, and all other fluxes of blood. *Thlasp.* is th white-man's faithful friend : "A native of Europe, it has accompanie Europeans in all their migrations, and established itself wherever the have settled to till the soil" (*Treas. of Bot.*). It does not refuse to gro in the poorest soils, but it luxuriates in the richest. Burnett notice that it flourished best in the neighbourhood of dunghills, and the odo of the tincture is much suggestive thereof. Some have seen in th seed-vessel the signature of the shape of the uterus, and Burnett foun in it an organ remedy of vast importance. The ϕ tincture, he said, is th best thing to give for menses that have been checked ; for uterine hæmo rhages he preferred the attenuations. He has observed it cause sexu excitement like *Cantharis.* It aided Burnett in the cure of a inveterate case of gall-stones, the origin of which he traced to th uterus. Dudgeon (*M. H. R.*, xxxii. 614) reports a case which revers this. He had treated a lady for jaundice, from which she made good recovery ; but there came on a peculiar discharge after th catamenial flux. It was of brownish-green blood and was attende with obscure abdominal pains. The cervix uteri was swollen and so but not ulcerated. Dudgeon failed to cure this ; but Rafinesque, c Paris, after trying other remedies, succeeded with *Thlasp.* The 6t had immediate good effect. Rafinesque afterwards gave the ϕ an then again the 6th, and in a few weeks the cure was complet Dudgeon's article on *Thlasp.* is the most complete we have. H quotes a case of Rademacher's showing the action of *Thlasp.* o uric acid excretion. A woman whom Rademacher had relieved te years before of a large quantity of urinary sand, again presente rself; her abdominal cavity was full of water, extremely swollen, d she was passing urine of a light red colour with bloody diment. *Thlasp.* φ, 30 drops five times a day, was given solely with e idea of stopping the hæmaturia. But the result was—a more pious discharge of urinary sand than ever before; the urine creased, the dropsy disappeared, and the woman was cured. udgeon also quotes a case of Kinil's: A woman had strangury ree weeks after confinement, she could not retain her urine, which ibbled away drop by drop. *Thlasp.* φ, 30 drops five times a day, noved the strangury at once, and in a few days the urine could be ained and became clear without sediment. "Dysuria of old rsons, when the passing is painful and there is at the same time asmodic retention of it" is an indication given by Heer. Dudgeon's n cases are no less striking: (1) A lady, 76, had rheumatic muscular ns in various parts, and the most abundant secretion of uric acid, ich passed away with every discharge of urine. Sometimes small culi formed and then there was much pain in their passage along ureter, but generally it passed in the form of coarse sand, which med a thick layer at the bottom of the utensil. This sand conued to pass after the cessation of the rheumatic pains, which lasted or seven weeks. *Puls.*, *Pic. ac.*, *Lyc.* had no effect. *Thlasp.* 1 ninished the sand to an insignificant amount. (2) A gentlemen, 57, addition to other dyspeptic symptoms had unusually large disrges of coarse uric acid, coming away in masses as large as a big 's head but without pain. *Thlasp.* 1 stopped this. (3) Lady, nearly was suffering from the presence of a calculus in left ureter. She l previously passed much sand. *Thlasp.* 1 caused a great discharge sand and a speedy relief of her pain. Dudgeon also refers to a e of Harper's illustrating the action of *Thlasp.* on the bowels. An erly lady had suffered for years from a copious discharge of muco-, sometimes mixed with blood, sometimes nearly all blood, which sed from the bowels after each evacuation. She had been under h homœopathy, oxygen treatment, and for a long time under rper himself without effect, when he gave *Thlasp.* φ in five-drop es and cured the case in a few days. With *Thlasp.* 1x I saved a y who had been curetted several times with small success from rther curetting, which was advised as being essential to the cure. *asp.* stopped the hæmorrhages, restored the periods to their proper n, and the patient immediately began to recover her strength, which been drained to the last degree. There has been no return of trouble. *Peculiar Sensations are:* As of needles or shocks from a ery between end of sternum and umbilicus. As if neck and left ulder would break with pain. Symptoms are > bending over. morrhages are profuse, periodic; blood dark, clotted. The toes affected along with cramping pain in stomach.

Relations.—*Compare:* Cruciferæ, especially Sinapis, Thios. oma; uterine tumours), Matthiol. (inspissated secretions; vs near sewage stream). Renal calculi, Oc. can., Uric acid; in shoulder, Urt. ur. Uterine hæmorrhages, Trill., Vibur., l., Senec. Hæmorrhages from bowel, Merc., Nit. ac., Sul., s., Merc. c., Pho.

SYMPTOMS.

2. **Head.**—Slight headache.

4. **Ears.**—Deafness and pain in l. ear.

5. **Nose.**—Frequent epistaxis, passive.—Free discharge of blood a mucus from l. nostril.—Dull pain at root of nose.

8. **Mouth.**—Teeth sore on closing jaws.—Gums sore ; neuralgic feeli in teeth.—Inside of gums feel as if full of blisters.—Ranula ; caused enlar ment of submaxillary duct.

9. **Throat.**—Soreness of upper part of throat.—Swelling of throat a face, < l. side.—Tonsils swollen.—Throat dry on swallowing.

11. **Stomach.**—Nausea.—Cramping pain in stomach ; toes hurt as v as stomach.—Sick, faint feeling in stomach.

12. **Abdomen.**—Gall-stone colic ; liver affection being secondary uterine condition (Burnett).—Pain between end of sternum and umbilicus, l needles or an electric shock.—Severe cramping pain > bending over.

13. **Stool and Anus.**—Passage of blood.—Obstinate and copious mu purulent discharge from bowels, more like pus than mucus ; discharge ne comes till fæces have entirely passed (cured in a few days with ϕ five drc after years of other treatment.—Harper).

14. **Urinary Organs.**—Hæmaturia.—Urine burning, passing frequen of strong odour.—Copious discharge of urinary sand, increased flow of ur relief of dropsy.—Renal calculus.—Increased quantity of urine with brickc sediment.—Strangury after accouchement ; dribbling of urine.—Dysuria old persons ; with dribbling.

16. **Female Sexual Organs.**—Sexual excitement.—Metrorrhagia ; v uterine colic ; in hæmorrhagic chlorosis ; in sequelæ of abortion or labou Premature menstruation ; first day she hardly had a show, second da hæmorrhage with severe colic and expulsion of clots, flow lasted eigh fifteen days, left a state of exhaustion which was not recovered from be the next period came on ; this proved very profuse, next less so.—Hær rhages : with violent uterine colic and cramps ; consequent on abortion critical age ; with cancer of cervix ; or fibroids.—Too frequent and cop menstruation, esp. in persons of a relaxed constitution.—Hæmorrhages d with clots.—Suppressed or checked menses.—Menses delaying from inerti Leucorrhœa : bloody, dark, fetid, before and some days after menses, w were profuse and dark.—Hæmorrhages after abortion.—Following an at of jaundice, after menses a discharge of brownish-green blood, with obs abdominal pains ; cervix swollen and soft but not ulcerated (*Th. b. p.* 6 immediate relief ; ϕ and again 6 completed the cure).

17. **Respiratory Organs.**—Hoarse in morning with slight sore th —Hæmoptysis.

18. **Chest.**—Pulsative pain in l. chest.

22. **Upper Limbs.**—Pain in l. shoulder so great, he thought neck shoulder would break.—Strong, almost painful pulsation in r. radial ar pulse 84, uneven.—Pains in fingers ; felon on tenth day.

Thuja.

Thuja occidentalis. Arbor Vitæ. *N. O.* Coniferæ (Tribe, Cupressineæ). Tincture of the fresh green twigs.

Clinical.—*Abdomen, distended.* Abortion. Angina pectoris. Anus, fistula in; fissure of. Asthma. Balanitis. *Cancer.* Catalepsy. Chorea. Clavus. *Condylomata.* Constipation. Convulsions. Coxalgia. Diarrhœa. Disparunia. Dysmenorrhœa. *Ear, polypus of.* Enuresis. Epilepsy. *Epulis. Eyes, tumours of; granular inflammation of.* Fatty tumours. Feet, fetid. Flatus, incarcerated. Frontal sinuses, catarrh of. Ganglion. *Gleet. Gonorrhœa.* Hæmorrhage. Hæmorrhoids. Hair, affections of. Headache. Hernia. Herpes zoster. *Ichthyosis.* Intussusception. *Jaw, growth on.* Joints, cracking in. Levitation. *Morvan's disease. Mucous patches.* Muscæ volitantes. Myopia. Nævus. Neck, cracking in. Onanism. Ovary, left, pain in. Ozæna. Neuralgia. Nose, chronic catarrh of; polypus of. Paralysis. Pemphigus. *Polypus.* Post-nasal catarrh. Pregnancy, imaginary. *Prostate, disease of.* Ptosis. *Ranula. Rheumatism, gonorrhœal.* Rickets. Sciatica. Seminal emissions, nocturnal. Sycosis. *Syphilis. Tea, effects of.* Teeth, caries of. Tongue, ulcers of; biting of. Toothache. Tumours. *Vaccination.* Vaccinosis. Vaginismus. *Warts.* Whooping-cough.

Characteristics.—The American Arbor Vitæ is a "spiry evergreen attaining a height of from 20 to 50 feet, though generally not above 40, and a diameter of about 10 to 20 feet through the greatest breadth of foliage." It abounds in the upper zones of North America, from Pennsylvania northwards, where it "often forms what are commonly known as cedar-swamps. It grows upon the rocky banks of rivers, and in low, swampy spots, blossoming from May until June and maturing its fruit in autumn. The Arbor Vitæ assumes a conical form with such true lines as to appear 'clipped,' thus forming one of our most valued high-hedge trees" (Millspaugh). *Thuja* was introduced to France from Canada in the reign of Francis I. of France, and it has now an honoured place in most of our gardens and shrubberies. The native habitat of *Thuja* is not without its importance in relation to therapeutics. It loves swamps; it is Hahnemann's typical antisycotic and Grauvogl's hydrogenoid. *Thuja* is one of Hahnemann's discoveries. Most of the remedies of his materia medica had been known in a fashion before his time. Of the therapeutic properties of *Thuja* practically nothing was known till Hahnemann proved it. Subsequent observers have only confirmed or added to Hahnemann's pathogenesis. Hahnemann found in *Thuja* the antidote to the miasm of the condition which he termed *Sycosis*, meaning thereby the constitutional disease resulting from constitutional gonorrhœa, and having as its characteristic manifestation excrescences, sometimes dry in the form of warts, more frequently soft, spongy, emitting a fetid fluid with a sweetish odour something like herring brine, bleeding readily and having the coxcomb or cauliflower form. Teste remarks that in the period when the doctrine of Signatures prevailed the "resinous callosities of the stems and leaves of *Thuja occ.* might have seemed an indication that the plant was the specific for sycosis and warts." Teste dismisses this idea, but he asks whether resinous substances which have the power of modifying vegetable juices in a peculiar way may not affect the animal fluids in the same manner. He includes *Castor.* in his *Thuja* group, and gives an instance in which it acted on fig-warts. *Castor.* is the product of an animal which subsists on the bark of resinous trees.—Hering gives this as the action of *Thuja* (1) on the fluids: "dissolution of fluids of the body, which become acrid, probably caused by *Thuja* perverting lymphatic secretions; disturbs digestion and sanguification"; and this (2) in the vegetative sphere: "A surplus of producing life; nearly unlimited proliferation of pathological vegetations, condylomata, warty sycotic excrescences, spongy tumours, and spongy pock exudates [which] organise hastily; all morbid manifestations are excessive, but appear quietly, so that the beginning of the diseased state is scarcely known." Bœnninghausen found *Thuja* both preventive and curative in an epidemic of small-pox. It aborted the process and prevented pitting. In veterinary practice *Thuja* has proved curative in farcy and in "grease." These facts open up another great branch of *Thuja's* homœopathicity—its anti-vaccinal action. This extension was made by Kunkel and Goullon following on Bœnninghausen's experience with small-pox. On this subject no one has written more forcibly or lucidly than Burnett (*Vaccinosis and its Cure by Thuja*). "*Arbor Vitæ: nomen omen*," says Burnett on his title-page. And in his hands *Thuja* has proved indeed a tree of life to numberless sufferers from the vaccinal taint. By "vaccinosis" Burnett means the disease known as vaccinia, the result of vaccination, *plus* "that profound and often long-lasting morbid constitutional state engendered by the vaccine virus." To this state *Thuja* is homœopathic, and therefore curative and preventive of it. Burnett makes the profound observation, which I can confirm, that the vaccine virus does not need to "take" (that is, to set up vaccinia) in order to produce the vaccinal dyscrasia: that "not a few persons date their ill-health from a so-called unsuccessful vaccination." So that vaccinosis may exist apart from vaccinia. The antivaccinal action of *Thuja* is part of its antisycotic action: vaccinia is a sycotic disease. Burnett gives the case of an infant ten weeks old, whom he was called to see as it was supposed to be dying. He found it ghastly white and in collapse. There was nothing to account for this except that the baby had had its wet-nurse changed two or three days before. The wet-nurse was questioned and declared herself quite well and looked it; but "her arm was a little painful." She had been re-vaccinated in the Marylebone Workhouse the day before she took charge of the patient. Burnett found the vaccine eruption just turning into the pustular stage. He concluded that the infant was sucking the vaccinal poison with its nurse's milk. He gave *Thuja* 6 to both infant and nurse. The baby gradually improved the same day, and next morning was, though still pale, practically well, and the vaccinal vesicles on the nurse's arm had withered. Burnett quotes a case of vaccinal rash in an infant following the vaccination of its mother, who was nursing it. The effects of chronic vaccinosis are protean. Prominent among them are neuralgias (of which Burnett gives many examples), morbid skin disorders, indigestion, and constipation; warts and new growths of many kinds. In these effects a favourite ıethod of Burnett's was to give a course of twenty-four numbered owders, only three or four of them medicated with *Thuja* 30; one to e taken at bedtime. With the same prescription he cured many ases of paralysis, his indications being: Left side of body; very chilly; : in morning, in wet weather, and in cold: with these indications resent he also found enlargements of the spleen to dissolve. In 889 I was consulted by Mr. A., 38, about a lump, or rather two ımps, in the right breast, which was like that of a girl approaching uberty, the left breast being quite flat and normal. There 'as a hard, not sharply defined lump to the right of the nipple, nd a smaller one to the left of it, but freely movable, the ırger somewhat tender and irritated by the pressure of the brace. 'he tumours had existed eighteen months and came on at a time f much anxiety when his wife died of consumption. His paternal randmother and two aunts had died of cancer. He had been twice accinated, but on the second occasion the arm did not "rise." As a mall boy his hands were covered with warts. At eight he had hingles. On August 15th *Thuja* 10m F.C. was given. October 21st.—f anything tumours a little less. *Thuja* 10m continued at intervals. 'ebruary 4, 1890.—Tumours can only be felt with difficulty. No ain. The medicine was repeated and when next seen some time ıter the patient was absolutely well. A very much vaccinated lady leveloped at the climacteric indurations in both breasts, especially he right. Menses were accompanied by severe neuralgic pains. '*huja* was given in 1m, 10m, and cm F.C. potencies. The last set ıp attacks of angina pectoris of such intensity that I did not repeat t. The indurations disappeared, but in the course of the cure an ruption closely resembling small-pox developed over her breasts on nore than one occasion. The first case I treated homœopathically vas one of new growths—a cluster of small warts on the forehead of a oy which had lasted eighteen months and followed the scratch of a :at. *Thuja* ϕ in fractional doses and *Thuja* ϕ painted on cured per-nanently in three weeks. A gentleman, about 50, consulted me recently ıbout a wart on the right side of his head. He was bald, and the wart vas black and unsightly. It had been growing some months, and he vas somewhat anxious about it as his father had had a similar wart levelop in the same locality at the same age, and it had never left ıim. My patient had been twice vaccinated. *Thuja* 30, twenty-eight owders, one in seven medicated, one at bedtime. In one month there was much reduction; *Thuja* was repeated, and in little over two nonths the wart was gone. Burnett says *Thuja* is the remedy for atty tumours, which he regards as sycotic in nature. *Thuja* not only produces symptoms of the secondary stage of gonorrhœal and vaccinal ıffections, it also produces urethritis and a variolous eruption. Dudgeon has reported acute urethritis with yellow discharge lasting ıltogether a fortnight as the result of chewing a *Thuja* cone. Mersch (*H. M.*, xxx. 686) gave *Thuja* 3 to a patient as a prophylactic against small-pox. This patient and another who took it for the same purpose developed simple urethritis. Mersch proved *Thuja* ϕ on himself and some others: (1) M. N. had rose-coloured blotches on the back, and several days after leaving off the medicine had warts develop on the outer side of the root of the thumb. These were sti present three years after, though smaller and softer. (2) Mersc himself, who took *Thuja* for fifteen days, had heavy sensation in th head on waking, an eruption of desquamative annular blotche and from the twelfth day a tearing along the right arm whic compelled him to keep the arm flexed for eight days, < attempt ing to extend the arm; slightly > by heat. A small soft war appeared at the external portion of right middle finger. Thi disappeared a month after the proving was ended. ("< By exten sion" is a characteristic of *Thuja;* it = cracking in joints. Th arm symptoms are also < when the limb hangs down, which i also an extension.) *Apropos* of the annular scaly blotches, I had case of psoriasis of the legs in a youth which was benefited by *Thuj* more than by any other remedy, though the *Thuja* was given for som other affection. A patient came to Raue (*H. R.*, ii. 162) complainin that his semen had a very offensive smell. Raue did not know of remedy producing the symptom, but selected *Thuja.* Two doses o the 200th and one of the 15th were taken. The man was at the tim in the hands of an eminent dentist for his teeth, which for five year had been a great trouble to him on account of their extreme sensitive-ness to cold; the gums were in a deplorable state and the teeth were encrusted with tartar. After receiving the *Thuja* the extreme sen-sitiveness of the teeth disappeared in one night; then the offensive odour of the semen. In four days the patient again saw the dentist, who was amazed to find his gums quite sound. Moreover, the patient had lost an oppression of the chest which had been troubling him some time. Goullon (*Leip. Pop. Zeit. f. H.*, translated *Rev. H. Belge*, September, 1895) relates the cure of a mental state by *Thuja* 30x. He remarks that, following the advice of Kunkel, he gives only a single dose of *Thuja*, one or two drops of the tincture on sugar or milk, at bedtime. When he has given a second dose the following night he has observed new symptoms: "*Thuja* in fact has a very marked action on sleep, and its symptoms appear by preference at night—the headache, for example." This is the case: Miss R., 40, complained of her head, especially at certain moments, when ideas which did not concern her in the least came to her *as if some one else was thinking by her side.* *Thuja* produces a confusion in the thoughts which patients cannot rid themselves of on account of great weakness and pain in the head. This patient had for months been attending on a paralysed sister, frequently getting up in the night and worrying herself about numberless things. Her nervous system was very impressionable, and for weeks had reached a point of extreme over-excitement. She could no longer calm herself, and in addition she sneezed and coughed much. The problem was to give her sleep and take away the pain in the head. Even when she was not obliged to get up she could not get sleep. Her eyes were also very much irritated. The patient afterwards described her condition thus: "I felt in the anterior part of the head, principally the forehead, a sensation as if lead were compressing my eyes; these were inflamed, < by light, > in open air. Before going to sleep I felt a congestion in the head with headache; at the same time queer, confused ideas which changed like a flash and fell upon the most odd things. These were > when I opened my eyes or sat up. Before my eyes images and statues arranged themselves. If I wished to think of something sensible, in the twinkling of an eye I lost the thread of my ideas. All this happened at night; during the day the wicked sprites did not appear. My head and eyes pained me when there was much movement, as when several people were speaking at once." The effect of the dose she described thus: "After having taken the *Thuja* I tasted a sweet repose; the next morning a complete transformation had taken place in the head, the weight was gone, the eyes were more fresh, the brain free." Goullon cured a lady who had had headache for a year; on waking felt as if a tight hoop enclosed forehead, not passing away till noon. *Eyelids heavy as lead.* *Thuja* 10x, one dose at bedtime, permanently cured. A. W. Holcombe (*Med. Vis.*, xii. 225) relates experiences bearing on the sleep and dreams of *Thuja.* (1) Mrs. E., 48, had a growth, wart-like, about the size of a sixpence, on left temple. It began as a slight roughness and itched at times. Also growth about the same size on a hard palate (left), very sore. Much headache, on left side of the head, throbbing in left temple, and the pains extend into left ear. *Cannot sleep after 3 a.m. Dreams much of falling.* Feels smothering in a warm room. Thirsty, < noon and afternoon. Feet sweat much, offensive; sweats much about groins. *Thuja* cm was given on October 25th. By November 15th the growths and all the rest of the symptoms had disappeared. (2) Led by this same symptom, "almost every night, dreams of falling from a height," Holcombe cured a man, 30, of tertian fever with *Thuja* cm when a large number of other seemingly well-indicated remedies had failed. Robert Farley (quoted *A. H.*, xxiii. 446) relates the case of two children, æt. 5, who had what he graphically terms "urinary tantrums." Two hours after being put to bed they would wake kicking, crying, and refusing to answer a question. This lasted an hour or more. Asked if they wanted to urinate they would refuse to answer, strike at attendant, or even say "No." Finally it was found that if they were taken up and put on the closet they would urinate and then go to sleep readily. One of the children developed signs of incipient inflammation of the left hip-joint. The totality led to the selection of *Thuja*, which was given in the 200th. After the first night there were no more "tantrums," and in two months the child was perfectly well. This child's father had had gonorrhœa, treated by injection, some years before the patient was born. But the other child's father had not had gonorrhœa. In the latter case, which was exactly like the former, the cure was immediate; in the former case relief occurred on the second night. C. W. Roberts (*H. R.*, xii. 137) found *Thuja* ϕ, in five- to seven-drop doses at bedtime, control nocturnal seminal emissions better than any other remedy. "Nocturnal seminal emission" is an emphasised symptom in *M.M.P.* Epulis is probably a malignant kind of sycotic hyperplasia. Percy Wilde (*H. W.*, xxi. 199) records the case of a young married lady who had a large epulis on the lower jaw, rapidly increasing in size, ulcerating on the surface, very painful, and filling the mouth with an ill-smelling secretion. The entire tumour was removed by operation, and also the subjoined bone. Three weeks later the tumour was as large as before and increased daily. *Thuja* 1x was now given. The growth stopped immediately; ulceration ceased; the pain disappeared. In three weeks the gum was healthy and remained so permanently. Villers (quoted *A. H.*, xxi. 421) relates a case of scalp tumour in a youth of seventeen. The tumour had existed two years, and had somewhat the appearance of a bean. It was situated about the posterior edge of the parietal bone, was devoid of sensation, and the hair had disappeared from it, making it very conspicuous. *Thuja* 30 was given, a dose every twenty days. In four months the youth was almost cured, in five months entirely so, the hair having grown again completely over the spot. George Royal (quoted *A. H.*, xxiii. 387) relates a case of persistent cough cured with *Thuja*. Miss X., 19, fair, had for three months a painless, dry cough. The irritation was only in the throat. There were six small growths at the back of the throat, and one near the vocal cord. She never had a cough before. Has leucorrhœa green and excoriating; menses a little too early. *Thuja* 30 cured the growths and the cough in about three weeks. Old-school observers (*N. A. J. H.*, xv. 63) have found in *Thuja* an efficient hæmostatic, locally applied, especially after tooth extraction. R. B. Johnstone (*H. P.*, ix. 257) gives some indications for *Thuja* in hernia: (1) Women of sycotic history who have a tendency to *left-side* inguinal hernia after labour (*Thuja*, high). (2) When babies cry much the umbilicus protrudes, growing red and sore; especially when the father has a sycotic history. (3) Left inguinal hernia in infants; child cries all the time, and is only quiet when the left inguinal region is relieved from pressure, or the thigh is flexed on the abdomen. Bœnninghausen observed this symptom of *Thuja*, which bears on the action of *Thuja* on the *sides* and *roots* of teeth (a sycotic symptom), rather than on the crowns: "on blowing nose, a pressing pain in the hollow tooth, at the side of it." The left ovarian pains of *Thuja* are remarkable. They are severe, sometimes burning, extend down thigh, any attempt at exercise and especially *walking* <; they occur with every menstrual period, and are generally < before and during the flow. The pain compels the patient to lie down; but lying on left side <. A keynote of *Thuja* is: "Frequent micturition accompanying pains." For example: "In evening, when in bed, terrible hammering and tearing in the ear, *accompanied with micturition every half-hour* and coldness of the legs up to the knees. The desire of *Thuja* is sudden and urgent, it seems impossible to reach the vessel or make the necessary preparations, but the patient *can* control it if compelled. There is severe cutting as with a knife at the end of micturition after the last drop has passed. *Thuja* also has chronic incontinence from paralysis of sphincter vesicæ. This is related to the general paretic weakness of *Thuja*. The patient feels she "could not go on exerting any longer." Burnett (*H. W.*, xxv. 487) records a case of lichen urticatus in a boy of fourteen, which came into his hands after a long course of treatment, external, internal, and dietetic, at the hands of allopathic specialists without result. The rash came periodically in warm weather; patient literally tore himself because of the irritation. The rash was < on the left (vaccinated side). *Thuja* 30 was given in infrequent doses. The spots continued to appear for a week and then disappeared. The skin remained clear in spite of the patient indulging in all kinds of previously forbidden foods. Among the skin effects of *Thuja* the marks and stains must be borne in mind. The skin is mottled and discoloured; brown or red mottled spots; discoloration of the backs of the hands and feet.—Villers (*J. of Hcs.*, iv. 408) treated a girl of twelve, who had had headaches going from front to occiput and sometimes in temples. Pains mostly came towards night, and were accompanied with an awful state of fear. The only account she could give of her fear was that she *saw green stripes.* Alone or in company, in the dark or in a well-lighted room the dread was always the same. Three years before, the child had had an abortive attack of scarlatina, treated with cold compresses. The urine had been abnormal all through the illness, but contained no albumen. *Thuja* 200, every tenth day. No more headache, nor fear. Patient slept well from the first dose, and in a few days the urine became clear. "Floating stripes" before the vision is a symptom of *Thuja. Peculiar Sensations* are: As if a strange person were at her side. As if soul and body were separated. As if under the influence of a superior power. As if whole body were very thin and delicate; as if its continuity would be dissolved; as if frail and easily broken; as if made of glass. As if a nail were pressing into vertex. As if vertex were pressed with a needle. As if a nail were driven from within outward in vertex. As if a nail were driven into right parietal bone and left frontal eminence. Lightning-like headache. As if a convex button were pressed on left ear. As if head were screwed asunder. As if forehead would fall out. As if bones of head were being knocked to pieces. Forehead, ears, and eyes as if stabbed. As if knives went tearing around in brain. Scalp as if beaten. As if insects on occiput and temples. As if eyes were swollen and would be pressed out of head. As of fine sand in eyes. As if a cold stream of air were blowing through eyes. As if a foreign body in eye. As if flesh were being torn from bones in left side and back. As if abdominal muscles were being pushed out by arm of a child. As if a living animal were in abdomen. Sudden bounding in right iliac region as if something alive. As if blood could not circulate in back opposite pit of stomach. As if boiling lead were passed through rectum. As if anus would fly to pieces during stool. As if skin of anus were cracked and chapped. Bladder as if paralysed. As if moisture running in urethra. As if a tape prevented urination. As of a single drop running along urethra. As if testicles moved. As if something were grown fast in region of left lower ribs. As of falling drops in chest. Legs as if made of wood when walking. As if lower limbs were elongated. As if muscles of thigh would break down. Lightness in body when walking. As if flesh were beaten from bones. As if skin were pricked with needles. As from fleabites. A keynote of Cooper's for *Thuja* is, "its pains keep extending from their original site." Another indication of his is, "pains > by wrapping up." *Thuja is Suited to:* (1) Hydrogenoid constitutions (possessing "an increased capacity to contain water; hence rain, cold, damp weather, beds, and food that increase the number of molecules of water in the system < the symptoms"). (2) Strumous and sycotic pains. (3) Lax muscles; light hair; children. (4) Lymphatic temperament, in very fleshy persons, dark complexion, black hair, unhealthy skin. (5) Ailments from vaccination or from suppressed or maltreated gonorrhœa. *Thuja* is a strongly left-sided medicine (the *left* arm is usually vaccinated). The symptoms are : < By touch (scalp ; vertex ; eruption ; anus ; condylomata ; = fingers to bleed) ; but > pain in eyebrow and in left malar bone. Pressure >. Rubbing >. Scratching >. Closing eyes <. Fall = wart-like growth in labium. Overlifting < headache. Rest > headache. Bending head backward > headache. Lying on left side = anxious dreams. Lying on affected side > asthma. Motion <. Extension <. Letting arms hang down <. Walking <. Looking up > headache. Throwing head back > headache. Talking < asthma. Ascending = palpitation. Riding = incontinence of urine ; < pain in ovary. < 3 a.m. ; early morning (the sycotic time). < Night. < Cold water ; cold ; damp weather ; change ; draught ; overheating ; sun's rays. < Bright light. < Warmth of bed. Warmth <. Cold > rheumatism. < After breakfast, after eating ; after tea ; coffee ; fat food ; onions. < By coitus. < Blowing nose (pain in side of teeth). < Increasing moon. < Sun ; bright light.

Relations.—*Antidoted by:* Cham. (nightly toothache) : Coccul. (fever) ; Camph., Merc., Puls., Sul. Teste found Colch. the best antidote in his experience. *Antidote to:* Merc., Sul., Iod., Nux. *Complementary:* Med., Sabi., Sil. ; Nat. s. in sycosis. *Compatible:* Nit. ac., Sabi. *Follows well:* Med., Merc., Nit. ac. *Followed well by:* Merc., Sul. (these follow best.—H. N. G.) ; also Calc., Ign., Lyc., K. ca., Puls., Sil., Vacc. *Compare:* Constitutional polychrests, Med. Syph., Pso., Sul., Merc. Bad effect of vaccination, Apis, Ant. t., Vacc., Var. Aversion to touch or approach, Ant. c. (Thuja on account of fixed ideas). Illusions of shape, Bapt., Petr., Stram. Imaginary conditions (Saba., imaginary diseases). Ozæna with thick green discharge ; gleet ; gonorrhœal rheumatism ; orchitis ; prostatitis ; Puls. (the discharge of Puls. is thicker than that of Thuja). Ozæna in sycotics, K. bi. Condylomata, balanorrhœa, greenish leucorrhœa, Nit. ac. (Nit. ac. has more aching in bones, especially when not covered with muscles). Long filiform condylomata, Staph. (Staph., especially after Mercury, system generally depressed). Balanorrhœa, Jacar. Red chancroid sores, Coral. Iritis ; green discharges ; rheumatism ; sweating, Merc. (Merc. < warmth of bed ; sweating more excessive ; Thuja, sweat on uncovered parts only). Condylomata, Sabi. (itch and burn, especially in women). Condylomata large, like cock's-comb, Euphras. Syphilis and sycosis, fig-warts fan-shaped, much itching, especially about joints, Cinnab. ("Cinnab. is preferable for warts on prepuce."—H. C. Allen). Sycotic eruptions, Sars. Ciliary neuralgia, Spi. (Spi. pains radiate downward ; Thuja, upward and backward). Nails grow soft, Fl. ac. (rapidly). Diarrhœa, &c., after vaccination, Sil. Affections of tea-drinkers, Sep. Urinary affections, Canth. Effects of fat food, Ipec., Carb. v., Puls. Fissure about anus, Nit. ac. Graph. Dry, whitish scales on skin, Ars., Calc., Dulc., Lyc.,

Sep., Sil. Vaginismus, extreme sensitiveness, Sil. Hissing or singing of kettle in right ear, Lyc. Violent movements of fœtus, Op., Croc., Sil., Sul. Sense of levitation, Calc., Can. i., Con., Gels., Sil., Sti. p., Tic douloureux, Spi., Coccin. Phimosis, Cann. s., Merc., Sul., Nit. ac., Sep., Rhus, Sabi. Left ovarian pains, Colo., Bry., Phos. Yellow-staining leucorrhœa, Agn. c., Carb. a., Chel., Kre., Nit. ac., Nux, Pru. s., Sep. Tongue: Ulcer on right border, Sil. (on left, Apis); semilateral swelling of, Calc., Sil., Lauro. (Lauro, left half with loss of speech), Semp. t. Piles < sitting, Lyc. Ph. ac. (> Ign.). Vertigo when closing eyes, Lach., Ther. Headache as if a nail being driven in, Coff., Ign. Headache from tea, Sel. Teeth decay at roots, Mez. (on edges, Staph.). Teeth crumble, turn yellow, Syph. Ranula, varicose veins on tongue, Amb. "On blowing nose, a pressing pain in the hollow tooth or at the side of it" (Culex, vertigo every time he blows his nose). Abdomen protrudes here and there as from the arm of a fœtus, Croc., Nux m., Sul. Left ovarian pain when walking or riding, must sit or lie down. Croc., Ust. (Thuja, < at each menstrual nisus). Stool recedes after being partly expelled, Sanic., Sel. Early-morning diarrhœa expelled forcibly with much flatus, Alo. Coition prevented by extreme sensitiveness of vagina, Plat. (by dryness, Lyc., Hdfb., Na. m.). Large, seedy, pedunculated warts, Staph. Feeling as if flesh beaten off bones, Phyt. (scraped off, Rhus). Severe cutting at close of urination, Sars. Sweat: all over except head (opp. Sel.); when he sleeps, stops when he wakes (opp. Samb.). Nails deformed, brittle, Ant. c. > Bending head back, Seneg. (Thuja, headache; Seneg., eye symptoms > bending head back and closing eyes; Thuja has < closing eyes). Fluids roll audibly into stomach, Cup. Enuresis when coughing, Caust. Desires cold things, Pho. Swelling and sensitiveness of breasts at menstrual period, Con. Calc. < Walking, Æsc. h. Discoloured skin, Adren. Cracking in cervical vertebræ (K. iod., grating). Cretinism, Bac., Thyr.

Causation.—Vaccination. Gonorrhœa, badly treated or suppressed. Sunstroke. Sexual excess. Tea. Coffee. Beer. Sweets. Tobacco. Fat meat. Onions. Sulphur. Mercury.

SYMPTOMS.

1. **Mind.**—Fixed ideas: as if a strange person were at his side; as if the soul were separated from the body; as if the body, esp. the limbs, were of glass and would break easily; as if a living animal were in the abdomen.—Sensation as if whole body very thin and delicate and could not resist least attack; as if continuity of body would be dissolved.—Insane women will not be touched or approached.—Imbecility after vaccination, restless, drivelling.—Mental dejection.—Anxious apprehensions respecting the future.—Disquiet, which renders everything troublesome and repugnant.—The merest trifle occasions pensiveness.—Music causes him to weep, with trembling of the feet.—Hurried, with ill-humour, talks hastily.—Indisposition to any kind of intellectual labour.—Mental depression after childbirth.—Very depressed, sad, irritable.—Scrupulous about small things.—Feels she cannot exist any longer; quiet, shunning everybody.—Aversion to life.—Moroseness and peevishness.

—Overexcited, quarrelsome; easily angered about trifles.—The child excessively obstinate.—In reading and writing he uses wrong expressions.- Talks hastily and swallows words.—Thoughtlessness; forgetfulness.—Slov ness of speech and of reflection; seeking for words when in conversation.- Incapacity for reflection.—Cretinism.

2. **Head.**—Head feels empty, as in intoxication, esp. in morning, wi nausea.—Weakness and confusion of head, as from torpor, or paralysis brain.—Vertigo, as from motion of a swing.—Vertigo when rising from a sea or when lying down, or else when looking into the air.—Vertigo on closin the eyes, disappears as soon as he opens them; or on stooping; or on lookin upwards or sideways.—Headache in morning, as after stooping, or after to profound a sleep, with redness of the face.—The headache is > from lookin upwards, and when turning the head backwards.—Headache: < from sexu excess, overheating, overlifting; > exercising in open air.—Dull, stupefyin headache.—Headache, < by stooping, > by bending head backwards.- Heaviness of head, esp. in morning on waking; in occiput (cerebellum), wi ill-humour and dislike to conversation.—Headache, as if forehead woul split, with internal shivering, > by walking in open air.—Pressive headach with shocks in forehead and temples.—Compressive headache, esp. in temple —Pain as if a tight hoop encircled forehead, on waking.—(Headache, as if tight hoop encircled forehead up till noon; eyelids heavy as lead.—Goullon.)- Pain in head as if a nail were driven into vertex (afternoon and 3 a.m.; when at rest, > after perspiration).—As if a nail driven in r. parietal bo and l. frontal eminence.—Boring pressing in head.—Headache on l. side as a convex button were pressed on part.—Neuralgia going from before bac ward.—Nervous, sycotic, or syphilitic headaches.—Meningitis of sycot children.—Sunstroke: everything seemed jumping, < from sitting up, from talking a long time, or closing eyes.—Semilateral tearing in the sincip and face, extending into zygomatic process, principally morning and evenin —Tearing jerking in occiput.—Lancinations across brain.—Congestion blood in head.—Pulsation in temples.—Excessively painful tenderness l. side of head, and also of the hair, at night, when lying down, and whe touched.—Hair becomes hard, dry, and lustreless, and falls out.—Hair thi grows slowly, splits; brittle, looks crimped.—Pressive drawing in th temporal muscles, esp. during mastication.—Shootings in temples.—Swellin of veins in temples.—He wants to have head (and face) wrapped up warm.- Itching and gnawing in scalp.—The scalp is very painful to the touch, an the parts on which one lies.—Cannot bear a hat on his head (agg.—R. T. C. —Dry herpes on the head, extending to eyebrows; dandruff.—White, scal peeling-off eruption over the scalp, extending over the forehead, temple ears, and neck.—(Flat black wart on r. parietal region.—J. H. C.)—Tinglin biting, stinging-itching on the scalp, > by scratching.—Perspiration, smel ing of honey (sweetish), on uncovered parts of head (face and hands), wi dryness of the covered parts, and of those on which one lies, mostly whe first going to sleep; > after rising.—(Pityriasis affecting forehead, face, ea and neck, < after washing in warm water.—R. T. C.)—Eczema comes out c glabella (after *Thuja* 30)—R. T. C.).

3. **Eyes.**—Pressure in eyes, and smarting, as if sand were in them.- Tearing in eyebrows.—Shootings in eyes, in a bright light, or in a keen air.-

Painful stitch through centre of l. eye, commencing in centre of brain.—Malignant balanorrhœa.—Wart-like excrescence on iris.—Inflammation of cornea.—Vascular tumour of cornea.—Small brown spots on cornea.—Episcleritis; sclero-choroiditis; staphyloma.—Ophthalmia neonatorum.—Phlyctenular conjunctivitis.—(Conjunctivitis of l. eye, with violent pain across forehead and in outer side of eyeball, constantly recurrent from childhood and due to suppressed eruption.—R. T. C.)—Fungous tumour in orbit.—Burning sensation in eyes.—Sclerotica inflamed, and red like blood.—Pupils dilated.—Inflammatory swelling of lids, with hardness.—Burning eruption on lids.—Granular lids with wart-like granulations.—Epithelioma of l. lower lid.—Feeling as if lids swollen, and a foreign body in eye.—Ptosis; lids fall down several times a day.—Lids heavy as lead.—Inflammatory softening of inner surface of lids.—Red and painful nodosities on margins of lids.—(Tinea ciliaris; dry and branny lids.—R. T. C.)—Styes; tarsal tumours; chalazæ; thick and hard knots.—Verrucæ and tumours like condylomata.—Purulent and itching pimples between eyebrows.—Condylomata in eyebrows.—Sensation of heat and of dryness in external canthi.—Lachrymation, esp. in l. eye, when walking in open air (the tears do not run off, but remain standing in the eye).—The eye must be warmly covered, when uncovered it pains at once, and it feels as if cold air were streaming out of the head through the eye.—Nocturnal agglutination of the lids.—Weakness of the eyes; obscure sight.—Clouded sight, when reading, with sensation of drowsiness.—Sight confused as if directed through a veil.—Diplopia.—Myopia.—Black dancing specks before the eyes.—Floating stripes.—(Sees green stripes which frighten her.)—Flames of light, mostly yellow; looking into light of day sees spots like bottles of water moving; a luminous disc shining like a firefly.—Sensation of dryness in eyes.—In the dark it seems as if falling down of luminous lights or sparks alongside of the eye, during the day and in the light it is as if dark drops were falling down.—The objects appear smaller before the r. eye.—Short-sighted.

4. **Ears.**—Otalgia, wtth squeezing compression and violent shootings, esp. in evening.—Stitches into ear from the neck.—Sensation as if inner ear were swollen, with increased difficulty of hearing.—(Vascular deafness with scurfy head.—R. T. C.)—Oozing from the r. ear, smelling like putrid meat.—Spasmodic pain in external ear.—Noise in the ear as from boiling water.—Roaring in l. ear, with cracking when swallowing saliva.—Hammering and tearing in ear, in evening, in bed, with frequent emission of urine, and coldness in legs and feet.—Pressive pain behind ears.—Orifice of l. meatus blocked up by a polypus, of raspberry-cellular vessels; pale red, bleeding readily when touched; muco-purulent discharge; deafness; shooting pains.

5. **Nose.**—Nose red and hot.—Red eruption on nose, at times humid.—Swelling in the alæ nasi, with hardness and tension.—Drawing tension in bones of nose.—Painful scabs in nose.—Painful pressure at root of nose.—Blowing of blood from nose.—Frequent epistaxis, esp. after being overheated.—Dry coryza, which becomes fluent in open air, with continued headache.—Fluent coryza, with cough and hoarseness.—Greenish and fetid discharge from the nose.—Blowing from the nose of a large quantity of thick green mucus, mixed with pus and blood; later of dry, brown scales, with mucus, which comes from the frontal sinuses and firmly adheres to the

swollen upper portion of the nostrils.—Accumulation of mucus in posterior nares.—Chronic catarrh after measles, scarlatina, variola.—(Ozæna.—Ussher.) —Warts on the nose.—Smell in nose as from brine of fish, or of fermenting beer.

6. **Face.**—Heat in face, sometimes only transient, or else with burning redness.—Heat and redness of whole face, with fine nets of veins, as if marbled.—Circumscribed burning redness of cheeks.—Dropsically bloated face.—Œdematous erysipelas of face.—Greasy skin of face.—Light-brown blotches (freckles) on face.—Faceache, originating in l. cheek-bone near the ear, extending through teeth to nose, through eyes to temples into head ; the painful spots burn like fire, and are very sensitive to the rays of the sun.—Neuralgia of trigeminus after suppressed gonorrhœa or eruption on ear.—Facial pains tending to spread to neck and head, chiefly l. side (many cases cured.—R. T. C.)—Large, hard, dark wart with large base.—Perspiration on face (esp. on side on which he does not lie).—Scabious, itching eruption on face.—Red and painful nodosities on temples.—Boring and digging pain in cheek-bones, > by touch.—Twitching of the lips.—Jerking sensation in upper lip, near corner of mouth.—Upper lip sensitive.—Wart on upper lip.—Thick upper lip with pea-sized tumour on its parenchyma, enlarging when taking cold.—Lips pale, swollen, peeling.—Flat ulcers on insides of lips and corners of mouth.—Eruption of pimples on lips and chin.—Shootings in lower jaw, which seem to pass outwards through the ear.—Cracking of articulation of jaw.—Fungus on l. lower jaw, more angry in damp weather —Swelling of submaxillary glands.

7. **Teeth.**—Toothache after drinking tea, with pressive pain extending into jaw.—Toothache with acute drawing pains, esp. during mastication.—The roots of the teeth become carious ; or the teeth become carious from the side ; the crown of the tooth remains sound.—On blowing nose, a pressing pain in hollow tooth at the side of it.—The teeth crumble off.—Teeth crusted with tartar ; extremely sensitive to cold water.—Dirty-yellow teeth.—Gnawing in (carious) teeth, with painful sensibility of whole side of head, greatly < by contact with cold things, or by mastication.—Gums swollen (inflamed, with dark red streaks on them), with pain of excoriation.—Alveolar periostitis where the pains come and go suddenly at short intervals (R. T. C.).—Epulis.

8. **Mouth.**—Flat, white ulcers on the inside of the lips, and on the corners of the mouth.—Aphthæ in mouth (ulcers ; mouth feels as if burnt).—Considerable swelling of salivary glands, with increased saliva in mouth.—Sanguineous, or bitter saliva.—Pain as of excoriation in tip of tongue, when touched.—Swelling of tongue (esp. on r. side ; bites tongue frequently), painful when touched.—Condylomata under tongue.—Varicose veins under tongue.—Ranula, on both sides of tongue, transparent, bluish red, grey, and, as it were, gelatinous.—Ranula and epulis with excess of venosity everywhere (Ussher).—Taste in mouth sweet as sugar, with gonorrhœa.—Slowness of speech.

9. **Throat.**—Roughness and scraping in throat.—Pressure and pain as from excoriation, in throat and palate, during deglutition.—A feeling of upward pressure in soft palate.—Necessity to swallow.—Shootings from gullet to ears.—Swelling of tonsils and throat.—Ulcers in throat and mouth, like chancres.—Accumulation of a large quantity of tenacious mucus in mouth,

which is hawked up with difficulty.—Painful swallowing, esp. empty swallowing, or that of saliva.—Throat feels raw, dry, as from a plug, or as if it were constricted when swallowing.—Hawking up of mucus of red colour, like blood.—(Exophthalmic goître.—C. Sargent, of Chicago.)

10. **Appetite.**—Mawkish and sweetish taste in the mouth, in the evening, and after a meal.—Taste : sweet ; of rotten eggs, mornings.—Bread has a dry and bitter taste.—Craves salt.—Food never seems sufficiently salt.—Thirst only at night, and in morning.—Appetite for cold drinks and food.—Unable to eat breakfast (a keynote of Burnett's).—Aversion to fresh meat and potatoes.—Speedy satiety, when eating.—Disagreeable sensations after eating fat food or onions.—While masticating food mouth becomes very dry.—After a meal great indolence, or dejection, with anguish, and palpitation of the heart, or great inflation and sufferings from flatulence.

11. **Stomach.**—Risings of food, after a meal.—Bitter or putrid risings.—Continuous eructations of air while eating.—Vomiting of mucus or of greasy substances.—Induration of stomach.—Swelling of pit of stomach.—The fluid which he drinks falls into the stomach with a gurgling noise.—Rancid risings, esp. after fat food.—Nausea and uneasiness in region of stomach.—Vomiting of acid serum and of food.—Cramp in stomach, with excessive < towards evening.—Pressure in scrobiculus after a meal, with pain when touched.—Throbbing in scrobiculus.—Anguish in scrobiculus, which extends upwards into head.

12. **Abdomen.**—Painful pressure in hepatic region.—After a dose of 30th headache comes on, and he feels on stooping forward as if liver overlapped the ribs (agg.—J. C. B.)—(Old rheumatism attacking bowels, liver, and kidneys.—R. T. C.)—Pressure in lumbar region.—(Soreness with swelling in hepatic region and violent pain under r. shoulder going through to breast and down to elbow < on getting out of bed in morning.—R. T. C.)—Inflation of abdomen, often with contractive and spasmodic pains.—Flatulence, as if an animal were crying in the abdomen.—Pot-belly.—Constrictive tension in abdomen.—Induration in abdomen.—The upper part of abdomen is drawn in.—Soreness of navel.—Pressive pains in abdomen, esp. towards the side (before evacuation).—Stitches in the hypochondria.—Sensation as if something alive were in hypogastrium (as if the abdominal muscles were pushed outward by the arm of a fœtus, but painless).—Soreness of navel.—Pain in abdomen, as from constriction of the intestines.—Grumbling and borborygmi in the abdomen.—Depressing pain in groins.—Drawings in groins, when walking and standing, with shootings along thighs when sitting.—Painful swelling of inguinal glands, sometimes with drawing as far as knee.—Intussusception of intestines.—Yellow or brownish spots on abdomen.—Zona.

13. **Stool and Anus.**—Constipation which continues several days (obstinate, as from inactivity or from intussusception of the intestines), sometimes after pollutions.—Tenesmus, with rigidity of the penis.—Stool in hard balls.—Difficult evacuation of hard, large fæces, covered with blood.—Discharge of blood, during the evacuation.—Diarrhœa : pale-yellow water is forcibly expelled, with much noisy discharge of wind ; with colic ; < after eating ; watery, painless ; bright yellow, watery ; streaming out with much gas, as if the cork were pulled out of a full jug, excessively exhausting, short

and difficult breathing, anxiety, intermitting pulse, acute pressive pain in back opposite pit of stomach, with feeling as if no blood could circulate there, rapid disappearance of fat.—In morning (after breakfast), periodically returning diarrhœa, always at the same hour.—Stools oily or greasy.—With stools, sensations in rectum as if boiling lead were passing through.—Burning soreness in anus, lasting all day.—Much flatus hard to expel, anus feels constricted, incarcerated flatus behind r. side of diaphragm.—Pains in anus < from motion.—Painful contraction of anus, during the evacuation.—Burning sensation in anus, and between buttocks.—Condylomata at anus.—Hæmorrhoidal tumours swollen, paining worse while sitting.—Swelling of hæmorrhoidal veins.—Pressing, itching, and burning in the hæmorrhoidal vessels, with dragging.—Offensive perspiration at anus and in perinæum.—Fistula in ano.—Fissure of anus.—Tearings along rectum.

14. **Urinary Organs.**—Kidneys inflamed; feet swollen.—Diabetes.—Stitch to bladder from rectum.—Violent burning in fundus of bladder.—Urging to urinate frequent and hasty.—Stream interrupted.—Frequent want to urinate, with profuse emission of a watery urine, also at night.—The urine foams; the foam remains long on the urine.—Involuntary secretion of urine; at night; when coughing; in drops after having urinated.—The bladder (and rectum) feels paralysed, having no power to expel.—Sediment of brown mucus.—The urine contains sugar.—Boring in region of bladder, with painful drawing up of testes.—Urine yellowish or wine-coloured.—Orifice of urethra agglutinated by mucus.—Cloudy sediment in urine.—Bloody urine.—Prolonged trickling of urine, after having urinated.—Sensation as if a drop were flowing into urethra, after emission of urine, and at other times.—Burning sensation in urethra, esp. in morning and during day; also after and during emission of urine.—Shootings in urethra, during emission of urine, and at other times.—Jerking, voluptuous formication in fossa navicularis.—Smarting in sexual part of females, during emission of urine.—Itching in urethra.—Stream small and split, next day yellowish discharge from urethra, with chordee.

15. **Male Sexual Organs.**—Venereal diseases.—Affections in general appearing in male or female genital organs, particularly on the external organs; affections on l. side particularly.—Profuse perspiration on genitals, esp. scrotum; sweet-smelling, like honey; staining linen yellow.—(Relaxed scrotum with sexual weakness and lethargy; unfit for strain.—R. T. C.)—Pseudo-gonorrhœa.—Painful spermatic cords from suppressed gonorrhœa.—Feeling in testes as if they moved.—Condylomata on glans and prepuce, moist, itching and suppurating, esp. while the moon is increasing.—Ulcers, like chancres, on prepuce.—Swelling of prepuce.—Red excrescence on inner side of prepuce; like fig-warts.—Smooth, red excrescence behind glans.—Many red pedunculated condylomata surrounding glans.—Round, unclean, elevated ulcers with red margins, moist and painful.—Sycotic cauliflower excrescences; fig-warts smelling like old cheese or herring brine.—Shootings in scrotum, in penis, and along spermatic cord, as far as navel.—Drawing in testes, with retraction of one of them (l.).—Continued painful erections, esp. night and morning, with lancinations in urethra.—Nightly painful erections causing sleeplessness.—Irresistible inclination to onanism even during sleep.—Nocturnal emissions; wake him; followed by heaviness and ill-humour.—Pollutions

with sensation of stricture in urethra.—Seminal emissions cured with 5-drop doses of ϕ (C. W. Roberts).—The semen has an offensive smell.—Flow of prostatic fluid. — Prostatic affections from suppressed or badly-treated gonorrhœa.—Blenorrhœa along with otorrhœa; penis constantly erect and prepuce inflamed (cured in boy, 12.—R. T. C.).—Gonorrhœa: scalding when urinating, urethra swollen; urinal stream forked; discharge yellow; green; watery; with warts; red erosions on glans; subacute and chronic cases, esp. when injections have been used and prostate is involved.—Gonorrhœa with a soft lump having an abrasion on it on l. side of frænum præputiæ, lump small and painless.—Profuse and watery discharge from penis.—Renewed gonorrhœa after coitus.

16. **Female Sexual Organs.**—Affections appearing on external organs, esp. l. side.—Warts, condylomata, and other excrescences about vulva.—Ulcers on internal surface of vulva; vulva has a sore, smarting feeling.—Itching and burning smarting, as from excoriation, in genital organs.—Burning and biting in vagina.—Vagina extremely sensitive during coition.—Recto-vaginal fistula (cured.—J. C. B.)—Pressure on genital organs.—Contractive and spasmodic pain in genital organs, extending to hypogastrium.—Ovaries, affections of. — Swelling and excoriation of labia. — Warts on orifice of uterus, with shootings and burning sensation when urinating. — Uterine polypus. — Cauliflower excrescences. — Prolapse.—L. ovary inflamed, < at each menstrual nisus; distressing pain, burning when walking or riding; must lie down; pain extends through l. iliac region into groin, and sometimes into l. leg, pain sometimes burning.—Cutting, squeezing, shooting pains in region of l. ovary.—Pain, located in ovaries or duct, from over-physiological action.—Menses: too early and too short; scanty, with terrible distressing pain in l. ovarian and iliac region.—Before menses: excitement and pulsation of arteries, back of head, headache and toothache; labour-like abdominal pains, tenesmus and fainting; much perspiration.—During menses: tiredness, palpitation, spasmodic weeping; restlessness in legs; retching, pressing in stomach, distension, pain in abdomen and back; bearing down out of genital organs; burning in varicose veins of genitals; sensitiveness and swelling of breasts; general coldness.—After menses: tiredness; rush of blood upward; toothache; sleeplessness; nightmare.—Bleeding fungus of breast (completed cure after *Phos.*).—Sycotic excrescences; moist, bleeding and offensive.—Leucorrhœa: mucous; is almost green.—Abortion at end of third month, commencing with a scanty discharge of blood for five days, then more and more profuse.—Bright red or clotted blood with bearing down in third month of pregnancy (cured with *Thujopsis dolabrata*.—R. T. C.).—During pregnancy child moves so violently it wakens her, causing cutting in bladder with urging to urinate; pains in l. sacro-iliac articulation, running into groin.—Labour: pains weak or ceasing; contractibility hindered by sycotic complications; pains in sacro-iliac articulation running into l. groin; pain from walking, insupportable, must lie down.

17. **Respiratory Organs.**—Voice low.—Sensation of a skin in the arynx.—Polypus of vocal cord.—Condylomata.—Hoarseness, as from contraction of larynx.—Shortness of breath from mucus in trachea.—Shortness of breathing from fulness and constriction in hypochondria and upper abdomen. —Asthma < at night, with red face; coughing spells, with sensation of

adhesion of lungs.—Asthma with gonorrhœa, without having been exposed to contagion.—Asthma with little cough, but with sensation of something growing fast in region of l. lower ribs.—Asthma of sycotic children (Goullon).—Respiration short and quick, < from deep inspiration and talking; > from lying on affected side, but pains compel him to lie on back.—Convulsive asthma.—Shooting and tingling in trachea.—Cough in morning, excited by a tickling in trachea.—Cough, excited by a choking sensation.—Sputa: green; taste like old cheese.—Expectoration of small grey, yellow, or green gobbets, when coughing.—Cough, with expectoration of yellow mucus, and pains in scrobiculus in afternoon.—Cough only during day, or in morning after rising, and in evening after lying down.—Cough as soon as one eats.—During evening cough after lying down, the expectoration becomes loose; easier when he turns from l. to r. side.

18. **Chest.**—Obstructed respiration, with violent thirst for water, and great anxiety.—Spasms of lungs from drinking cold water.—Stitching in chest, from drinking anything cold.—Hot rising into chest.—Pain in l. pectoral region extending to innominate bone.—Dyspnœa, with need to take full inspirations.—Oppression, at one time of l. side of chest, at another, of l. hypochondrium, with irritation which excites coughing.—Pain in chest, as from internal adhesion.—Pressure on chest, sometimes after a meal.—Agitation, and sensation of swelling in chest.—Hæmorrhage from lungs; quantity very great and terribly offensive.—Blue colour of skin round clavicles.—Brown spots on chest.

19. **Heart.**—Cramp in heart.—Ebullition of blood in chest, and violent and audible palpitation of heart, esp. when going up stairs.—Palpitation of heart, with nausea.—Painful sensibility in region of heart.—Anxious palpitation of heart when waking in the morning.—Visible palpitation without anxiety.—Stitches in region of heart.—Pulse slow and weak in morning, in evening accelerated and full.—In evening violent pulsations.—Swelling of the veins.

20. **Neck and Back.**—Uneasiness in nape of neck and chest.—Tension in skin on nape when moving head.—Greasy brown skin on neck.—Tension and stiffness of nape and l. side of neck.—Cracking in cervical vertebræ on making certain movements with head.—Small red pimples on neck close together.—Swelling of glands of neck.—Swelling of veins of neck.—Spinal curvature.—Boils on back.—Steatomatous tumours.—Pressing pain in region of kidneys.—Burning extending from the small of the back to between shoulder-blades.—(Pains from middle to lower back with tenderness of muscles on each side.—R. T. C.)—Painful drawing in sacrum, coccyx, and thighs, while sitting; after long sitting prevents standing erect.—Pain, as of a fracture, and stiffness in loins, back, and nape, esp. in morning, after rising.—(Weakness from injury to lower back followed by abscess, vesical weakness, enuresis with a clear gleet and balanitis.—R. T. C.)—Drawing in back and loins, when seated.—Boring in back.—Pulsation in spine.—Furunculi on back.—Violent stitch between coccyx and anus 7 p.m. when walking.—Itching burning in hollow below coccyx.

21. **Limbs.**—Cracking of joints when extended.—Trembling of hands and feet.—Limbs go to sleep.—Frozen limbs.—One-sided complaints; paralysis.—Rheumatism with numb feeling; < in warmth and on moving;

> from cold and after sweating.—Nails crippled; brittle or soft.—Hang-nails.

22. **Upper Limbs.**—Profuse perspiration under axillæ.—Brown spots under the arms, like nævus maternus.—Throbbing in shoulder-joint.—Sticking in shoulders.—Involuntary jerking of arm during day.—Atrophy of r. arm after revaccination.—Pain, as of ulceration, tearing, and throbbing, from shoulder to ends of fingers.—Wrenching pain in shoulder and arm, with cracking.—Digging drawing in arms, as if in bones or periosteum.—Sensation of coldness in arms at night.—Lancinations in arms and joints.—Cracking in elbow-joint when stretching arms.—Tearing pain along r. arm compelling him to keep it flexed.—Herpes on elbow.—Red marbled spots on forearm.—Wrist and elbow of r. arm feel as if gripped by a hand (agg.—*Thujopsis dol.*—R. T. C.)—Trembling of hand and arms, when writing.—Ganglion of wrist (cured by local use.—R. T. C.)—Sensation of dryness in skin of hands.—Brown colour on back of hand.—White scaly herpes on back of hand and on finger.—Perspiration on hands.—Swollen veins in hands.—Warts on hands; very numerous, esp. on dorsa; horny, painful.—Brown colour of dorsum of hand.—Coldness torpor, and paleness in fingers and finger-tips, extending sometimes to fore-arms.—(Erysipelatous swelling and) tingling and shootings in finger-tips.—Red and painful swelling in finger-tips.—Nails are crippled, discoloured, crumbling off.—Suppuration of finger-nails.—The pains in the arms are < when hanging down, or when exposed to heat; they are > by movement, cold, and after perspiration.

23. **Lower Limbs.**—Lower limbs feel like wood when walking in open air.—Tension from hip-joint to groin, and along back of thigh to knee.—Sciatica, l. side, leg atrophied.—Paresis and atrophy of r. leg with coldness.—Drawings in legs.—The hip-joint feels as if it were relaxed.—Coxalgia, the leg becomes elongated.—Brown skin on legs, esp. on inside of thigh.—Enlarged nævus on thigh of child, æt. five months.—Shootings in legs and joints.—Great weakness and lassitude in legs, esp. when going up stairs.—Heaviness and stiffness of legs, when walking (they feel as if made of wood).—Profuse perspiration on thighs and genital organs.—Itching in thighs.—Eruption of pimples on buttocks, thighs, and knees.—Ulcers on thighs.—Cracking in joints of knees and feet, when stretching them.—Suppurating pustules on knees.—Gonorrhœal rheumatism in fibrous part of knee-joint.—Pains in feet and ankles after suppressed gonorrhœa, could not walk.—Pain in heel as if gone to sleep.—Stitches above heel in tendo Achillis.—White nodosities, with violent itching in toes.—Inflammatory red swelling in ends of toes, or instep, with pain and tension when treading, and during movement.—Numbness of l. foot.—Nets of veins, as if marbled, on soles of feet.—Red, marbled spots on instep.—Perspiration (fetid) on feet, esp. toes.—Suppressed foot-sweat.—Chilblains on toes.

24. **Generalities.**—Emaciation and deadness of affected parts.—All manifestations excessive; their advent insidious.—Shootings in limbs (outer parts), and joints.—Burning darting pain.—Drawing in the blood-vessels.—Cracking in joints on stretching limbs.—Swelling of the veins in the skin.—Jerking of some of the limbs and of some of the muscles.—The flesh feels as if beaten off the bones.—Sensation of lightness of the body when walking.—Œdema about the joints; affects prominently epithelia, first causing harden-

ing, hypertrophy; then softening.—Stitches in various parts, changing to burning.—Tearing and pulsative pains, as if the parts affected were ulcerated.—Inflammatory swellings, with redness.—Sufferings after being overheated, drinking tea, or eating fat meat, or onions.—Bad effects from beer, fat food acids, sweets, tobacco, and wine; from the abuse of *Sulphur* and *Mercury*.—One-sided complaints—paralysis.—St. Vitus' dance.—Trembling of some of the limbs.—Easy benumbing of limbs, esp. at night, on waking.—Symptoms generally < in afternoon, or in night, towards 3 a.m.; they hinder sleep in evening.—Many of the symptoms are < during repose and by heat, esp. by that of the bed; they are > by movement, cold, and perspiration.—Many of the symptoms manifest themselves chiefly on l. side.—Affections of the r. abdominal ring; wings of the nose; loins; inguinal glands; fingers, tips of fingers; toes.—(Glandular cervical enlargements.—R. T. C.)—Stiffness and general heaviness over whole body, esp. in shoulders and thighs.—Physical weakness, with sustained mental powers.—Frequent jerking of upper part of body.—Violent ebullition of blood in evening, with pulsation in all the arteries, < by movement, > on sitting down.—Aneurism by anastamosis; swelling of the blood-vessels.—Dreams anxious, esp. of dead persons; of falling; of accidents.—Flushes of heat.—< In the afternoon; after midnight; while chewing; stretching the affected limb; while urinating.—> While drawing up the limb.

25. **Skin.**—Painful sensitiveness of skin.—Itching shootings in skin, esp. in evening and at night.—Purulent pimples, like variola.—Warts on any part of the body, with little necks, called fig-warts, tubular warts, same size all the way out; "mother's marks."—Warts, hard, cleft, and seedy.—Black sessile warts; on scalp.—Pustules.—Small-pox.—Eruptions only on covered parts.—The eruptions burn violently after scratching.—Universal psoriasis.—Sycotic excrescences, smelling like old cheese, or like the brine of fish.—White, scaly, dry, mealy herpes.—Sycosis of beard cured with single doses of ϕ after failure of much other treatment (R. T. C.).—Condylomata (large, seedy, frequently on a pedicle).—Flat ulcers, with a bluish-white bottom.—Zona.—Corns burning.—Crippled nails on fingers and toes.—Furunculi.—Chilblains.—Dirty-brownish colour of the skin.—Brown or red (or brown-white) mottled spots on the skin.—The majority of cutaneous symptoms are > by touch.

26. **Sleep.**—Urgent inclination to sleep in evening.—Sleep retarded, in consequence of agitation and dry heat.—Nocturnal sleeplessness, with agitation and coldness of body.—Unrefreshing nocturnal sleep.—Distressing, anxious dreams, of dangers and death, of falling from a height, soon after falling asleep, or else with starts and cries, esp. when lying on l. side.—When half asleep it suddenly seems as if a chair were standing in the middle of the bed; tries to move it but cannot stir, cannot utter a sound.—Continuous sleeplessness, with painfulness of the parts on which he lies.—Sleeplessness with apparitions as soon as he closes his eyes; they disappear on opening them.—Goes to sleep late on account of heat and restlessness.—Lascivious dreams, without emission of semen, with painful erections on waking.

27. **Fever.**—Shivering, with yawning, after midnight.—The warm air seems cold, and the sun has no power to warm him.—Shivering, every morning, without thirst.—Shivering and shaking, with internal and external coldness (and thirst), followed immediately by perspiration.—Chilliness in attacks

at various times in the day, but mostly in the evening.—Chilliness on l. side, which feels cold to the touch.—Chill without thirst after midnight and in morning.—Shivering every evening (at six o'clock), with external heat, dryness of the mouth, and thirst.—Heat in the evening, esp. in the face.—Dry heat of the covered parts.—Burning in the face without redness.—Perspiration at the commencement of sleep.—Perspiration on parts uncovered, with dry heat of covered parts.—Anxious, at times cold, sweat.—Perspiration after the chill, without any intervening heat.—Perspiration, at times oily (staining the clothes yellow), or fetid, or smelling sweet like honey.—General perspiration, but not on the head.—When walking in morning profuse perspiration; the most profuse on the head.—Perspiration only during sleep, disappearing at once as soon as he awakens.

Thyroidinum.

Thyroidin. Thyroid Extract. A Sarcode. Trituration of the fresh thyroid gland of sheep or calf. Attenuation of a liquid extract of the gland.

Clinical.—Abscess. Acromegaly. Albuminuria; of pregnancy. Amblyopia. Amenorrhœa. *Anæmia; acute pernicious.* Angina pectoris. Backache. *Chilblains.* Constipation. Convulsions, puerperal. Diarrhœa. Diuresis. Dropsy. Dysmenorrhœa. Ear, middle, affections of. Eczema. Fainting. Fibroma. Fractures, ununited. Goître; exophthalmic. Hair, new growth of; falling off. Heart, failure of; valvular disease of. Hysteria. Hystero-epilepsy. Ichthyosis. Idiocy. *Leprosy.* Mania. Milk, deficiency of. *Myxœdema.* Neurasthenia. Obesity. Œdema. Optic neuritis. Paralysis; of hands and arms. Paraplegia. Phthisis. Pityriasis rubra. *Psoriasis.* Puerperal fever. Rupia. Scleroderma. Syphilis. Tetanus.

Characteristics.—When the treatment of myxœdema and allied diseases by "Thyroid feeding" was introduced by Murray in 1892, many accidents occurred from overdosing. A large number of the pathogenetic effects I collected (*H. W.*, xxix. and subsequent volumes) and arranged in Schema form (*H. W.*, xxix. 251) along with cured symptoms, giving the authority and reference for each. In my subjoined Schema I have omitted the references. Cured symptoms I have bracketed, unless otherwise indicated. Marc Jousset collected other symptoms in *L'Art Médical*, and I have added some of these, together with others from later observers. The first published case treated with an attenuation was one of my own (*H. W.*, xxix. 111): Eleanor N., 17, suffered from fits of "hystero-epilepsy" for ten months, following a chill. At first the fits had been frequent, latterly only before the menstrual period. The fits sometimes lasted half an hour, were preceded by swelling of limbs and face, which sometimes occurred without the subsequent fit. She bit her tongue in the fits. Other symptoms were: pains in legs, back, and head (occiput and vertex); swelling of throat compelling her to loosen her clothes. Menses after an absence of four months returned excessively. Much left ovarian pain and tenderness. Despondent, feeble heart sounds; pulse 120; could not lie down for palpitation and headache. Legs so weak she could not stand. Thyroid very slightly enlarged. Constipation. Sleepless, has had to take hypnotics regularly of late. A brother of the patient was epileptic. *Lach.* did some good, especially improving the sleep; but no solid progress was made till *Thyr.* 3x, gr. ii. thrice daily, was given on November 1st. On November 4th she could lie down flat; on the 15th she could walk with assistance; on the 29th the headache had ceased; on December 6th she could walk alone quite well and the bowels acted without enema for the first time. The mental condition improved, the prominence of the eyeballs disappeared, and she left the hospital perfectly well before Christmas. With *Thyr.* 1m F.C. Skinner cured a case of dysmenorrhœa in a goitrous subject. In a case of valvular heart disease following rheumatism in a man, 24, *Thyr.* 3x, gr. ii. thrice daily, quickly relieved a squeezing pain at the heart with inability to lie down and materially hastened the patient's recovery. The action of *Thyr.* on the heart is most profound. Fatal syncope has occurred in a number of cases under "Thyroid feeding." Cyanosis was produced in many cases. Severe angina pectoris was produced by it in a patient to whom Burnett gave the 3x. The connection between the heart and the thyroid gland is very close, as seen in cases of exophthalmic goître. Many cases of the latter affection have been cured with *Thyr.* In myxœdema, cachexia strumipriva, cretinism and similar conditions the thyroid gland is absent or defective, and the idea of the Thyroid feeding is to supply a physiological want. A state of puffiness and obesity may therefore be regarded as a keynote indication for *Thyr.* As drugs act sometimes in opposite ways, I gave *Thyr.* 3x gr. ii. to a living skeleton of a child aged five, and looking not more than two, who had been kept in a box in a cellar all his life till brought into hospital, when he weighted $14\frac{1}{4}$ pounds. Under *Bac.* 200 and careful feeding he gained $\frac{1}{4}$ pound a week. When I commenced *Thyr.* he put on weekly $\frac{3}{4}$ pound, and gained the use of his legs, being able to stand by holding on to a chair. In a case of universal and very aggravated psoriasis in a schoolboy, fair, very chilly, cold, clammy hands and feet, *Thyr.* 3x and later 30 (which seemed to act better than the lower attenuation) completely cured after a prolonged course. An obese lady, æt. 60, developed diabetes. I cured her completely of the diabetes with *Thyr.* 3x and 30. She has now for many years been able to take any kind of food. (On her husband, a *spare* man, who also was diabetic *Thyr.* had no effect.) Skin cases in great variety have been cured with *Thyr.* in substantial doses: Pityriasis rubra, intense redness, and scaliness of legs, and also with intense itching; ichthyosis; syphilitic eruptions; scleroderma. The nutrition of the bones is affected, and acromegaly has been relieved and united fractures made to unite. *Thyr.* has increased the flow of milk in nursing women when the flow has been deficient. It has cured cases of tetany both operative and idiopathic. The keynote in these cases appears to have been "< of spasms by cold." Many cases of insanity have been cured with it, including a case of puerperal insanity with fever. H. O. Nicholson (*B. M. J.*, June 21, 1901) relates a case of eclampsia of pregnancy: A woman, 32, in her third pregnancy, had a fit on October 3rd. Thyroid feeding was begun next day. Marked improvement followed. Œdema of face and body diminished. On

October 23rd patient was about her usual duties. On November 6th she was delivered of a healthy boy without any untoward symptoms. *Thyr.*, according to Nicholson, is diuretic, like *Urea*; and Nicholson explains its action in eclampsia as being effected through its enabling the kidneys to carry off the toxins resulting from fœtal metabolism. *Thyr.* is antagonistic to *Adrenalin* in that the latter contracts, whilst the former dilates the arterioles. Among the pathogenetic effects of *Thyr.*, optic neuritis and accommodative asthenopia have been observed. Some curiosities have been noted in the action of *Thyr.* on the growth of hair. Myxœdema patients lose their hair as a rule, and *Thyr.* when successful restores the growth. But in some cases the opposite effect has been noted. In one case of myxœdema the hair had fallen off the head and face and a thick growth appeared on arms and chest. Under *Thyr.* the latter disappeared, and the hair on the head and face grew again (*L'Art Méd.*, lxxxii. 44). The pains of *Thyr.* are stitching, aching, or heavy pains, and tingling sensations. At the point of injection when administered subcutaneously brawny swelling occurred in one case (which may suggest scleroderma) followed by abscess of slow development. Persons suffering from skin diseases were found tolerant of much larger doses than myxœdemics. In a number of cases latent phthisis has been lighted up into activity. Syphilis, both secondary and tertiary, has been vastly relieved by *Thyr.* Hansen mentions fibroma uteri as having been cured by *Thyr.*, and Burford supports this. "Brawny swelling" is a keynote of *Thyr.* pointed out by Burnett. With *Thyr.* 3x gr. vi. thrice daily he cured a case of dropsy and albuminuria which had been given up by several doctors. Burnett noticed that the swelling was *brawny*. Soon after commencing *Thyr.* the patient passed a quantity of fluid from the feet and got quite well. The symptoms are: > By rest. < By least exertion; by stooping. (Heart was < lying down.) < By cold. (*Thyr.* treatment nearly always raises the bodily heat.)

Relations.—*Compare:* Myxœdema; psoriasis, &c., Ars. [I permanently cured a case of myxœdema with Ars. high, before the Thyroid method was introduced (*H. W.*, xxvii. 443); arsenic has been found to be a normal constituent of the healthy thyroid gland]. Phthisis, Bac. [I have found Thyr. follow Bac. well. Greenfield (see *H. W.*, xxix. 7) found tuberculosis very common in myxœdemics, in five out of seven fatal cases it was widespread and advanced; he also found it in one case of sporadic cretinism. Young, of Switzerland, has cured cretinism with Bac.] Syphilis, Merc., K. iod., Syph. Goître, exophthalmic, Spo., Iod., Spi. Diuresis, Urea. Optic neuritis, Tab., Carb. s. Dilated arterioles (Adren., opp.). Ununited fractures, Symph. Wakes with headache, Lach. *Follows well:* Lach., Bac.

SYMPTOMS.

1. **Mind.**—Acute stupor alternating with restless melancholia; at times could not be got to speak, but would lie on floor with limbs rigid; at other times would weep and undress herself; at times dangerous and homicidal, would put her arms round the necks of other patients so tightly as almost to

strangle them; (in this case the insanity was primary and the myxœdema secondary; both conditions were removed).—Evinced increased vivacity by quarrelling with another patient about a trifling difference of opinion —Depression.—Fretfulness and moroseness gave way to cheerfulness and animation.—"All progressed cases of myxœdema show some mental aberration which tends towards dementia, usually with delusions, the latter taking the form of suspicion and persecution. Occasionally actual insanity is present in the form of mania and insanity."—Delirium of persecution (three cases observed, one fatal, the result of taking *Thyr.* in tablets to reduce obesity).—Sudden acute mania occurring in myxœdema, perfectly restored mentally and bodily under *Thyr.*—Mental aberration dating three years before onset of myxœdema, subject to attacks of great violence, with intervals of depression and moroseness.—State of idiocy; fearful nightmares.—Excited condition, lasting all the rest of the day, grunting continuously and laughing in a way that was peculiar to herself.—Very excited; excited state followed by considerable depression.—For several hours in what can only be termed a hysterical condition.—Profound depression.—Irritable and ill-tempered.—Became a grumbler.—Angry.—Had frights.

2. **Head.**—Vertigo.—Feeling of lightness in the brain, scarcely amounting to giddiness.—Much giddiness and headache for twenty-four hours.—Awoke about 4 a.m. with sharp headache and intense aching in back and limbs, which continued for three days and compelled him to keep his bed.—Ever since taking the first thyroid [had had five glands altogether, at intervals] he had a strange heavy feeling in his head, with vertigo and palpitation on stooping.—Headache (with fever symptoms); disappeared on suspending treatment, reappeared seven days after recommencing. — Fronto-coronal headache about two hours after each tabloid.—Persistent frontal headache after taking one tabloid for four successive days.—(Constant headache, pains in occiput and vertex.)—(Headaches in case of acromegaly.)—Headache.—Headache and pains in abdomen.—Fresh growth of hair (many cases).—Black hairs growing among the grey.—In one case of scleroderma and in one case of myxœdema the hair fell off permanently.—In a case of myxœdema the patient lost all the hair of his head and face and had thick growth over his arms and thorax; under *Thyr.* the hair of the head and face grew again and that of the arms and chest fell off.

3. **Eyes.**—(Prominence of eyeballs — exophthalmic goître.) — Optic neuritis (in five persons, four of them women, under treatment for obesity; no other symptoms of thyroidism).—Accommodative asthenopia.

4. **Ears.**—Moist patches behind ears heal up (case of psoriasis).—Hyperplasic median otitis with sclerosis and loss of mobility of the ossicles (rapid amelioration—several cases).

6. **Face.**—Flushing: with nausea and lumbar pains; loss of consciousness, tonic muscular spasm; immediate; with rise of temperature, and pains all over; suddenly became breathless and livid.—Faintness, with great flushing of upper part of body and pains in back.—Swelling of face and legs.—In lupus of face, tight sensation, heat, and angry redness removed.—Burning sensation of lips with free desquamation.

8. **Mouth.**—Tongue became thickly coated.—Feverish and thirsty.—Great thirst.—(Ulcerated patch on buccal aspect on l. cheek near angle of mouth.)

9. **Throat.**—(Full sensation.)—Goître, exophthalmic, cured.—Goître reduced.

11. **Stomach.**—Loss of appetite.—Increased appetite with improved digestion.—Eructations.—Dyspeptic troubles.—Nausea, with flushing and lumbar pains.—Nausea, slight vomiting—Slight nausea recurring on thinking of it.—Nausea soon after taking the gland.—On five occasions the patient (a woman) vomited the thyroid.—Always felt a sensation of sickness after the injections.—Sensations of faintness and nausea (after a few injections).—Feels tired and sick.—Gastro-intestinal disturbance and diarrhœa.

12. **Abdomen.**—Flatuence increased, followed later in the case by amelioration.—Headache and pain in abdomen.

13. **Stool.**—Diarrhœa; with gastro-intestinal disturbance.—Relief of constipation with more natural actions.—Constipation.

14. **Urinary Organs.**—Increased flow of urine.—Increased urination, usually with clear, pale yellow secretion.—Slight trace of albumen found in urine.—Albuminuria.—Diabetes mellitus; caused and cured.

16. **Female Sexual Organs.**—Increased sexual desire.—Six days after commencement of treatment menstruation, which had been absent over a year, reappeared and continued profusely (in several cases of myxœdema with or without insanity).—Menses profuse, prolonged, more frequent; early amenorrhœa.—(Painful and irregular menstruation.)—(Constant left ovarian pain, and great tenderness).—Looks pale and feels ill.—Pain in lower part of abdomen, headache and sickness (in girl of sixteen, probably menstrual effort provoked by *Thyr.*; no catamenial flow appeared).—Acts as a galactagogue when milk deficient; when the deficiency is associated with a return of the menses it will suppress the latter.—(Puerperal insanity with fever.)—(Puerperal eclampsia.)

17. **Respiratory Organs.**—Slight attack of hæmoptysis, followed by cough and signs of phthisis at apex of l. lung.—(Voice became clear.)—Dormant phthisis; lighted up the disease in five cases.

19. **Heart and Pulse.**—Death, with all the symptoms of angina pectoris.—On trying to walk uphill died suddenly from cardiac failure.—While stooping to put on her shoes she "fainted" and died in half an hour.—On one occasion, after exerting herself more than she had done for a long time previously, "suddenly became extremely breathless and livid, and felt as if she was dying;" > by rest in recumbent position and stimulants.—Two fainting attacks.—Frequent fainting fits.—Complained occasionally of a feeling of faintness, not occurring particularly after the injections.—One patient showed extraordinary symptoms after the injection; the skin became so livid as to be almost blue-black.—Degeneration of heart muscle in animals.—A systolic cardiac murmur was less loud after the treatment than before.—Sensations of faintness and nausea.—Palpitation on stooping.—Weakness of heart's action.—Tachycardia and ready excitability of the heart persisting for several days after the feeding was stopped.—Pulse rose to 112.—Relaxation of arterioles.—(Rapid pulsation, with inability to lie down in bed.)—(Jumping sensation at heart.)

20. **Back.**—Flushing, nausea, and lumbar pains, lasting a few minutes.—Stabbing pains in lumbar region.—Intense aching in back and limbs, which continued for three days.—Flushing of upper part of body and pains in back.—(Backache.)

21. Limbs.—Quivering of limbs ; tremors.—Intense aching in back
limbs, lasting three days.—Pains in arms and legs, with malaise.—Skin
hands and feet desquamated.—(Acromegaly, subjective symptoms.)

22. Upper Limbs.—After injection, to a great extent lost the use of
hands for two days ; recurred later, lasting a few hours.—Felt queer
unable to raise her arms (after injection, another case).—Arms less
and painful (psoriasis).

23. Lower Limbs.—Tingling sensation in legs.—Œdema of legs
peared, and subsequently subsided and continued to reappear and sub
for a month.—Pain in legs.—Incomplete paraplegia.—Swelling of face
legs.—Feet repeatedly peel in large flakes, leaving a tender surface.—Pro
flow of fluid from feet (in case of dropsy cured by *Thyr.*).

24. Generalities.—Malaise > by lying in bed.—Stooping = palpitat
—Rest in recumbent position > extreme breathlessness with lividity, felt
dying.—Myxœdematous patients are always chilly ; the effect of the treatm
is to make them less so.—Loss of consciousness and general tonic musc
spasm for a few seconds.—Fainting attacks (many cases).—Tremors, quiver
of limbs, complete unconsciousness.—(Tetany.)—Epileptiform fit, after wh
he was unconscious for an hour ; next day felt better and warmer.—Mal
so great she refused to continue the treatment.—Agitation.—Incomplete p
plegia.—Hysterical attack.—(Hystero-epilepsy with amenorrhœa.)—Nerv
and hysterical, had to have nurses to watch her.—Feels tired and sic
Stabbing pains.—Aching pains (many cases).—Aching pains all over.—Diffu
pains.—Aching pains in various parts of body.—Pains over whole bod
Brawny swelling at point of injection, followed by abscess of slow deve
ment.—Myxœdema removed (many cases).—" A series of abscesses resul
from the injections, but probably originating from an accidental abscess q
independent of them."—A small abscess formed.—Increased suppuratio
case of lupus.—Gained a stone in weight.—Lost weight enormously (m
cases of myxœdema).—Rapid gain of flesh and strength.—Anæmia and debi
—Infiltration rapidly absorbed (psoriasis).—Persons suffering from
disease can bear much larger doses than those suffering from myxœde
—(Acromegaly, headaches, and subjective symptoms.)—(Fractures re
to unite.)—A peculiar cachexia more dangerous than myxœdema itsel
Syphilis secondary and tertiary.

25. Skin.—Flushing of skin.—Skin became so livid as to be almost b
black.—Skin has desquamated freely, but there has been no perspiratio
diuresis.—Psoriasis ; eruption extended and increased.—(Psoriasis ; red
and itching reduced ; eruption separating and being shed in great sc
angry, inflamed appearance completely gone.)—Moist patches behind
heal up.—Arms less stiff and painful ; swelling diminished.—Crusts separa
leaving faint red skin ; eruption not nearly so painful.—(Symmetrical
pigenous eruption ; dark red ; edges raised and thickened.)—Lupus :
feeling, heat, angry redness removed ; suppuration increased.—Ecze
irritation of skin markedly allayed.—Scattered pustules of eczema ma
quickly or abort.—(Teething eczema.)—(Syphilitic psoriasis.)—(Rupia
Scleroderma.—Peeling of skin beginning on legs and extending over w
surface ; skin has since become comparatively soft and smooth.—Pee
of skin of lower limbs, with gradual clearing (eczema).—Skin of h
and feet desquamated.

26. **Sleep.**—Continual tendency to sleep.—Awoke about 4 a.m. with sharp headache.—Fearful nightmares disappeared.—Insomnia.—Excited condition; could not sleep.

27. **Fever.**—Flushing: with nausea; with loss of consciousness.—Always felt hot, and had a sensation of sickness after the injections.—Felt better and warmer.—Flushing of upper part of body and pains in back.—Temperature never rose above 99° but she felt feverish and thirsty.—Temperature rose to 100° F., and remained there several days; pulse 112.—Rise of temperature; diaphoresis.—Profuse perspiration on least exertion.

Thyroiodinum.

Iodothyrinum. Trituration.

Clinical.—Goître. Obesity. Urine, increase of.

Characteristics.—*Thyroiodine* is now more generally named *Iodothyrine*, but I retain the former as more convenient. Hœnigschmied (*Aerz. Cent. Zeit.*, No. 6, 1900, quoted *A. H.*, xxvii. 211) says of it that it is present in only small quantities in the thyroid of the sheep. It is completely free from albuminous substances, stable, and directly assimilated. The iodine exists in organic combination, and *Thyri.* contains 0·003 parts of *Iodine* to every gramme. The general effects of the drug are—increased secretion of urine and corresponding loss of flesh. Hœnigschmied gives two cases: (1) Labourer, 42, for several years had enlargement and induration of all lobes of thyroid, the enlargement causing compression of the structures of the neck, dyspnœa, whistling respiration, hoarseness, short, dry cough, vertigo. *Thyri.*, 5-grain tablets, one every evening; at the end of a week twice daily. After using twenty-five tablets the gland was smaller and softer; the previously hard and resistant nodules were elastic; after two more weeks only remnants of the goître remained. (2) Man, 60, thyroid enlarged in all its lobes with a glandular cystic swelling in the right one; dyspnœa, loud whistling breathing. Two, three, and at last four tablets were given daily for two months, by which time the goître had vanished, but the cyst was not changed. (3) Man, 45, medium height, sedentary, suffered from obesity, vertigo, dyspnœa, weariness. Pulse feeble, 76; functions normal; appetite and sleep good; weight 230 pounds. With increasing doses of *Thyri.*, up to ten tablets daily, the weight steadily went down to 160 pounds, activity increasing in proportion. When the dose had reached four tablets daily the urine became very abundant, but was free from albumen. The daily dose was increased one tablet every four days. At one stage Fowler's solution of arsenic, four drops in wine, was given as well to prevent *Thyroidism*.

Relations.—*Antidoted by*: Ars. *Compare*: Thyr. Urine, Urea.

Tilia.

Tilia Europœa. The common Lime or Linden. *N. O.* Tiliaceæ. Tincture of fresh blossoms.

Clinical.—Dentition. Enuresis. Epistaxis. Leucorrhœa. Lichen. Neuralgia. Peritonitis. Rheumatism. Toothache. Urticaria. *Uterus, bearing down in*; prolapse of; inflammation of.

Characteristics.—The sap of the Lime contains sugar, and the flowers an abundance of honey, which makes the tree particularly attractive to bees. A tincture of the fresh blossoms was proved by the Austrian Society. The most striking characteristic is "an intense sore feeling about the abdomen and profuse warm sweat which gives no relief." This has led to its successful use in cases of peritonitis. In addition to this are marked bearing-down symptoms in the whole genito-urinary and rectal regions, especially in the uterus, and these combined with the others have indicated *Til.* in puerperal metritis and other disorders of the female generative sphere. An intense facial neuralgia was developed in the proving; and also a very aggravated condition of skin irritation with pimples of the lichen order. Some *Peculiar Sensations* are: As if a piece of cold iron pierced through right eye, causing burning. Burning as if a piece of ice were drawn over ear and face. As if something living were under skin of face. Tearing in anterior muscles of thigh, as if they were too short. There are a number of pains above the root of the nose; epistaxis of thin, pale blood which coagulated quickly. The left side was most affected. Great sensitiveness to draught of air was induced. The symptoms were: < Afternoon and evening; talking; walking; sneezing; stooping; cold water. > In cool room; walking about in open air; closing eyes (head); by coffee. Pain in head was > by application of cold water; pain in jaw <. Heat of bed < skin symptoms.

Relations.—*Compare*:—Puerperal metritis, Bell. Uterine bearing down, Lil. t. Sweat without >, Merc.

SYMPTOMS.

1. **Mind.**—Melancholy, disposed to weep.—Love-sick.—Dread of society.—Irritable.—Disinclined to work.

2. **Head.**—Vertigo, with staggering, and like gauze before the eyes.—Intoxication.—Stinging pain in forehead, with heat in head and face.—Extreme sensitiveness of head to draught of air.—Pressing-inward pains, as from a dull instrument, just above root of nose.—Tearing in r. temple extending down upper arm.—Pressure and burrowing in occiput.—Itching of scalp.—Eruption of small gritty vesicles, which itch and burn on scratching.

3. **Eyes.**—Hollow-eyed.—Sensation as if a piece of cold iron pierced r. eye, causing burning.—Vision: obscured; flickering.

4. **Ears.**—Stinging in ears.

5. **Nose.**—Bleeding from nose ; blood thin and pale, but coagulates quickly.—Frequent sneezing.—Tickling of nose.

6. **Face.**—Face pale ; or flushed ; frequent alternations.—Ulcerative, sore pain r. side of face from temple to jaw.—Cutting pains : starting from r. upper jaw ; near l. malar bone.—Sensation of something alive under skin of face.—Quivering of lips.—Sprained pain in l. jaw-joint.

7. **Teeth.**—Stinging pain in all the teeth, < by cold water.—Drawing pains in gums.

8. **Mouth.**—Much mucus in mouth, causing fuzzy feeling ; affecting speech.—Taste : bitter ; bitter-slimy ; pasty.

9. **Throat.**—Burning in throat.—Sensation of swelling of the palate, with desire to swallow, and hoarse voice.—Tickling in palate causing cough.

11. **Stomach.**—Unusual hunger.—Desires refreshing things.—Good appetite but speedy satiety.—Nausea after eating.—No desire for tobacco.—Putrid eructations.—Cramp-like pain in stomach.

12. **Abdomen.**—Bloated abdomen ; pains as from incarcerated flatulence ; repeated noisy discharges of it, with much >.—Circumscribed distension of abdomen.—Abdomen painful when touched, esp. round navel.—Constant rumbling and gurgling ; sometimes with colic.—Sensitiveness, soreness, and sensation of subcutaneous ulceration in upper part of abdomen.—Stitches suddenly appearing in abdomen, extending into pelvis, and impeding breathing.

13. **Stool and Anus.**—Pressure on rectum which seems to force out anus.—Sudden urgent desire.—Stool : early in morning ; soft, mushy, unsatisfactory ; pasty ; scanty ; delayed ; hard.

14. **Urinary Organs.**—Constant painful pressure on bladder and urethra.—Broad stitches in middle of urethra.—Frequent, copious micturition.—Enuresis twice towards morning when in a stupid slumber.

16. **Female Sexual Organs.**—Frequent pressing on uterus, as if everything would fall out of pelvis.—Spasmodic labour-like drawing from abdomen down small of back, as if catamenia would set in.—Great sensitiveness and soreness of whole uterus, as after parturition.—Redness, soreness, and burning of external parts.—Menstruation too late and very scanty (blood pale).—Profuse leucorrhœa ; pale mucus.

17. **Respiratory Organs.**—Tickling, scraping, irritating, provoking slight cough, esp. in l. side of larynx.—Fine stitches in larynx, < talking.—Hoarseness.—Frequent sighing.

18. **Chest.**—Oppression.—Whole chest weak ; acute pressure and pinching under sternum.—Throbs as from a dull stitch from thorax to back.—Bruised pain and swelling of l. sterno-clavicular joint.—Tearing from l. pectoralis major to axilla and also upper arm with weariness and sensation of paralysis in arm while in bed.

19. **Heart and Pulse.**—Tensive, sore pain in præcordial region.—Pulse accelerated ; small.

20. **Neck and Back.**—Tearing from nape to top of shoulder.—Sticking, drawing, and heat in r. back between liver and kidneys.—Heaviness in sacral and dorsal region.

21. **Limbs.**—Trembling ; weariness ; bruised feeling in limbs.

22. **Upper Limbs.**—Paralytic heaviness of arms, esp. upper arm.—

Weariness of l. arm even while hanging down.—Heaviness and painful lameness in l. shoulder.—Tearing : in forearm near wrist ; in r. wrist and l. half of skull ; in fingers.

23. **Lower Limbs.**—Weariness and prickling in limbs; cramps in flexor muscles.—Drawing in small spot l. hip whilst sitting.—Tension in anterior muscles of both thighs as if too short.—Sensation as if leg tightly bound while walking.—Cramp in l. sole.—Ulcerative pain in ball of l. great toe < by touch.

24. **Generalities.**—Esp. suitable for women after parturition, and for children during dentition.—L. side of body most affected.—< Afternoon and evening ; in warm room ; in heat of bed (skin symptoms) ; during motion (rheumatic symptoms).—> In cool room, and from motion.

25. **Skin.**—Skin red ; hard pimples ; burn like fire after scratching.—Burning itching at night.—(Urticaria.—Lichen simplex.)

26. **Sleep.**—Yawning ; sleepy ; exhausted.—Night disturbed by sudden waking.—Sleeplessness, with restlessness ; bed seems too hard.—Vivid frightful dreams ; skin of legs, esp. over tibiæ, bathed in perspiration.

27. **Fever.**—Pulse full, hard, and quick.—Chilliness in evening.—Heat all over, but most in head and cheeks.—Night-sweat.

Titanium.

Trituration of the copper-red crystals obtained from the slag at the bottom of a blast iron furnace, consisting of Titan. cyanide and Titan. nitride.

Clinical.—Hemiopia. Semen, too early ejaculation of.

Characteristics.—*Titanium* (Ti., A.W. 48·1) stands midway between Silicon and Tin in some of its relations ; and in other respects it is closely related to Iron, Chromium, and Aluminium. The crystals proved by Sharp (who took gr. ii. of the 1st trit. daily for a week) were originally believed to be the pure metal, but were proved later to be the cyanonitrid. One symptom of the proving is remarkable : "Imperfect vision, the peculiarity being that *half an object only* could be seen." Another symptom, which Burnett has turned to good account in cases of sexual weakness, is "Too early ejaculation of semen in coitus."

Relations.—*Compare :* Half-sight, Nat. c., Lyc., Aur., Lith.

SYMPTOMS.

2. **Head.**—Giddiness.

3. **Eyes.**—Desire to keep eyelids closed.—Only half an object could be seen at once.

11. **Stomach.**—Loss of appetite.—Nausea.—Discomfort in stomach.

24. **Generalities.**—Greatly disordered ; felt and looked wretchedly ill.

15. **Male Sexual Organs.**—Too early ejaculation of semen.

Tongo.

Dipterix odorata. Tongo, Tonka or Tonquin Bean. *N. O.* Leguminosæ. Tincture of the dried beans.

Clinical.—Hip, pains in. Migraine. Neuralgia of face. Toothache.

Characteristics.—*Tongo* was proved by Nenning. Its fragrant seed is much used by perfumers. *Dipterix odorata*, which yields it, is a native of Cayenne. The fruit is something like that of the almond-tree. Curiously in the proving it produced "Risings with taste of bitter almonds." The chief uses of *Tong.* have been in migraine and neuralgic affections. The symptoms are : < By rest ; when seated. > By movement. Pressure >.

Relations.—*Antidoted by :* Vinegar.

SYMPTOMS.

1. **Mind.**—Peevishness and ill-humour.—Dislike to labour and conversation.

2. **Head.**—Head confused, esp. in occiput, with drowsiness.—Heaviness of head, esp. on rising up after stooping.—Drawing headache.—Pressure, tearings, and shootings in head, esp. on coming into a room, with tearings on one side of the face and ill-humour.—Shootings in head, when laughing.—Pulsative headache, esp. on l. side.—The headaches disappear on taking vinegar.—Excessive sensibility of exterior of head.

3. **Eyes.**—Burning sensation and dryness of eyes, when reading in evening.—Drawing, tension, and quivering in eyelids.

4. **Ears.**—Tearing in ears.

5. **Nose.**—Coryza, with obstruction of nose.—Violent sneezing in the night.—Slight tearing in root of nose with irritation to sneeze and cough.

6. **Face.**—Paleness of complexion, with red cheeks.—Tearing in maxillæ.—Semilateral, tearing pains in face.

7. **Teeth.**—Toothache, with tearing pain, esp. in molars, < by pressing upon them, dissipated by the use of vinegar.—Acid blood from teeth and gums.

8. **Mouth.**—Copious accumulation of water in mouth.

9. **Throat.**—Roughness and scraping in throat.

11. **Stomach.**—Risings with taste of bitter almonds.

12. **Abdomen.**—Burning sensation and cuttings in the hypochondria, as if externally.—Movements and pinchings in abdomen.

13. **Stool.**—Tenesmus.—Hard fæces, evacuated with straining.—Diarrhœa, followed by excessive sensibility of abdomen.

14. **Urinary Organs.**—Scanty urine, with white sediment.—Urine of colour of white wine, with much slimy sediment.—Red urine, with abundant clay-coloured sediment.

16. **Female Sexual Organs.**—Catamenia premature.—Leucorrhœa,

when walking.—Discharge of thick mucus from vagina (when making an effort to pass a stool).

17. **Respiratory Organs.**—Hoarseness, with burning sensation in larynx.

18. **Chest.**—Shooting and burning sensation under sides of the chest.

20. **Back.**—Pains in loins, with excessive sensibility to the touch.

23. **Lower Limbs.**—Tearing in l. hip-joint 5 p.m. > rubbing.—Tearing in l. thigh and knee > pressure.—Violent stinging like the prick of a needle in fatty portion of r. great toe after dinner.

24. **Generalities.**—Tearing in the limbs, > by external pressure and also by movement.—The majority of the symptoms manifest themselves when seated, and during repose.—Vinegar dissipates many of the pains.

Toxicophis.

Toxicophis pugnax. Moccasin Snake. *N. O.* Ophidia. Trituration.

Clinical.—Œdema. Periodic neuralgia.

Characteristics.—Some effects of bites with this snake have been recorded. A peculiar feature of the cases was that the symptoms of pain and fever recurred annually at exactly the same period for many years with decreasing intensity each year. In one case the pains spread to other parts after some years.

SYMPTOMS.

23. **Lower Limbs.**—R. leg became painful and swelled rapidly.—For several years the pain was confined to the knee of the bitten limb ; in a few years it left the knee and seized the hip, and finally attacked the shoulder.

24. **Generalities.**—For the last eighteen years annual recurrence of symptoms with severe pain but without swelling ; occurred at precisely the same time of year ; decreased in intensity each year.

25. **Skin.**—Skin rather dry.

Trachinus.

Trachinus draco and T. vipera. The Great and Lesser Weever, Sting-bull and Sting-fish. Trituration of the poisonous fins.

Clinical.—Asthma. Blood-poisoning. Neuralgia. Ulcers.

Characteristics.—Some very serious effects have been recorded from wounds inflicted with the fins of *Trachinus*. Intolerable pains, swelling of the part, and in some cases gangrene, fever, delirium, and symptoms of hydrophobia have been observed. It should be indicated in cases of acute blood-poisoning with intense pains.

SYMPTOMS.

1. **Mind.**—Raving.—Hydrophobia.—Anxiety.—Fear of death.
2. **Head.**—Vertigo.—Violent headache.
11. **Stomach.**—Violent thirst.—Nausea.—Green, bilious vomiting.
17. **Respiratory Organs.**—Paroxysms of suffocation.
19. **Heart.**—Palpitation.
24. **Generalities.**—Swelling: of whole body; of wounded arm then of head and chest.—Stinging, burning, throbbing pain increasing to unendurable intensity lasting an hour and then decreasing.—Violent burning pain extending from wound to chest.
25. **Skin.**—Skin of whole body became yellowish green.—Gangrenous blisters on arms.
26. **Sleep.**—Sleeplessness.
27. **Fever.**—Constant fever with irregular pulse.—Cold, clammy sweat.

Tradescantia.

Tradescantia diuretica. *N. O.* Commelynaceæ. Tincture of fresh leaves.

Clinical.—Gonorrhœa. Orchitis.

Characteristics.—Mure proved *Trad.*, which belongs to a genus of lily-like plants. It produced disorder of the genito-urinary organs, urethral discharge. and inflammation of the scrotum; also embarrassed breathing.

SYMPTOMS.

2. **Head.**—Vertigo.
13. **Stool.**—Diarrhœa.
14. **Urinary Organs.**—Whitish discharge from urethra.—Pain when urinating.—Stream thin.—Urine: acid smelling; yellowish, copious, ash-coloured sediment.
15. **Male Sexual Organs.**—Scrotum inflamed, painful and red.
17. **Respiratory Organs.**—Breathing: very painful; embarrassed, difficult, sighing, as from want of air.
18. **Chest.**—Pain in l. side of chest.

Trifolium Pratense.

Trifolium pratense. Red Clover. *N. O.* Leguminosæ. Tincture of flower heads. [In the cancer cases an extract of the blossoms of the first crop is used. "This extract," says Cooper, "is made by boiling down the flowers till nothing but an inspissated residuum is left: in this condition it seems to be caustic and for this reason is used by herbalists: I doubt its utility."]

Clinical.—Cancer. Constipation. Cough. Mumps. Pancreas, affections of. Throat, sore; mucus in. Uvula, pain in.

Characteristics.—*Tri. p.* has a reputation among eclectics in whooping-cough, and coughs of measles and phthisis. T. C. Duncan and others proved it and elicited some very decided respiratory symptoms, dry, tickling cough, oppressed breathing with fever. One peculiar symptom was, cough followed by hiccough. Many symptoms of congestion appeared. The head felt full of blood. The lungs felt full of blood. Sensation in lungs as if breathing hot air; as if air full of impurities. There was persistent headache on waking. Sleep was unrefreshing. The pulse was weak and intermittent, showing an action on the heart; later it was full and bounding. Pharynx as well as trachea was irritated and there was: "Sharp pain through uvula causing tears to start." Dryness of trachea causing him to clear throat of some foreign substance. Secretion of urine increased. Dull, stupid feeling generally. Farrington gives as characteristic: Hoarseness and choking spells at night with cough; the neck is stiff, cramps in sterno-mastoid muscle > by heat and friction. Cooper says of *Tri. p.* that it causes salivation in horses, and diarrhœa if they eat much of it; and that it cures mumps and affections of the pancreas and salivary glands. Hale says it causes "heaves" in horses. Felter (*H. R.*, xiv. 431) gives it to persons disposed to cancer. He finds it retards the progress of cancerous tumours and improves the general condition of the patient. It keeps cancer from ulcerating. After ulceration has occurred *Tri. p.* does no good. Another indication of Felter's is "scaly and ulcerated conditions of the tibial region of the old." The symptoms are < in close room; > in open air. "When I became very warm (with the fever) my breathing stopped; lungs felt as if breathing hot air." < After sleep.

Relations.—*Compare:* Botan.; congestive symptoms, Meli. Headache on waking, Nat. m., Lach. Cough with pains in chest, Bry., Ranuc., Arn., Rhus.

SYMPTOMS.

1. **Mind.**—Confusion of ideas, morning.

2. **Head.**—Great headache in morning on waking.—Dulness in anterior brain.—Head feels full of blood.—Intermittent headache.—Pricking in forehead.

3. **Eyes.**—Eyes: dull and sore; heavy.

5. **Nose.**—Much mucus in nose; thin.

8. **Mouth.**—Whole mucus tract sensitive.—Taste of drug disgusting and always in mouth.—Salivation (horses).

9. **Throat.**—Much mucus in throat, constantly trying to clear it.—Throat irritated all the way down; as if scalded.—Irritation of pharynx and trachea causing dry cough.—Sharp pain through uvula causing tears to start.

11. **Stomach.**—Great thirst.—Hiccough.

12. **Abdomen.**—Rises at 5.45 a.m. with griping pains in abdomen and headache.—Colicky pains all day.

13. **Stool and Anus.**—Very costive, each stool followed by several drops of dark blood, attended by a bearing-down sensation as if bowel would prolapse by its own weight (this lasted fourteen days, after which bowels became regular).—Stool delayed several days, hard, covered with mucus; later bowels moved freely.

14. **Urinary Organs.**—Uneasiness in region of kidneys, and whole urinary tract.—Urine very profuse.—Vesical tenesmus after urinating.

17. **Respiratory Organs.**—Great dryness of trachea causing him to clear throat of some foreign substance at 11 a.m.—Irritation of pharynx and trachea causing short, hacking cough with accumulation of mucus which must be expectorated.—Incessant dry, hacking cough.—Seems as if trachea was loaded with impurities, after eating.—Dyspnœa > in fresh air.

18. **Chest.**—Lungs feel as if full of blood 2 p.m.; 10 p.m. had to leave a close room from oppression; on going into fresh air was obliged to cough much; this was followed by hiccough and profuse expectoration.—Chest tight; on lying down.

19. **Heart.**—Pulse slow and irregular; later full and rapid.

20. **Neck and Back.**—Neck stiff, cramps in sterno-mastoid muscles, > by heat and rubbing; with the cough.

22. **Upper Limbs.**—Tingling in l. palm; also in l. arm.

26. **Sleep.**—On waking in morning felt as if he had not been asleep.

27. **Fever.**—Immediately after retiring began to feel cold; pulse intermitting, later bounding; became very warm and breathing stopped; lungs felt as if breathing hot air.—Feet and hands cold, head hot.

Trifolium Repens.

Trifolium repens. White Clover. *N. O.* Leguminosæ. Trituration or tincture of flower heads.

Clinical.—Mumps. Salivation.

Characteristics.—The proving of *Tr. r.* produced a specific action on the salivary glands. Hale says it produces marked salivation in horses.

Relations.—*Compare:* Jabor., Pilo.

SYMPTOMS.

6. **Face.**—Feeling of fulness or congestion of all the salivary glands.—Discomfort and even pain in glands followed by copious flow of saliva.—One prover felt just as if she had mumps coming on.

Trillium.

Trillium erectum. Purple Trillium. Bethroot. Birthroot. Lamb's quarter. Rattlesnake root. Wakerobin. Three-leaved night-shade. [According to Millspaugh *T. pendulum* is the white variety of *T. erectum. Treas. of Bot.* gives the names as synonymous. The symptoms of H. Minton, the original prover, are given in Allen under *T. cernuum.* Minton obtained the tincture from a botanic physician and did not himself verify the plant. His symptoms are marked (M) in the Schema. Millspaugh considers *T. erectum* as the proper source of the homœopathic tincture.] *N. O.* Smilaceæ (or Trilliaceæ) of the Liliaceæ. Tincture of the fresh root.

Clinical.—Bladder, catarrh of. Climaxis. Diabetes. Dysentery. Fainting, with flooding. Fibroma, hæmorrhages from. Hæmorrhages; post-partum; ante-partum. Menorrhagia. Metrorrhagia. Writer's cramp.

Characteristics.—The chief uses of *Trill.* come to us from the eclectics, who learned some of them from the native Indians. The popular name Birth-root sufficiently indicates one part of its reputation. In hæmorrhage, ante-partum, post-partum, and climacteric, in fibroid tumours, and in hæmorrhages of all kinds *Trill.* has been found curative. Both the White and the Purple varieties have been used. Minton's proving of *T. cernuum* (?) brought out the hæmorrhagic property in the blood-tinged diarrhœa. One characteristic in connection with the hæmorrhages of *Trill.* is *faintness* and sinking at the stomach; also cold extremities and rapid, feeble pulse. "Flooding with fainting" is a keynote. Minton's proving brought out a symptom bearing on this: "Sensation of goneness in abdomen." He had also extreme debility; palpitation, and anxiety. *Trill.* has been used as a local hæmostatic in epistaxis and for bleeding after tooth extraction. *Peculiar Sensations are:* As if eyes too large (M). As if a crumb were in larynx (M). As if the chest was tightly bound and could not be expanded. As if hips and small of back were falling to pieces. As if sacro-iliac synchondroses were falling apart; wants to be bound tightly. As if bones were broken. Left side most affected. Restless, tossing agitation, fear of being sick, great anguish were experienced by Minton. The restlessness and exhaustion from hæmorrhages are typified in this. Blue vision; and craving for ice-water are other noteworthy symptoms. There is tendency to putrescence of fluids. The hæmorrhages of *Trill.* are copious; either active or passive; usually bright red and profuse. *Trill.* is *suited to* women who flood after every labour; flabby subjects. The symptoms of Minton's proving were: > Bending forward; < sitting erect. < By motion. < After eating. > By exercise in open air. Standing or walking = bearing down in pelvis. Motion < hæmorrhages.

Relations.—*Complementary:* Calc. p. (menstrual and hæmorrhagic affections). *Compare:* Anguish, restless tossing about, Aco. Hæmorrhages, Chi., Calc., Ham., Secal., Ust., Sang. Bright-red blood, Ipec.

Mill. Bleeding after tooth extraction, Ham., Kre. Menses profuse, every two weeks and lasting a week or longer, Calc. p. Flow profuse, gushing, light red, < least movement, Sabi. Flow dark, clotted, Ust., Thlasp. As if bones of pelvis broken, Æsc. h.

SYMPTOMS.

1. **Mind.**—Melancholy with sadness (M).—Repugnance to conversation (M).—Irritable (M).—Anguish; agitation and tossing about, impossible to keep still (M).

2. **Head.**—Vertigo, chiefly, on rising in morning (M).—Dull pain l. temple < least noise (M).—Pain in forehead > bending forward, < returning to erect position (M).—Headache < by least noise; walking; coughing (M). —Head and face feel hot (M).

3. **Eyes.**—Pain in eyeballs, feel too large and as if would fall from their sockets (M).—Burning in inner canthus with profuse flow of tears (M).—Vision blurred; everything looks blue (M).

5. **Nose.**—Profuse nose-bleed.

8. **Mouth.**—Bleeding from gums or after extraction of tooth.—Greasy feeling on tongue and gums (M).—Very offensive taste, esp. on rising in morning (M).—Profuse flow of saliva (M).

11. **Stomach.**—Disgust for everything except cold water (M).—Desire for ice-water (M).—Sickness; excessive pain; cramp of stomach (M).—Sinking in stomach with heat.—Hæmatemesis.—Stomach symptoms < after meals and in morning (M).

12. **Abdomen.**—Swelling of abdomen as in ascites, with sensation as if abdominal contents drawn back against vertebral column (M).—Flabbiness of parietes with sensation of goneness, a want of support in front, with at intervals of a few moments short, sharp, lancinating pains from before backward, compelling him to bend forward (M).—Much flatulence and grumbling.

13. **Stool and Anus.**—Dysentery, when passages are almost pure blood.—Diarrhœa thin, watery, tinged with blood; painless (M).—Constipation succeeded by thin, watery, very offensive diarrhœa (M).—Chronic diarrhœas of bloody mucus.

14. **Urinary Organs.**—Hæmaturia, passive.—Chronic catarrh of bladder. —Diabetes.—Sharp, cutting pain in urethra when urinating (M).—Urine copious, of strong disagreeable odour (M).

15. **Male Sexual Organs.**—Itching of genitals < by scratching.

16. **Female Sexual Organs.**—Hæmorrhage from uterus; with sensation as though hips and back were falling to pieces, > from a tight bandage. —Bearing down in pelvis when standing or walking; copious, yellowish, stringy leucorrhœa; period lingers several days beyond usual time.—Excessive flooding with fainting.—Metrorrhagia at climacteric; pale; faint; flow returns every two weeks.—Climaxis with weak sight; anxious look. —Displaced uterus, with consequent menorrhagia.—Menses come on after over-exertion.—Gushing of bright-red blood from uterus at least movement; later, blood pale from anæmia.—Hæmorrhages from fibroid tumours.—Threatened abortion; profuse hæmorrhages.—Pain in back and cold limbs, with hæmorrhages.—Too profuse menstrual flow after exhaustion by exercise.

—Profuse, exhausting leucorrhœa.—Hæmorrhage in abortion of third month. —Ante-partum hæmorrhage; os uteri dilated to size of half a dollar; no pains; flooding excessive.—Post-partum hæmorrhage.—Profuse, long-lasting lochial discharges.

17. **Respiratory Organs.**—Sensation of crumb in larynx, keeps up continual coughing (M).—Cough, with purulent or bloody sputum.—Hæmoptysis.

18. **Chest.**—Difficult breathing; feels as if chest bound up preventing it expanding (M).

19. **Heart.**—Palpitation with great anxiety (M).

21. **Limbs.**—Cramping pains in muscles of arms and calves (M).

22. **Upper Limbs.**—Pain in l. shoulder extending down arm to hand (M).—Cramping pains in fingers when writing (M).

24. **Generalities.**—Hæmorrhages usually bright red, profuse; also when sacro-iliac synchondroses feel as if falling apart; wants to be bound tightly. —Feels as if bones were broken, with hæmorrhages.--Crawling sensation in veins, like a tightening up of parts; < in legs and ankles.—Great debility (M).

25. **Skin.**—Skin hot and dry, with itching and burning, < by scratching (M).

26. **Sleep.**—Sleepless; rolling and tossing on bed (M).—Sleep disturbed by frequent dreams (M).—Dreams of festivities, sleigh-ride, &c. (M).

27. **Fever.**—Feverish during pain in abdomen, on the subsidence of which a profuse perspiration broke out (M).

Trimethylaminum.

Propylaminum. $N(CH_3)_3$. [Found in many plants, Chen. v., Cratæg. ox., Phal. imp., Pyr. com., Arn., Cotyl. u., Fag. syl., &c., and in herring-brine.] Solution.

Clinical.—Ankles, pains in. Rheumatic fever. Wrists, pains in.

Characteristics.—*Trimethyl.*, which is prepared from herring-brine among other sources, has a very unpleasant and penetrating fish-like odour. At one time it was regarded as a panacea in cases of acute rheumatism. Experiments on patients and others show that it diminishes the amount of urea excreted. Hansen gives these as characteristics: great pains in wrist-joints, also great restlessness, pains in ankle-joints from standing < slight movement. C. Carleton Smith (*H. P.*, vi. 432) gives these: "Rheumatism, when the needle held in the fingers gets so heavy she cannot sew." "Copious diarrhœa with pains in ankle-joints but not in wrists; thirst for large quantities of cold water (like *Bry.*)."

Triosteum.

Triosteum perfoliatum. Fever-wort. Horse-gentian. *N. O.* Caprifoliaceæ (Tribe, Lonicereæ). Tincture of fresh root.

Clinical.—Asthma. Backache. Fever; gastric. Headache; bilious. Influenza. Infra-mammary pain. Joints, stiff. Typhoid. Urticaria.

Characteristics.—*Triost.* is an energetically acting drug, and has been proved by Williamson, Neidhard, Gatchell, and other experienced provers. The name "fever-wort" tells its traditional reputation. Hale says it is one of the ingredients of the "fever powder" of the eclectics. Talmadge, one of the provers, found it of great value in typhoid and gastric fevers. It produced acute rheumatic symptoms and an intense urticaria. Talmadge says of the effect on himself: "It acted promptly and emphatically, causing aching pains in nearly every part of the body, especially of lower limbs and head." The right side of the head was more affected than the left. The stomach was very much disordered. The vomiting and pain in the stomach were very severe. At the anus there was itching and exudation of mucus. A peculiar concomitant of the evacuations was: numbness of the lower limbs after stool. Many symptoms came on in the early morning hours. One prover, though sleepy, could not sleep after midnight. The symptoms were: < Early morning, 3, 4, 5, and 7 a.m. < Sitting up; rising from bed; turning in bed; lying. < After sleep. < Drinking cold water.

Relations.—Gastric fever, Bapt. Rheumatism, Bry., Rhus. Load at epigastrium, Ab. n. Sleepy but cannot sleep, Bell.

SYMPTOMS.

1. **Mind.**—Greater cheerfulness.—Dulness and drowiness, with disinclination for active business.

2. **Head.**—Giddiness when rising at midnight, with extreme drowsiness.—Headache < sitting up.—Headache < r. forehead and r. temple.—Boring pain in r. temple 3 a.m.—Pain back of head with feeling of weight.

3. **Eyes.**—Slight pain in l. eyeball.

5. **Nose.**—Sneezing.

8. **Mouth.**—Soreness as if from swelling of pharynx, and pain in œsophagus on swallowing.

11. **Stomach.**—Increased appetite through day.—Loathing of all food.—Thirst.—Nausea; on rising, which was immediately followed by copious vomiting of very sour ingesta, attended with cramp in stomach and followed by sweat and pain in forehead which was < l. side.—Vomiting: 5 a.m. on rising to stool; drawing in calves.—Load and oppression in epigastrium 4 a.m., throbbing and undulating sensation all through system.—Pain in epigastrium, < by drinking water.—Soreness in epigastric region.

12. **Abdomen.**—Flatulence confined to stomach.—Sharp pains in bowels

and stomach.—Heat and sharp pain in r. side of abdomen in evening.—Th evacuations seemed to proceed from small intestines.

13. **Stool and Anus.**—Irritation of anus with exudation of mucus.—Stools most frequent in evening.—Stool 7 a.m. preceded by pain in abdome —Stool: watery, frothy, without pain, followed by exhaustion; at 7 a.n followed by numbness of lower limbs.

15. **Male Sexual Organs.**—Discharge of semen during sleep withou erection.

17. **Respiratory Organs.**—Asthmatic troubles.

19. **Heart.**—Audible beating of heart and slight pain under l. breast.

20. **Neck and Back.**—Pain in nape with perspiration.—Pain in nap and back.—Pain in nape and occiput with coldness and stiffness in feet.—Rheumatic pain in back from stooping.—Pain and stiffness in loins (l. side).

21. **Limbs.**—Stiffness in all joints of her upper and lower limbs.

22. **Upper Limbs.**—Pain in r. shoulder from lying on it.

23. **Lower Limbs.**—Remarkable stiffness in lower limbs, with sligh coldness and tingling sensation.—Stiffness in knees when attempting to rise —Pain in r. knee.—Drawing and shrinking sensation in legs; most decide pricking in soles.—Calves numb.—Penetrating pain under and behind l external malleolus, after sleeping.—Stiffness of all joints when lying.

24. **Generalities.**—Aching in all bones.—Acted promptly and ener getically, causing aching pains in nearly every part of the body, esp. lowe limbs and head.

25. **Skin.**—Vesicular eruption on forehead, over l. eye, on middle of chest and on r. arm.—Violent itching eruption on skin.—Great itching at night with welts all over surface.

26. **Sleep.**—Sleepiness with inability to sleep soon after midnight.

27. **Fever.**—Coldness and stiffness in the feet.—Fever.—Drying up of perspiration and development of fever, with hot skin and increased thirst.—General sweat.

Triticum Repens.

Triticum repens. Couch-grass. Cooch-grass. Cutch-grass. Quitch-grass. Twitch. *N. O.* Gramineæ. Tincture of fresh plant.

Clinical.—Bladder, irritation of. Dysuria. Urine, incontinence of.

Characteristics.—Burnett (*Organ. Diseases of Women*, 115) tells how he learned of a herbalist the use of *Trit. r.*, the herbalist having cured with it a patient of Burnett's, a man suffering from dysuria. Burnett has found it no less valuable for women than for men. "Frequently in dysuria from an inflamed state of the urethra, I found *Trit. r.* ϕ, ten drops in a little water, frequently repeated, of prompt effect, often giving complete relief in a few hours, and if the ailment is *primarily in the urethra* the relief is an abiding cure; if from a tugging of the heavy womb, it is only relief." He gives this case: A widow, suffering from complete procidentia uteri and very bad hæmorrhoidal bleeding, wrote

hat she was driven almost mad with painful micturition ; the burning
ınd straining were truly awful. *Trit. r.* φ, as above, was ordered, and
›rought a most grateful letter from the patient. She keeps a supply
ılways at hand.

Trombidium.

Trombidium muscæ domesticæ. *N. O.* Acaridea (Class, Arachnida).
Tincture of the animals.

Clinical.—Anus, prolapse of. Diarrhœa. Dysentery. Hip-joint, pain in.
.iver, pain in. Nose, catarrh of. Sciatica. Tibia, pain in. Toothache.

Characteristics.—*Tromb.* is "a parasite found singly or in groups
.pon the common house-fly, of a bright red colour, nearly circular in
hape. The alcoholic tincture, a brilliant orange in colour, was pre-
ared from specimens, about 115 in number, collected in Frankfort,
'hiladelphia, in September, 1864. The provings, under the super-
ision of Hering, were made by Harvey, Head, J. F. R., and Bancroft,
he potencies used 3x, 6x, 9, 18, and 30" (Hering, *Guiding Symptoms*).
'he grand keynote of *Tromb.* is "< by eating or drinking." The symp-
›m may be in the nose, teeth, or tonsils, this modality is characteristic.
n this indication I have cured some of the worst cases of diarrhœa ;
nd also intestinal pains coming on when the patient eats or drinks.
have used a 10m preparation of Fincke's given me by Skinner. A com-
rehensive keynote in diarrhœa and dysentery is : "Much pain before
nd after stool ; stool only after eating." *Tromb.* has cured dysen-
:ry with brown, thin, bloody stools and tenesmus. Congested liver
'ith urgent, loose stools on rising from bed ; during stool, sharp pain
left side, shooting downward." Skin symptoms were prominent,
specially itching of scalp and in whiskers. Fainting on rising up.
estlessness, inability to keep quiet. *Peculiar Sensations are :* As if
nere were no weight in head ; lightness. As from incarcerated
ıtus in abdomen. As if excoriated after tenesmus. As if everything
ere coming out of anus. As if hot air blowing over lower abdomen
ıd thigh. As if abdomen needed support. As if three toes on left
ot would be twisted off. As if her breath were leaving her. The
mptoms are : < By touch (pain in liver). < By pressure (pain in
›domen). Lying down : < toothache ; prevents fainting. Swallow-
g, or blowing nose = shooting in right ear. < Shaking head.
eading aloud = toothache. Rising up = fainting. Walking < pain
head ; = pain in hip-joint (which is, however, > after a few steps).
Moving. Warm drink > toothache. Open air > coryza. Cold
r < toothache. Cold bath < pain in abdomen. < Eating or
inking. < After stool.

Relations.—*Antidoted by :* Staph. (toothache) ; Merc. c. (diarrhœa),
mpare : Rheumatism, Ledm. Diarrhœa, Sulph. < Blowing nose.
ılex, Thuja. Stitches up anus, Ign., Nit. ac., Sul. ac. ; with pro-
›se, Pod.

SYMPTOMS.

1. **Mind.**—Talkative during day ; disposed to be contrary ; constan disposition to gape.—Inability to collect ideas, absence of ideas ; loss c memory.

2. **Head.**—Oppressive headache.—Dulness of head in forenoon.—Con gestion of head in evening, with red face and ears.—Lightness of head.- Dizziness ; on every attempt to rise from bed, with faintness.—Head heavy sometimes sharp pains in temples, extending over forehead, at 9.30 p.m., < l. side.—Pain : in l. mastoid process on waking at 7 a.m. ; in l. side of hea at 10 p.m., < shaking head and walking.—Shooting : above r. temple a 3 p.m. ; near r. parietal eminence at 11 a.m.—Intolerable itching at 7 a.m < vertex and occiput.

3. **Eyes.**—Redness of internal part of conjunctiva, similar to a pterygium —Lachrymation in open air.—Itching at r. inner canthus at 9 p.m.

4. **Ears.**—Shooting : in ears in afternoon, < r. ; frequently in r. durin day and evening ; in r. in forenoon, < swallowing or blowing nose.—Itchin in ears after rising.—Burning in both pinnæ, esp. r.

5. **Nose.**—Nose obstructed on rising.—Fluent coryza in open air an on eating.—Mucous discharge from nose, < during dinner.—Dryness of no in evening, with scabs.—Nose-bleed in morning ; afternoon.

7. **Teeth.**—Aching in l. decayed tooth : on waking at 7 a.m., renewe by breakfast, lasting till noon ; in evening ; in evening from reading alou preventing sleep almost all night, lasting next day, < lying down, eatin talking, and cold air, > warm drinks, > *Staph.*

8. **Mouth.**—Tongue coated white.

9. **Throat.**—Throat sore on r. side.

10. **Appetite.**—Appetite lost.

11. **Stomach.**—Eructations after meals ; tasting of ingesta.—(Vomiti after breakfast, thought it was from drinking coffee.)—Griping in pit stomach, < after dinner.

12. **Abdomen.**—Flatulent distension ; at 10 p.m. ; at 11 p.m., causi pain.—Shooting beginning in l. hypochondrium.—Griping on rising, obligi stool, which was brown and diarrhœic and which > the pain until aft breakfast, when it returned with greater violence and induced a second sto with tenesmus causing prolapsus, then burning about anus ; sudden gripi at 1.30 p.m., < l. side, which induced a stool, the stool passed quickly, th tenesmus and prolapsus, then pain as if excoriated ; stool > pain only te porarily, as it returned with such violence as to force sweat from all par abated gradually ; < by dinner, causing another stool of soft, brown fæc mixed with mucus, then tenesmus, prolapsus ; weakness, esp. in knees.—Pa in morning, with urging to stool.—Pain at 3 p.m., > diarrhœa ; on eati with desire for stool ; < pressure.—Darting pain, at 10 a.m., < above r. h —Pain as from incarcerated flatus at 3 p.m. ; sore, waking about 5 a.m., w urging to stool.—Heavy pain in forenoon, < drinking cold water and eati dinner, the same pain next day, < by pressure.—Pain in hepatic region j under ends of floating ribs ; in forenoon, sore to pressure ; sore in eveni with sensitiveness to touch.—Darting pain in liver at 10 p.m.

13. **Stool and Anus.**—Constipation after pappy stool.—Diarrhœa, with straining and expulsion of flatus.—Diarrhœa at 5 a.m., during day several small, loose stools, always preceded by sore pain in intestines, with the stool tenesmus and shivering along the back, on following days several stools daily, mostly small, consisting of mucus with tenesmus ; (> by *Merc. cor.*)—Before stool : pain in l. side of abdomen, with sweat ; griping pains ; sore pain in intestines.—During stool : pain in abdomen continues ; tenesmus ; chills on back ; much urging.—After stool : tenesmus ; prolapsus ani ; burning in anus ; great debility ; weakness in knees ; colic temporarily > but soon returns.—Light-brown diarrhœa at 10 a.m. and 2 p.m., preceded and followed by pain in abdomen, straining with the second stool.—Stitches upward along l. side of anus.

17. **Respiratory Organs.**—Hoarseness.—Hacking cough from irritation in throat.

18. **Chest.**—Cutting to r. of lower part of sternum at 7 a.m.—Sharp pain in lower part of chest at 7 a.m.—Throbbing all over chest from 9 till 11 a.m.

19. **Heart and Pulse.**—Shooting in region of heart at 7.30 a.m.—Pain in region of heart at 4 p.m., < by a long breath.—Darting rheumatic pain in heart region.—Pulse 100 and full at 9 a.m.—Intermittent pulse.

21. **Limbs.**—Shooting : in different joints during day ; in joints in afternoon and evening ; in l. heel and wrist ; in phalangeal joints of third finger and in l. knee in forenoon.

22. **Upper Limbs.**—Heaviness.—Shoulder : shooting in r. joint at 2 p.m. ; shocks in l. joint in afternoon and next forenoon ; pain in l. ; rheumatic pain in l.—Forearm : aching down l. ; pain in bones of l. at noon ; frequent pains in l., forenoon ; intermittent pain in l. at 11 p.m., then shooting.—Shooting : in a spot on inner side of dorsum of wrist at 4 p.m. ; in r. wrist at noon, intermittent at first ; in phalangeal joints of second l. finger at 8.30 a.m. ; in palmar surface of ungual phalanx of r. thumb ; intermittent in finger-joints, elbows, and wrists in forenoon.

23. **Lower Limbs.**—Pain in l. hip-joint on rising from a seat and beginning to walk, causing limping, usually > after taking a few steps.—Thighs : tearing in lower part of l. at 2.30 p.m. ; flying, sharp pains in l. at 9 a.m.—Knee : rheumatic pain in l. ; intermittent pain in r. at 9 a.m.—Boring in r. tibia in forenoon.—Pain in inner part of l. ankle at 12 p.m., < bearing weight on it.—Tearing in l. tarsus at 1 p.m.—Shooting : in r. ankle at 3 p.m. ; in l. tarsus at 6 p.m. ; in outer side of r. metatarsus at 3 p.m. ; in inner side of l. heel.

24. **Generalities.**—Rheumatic pains in l. shoulder, arm, knee, and region of heart.—Inability to keep quiet.—Weakness.—Felt > in evening ; > in open air.

25. **Skin.**—Pimples on nape in evening.—Itching : in spots on chin and among whiskers ; in evening, and about neck.

26. **Sleep.**—Constant inclination to gape through day ; in afternoon.—Sleepiness.—Restless sleep.—Wakefulness after 4 a.m., with restlessness.—Lewd dreams.

27. **Fever.**—Chilliness at night, < morning on waking.—Fever in afternoon, with pulsation in arteries of head and aching in occiput and small of back.—Burning in pinnæ of ears in evening, < r.

Tropæolum.

Tropæolum majus. Indian Cress. Garden Nasturtium. *N. O.* Tropæolaceæ. Tincture of fresh plant.

Clinical.—Urine, fetid.

Characteristics.—*Tropæolum* is a native of Peru. It was called "Cress" and "Nasturtium" because the taste of the leaves was considered like the taste of cress, and they have been used like cress in salads. The seeds make pickles, and are used as a substitute for capers. A patient to whom Cooper gave *Trop.* noted that it made the urine extremely fetid in smell. On this keynote Cooper has relieved several cases of urinary difficulty, giving single doses of the ϕ tincture.

Tuberculinum.

Tuberculin of Koch. A glycerine extract of a pure cultivation of tubercle bacilli (human). Liquid attenuations.

Clinical.—Acne. Albuminuria. Appendicitis. Asthma. Bones, caries of. Bronchitis. Catarrhal pneumonia. Chilblains. Cornea, opacity of; ulceration of. Dentition. Erysipelas. Erythema. Hæmaturia. Hæmoptysis. Headache. Heart, affections of; palpitation of. Influenza. Leprosy. Leucorrhœa. Lungs, œdema of. Lupus. Mania. Menses too early. Nephritis. Night-terrors. Œdema glottidis. Paralysis. Phthisis. Pleurisy. *Pneumonia, acute.* Tuberculosis.

Characteristics.—I consider it best to reserve the name *Tuberculinum* for this preparation of Koch, as it is universally known by that name. Burnett's "*Bacillinum*" is now accepted as the name of the original homœopathic preparation, and though its originator, Swan, named it *Tuberculinum*, it owes its present position in therapeutics to Burnett, and it will simplify matters if we make the term *Bacillinum* cover the homœopathic nosode and *Tuberculinum* the preparation of Koch. When Koch's *Tuberculinum* was first launched the medical papers were teeming with reports of cases undergoing the injection for various diseases. Of the reported effects, curative and pathogenetic, I made a collection. These will be found in *H. W.*, xxvi. 155. I have there given the authority for the observations and the nature of the cases in which the effects were observed. These symptoms will be found arranged in the Schema, and each symptom has appended to it the initial of the observer, or an indication of the disease from which the patient was suffering when the observation was made. Koch's own observations are marked (K); Virchow's, (V); Jonathan Hutchinson's, (H); Ewald's, (E); Albrand's, (A); Watson Cheyne's, (W C); Lennox Brown's, (L B). The names of other observers are given in full. Lupus cases are marked (lps.); observations made on a leper (lpr.). In *Jour. Belge d'H*, 1894, 236, Mersch published a pathogenesis of *Tub.* compiled mainly from the same sources as mine, but giving some additional symptoms. These I have included and marked (M). A few cured symptoms are put in brackets. The undistinguished symptoms are from a proving by Nebel, of Montreux (*H. W.*, xxxv. 397). The provers were tuberculous individuals, mostly workpeople, and only pathogenetic symptoms are recorded. *Tub.* 30 was used, the preparation having been obtained from Hausmann's Pharmacy, St. Gall. I do not find any appreciable difference between the action of *Tub.* and that of *Bac.* My own impression is that they are practically identical, and that the one will answer to the indications of the other. Nebel has used *Tub.* in exactly the same way as Burnett and others have used *Bac.*, on the indications Burnett laid down and with Burnett's results. In *H. W.* for May, June, and July, 1901, I have copied from *H. R.* of the same year articles by Nebel giving his experiences with *Tub.*: (1) Boy, 13, had diphtheria with fearful headache extending from neck to vertex, with swelling in back of neck and occiput, due, it was supposed, to an affection of the middle ear. Seven weeks passed without improvement. Paracentesis of the tympanum resulted in the evacuation of pus for a day or two. Nebel found the face bloated ; strawberry tongue coated white at the root ; mastoids not sensitive to even strong pressure. Swelling of occiput and neck down to fifth dorsal vertebra. The head is held fixed sideways towards the middle of the clavicle. If the boy wants to move his head he has to seize it with both hands and turn it slowly, with painful distortion of facial muscles, until it reaches the position desired. Even the slightest pressure on first, second, or third cervical vertebra was very painful ; the skin on them was reddened and the periosteum was swollen ; glands in neck enlarged. Tuberculosis of atlas and second and third vertebræ consequent on diphtheria was diagnosed. *Tub.* 1m. was given, five grains, during the day. Two days after the dose the boy could move his head more freely, the swelling of the neck diminished, appetite returned, and in a short time he was able to get up and run about. Five weeks after the dose, the swelling had altogether gone, and the boy's condition was altogether changed. (2) Swelling of tibiæ two inches below the knee, in a lady who had had cough for twenty years. Cured chiefly with *Tub.* 1m. This patient had offensive sweat in axillæ, strawberry tongue, lack of appetite. Distaste for milk, constipation, and bad sleep. [Mau, of Kiel, treated the following cases with *Bac.* (*H. W.*, xxxvi. 316)—I introduce them here for comparison : (1) Vigorous man, tall and of well-developed appearance, was very liable to get pneumonia in cold weather, and spent the winter in some sanatorium or other in order to escape. His father had died of pneumonia, his mother of consumption, and a sister was consumptive. He perspired much, took much fluid nourishment, partly alcoholic. Sleep poor. Almost constant fever. Enlarged glands. Three months' treatment with *Bac.* removed all the symptoms, and, moreover, made his tissues less watery and reduced his corpulence somewhat. (2) A distinguished author, 50, complained of dreadful pains in the head, almost total insomnia, and great debility. His brother and sisters had mostly died of dropsy of the brain ; he himself had congestion of the right lung, due probably to healed cavities, as he has frequently had hæmorrhages. For this he had had a lengthened treatment in the South, and had been pronounced cured of consumption. Softening of the brain and loss of reason were now feared. The headache was attended with a sensation as if his head was being tightly squeezed behind with an iron ring. Hands trembling; but he was most uneasy from a sensation in his back as if his clothes were moist. In less than a month, under *Bac.*, the headache, insomnia, and sensation in the back had all vanished. Another patient of Mau's, a child, had "screaming out in sleep and great restlessness at night," which were cured, along with peevish, irritable, taciturn disposition.] In 1892 B. S. Arnulphy (*Clinique*, xvi. 629) began giving *Tub.* 6x and 8x trituration internally in tubercular cases, acute and chronic, and with encouraging success, but with at times undesired aggravations; with 12x and 30x these were avoided. In one case, originating in grippe, both apices were affected, the right one breaking down; and abundant pleuritic effusion on the left side. Six weeks' treatment with *Tub.* brought about recovery, and seen a year later the patient was quite well except for retraction of the left side. Arnulphy considers (*Clinique*, xvii. 86) that *Tub.* is frequently the remedy for bronchitis, catarrhal pneumonia, lobular pneumonia, tubercular pleurisy, parenchymatous nephritis, and grippe. He gives (*Clinique*, xvii. 457) two cases of acute lobular pneumonia with characteristic symptoms and high temperatures quickly resolved by *Tub.* One was in a boy of three who received the 12x; the other was a man, 78, being a sufferer from chronic bronchial catarrh. The latter was taken with grippe, pneumonia developed, and he was in a very serious state. *Tub.* 30x made an almost immediate change for the better, and recovery followed. Arnulphy relates that in this case an abundant perspiration took place (the skin had been dry) during the night; and he has observed this in all cases of pneumonia when *Tub.* acted favourably. I have found *Tub.* 30, 100, 200, and 1m the best general antidote to the chronic effects of influenza poisoning. B. G. Clark (*H. W.*, xxix. 349) reports the case of a lady, 60, who had had for some time a mild form of tuberculosis of the skin of the face, and more recently a small growth (lupus) on the side of the nose on a line with the inner canthus of left eye. It had grown much in six months. *Tub.* 200 F.C., six powders given, one to be dissolved in twelve teaspoonfuls of water, one teaspoonful every two hours. The six powders were taken in this way on successive days. On the fifth day the growth began to dry up. On the tenth it fell off. Another dose of *Tub.* was given after this with marked improvement to the older affection of the face. A curious use has been made of *Tub.* by Jauregg, of Vienna, in a case of insanity (*H. W.*, xxx. 196). Having observed that cases of insanity are always benefited by an attack of an acute infectious disease, especially if it is accompanied with high fever, the idea occurred to him of utilising the fever produced by Koch's *Tuberculin* injections. He tried it on some patients, and though the decidedly favourable symptoms soon disappeared after the fever subsided, still there was a *steady clearing of the comfused sensorium.* Insanity is very frequently a manifestation of the consumptive taint, and there is something more than a pyrexial power in *Tub.* [Burnett has cured with *Bac.* a case of insanity, being led to give it by a ringworm-like eruption on the body.] Among the *Peculiar Sensations* noted under *Tub.* are: As if the brain were squeezed with an iron ring. As if the teeth were jammed together and were too many for the mouth. Of mucus in the throat; of a tumour in the throat. Pressure in stomach going to throat as if the clothes were too tight. As if the clothes on the back were wet (*Bac.*). Fatigue, faintness, profuse debility are frequent symptoms. Great weakness in the limbs after dinner: this at times amounts to paralysis. The circulation is always disturbed, chills and flushes alternating. "Shivering when beginning to sleep" is a peculiar and interesting symptom; also "cold feet in bed," which is common in persons of low vital reaction. "Sensitive to music" was observed in one of Nebel's patients; another had pains in the region of the appendix vermiformis, which should lead to serviceable action in appendicitis cases. The symptoms are: < By slightest exertion (it = excessive fatigue; sweat). Walking = pains in loins (fatigue). Raising himself up = palpitation. Every movement = sticking in chest and back. Rubbing = itching to change place. < Morning (much purulent expectoration; sickness and nausea; loss of appetite; thirst; fatigue). < From 10 to 3 p.m. (frontal headache). < Evening (heat in head; cough preventing sleep; severe pains in breast at beginning of menses. < Evening in bed (itching; feet cold). < Night (sweat; from 3 a.m. sleep disturbed). < Beginning to sleep (shivering). < After dinner (flushing; drowsiness). Sensitive to music.

Relations.—[Burnett recommends to give the Tuberculinum high if there is a strong tubercular element in the case; if that element is small, 30 is better.] *Compare:* Bacillinum (including Tuberculinum of Swan), Bacil. test., Aviaire. In tubercular meningitis, Iodf. Irregular distribution of circulation; constitutional remedy, Sul. Analogous constitutional remedies, Pso., Med., Syph., Thuja. Sensation of an iron band compressing brain (Thuj. hoop round forehead). Sensitive to music, Thuj. Phthisis, insanity, Thyroid. Pain in region of appendix, Ir. t., Ars., Lach. Pains in breasts at menses, Con., Calc. *Compatible:* Hydrast., "it actually seems to fatten up tuberculous patients" (Burnett; confirmed by Nebel), Calc., Calc. iod., Calc. ph., Phos., Thuj., Sep., Puls. Sensitive to music, Aco., Amb., Nat. c., Nux, Pho. ac., Sep., Thuj., Vio. o. (> by music, Trn.).

SYMPTOMS.

1. **Mind.**—Anxiety, gloomy, melancholy humour.—Has lost melancholy expression she formerly had (Ipr.).—Is disposed to whine and complain; dejected mind, anxiety.—She is very sad.—Nervous irritation; aversion to labour.—Indifferent.—Forgetful.—Aversion to all labour, esp. mental work.—Sensibility to music.—Does not like to be disturbed by people; trembling of hands.

2. **Head.**—Vertigo: esp. in morning; heavy with obscuration of eyes; is obliged to lean on something; by bending down, esp. by rising after

bending down; with palpitations; with headache; with nausea; with headache in morning; after dinner.—Great heat in head; flushes of heat after dinner; sensation of heat in head in evening.—Headache: deep in forehead; deep in temples; on vertex with sensation of heat; from neck to forehead; in morning, passing away in afternoon.—Sensation of heaviness on vertex.—Headache with obscuration of sight.—Headache with vertigo.—Piercing headache.—Piercing pain in forehead from 10 a.m. to 3 p.m.—Headache in evening; in afternoon.—Frontal headache in morning.—Headache with rushing in ears.—Headache in morning with bleeding of nose.—Headache from neck to forehead; burning, piercing.—Colossal hyperæmia of pia mater and brain substance; extreme engorgement of vessels on the surface, internally dusky red; tubercles presented no retrogressive changes (arachnitis.—V.)—(Sensation as if brain squeezed with iron band.—*Bac.*)

3. **Eyes.**—Swollen lids; headache with swollen lids in morning.—R. eye much swollen, conjunctiva inflamed (lps.).—Dulness and heaviness of eyes; darkness before eyes.—Obscuration of vision with vertigo.—Opens r. eye (which had been closed.—W C).—Breaking down of cicatrices of old corneal ulcers (Stoker).—Clearing of corneal opacity the result of old tuberculous corneitis (Stoker).—Tuberculosis of eyelids, small grey and yellow nodules, existing in conjunctiva of outer sections of lids, increased in size, ran together, then suddenly disappeared (A).—Phlyctenulæ appeared where none existed before (Maschke).—Conjunctivitis; herpes on lids (M).—Amblyopia with irregularity and complete paralysis of pupils (in an alcoholic).

4. **Ears.**—Tinnitus (lps.).—Rushing in ears with heavy head.—Sticking pain from pharynx to ears.—Headache with rushing in ears and pressure on vertex.—Great aching in ears and teeth.

5. **Nose.**—Coryza.—Secretion of mucus from nose, viscid, yellow-green.—Increased secretion of mucus, with frontal headache.—Aching of ears and teeth with coryza in evening, with headache.—Bleeding of nose.—Comedones on nose, surrounded with minute pustules (lps.).—The nose, which used to feel "hot and burning," has lost this sensation (lps.).

6. **Face.**—Œdematous, pale face.—Clonic convulsions of musculus orbicularis inferior, acute.—Convulsions in region of facial muscle, esp. buccinator.—In one case the inflammation of the lupus (on face) presented unquestionable erysipelas of a rather severe type, and the patient was for some time in danger (H).—Flushing of cheek of same side as lung affected, during the reaction (Borgherini).—Upper lip and nose become swollen during the first two or three reactions, the lip becoming cracked on inner surface (W C).—Herpes on lips and eyelids (Heilferich).—After the tenth injection his l. moustache, which was kept cut to prevent scabs from gathering, ceased to grow, every hair fell out, and for a month the l. upper lip was perfectly denuded of hair, and had all the appearance when seen under a lens of being depilated; however, the hairs began to grow well before he left the Home (lps., Hine).

7. **Teeth.**—Vague toothache.—Teeth felt loose (lps.).—"Feeling as if the teeth were all jammed together and too many for his head" (lps.).—Sordes on teeth (lps.).—Inflammation of gums, scurvy-like.—Gums turgescent, felt swollen (lps.).

8. **Mouth.**—Tongue foul, furred.—Tongue much coated (lps.).—Coating on soft palate and tongue (M).—Taste : salty, purulent.—Aphthæ on tongue and buccal mucosa.—Tongue dry (lps.).—Dryness of lips.—On lips black blisters.—Palate : granulations enormously swollen and vascular (lps.).—Breath offensive (M).

9. **Throat.**—Aching in pharynx and larynx.—Scratching in pharynx.—Tickling in throat exciting cough.—Sensation of mucus in throat.—Sensation of a tumour in throat.—Dryness in throat ; tonsillitis ; general inflammatory condition of pharyngeal mucous membrane (M).—Retropharyngeal abscess (M).—Burning pain in throat.—Sensation of constriction in throat ; in larynx. —Heaviness and sensation of rattling in throat.—Aching extending from throat to ears.—Dysphagia increased ; later diminished (in laryngeal phthisis.—L B).

10. **Appetite.**—Loss of appetite, esp. in morning.—Thirst : extreme, day and night ; burning in morning.

11. **Stomach.**—Eructations and sensation of fulness over stomach.—Nausea, vomiting (K, 5h.).—Vomited severely with > to headache (lps.).—Nausea and vomiting, nausea with efforts to vomit with colic and diarrhœa.—Transitory sickness and vomiting after dinner.—Vomiting after every meal.—Nausea and sickness in morning with heaviness in stomach region.—Pressure in stomach, going to throat, as if the clothes were too tight.—Cramping pain in stomach.—Nausea with pains in umbilical region with diarrhœa.—Nausea with racking and stirring in stomach and increased thirst.—Sickness in stomach and pressing.—Nausea in morning.—Sticking pains in stomach region.

12. **Abdomen.**—Cramping pains in stomach and abdomen.—Sensation of constriction in abdomen.—Colic with diarrhœa and heaviness in stomach. —Colic with great thirst.—Fatigue and sickness in region of stomach and abdomen ; sticking pains deep in spleen ; severe pain in region of liver.—Aching (sticking) in region of liver, spleen, ovaries, spermatic cord, testicles (esp. l.), in hip-joints, in rectum.—Pains in region of appendix vermiformis.—Mass of enlarged glands, in r. iliac fossa much smaller (W C).—Six pustules at different parts of skin of back and abdomen, and after discharging have healed (W C)—Discrete papular rash over chest and abdomen (W C).—Perforating ulcer in intestines (V).

13. **Stool and Anus.**—Obstipation ; stool hard, dry, with wind and colic.—Diarrhœa with pinching and burning pains.—Pressure and constriction in rectum.—Pain in rectum.—Itching sensation in anus.

14. **Urinary Organs.**—Diminished quantity of urine.—Is obliged to urinate very often, esp. during changes of weather.—One tenth albumen in height of reaction ; disappeared afterwards (W C).—Specific gravity of urine increases from 1016 to 1023 with an excess of urates and ropy mucus.—Peptonuria in man, 33 (Maregliano).—Hæmaturia with renal pain (M).—Excess of urates (M).—Abundant viscid mucous discharge.

15. **Male Sexual Organs.**—Pains in testicles, and cord of l. side.

16. **Female Sexual Organs.**—Severe pains in breast in evening at beginning of menstruation.—Menstruation with pains in lumbo-sacral and ovarian region.—Sticking pain in lower abdomen ; pains in lumbo-sacral region < when walking.—Weakness in genital region ; painful menstruation.—Blood

lumpy, menstruation lasting more days than usual ; menstruation antepones eight days.—Burning pains in external genitals ; sharp leucorrhœa ; pains in sacral and ovarian region to hip-joints.—Sensation of heat in genitalia externa, with increased leucorrhœa.—Cramps in uterine region with pains in sacral and ovarian region.—Burning pain in ovarian region.—Menstruation returns fourteen days after parturition.

17. **Respiratory Organs.**—Decided effect in laryngeal cases, mostly beneficial (L B).—After ten injections, larynx markedly affected, inflammatory swelling and ulceration (L B).—General infiltration of mucous membrane of larynx, high red colour, brighter than normal (L B).—Enormous swelling of arytenoids appeared (L B).—Tuberculous outgrowth (L B).—Exfoliation at r. vocal cord, appearance extravasated below its posterior part (L B).—Hyperæmia of cords intensified and covered with minute ulcerating points.—Cough and expectoration lasting four months, from a wetting (removed, no bacilli found).—Sensation of pressure on chest.—Cough and sputa.—Irritating cough, < in night.—Little cough in night with aching in side and blood-tinged sputa. —Severe cough in evening with pains below mamma on r. side.—Inclination to cough (K, 3 to 4h.).—Severe cough with muco-purulent secretion in morning. —Cough prevents him sleeping in evening.—Cough, secretion of phlegm, esp. by walking, with sticking pains in lungs and palpitation.—A sort of whooping-cough.—Dry cough ; in night.—Cough with viscid mucus.—After much cough sensation of mucus in pharynx, mucous secretion being easily ejected.—Expectoration diminished (Heron).—Palpitation and pains in back with cough.—Crackling râles at r. shoulder behind (lps.).—Copious watery expectoration usually seen during the reaction (Wilson).—With every increase of dose he suffered from asthmatic fits, lasting from three to seven hours.—Extreme rapidity of respirations without dyspnœa, 60 to 90 in the minute ; if the patient is spoken to, the rapid breathing ceases at once (as with a dog panting in the sun.—Heron).—Is obliged to take deep inspirations ; dyspnœa.—Difficulty in breathing speedily increased (K, 3 to 4h.).—Marked feeling of suffocation (lpr.).

18. **Chest.**—Sensation of pressure in chest.—Heat in chest (M).—Sticking pain in chest, esp. at the apex of l. lung.—Sensation of contriction in the præcordial region.—Pains in both sides of chest going to back.—Pains in l. side.—Sticking in side.—Nightly pains on chest.—Sticking pains : in lungs ; in l. side, pains between scapulæ.—Aching in side in night.—Sticking pain in chest, on r. and l. side.—Sticking pain in l. side in morning and afternoon.—Sticking pain in lungs when laughing.—Pain in axilla, esp. when elevating arm.—Sticking pain : in lungs with cough and palpitation.—Pressure in chest, sticking pain on both sides of chest, in back.—Palpitation, caused by deep inspirations, aching in back with pains under ribs.—Pains in subclavicular region with cough.—Sticking pain in l. lung.—Pain from clavicles to throat.—Pain in apex pulmonis radiating to axilla and arm.—Sticking pain in chest and in back, < from every movement.—Pain in l. lung to axilla.—Pain on l. side going to back.—Pain in l. apex and in region of the spleen.—Severe pain in back, in axilla and arms.—Pains in l. side, must take deep inspiration.—Bronchitic sounds in both lungs (W C).—Dulness r. apex (L B).—Sudden, profuse hæmoptysis, ends fatally (E).—Developed a cavity on side opposite to that first affected (E).—New deposit of tubercles on pleura (E).—Surface of

old pulmonary cavities showed unusually intense redness of granulation layers (V).—Hæmorrhagic infiltration of the walls (V).—Recent hæmorrhage observed in the cavities.—In fatal cases of ulcerative phthisis the lungs esp., and also the pleuræ, showed extensive and severe recent changes—pleurisy, for the most part very severe, simple and tuberculous, frequently hæmorrhagic, and not infrequently bilateral (V).—Caseous pneumonia or caseous hepatisation—the lung appearing like blood-pudding studded with pieces of lard; (the patient, an architect, 33, had six injections, the last four weeks before death. At the beginning he had induration of one apex only. The treatment was suspended because of persistent fever and infiltration of lower lobe.—V).—Catarrhal pneumonia was found, but it differed from ordinary catarrhal pneumonia (in which the alveoli when squeezed out have a gelatinous appearance) in that the contents of the alveoli were very watery and turbid—a turbid infiltration; it resembles a phlegmonous condition (V).—Soft hepatisation, which differs from ordinary catarrhal hepatisation in that in the midst of the patches foci of softening become developed, leading to rapid breaking down and excavation (V).—Development of fresh tubercles: small tubercles giving rise to new ulcers have suddenly appeared, esp. in pleura, pericardium, and peritoneum (V).—Metastasis, bacilli mobilised (V).—Abscesses in the lungs (V).—Perforating abscesses in respiratory organs (V).

19. **Heart.**—Palpitation early in morning.—Sensation of heaviness and pressure over heart,—Palpitation with cough and sticking pains in lungs.—By deep inspirations severe palpitation.—Aching in heart.—Palpitation in night, < when raising himself up.—Palpitation with pain in the back.—Death from paralysis of heart (Libhertz).

20. **Neck and Back.**—Glands in neck and scars swollen and very tender, various lupus points about them showing yellow fluid under epidermis (lps.).—Scars in neck softer and flatter; no lupus nodules now perceptible (lps.).—Glands cannot now be felt, except the largest, which is now reduced to size of a pea (lps.).—Cervical glands much smaller (W C).—Aching like needle-pricks in the back.—Prickly feeling in skin of back (lps.).—Weakness in lumbo-sacral region.—Sticking pain over both scapulæ; pain in region of spleen; vague pains in back and on chest, with sensation of pressure.—Sticking in back.—Pain in back with palpitation.—(Sensation on his back as if the clothes were moist.—*Bac.*)—Three red patches on l. side of back became much deeper (lpr.).—Violent reaction, during which severe pains in loins < by pressure; (case of Addison's disease; two injections given.—Pick.)—Tuberculosis of sacrum greatly improved (Kurz).

21. **Limbs.**—Sensation of formication in arms and legs.—Great weakness in limbs after dinner.—Sensation of fatigue and faintness in all limbs.—Pains in limbs, fatigue (K, 3 to 4h. after injection).—Pains in limbs (K, 2nd d.).—Pains in ulnar nerve and calves of legs and knees, l. great toe much affected, and became very red and turgid (lpr.).—Trembling of limbs (in an alcoholic).—Twitching in the limbs (M).

22. **Upper Limbs.**—Aching in forearms; vague, sticking pain.—Diminution of inflammation above elbow-joint; disappearance of abscess over olecranon; sinus connected with radius discharging freely a thick yellow pus (W C).—Sensation of luxation with severe pains in r. carpal joint; < by effort to move it; ceasing by rest.—Trembling of hands.

23. **Lower Limbs.**—During night pain referred to r. knee; r. leg rotated in and flexed slightly at hip and knee; movement of r. hip-joint free; 1 p.m., l. hip much more painful and tender, more flexed, abducted and rotated out (disease of l. hip in girl of five.—B. M. T.).—Aching in the hip-joints.—Pain in r. knee without swelling (Heron, a non-tubercular case).—The knee became easily movable and could be bent to a right angle (tuberculous affection of r. knee).—Swelling and tenderness of both knee-joints (Heron).—Tenderness in r. ankle-joint (Heron).

24. **Generalities.**—Feeling of fatigue (K, 2nd d.).—Malaise, depression, headache, somnolence, oppression of breathing, tightness of chest, nausea (lps.).—General fatigue in morning; sensation of faintness; great weakness in lower extremities, esp. from knees down to feet.—Terribly tired, so that she can scarcely walk.—General excessive fatigue after a short walk, so that he must lean on his companion.—Emaciation (lost six pounds in fourteen days, twenty pounds in five weeks).—In parts affected throbbing pain.—Leucocytosis; diminution of oxyhæmoglobin (M).—Oxyhæmoglobin first diminished then increased (Henoque).—Feeling well, but decidedly losing flesh (lps.).—Acts principally by very acute irritation of internal organs affected (in the same way as in external organs), causing intense redness and great swelling (V).—Actual inflammatory processes (not mere hyperæmias), and esp. active proliferations, occur to an intense degree, in (1) edges of existing ulcers; in (2) neighbouring lymphatic glands, esp. bronchial and mesenteric (V).—Lymphatic glands present a quite unusual degree of enlargement, and notably that form of medullary swelling, characteristic of acute irritations, which is caused by rapid proliferation of the cells in the interior of the glands (V).—Leucocytosis: various infiltrations of white blood corpuscles over affected parts, esp. round the tubercles themselves (V).—Enormous dangerous swellings in parts near ulcers (even where the surface of the ulcer becomes clean), causing dangerous constriction (V). — Phlegmonous swelling resembling erysipelatous œdema of glottis and retropharyngeal abscess (V).—Where tubercle is associated with any other specific disease, reaction is so slight as to be scarcely discernible (Heron).—Syphilitic cases are refractory to reaction Heron).—Children bear the treatment well (Wendt).

25. **Skin.**—Erythematous eruption like measles or scarlatina (M).—Erythema with subcutaneous indurated nodules (M).—Great bronze patches on the forehead and temples.—Bronze finger-points.—Finger-points as if touched by *Argentum nitricum*.—Itching all over the body in the evening in bed; changing place after rubbing.—" Rash on chest and abdomen similar, patient says, to what came out when disease first appeared" (lpr.).—Rash on abdomen and back, commencing very red; speedily becoming brownish, resembling ordinary skin eruption of secondary syphilis (L B).—Œdematous condition of upper lip.—Œdematous condition of eyelids.—Nose swollen, tense, erysipelatous-looking epidermis in lupus patch raised by yellow fluid.—In two cases, at least during the febrile action, old chilblains became again inflamed (H).—Slight attack of jaundice (several cases.—W C).—Site of injection slightly painful and red (K, 2nd d.).—Erythematous blush confined to lupus parts, which were the seat of throbbing pain.—It has repeatedly caused general erythematous eruptions on the skin, and, in some, nodular effusions into the cellular tissue (H).

26. **Sleep.**—Great desire for sleep; drowsiness during day; after dinner.—Inclination to sleep in mornings.—Shivering when beginning to sleep.—Cold feet in bed.—Troubled sleep; sleeplessness.—Sleep disturbed from 3 a.m.—Sleeplessness on account of constant coughing.—Many dreams; disturbed sleep, interrupted by fearful dreams; gloomy dreams; dreams of shame; cries out in dreams.

27. **Fever.**—Shivering, when beginning to sleep; cold feet in bed.—Freezing and heat alternately; cold and heat for moments.—Violent attack of ague, lasting almost an hour (K, 5h.).—Freezing on the back in evening.—Freezing during whole day.—Sensation of heat in evening in bed.—Flush of heat from back to head.—Feverish, nausea, thirsty, with headache, no vomiting (Heron).—Flushes of heat after eating.—High temperature, abating in twelve hours (K).—Lowering of temperature after each injection (Heron).—Lowering of temperature before a rise (Heron).—Temperature seven hours after injection, 103·8°, accompanied by thirst, rigor, increased cough, headache, and pains in joints (Heron).—Sweat in the night.—Much sweat, esp. on head in night.—Profuse sweat after light exertion.—A little walk and slight efforts produce sweats.—Short sweats in morning, while awaking.—Profuse sweats during slight exertion.

Turnera Aphrodisiaca.

Turnera aphrodisiaca. Damiana. *N. O.* Turneraceæ. Tincture of fresh plant.

Clinical.—Amenorrhœa. Dysmenorrhœa. Fatigue. Impotence. Leucorrhœa. Migraine. Prostate, affections of. Spermatorrhœa. Sterility. Urine, incontinence of.

Characteristics.—Hale has collected from old-school sources much experience respecting this drug, showing its power over the genito-urinary system. The herb *Damiana* (the local name of *Turn. a.*), has long been a domestic medicine in Mexico, where it is used to "invigorate the system." Indian hunters discovered that a decoction of it was a great invigorator after wearisome journeys; and they also found in it a cure for inability to exercise the reproductive functions in both sexes. Hale gives many cases illustrating the latter. Among the causes of the defect in the cured cases are injury to spine from a fall; sexual excess; syphilis or gonorrhœa, in the men; and amenorrhœa, dysmenorrhœa, and leucorrhœa in the women. Douglass (*Hahn Ad.*, xxxix. 660) reports three cases of incontinence of urine: Man, 63, for four years has had dribbling of urine day and night. *Turn.* 2x, in water, four times a day, cured in two months. Another use of *Turn.* is recorded (*H. R.* xii., 410) in severe migraine, "One or two doses given within an hour causes the headache to cease and induces sleep, from which the patient wakens free from headache and with good appetite." This is perhaps analogous to the power of *Turn.* to dispel fatigue.

Relations.—*Compare:* Impotence, injuries, over-exertion, fatigue, Bellis, Arn. Prostatic affections, Sabal., Solid. Migraine, Epipheg.

Tussilago Farfara.

Common Coltsfoot. British Herb Tobacco. (Waste, sandy, clayey banks.) *N. O.* Compositæ. Tincture of fresh plant.

Clinical.—Coughs. Scrofula.

Characteristics.—"*Tussil. farfara* is used to this day in the form of a confection for coughs. The leaves are mucilaginous and were much used in scrofulous affections. Smoking the dried leaves relieves coughs" (Cooper). *Tus. far.* has also a popular reputation in gonorrhœa.

Tussilago Fragrans.

Petasites fragrans. Italian or fragrant Tussilage. *N. O.* Compositæ. Tincture of whole plant.

Clinical.—Corpulence. Plethora.

Characteristics.—Demesnes proved *Tus. fg.* taking three drops of the ϕ tincture on the tongue. After first causing a disagreeable, spiteful mood, it set up, in a few days, an opposite condition, which lasted some time. A journey taken on the ninth day of the proving, which usually caused loss of weight, did not do so. Stoutness increased, and plethora was added ; later the abdominal protuberance permanently disappeared. A *Peculiar Sensation* induced was as if a morsel of food lay at the bottom of the cardia and would not pass.

SYMPTOMS.

1. **Mind.**—Complaining mood, fault-finding; spiteful (after a few hours).—Serenity ; benevolence ; calmness ; increased power of mind and expression (fifth to tenth day).

2. **Head.**—Transient headache as after spirituous liquors.

3. **Eyes.**—Dryness of eyes when looking in open air, compelling to wink.

8. **Throat.**—Acidity in œsophagus like heartburn, > after dinner.

11. **Stomach.**—Sensation at bottom of cardia as of a morsel that will not pass down.

23. **Lower Limbs.**—Weakness in legs.—Pain from side to side in tarsus (l.), below that and metatarsus, when walking ; (does not last long but frequently returns).—Pain in metatarsal joint as if caused by a blow.

24. **Generalities.**—Corpulency at first increased, later reduced.—Plethora.

26. **Sleep.**—Sleepless, and is none the worse for it.

27. **Fever.**—Sweat and heat from slight exertion.

Tussilago Petasites.

Petasites vulgaris. Bitter-bur (Sandy meadows on the banks of streams.) *N. O.* Compositæ. Tincture of whole fresh plant.

Clinical.—Gonorrhœa. Headache. Lumbago. Night-sweat. Pylorus, affections of. Throat, sore. Tibia, pain in. Uvula, burning in.

Characteristics.—*Petasites* is "a genus of Compositæ established for three or four species of *Tussilago*, which have the flower-heads partially diœceous in racemes, sometimes branching into panicles. The essential characters which separate them from the common Coltsfoot (*Tussilago farfara*) are very slight, and the foliage is the same" (*Treas. of Bot.*). I retain the name of *Tussilago petasites* under which it is best known. *Tussilago* grows on river-banks that are little trodden on. "The roots are an admirable medicine in the worst kind of fevers with boils or buboes" (Green's *Herbal*). Kuchenmeister and five others took substantial doses. Most noticeable among the symptoms are: a lumbago of very great severity. Tightness of the chest. (*Tussilago* means "cough-wort".) A headache shifting from one part of the head to another during two days. A pain about the pylorus. A urethritis, with yellow discharge. The last has been confirmed clinically. Hansen gives the indication: "Acute or chronic gonorrhœa, yellow or white, thick discharge." Crawling in urethra; jerking in spermatic cord, and drawing in r. testicle are additional symptoms of the proving. [Ivatt's (*H. W.*, xxxvi. 381) reports cures of gonorrhœa with *T. farfara*, common Coltsfoot.] Rosenberg (*H. R.*, ix. 501) gives some experiences: (1) An extremely violent gonorrhœa; penis swollen, painful; emission of urine extremely painful, mixed with blood, patient feverish and restless. *Tuss. p.* was given in water. There was a great aggravation of all symptoms in thirty-six hours. The remedy was discontinued and marked amelioration followed. Resumed again, much diluted, rapid cure followed. The remedy was used externally as well in this case. (2) Chronic ophthalmia, the result of gonorrhœa "cured" with turpentine. *Tuss. p.* restored the discharge and then cured. Rosenberg refers to a writer who says of the plant that if it is macerated in water, the water will not spoil even if kept for years. The symptoms are: < By pressure (pains in pylorus). < Standing; stooping; walking; going up stairs; especially < rising from a seat (lumbago). Drinking = eructations. < Walking.

Relations.—*Compare:* Pain in pylorus (Tus. fg. is as if a morsel had lodged at bottom of cardia). Lumbago, Ant. t., Act. r. gonorrhœa, Thuj.

SYMPTOMS.

2. **Head.**—Severe confusion of head, more l. side, in evening.—Vertigo; on waking.—Dulness and heaviness of head.—Headache l. upper forehead, thence extending slowly over vertex, as if under dura mater like a tearing pain; after two hours pain seated over r. eye, with sensation as if supraorbital

muscles would be drawn upward, obliging him to wink; in afternoon headache returned to vertex; in evening again in temporal region; next day on waking, in l. side of vertex extending forward to r. eye.

4. **Ears.**—(Otorrhœa with enlarged cervical glands.—R. T. C.)

8. **Mouth.**—(Toothache all day, < by cold drink, esp. violent in bed; > by *Merc.*).

9. **Throat.**—Pain and burning in uvula.—Sore throat and pain on swallowing.

11. **Stomach.**—Eructations; frequent; numerous always after drinking.—Nausea.—Pain in pit of stomach.—Burning in epigastrium.—Pain about pylorus, at the point where sternum and ribs form a triangle, < by pressure.

12. **Abdomen.**—Colic; > by emission of flatus.

13. **Stool and Anus.**—In afternoon, a second soft but formed stool followed by desire for stool.—Absence of usual stool after dinner.—Several unsatisfactory stools in one day.

14. **Urinary Organs.**—Pressed out a drop of yellow mucus from urethra before urinating, though the urethra was not congested.—Crawling in urethra, obliging scratching, with erections.—Urine very profuse; but not evacuated often.

15. **Male Sexual Organs.**—Jerking pain in spermatic cord causing him to bend backward.—Drawing in r. testis.

18. **Chest.**—Tightness of chest.—Oppression in r. chest.

19. **Heart.**—Sudden stitch in l. side of præcordium on deep breathing.

20. **Back.**—Pain in small of back: on standing or stooping; walking; going up stairs; esp. on rising from a seat.

21. **Limbs.**—Increased stiffness of limbs at night.

23. **Lower Limbs.**—Pain in middle of r. tibia confined to a small spot.

24. **Generalities.**—Weakness.

25. **Skin.**—Itching on forehead and in beard.

26. **Sleep.**—Restless sleep.—Many dreams.

27. **Fever**—Cold feet.—Morning sweat.—Sweat at night; profuse.

Ulmus Fulva.

Ulmus fulva. American Slippery Elm. Red Elm. Moose Elm. (Mountains of Canada and Pennsylvania.) *N. O.* Ulmaceæ of the Urticaceæ. Pounded dried inner bark. Decoction of dried bark. Tincture of fresh bark.

Clinical.—Constipation. Deafness. Hæmorrhoids. Herpes. Pain. Syphilis.

Characteristics.—A decoction of the viscous inner bark of *Ul. ful.* is much used as a poultice for lessening pain in inflammations. In a case in which the mucous membrane of the rectum was dry and extremely painful, Burnett relieved the sufferings with 20-drop doses of the tincture. The bark in trituration gives much relief as a snuff in old vascular deafness with tubal obstruction (Cooper).

Upas.

Strychnos tieuté. *N. O.* Loganiaceæ. Tincture of the inspissated juice obtained from the root and bark.

Clinical.—Amaurosis. Blepharo-conjunctivitis. Convulsions. Coryza. Hang-nails. Headache. Heart, palpitation of. Heels, pains in. Liver, affections of. Nails, affections of. Ptosis. Sciatica. Sexual excess. Spine, pains in. Tendo Achillis, pain in. Tetanus.

Characteristics.—The *Upas* of homœopathy is obtained from a *Strychnos* and must not be confounded with *Antiaris toxicaria*, the con-cocted juice of which forms the "Upas antiar" poison of the Javanese. *S. tieuté* is a climbing shrub. Pitet made a courageous proving of it, carrying it to the length of producing tetanic symptoms. A large proportion of the symptoms occurred in the head and eyes. A remark-able headache was this: "Superficial drawing pain traverses left temple from before backward, and ceases at outer angle of orbit; the part is hot and painful to touch." The pains generally are pressive and lancinating. In the eyes there is pressure and feeling of a foreign body under the lids; severe pains in orbits; inflammation of the conjunctiva of the lids; distorted vision. Drowsiness is a feature in *Upas.* "Every morning weakness of the eyes with lachrymation, the lids being so heavy that they close involuntarily as if from drowsi-ness." *Up.* is chiefly a left-side remedy. There is pain in the left side of the throat as from a splinter on swallowing; pain in left sciatic nerve; in left iliac fossa. Sensitiveness is a note of the remedy: irritability, crossness, moroseness; increased sensitiveness to cold; the least irritation brought on spasms; pressing in throat causing feeling of suffocation. Noteworthy symptoms are: Vertigo, ending in pressing headache. Twitching in brain and orbits. Pulsative headache with throbbing all over body. Smell of manure in nose. Sallow complexion was produced, and severe symptoms were felt in the liver and from the right lung to the liver (cutting as with knives). Itching in patella. Aversion to meat and eggs; the very thought of them = nausea. The tongue is coated white so thickly that it can be scraped off. Left half of face red and hot, right half pale and cold. *Peculiar Sensations* are: As if the brain were rudely shaken. As after sexual excess. As if a foreign body in eye; as if sand in eyes. As if a splinter in throat on swallowing. As if a foreign body in œsophagus preventing swallowing. As if an iron hoop round waist preventing breathing. The sexual function was depressed, coition was followed by distressing symptoms, and many of the symptoms were such as occur after sexual excess. Great exhaustion after convulsive seizures. The symptoms are: < By touch (pain in left iliac fossa). < Pressure (throat). < By motion; by walking. < Afternoon and evening. < Morning. > After rising. > Evening after dinner. > In open air (headache).

Relations.—*Compare:* Botan.; spasmodic symptoms, Nux, Ign. Gouty pain, Nux. Lancinations in rectum, Ign. Exaggerated sensitiveness; acid eructations, Nux. Foul smell in nose, Anac. Splinter pain in throat, Hep., Arg. n., Nit. ac.

Causation.—Sexual excess.

SYMPTOMS.

1. **Mind.**—Depression.—Melancholy; has to force tears back; cold and repelling to friends.—Morose; cross; irritable; quarrelsome.—Sensitive.—Great difficulty in concentrating attention.

2. **Head.**—Head muddled.—Vertigo as if falling; ends with pressing headache; great tendency to feel cold.—Severe twitchings in brain and orbits.—Pulsating pains all over head on waking, > in open air.—Constant dull tearing in fore-part of brain, r. side; sometimes sharp shootings.—Very sharp deep-seated shootings r. side of forehead.—Pulsating heaviness in forehead and through l. eye.—Pressure and drawing in both temples, < l.; part hot to touch.—Superficial drawing pain, which every few moments traverses left temple from before backward, and ceases at outer angle of orbit; parts hot and painful to touch; lasted all day, > next morning.—Heat of head with red face.—Shootings deep in brain and vertex.—In occiput: pressing inward pain; heaviness as after sexual excess.—Scalp numb.

3. **Eyes.**—Eyes sunken, bluish rings round them.—Pressure and dryness in eyes.—Sensation as if foreign body in eyes; in l. eye; pustule on inner surface of r. lid.—Eyes weak as after sexual excess.—Every morning weakness of eyes with lachrymation, lids so heavy they close involuntarily

as if from irresistible drowsiness.—Dull pain in orbital and nasal bones.—Prolonged and violent lancinations under orbits.—Flow of blood from the eyelids.—Intense smarting itching on margins of lids and canthi.—Lachrymation.—Vision: dim, letters run together; fog before eyes.—In open air dimness, and as if endless strings of white and transparent globules were floating in the air.—After rising from a stooping position, blackness before eyes, as if all the blood had rushed to the head, with vanishing of thought.

4. **Ears.**—Tearings in ear cartilages.—Twitchings in cartilage near orifice (l).—Ears stuffed without affecting hearing.

5. **Nose.**—Violent fluent coryza towards and during evening.—First r. nostril then l. stopped up, changing every few minutes, preventing sleep.—L. nostril stopped and discharging greenish mucus.—Smell of manure in nose.

6. **Face.**—Yellow complexion.—Face red with hot head.—L. side face red and hot, r. pale and cold.

8. **Mouth.**—Tongue: dry, burning; coated white; so thickly it can be scraped off.—Unable to open his mouth to speak.—Blisters inside under lip towards l.—Frequent itching in palate.—Increased saliva, which tastes sour.—Taste: sour; bitter on root of tongue; like old coryza.

9. **Throat.**—Hawking frequent mucus in morning cured in the prover.—Pains and acidity l. side throat on swallowing; the acid sensation extends to l. ear.—Scraping burning soreness in throat; cough with burning pain as if throat would burst; difficult expectoration of bronchial mucus.—Pain as from splinter in l. side of throat making deglutition painful, as if food were prevented passing into stomach by foreign body in œsophagus; swallowing of fluids becomes difficult: pressing l. side of throat = sense of suffocation.—Feeling of swelling of r. tonsil while writing.

11. **Stomach.**—Appetite totally lost.—Aversion to all food, esp. meat and eggs, the mere thought of which = nausea.—Hunger, but first morsel satisfies.—Urgent thirst.—Eructations: bitter after meals, tasting of ingesta, all day; violent, of wind.—Qualmish, as if going to faint.—In morning, while hiccoughing, pinching in a line with lumbar vertebræ.

12. **Abdomen.**—Pressing pain: in region of liver; in liver.—Outpressing in l. hypochondrium.—Stitches in region of liver and r. kidney.—Much flatulency pressing against both hypochondria, breaking it gives no >; flatus odourless.—Rumbling.—Sharp pains in l. iliac fossa, < drawing breath and by touch.

13. **Stool and Anus.**—Sharp colic in rectum > passing fetid flatus; shortly after, soft stool, preceded by renewed colic.—Lancinations or slow pinchings in cellular tissue extending to rectum, r. side.—Two soft diarrhœic stools daily.—Stools mushy, reddish, ending with brown jelly-like mucus.—Stool constipated, after much pressing, and insufficient; brown jelly-like mucus after stool.

14. **Urinary Organs.**—Pain in region of r. kidney during the night.—Frequent urging to urinate, with burning in urethra at 8 a.m.—Urine scanty, evacuated with great effort, light red.—Urine dark like brandy.

15. **Male Sexual Organs.**—Erections and diminished desire.—Virile function depraved.—Coition accompanied by painful and enervating uneasiness, and followed by great depression for several minutes.—Itching of pubes.

17. **Respiratory Organs.**—Roughness in air passages.—Hoarseness; aphonia.—Dry cough, from soreness in larynx and trachea, < towards evening; expectoration of colourless mucus.—Quickened breathing in morning.—Inability to breathe deeply from sensation of iron hoop round waist.

18. **Chest.**—Chest tight.—Pinching drawing all round base of chest.—Knife-thrusts through r. lung towards liver, stopping breathing.—Needle-thrusts across chest behind l. nipple.—Pinching l. side chest.—Stitches through r. lung, evening.

19. **Heart.**—After going to bed, severe palpitation and pulsation all over from vertex, where it is pulsative headache, to finger-tips.—While writing, severe palpitation and feeling as if r. tonsil swollen (which it is not).—Pulse: frequent; weak, small, slow.

20. **Neck and Back.**—Painful stiffness of posterior muscles of neck, morning.—Pain in r. trapezius.—Burning in r. side of nape.—Feeling of stretching along spine.—Pressive and beaten feeling in spinal column, most in region opposite stomach.

21. **Limbs.**—Hangnails, which become inflamed; itching and redness at roots of nails.—Weakness.—Numbness in hands and feet.

22. **Upper Limbs.**—Pinching along back of nerves of l. arm.—Drawings in r. wrist-joint.—Painful drawing in joint of l. middle ring-finger.—Sharp, deep-seated lancinating pains in palmar surface of l. middle finger.

23. **Lower Limbs.**—Pinching back of l. thigh along track of sciatic nerve.—Pains in knees; under patellæ, now one now the other.—Lancinations in l. calf.—Sudden cutting in l. tendo Achillis when stooping.—Violent and dull lancinations in l. os calcis.—Dull pains in heels, chiefly l.—Sharp pains in r. great toe-joint.

24. **Generalities.**—Clonic spasms of muscles of nape of neck or extremities, which were at one time extended, at another flexed, frequently repeated spontaneously on the slightest irritation, muscles relaxed completely in intervals.—Sudden jerking of whole body, followed by violent stitches in extensors and drawing back of head.—Great weakness after a paroxysm.—Uneasiness: in morning; in afternoon.—Increased sensitiveness to cold; pale face.

25. **Skin.**—Herpetic eruption: on upper lip, l. side; under lower lip near l. commissure.—At inner border of l. wrist-joint intense and obstinate itching, without eruption, > pressure.—Itching of pubes almost constant during several days.

26. **Sleep.**—Almost irresistible drowsiness in morning.—Restless nights; unable to sleep before 2 a.m.

27. **Fever.**—Feels chilly very easily, passing shivers.—Shivering; burning in palms after dark.—Shivering along spine and both arms.—Flashes of heat and redness of face and hands, evening after a meal, with drowsiness.—Night-sweat.

Uranium Nitricum.

Nitrate of Uranium. Uranyl Nitrate. $UO_2 2NO_3 6H_2O$. Solution in distilled water. Trituration.

Clinical.—Albuminuria. Anus, pruritus of. *Diabetes, mellitus and insipidus. Duodenum, ulcer of.* Enuresis, nocturnal. *Gastric ulcer.* Impotence. Milk, excessive secretion of. Ophthalmia. Phosphaturia. Seminal emissions. Sleeplessness. Stomatitis. Stye. *Urine, fishy odour of;* incontinence of.

Characteristics.—*Uranium* belongs to the *Chromium* group of elements. *Ur. nit.* was proved by E. T. Blake, whose monograph on the salt forms part of the *Hahnemann Materia Medica.* Blake's proving was suggested by the observation of an old-school experimenter, Leconte, who found sugar in the urine of dogs slowly poisoned with *Ur. nit.* Blake was not very successful in producing sugar, but his proving is not any less valuable on that account, and clinical use has filled out the picture. Many cases of diabetes have been relieved or cured by *Ur. nit.*, usually in the lower attenuations. In a case of diabetes insipidus of mine, in a young girl, *Ur. nit.* 30 gave more relief than any other remedy. Excessive thirst, polyuria, and dry tongue are the indications. Glycosuria is by no means an essential part of the indications for *Ur. nit.* In some of the animals experimented on by Blake the pylorus was found to be affected. With this the symptoms of the proving correspond, and *Ur. nit.* has cured both pyloric and gastric ulcer. One case (*N.A.J.H.*, Aug., 1890) in a married woman was cured with 5-gr. doses of the 2x. Patient was weak and emaciated; vomited mucus mixed with blood and coffee-ground matter, and passed dark, tarry stools; sensitive and tender over region of pylorus. *Sensations are:* As if blood were flowing to head. As if he had taken cold with headache. The left side was more affected than the right. Many symptoms were < at night. Head < walking. > Deep inspiration.

Relations.—*Compare:* Elemental relatives; gastro-duodenal affections, Chrom., and K. bi. Diabetes, Ph. ac., Syzyg., Thyr., Lac def., Lact. ac. Sinking immediately after meals, Ars., Cin., Lyc., Sil., Stp. Craves tea, Selen.

SYMPTOMS.

1. **Mind.**—Ill-humour; and not feeling well all day.

2. **Head.**—Vertigo twice in evening.—Head heavy on waking.—Pain: in forehead; over l. eye; in forehead and occiput in evening; in temple; in occipital protuberances; in occiput on walking.—Neuralgia on posterior edge of l. temporal bone (formerly on r.) from 2 till 4 p.m. leaving dull aching, neuralgia woke me at 1 a.m. that night, lasted an hour and prevented sleep, ill from the pain during next day, two days later pain in old place (r. side) came on gradually, > by dinner.

3. **Eyes.**—Stye in l. upper lid.—(Œdema of lower lids worse than

usual.)—Lids inflamed, agglutinated.—Shooting from r. orbit to occipital protuberance in evening.—Pain over l. eye.

5. **Nose.**—Itching in nose.—L. nostril stuffed.—Dry coryza.

8. **Mouth.**—Painless ulcer, with one elevated side, in mouth opposite l. anterior upper molar, < evening.—Acid saliva.

9. **Throat.**—Hawking of tenacious mucus.—Contracted feeling in throat.

10. **Appetite.**—Appetite lost; (during menses).—Craves raw ham and tea.

11. **Stomach.**—Eructations; tasteless; putrid at 11 and 3 o'clock.—Indigestion in afternoon a quarter of an hour before dinner, with gnawing sinking at cardiac end of stomach, not hungry nor faint.—Dyspepsia, flatus after food, acidity, pain from cardiac end of stomach to suprarenal region, > movement, lasted all day, bowels slightly moved, pale clay-coloured fæces (query, if from the drug, as I had had similar but slighter attacks), afterwards epigastric pain as above returned, > by food, with occasional twisting-screwing feeling lower down.—(Gastric and duodenal ulcers.—Recurring hæmatemesis.)

12. **Abdomen.**—Flatus; abdomen bloated.—Borborygmi.—Sharp colic, with tenesmus and with raw feeling in rectum, afterwards in sleep unconscious seminal emission.—Enteritis and peritonitis with meteorism; great prostration.

13. **Stool.**—Urging in rectum and bladder, waking me at 2 a.m., borborygmi, soft stool.—Stool twice in one day.—Constipation.—Pruritus ani.

14. **Urinary Organs.**—Sore pain in vesical region in evening,—Urine contained bile.—Urine high-coloured, a few lithates on standing.—"It produces acute parenchymatous nephritis; sugar is found in the urine, this generally does not come on until after albumen has appeared; glycosuria is very characteristic and persistent; it also produces at times a large amount of oxalate of lime."—Profuse nocturnal urination.—Urination profuse, painful, pale milky.—Acute and chronic diseases of adults.—Diabetes insipidus.—Diabetes mellitus.—Nocturnal enuresis.—Urine greenish and smelling fishy.

15. **Male Sexual Organs.**—Completely impotent with nocturnal emissions; organs cold, relaxed, sweaty.

16. **Female Sexual Organs.**—During menses: vertigo; faint; flushing of upper part of body.—No menstrual flow during diabetic attack; pale, anæmic; craves raw ham and tea.—Excessive secretion of milk.

17. **Respiratory Organs.**—Bronchitis, with copious mucous expectoration and much emaciation; chronic colds.—Cough with purulent discharge from l. nostril; lung infiltrated with grey tubercle.

18. **Chest.**—Intermittent pain radiating from l. side to ensiform cartilage; < fasting.

20. **Back.**—Loins stiff.—(Pain at lower angle of l. scapula < deep inspiration.)

21. **Limbs.**—White vesicles on arms and legs with red areolæ; burn and itch.

24. **Generalities.**—Extreme languor; on rising from bed.—Feeling as if he had taken cold.

25. **Skin.**—Epithelioma; lupus excedens; ecchymoses.

26. **Sleep.**—Night restless with shivering and heat.—Languor.

Urea.

Carbamide. The chief solid constituent of the urine of mammals. (White crystals.) $CO(NH_2)_2$. Trituration. Solution [also tincture or solution of the nitrate—Urea nitrica].

Clinical.—Albuminuria. Diabetes. Dropsy. Eczema, gouty. Gout. Liver, cirrhosis of. Tuberculosis. Uræmia.

Characteristics.—The failure of the kidneys to eliminate *Urea* from the blood leads to uræmic intoxication, delirium, convulsions, and coma. On general indications *Urea* has been used in medicine by both schools. Merck mentions that it is diuretic, and is used in cirrhosis of liver, pleurisy, renal calculus. Allen cites from Mauthner two cases of renal dropsy with symptoms of general intoxication in which *Urea nit.*, gr. ii., divided into three doses and given two hours apart, cured brilliantly. Burnett has used both *Urea* 6 and *Uric acid* 6 in gouty eczema, "where the gouty eczema has been the cutaneous outlet for the constitution." Burnett gave *Urea* in gouty cases where the urine was thin and of low specific gravity; "it thickens the urine and gives great relief to the patient." Arthur H. Buch (*Med. Press*, Aug 14, 1901) relates cases of tuberculosis cured, on the plan originated by Harper, of Nottingham, with *Urea* in 20- to 30-grain doses three times a day. *Urea*, Buch says, "is formed in the spleen, lymph and secreting glands, but principally by the liver." Under the treatment, lupoid nodules disappeared; tuberculous glands disappeared; tuberculous joints improved. No ill-effects of the treatment were noticed; "on the contrary, the action has evidently been in many cases that of a nervous tonic." Villers (*J. of Hcs.*, iv. 403) examined the urine of an intensely neurasthenic woman, suffering from severe asthma and found 4·5 per cent. of *Urea* instead of the usual 2·5. In order to find out the effect of *Urea* on the healthy he took for five days *Urea* 15 x., five drops thrice daily. He was then compelled to stop by the severity of the symptoms. He gave the same dose to a patient, a woman. She begged after a short time to be allowed to discontinue the medicine, as it affected her so painfully, causing constant urging to urinate; much sediment in the urine; intolerable sensation in abdomen and burning of the skin. The symptoms of Villers and this patient are marked (V) in the Schema.

Relations.—*Compare:* Urinum, Uric acid, Thios., Urt. urens. Diuresis, Thyr. Tuberculosis, Tub., Bac.

SYMPTOMS.

2. **Head.**—Head very dull, as if filled with a very heavy lump (V).

3. **Eyes.**—Itching and profuse watering of eyes (agg.—V).

12. **Abdomen.**—In r. hypochondrium, a steady, dull sensation (V).—Intolerable sensation in abdomen and burning of the skin (V).

14. **Urinary Organs.**—Constant urging to urinate, beginning at root of penis (V).—Constant urging, with much sediment in urine (V).—From bladder

to her groins a fatiguing, tearing pain < standing (V).—Profuse diuresis with rapid diminution of dropsy.—Albuminuria; bloody urine; general dropsy; intermittent heart (boy, 7, *Urea nit.* gr. ii., taken in three doses at two hours' interval, cured).—Delirium, nose-bleed, urine brown, very albuminous; œdema of pudenda; ascites; pulse small, slow; attacks of suffocation (girl, 6, *Ur. nit.* as above; urine increased; swelling decreased; albumen disappeared).

15. **Male Sexual Organs.**—Itching along sulcus of glans and a general tired feeling (agg.—V.)

24. **Generalities.**—General uneasiness; felt ill, poisoned (V).—Uræmia.—Acted as a nervous tonic in tuberculous patients.

Uricum Acidum.

Uric Acid. Lithic Acid. $C_5N_4H_4O_3$. Trituration.

Clinical.—Eczema, gouty. Gout. Lipoma. Rheumatism.

Characteristics.—*Uric ac.* has been used on inferential grounds in gouty conditions. Burnett gave it in 5th and 6th attenuations. It is most useful in cases where deposits persist; it stirs them up and helps to eliminate them. It is useful in gouty eczema where the eczema has been "the cutaneous outlet for the constitution." With *Uric ac.* 3x. Mersch (*H. W.*, xxx. 395) cured a case of lipoma situated on the left side between abdomen and breast, "as large as a man's head, only lengthened." Relief was immediate; the tumour disappeared in a month.

Relations.—*Compare:* Urea, Urtica urens.

Urinum.

Urine. Dilutions.

Clinical.—Acne. Boils. Dropsy. Ophthalmia. Scurvy.

Characteristics.—Under *Urea* Allen gives some symptoms observed on a man who, for a skin affection, drank in the morning the urine he had passed the night before. The symptoms were severe, consisting of general dropsy, scanty urine, and excessive weakness. These symptoms I have arranged under *Urinum.* Urinotherapy is practically as old as man himself. The Chinese (*Therapist*, x. 329) treat wounds by sprinkling urine on them, and the custom is widespread in the Far East. Taken internally it is believed to stimulate the circulation; and is valued as an active oxytocic. The parturient woman drinks the urine of a male child four to five years old, and the part voided in the middle of micturition. The child urinates into three vessels, the woman drinking the contents of the second. In the *Brit. Med. Jour.* of 1900 a number of instances of Western urinotherapy were given (collected *H. W.*, xxxv. 507). To these Cooper has made some additions (*ibid.*, p. 584). The cases are these: (1) A youth for crops of boils which nothing could remedy was recommended to drink every morning for three mornings a cupful of his own urine. Then after an intermission of three days to resume, and so on till cured. He was cured on the ninth day. (2) "Blackheads" cured in exactly the same way. This patient drank it when fresh. (3) Chronic bronchitis much relieved. This patient was deaf, and misunderstood the doctor's direction to *bring* some of his urine. He thought *drink* was the word and acted accordingly. (4) Ague (in the Lincolnshire fens). (5) Urticaria. (6) For thrush it is a custom in Yorkshire to wipe the baby's tongue with its own napkin. (7) For pimples and blotches the negroes of Barbados drink their urine and apply it locally. (8) For ophthalmia in children it is the custom in Switzerland to bathe the eyes in the children's own urine. Cooper mentions the case of a man who suffered very much from weak and inflamed eyes until he adopted this plan, which after a time cured him. Cooper also mentions that a celebrated breeder of cattle and horses succeeded in getting his animals' skin into an astonishing condition of fineness by giving them about a tablespoonful of old human urine with every meal. Kraft (*A. H.*, xxvii. 4) mentions that urine has been used as a remedy for croup. S. Mills Fowler (*M. A.*, xx. 281) mentions the use of urine as a remedy for scurvy in the Civil War. In Andersonville prison the starving prisoners were dying by hundreds of scurvy, and Mr. T. (who told the story) was one of the sufferers. His legs were flexed upon the thighs and the thighs upon the body in such violent contraction that it was impossible to extend them an inch, and any attempt to do so was attended with shocks of pain as from an electric battery. He could only move on his elbows and rump. Within the stockade were growing two large turpentine trees. Of the pitch from these trees the patients would take enough to make their urine "clear and white as crystal." The urine voided was allowed to stand till it began to sour, which took twelve to twenty-four hours. The patients then took a "good swallow" four or five times a day. They felt the good effect of every dose. The treatment cured Mr. T. and all his companions in misfortune who adopted it. These cures are to some extent analogous with nosode cures, as the patients drank their own urine; but *Urinum*, *Urea*, *Uric acid* are also medicines on their own account, and rank with the Sarcodes. The symptoms of uræmia may be taken as a pathogenesis of *Urinum* for the use of the attenuations. *Urea* cured renal dropsy, and *Urinum* produced it. The skin action of *Urinum* is remarkable in connection with its use in the dressing of leather; no substitute having been found for it in this.

Relations.—*Compare:* Urea (probably urine owes its chief effect to urea), Ur. ac., Urt. urens.

SYMPTOMS.

2. **Head.**—Heaviness of head, < on stooping.

6. **Face.**—Face very much swollen.—Countenance pale, expression heavy and vague.

11. **Stomach.**—Little thirst.

12. **Abdomen.**—Fluid in abdomen and in parietes of chest and belly.

14. **Urinary Organs.**—Urine scanty, thick, deep brown, and very offensive.

24. **Generalities.**—Anasarca ; generally more marked in upper than in lower parts of body.—Heaviness, heavy for work, having neither his usual life nor warmth in him.—Loses her breath if she walks quick, is obliged to stop.

Urtica Urens.

Urtica urens. Small Stinging-nettle. [Urtica dioica, the Common Nettle, has similar if not identical properties.] *N. O.* Urticaceæ. Tincture of the fresh plant in flower.

Clinical.—Agalactia. Anæmia. Bee-stings. *Burns. Calculus, prevention of.* Deltoid, rheumatism of. Dysentery. Erysipelas, vesicular. Erythema. *Gout.* Gravel. Hæmorrhages. Intermittents. Lactation. Leucorrhœa. Menorrhagia. Phlegmasia dolens. Renal colic. Rheumatism. *Spleen, affections of.* Throat, sore. Uræmia. Urticaria ; nodosa. Vertigo. Whooping-cough. Worms.

Characteristics.—Burnett may be said to have rediscovered *Urtica* as a remedy. The history of how he came to use it (*Gout*, p. 33) is one of the most fascinating passages of his works. As a remedy for a fit of the gout the discovery is entirely his own, and the result of great therapeutic acumen. Its use in gravel and urinary affections is very old. "Being eaten, as Dioscorides saith, boiled with periwinkles, it maketh the body soluble, doing it by a kind of cleansing faculty : it also provoketh urine and expelleth stones out of the kidneys : being boiled with barley cream it is thought to bring up tough humours that stick in the chest." Gerarde, from whom I quote, mentions these other uses : (1) The juice inserted into the nostrils stops nose-bleed ; it is "good against inflammation of the uvula." (2) Pleurisy, pneumonia, whooping-cough. (3) Antidote to Hemlock, Mushrooms, Quicksilver, Henbane, Serpents, Scorpions. "The leaves or seeds of any kind of nettle," says Gerarde, "do work the like effect, but not with that good speed and so assured as the Roman nettle" (*U. pilulifera*). "A bundle of nettles," says Cooper, "applied to a rheumatic joint or part, has long been a favourite country remedy. A leaf of the nettle placed on the tongue and pressed to the roof of the mouth stops bleeding from the nose." Burnett's tincture is made of the small nettle, *U. urens*, which is the correct one in homœpathy. Burnett had used *Urt. u.* a good deal in spleen affections, and found patients under its use often passed large quantities of gravel. To a middle-aged maiden lady who had enlarged spleen, and "who smelled so strongly of nettles that it almost nauseated me whenever it was my duty to examine her," Burnett gave *Urt. u.* ϕ. Whilst taking it she passed large quantities of gravel. But this did not attract much notice, as the lady was in the habit of passing considerable quantities of gravel *with her motions.* Localised abdominal pain preceding such an occasion by a number of days. The painfu spot, just under her spleen, she called her "gravel-pit." Putting this and other points together, the fever-action of *Urtica* among the number, Burnett concluded that *Urtica* was a remedy for acute gout, which would cut short the attack "*in a safe manner*, namely, by ridding the economy of the essence of the disease product, its actual suffering-producing material." He usually ordered five drops of the tincture in a wineglassful of quite warm water every two or three hours. Under its action the urine became more plentiful, dark, and loaded with uric acid. Burnett remarks of the nettle that it springs up everywhere near human habitations, and he has noticed it flourishing more by the side of ditches which carry off fluid sewage, "thus possibly living to some extent on uric food." A very severe case of uræmia was cured by him with *Urt.* His discovery of its fever action was through the cure of a lady patient of his of ague (which he had not succeeded in curing) by drinking nettle-tea on the advice of her charwoman. *Urt. ur.* was his sheet-anchor in cases of the fevers of the East—India, Burma, and Siam. This action of *Urtica*, as well as its antigout action, I have had abundant opportunity of verifying. *Urtica* causes fever as well as cures it, and one of Burnett's patients was obliged to stop taking it: "It sets all my pulses beating, makes me terribly giddy, makes me feel as if I was going to topple (forwards) on my head, and then a bad headache comes on; and when I take it *at night*, it makes me very feverish." When she took the dose in the morning she did not have the fever, and Burnett says, "The fever of gout generally comes on at night." He has often cured vertigo with *Urt.* The provings of *Urtica* are not very extensive; but supplemented by clinical observations, the picture is fairly complete. Headache, with spleen pain; rush of blood to head; soreness of abdomen; dysentery; burning and itching of anus; œdema; urticaria; rheumatic and gouty pains, and fever were all evoked. Among the rheumatic pains a pain in the right deltoid muscle is very striking. The relation of this symptom to Burnett's use of *Urt.* is illustrated by the case of Dr. W. H. Proctor (*A. H.*, xxvii. 126). The doctor was suddenly seized with agonising pain in right deltoid muscle, due, he believed, to retention of uric acid in the system. Hypodermic injections of Morphia and Atropia had to be resorted to. Then followed, for three weeks, scanty, pale urine, sour sweat, sleeplessness, restlessness, nervousness, loss of appetite, almost constant pain in deltoid with great soreness and lameness of the muscle, an intense sensation of general sickness and weakness *with continued fever.* Nothing did any good. Finally there appeared: An intense burning sensation in the skin after sleeping: he was *afraid to go to sleep* for fear of the suffering. *Urt. ur.* φ was now taken. After three doses he drifted into a quiet, refreshing sleep of two or three hours and woke absolutely free from all skin irritation. The nerves were quieted and all symptoms passed away. Soon after, Proctor had an opportunity of curing a patient of lameness of the deltoid of some standing in the same expeditious way. In this case there were no additional symptoms. J. L. Nottingham (*H. R.*, xv. 244) treated (1) Mrs. W., 38, tall, slender, with auburn hair, for eczema vulvæ with violent itching and burning, swelling and thickening of labia, smooth, pale, dry appearance of the mucous surface, a dry, scaly, fissured appearance of labia majora and skin. Thirteen years before, she had had a sinus from the right ovary emptying into the uterus. (The husband had sycotic warts on the glans penis.) *Urt. ur.* 1 x relieved all the symptoms and removed sexual excitement induced by the itching and uncontrollable desire to rub. (2) Mr. N., 21, had swelling, stinging, burning of face, hands, and feet, with redness. Rubbing with finger-tip would leave a white line for some time. When out in the cold, damp, snowy air, hands, feet, and face became purple red, puffed, and stinging cold ; going into a warm room he had increased swelling, stinging, itching all over him, especially of hands and face. *Urt. ur.* relieved in twenty-four hours. In four days he returned home better than he had been for years. (3) A woman with a lump in her left breast of some years' duration, was seen six weeks after childbirth, complaining of stinging pains in that part, entire absence of milk, stinging pains in whole right lower limb, with great soreness and stinging pains accompanying movements involving muscles of left side of head, cervical vertebræ, sacrum, and upper limbs, front of chest and both breasts, especially the left. She was very despondent. *Act. r.* relieved her, but the improvement ceased after a week. *Con.* improved the difficulty in moving the head but not the other symptoms. *Urt. ur.* was given, and after three days the breasts filled with milk and the pain was relieved. The breasts had now to be supported on account of their fulness. The right leg became natural. The action of *Urt.* in causing flow of milk has been often confirmed. In the case given in *Allen* it caused swelling of the breasts and profuse flow of milk in a woman years after the birth of her last child. *Urt.* is one of the best remedies for burns of the first degree, used locally and given internally. Gerarde mentions its antidotal action to snake-bites. A writer in *Monats. f. Hom.* of July, 1900 (*H. Envoy*, xi. 51) says it is *the* specific for bee-stings. An application of the tincture even on the most sensitive parts of the face or eyelid gives instant relief. In cases of stings about the eyes the application may have to be repeated every five minutes; and a compress must be kept on all night. Eclectics regard "profuse discharge from the mucous surfaces" as a specific indication for *Urt.* In Sweden nettles are regarded as a remedy for anæmia, and fresh nettles are cooked and eaten like spinach for the purpose, or a nettle-tea is prepared from dry nettles. The juice of nettles with sugar is in vogue for hæmorrhages of all kinds. *Sensations* of *Urt.* are : As from a blow in the eyeballs. As of sand in eyes. Muscles of right arm as if bruised. Burning, stinging, itching, and soreness are the principal pains. The right side very much affected ; but also the left hypochondrium (spleen). The symptoms are apt to return at the same season every year. This periodicity is a point in the correspondence of *Urt.* to ague. The symptoms are < by touch ; lying on arm. < Violent exertion (hæmoptysis). Lying down = soreness of bowels ; > nettle-rash. Burning in skin is < after sleep. < From application of water. (In the one observation with *U. crenulata*, an attack like lockjaw was induced in a man who lightly touched the plant, and this was renewed for some days in full force whenever *he put his hand in water*.)

< Exposed to cool, moist atmosphere.—Some new symptoms of Burnett's I have marked (B) in the Schema.

Relations.—*Antidoted by:* Dock leaves (Rumex obtus.) rubbed on the stung part lessen the pain; also the nettle's own juice, and the juice from the common snail. *Antidote to:* Apis (bee-stings). *Compare:* Gout, fever, spleen, Nat m. Dropsy, uræmia, gravel, gout, Ur. ac., Urea, Urinum. [The relation of Urt. to Nat. m. and Urinum is interesting in connection with the fact that nettles do not grow at any distance from human dwellings or away from parts where animals are fed. Schlegel asks (*H. R.*, xii. 179), is this due to the wetting of the soil with urine? He says yes; and queries further, if the *salt* in the urine is the efficient agent, recalling the fact that Barbarossa, after destroying Milan, strewed *salt* over the ruins "so that *nettles* might grow there." Schlegel remarks that the briny waves produce stinging nettles of their own in the shape of Medusæ.] Fever, vertigo, spleen, Querc. Spleen, Cean. Rheumatism of right deltoid, Sang. Secretion of milk, Ric., Puls. Urticaria, Apis, Nat. m., Ast. fl., Medusa, Homar, Pariet.

Causation.—Burns. Bee-stings. Blows. Suppressed milk. Suppressed nettle-rash.

SYMPTOMS.

2. **Head.**—Terribly giddy, as if I were going to topple forwards on my head; then headache (B).—Fulness in head, sensation of rush of blood and dulness; all day, with giddiness.—Headache < over eyes.—Headache with stitches in region of spleen.—Pain: in r. side of sinciput; and in r. side of face, extending to malar-bone; over r. eye and eyeball; over eyes during the day and evening; neuralgic, in r. side of forehead and face at 9 p.m.—Stinging pain in r. parietal bone forcing me to rub and press it.—Dull aching in occiput and over eyes.—Urticaria of scalp suddenly appearing and determining internally.

3. **Eyes.**—Pain: in r. eye; in l. at 3 p.m.—Pain in eyeballs as from a blow, with feeling as if sand were in eyes.—Eyes feel weak and sore.

9. **Throat.**—Burning in throat; with frequent hawking of frothy mucus; causing cough, expectoration scanty, frothy.

11. **Stomach.**—Nausea, with burning in throat.—Vomiting from suppression of nettle-rash.

12. **Abdomen.**—Soreness of abdomen at 10 a.m. when lying, and on pressure a sound as if bowels were full of water.—Pain in l. hypochondrium at 10 p.m.—(Tumour of liver; "stored gout."—Burnett.)

13. **Stool and Anus.**—Stool omitted in morning, but at 2 p.m. scanty, dysenteric stool, a greenish-brown slime, with urging and tenesmus, afterwards constipation, then small stool with straining, later dysentery, frequent urging, small painful stool, mucus mixed with white matter like boiled white of eggs, at times a little blood, pain in abdomen for a week.—Stool omitted for three days, then six hours after *Nux* 3 a natural stool, four hours later several dysenteric stools of whitish slime, with pain around umbilicus, then for the next five days, daily, two to four white and yellow stools mixed with mucus,

with colic and tenesmus.—A small hæmorrhoid, with raw burning in anus during and after stool, and in afternoon and evening itching and burning.—Ascarides with great rectal irritation.

14. **Urinary Organs.**—Urine suppressed for eight days, everything disappeared with desquamation.—Suppression of urine for twelve days ; œdematous swelling of whole upper body to umbilicus.—Strangury ; gravel ; disease of bladder and kidneys.—Hæmorrhage from bladder.

15. **Male Sexual Organs.**—Itching of scrotum, kept him awake at night and tormented him nearly all day ; scrotum swollen ; stinging and itching ; no moisture.

16. **Female Sexual Organs.**—Menorrhagia ; intense hæmorrhage.—Leucorrhœa, very acrid or excoriating.—Pruritus vulvæ with great itching, stinging, and œdema of the parts.—A woman who had had no children for three years and a half, and had nursed none of her children, had at first great swelling of breasts, which discharged serum, then copious milk (from a pint of hot infusion of the herb).—Arrested flow of milk after weaning.

17. **Respiratory Organs.**—Whooping-cough.—Not much expectoration, and what there is is frothy.

18. **Chest.**—Sore feeling as from a blow in l. side of chest.—Intermittent soreness in r. chest during day.—Hæmoptysis from least exertion of lungs.

19. **Pulse.**—Pulse accelerated.

21. **Limbs.**—Rheumatic pain in arms and ankles, < r. arm.

22. **Upper Limbs.**—Pain in r. deltoid, < 9 p.m., could not put on his coat alone.—Cramplike pain in r. deltoid in evening ; < rotating arm inward, with soreness to touch, with rheumatic feeling in l. arm ; next day pain in r. arm < by lying on it ; and on moving it a stitch darted through arm, extending over front of humerus.—At times pain in l. arm, muscles of r. arm feel sore as if bruised, cannot raise or stretch r. arm on account of pain, afterwards rheumatic stiffness and pain in r. wrist, later rheumatic pain in l. arm, wrist, and fingers.—Raised, red, itching blisters on skin of hands and fingers.—(Nodous joints of fingers.—R. T. C.)

23. **Lower Limbs.**—Stiff soreness on inside of l. knee.—Rheumatic pain in both ankles.

24. **Generalities.**—Symptoms returned at the same time every year.—Hæmorrhage from various organs.—Dropsy.—Sets all my pulses beating (B)

25. **Skin.**—Itching swellings all over fingers and hands, resembling "bold hives" ; lumps and red spots on hands and fever blisters on lips, itching.—Heat in skin of face, arms, shoulders, and chest, with formication, numbness and itching, lips, nose, and ears swollen, lids so œdematous that they could scarcely be opened, after awhile upper part of body as far as navel œdematous and pale, transparent blisters filled with serum and looking like sudamina, becoming confluent and making the skin look wrinkled, lids closed, forming transparent, here and there bluish shining swellings as large as hen's eggs ; disappeared on sixth day with desquamation.—(Intense burning in skin after sleep.)—Erythema.—Vesicular erysipelas.—Burns and scalds.

26. **Sleep.**—Drowsiness when reading.

27. **Fever.**—General heat on getting into bed, with soreness over abdomen.—When I take it at night it makes me very feverish (not when taken in morning.—B).

Usnea Barbata.

Usnea barbata. Tree-hair. Tree-moss. *N. O.* Lichenes. Tincture.

Clinical.—Headache, congestive.

Characteristics.—An article by M. B. in *U. S. Med. Invest.* (quoted *New, Old, and Forgotten Remedies*) gives an observation by the writer, who ate a little of the "moss" and had in consequence a severe congestive headache which compelled him to give up his work and go to bed. He got to sleep and woke very well next morning. Two young ladies out picking cranberries had headache from riding in the hot sun and were compelled to lie down. *Usn. b.* ϕ, one drop in a tumbler of water, a teaspoonful to be taken at once and repeated in fifteen minutes. The second dose stopped the pain. A young married lady subject to headache for five years; was almost frantic with the pain. *Usn. b.*, as above, cured in one or two doses.

SYMPTOMS.

2. **Head.**—Head began to ache; soon could feel the blood press into the brain; with domestic attentions he got to sleep, and woke next morning uncommonly well.—Pain over entire head or front head, with feeling as if temples would burst or eyes burst out of sockets.

Ustilago.

Ustilago maidis. Corn-smut. *N. O.* Fungi. Trituration.

Clinical.—Agalactia. Alopecia. Climaxis. Dysmenorrhœa. Fibroma. Galactorrhœa. Headache, menstrual. Masturbation. Menorrhagia, at climaxis. *Menstruation, excessive*; vicarious. Nails, affections of. Orchitis. Ovary, left, affections of. Rhinitis. Scald-head. Tonsillitis.

Characteristics.—Burt, who proved *Ust.* on himself and others, introduced the remedy to homœopathy. It had been observed that pregnant animals feeding on maize affected with smut were very liable to abort. Roullin had noted that shedding of the hair, and sometimes of the teeth, occurred in animals and men; that mules fed on it cast their hoofs, and that fowls laid eggs without shells. The provings brought out a specific affinity for the generative sphere of both sexes, and especially for the left ovary and uterus. *Ust.* congests the uterus and produces hæmorrhages, generally passive or in clots. It is in uterine hæmorrhages, menstrual, post-partum and climacteric that *Ust.* has been most successfully employed. It has also relieved vicarious menstruation, bleeding taking place from the lungs and bowels; and bleeding between the periods with left inframammary pain. Hurndall (*H. W.*, xxxvi. 27) relates the case of the small bitch which brings out many features of *Ustilago* action. About a fortnight before he saw the patient she had aborted five fœtuses, at about the fifth week of gestation. Since then there had been passive hæmorrhage of dark clots. Moreover, she was a *perfect specimen of alopecia*, not having a hair of any sort on her body and only a little about the head. Os uteri soft, spongy. Great tenderness about the posterior parts when manipulating the hind-quarters. *Ust.* 3x was prescribed, five drops three times a day. In two days the hæmorrhage was completely arrested, tenderness reduced, spirits revived, and general health improved. At the end of three months there was a nice coat of hair growing, which in due course became perfectly normal. Loss of hair and nails is a keynote for *Ust.*, and combined with the other symptoms made the correspondence perfect. Among the *Peculiar Sensations* are: As if head were being lifted off. As if forehead would burst open. As if something were under root of tongue pressing upward. As of a lump behind larynx. Excessively tired feeling. Bearing down, as if everything would come from her. Uterus as if drawn into a knot. As if intestines were being tied in knots. (This last symptom was produced in a patient of mine.) The symptoms are: < By touch (abdomen ; eyes). Pressure < (ovaries). Riding in carriage < backache. < Rising and motion (menorrhagia). Walking < frontal headache ; pain in left groin ; pain in loins. Warm room = oppression and faintness. Open air = lachrymation. Swelling < pains in tonsils. Colicky pains > by constipated stool.

Relations.—*Compare:* Botan., uterine affections, nails, Sec. Subinvolution, Na. hcl. Bearing down and prolapse of uterus, Sep. Left ovarian pain, Lil., Lach., Caul., Sul., Thuj., Vib. o. Vicarious menstruation, Bry., Ham. Millef. Intermittent flow, Ham., Bovis., Elaps. Crusta lactea, Vinc. m., Melit., Med., Mez. Pain in right shoulder, Urt. ur., Sang. Flying rheumatic pains, Puls. Faint at 11 a.m., Sul. Frequent emissions and lumbar pains, Cob.

SYMPTOMS.

1. **Mind.**—Depression of spirits in afternoon.—Very sad, cries frequently ; exceedingly prostrated from sexual abuse and loss of semen ; sleep restless.—Could not bear to see or talk with any one.—Irritability, < being asked a question or to repeat anything.—The day seemed like a dream.

2. **Head.**—Vertigo in attacks, sometimes with double vision, sometimes white specks blot out everything else, later attacks of vertigo with internal heat.—Vertigo at climaxis with profuse menstruation.—Headache: all the morning ; at 7 a.m. ; in evening, < forehead ; < walking.—Nervous headache from menstrual irregularities in nervous women.—Frontal pain: in morning; in forenoon, with smarting in eyes ; all day, with aching distress in eyeballs and with fulness in head in morning; with distress in epigastrium.—Scalp dry, head congested, with loss of hair.—Scald-head, watery serum oozing from scalp.—Prickling in l. temple.—Loss of hair.

3. **Eyes.**—Attacks of twitching in eyes, they appear to look (revolve) in

circles and dart from one object to another.—Continual watery flow from eyes and nose with occasional chills.—Spasms, with vanishing of vision and head seems to whirl.—Aching in eyes and lachrymation.—Hot feeling on closing lids.—Weakness of eyes.—Lachrymation in open air.—Lids agglutinated in morning.—Vision of spots dancing to and fro.

5. **Nose.**—Boil in r. nostril.—Dryness of nostrils in forenoon, with dry feeling in skin.—Bright epistaxis, > pressure.—Rhinitis, bitter taste, offensive odour noticeable to patient himself.

6. **Face.**—Sudden pallor in face when sitting, and in evening.—Burning of face and scalp from congestion.

7. **Teeth.**—Sometimes looseness of teeth.—Aching all day in decayed upper first and second molars.—Shedding of teeth (in animals).

8. **Mouth.**—Tongue coated in morning.—Prickling in tongue, with feeling as if something were pressing the roots upward, with dryness of nostrils.—Salivation : bitter ; thin, bitter.—Taste : coppery; in morning; slimy coppery; slimy coppery in morning; slimy; slimy, with burning distress in stomach.

9. **Throat.**—L. tonsil enlarged, congested, dark reddish, r. painful on swallowing at 2 p.m. ; l. painful at 9 p.m. ; next morning congestion of l. extending along Eustachian tube and causing pain in ear.—Lancinations in r. tonsil (fauces were somewhat inflamed when the medicine was taken), next day fauces hotter and more sensitive to motion.—Roughness of fauces.—Dryness of fauces, with burning dryness in stomach.—Dryness of fauces, with difficulty in swallowing, feeling of a lump behind larynx, later frequent efforts to swallow, with feeling as if something had lodged in fauces, afterwards irritation of fauces, and on swallowing feeling of a lump in larynx.—Burning in œsophagus at cardiac orifice.

10. **Appetite.**—Appetite : craving; poor.—Thirst at night.

11. **Stomach.**—Eructations : of sour fluid ; of sour food.—Cutting in stomach.—Pain in stomach : frequently in afternoon ; on full inspiration.—Pain in epigastrium with drawing pain in joints of fingers.—Burning in sternum and cardia.—Distress in stomach in forenoon ; in afternoon, > by supper.—Hæmatemesis, passive, venous, accompanied by nausea, which is > by vomiting.

12. **Abdomen.**—Periodical cutting in umbilical and hypogastric regions at 6 p.m., < at 8 p.m. by a constipated stool, afterwards grumbling pains in whole abdomen.—(Pain as if intestines were tied in knots.)—Pain : in r. lobe of liver ; in umbilicus ; in umbilicus before natural stool ; in l. groin when walking.—Drawing pain in r. hypochondrium all day.—Distress in umbilicus and r. hypochondrium.

13. **Stool.**—Natural stool at 4 a.m.—Loose stool at 4 a.m., with pain and rumbling in abdomen.—Light-coloured diarrhœa.—Soft stool, next day dry, lumpy, two days later black, dry, lumpy.—Constipated.

14. **Urinary Organs.**—Tenesmus of bladder and incontinence of urine.—Urging, urine light-coloured.—No desire, but uneasiness.—Urine : increased ; scanty, red ; acid, high-coloured.

15. **Male Sexual Organs.**—Genitals relaxed.—Erections : when reading at 4 o'clock ; frequently during day and night.—Scrotum relaxed and cold sweat on it.—Pain in testes, < r.—Pain in testes, sometimes neuralgic ;

in paroxysms, sometimes causing faintish feeling.—Desire depressed.—Chroric orchitis, irritable testicle.—Erotic fancies.—Seminal emissions and irresistible tendency to masturbation.

16. **Female Sexual Organs.**—Yellow and offensive leucorrhœa.—Tenderness of l. ovary, with pain and swelling.—Burning distress in ovaries.—Intermittent neuralgia of l. ovary ; enlarged, very tender.—Uterus : hypertrophied ; prolapsed ; cervix sensitive, spongy.—Menses : too scanty with ovarian irritation ; too profuse and too early ; blood clotted ; as if everything would come through.—Between periods constant suffering under l. breast at margin of ribs.—Oozing of dark blood, highly coagulated, forming occasionally long, black, stringy clots.—Extreme pain during period.—Suppression of menses.—Vicarious menstruation from lungs and bowels.—Constant aching distress at mouth of womb.—Menses that had just ceased returned, bright-coloured, soreness and bearing down in l. side preceding the flow and partially ceasing with it.—Menses copious, bright red, not coagulating easily (in a woman who thought she had passed the climacteric, as there had been no discharge for over a year), it stopped as suddenly as it began, no pain, only faintness and confused feeling in head.—Menorrhagia at climaxis.—Bland leucorrhœa.—Abortion.—Deficient labour pains.—Constant flooding.—Puerperal peritonitis.—Lochia too profuse, partly fluid, partly clotted ; prolonged bearing-down pains ; uterus feels drawn into a knot.—Hypertrophy and subinvolution.

17. **Respiratory Organs.**—Feeling as if there were a lump behind larynx, which produces constant inclination to swallow.

18. **Chest.**—Spasmodic tearing at top of l. side and passing to sixth or seventh rib, at 3 p.m. when standing or reading, < breathing.—Pain in l. infraclavicular region in morning.—Drawing pain in l. inframammary region, waking me at 3 a.m., > turning on back from r. side.—Aching, burning distress in sternum and under it in stomach, with neuralgic pains.—Oppression along median line.—Constriction, with pain.—Heat and pressure.

19. **Heart.**—Sudden flying pain from heart to stomach, arresting breathing.—Burning pain in cardiac region.

20. **Back.**—Pain in back extending to extreme end of spine.—Pain in lumbar region.—Pain in region of r. kidney, < sitting still ; next day in region of l. kidney, > moving about, with heat, fulness, soreness on deep pressure (but it relieved the pain), with uneasiness in l. thigh, frequent desire to urinate, stream very small, the following day it requires considerable effort of will to empty the bladder, which is done slowly, pain and soreness in l. loin continue ; heavy in lumbar region, in bed with uneasiness about bladder (had had no desire to urinate on going to bed), woke early in morning with distended feeling in bladder, micturition slow and difficult, urine scarcely coloured, pain in back < next night, < lying on face, > lying on r. side.—Bearing down in sacral region as in dysmenorrhœa, changing to l. ovarian region and gradually extending through hip.

21. **Limbs.**—Cutting in bones of r. hand and foot.—Frequent rheumatic symptoms in arms, fingers, and legs.

22. **Upper Limbs.**—Pain in shoulder-joints ; rheumatic, in muscles of r. shoulder.—Intermittent, numb tingling sensation in r. arm and hand every day.—Pain in r. elbow, < motion.—Stitching along metacarpal bone of r.

index.—Rheumatic drawing pain in finger-joints, < second joint of r. index, all afternoon.—Hypertrophy or loss of nails.

23. **Lower Limbs.**—Pain in l. knee when walking, increasing to cramp, obliging me to lean upon the arm of a friend, the pain, with occasional cramps, lasted all the evening, < raising foot so as to press upon toes.—Cramp-like stiffness in l. leg, < raising foot so as to press upon toes.—Feet swollen ; in morning.

24. **Generalities.**—Neuralgic pains in forehead, hands and feet.—Rheumatic pains all up and down l. side, with cutting in l. knee and calf if I pressed any weight upon toes or flexed knee with any weight upon it.—Rheumatic pains in muscles of arms, hands, fingers, and small of back, those in back < walking.—Symptoms of a cold.—Malaise as if I had taken cold ; felt sick with a cold, continual watery flow from nose and eyes, with occasional chills.—Languor : during the day, with headache, < noon, and with burning frontal headache at 9 p.m. ; in morning on rising ; at 2 p.m.—Faint feeling at 11 a.m. in a warm lecture-room.—Faint spells beginning in epigastrium, with small pains in hypochondrium and bowels.

25. **Skin.**—The scalp became one filthy mass of inflammation, two-thirds of the hair came out, the rest matted together, with oozing of watery serum from scalp, eruption like rubeola on neck and chest, gradually extending to feet, thickest on chest and joints, itching < night, rubbing any part brought out the eruption, on face and neck it was in patches like ringworm, but not vesicular.—Boils on nape.—Congested feeling in skin.—Skin dry and hot.—Painful, destructive disease of nails.

26. **Sleep.**—Difficult falling asleep and then unpleasant dreams.—Restless night ; with fever ; with troubled dreams.—Sexual dreams ; without emission ; and disgusting, waking him, arose and urinated with difficulty and tenesmus.

27. **Fever.**—Chills running up and down back.—Heat at night.—Internal heat ; with vertigo ; < eyes, which are inflamed and sensitive to light, eyeball sore to touch ; intermittent, < eyes.—Burning in face and scalp.—Skin dry ; at night ; and hot.

Uva-Ursi.

Arctostaphylos uva-ursi. Bearberry. *N. O.* Ericaceæ. Tincture or trituration of dried leaves and fruit. Tincture of fresh leaves gathered in autumn.

Clinical.—Cystitis. Dysuria. Hæmaturia. Urinary affections.

Characteristics.—A few experiments have been made with *Uva*, and these have seemed to accentuate its traditional reputation as an "astringent used to check excessive secretion of mucus, as in urinary and bronchial affections, and even in calculus." The keynote indications are : Painful micturition with burning sensation. Burning after the discharge of slimy urine. Slime passes with blood. In one cured case there were pains shooting through from hip to hip. The bladder symptoms are > lying on the back.

Relations.—*Compare :* Arbut., Gaulther., and Ericaceæ generally.

SYMPTOMS.

2. **Head.**—Slight vertigo and headache.

5. **Nose.**—Fluent coryza with rawness.

6. **Face.**—Flushing.

11. **Stomach.**—Weak, sick at stomach, sore all over as if bruised.

14. **Urinary Organs.**—Slimy urine ; slime passes with blood.—Painful micturition ; burning after the slime passes.—Hæmaturia ; slimy, purulent urine.—Green urine.—Constant urging and straining.—Shooting pain from hip to hip, bladder and urethra sensitive.

17. **Respiratory Organs.**—Hoarseness with pain in bowels ; stopped up in throat ; no appetite.—Throat tickles, feels like coughing all the time ; sore and bruised all over ; cough ; nose raw and burning ; cutting and burning on urinating.

Vaccininum.

Vaccininum. A Nosode. Trituration of vaccine matter.

Clinical.—Cheloid. Eczema. *Leprosy.* Nævus. Nephritis. Small-pox. Tumours. *Vaccinia. Vaccinosis.* Whooping-cough.

Characteristics.—Vaccinia, Small-pox, and Grease of horses are inter-related diseases, and the nosodes of each are available for the treatment or prevention of manifestations of all three. The vaccine poison is capable of setting up a morbid state of extreme chronicity, named by Burnett *Vaccinosis*. And it may do this without causing the primary symptoms: when the vaccination apparently does not "take." The symptoms of vaccinosis are protean, and are for the most part identical with the symptoms of the Sycosis of Hahnemann. Vaccinosis is a sycotic disease. Neuralgias, inveterate skin eruptions, chilliness, indigestion with great flatulent distension, are leading features of the vaccinal dyscrasia, and therefore indications for the nosode. There is another disease to which vaccinia is related, and that is whooping-cough. Some years ago an old-school observer vaccinated for some reason a child whilst suffering from whooping-cough, and the whooping-cough vanished. He repeated the experiment in other cases, and with such signal success that he wrote to the journals to recommend it as a routine practice in the case of unvaccinated children. On the other hand, homœopathic observers have seen whooping-cough follow immediately on vaccination, and have cured it with *Thuj.* 30. Turiansky (*B. M. J.*, December 12, 1891) tried hypodermic injections of freshly collected calf vaccine in a series of cases of tuberculosis of the lung apices, and states that they were "invariably, though somewhat slowly, followed by most decided amelioration both of the subjective and objective phenomena." The temperature became normal, appetite and sleep improved, night-sweats, dyspnœa, muscular weakness, and painful sensations decreased; cough lessened or disappeared; sputa became thicker and whiter, pulse slower; urine increased; body weight increased; bacilli decreased and degenerated. The exact amount and form of the injections is not stated. Here is a case in the potencies: Garrison (*N. A. J. H.*, quoted *H. R.*, x. 278) was consulted by a lady, 50, of phthisical family. She had consolidation of both apices; had been losing flesh for three months; severe night-sweats; almost constant, hacking cough, with considerable expectoration at times. *Vacc.* 200, one dose. In a week she reported that she had not had a severe coughing spell since the dose, and for the last three days hardly any cough at all. She received one dose of *Vacc.* a week, and at the end of six weeks returned to business. If a child has a nævus it is the rule, when possible, to vaccinate on the nævus. The inflammation and subsequent scarring destroy the growth. But that does not completely explain the cure : vaccinia is causally related to the production of new growths. Over a year ago a young lady came to me shortly after having been revaccinated under some Government rule. There had been nothing abnormal in the course of the vaccinia, but after the scabs fell off there was much pain in the arm, and each of the scars began to grow, and when I saw them were well-developed cheloids. *Thuja* removed the pains but did not arrest the growth. Under *Malan.* 200 they have now all but disappeared. Frölich (*B. M. J.*, October 15, 1898) relates the case of a child, 6½, who had well-developed nephritis seven days after vaccination with calf vaccine. The first symptom was puffed eyelids, then pain and swelling of scrotum ; on the fourteenth day the urine contained blood, inguinal glands enlarged and tender, slight œdema of legs. The urine contained blood and alumen for another month, when recovery took place. Other cases of this kind have been observed. The symptoms of the Schema are partly pathogenetic and partly cured. *Peculiar Sensations* are : As if forehead were split. As if heated or over-exerted in lower extremities. As if bones of leg were broken and undergoing process of comminution. Burnett says the < time of *Vacc.* is the early morning. One symptom is : "Waked in middle of night by pain in forehead and eyes as if split, and stinging in temples."

Relations.—*Antidoted by :* Thuj., Apis, Sul., Ant. t., Sil., Malan. *Compare :* In small-pox, Var., Malan., Thuj., Ant. t. Sarr. Nephritis, Apis, Merc. c. Phthisis, Bacil., Tub. Whooping-cough, Thuj., Meph., Coc. c., Coral.

SYMPTOMS.

1. **Mind.**—Crying.—Ill-humour, with restless sleep.—Nervous, impatient, irritable ; disposition to be troubled by things.—Morbid fear of taking small-pox.

2. **Head.**—Frontal headache.—Forehead felt as if it would split in two in median line from root of nose to top of head.—Stitches in r. temple.—Eruption like crusta lactea.

3. **Eyes.**—Tinea tarsi and conjunctivitis in a woman, æt. 28, remaining as result of variola in infancy, conjunctivæ painfully sensitive.—Weak eyes ; feeling in forehead as if it were split.—Inflamed eyelids.—Redness of eyes and face, with small pimples on face and hands.—Keratitis after vaccination

5. **Nose.**—Full feeling of head, with running at nose.—Bleeding at nose preceded by a feeling of contraction above and between eyebrows, soon after eating meat ; menses rather profuse and too frequent ; cured by revaccination.

6. **Face.**—Redness and distension of face, chill running down back.—Swelling of neck under r. ear (parotid gland) with sensation like being cut.

8. **Mouth.**—Tongue coated, dryish yellow, with papillæ showing through coat.—Dry mouth and tongue.

10. **Appetite.**—Appetite gone, disgust to taste, smell, and appearance of food.—Coffee tastes sour.

11. **Stomach.**—Aching in pit of stomach, with short breath.

12. **Abdomen.**—A stitch in hepatic region, at margin of last lower rib, axillary line.—Stitch in splenic region.—Blown up with flatulence.

14. **Urinary Organs.**—Nephritis with albuminuria, hæmatúria, and dropsy, developed eleven days after vaccination ; child recovered.

17. **Respiratory Organs.**—Short breath with aching in pit of stomach, and pressure in region of heart.—Whooping-cough.

18. **Chest.**—Stitch in l. side of chest, anteriorly, under short ribs.—Stitches in r. side under short ribs in front from r. to l., then at corresponding place in l. side, but from l. to r., lasting five minutes, felt in liver and spleen.

19. **Heart.**—Febrile action of heart and arteries.

20. **Back.**—Backache.—Aching pain in back, < in lumbar region, extending around waist.

22. **Upper Limbs.**—Severe pains in l. upper arm at vaccination mark, could not raise it in morning.—Rheumatic pains in wrists and hands.—Cheloids on re-vaccination marks.

23. **Lower Limbs.**—Tearing in l. thigh downward.—Soreness of lower extremities, as if heated or over-exerted.—Legs ached immoderately, hardly able to get about, a break-bone sensation, and a feeling as if bones were undergoing process of comminution.

24. **Generalities.**—Restlessness.—General malaise.—Languor, lassitude.—Tired all over, with stretching, gaping feeling ; unnatural fatigue.—Child wants to be carried.—Many persons faint when being vaccinated.

25. **Skin.**—Skin hot and dry.—A general eruption, similar to cow-pox.—Small pimples develop at point of vaccination with fourth dilution.—Red pimples or blotches in various parts, most evident when warm.—Eruption of pustules with a dark-red base and a roundish or oblong elevation, filled with pus of a greenish-yellow colour, resembling varioloid, some as large as a pea, some less, without depression in the centre, coming with a round, hard feel in the skin (like a shot), very itchy.—Tingling burning in skin over whole body, most intense in skin of forehead and in lower and anterior portion of hairy scalp, which parts are tinged with a scarlet blush, or efflorescence, similar to the immediate precursor of variolous eruption.—*Vaccininum* 6, in water, for one day with strict diet, repeated after eight days, acted as preventive in six hundred cases.—Treated a great many cases of variola and varioloid during last eighteen years, some of them of the most desperate character, and yet never lost a case when employing vaccine virus as a remedy ; moreover, none of the cases so treated were ever troubled with hæmorrhage, or with delirium, or secondary fevers, or were ever disfigured with pitting.—*Vaccininum* 200th quickly > severer symptoms of variola occurring in a child, æt. six months ; two days before appearance of eruption had been revaccinated (after an interval of eight days) on a nævus near r. nipple ; deglutition difficult through implication of tongue and fauces ; pustules, many of large size, scattered over scalp, face, body, and limbs.

26. Sleep.—Waked in middle of night by pain in forehead and eyes as if split, and stinging in temples.

27. Fever.—Fever, with heat, thirst, tossing about, crying, aversion to food.—Chill with shaking.

Valeriana.

Valeriana officinalis. *N. O.* Valerianaceæ. Tincture of the fresh root.

Clinical.—Asthma, spasmodic; nervous. Bed-sores. *Change of life.* Clairvoyance. Coxalgia. Headache. Heart, palpitation of. *Heels, pain in. Hypochondriasis. Hysteria.* Levitation. *Neuralgia.* Sciatica. Sleeplessness. Toothache.

Characteristics.—*V. officinalis* is usually found in moist hedgerows or on the banks of ditches and streams. The peculiar fetid odour of Valerians is probably due to the presence of Valerianic acid. It is especially agreeable to cats, who become, as it were, intoxicated with it. "Volatile oil of Valerian seems not to exist naturally in the plant, but to be developed by the agency of water" (*Treas. of Bot.*). *Val.* first appeared in homœopathic medicine in Stapf's *Additions*, the article on it was written by Franz, and Hahnemann and Stapf were among the provers. When Franz wrote, it was the custom among ladies in Germany to take *Valerian* almost as frequently as coffee, and to this practice he attributed no little of the nervous suffering then prevalent. "There is scarcely a drug," he says, "which communicates its primary as well as secondary action to the organism with more intensity than *Val.*" He instanced his own eye symptoms, which were both severe and remarkable, and of them he says that, though he had never had any tendency to anything of the kind before, they were excited at intervals for four months afterwards, the cause being frequently unknown, showing the deep action on the organism. "The many inveterate spasms of the stomach and abdomen; the incurable cases of hysteria and hypochondriasis; moral disturbances, passing from one extreme of emotion to another, from the highest joy to the deepest grief, from leniency, kindness, and mildness to grumbling impatience, obstinacy, and quarrelsomeness; from a *sinking of the vital forces accompanied by a painful craving for stimulants*, to the greatest liveliness and extravagance, and *vice versâ*"; tedious convalescence after nervous fevers; paralysis, and contractions of the limbs, &c.—these, in Franz's opinion, were much less owing to the original intensity of the disease than to the *Val.* with which the patients had been dosed; and they were only saved from worse effects by the fact that *Val.* was so frequently given in combination with one or more of its antidotes. Some notes by Franz are important: (1) The first and most rapid effect of *Val.*, which precedes any after symptoms, is an acceleration of the pulse and congestion of the head. (2) The symptoms of the upper and lower limbs alternate frequently. (3) The principal times of day when *Val.* produces its symptoms are noon and early afternoon and the hours before midnight. The abdominal symptoms especially are felt in the evening. (4) "*Val.* causes several kinds of darting, tearing pains *which come and go.* Similar to these pains are those which *appear* suddenly. If we compare with these two kinds of pains—the jerking pains which are scarcely felt in any other than muscular tissues and the cramping pains—we have a very easy and natural indication of the grounds on which Tissot's recommendation of *Val.* for epilepsy might be considered valid. The eye symptoms of Franz were burning, smarting, and pressure in the margins of the lids, which seemed sore and swollen. But in addition was this, which shows the exalted state of sensorum *Val.* can produce: "Shine before the eyes in the dark; the closed, dark room seemed to be filled with the shine of twilight, so that he imagined he distinguished the objects in the same; this was accompanied with a sensation as if he felt that things were near him even when not looking at them; on looking he perceived that the things were really there" (at 10 p.m., thirteen hours after the dose). There were also hallucinations of hearing and of sense. "Imagines she is some one else and moves to the edge of the bed to make room" was removed in one case. "Anxious, hypochondriac feeling, as if the objects around him had been taken from him; the room appears to him desolate, he does not feel at home in the room, he is compelled to leave it." "As if in a dream." The restlessness of *Val.* is a very prominent feature: Nervous irritation, cannot keep still; tearings, cramps, > morning. Constant heat and uneasiness. The digestion is disturbed. The taste caused by *Val.* is as disgusting as its odour. Before dinner a taste of fetid tallow; early in the morning on waking the taste is flat, slimy. Nausea begins in umbilical region, rising into pharynx. In the preface to his *Pocket Book* Bœninghausen gives a case which brings out many of the *Val.* characteristics: "E. N., 50, of blooming, almost florid complexion, usually cheerful, but during his most violent paroxysms inclined to outbreaks of anger with decided nervous excitement, had suffered for four months with a peculiar violent kind of pain in the right leg after the previous dispersion, allopathically, of a so-called rheumatic pain in the right orbit by external remedies which could not be found out; this last pain attacked the muscle of the posterior part of the leg, especially from calf to heel, but did not involve the knee or ankle-joint. The pain itself he described as extremely acute, cramping, jerking, tearing, frequently interrupted by stitches extending from within outward; but in the morning hours, when the pain was generally more endurable, it was a dull, burrowing with a bruised feeling. The pain became < towards evening and during rest, especially after previous motion, while sitting and standing, particularly if he did it during a walk in the open air. While walking the pain often jumped from the right calf to the left upper arm if he put his hand into his coat pocket or his breast and kept the arm quiet, but it was > while using the arm, and then the pain suddenly jumped back again into the right calf. The greatest relief was experienced while walking up and down the room and rubbing the affected part. The concomitant symptoms were sleeplessness before midnight, frequently recurring attacks during the evening of sudden flushes of heat with thirst, without previous chill, a disgusting, fatty taste in the mouth with nausea in the throat, and an almost constant pressing pain in the lower part of the chest and pit of the stomach as if something were there forcing itself outward." Of course *Val.* was the remedy. *Val.* has a strong affinity for the tendo Achillis, and I have cured with it many cases of painful affection of this tendon and heel when the *Val.* conditions were present. Nash cured with it a severe case of sciatica in a pregnant woman on the symptom, "pain < standing and letting the foot rest on the floor." She could stand with the foot resting on a chair or lie down in comfort. *Val.* is a leading member of the group of remedies which meet lack of reaction. It is *Suited to:* (1) Hysterical women who have taken too much chamomile tea. (2) Nervous, irritable, hysterical subjects in whom the intellectual faculties predominate and who suffer from hysteria and neuralgia. It meets "nervous affections occurring in excitable temperaments; in hypochondriasis it calms the nervousness, abates the excitement of the circulation, removes the wakefulness, promotes sleep, and induces sensation of quietude and comfort; sadness is removed; in globus, in all asthmatical and hysterical coughs, nervous palpitation of the heart, profuse flow of limpid urine" (quoted by Hering). "Red parts become white" is another indication of Hering's. Among *Sensations* are: As if flying in air. As if eyes would be pierced from within outward. As if smoke in eyes. As if a thread were hanging down throat. As if something forcing a passage through pit of stomach. As if something warm were rising from stomach. As if something pressed out in lower chest. As from cold or over-lifting, pain in loins. As if he had strained left lumbar region. As if an electric shock through humerus. As if thigh would break. As if strained in right ankle. As if bruised in outer malleolus of right foot. Lightness in leg. Like lead in limbs. The symptoms are: < By touch (blisters on cheek and lip). Rubbing > cramp in calf. Pressure of hand or covering with hat = icy coldness on vertex. Early decubitus in typhoid. Slight injury = spasms. Rest; sitting; standing <. Motion >. Moving eyes < headache. Bending head back < pain in occiput. Straightening out limb < sciatica. < Noon. < Before midnight (cannot sleep before midnight). Profuse sweat at night. < Open air; draught of air. > After sleep. < Fasting. > After a meal.

Relations.—*Antidoted by:* Bell., Camph., Cin., Coff., Puls. *Antidote to:* Merc., abuse of Chamomile tea. *Compare:* Hysteria, Mosch. (Mosch. has more *unconsciousness*), Ign., Asaf. Alternating mental states, Croc. Defective reaction, Ambra., Pso. (despair of recovery), Chi., Lauro. (chest affections), Caps., Op., Carb. v. Periodical neuralgia, Ars. (Val. hysterical patients). Pain = fainting, Cham., Hep., Ver. Rheumatism > motion, Rhus. Pains come and go suddenly, Bell., Lyc. Infant vomits curdled milk, Æth. Over-sensitiveness, Nux. Averse to darkness, Stram., Stro., Am. m., Ars., Bar. c., Berb., Calc., Carb. a., Carb. v., Caus., Lyc., Pho., Pul., Rhus. As if in a dream, Ambr., Anac., Calc., Can. i., Con., Cup., Med., Rhe., Ver., Ziz. Levitation, Nux m., Sti. p., Ph. ac.

Causation.—Injuries (slightest injury = spasms. Bed-sores form soon in typhoid).

SYMPTOMS.

1. **Mind.**—Extremely delirious, attempting to get out of the window, threatening and vociferating wildly.—Anxious, hypochondriacal sensation, as if all around were desolate, disagreeable, or strange (very changeable disposition).—Joyous, tremulous excitement; mild delirium.—Intellect clouded.—Fear, esp. in evening, and in the dark.—Despair.—The most opposite moral symptoms appear alternately.—Extreme instability of ideas.—General illusions and errors of the mind.—Hallucinations: esp. at night; sees figures, animals, men; thinks she is some one else, moves to edge of bed to make room.—Great flow of ideas, chasing one another.—Felt like one who is dreaming.—Hysteria, with nervous over-excitability of the nerves.

2. **Head.**—Head confused, as after intoxication.—Intoxication and dizziness, with absence of ideas.—Whirling in head when stooping forwards.—Headache, which appears suddenly or in jerks.—Fulness as from rush of blood to head.—Pressive headache, or with pressive shootings, esp. in forehead, towards orbits, often alternating with confusion and dizziness in the head.—Headache; < in evening, when at rest, and in the open air; > from movement in the room and when changing the position; the pressure over the orbits alternates between a pressing and a sticking; the sticking is like a darting, tearing as if it would pierce the eyes from within outward.—Headache an hour after dinner, pressure over eyes as if they would be pressed out, < moving them.—Drawing pain on one side of head, from a current of air.—Headache in the sunshine.—Stupefying contraction in head, as from a violent blow on vertex.—Sensation of icy coldness in upper part of head, from pressure of hat.—Pressure and drawing into side of occiput.—Piercing drawing, with pressure from nape to occiput, when bending head back.—Sweat in hair of forehead and on forehead about noon.

3. **Eyes.**—Eyes downcast, as after a nocturnal debauch, esp. after a meal.—Pressure, burning sensation, and smarting in eyes as from smoke; morning after rising.—Tearing in r. eyeball, sight dim in morning, and pain as from insufficient sleep.—Sees things at a distance more distinctly than usual.—The eyes shine.—Redness, swelling, and pain as from excoriation in margin of eyelids.—Swelling and painful sensibility of eyelids.—Myopia.—Brightness and light before eyes when in the dark, so that objects become almost distinguishable; with this a sensation as if he felt that things were near him even when not looking at them; on looking, he perceives they really were there (10 p.m.).—Sparks before eyes.

4. **Ears.**—Otalgia, with spasmodic drawings.—Jerking in the ears.—Tinkling and ringing in the ears.—Illusions of hearing; imagined he heard the bell strike.

5. **Nose.**—Violent sneezing.

6. **Face.**—Pain in face, with spasmodic twitching and drawing in zygomatic process.—Redness and heat of cheeks in open air; a quarter of an hour later sweat breaks out over whole body, esp. in face.—Twitching of muscles of face.—Darting like electricity in r. ramus of lower jaw.

7. **Teeth.**—Toothache, with shooting pain.

8. **Mouth.**—White blisters on tongue and upper lip, painful when touched.

10. **Appetite.**—Taste in mouth (and smell before nose) as of fetid tallow (early in the morning after waking).—Bitter taste on tip of tongue when passing it over the lips after a meal.—Insipid and slimy taste in mouth after waking in morning.—Bulimy, with nausea.

11. **Stomach.**—Risings, with the taste of rotten eggs, on waking in morning.—Frequent, empty, or rancid and burning risings.—Voracious hunger with nausea.—Nausea and a sensation as if there were a thread from gullet to abdomen (arising from umbilicus and gradually rising to fauces), with copious accumulation of saliva.—Nausea, with syncope, lips white and body cold.—Disposition to vomit.—Vomiting of bile and of mucus, with violent shivering and shaking.—Nocturnal vomiting.—Weak stomach and digestion.—Pressure at scrobiculus, appearing and disappearing suddenly, with a gurgling in abdomen.

12. **Abdomen.**—Pains in hepatic region and epigastrium when touched.—Painful shocks in r. hypochondrium.—Abdomen inflated and hard.—Powerful sensation of expansion in abdomen, as if about to burst.—Tendency to retract abdomen.—Spasms in abdomen, generally in evening, in bed, or after dinner, allowing no > in any position whatever.—Hæmorrhoidal colic ; from worms.—Gripings and painful pinchings in abdomen when retracting it.—Pains in l. side of abdomen in evening, as from subcutaneous ulceration.—Drawing, pressure, and pains as from a bruise in hypogastrium, inguina, and abdominal muscles, as after a chill or strain.—Digging pains in abdomen.

13. **Stool and Anus.**—Loose evacuations.—Greenish fæces of consistence of pap, mixed with blood.—Painful borings in rectum.—Bubbling pressure above anus in region of coccyx.—Discharge of blood from anus.—Ascarides from rectum.

14. **Urinary Organs.**—Profuse and frequent emission of urine.— Urine contains a white, red, or turbid sediment.—During urination much straining and prolapsus recti.

15. **Male Sexual Organs.**—Creeping and drawing in penis as if it had gone to sleep ; frequent erections the day previous, early in morning.—Tensive gurgling in r. testis when sitting.

16. **Female Sexual Organs.**—Menses too late and scanty.—Neurasthenia of sexual organs of women.—Child vomits as soon as it has been nursed, after mother has been angry.—Child vomits curdled milk in large lumps, the same in stools.

17. **Respiratory Organs.**—Choking in throat-pit on falling asleep ; wakens as if suffocating.—Inspirations grow less and less deep and more rapid till they cease ; then catches her breath by a sobbing effort in spells.—Sensation as if something warm were rising from stomach, arresting breathing, with tickling deep in throat and cough.

18. **Chest.**—Obstructed respiration and anguish in chest.—Oppressed respiration, with pressure on lower part of chest.—Frequent jerks and stitches in chest (with the sensation as if something were pressed out), sometimes on l. side (in region of heart) when drawing breath.—Sudden stitches in chest and liver from within out.—Eruption of small, hard nodosities on chest.

20. **Back.**—Drawing pains in the loins and back.—Pain in the region of

the loins as from a chill or a strain.—Lancinations in l. lumbar region above hip, worse when standing, and esp. when sitting, than when walking.—Rheumatic pains in the shoulder-blades.

21. **Limbs.**—Painful drawing in upper and lower extremities when sitting quietly, > by walking.

22. **Upper Limbs.**—Spasmodic drawings and jerkings, or else tearing in arms.—Crampy drawing in region of biceps, in r. arm from above downward while writing.—Crampy, darting tearing like an electric shock, repeatedly through the humerus, intensely painful.—Paralytic pain in joints of shoulder and elbow towards the end of a walk.—Eruption of small, hard nodosities on arms.—Trembling of hands when writing.—Painful shocks across the hand.

23. **Lower Limbs.**—Burning pain in hips when in bed in evening.—Crampy tearing in outer side of thigh, extending into hip.—Pain in hip and thigh intolerable when standing, as if thigh would break.—Spasmodic drawing and jerking in thighs.—Great heaviness and lassitude in legs, but esp. in calves.—Twinging pain in outer side of calf when sitting.—Pulsative tearing in r. calf when sitting in the afternoon.—Pain, as of a fracture, in the thighs and tibia.—Paralytic pain in the knees towards the end of a walk.—Violent stitch in knee.—Tensive pain in the calves of the legs, esp. when crossing the legs.—Drawing and weak feeling along tendo Achillis, toward heel, as if the part had lost all strength, when sitting; disappearing when rising from a seat.—Constant pain in heels.—When sitting heels, esp. r., painful.—Drawing in the joints of the feet when sitting down.—Sudden pain, as if bruised, in outer malleolus of r. foot, < when standing, > when walking.—Wrenching pain in the joints of the foot and ankles.—Transient pain in r. ankle, < while standing, but seems to disappear when walking.—Lower limbs contracted.—Pains and shootings in heels, esp. when seated.—Tearing pains in the soles of the feet and in the toes.

24. **Generalities.**—[This remedy is like *Puls.* in many of its aggravations, &c., but it has a different temperament—patients get "raving, tearing, swearing" mad; get < toward evening from being still; great sleeplessness in early part of night—all like *Puls.*, but the temper decides.—Affections in general of the orbit of the eye; margins of the eyelids; calves of the legs.—Fatty taste; sediment in the urine; reddish urine; hysterical condition; pains darting from within outward.—< On stooping; after moving and being at rest; while resting; standing.—> From moving, from walking.—H. N. G.]—Rheumatic tearing in limbs, but not usually in the joints, chiefly during repose, after exercise, and mostly > by movement; or which gives place to other sensations in other parts of the body during a walk.—Jerking and shaking pains, appearing (in many places) suddenly and by fits.—Pains which manifest themselves after resting a long time in any position, and are > by changing it.—Drawing and jerking in limbs, as if in bones.—Pain, as from paralysis in limbs, towards the end of a walk.—Periodical symptoms, which reappear after two or three months.—Epileptic fits.—Paralytic torpor in limbs.—The majority of the symptoms manifest themselves in the evening and after dinner.—Over-sensitiveness of all senses.—General morbid excitement and irritability, with lassitude in the limbs, great gaiety, and appearance of vigour.—Painful weariness, esp. in lower extremities, after rising in morning.

25. **Skin.**—Eruption of small nodosities, at first red and confluent, the white and hard.—Painful eruptions.—Skin too dry and warm.

26. **Sleep.**—Sleeplessness.—Disturbed sleep (could fall asleep only towards morning), with tossing and anxious and confused dreams.

27. **Fever.**—The chilliness generally begins in neck and runs down back. —Sensation of icy coldness.—Fever, with constant heat, after a short fit of shivering, accompanied by confusion in head and thirst.—Heat < in evening and when eating.—Accelerated pulse.—Pulse irregular ; generally rapid and somewhat tense, sometimes small and weak.—Frequent perspiration, esp. on face and forehead (often appearing and disappearing suddenly).—Profuse perspiration, esp. at night and from exertion, with violent heat.

Vanadium.

Vanadium. The Metal. V. (A.W. 51·2). Trituration. (Burnett used the "soluble ammonium salt.")

Clinical.—Addison's disease. Atheroma. Fatty degeneration. Innutrition.

Characteristics.—Burnett (*Fifty Reasons*) tells how he came to use *Van*. through reading the result of some experiments on animals in which the Salts of Vanadium produced "true cell destruction, the pigment escaping, the liver being hit hardest." Burnett had at the time a case of "fatty liver, atheroma of the arteries, much pain corresponding to the course of the basilar artery, large, deeply pigmented patches on forehead, profound adynamia." *Van.* restored the patient, who was seventy, and at eighty he was "hale and hearty." Marc Jousset (*L'Art Méd.*, lxxxix. 217) tells of experiments with salts of *Van.*, chiefly the meta-vanadate of sodium, by Lyonnet and others. Animals poisoned by intravenous injections rapidly develop Cheyne-Stokes respiration ; with little or no action on circulation or blood. These observers gave *Vanadates* to two hundred patients (suffering from tuberculosis, chlorosis, chronic rheumatism, neurasthenia, &c.), and produced in nearly all cases increased appetite, strength, and weight. The amount of urea was also increased. They regard *Van.* as "an energetic excitant of nutrition," and probably an oxydant stimulating organic combustion. The dose was 2–5 mgr. in twenty-four hours, and only on three separate days in the week.

Relations.—*Compare :* Fatty degeneration, Phos., Ars. Addison's disease, Adren. Tuberculosis, Tub., Bac.

Variolinum.

Variolinum. Nosode of Small-pox. Trituration of matter from small-pox vesicle.

Clinical.—Asthma. Backache. Chill. Fever. Headache; occipital. Herpes zoster. Neuralgia. Small-pox. Testicle, swelling of.

Characteristics.—The cardinal symptoms of small-pox are the keynote symptoms for the use of *Variolinum*. The backache of small-pox is about the worst backache known, and *Var.* has cured in my practice a number of bad backaches that nothing else seemed to touch. *Var.* was Burnett's chief remedy in shingles; it generally, as he expressed it, wiped out the disease, eruption and pain as well. It will also cure neuralgia left by herpes. *Var.* has aborted many cases of small-pox, and has proved an efficient preventive against small-pox contagion and vaccinal infection. G. M. H. (*H. W.*, xxxii. 546) records this experience: *Var.* 6 (three pilules) was given to the mother and children of a family, one of whose members was taken with small-pox and removed to an isolation hospital, with his mother to nurse him. The patient (who did not receive *Var.*) was dangerously ill for a month. Neither the mother who nursed him nor any of the other children took small-pox. Vaccine was sent by the Government and all the family were vaccinated, but it did not take with any of those who had taken *Var.*, although the vaccination was repeated. Moreover, G. M. H. himself, who had taken a dose of *Var.*, submitted to vaccination, but "although four thorough inoculations were given, they healed up immediately, and did not even itch or smart."—These are cardinal indications for *Var.*: Severe cold; chill; chilly creepings as if cold water were trickling down the back; violent fever with extremely hot skin, with or without high pulse. Violent headache. Nausea. Pain in epigastrium. Pain in limbs as if in bones. Severe backache. There may be rash or there may not. Here is a case of Swan's, who is a pioneer with nosodes (*H. W.*, xviii. 205): Miss H., 21, healthy, hearty; complained of the following symptoms: Confusion of head as if going crazy, with a sensation as if it was all in the back of the head and running down spine, followed by intense, heavy, hot headache in back of head and neck and region of medulla; sensation as if head weighed a hundredweight, with a tendency of it to fall backwards; deathly nausea in throat-pit during headache. During headache hands and feet icy cold, particularly the hands; tongue coated yellow in morning, with bad, disgusting taste in mouth; no appetite; knees feel weak as if they would give way, especially on going down stairs; pains in thighs and hips; severe aching, burning pain in small of back; skin hot and dry; pulse not feverish. *Var.* cm (Swan), in water, cured in six hours, the confusion of the head ceased after the pain did. A school of two hundred children was "internally variolated" with *Var.* cmm (Swan) on the evening of February 18th and the morning of February 19th. Of two schoolmistresses one was not at all affected; the other was two days in bed ill. On 21st many of the children were ill; by the 23rd all except forty were, the symptoms being the usual preliminary symptoms of small-pox, and later Swan found pustules on many. After the varioloid had passed off, but before the patients had recovered their vitality, twenty-three children were vaccinated without Swan's knowledge. All but one took and had terrible ulcers on the arms, and had to be remedied by *Vacc.* (cmm, Swan). *Sensations* of *Var.* are: As if a band tightly encircled head. Crazy feeling through brain. As if throat were closed. As of a lump in right side of throat. Like streams of ice-water running down back. Pain as if back were broken. The symptoms are < By motion.

Relations.—*Antidoted by:* Malan., Thuj., Ant. t., Vacc., Sarr. *Compare:* Herpes, Mez., Rhus, Ars.

Causation.—Contusion (enlarged testicle).

SYMPTOMS.

1. **Mind.**—Delirium with the initial fever.

2. **Head.**—Vertigo.—Syncope in attempting to rise.—Forehead very hot, face red and bloated, carotids pulsating violently.—Headache: with or after a chill; all over head; particularly in forehead; severe in vertex; as if a band tightly encircled head; severe lancinating, throbbing; < with every pulsation.—Intolerable pain in occiput.—Crazy feeling through brain, hard to describe.

3. **Eyes.**—Keratitis, with small-pox and after vaccination.—Chronic ophthalmia with loss of sight.—Pupils contracted.

4. **Ears.**—Deafness.

6. **Face.**—Skin of face and neck deep dark-purple hue.—Jaw falling when asleep, with trembling when aroused.

7. **Teeth.**—Teeth covered with thick brown slime.

8. **Mouth.**—Thick, dirty yellow coating on tongue.—When asleep tongue protruded, black coating, when raised it is with difficulty drawn back; looks like a mass of putrid flesh.

9. **Throat.**—Throat very sore, redness of fauces.—Pharynx and fauces deep purplish crimson, with gangrenous appearance; breath horribly offensive.—Painful deglutition.—Sensation as if throat were closed.—Sensation as of a lump in r. side of throat.—Diphtheria with horrible fetor oris.

10. **Appetite.**—Food, esp. water, tastes sickish sweet.

11. **Stomach.**—Soreness in pit of stomach and across epigastric region.—Severe pain in præcordial region, frequent nausea and vomiting of bilious and bloody matter.—Frequent bilious vomiting.—As soon as he drinks milk he vomits it up.

13. **Stool.**—Thin, bloody stools.—Several brown, green, at last grass-green stools, painless, loose, of intolerable fetid odour; no thirst; last stool slimy, with small quantity of blood.—Dysentery.—Constipation.

14. **Urinary Organs.**—Urine: high-coloured, like brandy; turbid and offensive; stains a rose tea-colour, difficult to remove.

15. **Male Sexual Organs.**—Enlargement of testicle.—Hard swelling of l. testicle in consequence of a contusion.

17. **Respiratory Organs.**—Oppressed respiration.—Asthma.—Troublesome cough, with serous and sometimes bloody sputa.—Hawking up thick, viscid slime, smelling bad.

20. **Neck and Back.**—Stiffness of neck, with tense drawing in muscles, < on motion.—Pain in base of brain and neck.—Chills like streams of ice-water running down from between scapulæ to sacral region.—Intolerable aching in lumbar and sacral region.—Pain in muscles of back like rheumatism; < on motion.

22. **Upper Limbs.**—Hands icy cold during invasion.—Swelling of arm which had been half-paralysed.

23. **Lower Limbs.**—Muscular rheumatism; < on motion.

25. **Skin.**—Exanthema of sharp, pointed pimples, usually small, seldom large and suppurating, dry, resting on small red areolæ, frequently interspersed with spots of red colour, sometimes severe itching.—Petechial eruptions.—*Var.* 30 warded off an attack of small-pox after intense sickness of stomach had been caused by the smell of a case.—*Var.* 1m in water every two hours, given on third day of eruption of a confluent case cut short the attack.—Shingles.

27. **Fever.**—Very severe chill, followed by hot fever.—Intense fever, commencing with chills running down back like streams of cold water, causing shivering and chattering of teeth.—Fever with intense radiating heat, burning hot to touch.—Hot fever, no thirst.—Very profuse, bad-smelling sweat.

Veratrinum.

Veratria. (An alkaloid obtained chiefly from seeds of Sabadilla and roots of Veratrum.) $C_{32} H_{52} N_2 O_8$. Trituration.

Clinical.—Colic. Diarrhœa. Dysentery. Dysuria. Intestines, catarrh of; neuralgia of. Jaw, snapping of. Neuralgia. Œsophagus, stricture of. Paralysis. Spine, neuralgia of. Tetanus.

Characteristics.—"Large doses of *Veratrinum* cause violent sneezing and great gastro-intestinal irritation, vomiting, purging, and symptoms of collapse, the pulse being rapid, small, and irregular; and often involuntary muscular tremors come on. A peculiar creeping and prickling sensation in the skin generally accompanies these symptoms. Externally applied to the unbroken skin it has no marked action, but if rubbed on with some fat, it passes through the epidermis and acts on the true skin, causing first irritation and then paralysis of the ends of the sensory nerves, and producing a prickly and creepy sensation, succeeded by numbness. This effect is produced whether applied locally or taken internally. Its irritating action in the sensory nerves is also observed if it be inhaled through the nose, when it causes violent sneezing, which also occurs after absorption through the stomach" (Brunton). A large number of the effects of *Vern.* were the result of inunctions. *Vern.* is both a paralyser and a great pain producer. It causes electric pains; sensation like electric streams in nerves; shooting pains like electric-shocks in veins, muscles and joints. *Vern.* causes tetanus, which Farrington distinguishes from the convulsive action of *Nux* in that *Vern.* causes purgation and vomiting with the spasms, and that general paralysis does not take place from exhaustion as with *Nux*, but from devitalisation of the muscles. Twitchings, subsultus tendinum, fibrillary twitchings are marked. Startings and tremors occur in limbs previously affected by paralysis or pain. The pains are tingling, sparkling, prickling, burning. There is a drawing pain along the spine. *Sensations :* of oppression in head, suffocation ; of boiling water running over the back. As if a stream of warm air or drops of hot water issued from various parts. As if a frozen atmosphere round feet to knees ; or cold water poured on them. Shocks in head. Twitching of facial muscles. Snapping, closure of lower jaw. One *Peculiar Symptom* is : " Dull pain, afterwards burning, in lower part of spinal column, followed by pain in bowels and prepuce, accompanied with jerking in lower limb."

Relations.—*Antidoted by :* Coffee mixed with a little lemon-juice. *Compare :* Sabad., Acon., Coniin.

SYMPTOMS.

1. **Mind.** — Delirium with illusions. — Great anxiety. — Loss of consciousness.

2. **Head.**—Vertigo.—Peculiar sense of oppression and anxiety in head, a sense of suffocation.

3. **Eyes.** — Conjunctiva red. — Lachrymation. — Pupils extremely contracted.

5. **Nose.**—Frequent sneezing. —After vomiting had been produced, violent sneezing came on and lasted half an hour.

6. **Face.**—Twitching of muscles of face.—Violent shocks, tearing pain, extending from face (place of application) to vertex.—When eating or laughing heartily, or talking animatedly, frequently spasmodic closure of lower jaw, shuts suddenly with a loud snap.

8. **Mouth.**—Tongue much swollen.—Peculiar biting and creeping in tongue.—Mouth dry.—Mouth and throat very sore as if she had swallowed boiling water.—Intense irritation of mouth and pharynx.—Salivation very profuse, lasting weeks ; nausea and vomiting.

9. **Throat.**—Constriction of throat.—Sense of constriction in fauces rendering swallowing difficult.—Prickly sensation in pharynx and throat, sometimes irritable.

11. **Stomach.**—Appetite lost.—Violent, unquenchable thirst.—Frequent bitter eructations.—Nausea : violent ; and vomiting.—Copious vomiting.—Slight transient burning in stomach.—A peculiar feeling increases to a burning.—Cramp.

12. **Abdomen.**—Electric streams along nerves of abdomen and breast (inunction to back).—Great pain extending over all the nerves of the abdomen.—Colic.—Sensation as if whole intestines were tied together with a strong cord continually tightened.

13. **Stool and Anus.**—Diarrhœa : slimy ; profuse watery ; of bloody mucus ; of mucous substances ; with tenesmus.

14. **Urinary Organs.**—Spasmodic contraction of bladder with evacuation of watery urine.—Continual calls to urinate.—Ineffectual efforts to urinate (primary effect).—Urine : increased ; scanty, red, thick.

17. **Respiratory Organs.**—Breathing hurried.

19. **Heart.**—Burning pain in præcordial region.—Excessive feebleness, beats weak.—Sinking of pulse.

20. **Back.**—Dull pain in back.—Dull pain, afterwards burning, in lower part of spinal column, followed by pain in bowels and prepuce, watery and mucous evacuation, accompanied with jerking in lower extremities.—Drawing pain along spine.—Sensation of boiling water running over back.

21. **Limbs.**—Paralysis and numbness of limbs.

23. **Lower Limbs.**—Painful jerking in toes.

24. **Generalities.**—Trembling and uncertain movements when he wants to lay hold of anything, he misses his grasp.—Subsultus tendinum.—Twitchings : slight in various muscles ; starting or tremors in paralysed or previously affected parts.—Faintness : collapse.—After an excellent night's rest felt dreadfully tired and weak.—Great agitation with violent vomiting.—Tingling, sparkling, prickling in parts remote from stomach half an hour after dose ; sometimes with sense of warmth ; sometimes with coldness.—Warmth in stomach extending to other parts, cold or tingling exactly as after local application of *Veratria.*—Electric streams in nerves.—Electric shocks in muscles.

25. **Skin.**—Erysipelatous inflammation with violent pain, nettlerash eruption (from inunction).—Heat and tingling extend from parts rubbed over rest of body.—Parts rubbed very sensitive to stimuli, esp. electricity and galvanism.—Itching followed for weeks after by tingling.

27. **Fever.**—Coldness, warmth, sticking, and prickling.—Cold extremities ; must use foot-stove.—Sweat.

Veratrum Album.

Veratrum album. White-flowered Veratrum. White Hellebore. *N. O.* Melanthaceæ (of the Liliaceæ). Tincture of the root-stocks collected (in the Alps and Pyrenees) early in June before flowering.

Clinical.—Amenorrhœa. Anæmia. Anasarca. Angina pectoris. Apoplexy. Asthma. Bronchitis. *Cholera asiatica. Cholerine. Colic.* Collapse. *Constipation.* Coprophagia. Cramps. *Debility.* Diaphragm, affections of. *Diarrhœa.* Dysmenorrhœa. Emphysema. Epilepsy. Fainting. Gastric catarrh. General paralysis. Headache ; sick ; nervous. Hernia. Hydrocephaloid. Hysteria. *Influenza. Intermittent fever.* Intussusception. *Labour, constipation after.* Lips, cracked. Liver, hyperæmia of. Lock-jaw. Lungs, œdema of. *Mania.* Measles. Mendacity. *Melancholia.* Meningitis. *Menstruation, nausea before ; diarrhœa before.* Neuralgia, palpebralis. Nyctalopia. Œsophagus, stricture of. Peritonitis. Pernicious fevers. Plica polonica. Pneumonia. Pregnancy, imaginary. Ptosis. Pyæmia.

Rheumatism. Salivation. Scarlatina. *Sleep, whining in.* Spleen, swollen. Sternum. *Throat.* Toothache. Typhoid fever. Vertigo. *Water-brash.* Whooping-cough. Yellow fever.

Characteristics.—In his *Helleborism of the Ancients*, Hahnemann showed that *Verat. alb.* was the principal agent used at Anticyra and other places in Greece to produce the evacuations which were regarded as an essential of the "cure." Spring was deemed the most favourable season and autumn the next. Among the diseases in which the treatment was employed were "mental derangements, epilepsy, spasms of the facial muscles, hydrophobia, ptyalism of the pancreas, diseases of the spleens, goitre, hidden cancer," &c. (Hahnemann quoted by Teste). Hahnemann says (*M. M. P.*) that doubtless many patients were cured, but not a few succumbed to the enormous doses given. These doses he showed were quite unnecessary, when the symptoms of the proving are taken as guides. The "evacuant" use of *Ver.* gives one of the keynotes for its homœopathic use—its discharges are *copious;* copious stools, copious vomiting, copious urine, copious salivation, and copious sweat. The discharges drain the tissues like cholera, in which disease its pathogenetic effects render it one of the first remedies, ranking with *Camp.* and *Cupr.* in Hahnemann's trio. The discharges exhaust the vitality as well as the tissues and cause vertigo; blackness before the sight, fainting, collapse: "Rapid sinking of forces; complete prostration; cold sweat and cold breath." "Skin blue, purple, cold, wrinkled; remaining in folds when pinched." "Face hippocratic, nose pointed." "Hands icy cold." "Face and legs icy cold." This *coldness* is another of the keynotes of *Ver.* It is one aspect of the fever-producing power of the drug: "Coldness of the whole body." "Coldness running over whole body soon after taking it." "Feeling of internal chill ran through him from head to toes of both feet at once." "Continued rigor in back and over arms." Very characteristic are: "Cold feeling in abdomen;" "coldness as of a piece of ice on vertex;" "cold nose;" "face cold and collapsed;" "cold tongue;" and most characteristic of all, "cold sweat on forehead." Along with the coldness is blueness of face and extremities. *Ver.* is like cholera in that coldness predominates in its fever, but it has also "heat and redness of face and hands." With the fever there is apt to be delirium and prolonged sleep. The delirium may develop great intensity and violence: "Fury: tears his clothing; bites her shoes to pieces and swallows the fragments; cursing; stamping; wants to run away; makes a great noise." These and kindred symptoms seem to indicate *Ver.* in acute affections attended with delirium; and also in cases of mental alienation, which was prominent among the affections treated with the drug by the ancients. Hahnemann says of *Ver.* that it has the power "to promote a cure of almost one-third of the insane in lunatic asylums (at all events as a homœopathic intermediate remedy)." One of the symptoms taken by Hahnemann from Grading is this: "He swallows his own excrement," which Goullon has verified (*Z. Berl. V. H. A.*, xix. 156): a child had a craze for eating its own fæces, or dung lying in the street. *Ver.* 2., thrice daily, cured in a month. The mania of *Ver.*

may be of the exalted kind, religious or sexual. Imagines she is pregnant and will soon be delivered; nymphomania; puerperal mania; mania for kissing everybody have been cured by *Ver.* Generally there will be collateral *Ver.* symptoms to confirm the choice: coldness, blueness, collapse, fainting, vomiting, or diarrhœa. *Ver.* is a great *fainting* remedy. There is fainting from emotions, from the least exertion, from retching, from stool. Sinking feeling during hæmorrhage. The gastric conditions are characterised by extreme hunger; craving for cold food and refreshing things; thirst for ice-cold water. This last is very characteristic, and appears in the chill and heat of fever. The copiousness of the stools distinguishes *Ver.* from *Camph.* The evacuations are apt to be *green*, vomit, stool, urine. The characteristic diarrhœa of *Ver.* is: frequent, greenish, gushing; mixed with flakes; cutting colic, with cramps commencing in hands and feet and spreading all over; prostrating, after fright; < least movement; with vomiting, cold sweat on forehead during stool and prostration after. "Violent vomiting with profuse diarrhœa" is a keynote of *Ver.* The constipation of *Ver.* is no less characteristic: no desire; stools large, hard; in round black balls; from inactive rectum; frequent desire felt in epigastrium; painful of infants and children; of women after confinement. *Ver.* is a great pain producer, and the pains of its neuralgias (dysmenorrhœa, migraine) are often accompanied by diarrhœa, vomiting, cold sweat, fainting, or prostration. This case was reported in *P. C. J. H.* (vii. 150): Prosopalgia, right-sided, kept an anæmic woman awake and in misery for several days and nights from the crushing paroxysmal pain, causing sweating and prostration. *Ver.* cured at once. E. F. Watts (*A. H.*, xxi., 317) had this case: Mrs. C. had severe nervous headaches for years. Any over-exertion, as riding or working on hot days, would excite them. They frequently began in occiput, settling sometimes in one eye sometimes in the other. *Spi.* and *Sil.* gave no relief. One day Watts noticed that the brow contracted and eyelids nearly closed with the intensity of the pain. *Ver.* was now given and relieved at once. Gee (*M. A.*, xxv. 22) cured this case with one dose of *Ver.* 200: Mrs. L., widow, 43, had sciatica four years. Pain sharp, transient, darting upwards and downwards and from both sides to centre. Heat <; "the cooler the better." Cold sweat with the attacks. Headache from both temples to base of brain < by heat. Vertex itches during attacks. Pain compels her to move about, but no > from motion. The cramps of *Ver.* are part of its general convulsant properties. The convulsions of *Ver.* may be tetanic, with lockjaw, or epileptic. The eyes are particularly convulsed or the lids paralysed. There may be vanishing of sight or sparks before the sight or night-blindness. *Dryness* and *burning* are leading sensations as in other parts. Dryness is felt in nose, mouth, palate, throat. *Ver.* has a sharp action on the respiratory organs and has cured many cases of pneumonia when the mental and other symptoms of *Ver.* have been present. A leading local sympton is *tickling:* Tickling deep in trachea and bronchi. "Tickling in chest, as if it would provoke cough, in middle of sternum." This symptom helped me to the remedy in the following case: Mrs. W., 30, had much pain inside throat. Painful ulcer in mouth. Throat sore and inclined to be ulcerated. *Tickling all over inside of chest and throat;* outside tender. No pain on swallowing. Has had cold and cough some time, cough hurts chest. *Stan.* had no effect. *Ver.* 1m thrice daily gradually removed all symptoms. *Ver.* meets cardiac debility, following acute diseases ; pulse thread-like ; faints in morning ; face red when lying down or sitting up, deadly pale ; hands cold, clammy. *Ver.* is *Suited to* (1) the extremes of life—children and old people ; (2) lean, choleric, or melancholy persons ; (3) young people and women of a sanguine or nervo-sanguine temperament (of mountaineers. —Teste) ; (4) people who are habitually cold and deficient in vital reaction ; (5) persons of gay disposition ; (6) of fitful mood ; (7) anæmic persons. *Peculiar Sensations are:* As if pregnant or in throes of child-birth. As if he had a bad conscience, or had committed a crime. As if in a dream. As if things whirled in a circle. As if a lump of ice on vertex. Burning in brain. As if head would burst. As if heat and cold at same time on scalp. Hair as if electrified. Eyelids as if rubbed sore. As if inner surface of lids too dry. As if hundreds of fine needle-points were thrust into eyelids. As if ears were stopped. As if alternate current of cold and warm air coming out of ear. As if nose dry. As if teeth were filled with lead. As if tongue too heavy. As of dust in throat. As if mouth lined with mucus. As if something alive running from stomach into throat. As from ravenous hunger, pain in stomach. Radiating pain from abdomen. Distress over heart and epigastrium. Sinking, empty feeling in abdomen. As of knives cutting bowels. As of hot coals in abdomen. Pinching as with pincers in abdomen. As if intestines twisted into a knot. As if cold water running through veins. Arms as if bruised or broken. As if bones of l. forearm were pressed. As if arms too full and swollen, feel cold when raising them. As if hands had been asleep. As if a heavy stone were tied to feet and knees. Limbs pain as if exhausted by excessive fatigue. As if she would have to fly away. Electric pains occur in various parts. The symptoms are: < By touch ; pressure ; shock of injury. Slight wounds = fainting. Rest > palpitation. Horizontal position > vomiting, cough, and general condition. Stooping < headache ; = rush of blood to head. Motion <. Throwing back head > asthma. Walking > jerks in limbs ; neuralgia of arms and legs ; pain in feet and knees. Least exertion = fainting ; cough ; sweat. < Night ; and morning on waking. Warmth <. Hot water <. Drinking <. Cold food and drink < cough. Drinking cold water on a hot day = diarrhœa. < Damp weather. < Change of weather. (Rheumatism < in wet weather which drives patient out of bed.—Nash.) < Sharp, cool air = dry tickling cough. < Before and during menses ; before and during stool ; after stool ; during sweat. < from fright.

Relations.—*Antidoted by:* (Poisonous doses) Strong Coffee ; Camph. (pressive pain in head with coldness of body and unconsciousness after.—Hahn.) ; Acon. (anxious, distracted state with coldness of body or burning in brain.—Hahn.) ; Chi. (other chronic affections from abuse of Ver.—*e.g.*, daily forenoon fever.—Hahn.) ; Staph. (most cases.—Teste). *Antidote to:* Ars., Chi., Cup. (colic), Op., Tab. ; removes the bad effects of Opium and Tobacco. *Follows well:* Ars.,

Arn., Chi., Cup., Ip.; Camph. (cholera); Am. c., Carb. v., Bov. (in dysmenorrhœa with vomiting and purging). Lyc. and Nux in painful constipation of infants. *Followed well by:* Puls., Aco., Bell., Cham., Rhus, Sep., Sul. *Compare:* Electric sensations; tickling, prickly sensations, Veratrin. Cold sweat on forehead (Tab. over entire body). Mania with desire to cut clothes, Trn. Lascivious talk, amorous or religious, Hyo., Stram. Fainting from least exertion, Carb. v., Sul. Sinking during hæmorrhages (Trill., fainting). Sensation of lumps of ice on vertex with chilliness, Sep. Facies hippocratica, Aco. Craves acids or refreshing things, Ph. ac. Cold feeling in abdomen, Colch., Tab, Vomiting < by drinking. Ars. Vomiting < by least motion, Tab. Cholera after fright, Aco. Prostration after vomiting, Ars., Tab. Large hard stools, Sul., Bry. Round black balls, Chel., Op., Pb. Frequent desire for stool felt in epigastrium, Ign. (Nux, in rectum). Weakness at menses, Alm., Carb. an., Coccul. Collapse, cholera, coldness, < by heat, Camph. (Camph. has scanty, Ver. copious stools). Rheumatism < in wet weather, which drives patient out of bed, Cham. Delirium, Bell., Stram. (these have not the cold surface and cold sweat of Ver.). Fright = Diarrhœa, Gels. Cholera, Jat. c. (vomits ropy, albuminous matter with purging); Pod. (painless); Ir. v. (better for summer complaints; excoriated, raw feeling at anus); Crot. t. (single gush; every attempt to eat or drink = stool); Elat. (olive-green stools). Suppressed scarlatina, Zn. (Ver. has succeeded when Zn. has failed to = reaction). Emaciation about neck, Nat. m. (Ver. especially in whooping-cough). Weak from talking, Stan., Coccul., Sul., Calc. Collapse, diarrhœa, vomiting, Ant. t. (Ant. t., more drowsiness; Ver., more cold sweat). Neck muscles too weak to hold head up, Ant. t. Craves cold drinks, Ars. (Ver. is between Ars. and Nux.—Teste.) Purging and collapse, Hell. (Hell., apathetic). Pressure in vertex with pain in stomach > pressure < motion, Puls. Abdominal pains, Coloc. (Ver. must walk about). Pain = fainting, Cham., Hep., Val. Convulsion after sudden emotions, Ign. Convulsions with spasm of glottis, Nux (Ver. secondary to exhausting diseases). Intermittent fever, Lach. Cough followed by belching, Amb., Sul. ac. Alarmed about soul's salvation, Sul. Windy colic and spasms of women, Castor. (with yawning), Diosc. (> moving about). Desire to ramble hither and thither, Bell. As if in a dream, Amb., Anac., Calc., Can. i., Con., Cup., Med., Rhe., Val., Ziz. Umbilical hernia with absence of urging, Bry., Nat. m.; (with urging, Nux, Coccul.). Faintness connected with evacuations, Ap., Nux m., Pul., Spi. (with scanty stools, Crot. t., Dulc., Ox. ac., Pet., Sars., Sul.). > Uncovering, Aco., Calc., Camph., Fer., Iod., Lyc., Pul., Sec., Sul. Griping, cutting, tearing, and spasmodic pains in body, Col., Dulc. Laughing and weeping by turns, Aur., Pul., Lyc., Stram., Alm., Pho., Sep., Sul. Loquacity, Cup., Hyo., Lach., Op., Stram. Gossiping, babbling, Hyo. (Ver. on religious subjects). Kisses everybody, Agar. Averse to hot food, Pho. Cold drink < cough (> Caust.). Night-blindness, Nux, Bell. Smell of manure or smoke before nose, Anac. "Evacuant" action, Lobel.

Causation.—Fright. Shock of injury. Disappointed love. Injured pride or honour. Suppressed exanthema. Opium. Tobacco. Alcohol.

SYMPTOMS.

1. **Mind.**—Affections of the mind in general; tired of life, but fear to die; amativeness; haughtiness; delirium; madness; sensitiveness; memory weak, or entirely lost (H. N. G.).—Melancholy dejection, sadness, and inclination to weep.—Inconsolable affliction, with howlings and cries on account of imaginary misfortunes.—Melancholy, head hangs down, sits brooding in silence.—Excessive anguish and inquietude, with apprehension and troubled conscience, esp. at night, or in morning, often also when getting out of bed, or rising from a seat.—Strong tendency to be frightened, and timidity.—Deadly anguish.—Discouragement and despair (hopelessness of life).—Busy restlessness, constant motion, with great inclination for labour.—Disposition to be angry at the least thing, often followed by anxiety, and palpitation of the heart.—Woman, 66, after paralytic seizure became maniacal, extremely angry, constantly accusing her nurses, pupils contracted, continual excitement, often incoherent: a dose of *Ver. a.* increased these symptoms, and then a single dose of *Ver. v.* φ calmed all down (R. T. C.).—Loquaciousness, he talks rapidly.—Swearing, inclination to run away, tearing things.—Is conscious only as in a dream.—Cannot bear to be left alone; yet persistently refuses to talk.—Strong disposition to silence, with abusive language on the slightest provocation; if he talks he scolds, and the voice is weak and scarcely audible.—Disposition to converse about the faults of others.—(He hunts up other people's weak sides and reproaches them.)—She is continually accusing and scolding her husband when dying of phthisis.—Never speaks the truth; does not know herself what she is saying.—Erroneous and haughty notions.—Thinks himself distinguished; squanders his money, proud of his position.—Imagines he is a hunter.—Immoderate gaiety and loquacity.—Fury, with impulse to bite, to tear everything, and to run away.—Loss of memory.—Absence of ideas.—Loss of sense.—Insanity, he wants to cut up everything.—Unusually joyous mood.—Mild delirium, with trembling excitement.—Mental alienation and insanity, with singing, whistling, laughing, inclination to run from place to place, extravagant and haughty ideas and actions, or else a disposition to ascribe to one's self diseases which are altogether imaginary (thinks herself pregnant, or that she will be delivered soon).—Persistent raging with great heat of body.—Swallowing his own excrement.—Paroxysms of amorous or religious alienation.—Mental disorders, with lechery and obscene talk.—Kisses everybody; before menses.—Puerperal mania and convulsions.—Nymphomania with violence and destructiveness.—Violent delirium (religious or exalted).—Suicidal tendency from religious despair.

2. **Head.**—Confusion in head, as if all within it were in motion, esp. in morning.—Dulness of all the senses.—Whirling vertigo.—Intoxication and dizziness.—Vertigo, esp. when walking.—Vertigo: with cold sweats on forehead; with loss of vision; sudden fainting; from opium eating; from abuse of tobacco and alcohol.—Fainting from least exertion, turning in bed, straining at stool, retching, slight wounds, pains; loss of fluids; anxiety, nausea, convulsive, twitchings.—Fainting with lockjaw, convulsion of eyes.—Fits of headache, with paleness of face, nausea, and vomiting (of green mucus).—Headache with painful stiffness of nape of neck.—Headache with (profuse)

flow of urine.—Sick-headache in which diuresis forms a crisis.—Headache, by paroxysms, as if the brain were bruised or torn (with pressure).—Heaviness of the whole head.—Pressive headache, often in vertex, or else semilateral, with pain in stomach.—Violent headache which disappears on appearance of menses.—During menses (which had not occurred for six weeks) headache, esp. in morning, with qualmishness ; > evening.—Headache, with nausea and vomiting.—Neuralgia of head with indigestion, features sunken.—Constrictive pain in head (and gullet).—Incisive pain in vertex.—Shaking in head, with jerking in arms and paleness of the fingers.—Blood rushes violently to head when stooping.—Hyperæmia of brain from whooping-cough.—Pulsative headache.—Burning pain in brain.—Sensation of a cold wind blowing through head.—Headache as if brain were broken.—Sensation of coldness and heat in the exterior of head, with painful sensibility of the hair.—Crawling, bristling sensation (r. side of head) as if the hair were electrified ; with slight shivering of skin under hair.—Plica polonica.—Coldness at vertex as if there were ice upon it (with icy-cold feet and nausea ; < when rising from the bed ; > from external pressure, and when bending head backward).—Sensation of warmth and coldness on head at same time.—Head burning hot ; limbs alternately hot and cold.—Head hot and covered with sweat ; children rub head, cannot bear to be left alone ; put hands to head (typhoid).—Scalp very sensitive, with headache.—Cold sweat on forehead.—Sensation of soreness of the head, with nausea.—Neck too weak to hold head up.

3. **Eyes.**—Pain in the eyes, as if the eyeballs were bruised.—The eyeballs are turned upwards.—Painful tearing or compression in eyes.—Permanent burning in eyes.—Redness of eyes.—Painful inflammation in eyes, esp. r., and sometimes with violent headache, and nocturnal sleeplessness.—Eyes dull, clouded, yellowish.—Blueness of eyes.—Eyes surrounded by blue or black rings.—Eyes fixed, watery (sunken, with loss of lustre), and as if they were covered with albumen.—Excessive dryness of eyelids.—Profuse lachrymation, often with burning, incisive pains, and sensation of dryness in eyes (and lids, with redness).—Agglutination of the eyelids during sleep.—Trembling of upper eyelids.—Neuralgia palpebralis.—Paralysis of eyelids.—Eyes convulsed and prominent.—Pupils strongly contracted ; or perceptibly dilated.—Loss of sight.—Diplopia.—Nocturnal blindness.—Sparks and black spots before eyes, esp. when rising from a seat, or getting out of bed.

4. **Ears.**—Shootings in ears.—Pressure and constrictive sensations in ears.—Alternate sensation of coldness and heat in ears ; as if an alternate current of cold and warm air were coming out of the ear.—Deafness, as from obstruction in ears.—Sensation as if a membrane were stretched over ear.—Humming, with sensitiveness to noise.—Roaring in ears, esp. when rising from a seat.

5. **Nose.**—Nose grows more pointed ; seems longer.—Icy coldness of nose.—Inflammation and pain, as from ulceration, in interior of nose.—Contractive or depressing pain in nasal bone.—Nose-bleed : at night ; during sleep ; from one nostril only ; before menses.—Smell of manure, or smoke, before nose.—Distressing sensation of dryness in nose.—Violent and frequent sneezing.—Coryza.

6. **Face.**—Face pale, cold, hippocratic, wan, with the nose pointed, and a blue (or green) circle round eyes.—Bluish colour of face.—Yellowish

colour of face.—Redness of one cheek, the other is pale.—Alternate redness and paleness of face.—Redness of face when lying down, paleness when getting up.—Burning heat, deep redness, and perspiration on face.—Cold perspiration on face (esp. on forehead).—(Periodical neuralgia of face and head, with coldness of hands and tendency to faint.—R. T. C.)—Drawing and tensive pains in face, on one side only, and extending to ear.—Jerkings and pinchings in muscles of face (when masticating). Lockjaw.—Risus sardonicus.—Pustules in face, with pain, as from excoriation, when touched.—Acne.—Military eruption on cheeks.—Bloatedness of face.—Lips : bluish or hanging down ; dry, black, parched ; wrinkled, pale or black and cracked.—Froth from mouth.—Eruption on the commissures of the lips.—Acne round the mouth and chin.—Cramp in the jaw.—Pain and swelling of the submaxillary glands.

7. **Teeth.**—Toothache with headache, and red, bloated face.—Toothache (sometimes pulsative), with swelled face, cold perspiration on forehead, nausea, and vomiting, painful weariness, and coldness of whole body, prostration of strength, even to fainting, internal heat, and insatiable thirst.—Aching, and sensation of extreme heaviness in teeth, with drawing pain during the mastication even of soft food.—Grinding of teeth.—Looseness of teeth.

8. **Mouth.**—Mouth dry and clammy.—Burning in mouth and throat.—Salivation, with nausea, or with acrid or salt taste.—Much flow of saliva from the mouth like water-brash.—Froth before mouth.—Sensation of coldness, or burning in mouth and on tongue.—Inflammation of interior of mouth.—Tongue, dry, blackish, cracked, or red and swollen.—Tongue loaded with a yellow coating ; or cold and withered.—Biting taste as from peppermint in the mouth.—Stammering.—Loss of speech.—Sensation of torpor, and great dryness in palate (with thirst).

9. **Throat.**—Sore throat, with constrictive pain of contraction (as by a pressing swelling) esp. during deglutition.—Contraction of gullet, as from a pressive swelling.—Swelling of the gullet, with danger of suffocation.—Sensation of coldness, or burning in back of mouth and gullet.—Dryness in throat, which cannot be mitigated by any drink.—Roughness, dryness, and scraping in throat.—Exophthalmic goître (Kirsch).

10. **Appetite.**—Insipidity of the saliva in the mouth.—Bitter, bilious taste in mouth.—Water tastes bitter.—Putrid taste in mouth, like manure, also herbaceous taste.—Cooling, or sharp taste in mouth and throat, as from peppermint.—Insatiable thirst, with craving, principally for cold drinks.—Craves ice.—Appetite and craving for food, also in intervals between vomiting and evacuation.—Raging and voracious hunger.—Hunger and thirst with profuse flow of urine.—Bulimy.—Ardent and continued desire for acid or cool things (fruits).—Craves : fruits ; gherkins ; citric acid ; salted things ; herrings ; sardines.—Aversion to hot food.—After eating, however little may be taken, immediate vomiting and diarrhœa.—Nausea, with hunger, and pressure at the stomach, when eating.—After a meal hiccough, inclination to vomit, and regurgitation of bitter serum (of bile ; of bitter substances ; greenish).—> From eating meat and drinking milk.—< From potatoes and green vegetables.

11. **Stomach.**—Risings with taste of food.—Violent empty risings, also after a meal.—Bitter or sour risings.—Frequent and violent hiccough.—

Qualmishness and salivation with closure of the jaws.—Violent nausea, which frequently almost induces syncope, and generally with excessive thirst (and increased flow of urine).—Frequent or continued nausea, also in morning.—Extreme nausea causing one to retch and strain with great violence, sometimes with vomiting, sometimes not.—Great nausea before vomiting.—Water-brash.—Violent vomiting, with continued nausea, great exhaustion, and want to lie down, preceded by coldness of hands, with shuddering over whole body, accompanied by general heat, and followed by ebullition of blood and heat in hands.—Vomiting of food.—Bitter, or sour vomiting.—Vomiting of froth and of yellowish green or white mucus; with cold sweat.—Green vomit.—Vomiting of green mucus.—Vomiting of mucus at night.—Vomiting of black bile and of blood.—Continued vomiting, with diarrhœa, and pressure in the scrobiculus.—The least drop of liquid, and the slightest movement, excite vomiting. — Painful contraction of abdomen, when vomiting.—Pain in stomach, with hunger and burning thirst.—Excessive sensibility in region of stomach and scrobiculus.—Pyloric end of stomach affected (Bayes).—Pains come some minutes after eating.—(Severe gastralgia an hour or two after meals, a pain extends from middle of sternum to below ribs, must hold stomach from the violence of the pain, but the pressure does not >, the pain then extends to above hip, is accompanied by distressing vomiting, brings up a quantity of stuff like vinegar; the pain = thirst, and lasts eight to ten hours; she trembles with it.—R. T. C.)—Excessive anguish in pit of stomach.—Intermittent neuralgia in girl, 11, about 4 p.m. throws up quantity of wind, about 5 p.m. agonising pain sets in like knives cutting the bowels every few minutes, lasting one or two minutes; so intense that it took three or four men to hold her; attacks end by sighing (Kitching).—Painful distension of pit of stomach.—Emptiness and uneasiness in stomach.—Cramp in stomach.—Pressure in scrobiculus, extending sometimes into sternum, hypochondria, and hypogastrium, esp. after a meal.—Acute pains in stomach and epigastrium.—Burning sensation in pit of stomach.—Inflammation of stomach.

12. **Abdomen.**—Tensive pain in hypochondria as from flatulence.—Shaking in spleen, while walking, after a meal.—Spleen swollen.—Hyperæmia of liver with cholera-like symptoms, or with asthma.—Diaphragmatis with peritonitis, vomiting, and coldness.—Colic in umbilical region.—Excessively painful sensibility of the abdomen when touched.—Nocturnal pains in abdomen, with sleeplessness.—Swelling of the abdomen.—While vomiting abdomen is painfully contracted.—Abdomen hard and inflated.—Tension in the hypochondria and umbilical region.—Cramps in abdomen, and colic.—Colic: cutting; griping and twisting, esp. about navel, > after stool; as if intestines were twisted in a knot; flatulent; cold sweat; < after eating.—Pressive, drawing pains in abdomen, when walking, in evening.—Cuttings (in abdomen) as by knives, accompanied by diarrhœa, and thirst, with flow of urine.—Burning sensation throughout abdomen, as from hot coals.—Cold feeling in abdomen.—Pain in entrails, as if they were bruised.—Inflammation of intestines. — Inguinal hernia.—Incarcerated hernia.—Protrusion of hernia during cough.—Flatulent colic, with noisy, gurgling borborygmi in abdomen.—The longer the flatus is retained, the greater the difficulty with which it is expelled.—Violent expulsion of flatus upwards and downwards.

13. **Stool and Anus.**—Constipation, sometimes obstinate, mostly from

inactivity of rectum, and often accompanied by heat and headache.—Fæces hard, and of too large a size.—Unsuccessful urging to stool.—Constipation of nursing infants.—Violent and painful diarrhœa, often with tension of abdomen, preceded and followed by gripings.—Watery diarrhœa, < from motion; desire for very cold drinks.—Complaints before stool, during, and after.—Copious evacuations.—Rice-water stools with tonic cramps.—Simultaneous purging and vomiting.—Cholera, cramp, cold tongue and breath, feeble, hoarse voice, wrinkled fingers, retention of urine.—Sudden vomiting and purging.—Diarrhœa of acrid matter, with burning sensation in anus.—Nocturnal diarrhœa.—Loose blackish, greenish, brownish, evacuations.—Flaky, green stools, like spinach.—Loose, sanguineous evacuations.—Sudden involuntary evacuation of liquid fæces; when expelling flatus.—Diarrhœa of phthisis.—During the evacuation, great lassitude, shivering, with shuddering, paleness of face, cold perspiration on forehead, and anxiety, with fear of apoplexy.—Fainting during stool.—Burning sensation in anus, during evacuation.—Pain, as from excoriation in anus.—Pressure towards anus, with blind hæmorrhoids.—Verminous symptoms.

14. **Urinary Organs.**—Retention of urine.—Want to urinate, while bladder is empty, with pain as if urethra were constricted behind the glans.—Urine diminished, yellow and turbid even during emission.—Flow of urine, with raging hunger and thirst, headache, nausea, colic, hard fæces, and coryza.—Involuntary emission of urine; during cough, in typhoid.—Acrid urine.—Deep-coloured or greenish urine.—Dark red urine, discharged frequently, but in small quantities.—Pressive pain in the bladder, and burning sensation when urinating,

15. **Male Sexual Organs.**—Excessive sensibility of the genital organs.—Excoriation of prepuce.—Drawings in testes.

16. **Female Sexual Organs.**—Catamenia premature and profuse.—Catamenia suppressed.—Before catamenia: headache, vertigo, epistaxis, and nocturnal perspiration.—At commencement of catamenia: diarrhœa, nausea, and shivering.—During catamenia: headache in morning, with nausea, humming in ears, burning thirst, and pains in all limbs.—Towards end of catamenia: grinding of teeth, and bluish colour of face.—Nymphomania: before menses: from unsatisfied passion or mental causes; from disappointed love; puerperal mania; during confinement.—Metritis.—Menorrhagia.—Dysmenorrhœa: with prolapse; nausea, vomiting, diarrhœa, exhaustion; cold sweat; chilliness; pain in kidneys and uterus before and during menses.—Amenorrhœa.—Strangulated, prolapsed vagina, with cold sweat, exhausting vomit and diarrhœa.—Suppressed catamenia, lochia, and secretion of milk, with delirium.—Sexual desire too strong, particularly in childbed; < at night; nymphomania (of lying-in women); complaints during menstruation, as, *e.g.*, vomiting and diarrhœa, which may occur at these times.—Threatened abortion, with cold sweat, nausea, and vomiting.—During pregnancy wants to wander about the house; taciturn; haughty; thirsty; hard fæces, inactive rectum.—Vomiting of pregnancy.—Labour pains exhaust.—Suppression of lochia or milk with nymphomania.—Puerperal mania, wants to kiss everybody.—In childbed: impudent behaviour; nymphomania; exhaustion.—Eclampsia.—Painfulness of breasts.

17. **Respiratory Organs.**—Respiration oppressed; voice hollow;

weak.—Chest loaded with mucus, with roughness and scraping in the throat. —Spasmodic contraction of glottis with dilated pupils.—Suffocative constriction in larnyx.—Tickling very low down in trachea, provoking cough without expectoration.—Cough, excited by a tickling, deeply seated in the bronchia, with easy expectoration, or else dryness.—Cough, irritation referred to lowest part of sternum; pressure at stomach-pit, or over abdomen = cough immediately (Bayes).—Dry, tickling cough, after walking in sharp, cold air.—Cough provoked by drinking, esp. cold water.—Violent cough, with continued risings, as if about to vomit.—Cough in the evening, with salivation.—Dry, burning cough, generally in evening and morning.—Cough, with pain in side, weakness and obstructed respiration.—Hollow, deep cough, always in three or four shocks, as if proceeding from abdomen, with incisive pains in abdomen.—Lancinations towards inguinal ring, when coughing.—Cough, like whooping-cough, with vomiting. — Cough, with yellowish expectoration, on entering a warm room, followed by pain, as from a bruise in chest.—Cough, with copious expectoration.

18. **Chest.**—Obstructed respiration, often to the verge of suffocation, generally produced by a spasmodic constriction of throat and chest.—Shortness of breath on least movement.—Dyspnœa and impeded respiration, also when seated.—Chest very much oppressed, with pain in side, during an inspiration. —Pressure at chest, esp. in region of sternum, and principally after eating or drinking.—Sensation of fulness in chest, which induces frequent eructations. —Squeezing in chest, esp. after drinking.—Cramp in chest, with painful constriction.—Spasmodic contraction of muscles of chest.—Incisive pain in chest.—Tickling in chest, as if it would provoke cough, in middle of sternum. —Shootings, by paroxysms, in chest, with obstructed respiration.—Slow, sharp stitches near nipples, which at last itch.

19. **Heart.**—Violent palpitation of heart, which pushes out the ribs, with choking, and severe fits of anxietas præcordium.—Pulse slow, almost lost.—Great activity of arterial system.—Angina pectoris.—The blood runs like cold water through the veins.

20. **Neck and Back.**—Rheumatic stiffness in nape, extending to sacrum ; with vertigo, moving.—Paralytic weakness of the muscles of neck (esp. in whooping-cough) which become incapable of supporting head.—Muscles of nape paralysed.—Pain (back and small of back feel sore and bruised) as of a fracture in loins and back, with drawing pressure, esp. when stooping and rising.—Squeezing (tension like cramp) between shoulder-blades. —Pain in scapulæ, extending over whole back, with diuresis, thirst, and constipation.

21. **Limbs.**—Painful paralytic weakness in all limbs. — Numbness, tingling, or falling asleep of the limbs.—Stiffness of limbs, < morning and after a walk.—Trembling of limbs.—Shooting in limbs as from electric sparks. —Pain as from fatigue.—Nails blue from coldness.—Pains in limbs resembling a bruise, < during wet, cold weather ; < in warmth of bed ; > walking up and down.—Icy coldness of limbs ; of hands and feet.

22. **Upper Limbs.**—Paralytic pain, as of a fracture in arms, from shoulder-joint to wrist.—Jerking in arms.—Coldness or sensation of fulness (heaviness) and of swelling in arms.—Constant sensation of numbness in arms.—Pain in middle of l. forearm as if bones were pressed together.—

Trembling of arms, on grasping an object.—Shocks in elbow, as from electricity.—Dry tetters on hands.—Tingling in hands and fingers.—The hands go to sleep and feel like dead.—Numbness and paleness of fingers.—Icy coldness and blueness of hands.—Drawings and cramps in fingers.—Nails blue.

23. **Lower Limbs.**—Paralysis in hip-joint (first r. then l.), with difficulty in walking.—Paralytic pain, as of a fracture in legs.—Arthritic tearing and drawing in legs and feet.—Constant sensation of numbness in legs.—Tension in tendons of ham, as if they were too short.—Pain, as of a fracture in knees, when going downstairs (or when stepping).—Shocks in knee, as from electricity.—Extreme and painful heaviness in knees, legs, and feet, with difficulty in walking.—Violent cramps in calves and feet.—Rapid swelling of feet.—Icy coldness of feet.—Trembling of feet, with coldness, as if cold water were circulating in the part.—Shootings (stitches) in (great) toes.—Stinging in toes when standing.—Painful gout in feet.—Lancinations, and pain as from excoriation, in the corns of the feet.

24. **Generalities.**—[We may think of this remedy where there is a marked debility or exhaustion from functional or physical disturbance, as *e.g.*, in whooping-cough, patient will cough until completely exhausted, and then have a cold perspiration on the forehead ; or there may be a great exhaustion obliging one to lie down after the passage of a stool, even though it be soft, with cold sweat on the forehead.—Affections in general of the sexual organs, principally on r. side ; on crown of head, esp. for sensations felt there ; appearing in the rear of the navel ; small of the back.—Countenance is almost always changed presenting an unnatural appearance.—Dry mouth.—Inguinal hernia.—Flatus in general ; flatulent colic.—Urine very dark ; blackness of outer parts, staggering when walking, from debility ; drowsiness ; dry exanthema.—< After drinking ; before and during menstruation ; before and during stool (feeling very weak and turn pale during stool) ; often after stool ; during perspiration.—H. N. G.].—Paroxysms of pain, which always occasion, for a short time, delirium and dementia.—Drawing pain in limbs, esp. during a long walk.—Pressive pain, as of a fracture, in limbs, muscles, and bones.—Paralytic pain in limbs, as after great fatigue or exhaustion.—Tearing in extensors, when seated.—Pains (rheumatic) in limbs, which are rendered insupportable by the heat of bed, > on getting up, and which disappear completely when walking, generally manifesting themselves towards 4 or 5 a.m.—Pains in limbs, < in spring and autumn by bad weather, when it is cold and damp.—Pain < by hearing another speak.—Relaxation of muscles.—Continuous weakness and trembling.—Fits of cramp, and convulsive movements of limbs.—Tetanic stiffness of the body.—Attack of spasm, with clenching of jaws, loss of sense and movement, and convulsive jerking of eyes and eyelids ; before the attack, anguish, discouragement, and despair.—(Epileptic fits.)—Tonic spasms, sometimes with contraction of palms of hands, and soles of feet, which are spasmodically drawn inward.—Several of the symptoms are renewed by rising up, and > by lying down.—Sudden, general, and paralytic prostration of strength.—Excessive chronic weakness, which does not permit to be seated, nor to remain lying down, or else excited by the least movement.—Tottering gait.—Syncope, sometimes also on the least movement (characteristic).—General emaciation.—Tingling

in whole body, as far as ends of fingers and toes.—The patient is affected by the open air.—Inflammation of inner organs, esp. those of digestion.—Sporadic and Asiatic cholera.

25. **Skin.**—Miliary eruption, which itches in the heat, and burns after being scratched.—Measles, tardy and pale ; skin livid ; hæmorrhages but no relief ; drowsy, weak, vomiting.—Scarlatina in hot weather, eruption bluish, burning heat of limbs alternating with coldness.—Nettle-rash.—Dry eruption, resembling scabies, with nocturnal itching.—Dry tetters.—Desquamation of the epidermis (of indurated or thickened portions of the skin).—Skin flabby and without elasticity (the folds remain in the state into which the skin has been pressed).—Whitish colour of the skin.—Skin anæmic or cyanotic.—Skin blue, purple, cold.

26. **Sleep.**—Yawning.—Drowsy insensibility, or coma vigil, with incomplete consciousness, starts with fright, and eyes half open, or shut only on one side.—(Drowsy in evening, yet cannot sleep at night.—R. T. C.).—Nocturnal sleeplessness, with great anguish.—Sleep, long, uninterrupted, heavy, too profound.—Sleep, with the arms passed over the head.—Dreams : anxious, of being bitten by a dog and cannot escape ; of being hunted ; of robbers, with frightened awakening and a fixed idea that the dream is true ; of quarrels ; frightful, followed by vomiting of a very tenacious, green mucus.—Moaning or whining during sleep.—Sleep with thirst and diuresis.

27. **Fever.**—General coldness of whole body, and cold, clammy perspiration, esp. on forehead.—Coldness of the skin even when covered up warmly.—Coldness of single parts.—Shuddering, and shivering, with thirst for cold water.—Coldness over the back.—Shivering with sensation of coldness in the limbs, esp. shoulders and arms, as if ice-cold water streaming through the bones, in a warm room.—Coldness of the feet as if ice-water running into them, with trembling.—Shuddering, and cutis anserina, after drinking.—Chill < by drinking.—Fever, with external coldness.—Violent shivering and shaking (followed by heat and slight thirst), then perspiration, which soon changes to coldness.—Chilliness and coldness predominate, and run from below upwards.—Shiverings, at first with much thirst, followed by shivering alternately with heat, then permanent heat, with thirst.—Fever, with internal heat only, and deep-coloured urine, or with vomiting and diarrhœa, or with constipation ; during the shivering, vertigo, nausea, and pains in loins and back.—During the heat, continual coma, or delirium, with redness of face.—Heat only internal, with thirst, but without desire to drink.—Heat in the evening, with perspiration.—Heat suddenly alternating with chilliness.—Fever before midnight, and in morning quotidian, tertian, or quartan.—Creeping running from head to toes.—Pulse slow, and almost extinct, or small, quick, and intermittent.—The blood runs like cold water through the veins.—Perspiration in general ; complaints concomitant with.—Perspiration easily excited during day, by least movement.—Violent perspiration in morning, in the evening, or all night, as well as during every stool.—Cold, sour, or putrid perspiration, sometimes colouring linen yellow, always with deathly paleness of face.—Intermittent fever : external coldness, with dark urine and cold perspiration, desire for cold drinks, and chill with nausea ; afterwards heat with unquenchable thirst, delirium, redness of face,

constant slumber; finally perspiration without thirst, and very pale countenance.—Sweat only on hands.

Veratrum Nigrum.

Veratrum nigrum. Dark-flowered Veratrum. *N. O.* Melanthaceæ. Tincture of fresh leaves and succulent flower-stalks.

Clinical.—Headache. Menstruation, protracted. Tinnitus aurium.

Characteristics.—Cooper has given me a few observations with *Ver. nig.*, which I have arranged in Schema form. The plant, he says, has much the same botanical characters as *Ver. alb.*, but the flowers are dark-coloured. It is native to Austria and Siberia.

SYMPTOMS.

2. **Head.**—Constant headache when attempting to move or exert the brain (cured).—Fierce headache threatening acute mania (cured).

4. **Ears.**—Constant buzzing of l. ear for two weeks with tenderness of meatus and intense sensitiveness of the head to the motion of an omnibus with beclouding of the brain; can hardly tell which instrument to take up (in his work as a dentist), and pain in nape of neck (agg.).

16. **Female Sexual Organs.**—Period continually returning; sometimes light-coloured and slight in quantity, and sometimes profuse; with weak feeling in back.

Veratrum Viride.

Veratrum viride. American White Hellebore. Indian Poke. *N. O.* Melanthaceæ (of the Liliaceæ). Tincture of fresh root gathered in autumn. [Burt proved Squibb's liquid extract and says he found no other preparation satisfactory.]

Clinical.—Amaurosis. Amenorrhœa. Apoplexy. *Asthma. Bunions. Cæcum, inflammation of. Chilblains. Chorea.* Congestion. Convulsions. Diplopia. Diaphragmitis. Dysmenorrhœa. *Erysipelas.* Headache, nervous; sick. Heart, affections of. Hiccough. *Hyperpyrexia.* Influenza. Malarial fever. Measles. Meningitis. Menses, suppressed. *Myalgia. Œsophagus, spasm of.* Orchitis. Pneumonia. Proctalgia. Puerperal convulsions. Puerperal mania. *Sleep, dreamful.* Spine, congestion of. Spleen, congested. Sunstroke. Typhoid fever. *Uterus, congestion of.*

Characteristics.—*Verat. v.* is the American *White* Hellebore. Growing side by side, *Verat. a.* and *Verat. v.* are scarcely distinguishable when not in flower. Millspaugh, however, says that though much like *Ver. alb.* in its minor points, *Ver. v.* is strikingly different in general appearance, having a much more pointed leaf, panicles looser and more compound; the racemes of *Ver. a.* being more compact and as a whole cylindrical, those of *Ver. v.* scattered, compound, and scraggy. *Ver. a.* flourishes in mountain meadows, *Ver. v.* grows in swamps, and wet meadows, and along mountain creeks from Canada to the Carolinas. Cooper has pointed out (*H. W.*, xxxvi. 153) a confusion which exists through the Veratrums being also called Hellebores. *Ver. v.* is "American White Hellebore" and not "Green Hellebore" (which is *Helleborus viridis*). Through this confusion an accidental proving of the latter (G. C. Edwards, No. 11. in *Allen*) has been included in the pathogenesis of *Ver. v.* The plants belong to different orders, though it must be admitted there is a close resemblance in their effects. The root of *Ver. v.* contains *Veratrin*, and the other alkaloids found in the root of *Ver. a.*, but in different proportions. Hale was chiefly instrumental in introducing *Ver. v.* to homœopathy, using it in fevers and particularly in pneumonia. Burt made a heroic proving of the liquid extract; and his infant daughter (twenty-one months) very nearly died from taking a few drops of the tincture from a phial. In two minutes she began vomiting. Coffee and *Camphor* were given as antidotes. In five minutes her jaws were rigid; pupils widely dilated; face blue; hands and feet cold; no pulse at wrist. Abdomen and back were rubbed with *Camphor*, when she went into spasms with violent shrieks. These spasms were frequently repeated, a hot bath being most effective in relaxing the muscles. Vomiting ropy mucus kept up for three hours. Pulseless; hands and feet shrivelled. After three and a half hours she slept quietly and soundly and next morning was well but a little weak. Burt recalls his own symptom, "constant aching pains in back of neck and shoulders," and concludes that *Ver. v.* acts on the cervical portion of the spinal cord and base of brain. He also regards it as acting on the vagus, and paralysing the circulatory apparatus. The great keynote of *Ver. v.* is *congestion*, and it is in resolving congestive states that its chief successes have been scored. The correspondence is rough and the lower potencies have been mostly used. D. McLellan told me of a case of his. He was sent for in the middle of the night to see an old lady whom he found sitting up in bed gasping for breath, and blue. Rapid congestion of the lungs had occurred. The attack had come on suddenly. *Ver. v.* quickly rescued the patient from a condition of imminent peril. The concomitance of congestive symptoms, and also of nausea and vomiting, form one of the leading indications of *Ver. v.* in a great variety of cases. Sensations of fulness ("Head feels full and heavy;" "rush of blood to the head;" "face flushed;" buzzing in the ears;" "chest constricted; or oppressed as from a heavy load;" point to the congestive tendency. The localities most congested by *Ver. v.* are: Base of brain; chest; spine; stomach. Slowing of the heart's action is a leading effect of the provings (from its action on the heart muscle and cardiac ganglia—*Dig.* on the pneumogastric); and *Ver. v.* has been used to "knock down" fever in the same way as *Acon.* Nash points out that there is some risk in this. When *Ver. v.* was first introduced he used it largely and successfully in a number of cases; but in one case which appeared to be going on favourably, the patient died *suddenly*. This he attributes to the *Ver. v.* In chorea *Ver. v.* has had many successes: "twitchings during sleep" was a characteristic of some cases. "Constant jerking or nodding of the head," "jerking and trembling, threatened with convulsions," are other leading symptoms. In puerperal convulsions *Ver. v.* has only succeeded when nauseating doses have been given. In muscular and articular rheumatism it has been used locally as well as internally; and in chorea an application to the spine of the tincture, diluted with spirit, has proved a serviceable adjunct. Among other indications for *Ver. v.* are: "Violent pains attending inflammation." "Head full, throbbing of arteries, sensitive to sound; double or partial vision." *Suddenness:* Sudden fainting; prostration; nausea. A keynote symptom is: Red streak down the centre of the tongue. *Ver. v.* has a pronounced action on the œsophagus; it causes a sort of ruminating action or reversed peristalsis. Numbness is prominent among the effects of *Ver. v.* With the 30th I cured a man, 56, of these symptoms: Dim sight as if scales over it; numbness; pain in head as if a tight band were round it; rush of blood to head; sleeplessness. *Peculiar Sensations are:* Confused feeling in head as if head would burst. As if boiling water poured over parts. Tongue as if scalded. As if a ball rising into œsophagus. As if stomach tightly drawn against spine. As of a load on chest. As if ankles distorted. As of galvanic shocks in limbs. As if damp clothing on arms and legs. *Ver. v.* is *Suited to* full-blooded, plethoric persons. Dreaming about water is a characteristic which I have confirmed. The symptoms are: > By rubbing. > By pressure (pain in head). Motion <. Sudden motion = faintness and blindness. Rising <. Walking <; = blindness. Lying < (headache, breathing, &c.); > faintness and blindness. Closing eyes and resting head > vertigo. < Going from warm to cold. < After exposure. The least food = vomiting. < Morning on waking; also evening.

Relations.—*Antidoted by:* Hot Coffee. *Antidote to:* Strychnine. *Compare:* Puerperal convulsions, Gels. (Gels. has dull, drowsy state of mind); Ver. v., apoplectic condition between the fits, face red, eyes congested, violent convulsive twitches). Congestions, Fer. ph., Bell. Plethora, Aco. Chorea, Hyo. Pneumonia with engorgement, Sang. (Ver v. more marked arterial tension). Scalded tongue, Sang. Tetanus, Nux, Hyperic. Rheumatic fever, Bry., Sal. ac. Sunstroke; double or partial vision, Glon., Gels. Slow, irregular intermittent pulse, Dig., Tab. Aching in gall-bladder, Bap. Heat in heart, Lachn., Rhod., Kalm. Clumsiness, Bov. As if damp clothing on legs, Calc. (Ver. v. and arms). Nodding of head, Lyc., Stram. Neck muscles weak, Ant. t., Ver. a.

Causation.—Sun. Suppressed menses. Suppressed lochia.

SYMPTOMS.

1. **Mind.**—Stupefaction; congestion.—Mental confusion, loss of memory.—Temporary delirium.—Quarrelsome and delirious, striking and kicking with r. hand and foot (at times these movements seemed to be involuntary); changed to a happy and comical delirious state.—Depression

and prostration.—Great fear of death.—When not vomiting lay in a stupor. —Puerperal mania : silent, suspicious; fears being poisoned.—Loquacity with exaltation of ideas.

2. **Head.**—Vertigo : with nausea and sudden prostration; with vomiting as soon as he rises; with photophobia, > closing eyes and resting head.—Sunstroke with prostration, febrile motion, accelerated pulse.—Headache with vertigo, dim vision and dilated vessels.—Head feels full and heavy.—Fulness in head, throbbing, aching, buzzing in ears, double or partial vision.—Constant dull frontal headache, with neuralgic pains in r. temple close to eye.—Rush of blood to head.—Pain in head as if tightly bound.—"A principal headache remedy" (Cooper).—[Cooper gives me the following cured cases : Sick-headache; eyes ache and burn, fearful headache and pain in lower back on waking in morning, digging in shoulders.—Headache generally before menses, and much sensitiveness of nerves, has to keep in a dark room; pain < behind eyelids; unable to bear sounds.—Sick-headache dating from childhood, often at beginning or end of menses, with great depression and lasting two days.—Headache in girl, 23, for two years, on getting up in morning is very giddy and weak on her knees, falls down faint in the street, vertigo and sickness and pains all over head, < on vertex, behind ears and in occiput, can't bear to talk or be in noise.—Painful swelling of sides of neck, head also feels swollen with suffocative feeling and sneezing and chills down back (*Ver. v.* cured after *Apis* failed).—Sick-headache, vomiting, < from fatigue.]—On waking after a short sleep indescribable sensation rising from forehead to crown and seems to grasp vertex and occiput.—Dull occipital headache.—Constant jerking or nodding of the head.—Congestive apoplexy.—Basilar meningitis.—Cerebral irritation; threatened hydrocephalus.—Erysipelas of r. side of head and face, with swelling.—Phlegmonous erysipelas of scalp.

3. **Eyes.**—Full, pressing heavy feeling in eyes.—Severe shooting, suddenly stopping pain in l. eye.—Aching : upper part of r. orbit; directly over r. eye.—Fulness about lids as after crying.—Lids heavy and sleepy.—Profuse lachrymation.—Vision : dim (as if scales over eyes); unsteady; double; dim with faintness on rising up.—Green circles round gas-light.—Immense green circles round candle, which as vertigo came on and I closed my eyes turned to red.—Suddenly blind in upper half of visual field.—Cannot walk; if attempts it very faint and completely blind; obliged to keep horizontal position 2.20 p.m.—Photophobia and vertigo > closing eyes and resting head, morning.

4. **Ears.**—Fulness and throbbing in ears (esp. l.).—Used locally relieves earache (R. T. C.).—Earache with sleeplessness and restlessness, sometimes leaving l. ear and passing up to vertex causing eyeballs to ache and back of head to be painful; chills down back and electric twitches in fingers of both hands, and affecting tongue; temperature and pulse high (great relief.—R. T. C.).—Deafness from moving quickly with faintness.—Ringing; humming with sensitiveness to noise.

5. **Nose.**—Nose pinched and blue.—Catarrh and sneezing.—Profuse secretion of mucus from nose.—Itching first of r. then l. ala.

6. **Face.**—Face : very pale; with cadaverous look; blue; hippocratic; flushed.—Stinging in r. malar bone.—Pains in r. angle of lower jaw.—Lock-

jaw.—Convulsive twitchings of facial muscles.—Mouth drawn down at one corner.—Lips dry, and mucus of mouth thick.—(Phlegmonous erysipelas of face and head.)

8. **Mouth.**—Tongue : white as if bleached (not coated); white centre, red edges and tip ; strawberry ; red centre, edges yellow, feels scalded ; red streak down centre ; inclined to be dry.—Acrid burning sensation in mouth. —Faint odour of chloroform or ether in mouth.—Great increase of saliva ; and mucus from stomach and nose.—Taste : flat ; like lime water ; bitterish and peculiar, like odour of semen.—Loss of speech.

9. **Throat.**—Dryness and heat in throat, with severe hiccough.—Burning in fauces and œsophagus, with constant inclination to swallow.—Numbness of fauces.—Spasms of œsophagus constant, violent, with or without rising of bloody frothy mucus ; with violent hiccough.—Sense of ball moving into œsophagus as far as top of sternum.

11. **Stomach.**—Ravenous appetite ; on waking.—Very thirsty, drinks little, which > for a short time.—Hiccough : constant ; exceedingly painful and violent.—Eructations : frequent of wind : acrid, sour risings.—Nausea and dizziness, followed by heat of surface.—(Continual nausea and sick feeling with dread of food in a bronchitis patient.—R. T. C.)—Contents of stomach thrown off with a rumbling action without nausea.—Sensation as if stomach slowly contracting on its contents and forcing them into œsophagus, producing sensation as of a ball rising up to top of sternum.—Retching with agonising pain.—The least quantity of food = violent vomiting.—Vomiting : profuse, of thick, glairy mucus ; of food ; of bile ; with collapse and cold sweat.—Twisting-tearing pain in stomach < by least motion.—As if waves rising from stomach to chest, on waking.—Pains in stomach, sharp ; flying.—Great irritability of stomach.—(Choked spleen.—R. T. C.)

12. **Abdomen.**—Dull, heavy aching in region of gall-bladder ; and umbilical region.—Neuralgic pain r. side of navel to groin.—In umbilical region : severe cutting aching pains, with rumbling ; dull aching ; distress.—Peritonitis when pulse is hard and firm (A. C. Clifton).—Pain and soreness across abdomen just above pelvis.—Pain in bowels ran into scrotum ; pain in scrotum last to disappear.

13. **Stool and Anus.**—Crawling in anus.—Tenesmus and diarrhœa, copious and offensive stool, with burning of anus and pale face ; tenesmus and burning before and up to stool, not during and after ; > after stool.—Sudden excessive tenesmus.—Stools : copious, light, mornings ; mushy, with enesmus and burning ; bloody (black in typhoid) ; doughy, stringy, hard to xpel ; alternately soft and hard every two hours.

14. **Urinary Organs.**—Smarting in urethra on urinating.—Urine : nty ; very clear ; turbid, with reddish sediment, and scum.—Hæmorrhage fungus hæmatodes vesicæ.

15. **Male Sexual Organs.**—Pains in both testicles, < l., morning ; etimes shoots up into abdomen.—Severe pain in l. testicle all through the ing.

. **Female Sexual Organs.**—(Congestion of pelvic organs, tender-of uterus ; fever ; heat ; restlessness ; palpitation ; local or general nesia.—Menstrual colic or dysmenorrhœa ; much nausea and vomiting ; a ; cerebral congestion.—Membranous dysmenorrhœa, soreness as of a boil in uterine region.—Suppressed menses with cerebral congestion; plethora.—Amenorrhœa from exposure; chill, complete suppression of discharge, heavy pressive aching in uterine region; intense pain in head with heat and throbbing arteries; mind wandering, sobbing; tendency to hysteric spasms.—Vomiting during pregnancy.—Rigid os.—Puerperal convulsions with arterial excitement; cold, clammy sweat.—Puerperal fever, sudden suppression of milk and lochia; quick, weak, or hard, bounding pulse.—After abortion retained placenta.—Mastitis with great arterial and nervous excitement.)

17. **Respiratory Organs.**—In evening, tickling, spasmodic cough from just above sternum.—Respiration: difficult; with nausea: slow between the vomiting spells; convulsive almost to suffocation.—Oppressed breathing on attempting to walk, irregular bowels, sleepless; fulness and heaviness in splenic region, history of ague in early life; profuse diarrhœa followed *Ver. v.* with great relief (R. T. C.).—(Membranous croup, after *Acon.*)—Cough: short; dry; hacking; loose, rattling; < going from warm to cold.

18. **Chest.**—Constriction of chest; when vomiting ceases.—Chest oppressed as from heavy cold.—(Oppression of chest with phlegmmy sickness in woman, 83.—R. T. C.)—Feeling of dislocation in chest when walking.—Throbbing in r. side of chest.—Pains about l. nipple.—(Congestion of chest with rapid respiration, nausea, vomiting; dull burning in region of heart.—Pneumonia and pleurisy: pulse hard, strong, quick, or slow and intermitting; lungs engorged; faint feeling in stomach; high fever, face flushed.)—(Old pneumonic congestion with superadded acute pleurisy.—R. T. C.)

19. **Heart.**—Pricking pains in region of heart with the headache.—Constant burning distress in region of heart.—Burning under sternum.—Dull, hot, aching pain in heart region 3 p.m.—Neuralgic pains in heart.—Slow action of heart.—Palpitation and dyspnœa.—Violent palpitation of heart and faint feeling (agg.—R. T. C.).—Faintness and biliousness; when rising from lying; from sudden motion; lying quietly.—Pulse: slow, soft and weak; irregular, intermittent; suddenly increases and gradually decreases below normal.

20. **Neck and Back.**—Aching in neck and shoulder, almost impossible to hold head up.—Muscles of back contracted, drawing head back.—Pain in r. and l. sides of neck.—Throbbing and crawling in l. back.—Pain in r. of sacrum where it joins pelvis.

21. **Limbs.**—Rheumatism esp. l. shoulder, hip, and knee; high fever, scanty red urine.—Clumsiness.—Loss of power of gastrocnemii and muscles of forearm.—Slight drawing in r. elbow and calves.—Throbbing in l. radius and r. femur.—Sensation as of galvanic shocks in limbs.

22. **Upper Limbs.**—Aching: top of l. shoulder above scapular ridge; in arms and neck.—Shuddering in l. and r. shoulders in succession.—Pain: in outer condyle of r. humerus; in r. elbow; in r. and l. ulna; in fingers and thumb.

23. **Lower Limbs.**—Total loss of locomotion for some hours.—Pains in either great trochanter when lying on it.—Much pain in hip-joints and about condyles.—Cramps in legs.—Sensation of cramp in gastrocnemii with inability to exert them.—Drawing in r. calf while walking.—Lancinating pain in r. hip.—Joints swollen, very tender, high fever.—(Knee tender, swollen after a wrench.)—R. ankle feels dislocated, can scarcely walk; later, l.

24. Generalities.—Pallor with syncope.—Tremor.—Spasm with violent shrieks; opisthotonos; face dark blue; breath suspended; lasting two minutes and recurring after few minutes' interval.—(Epileptic fits in a child, bad case.—R. T. C.)—Nervous attack with shaking trembling and chilliness (agg.—R. T. C.).—Numbness.—Clothes irritate as if they did not fit well. —Convulsions.—Chorea, movements continuing in sleep.—Often indicated in hæmorrhage from various organs (R. T. C.).—The pains of influenza; headaches, gastralgia, pains in calves of legs (R. T. C.).

25. Skin.—Itching in many parts.—(Erythema.—Erysipelas.—Congestive stage of exanthema.)—Used locally, relieves pain in erysipelas (R. T. C.)—(Measles, with intense conjunctivitis and high fever.—R. T. C.)

26. Sleep.—Very sleepy.—Coma; blue face; spasms.—Restless and sleepless.—Dreams: frightful; of being on the water; of people drowning; about water, fishing, &c.; lively in which he was continually baffled and provoked.

27. Fever.—Chilly; body cold but moist skin.—Cold shivers, head and feet cold and numbed, crept up arms and legs as if enveloped in damp clothing.—Heat followed dizziness and nausea; icy coldness followed the heat.—Feverishness; depressed in mind and body, weak, pains in shoulder and over body as from influenza, with prickling irritating rash on forehead, face, and chest (agg.—R. T. C.).—Profuse diaphoresis and sense of utter prostration.—Bathed in cold sweat.—Cold, clammy sweat on forehead.—(Irritative fever with cerebral congestion.—Streptococcus fever; rapid and violent alternations of temperature.—Ephemeral fevers with nausea and retching.—Cerebro-spinal fever.—Typhoid.—Yellow fever.)—(Typhoid fever, fourth week, beef-steak tongue; sickness, unable to retain any food, great prostration and sinking at epigastrium.—R. T. C.)

Verbascum.

Verbascum thapsus. Great Mullein. *N. O.* Scrophulariaceæ. Tincture of fresh plant at the commencement of flowering. ["Mullein Oil" is prepared by placing the crushed yellow blossoms in a bottle, which is corked and allowed to stand in the sun (Cushing); or by steeping the blossoms in oil and keeping in a warm place till the oil has absorbed them (Gerarde)].

Clinical.—*Anus, itching of.* Colic. Constipation. *Cough.* Deafness. Enuresis. *Hæmorrhoids. Neuralgia.* Prosopalgia. *Urine, incontinence of.*

Characteristics.—"The thick woolly leaves of *V. thapsus*, the Great Mullein, have a mucilaginous, bitterish taste, and a decoction of them is employed in domestic practice in catarrhs and diarrhœa. They are also used as emollient applications to hard tumours and in pulmonary complaints in cattle—hence one of its popular names is Bullock's Lung-wort. It is also called Adam's flannel, from its flannel-like leaves" (*Treas. of Bot.*). Hahnemann proved *Verbascum*, and his proving confirms many of the old uses. It produced neuralgic pains of very great intensity, pressing and lancinating, and especially in the facial bones, navel, and limbs, and a peculiar cough. "Cough, deep, hollow, hoarse, in sound like a trumpet," is Nash's description. He has cured many cases and always used it low. It is more especially a night cough. It occurs in children during their sleep. Some years ago Mullein was brought forward as a popular specific for phthisis, the leaves being boiled in milk, which was then strained and given warm. Among its traditional uses Gerarde mentions it as a remedy for piles, and I do not know a better application for itching hæmorrhoids or pruritus ani than an ointment made of the φ tincture in the proportion of ʒi to the ℥i of Cetacean ointment. I generally direct it to be applied at bedtime. Gerarde says that the oil of the yellow flowers is also curative in piles. The flowers contain "a yellow volatile oil, and fatty acid, free malic and phosphoric acids, and their -ate salts of lime, a yellow resinous colouring matter, and the general plant constituents including an uncrystallisable sugar" (Millspaugh). Cushing prepared from the flowers an "oil" (1) by putting the blossoms in a bottle and laying the bottle in the sun; and later (2) by expression. This "Mullein Oil" has found many uses, and especially for instilling in the ears in cases of deafness, or earache; in cases of enuresis nocturna (Cushing had good success with the 3x), and painful micturition. The provings brought out some very marked symptoms in the ears, especially the left ear (*Verb.* is predominently left-sided). W. B. McCoy (*Hom. News*, xxviii. 36) gives several illustrations. According to him *Verb.* (*i.e.*, the "oil") has a "soothing effect on the entire nervous system, in many cases acting as a soporific." In summer diarrhœa he gives one to four drops in two ounces of warm water, a teaspoonful every hour. In enuresis or dribbling of urine one-drop doses in warm water three or four times a day. Among his cases were those of two boys who had become deaf from getting water in their ears when swimming. They were cured by having three drops of the oil instilled "in each ear alternately night and morning." O. S. Laws cured a youth, of 16, of enuresis with fifteen drops of the oil three times a day (*N. Y. Med. Times*, xxiv. 318). The oil plainly acts on the indications of the proving, and may be regarded as an alternative preparation to the official tincture. It might be called *Verbasci oleum*. E. E. Case reports a case of neuralgia cured by *Verb.* (*Med. Adv.*, quoted *A. H.*, xxvii. 234): A widow, 36, black-haired, had been for a long time overworked, sewing, and her life made miserable by neuralgia. The symptoms were: Tearing, stitching pain above left ear, downward and inward; outer ear numb; dulness of hearing left side; heavy pressure in vertex. Shivers run up back and left side with the pain. Irritable and despondent. *Verb.* 1m, one powder taken in four doses at three-hour intervals, cured. Among the *Sensations* are: As if everything would press out at forehead. As if left ramus of jaw were pressed against upper jaw. As if temples were pinched and crushed. As if ears were stopped up. As if nose and larynx were stopped up. As if something had fallen before ear. As if one were violently pressing on left malar bone. As of a crushing with tongs. Pressure as from a stone on umbilicus. As from needles from umbilical region to back. As if intestines were adherent to wall of abdomen and were being torn away. As of a twist around navel. As if a weight were hanging on lower extremities. As if cold water were poured over side of body from shoulder to thigh. "Salt water collects in mouth" is a guiding symptom. The symptoms are < By touch; by pressure. Rest = sticking in left metatarsal bones. Lying = tension across chest, stitches in region of heart. Sitting = pains; sitting up >. Motion > some pains; < prosopalgia. Stooping <; (> pressure in forehead). Walking <. < Night; no sleep after 4 a.m. < Draught of air; exposure to cold; change from cold to warm and *vice versâ*. Attacks appear at 9 a.m., reach their height at noon, gradually diminish till 4. Many pains are intermittent.

Relations.—*Compare:* In neuralgia, Plat. (pressure); Stan. (gradually increasing and decreasing). Deep cough, Coral., Dros., Spo., Sul. Sheep-dung stools, Mg. mur. Cough from tickling in chest, Ver.

SYMPTOMS.

1. Mind.—Apathy.—Moroseness, ill-humour, and irascibility.—Excessive gaiety, with laughter.—Mental excitement, with voluptuous images.—Weakness of memory.—Distraction.—A great concourse of ideas, and liveliness of imagination.

2. Head.—Dulness and confusion in the head.—Vertigo: when pressing one (l.) cheek while supporting the head; sudden, as from pressure on whole head.—Headache, with a forcing outwards at forehead.—Pressive, stupefying headache, principally in forehead; or semilateral, and mostly when passing from a warm into a cold temperature (and *vice versâ*).—Heaviness of head, with dull pain.—Pinching in temples.—Deep, stupefying stitches in brain (pressing, slow stitch from behind forward through l. hemisphere of brain).—Stupefying shooting in temples (in r. temple when eating; < from pressure; extending into upper teeth of r. side).—Resonance in head, when walking.

3. Eyes.—Pains in eyes, as from contraction of the sockets, with burning in eyes.—Sight confused, as if directed through a veil.

4. Ears.—Tearing in ears, sometimes when eating, with lancinations.—Sensation as if ear were drawn inwards.—Deafness as from stoppage of ear.—Sensation of a stoppage of ears (first l., then r., also of nose and larynx) when reading aloud; hearing unaffected.—Numbness in l. ear.—Oil of Mullein (*Verb. ol.*) relieves earache at once.—*Verb.* is said to meet many cases of deafness (R. T. C.).

5. Nose.—Sensation of stoppage of larynx and ears.—Profuse coryza from frontal sinuses, with hot, burning, profuse lachrymation.

6, 7. Face and Teeth.—Facial neuralgia (esp. caused and < by a change of temperature), generally with stupefying, pressive or tensive pains, principally in cheek-bones, and commencing from maxillary joint, < by clenching teeth, and by external pressure.—Violent pressure in l. malar bone and zygoma.—Stitches in l. zygomatic arch.—Shootings in the cheek-bones, with dull pressure.—Violent tension in integuments of chin, masseters, and throat.—Toothache, with tearing pain in the molars.—Pinching pressing pain on lower side of jaw.

8. **Mouth.**—Copious accumulation of salt saliva in the mouth.—Root of tongue brown, without bad taste, in morning and during forenoon.—Tongue of a brownish yellow colour, loaded with viscid mucus in morning and after dinner.

9. **Throat.**—Very severe pain in throat on swallowing.

10. **Appetite.**—Mawkish taste, with fetid breath.—Hunger, without relish for food.—Insatiable thirst.

11. **Stomach.**—Regurgitation of insipid serum.—Empty, or else bitter risings, with nausea.—Frequent hiccough.—Aching of stomach.—Sensation of emptiness at pit of stomach, which disappears with a rumbling below l. ribs.

12. **Abdomen.**—Cuttings and shootings in l. hypochondrium.—Incessant gurgling and rumbling beneath l. ribs.—Inflation of the abdomen, violent and painful pressure on navel, as by a stone, < by bending double.—Spasmodic constriction of the hypogastrium, towards the umbilical region.—Pains in abdomen, which extend deeply downwards, with want to evacuate, and spasmodic contraction of anus.—Pinchings and gripings in abdomen.—Shootings in abdomen, principally in umbilical region, sometimes tearing and tending downwards.—Sensation as if intestines had adhered to umbilical region, and were torn away.

13. **Stool and Anus.**—Fearful diarrhœa ; griping ; much pain as if pierced with a lance through inside of l. ankle-joint ; pain in both cheek-bones and above eyebrows ; menses came on early this time, and she has coughed a good deal.—Suppressed evacuations. — Fæces hard, like sheep-dung, and expelled with effort.—(Itching hæmorrhoids.—Pruritus ani.)

14. **Urinary Organs.**—Frequent want to urinate, with profuse emission (afterwards scanty).—Enuresis nocturna ; (obstinate, with seminal emissions. —Cushing).

15. **Male Sexual Organs.**—Pollutions without lewd dreams.

17. **Respiratory Organs.**—Sensation of obstruction in the larynx and nose, with hoarseness when reading aloud ; deep voice.—Catarrh, with hoarseness and stuffed chest.—Cough esp. in evening, and at night, when sleeping, generally rough and dry, or hollow and dull.—Dry, hoarse cough < at night —Frequent attacks of deep, hollow, hoarse cough, with sound like a trumpet, caused by tickling in larynx and chest.—The cough is lessened as soon as the patient succeeds in taking a breath.

18. **Chest.**—Shooting in chest, sometimes with oppression and obstructed respiration.—Tension in chest, with lancinations in region of heart, in evening, after lying down.—Stitches in the chest.—Red nodosity near xiphoid cartilage, painful when pressed upon.

20. **Back.**—Lancinations in the back and shoulder-blades.—Sharp intermittent stitches in l. scapula.—Fine persistent stitch in last dorsal vertebra.—Between r. loin and spine deep, knife-like stitches quite intense in intestines.—Backache < from pressure.

21. **Limbs.**—Stitching in the limbs.

22. **Upper Limbs.**—Tearing pain in the shoulder, back of hand, and elbow.—Spasmodic pressure in forearm, hand, and thumb.—Tearing shootings

in hand and fingers.—Tensive pain in wrist.—Wrenching pain in joint of hand.—Stitches like a sprain (or paralysis), where carpal bone of thumb articulates with radius.—Paralytic pain in joints of fingers.

23. **Lower Limbs.**—Excessive heaviness and lassitude in legs and feet, esp. when going up stairs.—Cramp-like pain in muscles of r. thigh, while walking in open air.—Spasmodic pressure in thighs, legs, and soles.—Cramp-like pressure in sole of r. foot, while standing, disappears when walking.—Trembling of knees.—Dull lancinations in patella, bones of feet, and toes.—Violent, intermittent, dull sticking in metatarsal bones of great and adjacent toes of l. foot during rest.—Tearing along legs.

24. **Generalities.**—General indolence, and disposition to sleep, after rising in the morning.—Stretching and frequent yawning.—Hæmorrhoids ; affections of the inner navel region ; obstruction from induration of stool.—Darting pains in inner parts ; want of perspiration.—< When sitting ; from change of temperature.—> On rising from a sitting posture.—Stinging pains in the limbs.—Benumbing sensation with almost all the pain.—Tearings, sometimes lancinating, in different parts (going downwards).—Tottering when walking.

26. **Sleep.**—Strong disposition to sleep after a meal.—Disturbed sleep, at night, with tossing.—Short sleep at night, lasting only till 4 a.m., with anxious, frightful dreams of wars and dead bodies.

27. **Fever.**—Internal coldness of whole body, of hands and feet, perceptible also externally.—Shuddering, esp. on one side of body, as if it were bathed in cold water.

Verbena Hastata.

Verbena hastata. Ironweed. *N. O.* Verbenacæ. Tincture of entire fresh plant.

Clinical.—Ague ; chronic. Epilepsy. Rhus poisoning.

Characteristics.—According to Hale *Verbena h.* grows profusely on the prairies and low bottom lands all over U.S. It is a popular domestic remedy for ague, especially when chronic. The root is intensely and disagreeably bitter. Dr. Griffin, of New York, suggests its use as a remedy for *Rhus* poisoning. Richey Horner (*Med. Cent.*, vi. 324) mentions a case of epilepsy developing during whooping-cough, treated with 12-drop doses (" presumably of the tincture ") every four hours. Improvement set in from the first and proved permanent ; though during the first two weeks there were attacks of petit mal. The patient took the remedy at increasing intervals during six weeks.

Vesicaria.

Vesicaria communis. *N. O.* Cruciferæ (Tribe, Alyssineæ). Tincture of whole fresh plant.

Clinical.—Albuminuria. Cystitis. Dropsy. Gleet. Gonorrhœa. Gravel. Hæmaturia. Nephralgia. Prostatitis.

Characteristics.—*Vesicaria* is a "genus of *Cruciferæ*, natives of the Northern Hemisphere, distinguished by the globose or ovoid inflated pouch, with hemispherical valves and numerous seeds (generally four to six) in each cell. They are herbs, sometimes shrubby at the base, with oblong or linear entire or repand leaves, and terminal racemes of yellow flowers" (*Treas. of Bot.*). George R. Shafer (*Chic. Med. Times*, quoted *H. News*, xxx. 117) says *Ves. com.* is an old remedy much used in some parts of Germany for all forms of urinary and kidney difficulties; for gravel; for gonorrhœa, both in the male and female. Shafer's indication for the remedy is "a smarting, burning sensation along the course of the urethra and bladder, with frequent desire to void urine, often accompanied with strangury." The conditions he has found particularly amenable to *Vesic.* are: Nephralgia; acute cystitis; irritable bladder, following acute cystitis; chronic cystitis. He mentions these cases: (1) T. S., 67, suffering from nephralgia, for which he had received *Morphia* injections in former attacks. *Vesic.* φ, in 15-drop doses every fifteen minutes, gave marked relief in two hours, which in six hours was complete. (2) S. B., 57, cystitis from cold; high fever, sweating, burning pain on voiding urine, which was drop by drop. *Vesic.* φ, in 10-drop doses. cured in two days. (3) Lady, 39, pain in back, brick-dust sediment in urine; hands and feet swelling so she could hardly close her hands or walk. *Vesic.* φ cured. (4) Man, 65, irritable bladder, had to rise twenty to thirty times in the night. *Vesic.* φ, in 20-drop doses, relieved quickly and cured in six weeks. (5) C. M., 89, chronic cystitis, passing large quantities of muco-pus. The bladder was at first washed out with Boric acid solution, then *Vesic.* φ, 20 drops every two hours, were given. Improvement followed, and in two hours the Boric acid washing was stopped and *Vesic.* given every four hours. This finally cured. (6) Gonorrhœa with smarting and burning on micturition and thick creamy discharge. *Vesic.* φ, a drachm every four hours, soon cured. (7) Gonorrhœa, female, after being treated for two weeks with injections, was cured in seven days with *Vesic.* φ in drachm doses. Cowperthwaite (*H. M.*, July, 1900, 477) has succeeded in causing albumen to disappear from the urine even in cases of actual Bright's disease. He adds that "it is necessary to use only the imported [*i.e.*, European] tincture, 15 drops every four hours." (There are several Vesicarias native to North America.) A. L. Davison (*H. News*, Dec., 1892, 568) treated Mrs. P. for general dropsy of a year's standing; was in uræmic spasms when first seen; the kidneys having ceased to secrete urine. *Vesic.* φ was prescribed, 15 drops in a teaspoonful of water every hour till urine was freely secreted, then three times a day. The second day the kidneys were pouring out urine, and watery stools were passed. In a week all dropsy had disappeared. Bancroft (*ibid.*, 557) treated Mrs. T. for irritable kidneys and bladder with polyuria. After a time the urine became bloody, with occasional thin clots; previously there had been for some months a thick, yellow sediment. *Vesic.* φ, 6 drops four times a day and later 15 drops three times a day, taken persistently, effected a cure. Halbert (*Clinique*, xx. 107) reports the case of Mr. H., a young man whose occupation involved much outdoor exercise, and who contracted a chill and had lumbago in consequence. Under an "orificial" surgeon his rectum was operated on and the sphincter stretched. Thereafter he had fever, rigors, and acute prostatitis. Micturition was painful and difficult, and soon hæmaturia ensued. The pain and nervous exhaustion were so extreme that he was put into hospital, and for a time only relieved by injections of *Morphia*. The urine contained albumen, blood-clots, much pus. Urine was only passed by means of the catheter, and defecation was extremely painful. *Vesic.* 1 x was given hourly, and great relief followed. The painful tenesmus was alleviated, and he was soon able to pass urine without the catheter. In three weeks he was able to go home.

Relations.—*Compatible:* Cact., Thlasp. b. p. *Compare:* Botan., Thlasp. b. p. In Gravel, Coc. c., Urt. ur., Thlasp. b. p. Hæmaturia, Chi. s., Fic. r. Phos. Prostatic affections, Hydrang., Solid., Sabal. Cystitis, Chimaph. u. [Shafer gave Cact. and Thlasp. b. p. in a case of dropsy from heart disease in a lady, 48. These gave little relief. He then gave Vesic. *in combination with* the others. There was marked relief in twenty-four hours, and in ten days the dropsy had disappeared.]

Vespa.

VESPA VULGARIS, the Wasp; VESPA CRABRO, the European Hornet; and VESPA MACULATA, "Yellow-jacket," the American Hornet. *N. O.* Hymenoptera (Sub-order Vespidæ). Tincture of the living insects.

Clinical.—Abscesses, multiple. Alopecia. Chemosis. Enuresis. Fainting. Flushing. Glottis, spasm of. Indigestion; with flushing. Œdema. Ophthalmia. Ovary, left, pain in. Quinsy. Tongue, swelling of. Uterus, ulcerated. Vertigo.

Characteristics.—*Vespa* was introduced into the materia medica by Hering. The symptoms of the Schema are mostly the results of stings. Berridge proved *Vesp. crabro* 30 on three persons. Low spirits; pain in right ear; nausea with faint feeling and trembling; pain in left side of the neck on waking—these were the chief symptoms experienced by them. Berridge demonstrated that the poison of the hornet and the wasp may answer to each other's indications by curing with *Vesp. c.* cm. (Fincke) a symptom produced by *Vesp. vulgaris*, namely, chemosis of the right eye. Mr. X., 66, had had his right eye inflamed for six days. When seen there was redness of right lower lid; baggy swelling of conjunctiva partly covering the cornea when pressed upward; lachrymation of right eye < in open air; right lids adhere in morning. *Vesp. c.* thrice daily cured in a few days (*Org.*, ii. 319). E. T. Blake (*M. H. R.*, xxii. 370, quoted *Org.*, i. 320) cured with *Vesp.* 1. the following group of symptoms: Face swollen and puffy, skin transparent and blanched; scalding urine followed by itching; itching of right arm. Blake also related (*M. H. R.*, xix. 418, quoted by Allen) the case of Miss C. J., who at the age of thirty-one was stung on the left thumb, through some calico, and was never well after, dying at the age of thirty-eight. She was prone to constipation all her life, and at twenty-three had had "congestion of the left lung." Most of the abdominal, urinary, ovarian, and uterine symptoms were hers. Among the latter was an irritable ulcer surrounding the *os tincæ*. W. Rowbotham (*Org.*, ii. 79) was stung on the right cheek. Next day, about 4 a.m., was *suddenly* awakened by burning, stinging pain in cheek, "as if pierced with red-hot needles," and soreness and smarting along the lymphatics. After bathing the face he got to sleep and was again *suddenly* awakened by the pain two hours later, which recurred *periodically*, in *paroxysms*, throughout the day. Burnett observed a case of sting on the tongue in a woman. The tongue entirely filled the buccal cavity. The patient's appearance was exactly like one suffering from severe cynanche. The swelling was diffuse and deep-seated. There was not much redness. *Peculiar Sensations* were: As if a harpoon were sticking deep in and were drawn on. Cold, chilly sensation round sting. As if pierced with red-hot needles. As if about to suffocate. As if left shoulder-joint were sprained. As if a cutting instrument were piercing all joints like an electric shock. As if dying. The symptoms were: < By motion. Cold water applied, first >, then <. Open air < lachrymation. Feet were cold except in summer, when they burned uncomfortably. < After sleep. < After eating (indigestion with flushes).

Relations.—*Antidoted by:* Apis, Led., Camph., Salt-water, Vinegar. *Incompatible:* Arg. n. *Compare:* Pains as if pierced with red-hot needles, Ars., Apis. Ulcers around os uteri, Mitch., Eu. pu., Apis., Hydrocotyle.

SYMPTOMS.

1. **Mind.**—Terrible anxiety. — Low-spirited.—Insensibility. — Unconsciousness, with inability to move.

2. **Head.**—Fainting and loss of consciousness.—A violent heat came over him, felt sick; then turned giddy and spun round and round like a top till he fell; staggered to the house, got into a chair, in a moment, fell out of it, almost fainting; dashed water into his face, at length was able to lie down on his bed.—Headache.—Face and head swollen and inflamed.—Alopecia.

3. **Eyes.**—Injection of r. conjunctiva.—Itching of r. lid in evening, with swelling, afterwards pain in lid and ball, erysipelatous inflammation of lid, whole side of face painful and swollen, almost complete chemosis of conjunctiva, it being raised up on the sclerotic membrane, more than half over

eye to border of cornea, as if fatty matter were under it, caused by effusion of lymph, an abscess opened upon inside of upper lid about its centre, later the chemosis became reddish.—Inflammation of r. eye, with baggy swelling of conjunctiva.

4. **Ears.**—Sticking deep in r. ear.—Purulent catarrh of middle ears.

6. **Face.**—Face livid.—Face smooth, dark red, bloated.—Anxious expression.—Face and eyes œdematous, face, mouth and throat appeared as in severe cynanche (after a sting on tongue).—Pain in cheek (part stung) as if pierced with red-hot needles, suddenly awakening him from sleep, and recurring periodically.

8. **Mouth.**—Tongue : swollen and tense, swelling below chin, between that and hyoid bone, pain in a point in middle line of tongue, ¾-in. from apex ; swollen, red, rounded, filled the mouth, immovable, could not speak, only mumbled, swallowing was painful and difficult.—Swelling of palate, with inflammation, so preventing respiration that he died.—Swelling of mouth and throat, with burning pain, nausea, vertigo, after two hours fever, delirium, face, neck, arms, and chest swollen and shining red, respiration impeded, swallowing difficult, pulse 126, heart's action irregular and tumultuous (cured by *Camph.*).—Peculiar taste, a combination of palatal and nasal sensation, as when a nest of wasps is disturbed, < heat.

9. **Throat.**—Swelling of throat ; soreness ; heat of throat.—Difficulty of swallowing.—Hypertrophied tonsils which secreted a cheesy matter.—Pharyngeal varicosis.

10. **Appetite.**—Hunger.—Thirst.

11. **Stomach.**—Eructations.—Nausea : in evening after coming indoors, with weight in stomach ; with faint feeling and trembling.—Vomiting, with swelling of head.—Cold feeling in stomach.—Heat in stomach.

12. **Abdomen.**—Uneasiness in abdomen.

14.—**Urinary Organs.**—Marked tenderness to deep pressure in renal region.—Incessant enuresis (after five years).—Burning micturition in women.—Remittent dysuria with backache.—Hæmaturia.

15. **Male Sexual Organs.**—Swelling of scrotum and penis.

16. **Female Sexual Organs.**—(Valuable in affections of l. ovary, with tenderness, frequent micturition, pain in sacrum extending up back.)—Pain in l. ovarian region.—Menses : intermittent ; sometimes brown ; always accompanied by pain and flatulence, preceded by mental depression, pain, pressure and constipation.—An irritable ulcer surrounded os tincæ.—Irritation (< in groins), passing into pudenda = ulceration.

17. **Respiratory Organs.**—Hoarseness.—Voice lost.—Spasm of glottis (after application of diluted ammonia to tongue), face pale, drops of sweat on forehead, arms thrown out to gasp for air, he got out of bed, sank back on bed, face livid, breath and pulse stopped.—Dyspnœa.—Respiration hurried.

19. **Heart and Pulse.**—Aching in heart.—Slow beating of heart, almost imperceptible.—Pulse : rapid and small ; rapid and feeble ; rapid with violent beating of carotids.

20. **Neck and Back.**—Pain in l. side of neck, waking her at night, preventing her from turning it to l. side, felt least when lying on back, best on r. side.—Pain in scapula (place of sting), with soreness.

22. **Upper Limbs.**—Pain in shoulder, in region of stings, axillary glands

swollen.—Sprained pain in l. shoulder-joint on moving it, < lifting arm or twisting it.—Aching in hand and arm.

24. **Generalities.**—Trembling, quaking, with chattering of teeth.—Nervo-muscular excitement.—Stinging piercing deeply, as if a hook were pulled out.—Sudden stinging and burning in cheek waking me at 4 a.m. (after a sting on the cheek).—Burning of the part, then swelling, red, with burning pain.—Sudden tearing.—Cutting like electric shocks through all joints, arm, head and face swollen, eyes red and twitching, red lines along absorbents, itching over whole body, insensibility, vomiting, pulse slow, heart's action scarcely perceptible.—Feeling as if dying at night.—Weakness; with enuresis somni, heat esp. overpowers him.—Faintness; all day with trembling and nausea.

25. **Skin.**—Redness of hands, feet, and chest.—Swelling: of face, body, and limbs; of cheek, skin soon became bright red, the redness spread over head and down neck, shoulders, back and front of chest, with pain and tenderness; of the stung part (r. side of neck), with aching, redness, and burning, the burning > then < by cold water.—Swelling of thumb and face, soon became red as if covered with scarlet rash; restlessness at night, heat, irritation, and wherever he scratched himself there arose spots like nettle-rash, swelling and redness of l. arm and hand, after forty hours œdema of lids (esp. lower), face pallid and puffy.—Prurigo-like, pinkish, lentil-shaped spots on hand and forearm, on neck, and all over, down to feet.—Ulcer.—Desquamation of whole surface.—Abscesses over whole body, causing emaciation.—Itching: of whole body; of the part every day about 3 or 4 a.m., slightly > by application of vinegar, always burning after scratching; also the same every day about 8 or 9 a.m. and at 3 p.m., the itching > by applications of salt and vinegar.

26. **Sleep.**—Night restless.—Sleepless all night.

27. **Fever.**—Heat, with sick feeling, vertigo, almost faintness.—Burning (after the sting) as if something were sticking and drawing out, the part stung was bright red, elevated, with hard swelling, the redness surrounded by a circle of chilliness, soon changing to a general chill, intermittent, extending in waves over whole body.

Viburnum Opulus.

Viburnum opulus. High Cranberry Bush. Cramp Bark. Water Elder. (The Gueldres Rose, or Snowball-tree of our gardens, is the cultivated and sterile variety.) *N. O.* Caprifoliaceæ. Tincture of the fresh bark.

Clinical.—After-pains. Cough, of pregnancy. Cramps. Dysmenorrhœa; spasmodic; neuralgic; membranous. Ears, painful. Epididymitis. Headache. Hysteria. Labour pains, false. Lumbago. *Menstruation, painful.* Miscarriage. Ovaries, pain in. Paralysis. Uterus, cramps in; bearing down in.

Characteristics.—*Viburnum opulus*, a native of Great Britain, is widely distributed over the northern parts of the continent and America. In America (says Hale) the wild species is called "Cramp bark," and the knowledge of its curative virtues in painful spasmodic diseases, especially in dysmenorrhœa, is derived from the American aborigines. The tincture has a strong odour of *Valerianic acid* (as also has that of *Vib. tinus*). Hale derived his knowledge from domestic sources. He gives these indications and directions: (1) In spasmodic dysmenorrhœa he gives a few drops of φ to 3x thrice daily for a week before the period, every hour when the pains set in, or every fifteen minutes if the pains are severe. (2) False pains preceding labour. (3) After-pains, a dose after each pain. (4) Cramps in abdomen and legs of pregnant women. (5) To prevent miscarriage when the pains are spasmodic or threatening. Hale considers it acts like galvanism; he cured with it cases exactly resembling a series cured with galvanism by Neftel. The first provings were by H. C. Allen, assisted by eleven provers, male and female, with φ and 1st and 30th dilutions. Their symptoms constitute the basis of the Schema. Dr. Susan J. Fenton, of Oakland (*Pac. C. J. H.*, reprinted *New Eng. M. Gaz.*, xxx. 405), proved *Vib. o.* on six provers. One of the six took the tincture up to drachm doses without obtaining a single symptom. One prover was cured of a number of symptoms, but developed no new ones. The other four had very pronounced symptoms, which I have marked in the Schema (F_1), (F_2), (F_3), and (F_4). They were: (1) Mrs. A., 49, tall, slender, rigid fibre, dark hair and eyes, nervo-bilious, (F_1). (2) Miss B., 21, short, plump, dark hair, grey eyes, phlegmatic, (F_2). (3) Miss D., 24, nurse, short, plump, dark hair and eyes, bilious, good health, (F_3). (4) Miss E., 21, nurse, medium height, dark-brown eyes, dark hair, bright, lively temperament, (F_4). All took potencies at first without eliciting any symptoms. Taking the tincture all had these symptoms with variations: severe backache going through to the front or round the abdomen to uterus. Cramping pelvic pain. Temporal headache. Three had nausea with the pains. All had "sick feeling all over." One had omission of a period; two had menses too early. The cured case was the following: Miss F., 25, housekeeper, medium height, rather slender, blonde, sanguine, was strong till late in 1891 (*i.e.*, 3½ years before the proving), when she had severe pelvic congestion and was fifteen months under treatment and most of the time in bed. In June, 1892, double oophorectomy was performed with great relief; but attacks of pelvic congestion with severe pain still persisted, at first every two to four weeks, later less frequently, causing impairment of general health and strength. The symptoms were: excruciating pains through lower abdomen, with bearing-down sensation and a feeling as if the body from the waist to lower part of pelvis would collapse; an indescribable sick feeling all over with severe aching in rectum; great depression of spirits; symptoms > when lying down. *Vib. o.* φ was taken in three-drop doses thrice daily. After taking it for three days she lost all her symptoms and felt "perfectly well for the first time in over four years." It is evident that "sick feeling all over" in connection with pelvic complaints; and "< from movement, > by rest" are keynotes of *Vib. o.* *Peculiar Sensations are:* As if she could not tell where she was or what to do on awaking. Crushing pain in head. Opening and shutting in left parietal region. As if stabbing with a knife in eyes and ears. Ear as if bruised; as if pinned to head. As if she could not live, sick feeling at stomach. Sick feeling all over. Goneness as if stomach empty. As if body from waist to lower pelvis would collapse. As if a hot fluid running through splenic vessels. As if urine continued to flow after urinating. As if menses coming on. As if pelvic organs were turning upside down. As if parts would be forced through vulva and she must support the part. Pain in back and across lower abdomen. As if breath would leave body and heart would cease beating. Bruised feeling in back as after severe exertion. Buzzing in hands as if they would burst. Left side as if strained or bruised by over-lifting.—The *left* side is much more powerfully affected than the right. *Vib. o.* is *Suited to* tall, slender, dark- or fair-haired hysterical subjects. The symptoms are : < By sudden jar. > By pressure. < By motion. Rest ; lying down >. Lying on left side impossible. Straining at stool < headache. Stooping = dizziness. Rising = fainting, nausea, and dizziness. < At night. < In close room. Open air >.

Relations.—*Antidoted by :* Acon. (epididymitis), Ver. (diarrhœa). *Compare :* Botan., Samb., Vib. p., Vib. t. Chemical, Valer. Nervous, rheumatic diathesis, Act. r. Cramplike abdominal pains and menstrual symptoms, Caulo. Threatened miscarriage, pains go down into thighs, Cham. (with Cham. pains are intolerable, and there is flow of dark blood). Pains coming round pelvis to uterus ; goneness ; bearing down ; feeling that organs will escape from vulva, and wants support ; nervousness, Sep. (with Vib. the bearing down is more violent and culminates in uterus in cramps). Uterine cramps, Caul., Sec., Act. r. Aching eyeballs, Act. r. Bearing-down pains, Bell., Calc., Gossyp., Lil., Pul., Sul. Left ovarian and left inframammary pain, Lil., Lach., Caul., Sul., Ustil. > Menses coming on, Lach.

SYMPTOMS.

1. **Mind.**—Exaltation of spirits, in some cases followed by depression. —Depressed.—Irritable, wishes to be alone.—Very nervous and excessively irritable, lasting all day (F_3).—Confusion ; and inability to concentrate thoughts. —Stupid feeling as if I could not tell where I was or what to do in morning on waking.—Inability to perform mental labour.

2. **Head.**—Vertigo : in afternoon on closing eyes ; < descending stairs or walking in a dimly-lighted room ; with inclination to turn to left ; as if he would fall forward on rising from a seat.—Head hurt by every cough.—Pain in head : beginning about 3 p.m., < at night ; with red face.—Throbbing in head, all the evening, so severe on retiring that I felt sick all over.—Heavy headache, < over eyes, < l. side, at times extending to vertex and occiput (< when delayed menses should appear), < a sudden jar, bending over, false step or movement.—Dull, heavy pain r. side of head, throbbing on movement, > by rest ; with dizziness and nausea (F_2).—Very painful shootings from temples (< r.) to base of brain (F_3).—Head dull and sluggish.—Frontal headache : over l. eye ; in r. supraorbital region ; in forenoon over eyes on opening them, the soreness extending back into head ; with occasional vertigo, almost incapacitating him for study, with profuse and frequent micturition ;

and in supraorbital region, with profuse, clear, watery urine.—Headache beginning over r. eye and extending to vertex, with fulness in head and pressure on vertex.—Throbbing pain in forehead, extending to eyeballs, < by mental exertion, > moving about.—Terrible crushing pain in head, < l. parietal region where there is sensation as if head opening and shutting; < by motion; by mental exertion; > by rest (F_1).—Confusing, dull frontal headache extending to temples as after night-watching, compelling cessation of mental exertion.—Pain in l. temple, with pinching.—Pain in l. side of head.—Sharp pain in parietal region penetrating into brain, < coughing, moving head, and at stool.—Pressive pain in r. supraorbital region.—Hair feels as if pulled.—Scalp sensitive to touch.

3. **Eyes.**—Swelling about r. eye with induration.—Sclerotica streaked with blood.—Sensation of sand in eyes.—Pain in r. eye with congestion.—Sore feeling on closing lids.—Burning and lachrymation.—Heaviness of eyes; feels almost sick enough to go to bed.—Heaviness over eyes and in balls, at times had to look twice to be sure of seeing an object.—Eyeballs feel sore; (also F_1).—Lids swollen.

4. **Ears.**—Stabbing in ears.—Pains in bone waking at night.—External ear sore as if bruised, cannot lie on affected side of head; had to rub ear and it seemed as if I must straighten it out, sensation as if pinned to head; lay on other side, and was awakened by same feeling in that ear, in consequence compelled to change position often.

5. **Nose.**—Sneezing.—Watery coryza.

6. **Face.**—Very pale with dark circles under eyes (F_4).—Face and lips pale; dark circles under eyes (F_2).—Face swollen and congested with dark circles under eyes.—Face flushed and hot.—Lips dry.

7. **Teeth.**—Tooth sore on pressure.

8. **Mouth.**—Tongue broad and white, with brown centre and imprints of teeth.—Dryness of tongue; of mouth.—Taste disagreeable; coppery.

9. **Throat.**—Tickling in r. side of pharynx, causing cough.

11. **Stomach.**—No desire to eat; stomach feels full (F_3).—Nausea: every night; during menses; for ten days after menses, with faintness at stomach; > eating, with faintness, both returning; in pit of stomach, > lying perfectly quiet, faintness always on trying to get up; with faintness; (without inclination to vomit), > eating; then vomiting.—Pain in stomach in afternoon, > stretching body and throwing stomach forward.—Cramp-like pain in stomach and abdomen, doubling him up.—Cramping pain in stomach (F_1).—Sensitiveness of stomach region.—Indigestion, food lies heavy.—(Dyspepsia, habitual, with flatus, nausea and distension, and general catarrhal tendency.—R. T. C.).—Goneness.

12. **Abdomen.**—Rumbling and darting and flying pains in abdomen.—Darting pains, which settle about navel.—Bearing-down pains as during menstruation, with heavy pain over pubes.—Bearing-down pain, with drawing pains in anterior muscles of thighs and occasional shootings in ovarian regions.—Soreness of abdomen (F_3).—Sensitiveness to pressure, < about umbilicus.—Pressure of flatus in l. side.—Throbbing pain under l. floating ribs from 11 p.m. till 3 a.m., > hard pressure and walking about the room.—Throbbing in l. hypochondrium when lying on l. side.—Sticking in spleen in evening, > walking about the room, with sensation as if a hot fluid ran through

its vessels.—Pain in region of spleen causing faintness, > sweat.—Cramping pain in hypogastrium during menstruation.—Sudden cramping pain; as before menstruation, < night.—Constant bearing down from back through to front in ovarian and uterine region (F_3).—(Feeling as if the body from the waist down to lower pelvis would collapse.)

13. **Stool and Anus.**—Stools watery, profuse, frequent, at menstrual period, with chills and cold sweat rolling off forehead.—Hæmorrhage of dark red blood during and after stool.—Inactivity, no inclination for stool.—Constipation; with tenesmus; when bowels moved pain in l. orbital region.—Desire with much straining.—Constipation alternating with diarrhœa.—Stools: hard, large, with cutting in rectum and anus when passed; hard, large, painful and so difficult that mechanical assistance was necessary; scanty, in balls; long, large, hard and difficult, having a desire to evacuate, but on attempting feels as if nothing were there, evacuation occurs slowly and only after long straining.—Large stool, difficult, with urging.—Irregular.—Omitted two days, then hard stool, with blood and soreness of anus.—Frequent desire for stool with aching hæmorrhoids, frequent urination (F_1).

14. **Urinary Organs.**—Sensation after micturition as if urine continued to flow.—Frequent, profuse urination (F_1).—Copious urine; in morning, clear, watery, sp. gr. 1019, frequent micturition; every hour in afternoon and evening; at night, and pale, sp. gr. 1021; every hour or two during menses, and clear, light-coloured; and watery; in afternoon, watery, clear, micturition frequent.—Spurting of urine when coughing (J. C. B.).—Light-coloured urine.

15. **Male Sexual Organs.**—Pain and swelling of epididymis and testicle of l. side; next day epididymis of r. side so painful and swollen he was compelled to wear a suspensory bandage.—Emission without dream.

16. **Female Sexual Organs.**—Leucorrhœa: thick, white, and copious; thin, yellowish white after menses; thin, colourless, except with every stool, when it was thick, white, inodorous, blood-streaked; causing redness, smarting and itching of genitals.—Sudden pain in womb and hypogastrium before menstruation.—Pain in ovarian region.—Congested feeling in pelvic organs, as before menses.—Bearing-down pains: in pelvic region, with uneasiness; as before menses; as during menses, with heavy aching in sacral region and over pubes; as during menses with drawing pains in anterior muscles of thighs, every day after 3 p.m., with occasional shooting over ovaries, later the same, with nervousness, could not sit or lie still on account of the pains.—Menstrual pain, with feeling as if the breath would leave her body and heart would cease to beat.—Crampy, colicky pains in both ovarian regions, extending down thighs (F_1).—Slight, deep-seated pain in r. ovarian region, extending down thigh and < by walking or exertion (F_2).—Bearing down as if menses would appear (F_2).—Whole pelvis feels full and congested (F_2).—At 4 a.m. heavy bearing-down pains running from back around abdomen to uterus where pain is cramping; pressure on bladder; surprised to find herself menstruating (eight days after previous period ceased—F_3).—At intervals, distressing, grinding pains in ovaries and uterus, with sensation as if organs were turning upside down; and as if parts were being forced through vulva; desire to support the parts (F_3).—Menses began ten days early (always regular before); pain in back and cramps lasted throughout the period (F_4).—Menses:

too early, profuse and offensive; too late, scanty, thin, light-coloured, lasting but a few hours, with lightness of head, faintness on attempting to sit up; look like jelly; stain permanently; ceased for several hours, then four large clots of the colour of raw beef, but as solid as liver; for two days flow like normal menses, but with cramping pain and nervousness.—(Dysmenorrhœa, excruciating colic through the uterus and lower part of the abdomen, just preceding menstruation.—After-pains.—Membranous dysmenorrhœa.—Cramps in the calves always between the menses, < just before the period, with scanty, delayed menstruation, dysmenorrhœa.—Cramps in abdomen and legs in pregnant women, &c.)

17. **Respiratory Organs.**—Hoarse.—Suffocating spells at night.—Cough during second month of pregnancy; < night and morning and on lying down; urine spurting out when coughing (J. C. B.).

18. **Chest.**—Shooting over l. sixth rib near sternum.—Feeling of oppression over whole chest (F_4).—In lungs sensation as if muscles of chest failed to act, causing dyspnœa.

19. **Heart.**—Clutching pain in region of heart < by any exertion (F_4).—Excruciating, cramping pain in heart (F_4).—Palpitation, with sensation of lack of air after each severe pain (F_3).—Heart's action increased.

20. **Back.**—Pain as if back would break during menses.—Lame and bruised feeling in muscles of back.—Wandering, tired pains in muscles, < l. side.—Terrible clutching, cramping pain beginning in back, extending round lower abdomen to uterus with bearing down, as if menses would appear (lasted six days, > only when menses appeared, having missed the previous month—F_1).—Tired, bruised pain in muscles from point of scapula to wing of ilium, on both sides of spine, > firm pressure.—Pain: in lumbar region; between l. floating ribs and wing of ilium, > pressure, but must keep moving; in kidney region, < working in laboratory, > pressing across back with arms crossed; in l. loin and l. hypochondrium, causing faintness, > warm sweat though the night was cool; throbbing in l. loin, < lying down, > walking with cane pressed across back; in back, loins, and hypogastrium as if menses were coming on, < early part of evening and in a close room, > open air and moving about.—Pain in back in region of sacrum, an "unjointed feeling" (F_4).

21. **Limbs.**—Aching in limbs (F_2).—Aching of arms and thighs; feet somewhat swollen (F_3).

22. **Upper Limbs.**—Pain in r. shoulder.—Soreness of l. shoulder in region of subclavian muscle, < rest and wet weather, > motion, with lameness.—Pain in l. biceps.—Numbness of l. arm and hand.—Buzzing feeling in hands as if they would burst.—Swelling of fingers, < washing in cold water, with numbness.

23. **Lower Limbs.**—Weakness of lower extremities with heaviness.—Wandering, tired pains extending to hips and knees, with disinclination to move about.—Cramps in legs in pregnant women.—Feeling in feet as from the starting of circulation after constriction is removed.—Cramps in feet after long walking.

24. **Generalities.**—Pains flying from one part to another; wandering, tired pains extending to hips and knees.—Felt bloated all over (F_3).—Sick feeling all over ($F_{1, 2, 3, 4}$).—Pains = perspiration; during the pains felt she could not move (F_3).—Great exhaustion (F_3).—Paralytic condition coming on

after convulsions.—Hysterical convulsions from uterine conditions.—Cramps and contractions of limbs, esp. during pregnancy.

26. Sleep.—Retired early, very restless sleep, felt sick all over ; when asleep, sensation of falling and awakened frequently with a start (F_3).—Desire to sleep between severe pains from exhaustion, but could not (F_3).

27. Fever.—Chill followed by severe headache.—Dripping wet all over, with the pains.

Viburnum Prunifolium.

Viburnum prunifolium. Black Haw. (An American species.) *N. O.* Caprifoliaceæ. Tincture of fresh bark ("gathered in October and November from trees grown in open situations."—Phares, quoted by Hale).

Clinical.—Abortion, threatened. Dysmenorrhœa. Menorrhagia. Tetanus. Tongue, cancer of.

Characteristics.—Hale quotes experiences showing a close resemblance between *Vib. p.* and *Vib. o.*, with some additional uses of *Vib. p.* E. P. Fowler cured two cases of cancer of the tongue with the decoction of *Vib. p.* bark, used topically. Phares thinks it perhaps "the best remedy in the world for tetanus." Hale used the tincture in threatened miscarriage, dysmenorrhœa, and spasmodic uterine pains. Phares says of it, "It is particularly valuable in preventing abortion and miscarriage, whether habitual or otherwise ; whether threatened from accidental causes or criminal drugging," and he gives cases in support of each. It entirely antidotes the effect of *Gossyp.*, which is much used for procuring abortion in some of the States ; one pint of a strong decoction of the cotton-root being sufficient. *Vib. p.* taken regularly completely neutralises this. Here are some of Phares' cases : (1) Mrs. W. had never gone to full term ; had had several children at eight months, all of them dying one month after birth. Frequent pregnancies and hæmorrhages had seriously impaired her health. When next pregnant *Vib. p.* was ordered, and at the eighth month when pains set in vigorously with copious sanguineous discharge, *Vib. p.* was given freely, and she went to term, giving birth to a healthy boy, who survived. (2) Mrs. L., married eighteen months, had miscarried, and suffered long and much in consequence. Being again pregnant, Phares gave *Vib. p.* φ, a teaspoonful thrice daily. At the third month she was severely injured by a fall from her carriage. Strong uterine contractions ensued, but were arrested by *Vib. p.*, which had to be given freely for several days, the dose being gradually diminished. For nearly a week abortion was threatened whenever *Vib. p.* was too long suspended. The patient went to term and gave birth to a large boy.

Relations.—*Antidote to :* Gossyp.

Viburnum Tinus.

Viburnum tinus. Laurustinus. *N. O.* Caprifoliaceæ. Tincture of fresh leaves.

Clinical.—Deafness. Diaphragm, cramp in. Hypochondriasis. Ovary, pain in.

Characteristics.—*Viburnum tinus* is the beautiful evergreen shrub known in our gardens as *Laurustinus*. Cooper has investigated it, giving always single doses of the ϕ tincture in cases analogous to those for which *Vib. o.* is given. He has cured with it : (1) Pain in ovary with depression. [He considers hypochondriasis an indication for *Vib. t.*] (2) Deafness, with sufferings in lower segment of abdomen and dysmenia ; erosions about the os uteri. (3) Cramp in diaphragm. (4) Horrible headache all over head, < on right side with right-sided deafness, coming on at 7 and 11 a.m. and 4 and 7 p.m., with great sinking in pit of chest. (5) Waking at 4 a.m. with horrid depression of spirits that lasts till noon, with a weight on chest and back ; has to hold herself up in order to breathe.

Vichy.

Mineral springs at Vichy, in France. [Grande-Grille springs, containing in 100 parts : Carbonic acid 4·418, Mur. ac. 0·344, Sulphuric acid 0·164, Sil. ac. 0·070, Phos. ac. 0·070, Arsenic acid 0·001, Ferric oxide 0·002, Sodium 2·488, Potassium 0·182, Calcium 0·169, Magnesium 0·097.] Dilution.

Clinical.—Bladder, catarrh of. Constipation. Diabetes. Gall-stones. Gout. Gravel. Heartburn. Indigestion. Intermittent fevers. Liver, affections of. Neck, stiff. Rheumatism. Salivation. Skin, affections of. Uterus, affections of.

Characteristics.—The springs of Vichy are alkaline, both hot and cold. They are used in a large number of maladies, especially (1) diseases of the digestive tract ; (2) diseases of the liver with or without calculi ; (3) abdominal engorgements consequent on paludal fevers ; (4) chronic engorgements of the uterus ; (5) catarrh of the bladder ; (6) gravel ; (7) gout and rheumatism ; (8) diabetes mellitus ; (9) skin diseases (Constantin James). Croserio proved *Vichy*, taking the water, and triturations of the salt and dilutions. His symptoms make up the Schema. Among the most prominent symptoms were *stitches :* stitches below mastoid ; in chest ; in right loin and in heart. Across the chest there was a sensation as of a bar impeding breathing. Sinking sensation ; and sensation as if about to be sick. Burning flatulence. In the nose there were illusions of smell ; corpse-like odour ; odour of cucumbers. After coitus there was excessive weakness as if from hunger. The symptoms are : < From cold ; from draughts of air. < After eating ; when eating. (Uneasiness is > by dinner.) < When seated. < After coitus.

Relations.—*Compare :* Nat. mur. Stitching pains, K. ca. Bar sensation, Hæmatox., Ars., Ox. ac. < From coitus, K. ca., K. bi., Staph. Illusory smells, Anac.

SYMPTOMS.

1. **Mind.**—Very low-spirited ; felt as though some misfortune about to happen ; causelessly anxious about the future.

2. **Head.**—Slight compressive pain in forehead and temples.—Painful stitching in r. temple for some minutes.—Stitching below r. mastoid process, followed by griping in middle abdomen, then return of stitching.—Stitches in petrous portion of temporal bone.—Pressure at occiput with general uneasiness, as if fever were coming on.—Stitches in occiput below l. tuberosity.—Itching of head : violent in morning on rising ; in forehead.

3. **Eyes.**—Stinging in eyes with lachrymation.—Pain below l. eye like pressure after breakfast.—Different coloured sparks before eyes in morning.

4. **Ears.**—Stitches in bones below ears.

5. **Nose.**—Coryza.—Fetid, corpse-like odour in nose, morning on rising.—Very strong smell of cucumbers in nose, morning.

6. **Face.**—Sharp stitching between articulation of jaw and l. temple.—Twisting pain in lower jaw, near ethmoid process, as if jaw was swollen, when masticating on that side.—Red and sore pimples on upper lip.

8. **Mouth.**—Mouth very dry, with very bitter taste all day.—Saliva : abundant, immediately ; salty, with burning in stomach.—Taste : bitter and clammy ; bitter in evening with thirst ; bitter, morning on rising.

11. **Stomach.**—Great hunger.—Keen relish.—Diminished thirst (in spite of hot weather).—Longing for wine.—Craving for food as from feebleness of stomach, with sick feeling without hunger.—Heartburn.—Transient nausea while eating.—Acidity.—Belching.—Pinching ; griping ; burning in stomach.—After the first swallow, cutting pain throughout whole stomach.—Burning in stomach < afternoon.

12. **Abdomen.**—Shooting in liver.—Compressive pain in l. hypochondrium.—Emission of burning flatulence, with slight urging to stool.—Borborygmus, with gripings, during day.—Distension and uneasiness.—Burning borborygmi.—Griping and colic.—Feeling of desire for stool, only wind passes.—In evening sensation as if diarrhœa would come on, with sensation of hunger at an unusual hour.

13. **Stool and Anus.**—Ineffectual urging to stool, only wind passes.—Very difficult stool with copious flatulence, followed by burning and uneasiness in rectum.—Large, soft stool.—Copious diarrhœic stool.

14. **Urinary Organs.**—Griping in bladder, morning.—Frequent urination during night.—Urine : abundant, watery, foamy.

15. **Male Sexual Organs.**—Strong and long-lasting erections without desire.—Excessive itching : at orifice of glans, fossa navicularis, scrotum.—Desire diminished.—Excessive weakness after coition, as if suffering from hunger.

17. **Respiratory Organs.**—Dry cough produced by a pricking or tickling in the neck ; followed by fluent coryza.—Cough at night with difficult expectoration.

18. **Chest.**—Painful uneasiness in chest followed by expectoration of purulent matter.—Sensation in chest as if a bar across it preventing respiration, followed by a cough with expectoration of thick mucus.—Tearing pain at border of false ribs on both sides.—Stitches in r. chest, evenings.—Very painful stitches in r. chest, corresponding to commencement of cartilaginous portion of two first false ribs, and extending below and behind breast towards back.

19. **Heart.**—Stitch in heart followed by stitch in r. lumbar region, when seated.

20. **Neck and Back.**—Painful stiffness of muscles of back of neck and l. scaleni as after making a false step ; moving these parts is very painful.—Stitch in r. loin when seated, following stitch in heart.

22. **Upper Limbs.**—Bruised pain in arms.—Bruising pain in fingers and uneasiness as if a fever were coming on, after lunch.

23. **Lower Limbs.**—Stitch in r. tibia, extending from upper part of instep.

24. **Generalities.**—Uneasiness as if fever coming on.—Weakness after coition.—Very sensitive to cold and draughts.

25. **Skin.**—Pimples : on lip ; back of neck, with pricking.—Pricking and itching compelling scratching, which >, but itching returns.

26. **Sleep.**—Sleepy : after dinner ; in evening; fatiguing dreams, but sleep more prolonged than usual.

Vinca Minor.

Vinca minor. Lesser Periwinkle. (Woods and shady places.)
N. O. Apocynaceæ. Tincture of whole fresh plant.

Clinical.—Acne. Alopecia. Crusta lactea. *Eczema.* Favus. Neck, stiff. Nose, redness of. *Plica polonica. Seborrhœa.* Throat, sore. *Uterus, bleeding from.*

Characteristics.—*Vinca* was proved by Rosenburg on four healthy persons, who took the tincture in 20- to 60-drop doses. It produced a deep impression on the organism and tissues. Weakness and prostration accompanied many of the sufferings ; the stool caused exhaustion ; great debility accompanied the uterine hæmorrhage. There was "weakness as if he would die" ; inclination to stretch ; tremulousness and tendency to start, especially on exciting the mind ; and tremulousness in all the blood-vessels. Allied to this an empty, all-gone sensation appeared in the stomach and chest. A corresponding deep impression was made on the tissues : blood and blood-vessels ; skin, hair, and nails ; bones. In passive uterine hæmorrhages *Vinca* has a wide range. This case is related in *Ind. H. R.* (ix. 113) : Uterine hæmorrhage, blood dark red, flow copious, uninterrupted, with extreme debility. *Chi.* and *Helon.* failed to relieve ; *Vinca* 1 x effected a rapid and permanent cure. Frequent nose-bleed is another effect of *Vinca.* And there is a curious symptom in connection with the nose which it is well to remember : it "becomes red from the slightest cause ; *when the least bit angry.*" There are scabby eruptions about the nose and on the septum, which are part of the general skin effect of the remedy. It causes corrosive itching of the skin provoking scratching ; moist spots, and burning in ulcers. The most characteristic effect is on the scalp, where it produces a condition having many features of crusta lactea, favus, and plica polonica. I have cured with *Vinca* "sore spots on the scalp" in a young lady. A number of symptoms were produced in the throat and œsophagus. C. M. Boger records this case (*M. Coun.*, xvi. 265) : Woman, 31, had a cutting sensation in lower part of œsophagus while swallowing food, continuing after. Empty faintness in stomach > by eating. Stomach sore to touch or pressure of clothing. Constipation from induration of fæces. Hæmorrhoids constantly sore, smarting after stool. *Vinca* 41m (Fincke) cured. *Peculiar Sensations* are : As if a hammer were beating from within outwards in vertex. Cold wind in ears. As if something sticking low down in œsophagus. As if a weight lying on cervical muscles. As if he would die from weakness. The left side was most affected. A peculiar symptom was distension of abdomen *after stool.* "Toothache > in warmth of bed" is unusual. The symptoms are : < On stooping. < Walking. < Reading. > Moving in open air. Toothache > by warmth of bed. Drinking < : liquids (esp. beer) = eructations ; coffee = nausea. Mental exertion < ; = tremulous feeling and tendency to start.

Relations.—*Compare :* Peevishness with repentance, Croc. Crusta lactea, Med., Melit., Mez., Jug. r., Olean., Viol. t. (with strong-smelling urine), Arct. l. (glands swollen ; axillary glands even suppurate), Staph. (sickly children, pale face, dark rings round eyes), Ustil. (filthy eruptions, part of hair comes out, part matted). Alopecia, Bacil., Pho.

Causation.—Anger (red nose). Mental exertion (tremulousness and starting).

SYMPTOMS.

1. **Mind.**—Sadness with fear of death.—Lachrymose.—Peevish and quarrelsome, soon followed by repentance.

2. **Head.**—Whirling vertigo with flickering before eyes.—Pressure on head ; in temples.—Dulness of sinciput with slow pressure towards eyes and dimness of vision, < stooping when writing.—Sticking in l. temple extending to malar bone.—Tearing in vertex with feeling as if a hammer beating from within out.—Corrosive itching on the hairy scalp.—Badly-smelling eruptions on the head, in the face, and behind the ears (breeding vermin).—The hairs are entangled, as in plica polonica.—Hair falls out and is replaced by grey hair.—Bald spots, covered with short, woolly hair.—Humid eruptions on the head, with much vermin, and nightly itching, with burning after scratching.

3. **Eyes.**—Itching and burning of lids, which become red.—Eye dry, on getting snuff into it there was so little secretion he was obliged to wash it out.—Obscuration of vision (fog before eyes) while reading ; at times also while walking.

4. **Ears.**—Ringing and whistling in ears, with feeling of cold wind, esp. l.

5. **Nose.**—Nose becomes red on becoming the least angry.—Tip of nose becomes red from slightest cause.—Frequent nose-bleed.—Stoppage of nose, mostly of one nostril, with discharge of much mucus through posterior nares.—Distressing dryness and heat in nose extending into frontal sinuses.—Itching in nose.—Moist eruption on septum exuding moisture which forms light-brown scab ; skin dirty white, elevated, with red areola.

6. **Face.**—Bloated face, with pimples.—Tearing in malar bones.—Dry lips.—Swelling of upper lip and corner of mouth.

8. **Mouth.**—Tearing in teeth > by warmth of bed.—Aphthæ.—Increased secretion of saliva.—Insipid taste in mouth ; to all food.

9. **Throat.**—Frequent hawking through day.—Ulcers in throat (?).—Sore throat, with difficulty in swallowing.—Sensation as if something was sticking low down in œsophagus, which provokes swallowing.

11. **Stomach.**—Hunger alternating with loss of appetite before the hunger has been satisfied.—Scarcely any thirst.—Empty eructations after drinking beer, and generally < from taking liquid.—Nausea after coffee.—Violent, bitter, copious vomiting of yellowish-green liquid.—Gastric disturbance.—Emptiness in stomach.

12. **Abdomen.**—Distension after a stool.—Abdomen full, tense but painless.—Rumbling and gurgling, with passage of much offensive flatus.—Griping.

13. **Stool and Anus.**—Urging to stool.—Stool first hard, then soft.—Stool exhausting, with burning in anus.

14. **Urinary Organs.**—Diminished secretion of urine.—Urine pale yellow.

16. **Female Sexual Organs.**—Excessive, profuse menses, flowing like a stream, with great weakness.—Passive uterine hæmorrhage from fibroid tumour.—Passive uterine hæmorrhage in women long past their climacteric.

17. **Respiratory Organs.**—Hoarseness.—Tenacious mucus in trachea.—Spasmodic cough, with little tickling in larynx.—Rapid respiration.

18. **Chest.**—Pains in chest, with sticking and dyspnœa.—Pressure on sternum, with feeling of emptiness in chest.—Stitching in sternum.

20. **Neck.**—Painful tension and stiffness of cervical muscles, with an illusive sensation as if a weight were lying on them.

21. **Limbs.**—Inclination to stretch limbs.—Tearing pains in limbs.—Arthritic tearing in bones.

22. **Upper Limbs.**—Cramp-like drawing in upper arm and tips of fingers.—Swelling and stiffness of first joints of fingers, with burning pain in the nails.

23. **Lower Limbs.**—Cramp-like drawing in feet and toes.

24. **Generalities.**—Weakness as if he would die.—Tremulous feeling : in all the vessels ; in upper extremities, with tendency to start, esp. on exerting the mind.—Emptiness or hungry feeling.—Most symptoms > moving about in open air.

25. **Skin.**—Great sensitiveness of skin, with redness or soreness even from slight irritation.—Burning in the ulcers like bed-sores on l. buttock.—Corrosive itching provoking scratching.—Itching, moist spots on upper part r. ankle.

26. **Sleep.**—Frequent yawning.—Sleeplessness and restlessness at night.—Lascivious dreams.

27. **Fever.**—Sudden paroxysms of shivering.—Heat with firm, hard pulse.—Great warmth in scalp with prickling.—Heat of cheeks with redness.—Tremor in every blood-vessel.

Viola Odorata.

Viola odorata. Sweet-scented Violet. *N. O.* Violaceæ (an order most members of which contain Emetin, and under which *Ipec.* is sometimes placed : allied to Cinchonaceæ). Tincture of fresh plant in flower.

Clinical.—Cancer. Choroiditis. Cough, spasmodic ; by day. Hoarseness. Hysteria. Neuralgia, supra-orbital. Otorrhœa ; suppressed. Rheumatism. Seminal emissions. Styes. Whooping-cough. Wrists, rheumatism of.

Characteristics.—The Violet was introduced by Gross and proved by Hahnemann, Gross, and Stapf. Gross says of his symptoms that they recurred equally in all positions, were mild, yet more definitely felt than from other drugs. Hahnemann had bruised pain in all the bones in the morning, in bed after waking, > after rising. Stapf had relaxation of all the muscles. The mind was greatly excited and disturbed, and *V. od.* found its first uses in hysterical cases. Aversion to music, especially the violin, is one of the peculiar symptoms. There is increased activity and rush of ideas, generally confused : "Can only grasp half an idea ; puts it in its proper place but cannot hold it." A keynote symptom of *V. od.* is *Tension :* "Tension of the occiput and forehead" ; "Tension of the scalp of occiput even when not moving, though < bending head forward and backward ; painful, compelling him to wrinkle forehead ; lasting several days." Gross experienced the former and Stapf the latter of these. The following is from Gross : "Tension which at times extends to upper half of face, especially of nose, thence to forehead and temples, as far as ears, alternating with a similar sensation in occiput and cervical muscles." Cooper (*H. M.*, xxix. 154 and 640) has illustrated the action of *V. od.* on the head and eye by a case : Miss X. had for twenty years attacks of fearful headache which began suddenly and without apparent cause at intervals of a week or more. The pain was throbbing under right temple and eye, sometimes flying for a short time to the other side. Vision very defective, especially on dull, wet days ; chronic choroiditis had been diagnosed by one prominent oculist. On September 11, 1893, a single dose of *V. od.* φ was given. Next day the patient had a headache, not in the usual place, but quite at the vertex. After this there were no severe headaches and very few threatenings. General health improved and the sight also ; the pain and irritation, which were formerly distracting, disappeared. Cooper ordered discontinuance of glasses. On March 10, 1894, there was a rather pronounced attack of headache, with sick feeling, at the time of the period ; "the first day the pain was through my head, the second day about an inch or two above the right ear." Another dose of *V. od.* φ was sent. From this time the cure went steadily forward.

Appetite and strength increased, and sight gradually became normal. On May 11, 1894, the patient wrote, "I am quite well, and my sight is in splendid order." Cooper considers *V. od.* has a very specific relation to the lateral sinuses and their vasomotor nerves. Symptoms of the proving show a "decided pitch" on the interior of the eyes: "Oppression in the eyeballs; heat and burning of the eyes"; "Fiery appearances (a fiery semicircle) before the eyes"; "Stinging in the eyes." Cooper has also published an ear case treated with *Viola* (*H. M.*, xxix. 154): A child of seventeen months had been affected with recurring otorrhœa of both ears (< right) from birth; and two other children of the same parents were said to have died from discharges of the ears, coming on in the same unaccountable manner. *V. od.* ϕ, one dose, was given, and the next day a great quantity of ill-smelling discharge came from the right ear, with immediate improvement in the child's condition; from being drowsy and listless she became bright and intelligent. Thereafter both discharge and deafness disappeared. Ear affections with pain about the orbits indicate *V. od.* *V. od.* has cured a number of cases of rheumatism, chiefly right-sided. It has a marked affection for the wrists, especially the right. Cooper considers it *Suited to* "dark-complexioned people of the *Fer. pic.* type"; Hering says to: "tall, thin, nervous girls"; to "mild, impressive girls of fair complexion"; and to "tuberculous patients." Teste, who used *Viola* frequently, described the type as "a lymphatico-nervous temperament, a mild disposition, dry and cool skin." Many patients cured by him were tall and slender. [The cure of Lady Margaret Marsham, 67, of an affection of the throat pronounced to be malignant (apparently epithelioma of tonsil), with an infusion of Violet leaves is on record (*H. W.*, xxxvi. 556). Boiling water was poured on the fresh leaves and allowed to stand twelve hours. Compresses moistened with this were applied externally to the throat and covered with oil-silk. Relief of pain, dysphagia, and suffocative symptoms was immediate. The external swelling disappeared in a week, the growth on the tonsil in a fortnight.] *Peculiar Sensations* are: As if everything in head whirled around. As if eyeballs were compressed. As if nose had been beaten and blood were pressing out. As if hard palate were dried up. As if a stone were lying on chest. Burning like a small, transient flame in spots here and there. The symptoms are: < Bending head backward and forward. < By day (cough). < From music. Bone pains > after rising in morning. < Cold room (hoarseness). < Dull wet day (vision).

Relations.—*Antidoted by:* Camph. *Compatible:* In whooping-cough, Coral.; in helminthiasis, Cina. *Compare:* Pain in right wrist, Act. spi., Bry. Ropy sputa, K. bi. Weakness of muscles of neck, Ver., Ant. t. < Music, Nux, Sep., Ph. ac., Aco., Nat. c., Puls. [Cooper has pointed out a close relationship between the Violaceæ and the Rubiaceæ, notably between Viola and Ipecac. Both Viola and Ipec. have been used externally as remedies for stings and snake-bites (*H. W.*, xxxvi. 249).] Teste puts Viola in the Chelidonium group, and finds a striking analogy between these two remedies.

Causation.—Suppressed discharges.

SYMPTOMS.

1. **Mind.**—Sombre melancholy and sadness.—Hysterical humour, with constant weeping, without knowing why.—Aversion to conversation.—Great weakness of memory and forgetfulness.—Great concourse (excessive flow) of unsettled and confused ideas.—Insane confusion, childish behaviour, disobedience, refusing nourishment, talks in a low, soft voice.—Remarkable perspicuity and great activity of brain.—Predominance of intellect over feeling.—Increased activity of the intellect.

2. **Head.**—Dull and painful confusion in the head.—Turning vertigo, also when seated.—Headache, sometimes with cramps in eyes and luminous circles before sight.—Drawing in l. frontal eminence.—The head feels heavy and sinks forward ; sensation of weakness in muscles of nape.—Rush of blood to head, with prickings in sinciput (forehead).—Tension in integuments of the head, extending into face, nose, and ears, frequently causing a knitting of the brows.—Burning in forehead.

3. **Eyes.**—Cramps in eyelids.—Closing of eyes as from drowsiness.——Heaviness of eyelids.—Sensation as if eyeball were compressed.—Pupils contracted.—Heat and burning sensation in eyes.—Myopia.—Flames before eyes.—(Chronic choroiditis with fearful throbbing headache under r. temple.—R. T. C.)—Caused styes on r. eyelids in a case of Cooper's.—(Vision dim, < on dull, wet days).

4. **Ears.**—Shootings in (and around) ears.—Aversion to all kinds of music, principally violin.—Murmuring and tinkling before ears.—(Discharges of both ears with deafness disappeared after one dose of φ.—R. T. C.)—Brings on a discharge that has stopped ; or heals a discharge in a few days (R. T. C.).

5. **Nose.**—Numbness of tip of nose as from a blow, and as if blood were pressing out.

6. **Face.**—Hot forehead.—Pain in face, with drawing pressure in zygomatic process.—Tension in integuments of face, esp. above eyes.—Tension below eyes and above nose, extending to temples.—Tearings in (l.) lower jaw in direction of ear.

7. **Teeth.**—Tearing pain in (r.) lower teeth.

8. **Mouth.**—Sensation in hard palate as if it were completely dried up.—Aphthæ.

12. **Abdomen.**—Distension of abdomen.

13. **Stool and Anus.**—Constipation, with ineffectual want to evacuate.—Helminthiasis.—Itching of anus every afternoon.

15. **Male Sexual Organs.**—Pollutions, followed by headache.

16. **Female Sexual Organs.**—During pregnancy, dyspnœa.

17. **Respiratory Organs.**—Hoarseness, followed by coryza.—Dyspnœa with violent cough ; < in daytime.—By day chiefly, in long-lasting spells, dry, short, violent cough, with much dyspnœa.—Whooping-cough in nervous, thin little girls.—Sputum profuse, clear, ropy, jelly-like.—Respiration difficult, and scarcely perceptible, with painful expiration, excessive anguish, and violent palpitation of heart.—Shortness of breath.

18. **Chest.**—Violent oppression of the chest and dyspnœa, with pressure on the chest, as by a stone.

20. **Neck and Back.**—Tension in muscles of the neck.—Jerking drawing in cervical muscles, near nape, extending down, < lying on opposite side.

21. **Limbs.**—Rheumatism of r: side ; motion of r. side almost impossible. —Bruised pain in all bones in morning in bed, after waking, disappears after rising.—Relaxation of all the muscles.—Drawing pains in limbs.—Pain as if broken in all joints on waking in morning.—Trembling of limbs.

22. **Upper Limbs.**—Slight trembling of arms ; dyspnœa.—Rheumatism of upper limbs ; deltoid ; of r. carpal and metacarpal joints.—Drawing pain in elbow-joint and back of hand.—Pressive, aching pain in the wrists, esp. r.

23. **Lower Limbs.**—Œdematous swelling of lower limbs with stitching pains.

24. **Generalities.**—Congestion of blood to single parts.—Troubles of or on l. ear.—Burning and flushes of heat in different parts.—Great nervous debility.—The sufferings are mild, but still well defined, and the same in all positions.—Yawning every morning, with lachrymation.—The patient lies on the back while asleep at night, with the l. hand passed above the head and the knees bent ; contrary to his habit.

25. **Skin.**—Dry, warm skin, want of sweat ; only palms moist ; measles running an irregular course.—Transient burning here and there in small spots.

26. **Sleep.**—Yawning : and stretching without sleepiness ; every morning so that eyes fill with water.—Sleepiness in eyes, lids will close. —Lies on back in sleep with l. hand over head, knees bent and lying far to side.

27. **Fever.**—Chilly disposition.—Forehead hot.—Transient burning, here and there, as if it concentrated in a small spot and burned there like a small flame.—Febrile shuddering.—Night-sweats.

Viola Tricolor.

Viola tricolor. Jacea. Pansy. Heartsease. *N. O.* Violaceæ.
Tincture of fresh plant in flower.

Clinical.—Crusta lactea. *Eczema.* Enuresis. Gonorrhœa, suppressed. Gout. *Impetigo.* Leucorrhœa. Ophthalmia, scrofulous. Orchitis. Plica polonica. Rheumatism. Ringworm. Seminal emissions. Syphilis. Throat, ulceration of.

Characteristics.—The Pansy was proved by Hahnemann and his provers. It had an ancient reputation in asthma and epilepsy, and especially in obstinate skin diseases. Teste quotes from old observers (Starck, Haase, Murray, &c.) the following as cured by *V. tri.* : (1) Milk-crust in children at the breast, [or] recently weaned. (2) Milk-crust with violent cough and excessive oppression. (3) Impetigo of hairy scalp and face in children and adult females. (4) Favus and serpiginous crusts in children and adults, with swelling and induration of cervical glands. (5) Large boils all over body in a scrofulous child. (6) Pustules and ichorous exanthema of feet. (7) Squamous spots on skin. (8) Rheumatism and gout ; articular rheumatism with itch-like eruption round the joints. (9) Impetigenous exanthema on forehead. (10) Ichorous ulcers with violent itching. In Russia a decoction of Pansy is a popular remedy for scrofula; and Schlegel, of Moscow, used it with good effect in syphilitic affections, especially venereal ulcers. Teste (from whom I take all the above) puts *V. tri.* in two groups, whose types are *Lyc.* and *Cham.* Homœopathy has brought out some characteristics of *V. tri.* which single out its cases. One of these is concomitance of urinary symptoms with skin affections: Tinea capitis with frequent involuntary urination. Eczema with urinary disturbances; too copious urination; or sudden arrest of secretion. "*Urine smelling like cat's urine*" is a keynote. The male sexual organs were much excited. Emissions with vivid dreams occurred; swelling, itching, and pains in prepuce and glans, with erections. *Peculiar Symptoms* are: Face hot and sweating after eating. Dyspnœa after eating. Hands twitch and are clenched in sleep. Nervous paroxysms followed suppressed milk-crust. The axillæ and clavicular regions were noticeably affected; and stitches and burning stitches were prevailing pains. The symptoms are: < By pressure on side opposite to painful side. < Lying on unpainful side. Lying = anxiety about heart. Raising head =, and stooping >, heaviness in head. Walking = vertigo; stitches through chest and abdomen. Sitting = stitches in abdomen and groin (standing > them). < At 11 a.m.; at night. Open air > headache; = chilliness. Aversion to open air. < In winter when walking in cold air.

Relations.—*Antidoted by:* Camph., Merc., Puls., Rhus. *Compatible:* Puls., Rhus, Sep., Staph. *Compare:* Tension of integuments of face and forehead, V. od. Crusta lactea, Vinca m. (V. tri. has urinary concomitants). Eruptions, ulcers, &c., Cham., Graph., Hep., Merc., Olean., Petrol., Staph. Stitches, K. ca. Botan., see *Viol. od.*

Causation.—Suppressed milk-crust (nervous paroxysms).

SYMPTOMS.

1. **Mind.**—Sadness respecting domestic affairs.—Precipitation as from internal anguish, with sensation of great weakness.—Tendency to shed tears.—Ill-humour, moroseness, with dislike to conversation.—Great sensitiveness, inclination to scold, and combativeness.—Disobedience.—Aversion to labour.—Great dulness of the intellect.

2. **Head.**—Head bewildered and perplexed.—Vertigo and dizziness when walking.—Headache from root of nose to brain, disappearing in open air.—Heaviness of head, which draws it backwards, principally when getting up, > by stooping.—Pressive headache, esp. in forehead and temples (extending outward).—Shootings in occiput day and night.—The brain shakes when walking.—Burning stitches in scalp, esp. in forehead and temples (tearing stitch externally in l. temple).—Scurfs on head, unbearable burning, most at night.—Impetigo of the hairy scalp and face.—Crusta lactea in children recently weaned.—Thick incrustations, pouring out a large quantity of thick, yellow fluid, which mats the hair.

3. **Eyes.**—Pain in eyes, as if a hard body were between upper eyelid and eyeball.—Smarting and incisive and itching shootings in eye.—Contraction and closing of eyelids, with inclination to sleep.—(Myopia.)

6. Face.—Heat in face at night in bed, sometimes semilateral, and in cheek on which patient is not lying.—Heat and perspiration of face after eating.—Thickness and hardness of skin of face.—Scabs on face with burning itching, esp. at night, and running of a yellow and viscid pus; also behind ears.—Tension in integuments of face and forehead.

8. Mouth.—Tongue loaded with whitish mucus of a bitter taste.—Accumulation of saliva in the mouth, with sensation of dryness.

9. Throat.—Sore throat in evening.—Swelling of cervical glands.—Much phlegm in throat = hawking, 11 a.m.—Swallowing difficult and very painful (syphilis).—Chancroid ulcer on posterior surface of fauces and soft palate (syphilis).

12. Abdomen.—Stitches and cutting pain in abdomen, with urging to stool and crying and lamentations, followed by discharge of lumps of mucus and flatulence.—Pressing-stinging in diaphragm.

13. Stool.—Chopped soft stools.—Stool with mucus and much flatus.

14. Urinary Organs.—Urging (frequent) to urinate, with profuse discharge of urine.—Fetid urine; it smells like cat's urine.—Very turbid urine.—Stitches in the urethra.

15. Male Sexual Organs.—Swelling of the prepuce with itching.—Stitching in penis or pressing in glans; burning of glans.—While standing voluptuous itching of prepuce, accompanied by an erection which prevented scratching.—Itching stitches in scrotum.—Involuntary seminal discharges, with vivid dreams.—Loss of seminal fluid at stool.—Suppressed gonorrhœa; indurated testicle.

16. Female Sexual Organs.—Stitch in region of mons veneris, r. side.—Painful pustules on labia.—Leucorrhœa: with stitching pain; in children; in syphilis.—Chancroid ulcers about breasts.

17. Respiratory Organs.—Stitches in l. side of chest; < during inspiration and expiration.

18. Chest.—Syphilitic ulcers on clavicles.—Shooting in chest.—Stitches in the chest, on the ribs, sternum, and intercostal muscles.

19. Heart.—Oppression and lancinations in region of heart on bending forwards while sitting.—Anxietas præcordium, with palpitation of heart when lying down (with beating like waves).

20. Neck and Back.—Swelling of glands of neck.—Spasmodic pain and contraction, with pinching between shoulder-blades (with cutting, tingling, and crawling in the skin).

22. Upper Limbs.—Lancinations in joints of shoulder, elbows, forearms, and fingers; > on motion.—Painful pustules in axillæ (syphilis).—Cutting stitches with itching in axillæ.

23. Lower Limbs.—Pain, as of broken thighs, on waking in morning.—Flexion of knees when walking; with drawings in thighs and calves.—Jerking of muscles in calves.—Fine stitches in r. tibia when walking.—Shootings in patellæ, tibiæ, and feet.—Pustulous and ichorous exanthema on feet.

24. Generalities.—[The principal use for this remedy is for nocturnal emissions accompanied by very vivid dreams; they are not very exhausting, but cause an uneasy and "played-out" state of the mind.—Loss of seminal fluid at stool and in the urine, trembling, poor appetite, feels dull, sleepless.—Very vivid, amorous dreams.—Pricking in skin; pricking itching.—< When sitting.—> After rising from a seat.—H. N. G.]—Dejection, sometimes as from insufficient sleep.—Lancinating pains in the limbs.—Miliary eruption over whole body, with lancinating, gnawing sensation.

25. **Skin.**—Stinging-biting rash.—Dry scabs over the whole body; when they are scratched they exude yellow water.—Eruption over face (except eyelids) and behind ears, with burning, itching, < at night, a thick, hard scab formed, cracked here and there, from which a tenacious yellow pus exuded, and hardened into a substance like gum.

26. **Sleep.**—Inclination to sleep in afternoon.—Disturbed sleep, with frequent waking.—Awakens frequently without cause.—Sleep retarded by a concourse of ideas, with difficulty in waking in morning.—Vivid and amorous dreams.—Jerking of the (child's) hands and retraction of thumbs when sleeping, with redness of face and general dry heat.

27. **Fever.**—Chill, or chilliness in forenoon and in open air.—Dry, anxious heat at night in bed, with red face.—General heat, esp. in face, with anxiety; dyspnœa immediately after eating.—Night-sweats.

Vipera.

Vipera communis. Pelias berus. Common Viper [with other varieties, especially V. redi (Italian Viper) and V. torva (German Viper)]. *N. O.* Ophidia (Family, Viperidæ). Attenuations of the venom.

Clinical.—Epistaxis. Goître. Hæmorrhages. Jaundice. Liver, enlargemen of. Neurasthenia. Phlebitis. Senility, premature. Tongue, swelling of. Vari cosis.

Characteristics.—The effects of bites by the Common Viper and related species have been collected, and have furnished the data for homœopathic prescribing. *Vipera* affects the blood and blood-vessels, conducing to hæmorrhage and inflammation of the vessels themselves. A keynote for *Vip.* in cases of phlebitis and varicosis is "< on letting the limb affected hang down"; as if it would burst with fulness. The region of the vessel affected is inflamed and sensitive. Allen (*Handbook*) relates this case: A goldbeater found the veins of his right arm become exceedingly swollen and painful, so that he could no longer work, or *let his hand hang down. Vip.* cured immediately. A case (quoted from *Med. Adv.* in *Med. Cent.*, ii. 79) of varicose vein of the popliteal space, with the sensation as *though the leg would burst*, and a nervous, fidgety condition of the feet which kept them in constant motion, was cured with *Vip. torva* 30. The *bursting* feeling appears to be at the root of this characteristic. Swan said *Vip.* was a remedy for all forms of epistaxis. *Vip.* has a chronic and periodic action; the symptoms return annually for years. Patients resist the cold badly. The parts may be paralysed and ulcers and gangrene follow. A *Sensation* as if something ran up the thigh occurred in the bitten limb in one case. In one case there was sweat over the whole body *except the bitten limb.* Leonard (*M. A.*, xxvi. 103) gave *Vipera* *acontica carinata* (1) to a lady suffering from climacteric hæmorrhage; flow red with dark clots; excessive to prostration and faintness. She had a small uterine fibroid. A few doses relieved, and the excessive hæmorrhage did not return. (2) A lady nursing a child a year old was much prostrated by hæmorrhage lasting several weeks, not profuse, but continuous: Nose-bleed nearly every day; weaning brought no relief. *Chi.* 200 did no good. *Vip. ac.* cm cured in three doses. The symptoms are: < By touch; by pressure; on change of weather. < Letting limb or part hang down.

Relations.—*Compare:* Hæmorrhage of fluid blood, Sanguisuga. < Hanging down limbs, Calc., Alm., Am. c., Sbi., Thu.

SYMPTOMS.

1. **Mind.**—Delirium; and raving; with vomiting; alternating with sopor.—Coma, with thirst for water.—Loss of mental functions with drawn features.

2. **Head.**—Vertigo: with falling forward, with nose-bleed and anxiety; with nausea and vomiting, so that he fainted; with loss of vision.—Ecchymoses in membranes of brain, effusion of bloody serum into ventricles.—Tearing at every change of weather, with sticking.—Headache: with coated tongue and bad appetite; with inclination to sigh.

3. **Eyes.**—Eyes: dark yellow; red, inflamed, and watery; staring; sunken.—Pupils: dilated; l. dilated, r. contracted.—Paralysis of lids; dropped over eyes.—Vision: dim; dim in l. eye, lost in r.; lost.

5. **Nose.**—Bleeding from nose; with vertigo.

6. **Face.**—Face: swollen (and neck), with pressing out of eyes; tense and blackish, with closure of throat; convulsed; red; pale and hippocratic, with cold sweat on forehead; covered with drops of sweat.—Lips: blue; lips and tongue swollen, covered with saliva and pale; livid and protruding. —Acid burning in lips, mouth, and throat.

8. **Mouth.**—Scorbutic line on gums.—Sensation of swelling in the teeth (*H. W.*, xxviii. 25).—Swelling of salivary glands; of mouth; of mouth and throat, with dryness, so that swallowing was impossible.—Tongue: swollen; and brownish-black, protruding; so that he could not speak; with closed jaws and difficult speech.—Tongue: black; fuliginous and breath fetid; yellow, tip red; white, tremulous; white in middle, moist on edges, with thirst.—Speech: inarticulate; and thick; lost on account of weakness.

9. **Throat.**—Swelling like a goître.—Closure of throat so that she could swallow only water and milk, afterwards biting in fauces, the swelling of which became blackish.—Viscid mucus adheres to pharynx.

10. **Appetite.**—Appetite lost.—Thirst: with moist tongue, for cold drinks.

11. **Stomach.**—Nausea: with shuddering; with attack of faintness.—Retching; with suffocative sensation.—Vomiting: after milk; of all food and drink; with weakness; faintness; shivering and thirst; coldness of body; with colic; with colic and thirst; bilious diarrhœa of bitter yellow fluid; green substances; green liquid; viscid greenish fluid.—Pain: in epigastrium;

< pressure ; in epigastric or umbilical region.—Uneasiness in epigastrium.—Digestion slow.

12. **Abdomen.**—Hypochondria tense ; sore.—Abdomen tense, pressure causes distension of facial muscles.—Swelling with raging pains and spasms even to faintness, and after drinking milk vomiting of a mass of round worms, then freedom from worm troubles which he had before.—Sudden flatulent distension, with colic, pain in back, and vomiting.—Rumbling.—Pain in abdomen ; in umbilical region, < pressure.

13. **Stool and Anus.**—Diarrhœa : frequent ; bilious.—Fetid ; and black.—Bloody stools ; in masses of dark, offensive blood (apparently from the tongue, which had been scarified).—Stools : copious ; numerous, with shivering, urging, and thirst ; involuntary ; and frequent, mixed with blood and mucus ; and involuntary micturition.—Discharge of black, coagulated blood ; of blood just before death.—Pain and tenesmus.—Urging to pass stool and urine ; desire for stool, with coldness to touch.—(After diarrhœa, greenish and bloody, most violent pain in the enlarged liver, with jaundice and fever, pain extending from liver to shoulder and down to hip ; *Vipera* immediately removed the pain and reduced the liver to its normal size.)

14. **Urinary Organs.**—Ineffectual desire.—Strangury.—Involuntary micturition.—Urine : increased ; suppressed ; dark yellow, as in jaundice.

17. **Respiratory Organs.**—Suffocation.—Dyspnœa ; with sticking in heart.—Anxious breathing, as in croup, threatening asphyxia.—Breathing ceased suddenly, heart stopped, face became livid, &c., tracheotomy was performed, blood drawn from arm flowed scantily, was dark, mixed with bright streaks.

18. **Chest.**—Veins of chest and abdomen thick and hard.—Swelling of chest as far as umbilicus after bite on face.—Œdema of lungs before death.—Pain : in l. side ; over four or five r. ribs on pressure.—Oppression, with anxiety ; with violent efforts to breathe and swallow.

19. **Heart and Pulse.**—Sticking in heart ; with cold sweat and faintness.—Pain in heart with faintness.—Dragging pain so that he tears his clothes, becomes faint.—Anxiety at same time for four years, with soreness of the bitten foot and paralysis of r. arm.—Heart's action : slow ; feeble ; and no pulsation in radial or carotid arteries, but that in crural was very strong.—Pulse : rapid ; interrupted ; slow, febrile ; irregular ; weak.—(*Vip.* is a very valuable remedy for varicose veins and for acute phlebitis, the vein is swollen, bordered by an area of inflammation, which is very sensitive to touch, but particularly with the sensation, on letting the leg hang down, as if it would burst from the fulness of the veins.—Phlebitis of r. arm, < hanging arms down.)

20. **Back.**—Sticking in kidneys.—Pain in loins.

21. **Limbs.**—Limbs swollen and red.—Livid spots on the bitten limb every year at the time of the bite.—Yellowish, livid, mottled spots.—Trembling.—Pain in limbs : < touch ; alternating with pains in abdomen.—Limbs : benumbed : relaxed.—(Burning feeling in limbs in three cases—neurasthenia, an old sprain, and varicose veins.)

22. **Upper Limbs.**—Pain : in shoulders ; in arm, extending to chest.—Arm swollen ; livid red ; red, covered with spots ; painful.—Paralysis of r. arm recurring for years after a bite on foot.—Swelling : of the hand not

bitten; of hand, not pitting on pressure, with pain as if it would burst, with pain on touch; and stiffness.—Hands violet-coloured, covered with phlyctenules.—Skin of hand dead and detached in large plates, subjacent tissues livid.—Stitches in finger-tips after bite on arm.

23. **Lower Limbs.**—Shuffling gait caused by paralysis.—Convulsive movements.—Cramps.—Weakness.—Feeling as if something moved up along thigh (after bite on ankle).—Tension in knees and ankles.—Knees stiff.—Leg swollen, cold, and insensible.—Paralysis of foot with shuffling gait.—Paralysis, then ulcers.

24. **Generalities.**—Persons become prematurely old; the development of children is arrested.—Blood altered, tending to hæmorrhages, coagulability lost; blood black.—Symptoms periodic, return every year.—Persistent œdema with tendency to ulcers.—Faintness.—Reeling.—Prostration.—Collapse.—The bite was felt through the whole body like a streak of lightning, she sank to the ground.—Bitten part seat of violent pain.—The swelling was insensible.

25. **Skin.**—Skin: pale; yellowish; jaundiced on face and trunk, with red patches on limbs; livid; in spots; black petechial spots over whole body, which was cold to touch.—Herpetic eruption, with itching about the wound.—Roseola-like eruption on inside of arm and down side of body.—Ulcers.—Blisters about the bite, bursting and leaving ulceration, muscles were laid bare, were dark red, dry, looked like smoked meat, insensible to touch, the sore was offensive.—Gangrene.—Crawling in soles, then also in palms.

26. **Sleep.**—Disposed to yawn.—Sleepiness; and heaviness; with inability to sleep, and also almost constant necessity to change the position.—Sleeplessness; from pain.—Night restless.

27. **Fever.**—Chilliness: with sweat; with cold sweat; with rigidity and clammy sweat; then fever.—Temperature diminished, resists cold badly.—Heat: in morning, with thirst, restlessness, and moderate pains; towards evening; at night, with delirium; then shivering.—Fever of irregular type; intermittent fever.—Burning: running up arm; rising from heel to tongue; on chest and abdomen, with longing for cold applications though skin was cold to touch; of fingers (from rubbing a stick with which a snake had been bruised), with swelling.—Sweat: after vomiting; after chamomile tea, copious sweat from abdomen to toes except over the bitten limb; cold; cold, clammy.—Skin dry.

Viscum Album.

Viscum album. Mistletoe. *N. O.* Loranthaceæ. Tincture of ripe berries. Tincture of bruised leaves. Tincture of whole plant.

Clinical.—Aura epileptica. Chorea. Deafness. Dysphagia. Endometritis. Epilepsy. Labour, slow. Levitation. Lumbago. Menorrhagia. Metrorrhagia. Orchitis. Otalgia. Otorrhœa. Ovaritis. Retained placenta. Sciatica. Spleen pain in. Struma. Throat, sore. Whooping-cough.

Characteristics.—In a pamphlet on "*Viscum Album*" Dr. George Black, of Torquay, has put together most of the facts relating to this plant, including four new provings, by himself and three female provers. The symptoms of these provings I have marked in the Schema—(B) Dr. Black, 43, from 3x and ϕ; (B_1) Miss F., 20, from 2x and ϕ; (B_2) Mrs. X., 37 from 3; (B_3) Miss S., 27, from 3x, 2x, 1x, and ϕ. Proell made a proving of the tincture, and developed symptoms resembling epileptic aura and petit mal, which had the additional epileptic feature of recurrence—they recurred frequently for two years. Belcher gave to a girl, 17, suffering from chorea, 5-drop doses of a tincture of leaves and berries. On the second day he was called to see her, and found her suffering as if under the influence of an opiate. Two women took *Visc.* to procure abortion. Every muscle save those of the eyes became paralysed, as did also the intestinal tract. They could not swallow, and died of starvation in consequence, the bowels being obstinately constipated. The muscles of speech were also paralysed. A boy, 14, ate some berries; soon after began to feel giddy, and then became insensible. He was found with suffused countenance, lips livid, conjunctiva injected, pupils slightly dilated and fixed, pulse slow and full, bounding; breathing slow, stertorous. On pricking the soles the feet were quickly drawn up. Cold affusions roused him, when he began to talk incoherently, had spectral illusions, and was inclined to be violent. Laville (*Epilepsy and Mania in Men and the Lower Animals*) isolated (1) *Viscine*, a soft substance, yellowish blue, of poisonous odour and bitter taste; (2) *Visco-resin*, a bluish resin, pitchy, saccharine, odour at first agreeable, then fetid. *Viscine* is most abundant in the mistletoe of the apple-tree; *Visco-resin* in that of the oak and acacia, which last excites the sexual appetite. The mistletoe of the hawthorn possesses, like all the rest, but in a higher degree, the contractile properties of *Secale* on the uterus in uterine inertia. That of the oak has a remarkable anti-epileptic power on horses. A breeder had a very fine stock which became epileptic at four or five years old. He cured them with a tincture of the fresh leaves bruised in a mortar. According to Laville, all mistletoes are useful in epilepsy and rabies (Ozanam's account of Laville's work, *B. J. H.*, xxv.). Black also quotes from *B. J. H.*, xxii. 637, William Huber's experience with *Visc. a.*: (1) Case of retained placenta with constitutional symptoms after miscarriage at sixth month. Expulsion rapidly effected by *Visc. a.* 3. (2) Man, 22, robust, fair, took a chill from travelling in ice-cold wind. Got a drawing-tearing pain in left lower jaw, lasting some hours, succeeded by loud buzzing, and stopped-up feeling, ending in complete deafness of that ear. *Visc.* 3 cured. (3) Metrorrhagia following suppression from a cold foot-bath. *Visc.* 3 cured. (4) Metrorrhagia following suppression from working in water. (5) Sciatica left side. *Visc.* 3 cured. (6) Rheumatism from wading ill-shod through great tracts of snow. *Visc.* 3 cured. (7) Hydrothorax (right) from chill, with shooting in spleen. *Visc.* 4 and 3 cured. John Wilde (*M. H. R.*, xii. 144) made a tincture of the bruised leaves, and gave 5-drop doses to a boy, 14, who had chorea affecting face and limbs. There was improvement in two days, and in a few weeks a complete cure. A boy, nine, strumous, with tendency to skin disease, was affected with chorea after a fright. He was completely changed in expression, speech quite inarticulate, look idiotic. The movements continued at night, and the boy was worn out for want of sleep. *Visc.* ϕ, 1 to 2-drop doses, did no good. The dose was then increased to 15 drops. Improvement set in at once, and a perfect cure was effected; the doses being diminished after a time because soreness of the tongue and redness of the conjunctiva were set up. Black removed with *Visc.* 3 the following: (1) Lumbago, from chill, tearing pain, wants something to press against it. (2) Lumbago, right, extending to right buttock, < by slightest movement. (3) Pain in sacral region, unable to turn either side, < slightest movement; "pain of a terrible clutching nature, as if her vitals were affected." [Cooper has given great relief with *Visc.* in "old spinal-irritation pains." He names also "spinal symptoms due to uterine causes" as indicating it.] (4) Rheumatism; "the weight of my body on the joint causes it to be very sore"; excessive perspiration. (5) Sciatica associated with otorrhœa. Burning pain from centre of left buttock to inner ankle; heel as if red-hot coal applied; leg feels heavy as lead. In addition a number of cases of catarrhal deafness with noises in the ears were cured or greatly improved. C. M. Boger (*Med. Couns.*, xvi. 266) relates this case: Persistent vertigo after epileptic seizures, lasting a month at a time. *Visc.* cm cured. Huber (*H. R.*, ii. 74) used the 3x and 6x. He considered it applicable to all kinds of rheumatism, acute and chronic, especially when characterised by *tearing* pains; in cases occurring in winter, the result of exposure to sharp winds; and in cases of rheumatic deafness. The symptoms are < By movement; by slightest movement. The lumbago cured in one case was > by pressure.

Relations.—*Antidoted by:* Camph., Chi. *Follows well:* Aco. (rheumatism). *Compare:* Epilepsy, Bell., Stram., Plumb. Effects of working in water, Calc. Chill, fright, Aco. Uterine action, Secale. Rheumatism, Aco., Bry., Puls., Rho., Rhus, Spi.

Causation.—Chill. Wetting. Fright. Suppression of menses.

SYMPTOMS.

1. **Mind.**—Incoherent talk and spectral illusions; inclined to be violent.—Insensibility.—Stupor, succeeded by almost entire insensibility, lying motionless, with her eyes closed, as if in a sound sleep, but easily roused by a loud noise, and then would answer any question, but when she relapsed into her former condition there was a slight disposition to stertorous breathing (2nd d.).—Feels as if going to do something dreadful while the tremblings are on (B_1).—Keeps waking in night thinking the most horrible things imaginable (B_1).—If awake seemed to be dreaming, if asleep she was dreaming (B_3).—Felt in bad temper when pain in chest was on (B_3).—Great depression (B).

2. **Head.**—Giddiness (2nd d.).—Intense throbbing headache (B_1).—Sharp pain in head and face, leaving them sore (B_1).—Numb feeling in head (B).—Tightening sensation of the brain once or twice (B).—Sharp shooting in l. occipital bone (B).—Twinges of pain in l. supraorbital region and r thigh (B).

3. **Eyes.**—Conjunctiva injected.—Pupil slightly dilated and fixed.—Pupils contracted, and at first insensible to light (2nd d.).—Spectral illusions.—Eyes sleepy, difficult to open, lids heavy (B_3).—Neuralgic pain lower part r. orbit (B).

4. **Ears.**—(Deafness in l. ear.)—Hearing in l. ear impaired, sounds muffled (B).—Dulness of hearing, l. ear; sharp twinges of pain in r. ear; later in l. (B).—Sound as of wind in trees (B).—Singing in r. ear, crackling in l. (B).

5. **Nose.**—Dryness back of nose, extending to larynx (B).

6. **Face.**—Countenance suffused.—Lips livid.—Face flushed (after palpitation, B_1).—Face hot and flushed (B).

8. **Mouth.**—Teeth have bled (B_1).—Teeth chattered.—Mouth suddenly fills with saliva (B).—Unpleasant taste on waking, tongue coated to tip with ochre-yellow fur (B).—Tongue sore.—Felt starving at supper-time (B_1).—Appetite ravenous (B_1).

11. **Stomach.**—Squeamish before breakfast and dinner (B_1).

12. **Abdomen.**—Whole alimentary canal paralysed.—When out at times feels as if some one were dragging her down from the waist; and directly after as if upper part of body floating in air (B_1).—Hot feeling and constant ache in l. groin; followed by sick feeling and shivering (B_3).—Aching in hypogastrium as if menses coming on (B_3).—Sharp twinges of pain about r Poupart's ligament, inner aspect, shooting along spermatic cord (B).

13. **Stool and Anus.**—Bowels obstinately constipated.—Copious action of bowels and very offensive (cadaverous) flatus (B).—Stinging, stitching pains l. side of rectum near anus, on lying down soon after midnight; coming and going (B).—Constipated stool following itching of anus (after leaving off *Visc. a.*—B).—Acute aching l. side of anus for hours, $<$ evening (B).

14. **Urinary Organs.**—Frequent urination; urine pale, increased in quantity (B_1).—Urine milky-white after standing (B_3).—Urine turbid after standing, pink deposit (B).

15. **Male Sexual Organs.**—Erotic dreams and seminal emissions (B).—Sharp twinges of pain along r. cord to testicle, which was drawn up close to inguinal ring.—During coitus rather severe palpitation of the heart (B).—Pain in r. testicle (B).

16. **Female Sexual Organs.**—Sharp pains in ovarian region coming and going for two weeks, $<$ morning in bed (B_1).—Shooting pains in l. ovarian region, and on movement lumbar pain and stiffness (B_2).—Shooting pains in l. ovarian region, $<$ lying on l. side; with dead ache after (B_3).—Felt faint, and actually fainted before menses (B_3).—(Numerous cases of retained placenta.)—Metrorrhagia, partly bright, partly clotted and dark, with dull headache, stitches in temples, numbness of extremities, blue rings round eyes, sunken eyes.—It causes uterine contractions and stops hæmorrhages.—[Chronic (granular) endrometritis characterised by enlargement; either subinvolution, alveolar hyperplasia or hypertrophy.]

17. **Respiratory Organs.**—Spasm of glottis, came with dry sensation in throat, followed by efforts to swallow, then a sort of complete block, causing efforts to swallow and eyes to fill with tears (B).—Breathing slow and stertorous.—Slight disposition to stertorous breathing (2nd d.).—(A case of whooping-cough was cured in two days.)

18. Chest.—Pain across sternal region, below breasts, coming and going, < by deep breath or lying on l. side (B_3).—Stitching pain at upper part of l. breast (B_3).—Stabs under l. false ribs and constriction upper part of l. lung, < taking deep breath.—Stitch in chest below l. breast, again above r. knee (B).—Creepy, chilly feeling l. side of lower outer chest (B).

19. Heart.—Just when going off to sleep heart gave two severe thumps, then went off beating at a great rate (B_1).—Heart gave a throb and then a pause (B).—Palpitation during coitus (B).—Pulse small, quick, and very irregular.—Pulse slow, full, and bounding.

20. Neck and Back.—Sudden, momentary pain r. side of neck, two inches above clavicle (B).—Pain in l. side of neck on turning head to l. (B).—Aching between shoulders (B_1).—Aching and burning in sacral region (B_1).—Lumbar pain and stiffness < on movement (B).—Creepy shivering lumbar region (B).

21. Limbs.—Twitching in hands and legs like chorea (B_3).

22. Upper Limbs.—Severe pain in r. shoulder-joint while sitting think-ng, 9 p.m.; < on raising arm.—Felt in dorsum of l. hand as if a large spider were crawling over it; soon afterwards felt same sensation in dorsum of the r. hand (Proell, after 40 drops).

23. Lower Limbs.—(Several cases of sciatica.)—In same winter suddenly felt in r. foot a violent aching pain from within outwards, that compelled him to take off his boot, as it felt too *tight*; this sensation went off in an hour (Proell).—Sharp pain in r. buttock (B).—Unable to sleep till 4 a.m. for pain in r. leg, in popliteal space and edge of tibia, as during catamenia; > moving leg about (B_3).—Burning in centre of calf, changing position of limb > but does not remove the pain (B_3).—Aching at upper and outer aspect of both calves, must keep moving them (B_3).—Sharp shoot centre r. thigh at back (B).—Sharp twinge of pain in l. tibia (B).—Sharp twinge of pain in ball of l. great toe (B).—Stitch above r. knee (B).—Sudden twinges of pain in lower r. thigh and l. supraorbital region (B).

24. Generalities.—About 10 a.m., when he was going to see a patient, he felt very queer, as if he must fall down; he felt a glow that rose up from the feet to the head, and it seemed to him as if he were on fire, at same time his face became very pale; this kind of aura epileptica recurred three times during the winter (Proell, after 40 drops).—Every muscle of body, except those of eyes, were paralysed; could not speak or swallow, and both died about eighth or ninth day, literally starved.—Frequent recurrence of the symptoms during two years.—(Chorea from fright.)—Trembling in limbs, teeth chattered, got generally shaky (B_1).—Unable to keep any part of body quiet at night, jerking first in one part then in another (B_1).—Jerking and twitching of muscles (B_2).—Fearfully tired as after hard work, evenings (B_3).—Shooting pain in various parts of body (B).—Tremor through body as if all muscles in fibrillary contraction (B).

25. Skin.—Skin warm and moist.—Skin felt dry and burning (B_3).—Red spots on neck and chest (B_3).—L. side of neck large papule or small blood-boil (B).

26. Sleep.—Drowsiness (2nd d.).—Wakes thinking of horrible things; gets to sleep again soon by changing thoughts (B_1).—Sleep dreamful; worrying dreams of affairs of day (B_3).

27. Fever.—Chilly even near a stove; cold, chilly feeling creeps over him frequently (B).—Skin warm and very moist (2nd d.).—First cold and then hot feeling without being actually hot (B_1).—On waking always very hot except on knees, legs, and feet, which are very cold.—Hot feeling at night during micturition (B).

Voeslau.

Mineral Spring at Voeslau, in Austria. (Contains in 100 cubic inches 15·2 gr. of solid constituents: Calc. c. 4·9, Calc. sul. 2·7, Calc. mur. 0·5, Mag. c. 2·7, Mag. sul. 1·8, Mag. mur. 0·4, Nat. sul. 0·9, Nat. m. 0·4, Alumina and Silica 0·4, Fer. c. 0·2, gummy substance 0·1.) Dilution.

Clinical.—Menstruation, disorders of. Seminal emissions. Urticaria. Vertigo.

Characteristics.—Rosenberg observed the effects of *Voeslau* on the healthy. His symptoms constitute the Schema. The waters produce: Orgasm of blood; pressure and tension. The throat was sensitive to swallowing warm food and drink. Nettlerash with desquamation. In males there was sexual excitement and emissions; and in females increased secretion of mucus in genitals and many troubles connected with menses.

SYMPTOMS.

1. Mind.—Mind restless and excited.—Irritability, peevishness.

2. Head.—Vertigo and whirling in head.—Reeling and tottering of whole body two or three hours after a bath.—Congestion to head and orgasm of blood.—Heaviness of head.

9. Throat.—Hoarseness and dryness in throat, painful sensitiveness swallowing warm food or drink.

11. Stomach.—Appetite is increased after the first bath.—Heaviness and sensation of fulness in stomach.—Sensitiveness and pressure in stomach after eating.

12. Abdomen.—Pressure and tension in hepatic region, extending to r. shoulder.

13. Stool and Anus.—Thin stools, increasing to diarrhœa, with a slight degree of tenesmus.

14. Urinary Organs.—Frequent desire and frequent micturition.—Urine: first days red, afterwards watery and copious.—Increased secretion from prostate.

15. Male Sexual Organs.—Erections.—Rush of blood to genitals.—Nocturnal emissions.

16. Female Sexual Organs.—Increased secretion of mucus from genitals.—Menses: delayed; diminished, accompanied with numerous troubles; offensive; too frequent and copious.

17. **Respiratory Organs.**—Hoarseness and dryness in throat, painful sensitiveness on swallowing warm food and drink.—Dry cough with slight pains in chest.

18. **Chest.**—Congestion to chest and other organs.—Oppression ; respiration difficult, rapid, short.

21. **Limbs.**—Weakness and falling asleep of limbs.

24. **Generalities.**—Emaciation of young people.—Uneasiness and unsteadiness at work.—Increased sensitiveness, esp. to external air.

25. **Skin.**—Itching nettlerash on whole body after fourteen baths, ending in desquamation.—Itching, heat, biting, esp. towards midnight, previous to the outbreak of perspiration.

26. **Sleep.**—Overpowering sleepiness during day ; esp. afternoon.

27. **Fever.**—Coldness and chilliness at times changing to heat, with increased thirst.—Flushes of heat without thirst.—Perspiration in bed towards morning.

Wiesbaden.

The Spring at Wiesbaden, in Prussia. (Contains in sixteen ounces Carbonic acid 6·416 cubic inches, Nitrogen 0·103 cubic inches; of the following solids, in grains, Nat. m. 52·49, K. mur. 1·119 Li. mur. 0·00138, Am. mur. 0·128, Calc. mur. 3·617, Mag. mur 1·566, Mag. bro. 0·027, Calc. sul. 0·692, Calc. ph. 0·0029, Calc ars. 0·0015, Calc. c. 3·210, Mag. c. 0·079, Fer. c. 0·043, Mang. c. 0·004, Silicic acid 0·46, Alumina silicica 0·603; traces of Mag. iod., Stro. c., Cup. c.) Dilution.

Clinical.—Amenorrhœa. Angina pectoris. Body, odour of, offensive. Constipation. Corns. Diarrhœa. Ear-wax, excessive. Epistaxis. Glaucoma. Gout. Hæmorrhage. Hæmorrhoids. Hair, rapid growth of; falling of; grows darker Hernia, inguinal; femoral. Indigestion. Miscarriage, prevents. Rheumatism. Sterility. Vertigo; caduca. Whitlow.

Characteristics.—The hot, chlorinated saline springs of Wiesbaden (Fontes Mattiaci of Pliny) contain 8·176 grammes of solids to each litre, and of these *Nat. mur.* makes up more than seven grammes. The baths, which constitute the chief part of the treatment, are extremely excitant. The baths, combined with drinking the water, generally determine at the commencement of the cure certain phenomena of saturation which disappear on temporary suspension of the treatment. The most common of these is a saburral state of the stomach, and a feeling of fulness and tension in the whole abdomen. Gout and rheumatism are the chief affections for which Wiesbaden is sought. Passive or atonic gout is the only kind for which *Wiesb.* is suited, and these cases usually pass through a period of aggravation before improvement sets in. Torpid and nodous rheumatism are benefited, the douche being employed as well as the bath. Paralysis; muscular and tendinous contractions; sprains; in complete anchyloses; stiffness from old fractures; gunshot wounds which are slow to heal, are also benefited by *Wiesb.* "Abdominal plethora and portal obstruction are relieved. "By the artificial congestion which they set up in the venous plexus of the rectum they have for an almost constant effect the disengorgement of the viscera under the diaphragm, and the prevention of stasis in their parenchyma" (Constantin James—to whom I am indebted for the whole of the above facts). Apelt observed the effects of drinking the water and excessive bathing. Magdeburg observed the effects on eight healthy persons. The excitant, congestive, and evacuant effects mentioned by James appear in the provings. Blood rushes to the face. There is vertigo when lying in bed; and vertigo which causes falling. Hæmorrhages occur from anus and nose which relieve other symptoms. Fermentation occurs in the abdomen, and there is great exhaustion after diarrhœa. Hæmorrhoidal flow occurs with > of abdominal plethora. In one case nose-bleed occurred persistently for six weeks, at the end of which a weakness of vision bordering on blindness was cured. During the menses there is great weakness; also constipation. A number of remarkable symptoms appeared in reference to the skin and nails. The hair grew rapidly and became darker. Nails also grew rapidly. Corns and callosities dropped off. Berridge cured with *Wiesb.* 200 a Miss B., 21, of a soft corn between fourth and fifth toes of right foot. There was burning and shooting pain in the corn (*H. P.*, vii. 477). With the sweat of *Wiesb.* there is itching. The sweat on the diseased parts made a brown stain. The urine stiffened linen. The symptoms were: > By nose-bleed; by hæmorrhoidal flux. < During menses. < From coffee (frequent micturition). < Lying in bed (vertigo).

Relations.—*Compare:* Nat. m. Corns, Fer. pic. Callosities, Ant. c. Hair turns darker, Jabor., Pilo., Wild.

SYMPTOMS.

1. **Mind.**—Becomes more cheerful (after 7th d.).—Impatient, depressed, hopeless.—Anxiety and uneasiness prevent sleep.—Apprehensive.—Ill-humour.—Peevish, talks to no one.—Disinclined to think.

2. **Head.**—Vertigo: falls while walking; whirling in head, kind of insensibility, trembling faintness, spasmodic hiccough, alternations of chills and heat, thirst, hæmorrhage while riding in a carriage.—Dizziness and heaviness of head while lying in bed, sensation as if she would fall.—Reeling and tottering, objects move before the eyes.—Head heavy, dull.—Hair: grows much more rapidly than usual; falls out and grows again rapidly; new growth darker; formerly soft, becomes hard and brittle.—On scalp: large boils; desquamation; itching, as from vermin; intolerable; incessant.

3. **Eyes.**—Glistening of eyes without clearness; slimy moisture is wiped from them.—Copious secretion: tenacious; slimy; purulent.—Moisture in canthi.—Eyes ache.—Pressure deep in eyeballs.—Eyeballs painful.—Increased tension.—Falling of eyebrows and lashes, with rapid secondary growth.—Itching of lids and margins.—All things seem to move before eyes when walking; reeling; staggers to and fro.—Weakness of vision > by persistent nose-bleed.

4. **Ears.**—Copious secretion of ear-wax; soft; slimy; pale brown; thin, almost fluent.—Tickling sticking in meatus.—Much itching of ear, > after copious flow of ear-wax.—Pains in ears.—Roaring in ears with diminished hearing.

5. **Nose.**—Frequent sneezing, secretion of thick mucus.—Secretion from nose: watery; tenacious, like isinglass; yellow mucus for four months.—Nose-bleed for six weeks, with which weakness of vision, bordering on blindness, disappeared.—Inclination to nose-bleed.—Frequent itching of nostrils.

6. **Face.**—Expression of suffering.—Face: sunken; emaciated; red and hot, with itching; circumscribed redness.—Blood rushes violently to face.—Sensation of cobweb lying on skin of l. cheek (2nd d.).—Profuse sweat on face compels rubbing.

8. **Mouth.**—Teeth seem too long.—Drawing tearing in teeth, so he could scarcely eat.—Gums: became scorbutic after long bathing; blistered; loose and painful; sore while eating.—Tongue: fuzzy with nauseous taste; white on edges; middle brown.—Injected veins under tongue.—Mouth dry. —Skin forms folds on inner side of mouth, lips, and cheeks, after which it peels off.—Tickling in posterior part of palate.—Very bad taste in morning.

9. **Throat.**—Inclination to clear throat.—Swollen cervical and parotid glands.

11. **Stomach.**—Appetite: great; at first increased, afterwards diminished. —Thirst: great, with chilliness; for refreshing drinks.—Qualmish; inclination to vomit; vomiting.—Promotes digestion.—Pressure in stomach, feeling of fulness and visible swelling of epigastric region.

12. **Abdomen.**—(Inflammation of the liver.)—Violent pain in region of spleen.—Emission of much flatus; preceded by much rumbling and fermentation in abdomen.—Fermentation < after drinking the water.—Heaviness.—Colic.—Dragging from abdomen, half-way down r. thigh, at the point where a femoral hernia had protruded, with a sensation as if the hernia would protrude (lasting several days, very distressing).—Swelling of r. inguinal region, with a sensation of an inguinal hernia.

13. **Stool and Anus.**—Hæmorrhage from rectum.—Hæmorrhoidal flow (curative of abdominal plethora).—Burning in rectum and bowels.—While urinating very urgent desire for stool.—Diarrhœa: early in morning, after drinking the water; scanty; copious, slimy; then liquid, mixed with lumps, great exhaustion; then pasty; involuntary; black; grey; slimy; smells like rotten eggs.—Stools more seldom as activity of skin or kidneys increases.—Constipation.—Retained stool.—No stool during menses.—Stool lustreless, like hardened membranous bile.

14. **Urinary Organs.**—(Inflammation of the kidneys.)—Pressure in region of kidneys.—Urination frequent; during night; < after coffee; scanty with perspiration.—Urine: copious, becoming dark, with a greenish-yellow sediment; clear, light yellow, fatty; sediment in urine with "hæmorrhoids of the bladder."—Urine stiffens linen.

15. **Male Sexual Organs.**—Genitals turgid, excited.—Intolerable itching on genitals.—Emissions.

16. **Female Sexual Organs.**—(A woman, married for several years, became pregnant for the first time.)—Miscarriage, that had taken place several times, was avoided.—Oozing of slimy moisture from the vagina.—Menses profuse, like hæmorrhage for several days, then scanty, but continued fourteen days.—Scanty menses increased.—Menses return after climacteric.—Menses, usually late, became earlier and more profuse.—Menstrual flow, that had been long absent, returned on sixteenth day after drinking the water, with whirling in head, trembling, faintness, colic, alternations of chill, heat, and sweat, with thirst, cramp in thighs, calves, feet, with cramp-like hiccough; menses very profuse.—Menstrual blood: seems like mucus; slimy dark-coloured, not watery.—During menses, great weakness.

17. **Respiratory Organs.**—Loose cough in morning.—Expectoration: lumps of mucus; firm, tenacious mucus; sweetish after drinking the water; salt.—Respiration in the bath, at first accelerated, gradually becoming slow, after which gradually increases.—Short breath on walking, on ascending.

18. **Chest.**—Oppression of the breath, constriction of chest in region of diaphragm as soon as that region is bathed; obliged to raise chest out of water; returned whenever the water reached the region of diaphragm.—Chest seems constricted by clothes, which are not tight.

19. **Heart.**—Slight angina pectoris.—Becomes very weak about the heart.—Beat of heart accelerated, violent.—Palpitation.—Pulse: slow; irregular; accelerated; intermittent.

20. **Neck.**—Tension and stiffness in nape.—Drawing in nape.

21. **Limbs.**—Trembling of limbs with weakness.—Very rapid growth of nails.—Limbs: feel light, with desire to move; heavy; indolent; weary; exhausted.—Swelling of hands and feet disappeared after copious sweat.—Sweat of hands and feet.

22. **Upper Limbs.**—Trembling of hands.—Inclined to panaritia.

23. **Lower Limbs.**—Great weariness of lower limbs, with pain in toes.—Cramp in thighs.—Rheumatic pain in r. thigh for several days, < walking.—Pain in r. thigh-bone as if hernia would protrude.—Feet: painful and sensitive; burning.—Corns become raised, softened, and drop off.—Strong odour of sweat on feet.

24. **Generalities.**—Body smells like rotten eggs.—Great ease and vigour of motion.—Feeling of comfort with very profuse sweat.—(Less weakness.)—Weariness; fatigue; exhaustion; uneasiness.—Faintness.—Dormant rheumatism reappears.—Aversion to the water, sometimes causing cramp-like sensations when coming near the bath.—Much inclined to take cold.—Whole body feels bruised.

25. **Skin.**—In the bath the skin becomes thick, parchment-like, after a while rough like sand between the fingers, feeling wrinkled.—(Parchment-like skin becomes soft.)—Cracks.—Desquamation.—Callosities come off.—Pimples, vesicles, boils; red, elevated points; moist tetter.—Very painful abscesses develop towards surface from deep in flesh, with long-continued suppuration.—Itching: biting, burning; intolerable.

26. **Sleep.**—Sleepiness.—No desire to rise; weary, with sleep in morning.—Sleep sound but not refreshing.—Sleep disturbed by dreams.

27. **Fever.**—Chills: from slightest air on the clothes or under bedcovers; while dressing after bath.—Alternations of chill and heat.—Orgasm of blood disturbing sleep.—General heat of body with a hard stool.—Sensation of burning heat over whole body.—Constant sensation of heat with qualmishness.—Burning heat of hands.—Sweat: profuse, and urine; copious on a long walk, with itching; clammy, itching; trickles from head; on neck, with disappearance of the yellow spots; profuse on face, compels rubbing.—Sweat on palms and soles, wrinkling of skin of hands as washerwoman's.—The sweat on diseased parts colours linen brown.

Wildbad.

The Springs at Wildbad, in Würtemburg. (The water contains in 16 ounces, Carbonic ac. gr. 0·972, Nat. m. 1·808, Nat. c. 0·837, Nat. sul. 0·291, K. sul. 0·108, Calc. c. 0·738, Silicic acid 0·480, Mag. c. 0·079, Fer. c. 0·002, Alumina 0·004, and traces of Mang.) Dilution.

Clinical.—Bones, pains in. Catarrh. Gout. Hair, affections of. Indigestion. Knees, creaking of. Nails, soft. Paralysis, spinal. Paraplegia. Rheumatism. Shoulder, rheumatism of.

Characteristics.—In spite of its very slight mineralisation, says Constantin James, the water produces very distinct effects in a graduated series. The first impression of the bath is delicious ; this is succeeded by sensations more clear and distinct : a slight degree of excitement ; at times luminous sparks before the sight ; a finer (*plus subtil*) blood seems to flow to the brain. "One would like to remain in the bath, but something unusual and strange warns you that it is time to get out." It is chiefly, says the same authority, for affections of the spinal cord that Wildbad is frequented, more than half the patients being paraplegic. Hartlaub, Kallenbach, and others proved the water. Among the symptoms were : Sensation as if the brain were over-filled. Gnawing, sinking, empty sensation. Pain as if sprained. Sensation of looseness in the joints ; ankles loose ; knees loose ; the bones seem as if they did not fit. Teeth seem too long. In one prover the hair, which had been greasy, became dry ; and the beard became of a darker colour. Desire to stretch. The symptoms were : < On waking at night. < Lying down (throbbing and heat in occiput). < Walking (pain in sciatic nerve ; looseness of knees).

Relations.—*Compare :* Uric acid in urine ; pain in right shoulder, Urt. ur. Right shoulder, Sang.

SYMPTOMS.

1. **Mind.**—Great depression with anxiety.—Memory weak.

2. **Head.**—Rush of blood to head.—Head : dull, heavy, esp. occiput.—Sensation as though whole brain overfilled, intolerable lying with head on pillow.—Throbbing headache on waking at night.—Tearing pains in forehead, extending from middle of r. eyebrow.—Violent pulsation on vertex and occiput.—Heaviness in vertex on waking at night.—Throbbing and warmth in occiput, < lying down.—Hair lost its oiliness ; hair of beard grew darker.—Moving scalp was difficult, as though frontal muscles too short.

3. **Eyes.**—Pain and pressure in eyes on writing in evening.—Fine sticking pain in eyes (< l.) and above eyes (eyebrows, below eyes, and also in eyeballs), without affecting vision.—Acute pain in l. upper eyebrow, spot remained sensitive after.—Pain in l. (and r.) supraorbital foramen.—Itching in canthi.

4. **Ears.**—Sensation in ears as after taking cold, first r., then l.—Sensation of warmth in r. ear.—Pressing stitches in l. ear as if deep in meatus.

5. **Nose.**—Blood from r. nostril in morning.

6. **Face.**—Violent painless twitching in face.—Pain l. jaw-joint, lower jaw, and in top of shoulder.

8. **Mouth.**—Teeth, esp. r., painful, as if too long, or as after taking cold. —Dryness of mouth; without thirst, and with coated tongue in morning.—Mouth and tongue dry toward morning.—Burning point in r. corner of mouth or wing of nose.—Bloody saliva, apparently from fauces, after talking in open air.

9. **Throat.**—Expectoration of mucus from throat, larynx, and posterior nares.—A retching, spasmodic, or drawing pain in œsophagus, above the stomach, with some nausea.

11. **Stomach.**—Hunger: ravenous; as from an empty stomach in morning, also in evening after supper.—Gnawing emptiness in stomach and whole abdomen.—Emptiness without hunger.—Eructations; empty.—Nausea; on waking.—Feeling of indigestion or disordered stomach.—Pressure in stomach.

12. **Abdomen.**—Colic in umbilical region, as before a stool, without an evacuation.—Sticking, drawing pains in both hypochondria.

13. **Stool and Anus.**—Spasmodic pressure in anus and perinæum.—Great urging to stool, which was at first dark and thin; afterwards brown with mucus, and at 11 a.m. very watery, yellowish grey, with some colic.—Stool: dark, with tenacious mucus; lumpy, covered with mucus of a dark blackish-brown colour; retained, hard, lumpy, dark; constipated, after a few days natural with colic.

14. **Urinary Organs.**—Frequent urgent desire to urinate.—Mucus in urine with large uric acid crystals.

15. **Male Sexual Organs.**—Erections: painful on waking; more easy than natural.—Painful drawing in cords on waking, after an emission.

16. **Female Sexual Organs.**—Menstruation usually hastened.

17. **Respiratory Organs.**—Dry cough.—Breathing oppressed; on ascending stairs.

18. **Chest.**—Pain and cracking in upper part of sternum at junction with first r. rib.

20. **Neck and Back.**—Tearing pain, as if sprained, transversely through nape.—Constant pulsation in nape and occiput at night.—Drawing in back as though a hot sponge drawn along skin on waking in morning.—Prickling on back, followed by nettlerash.—Disagreeable sensation of warmth along lumbar vertebræ.

21. **Limbs.**—Joints weak.—Fulness and heaviness in limbs.—Drawing pains here and there in limbs; drawing pain in l. upper arm and r. thigh.

22. **Upper Limbs.**—Violent drawing tearing about r. shoulder.—Shuddering jerking about r. upper arm.—Drawing in l. upper arm.—Acute pain in l. arm above elbow, outer portion, as if in bone or tendon, as if sprained.—Drawing burning beneath r. elbow, in bone.—Rheumatic pain in forearm from back of wrist to elbow, near wrist arm painful.—Nails became so soft he could not open a watch with them.—Hang-nails.—Stiffness and painfulness of all fingers on opening and closing hand.—Painful swollen sensation in l. thumb.

23. **Lower Limbs.**—Weariness of hips after a slight effort.—Pain in

nates, r. and l., as if in sciatic nerve, esp. on walking.—Pain in muscles of r. thigh, on posterior and inner surfaces.—Drawing pain in r. thigh, a hand's-breadth above knee, below anterior and outer portions.—Violent cracking : in both knees on rising ; r. knee.—Pain and stiffness in r. knee, as if contracted, on waking in morning.—Knees feel loose, as if bones did not fit ; must be supported in walking.—Violent itching in l. calf and on tibia.—Pain in r. calf on walking.—Ankles feel loose.—Drawing : in ankles ; in l. sole behind toes. —Sprained sensation : in first joint of r. great toe ; in r. and l. great toes.—Acute pain in l. little toe.

24. **Generalities.**—Weak, weary, wants to keep quiet.—Weary : after walking ; esp. knees and ankles ; sudden, ankles seem loose.—Great desire to lie on back and stretch, with feeling of comfort and warmth through whole body, and averse to business, esp. after a bath.

25. **Skin.**—Crawling itching about l. half of mouth, around red of lip, esp. lower lip.—Itching on : one finger of r. hand ; r. thumb, in small spot as if in periosteum, > (but not removed) by rubbing ; l. calf and tibia ; l. index finger, with development of a small vesicle ; middle knuckle of l. ring-finger ; r. natis.

26. **Sleep.**—Very sleepy in evening.—Unusual desire to sleep after eating. —Complete sleeplessness till 4 a.m., with constant excitement and uneasiness, dry, burning heat ; > sitting erect with head against hard pillow.—Sleep : restless ; full of confused dreams, wakes every few minutes feeling as if he had slept for hours.—Dreams : disagreeable ; forgetful ; anxious ; confused. —Violent weeping in a dream, waking in perspiration.

27. **Fever.**—Hands quite cold, with weakness and sweat on waking. —Feet cold.—Violent, dry heat over whole body.—Prickling heat over whole body, with some sweat.—Very disagreeable heat in occiput, intolerable on lying down, and amounting to violent pulsation.—Sweat : easy ; free at night and during day after any exertion.

Wyethia.

Wyethia helenoides. Alarconia helenoides. Melarhiza inuloides. Poison Weed. *N. O.* Compositæ. Tincture of the root.

Clinical.—Amenorrhœa. Asthma. Constipation. Cough. Debility. Diarrhœa. Dysmenorrhœa. Epiglottis, affections of. Fever. Hæmorrhoids. Headache. Hiccough. Indigestion. Influenza. Nervousness. Ovaries, pain in. Post-nasal catarrh. Salivation. Throat, sore. Uvula, affections of.

Characteristics.—*Wyethia* was introduced and proved, with the fresh root or the ϕ tincture, on seven men and two women, by J. M. Selfridge. Their symptoms make up Allen's pathogenesis. A later proving ((*Pacif. C. J. H.*, vii. 127) was made under Selfridge's direction with the 1x on Dr. A. McNeil, the 15x on Dr. M. F. Underwood, and the 30x on Dr. Eleanor F. Martin. Their symptoms I have marked respectively (M), (U), and (E M) in the Schema. The first proving gave *Wyeth.* a definite and important place in throat affections.

These symptoms have been confirmed: "Throat feels swollen; epiglottis dry, and has a burning sensation; constant desire to swallow saliva to relieve the dryness yet affording no comfort; swallows with difficulty.—Prickling, dry sensation in posterior nares; sensation as if something were in nasal passages; an effort to clear them through the throat affords no relief. Burning sensation in bronchial tubes. Dry, hacking cough, caused by tickling in epiglottis." The following case was reported to me: A boy had been kept awake many nights by a persistent, dry, hacking, nervous cough. *Wyeth.* 30 cured in one dose. Hale gives these cases from Selfridge: (1) Dry asthma in a lady; *Wyeth.* gave prompt relief in several paroxysms. (2) Chronic follicular pharyngitis with dryness of pharynx and burning in epiglottis. In a severe epidemic of influenza Hale found *Wyeth.* most successful. Other noteworthy symptoms are: Tough, ropy saliva. Pain over left ovary, shooting down to knee. In one case menses, which had been in abeyance since confinement a year before, returned with much pain. *Peculiar Sensations* are: Mouth as if scalded. Uvula as if elongated. Epiglottis feels dry and burning. Weight in stomach as if something indigestible had been eaten. Uterus feels as if it enlarged in order to contain all the pain. There is belching alternating with hiccough. The symptoms are: < After eating. < By motion. < By exercise; it = perspiration. < Afternoon.

Relations.—*Compare:* In throat affections, Ar. dracon., Caust., Hep., Stict., Rumex, Penth., Pho., Sul. Tough, ropy saliva and headache, Epipheg. Sensation as if something indigestible eaten, Ab. n. Scalded mouth, Ran. sc.

SYMPTOMS.

1. **Mind.**—Nervous, uneasy; apprehensive of calamity.—Depressed; incapacitated for mental work; averse to company; impatient, quarrelsome (U).

2. **Head.**—Dizziness.—Rush of blood to head.—Severe headache.—Sharp pain in forehead over r. eye, followed by feeling of fulness.—At 10 a.m. headache in l. anterior part of brain, as if radiated from l. inner canthus; 12.30 in l. occipital protuberance (M).—Terrific headache during the sweat; intense, congestive; eyes sensitive; bones of face sensitive; least movement intolerable.

3. **Eyes.**—Itching in l. inner canthus (M).

4. **Ears.**—Itching in r. ear.—Pain in l. ear (M).

5. **Nose.**—Sensation as if something in nasal passages.

8. **Mouth.**—Mouth feels as if scalded.—Increased flow of tough, ropy saliva.—Mouth full of sweetish saliva (M).

9. **Throat.**—Throat feels swollen; epiglottis dry and has a burning sensation; constant desire to swallow saliva to relieve the dryness; swallowing with difficulty.—Prickling, dry sensation in posterior nares; sensation as if something were in the nasal passages; an effort to clear them through the throat does not >.—Uvula feels elongated.—Dryness of fauces; constant

desire to clear throat by hemming.—Sensation of heat down œsophagus into stomach, < while eating.—After restless night waked with sharp pain in r. tonsil, throat swollen and sore, glands externally swollen and sore (E M).

11. **Stomach.**—Belching of wind alternating with hiccough.—Nausea and vomiting.—Sense of weight in stomach as if something indigestible had been eaten.

12. **Abdomen.**—Pain and bearing down in abdomen, r. side.

13. **Stool and Anus.**—Itching in anus.—Itching in rectum (M).—Stools: diarrhœic, dark brown, came on at night, lasted five days; small, dark brown, look burned; previously light-coloured, irregular, and constipated, became dark, regular, and soft.—Great constriction, hæmorrhoids, not bleeding (never had them before or since—several provers).

16. **Female Sexual Organs.**—Pain in l. ovary, shooting down to knee. —Menses appear for first time after birth of last child, a year before; purple, scanty, great pain.—Leucorrhœa.—Menses commenced with intense burning pain, constant, but increasing in paroxysms, with sensation as if uterus expanded in order to keep all the pains within its walls (E M).

17. **Respiratory Organs.**—Burning sensation in bronchial tubes.—Dry, hacking cough, caused by tickling in epiglottis.—Persistent, dry, hacking, nervous night cough (in boy, cured with 30th).

18. **Chest.**—Sharp pain just below r. ribs, deep-seated, followed by soreness.

19. **Heart.**—Pulse slowed (from 72 to 58, in 10 h.).

20. **Neck and Back.**—Glands r. side of neck swollen and sore (E M).

22. **Upper Limbs.**—Pain in r. arm, with stiffness of wrist and hand.—Neuralgic pain commenced in l. arm and hand, spreading to back and other parts (E M).—Sore hang-nail on r. third finger (M).

23. **Lower Limbs.**—Tingling in r. foot when standing (M).

24. **Generalities.**—Feels weak, nervous, uneasy; apprehensive.—Feels as after a severe illness.—Irritability from exertion; least exercise = sweat.—All symptoms < afternoon.—Aching all over body, with chill and fever (E M).

26. **Sleep.**—Wakes frequently and too early (M).

27. **Fever.**—Chill 11 a.m.; thirst for ice-water during chill; no thirst with heat; profuse sweat all night; pains in back and limbs, at times jerking; chill recurred at 1.30 p.m. six days later, with intense headache (E M).—Cold sweat over whole body, which soon dies off, and comes again and goes as if by flashes.—Fever and pains all over body, with inflamed r. tonsil (E M).

Xanthoxylum.

Xanthoxylum americanum. X. fraxineum. Prickly Ash. Toothache-tree. *N. O.* Rutaceæ. Tincture of fresh bark.

Clinical.—After-pains. Asthma. Coccygodynia. Dysmenorrhœa. Earache. Fibroma. Headache. Hemiplegia. Hysteria. Jaw-joint, pain in. Levitation. *Menstruation, painful.* Nerves, injured. Nervousness. Neuralgia; crural. Ophthalmia. Sciatica. Toothache. Ulcers.

Characteristics.—According to Hale, Rafinesque was the first to investigate *Xanthoxylum*, which was known to him as "a great article in the materia medica of our Indians"; who use the root bark in decoction for "colics, gonorrhœa, syphilis, inward pains, toothache, ulcers, &c. It is a great topical stimulant," he continues, "changing the nature of malignant ulcers." *Xan.* contains *Piperin*. T. C. Duncan (*Minn. H. M.*, ix. 340), recounting reminiscences of his boyhood, says: "There was another drug that set my youthful mouth and stomach on fire, and that was Prickly Ash. You wanted to open the mouth to let the cool air get in." This warmth is felt as a warm glow through the entire system, with a sensation in the nerves as if gentle shocks of electricity were passing through the body. In one of Cullis' provers, Miss D. (there were six provers, three of them women; all took the ϕ tincture), the entire left half of the body became numb, the left half of the head being sharply divided in sensation from the other half. These symptoms, with the many head pains and fulness in the head, give the correspondence in hemiplegia, in which *Xan.* has been given with success. Two additional provings on women appear in *C. D. P.* (quoting from *Publ. Mass. Hom. Soc.*). In these provings 20- to 100-drop doses of the tincture were taken, and symptoms of great severity were produced. Both provers had severe dysmenorrhœal pains, with increased and anticipating flow. This is the characteristic of *Xan.* The symptoms in each case roused the prover from sleep with pain and suffocation; the pain being confined to head, heart, throat, and pelvis. Many of the pains were radiating—from above right eye over head; from right ovary down thigh and in other directions. Left-sided numbness was present in one; who also had symptoms of levitation and disordered sensation. In dysmenorrhœa *Xan.* has a wide range. Cullis, who had most success in cases of *dysmenorrhœa and amenorrhœa*, relates these cases: (1) Miss A., 25, brunette, had menstrual irregularity since commencement; would go three, four, or five months, and then her sufferings were excruciating. When she came under treatment had had no menses for two months. *Xan.* 1 was given, 5 drops thrice daily. Menses appeared in three days and were painless. (2) Miss B., fair, nervous, had menses suppressed by getting feet wet, being then a week over time. *Xan.* 1 x, 5 drops every three hours, brought on menses next day. Cullis thinks *Xan.* especially *Suited to* women of spare habit, nervous temperament, and delicate organisations. Leucorrhœa with amenorrhœa he regards as a strong indication. P. C. Majumdar (*Ind. H. R.*, viii. 21) cured a case of uterine fibroid with *Xan.* 3x: An emaciated, feeble, wrinkled woman, 56, widow, had been advised by allopaths to have an operation for tumour. Menstruation had ceased fifteen years before. It had always been profuse and painful, and preceded and followed by leucorrhœa. She had neuralgic pain in right ovarian region; a hard nodular tumour size of a small orange, painful on deep pressure. Fetid, yellowish white discharge from vagina. Patient was nervous, depressed; lazy and sleepy even in the daytime. Appetite poor; disgust for food. *Xan.* 3x was given night and morning. In a week the pain was better and discharge less. In four weeks Majumdar found the patient a changed person. The tumour was much softer and reduced by half. In six months the tumour had gone, and the patient was quite well, *Xan.* having been taken intermittently all the time. *Xan.* belongs to the Rutaceæ, and, like *Ruta*, has a vulnerary action, as I discovered in this case: Miss X., 28, injured her right ulnar nerve at the elbow by repeatedly striking it against the edge of a bath whilst washing some articles. For two months she had had to keep the arm in a sling. A few weeks after that the arm swelled. Some eight months after the injury I saw her. The pain centred in the ulnar nerve where it crosses the inner condyle of the humerus, though there was pain above and below as well. I gave *Ruta* 30, which gave some relief to the pain, and relieved a frontal headache to which the patient was subject. The arm becoming less well, I gave *Xan.* 12 four times a day. This made a distinct improvement in the arm, and also relieved a dysmenorrhœa to which Miss X. was subject. After persistent treatment with various attenuations of *Xan.* the nerve lost its sensitiveness, and the patient could use her arm freely. *Xan.* 1 in five-drop doses night and morning, with a liniment of *Xan.* φ, proved most effective. A patient to whom I gave *Xan.* 3x had immediately a hot pricking pain in right ovary. Among the *Peculiar Sensations* are: As if top of head would be taken off by flashes of throb-like pain. As if bewildered with pain in back of head. Feeling of looseness or quivering of brain. As if head falling to pieces. As if head surrounded by a tight band. Eyes as if full of sand. As if pepper in mouth and throat. As of a bunch in throat. Tongue as if expanding and contracting. As if throat swollen and enlarged. Throat as if in a vice. Back of neck as if stiff. Coccyx as if elongated. As if floating in the air. As if walking on wool. As if sunk deep in bed. As if body expanded. Many pains are radiating; some are sudden, arouse from sleep, and cause the patient to catch her breath. Pains are excruciating, unbearable, and are accompanied with red, hot face; but the heart pains = pallor. The symptoms are: < By moving head suddenly. Neck pain is > by pressure and by throwing head back. Lying down >. Drink of ice-water >. Headache is > by cold water and in open air. Pains are < in morning ; 4 a.m.

Relations.—*Compare :* Head, heart, and uterus, Act. r. Lack of eruption in measles, Bry. Dysmenorrhœa with reflex neuralgia, Coloc. Dysmenorrhœa and sciatica ; numbness, Gnaphal. Dysmenorrhœa, Vib. o., Caulo. After-pains, Pul., Cham., Cup. Pains increase and decrease gradually, Stan. Levitation, Can. i., Stic. p., Ph. ac. Headache over root of nose, Ign. Headache over right eye, Sang. Heart and uterus, Cact.

Causation.—Injury to nerve. Wetting (getting feet wet). Suppression of menses.

SYMPTOMS.

1. **Mind.**—Nervous, frightened feeling.—Easily startled, hysterical.—Depression and weakness.—Indifference and malaise.—Did not care if she lived or died.—Seemed entirely void of ideas.

2. **Head.**—Giddiness with nausea, < after rising, had to go to bed.—Pain over eyes, with throbbing above root of nose.—Head dull and aching.—Frontal headache.—Intense burning, pressing, frontal headache, waking her at 4 a.m. ; < moving head suddenly ; extending into vertex and orbits ; with hot flushes over head and face.—Severe frontal headache ; with dizziness.—A dull headache, in a space not larger than half a dollar, over nose.—Diffused pain in upper part of forehead ; < in r. side ; pain extends to base of brain, with soreness.—At 6 p.m. sudden and violent pain over r. eye, with burning through temples ; after it, vision blurred.—Throbbing headache over r. eye, with nausea.—Darting pain in l. temple, recurring again and again.—A tightening of scalp and heavy pain in temples ; increase of head difficulties, with a great heat and quiet flowing (menstrual), being two days in advance of proper time ; some headache.—Pain in l. side of head and l. elbow.—Heavy feeling in top of head.—About upper part of cranium an aching feeling, accompanied by flashes of throb-like pain, as if top of head were about to be taken off.—Pain in back of head, also a bewildered sensation.—Head feels full.—Pressure in head, with fulness of veins.—Tightness of head, with pain increasing over eyes.—L. side of head (and body) numb, the division made perceptible in head, affecting half the nose.—Headache, with sleepy feeling in morning.—Shaking head produces a feeling of looseness or quivering of brain, followed by dizziness.—As if head were surrounded by a tight band (dysmenorrhœa).—Head seemed falling in pieces.

3. **Eyes.**—Watering of eyes and nose.—Eyes bloodshot, with red margins, and feel as if full of sand.—Lachrymation, pain in lid of r. eye.—Eyes twitched, pupils dilated.—Dull, heavy, grinding pain in l. eye.—Ophthalmia.—Vision blurred, as if looking through blue lace.—Atmosphere appeared blue, and there were flashes of (blue) light before eyes.—Objects seem a long way off.

4. **Ears.**—Ringing in ears, esp. in r.—Loud noise in r. ear, as of a valve constantly opening and shutting.—Loud noise like a windmill in l. ear.—Dull pain in r. ear, seeming to affect jaw socket ; does not know whether his tooth or his ear aches.—Darting pain under and back of r. ear.

5. **Nose.**—R. nostril seems filled up; discharge of dry and bloody scales of mucus.—Numbness throughout l. side of body, division felt in nose.—Dryness of both nostrils.—Discharge of mucus from nose, with congested feeling, as if it were about to bleed.—Slight nose-bleed.—Fluent coryza.

6. **Face.**—Pain in r. jaw-socket.—Dull pain in l. side of lower jaw.—Hot flushes over face and head.—Face much flushed.—Pallor even to lips, with heart pains.

8. **Mouth.**—Ptyalism; tongue coated yellow.—Peppery taste in mouth, fauces, and throat.—Burning and dry feeling in mouth and tongue.—Tongue seemed to alternately expand and contract.

9. **Throat.**—Peppery sensation in throat; soreness, with expectoration of tough mucus.—Feeling of a bunch in l. side of throat when swallowing, shifting to r.—Throat felt as if in a vice.—Pain and soreness in r. side of throat.—Throbbing in throat and sensation of swelling.—Intense burning and stinging in œsophagus, with slight nausea.—Throat dry, very difficult to talk.

10. **Appetite.**—Very thirsty, drank much at a time.—Unusually hungry.—No appetite.—Anorexia, could eat but a few mouthfuls at breakfast, and could only drink half a cup of coffee, which was vomited soon afterward.

11. **Stomach.**—Faintness at stomach as if after fasting; when food was brought cared to eat only a few mouthfuls, which nauseated her.—Empty eructations, with slight taste of ingesta.—Nausea with headache.—Slight nausea, with sense of oppression at stomach; nausea increased, accompanied by frequent chills.—Feeling of fulness or pressure in epigastrium; fluttering.

12. **Abdomen.**—Some pain in r. side below ribs.—Colic pain in r. iliac region.—Rumbling, with soreness on pressure.—Flatulence.—Griping pain on waking in morning, continued at intervals through day, with general feeling of indifference and malaise.

13. **Stool and Anus.**—Constipation in morning.—Griping pains 7 a.m. with thin, brown stools, mixed with mucus.—Burning and pressure for an hour or two after stool.—Epidemic dysentery, characterised by spasmodic tenesmus, intestinal spasms, tympanitis, &c.—Inodorous discharges with tenesmus.—Cholera, in stage of collapse.

14. **Urinary Organs.**—Urine at night and next morning scanty and high-coloured.—Profuse, light-coloured urine; nervous women.

16. **Female Sexual Organs.**—Ovarian pain: with scanty and retarded menses; extending down genito-crural nerves; and sacral pains during pregnancy.—Menses appeared one week before usual time; attended with a good deal of pain.—Menses eight days before time; flow increased, bright red; bearing-down pain and pain in r. ovarian region.—Severe constant aching pain in r. ovarian region, radiating to hip, thighs, and back, with occasional shoots, making her catch her breath.—Sharp, cutting pain in r. ovarian region, extending about hip and down thigh, awoke her.—Cramp-like pain in l. groin, menses five days early.—Pain in l. ovarian region gradually increasing and gradually decreasing.—Dysmenorrhœa: with agonising pains, driving patient almost distracted; neuralgic pain runs along course of genito-crural nerve; in women of spare habit and of a delicate, nervous temperament; with headache, esp. over l. eye, commencing day before menses; fulness in head; eyes congested, with photophobia; face flushed and feverish; agonising bearing

down ; abundant discharge ; excruciating pain in loins and lower abdomen. —Menstrual flow : too early and profuse; pains down thighs; scanty and retarded.—Constant headache, < during menses, at which time she also suffered agonising pains in pelvic region.—Amenorrhœa for five months; face and legs œdematous ; very nervous, sensitive to least noise, hysterical mood ; voice tremulous ; fears she is going to die ; general chlorotic appearance, constipation, scanty, frequent, and dark urine.—Amenorrhœa for five months, with severe pains in r. ovary ; constant headache ; bearing down and tension in hypogastric region.—Amenorrhœa from getting feet wet ; lasting six months ; emaciation with cough ; dirty-grey expectoration ; pale face, night-sweats.—Leucorrhœa ; profuse, milky-white.—Great increase of leucorrhœa during the time when menses should appear.—After-pains.—Profuse lochia.—Violent hot pricking in r. ovary (produced immediately by a dose of 3x).

17. **Respiratory Organs.**—Hoarseness, with husky feeling in throat ; obliged to clear throat frequently.—Aphonia from cold or general debility.—Aphonia and pain in lower r. lung on deep inspiration or coughing.—Shortness of breath.—Constant desire to take a long breath.—Cough : slight hacking cough ; in spells, only in open air.—Dry cough night and day, from sheer exhaustion could scarcely turn herself in bed ; face pale, bloated ; dark rings about eyes ; head full and heavy ; lips colourless ; tongue pale and flabby ; shortness of breath ; no appetite ; bowels constipated ; urine light-coloured, alkaline, sp. gr. 1025 ; fluttering in stomach, pain in l. side ; limbs weak and bloated.—Had to sit up in bed and turn first one way, then another, as in a severe fit of asthma, with several spasmodic coughing spells.—Thought she could not get air enough into lungs, inspiration was so difficult.

18. **Chest.**—Tightening about chest, with inclination to gape.—Pain in l. side, under fourth rib.—Sharp pains in r. side of a neuralgic character.—Oppression of chest, with desire to take a deep inspiration.—Sharp, shooting pains in r. side (like pleurisy pains), occasionally extending through to shoulder-blade, continual desire to take a long breath.—Menses irregular and scanty ; tight, dry cough, which hurts chest and shoulders ; bowels almost constantly loose, profuse night-sweats.

19. **Heart.**—Severe momentary pain in region of heart, making her catch her breath, and turn pale even to lips ; recurred at irregular intervals of from five to thirty minutes ; the pain was cutting, < during inspiration, passed directly through thorax in heart region ; immediately after each attack thirsty, flushed, exhausted.—Pulse irregularly intermittent.—Startled from sleep by severe pain in heart region, followed by violent action of heart and feeling of suffocation.

20. **Neck and Back.**—(With headache) pain and stiffness in nape, somewhat > by hard pressure or throwing head back.—Very severe pain in cervical and upper sacral region.—Back of neck numb.—Slight pain in l. side and under l. scapula, also in l. hip.—Dull pain from nape to r. scapula.—Dragging pain in lower part of pelvis and back.—Coccyx seemed elongated, extremely sensitive to pressure and ached all the time ; could not sit except on cushion.

21. **Limbs.**—Suddenly taken with cramp-like pains in wrists and knees. —Pain in limbs, neuralgic, shooting ; numbness and weakness.—Dull pain in l. knee ; also in l. elbow, extending to hand, then in l. side and top of l. foot.

22. **Upper Limbs.**—Pain in r. shoulder and arm.—Pain and pricking feeling in arm, extending to third finger.—Pricking and throbbing sensation in l. arm and fingers.—Severe pain in r. arm, commencing just above bend of elbow.—Whole l. arm and shoulder numb.—Pain in l. elbow and l. side of head.—Dull pain in l. elbow, passing to palm of hand, then to shoulder.—Pain in both elbows.—Severe pain in wrist, extending to thumb.—A flash of pain in r. thumb, extending to hand.

23. **Lower Limbs.**—Severe neuralgic pains in course of genito-crural nerves (dysmenorrhœa).—Excessive weakness of lower limbs (chlorosis).—Pain in l. leg, between hip and knee.—Weakness in lower limbs, with pain in knees; pain of extremities increased, accompanied by frequent chills.—Legs and feet feel tired.—Pain in l. knee very severe; pain has lasted, without cessation, a little more than half an hour.—Dull pain in r. knee.—A flash of pain in calf of r. leg.—Pain in ankle.—Pain in l. heel.—Pain in both feet, shooting up to knees.—L. foot numb.

24. **Generalities.**—Nerves: acts upon nervous system, mostly upon sensory nerves, but causes a marked depression of vitality, a non-reactive state; hence its use in chlorosis, measles, neuralgia, &c., when there is sensorial and bodily depression.—Paralysis of single members.—Hemiplegia (after *Nux vom.* failed).—Pricking sensation, shocks as from electricity.—Feeling of numbness through whole l. side of body from head to foot, the division made perceptible in the head, affecting half the nose.—Whole l. side, esp. l. foot, numb.—Body felt as though it were elastic and stretched itself out.—Seemed as if floor were soft like wool on walking.—As if floating through air on sitting; as if sunk deep in bed on lying down.—Mucous membrane smarts as from pepper.

25. **Skin.**—Measles, dulness, bewilderment, drowsiness, want of sufficient development of the eruption.—Old and indolent ulcers.

26. **Sleep.**—Continued gaping; drowsiness.—Slept hard and heavy; dreamed of flying about over tops of houses.—A dream of suffocation woke her.—Dreamed the throat grew up, and woke with fright, finding it difficult to breathe.—Awoke in morning languid and depressed.

27. **Fever.**—Sense of heat all over veins, with a desire to be bled; flash of heat from head to foot.—Slight chill accompanied by death-like nausea.—Frequent chills, with pains in extremities; nausea.—Typhoid fever in stage of collapse.

Yohimbinum.

Johimbin. A crystalline alkaloid obtained from the bark of the Yohimbeha, or Yumbehoa tree, of the Cameroons. *N. O.* Rubiaceæ (?). $C_{23}H_{32}N_2O_4$, or $C_{22}H_{30}N_2O_4$. Trituration.

Clinical.—Diuresis. Heart, palpitation of. Impotence. Priapism.

Characteristics.—The natives of West Africa discovered a potent aphrodisiac in the bark of the Yohimbeha tree, and from this an active principle, *Yohimbin*, has been isolated and tested in Europe (*Therapist*, December 15, 1900). It is a powerful stimulant of the genital function in males. In animals it causes increased liveliness and cheerfulness, hyperæmia of the conjunctiva, heat and redness of the ears, and of the nose also in dogs. Lambreghts (*J. Belge d'H.*, viii. 188) relates the case of a young man, 28, "thin, anæmic, nervous, and partially impotent," who took a 5-mgr. tablet one morning, another in the evening, and a third the following morning. The symptoms of the Schema are his, and they were so severe that he discontinued the drug in spite of a certain amelioration of the sexual neurasthenia. *Yohim.* set up symptoms of fever, disordered the digestion, caused agitation and tremors, and increased the action of the heart. Eulenburg (*Deut. Med. Woch.*, April 25, 1901, quoted *B. M. J.*) used *Yohim.* in 10-drop doses of a 1 per cent. solution, and in 5-mgr. tablets, "in cases of neurasthenic impotence with excellent results." *Yohim.* should be a homœopathic remedy in priapism and congestive states of the sexual organs.

Relations.—*Compare:* Erections, Pic. ac., Pho., Graph., Canth., Hdfb.

SYMPTOMS.

1. **Mind.**—Intense agitation, with trembling.

6. **Face.**—Flying sensations of heat, heightening the colour.

8. **Mouth.**—Tongue covered with a yellow coat.—Disagreeable metallic taste.

11. **Stomach.**—Appetite almost completely disappeared.

12. **Abdomen.**—Flying heats in abdomen.

13. **Stool and Anus.**—Stools frequent, liquid, black, and bilious.

14. **Urinary Organs.**—Urine clear, abundant, foamy, no trace of albumen ; had to rise three times in the night.

15. **Male Sexual Organs.**—In the morning strong and lasting erections without increase of desire.—Sexual neurasthenia, with impotence, is relieved.—Enlargement of testicles and epididymis (animals).

19. **Heart.**—Flying sensation of heat in heart.—Heart-beats more intense and more frequent ; pulse, normally 80, became 108.

20. **Back.**—Flying heat in back.

22. **Upper Limbs.**—Hands trembled, he could scarcely write, and his writing was illegible.

26. **Sleep.**—No sleep all night.

27. **Fever.**—Three hours after the dose (5 mgr.), flying sensations of heat, true vapours (*vapeurs*) which heightened the complexion ; afterwards the same phenomena in the back, heart region, and lower abdomen, so that in spite of the cold weather the prover was inconvenienced by the intense heat and tendency to sweat.

Yucca Filamentosa.

Yucca filamentosa. Bear Grass. *N. O.* Melanthaceæ (Liliaceæ). Tincture of root and leaves when not in flower. Tincture of flowers.

Clinical.—Biliousness. Coryza. Diarrhœa. Flatulence, odourless. Headache ; temporal. Post-nasal catarrh. Throat, granular.

Characteristics.—*Yucca* was proved by Rowell and four others in the 30th. Farrington gives these indications : Biliousness with pain going through upper part of liver to back. Bad taste in mouth. Stools diarrhœic, and contain an excess of bile. Much flatus passed by rectum. Frontal or temporal headache with frequent flushing of face. Face sallow. Tongue coated yellow and taking imprint of teeth. Dull ache in centre of liver. Abdomen sensitive. Frequent passage of flatus and of watery, yellowish-brown stools. The tongue of *Yuc.* is usually a bluish white. As with many liver disorders, there is chilliness : cannot bear to be away from the fire. Among the *Sensations* are : As of something hanging down from back of nares. As if cold air blowing on left side of scalp. The symptoms are : < By noise ; motion ; pressure. Griping pain is > bending forward.

Relations.—*Antidoted by :* Coccul. *Compare :* Constriction in heart, Lil. t. Biliousness, Bry. Tongue imprinted with teeth, Merc., Pod. Blue tongue, Gymnocl.

SYMPTOMS.

1. **Mind.**—Very despondent.—Irritable.—Irresolute.—Disinclined to study.—Mind wanders ; uses wrong words.—Unable to remember anything read, with severe pains, which appear first on r. side, then in apex of heart.—Dull sensation in head 1.30 p.m. when others talking to him, hears but doesn't seem to understand, and two minutes after doesn't know what was said.

2. **Head.**—Headache : frontal, heavy, pressing ; throbbing.—Temples : pressing pains in both all day ; < r., and cringing feeling in both, < by motion ; dull, heavy pain extending to eyes, with aversion to light ; intense aching, < by noise, motion, and heat, but at same time chilly when away from stove.—Headache somnolent, > sitting still ; throbs with every step.—Strange feeling in temporo-maxillary joint.—Temporal arteries throb.—Head itches all evening, very annoying.—Sensation of cold air blowing on l. side of scalp.

3. **Eyes.**—Dark rings under eyes.—Eyes feel hot and inflamed.—Itching and smarting l. eye ; l. inner canthus.—Dull pain over l. eye (momentary).

4. **Ears.**—Pain behind r. ear, 6.30 p.m.—Very sensitive to least noise.

5. **Nose.**—Nose red.—In evening r. side of nose constantly running, l. dry.—Profuse, bloody, watery discharge.—Some coryza.

6. **Face.**—Face : pale ; flushed ; burning ; yellow.—Momentary aching in zygoma, recurring several times.—Pain in jaw-joints.

8. **Mouth.**—Tongue : coated white evening, with raised, scattered papillæ ; looks parboiled ; white at root ; bluish white ; raised papillæ, teeth-marks on edge ; pale, flabby.—Bad odour from mouth.—Back of mouth dry.—Soft palate dry, had to drink to moisten it.—Taste of rotten eggs.

9. **Throat.**—Sensation as if something hanging down from posterior nares, cannot get it up or down.—Tonsils dark red, not sore.—Pharynx seems covered with granules, is dark red.—Strings of mucus hang from mouth to root of tongue.—Stringy, greasy-looking mucus back of throat.

11. **Stomach.**—Appetite : increased, food relished ; lost.—Aching and sharp pains in stomach.—Region of stomach sore and sensitive.

12. **Abdomen.**—Abdomen bloated ; after dinner, and feels sore.—Much flatus emitted ; odourless.—Rumbling.—Colic.—Crampy pains in abdomen after breakfast, > lying down, < by movement ; followed by diarrhœa.—Throbbing, painless, r. side about twelfth rib.

13. **Stool and Anus.**—Constant desire.—Sudden, violent tenesmus, followed by discharge of wind, which > the pain.—Tenesmus after stool.—Diarrhœa following pains in abdomen, several yellowish stools in an hour.—Stools : increased in number, but natural though small ; at 6.30 a.m. ; hard and large at first, later thin and watery ; copious, thin, yellowish brown, with smarting at anus.

14. **Urinary Organs.**—Irritable bladder, frequent urination.—Round meatus circumscribed œdematous red swelling, raw sensation.—Burning when urinating.—Urine increased, high specific gravity.

15. **Male Sexual Organs.**—Erections ; all night long but no emissions ; all forenoon, cannot study, mind runs on sexual subjects.

17. **Respiratory Organs.**—Hard, rattling cough.

18. **Chest.**—Constriction in whole chest and in heart.—Pain in upper intercostal muscles, 9.15 p.m.—At 3.30 p.m. extremely severe cramping pain in r. chest, < stooping, partially > sitting straight or leaning a little back ; lasted five minutes.

19. **Heart.**—Constriction in heart.—Momentary aching in heart region.—Visible throbbing in arteries of hand.—Pulse : full and heavy ; a little irregular.

20. **Neck and Back.**—Constriction of neck muscles, seems to draw

head backward.—Tight feeling round neck, evening, had to take off collar.—Severe pain in l. scapula, 9 p.m.—Backache ever since she took the drug.

23. **Lower Limbs.**—Crampy pains in knees.—Sore, crampy pains in muscle of back of l. leg, just above ankle ; as if sprained.

24. **Generalities.**—Restless, feverish.

26. **Sleep.**—In evening very sleepy.—Restless night.—Lewd dreams.

27. **Fever.**—Coldness of scalp, l. side, as if cold air blowing on it.—Coldness ; cannot bear to be away from fire.—Hot ; feverish.—Face sweats, evening

Zea.

Zea mays. Maize. Indian Corn. *N. O.* Gramineæ (Tribe, Phalarideæ).

1. STIGMATA MAIDIS. Corn Silk. Green pistils. Tincture : One part, by weight, of the Silk to two of alcohol. Fluid Extract. (Z. st.)
2. SHUCKS. Decoction or tincture of the husks of Maize after the removal of the grain. (Z. sh.)

Clinical.—Albuminuria (St.). Cystitis (St.). Dropsy (St.). Gonorrhœa, chronic (St.). Heart, failure of (St.). Malaria, chronic (Sh.). Renal colic (St.). Pyelitis (St.). Urine, retained ; suppressed (St.).

Characteristics.—Two parts of Maize have been used in medicine, the pistils (*Stigmata maidis*) and the husks (*Shucks*), but I think it best to take them together. I have distinguished them under the heading CLINICAL by (St.) and (Sh.). The grain of Maize in bulk appears to be capable of generating a poisonous gas, as four men were suffocated, one fatally, on opening a cargo of maize for the purpose of discharging it in the London docks (*H. W.*, xxxv. 436). Corn silk has been used in : (1) Irritable conditions of the urinary tract ; ureters, bladder, urethra. (2) As a powerful diuretic in renal disorders unconnected with cardiac involvement. (3) Heart and urinary conditions combined. J. H. Cook gives an account of it in *Med. Cent.* (iv. 589). He quotes the results of Dumont's investigation of its action on the heart : (1) It makes the heart's action slower and stronger. (2) Regulates its rhythm. (3) Its diuretic action is manifested first. (4) Its action is more powerful and evident in cardiac affections with dropsy. (5) With the disappearance of the dropsy arterial tension increases and venous tension diminishes. Cook gives this case : Mr. X., 63, florid, robust, temperate, had been many months under treatment with the following condition, traced originally to cooling off too rapidly when perspiring : Intense prostration, intermittent pulse, dyspnœa. The urine contained much albumen, mucus, and some blood ; specific gravity 1010. Great tenderness over entire abdomen, especially in region of ureters. Under remedies he would improve for a few days, when a slight chill would be followed by fever, and the symptoms would come back in full force. The microscope revealed pus cells and granular epithelial cells in abundance. *Z. st.* was now given, a teaspoonful of the fluid extract every four hours. In less than a week there was visible improvement. The constant calls to urinate (every forty-five minutes) ceased, and the patient could go through the night without being disturbed more than once or twice. The specific gravity of the urine increased, and pus, blood, and albumen disappeared. Only a little abdominal tenderness remained, which did not prevent the patient from attending to his business and enjoying life. Hansen has confirmed the value of *Z. st.* in 20-drop doses of the fluid extract in organic heart disease with dropsy, much œdema of lower limbs, and scanty urination. He mentions also as suitable cases: (1) Renal lithiasis with nephritic ulcer and discharge of small calculi, red sand, and blood. (2) Chronic pyelitis from catarrh. (3) Chronic retention of urine with great tenesmus after urinating. (4) Suppression of urine with lack of solids and low specific gravity. (5) Vesical catarrh, tenesmus of neck of bladder, ammoniacal urine, much mucus. (6) Chronic gonorrhœa, prostate involved, painful urination. The other use of *Zea* (*Z. sh.*) was communicated to the profession by Dr. J. W. Pruitt (*Arkansas Eclect. Med. J.* quoted *H. R.*, viii. 494). Pruitt learned it from the people. "Shuck tea" is a popular remedy for chronic malaria. Pruitt's son took a chill in the Arkansas river bottom. The chills were stopped with the usual remedies, *Cinchonidia, Iron, Piperine,* &c., but every fourteen days would come back with increased severity. Presently gastric symptoms set in, with anæmia, and other symptoms of chronicity. "Shuck tea" was recommended by a lay friend, and was taken for one day only. There was never a chill after. Pruitt thenceforward used *Z. sh.* largely, and he found it was in the *chronic cases only* that it was beneficial.

Relations.—*Compare:* In bladder affections, Trit. r., Sabal ser. Renal colic, Oc. c. Heart, Dig., Stroph. Malaria, Malar.

Zincum.

Zincum metallicum. Zinc. An Element. Zn. A. W. 64·9.
Trituration of the metal.

Clinical.—*Alcoholism.* Amblyopia. Asthma. Brain-fag. Brain, paralysis of. Breasts, affections of. Cataract. Chilblains. Chin, eruption on. Chlorosis. Cholera. Chorea. *Constipation.* Cracks. Dentition. Diarrhœa, nervous; with stupor. Diphtheria. Dysentery. Dysuria. Earache. Eczema. Enuresis. Eruptions; suppressed. *Eyes, affections of;* granular lids. Fag. Foot-sweat; suppressed. Gastralgia. Headache; nervous; chlorotic. Heels, pains in. Hernia, inguinal. Hiccough. Hydrocephalus. Hyperpyrexia, nervous. Hypochondriasis. Hysteria. Inframammary pain. *Joints, creaking in.* Lips, affections of. Lochia; suppressed. Malar bones, neuralgia in. Masturbation. *Memory, weak. Meningitis. Mental weakness.* Milk, defective; suppressed. Neuralgia; intercostal; subcostal. Neurasthenia. Nipples, sore. Nose, redness of. Nymphomania. Œsophagus, spasm of. Otorrhœa. Photopsia. Prostatorrhœa. Ptosis. Reaction, defective. Rheumatism. *Screaming.* Sleepiness. Somnambulism. Spermatorrhœa. Spinal irritation. Spine, affections of. Spleen, neuralgia of. Strabismus. Suppressions. Tarsal tumours. Throat, sore. Tibia, burning in. Typhoid fever. Ulcers. Urine, hysterical retention of. Varicosis; during pregnancy; of external genitals. Whooping-cough. Worms.

Characteristics.—*Zincum* belongs to the *Magnesium* group of metals, comprising also *Cadmium* and *Glucinum.* It has long been known in the arts, especially in its combination with *Cuprum* in the manufacture of Brass. *Zn.* was proved by Hahnemann and his associates, and it appears among the remedies of his *Chronic Diseases*. *Zn.* poisons the brain and nerve, and it corresponds to nerve-poisoning of various kinds. The word "fag" covers a large part of *Zn.* action ; it may be nerve- or brain-fag ; or it may be muscle-fag. Fag means that tissues are worn out faster than they can be repaired. This leaves them poisoned by waste products. *Zn.* meets the effects of brain-fag from over-study ; from night-watching ; fatigue. But there is another kind of nerve-poisoning met by *Zn.*: the poisoning of suppressed eruptions or discharges. The common old-school use of Zinc ointment to suppress eruptions, and Zinc injections to suppress discharges, is based on fact : *Zn.* does suppress them, and it transfers the morbid action to the nervous system, setting up a poisoning there ; and, conversely, in homœopathic attenuations *Zn.* can reverse the process. It can restore suppressed eruptions, can cure the consequences of suppressions, and can set free the reactive power in conditions of undeveloped disease. Some of the keynotes of *Zn.* will be present to give the clue. The most important of these is : "Incessant and violent fidgety feeling in feet or lower limbs ; must move them constantly ; cannot keep them quiet." These movements may continue even during sleep. Another is : "Too weak to develop exanthemata or menstrual function, to expectorate, to urinate ; to understand, to remember." Corresponding to these is : "Relief to all suffering as soon as menses begin to flow," or as soon as other excretory functions are restored. In asthma "the patient cannot expectorate, but as soon as he can he is relieved" (Nash). General twitchings and *general trembling* are, according to Nash, equally characteristic of *Zn.* He records this case : Miss X., 20, had been ill for a week with headache, loss of appetite, and especially prostration. Over-study was the cause. Under *Gels.*, and later *Bry.*, she was improving, when she threw off the bedclothes whilst sleeping and perspiring, and took a chill. [*Zn.* has "cannot bear any covering during the sweat."—J. H. C.] The bowels became enormously distended ; profuse hæmorrhage occurred (finally controlled by *Alumen*), a low form of delirium came on, and prostration increased in spite of the cessation of hæmorrhage. This was the condition : Staring eyes rolled upward, head retracted ; complete unconsciousness, lying on back and sliding down in bed ; twitching, "or rather intense, *violent trembling all over so that she shook the bed,*" her hands had to be held constantly night and day by nurses ; hippocratic face, extremities deathly cold to knees and elbows ; pulse intermittent, uncountable ; all signs, in short, of impending paralysis of the brain." Two drops of *Zn.* 200 were mixed in two teaspoonfuls of water. One teaspoonful was worked, a little at a time, between the set teeth ; and the rest half an hour later. About an hour after the latter dose the patient turned down her eyes and said "Milk." Through a bent tube she swallowed half a glass of milk, the first nourishment she had taken for twenty-four hours. From that time she improved steadily, and received no more medicine for four days. Afterwards she had a dose of *Nux*. Recovery was perfect. A. W. Holcombe (*Hahn. Ad.*, xxxviii. 27) reports this case : Man, 40, had gonorrhœa suppressed by local treatment three months previously. A week before Holcombe saw him first he was unable to pass water, and had to resort to the catheter. Since then could pass urine, but passed almost pure blood with it. Could only urinate when sitting down with knees spread apart. Great soreness of perinæum ; on sitting down had to sit sideways on chair. *Zn.* cm one dose. Five days later perinæal soreness gone, could urinate freely in any position, and had a profuse whitish discharge from the urethra. Suppression of foot-sweat ; of lochia ; of milk, are all caused and cured by *Zn.* Weyner (*H. R.*, x. 152) relates the poisoning of cows pasturing near a cadmium mine, near which Zinc-smelting was carried on. These were some of the effects : General emaciation, skin clinging tightly to the body ; eyes pale bluish, *drawn back into the orbits ;* horns and ears unequally warm, mouth hot and shiny and hanging down, at times dry ; appetite undisturbed ; rumination slower ; dung grass-green, thin-flowing and fetid ; at times cough. As the disease progressed emaciation increased, the horns became rough, *milk dried up*, and diarrhœa increased till the animals could no longer rise, and died of total prostration. *Zn.* meets these suppression-effects : paralysis and vertigo from brain softening following suppressed foot-sweat ; chorea from eruptions suppressed by gout ; puerperal convulsions from suppressed eruption ; nymphomania from suppressed lochia. *Zn.* has a strong action on the generative sphere, it excites both sexes and causes seminal losses and prostatorrhœa of the male, and nymphomania and masturbation in the female. This may be associated with varicosis or pruritus of the external genitals. A notable symptom of *Zn.*, and one which may indicate it in children and in delirious cases, as well as in affections of the genitals themselves, is that the patient is continually pressing on the pubes or applying the hand to the genitals. With the emission there is backache, which is temporarily > by the emission ; and with the female sexual disorders there is also backache and spinal irritation. Dull aching in spine, < when sitting. Burning pains all along the spine. The burning pains of *Zn.* appear in many parts. Pricking, pressive, cramp-like pains, tension and constriction are also present. Neuralgia in malar bones with pressive pains. Pressure at root of nose as if it would be pressed in. The constriction is especially felt in the chest, and is connected both with respiration and the heart. "Sudden, spasmodic, bursting sensation about heart ; it appears to be beating regularly, when it suddenly seems as if it would burst through the chest." *Zn.* affects the blood-vessels and corresponds to varicosis : varices of the labia ; of the thighs, running into the labia ; of the legs, with fidgety feet. Numbness, tingling, formication, and fainting spells are other nervous effects of *Zn.* It has an insatiable craving hunger and goneness, notably at 11 a.m. ; thirst quite as great ; and "hasty eating" and "hasty drinking" are among the keynote symptoms. Another of the first importance is *intolerance of wine :* wine aggravates all symptoms. This is noteworthy in states of nervous exhaustion, which usually crave stimulants. There is the aversion to wine. Other characteristic aversions are : Meat (especially veal) ; sweets ; cooked or warm food.

Eating as well as wine-drinking < the pain. There is a tearing headache, most in side of head, < from wine, < after dinner. In meningitis there are sharp, lancinating pains in the head, < from the least stimulant. Pain may account for the anxious scream which accompanies the convulsions of *Zn.* The child springs up in bed, gnashing teeth, eyes rolled up. A characteristic of brain affections of children is "crossness in the evening." On waking there is delirium as if frightened, knows no one. "Child repeats everything said to it" is another leading symptom. "Grits teeth" occurs in these conditions, and will often give *Zn.* a place in worm cases. Among the symptoms indicating lack of power is "teeth fail to develop." The "fidgety feet" of *Zn.* are not the only automatic movements of the remedy, though the most characteristic. There are automatic movements of mouth, arms, and hands, and general restlessness. Among other features of *Zn.* is blueness of surface. Related to this is the tendency to chilblains, which are swollen and painful, and easily made worse by rubbing. There is sensitiveness to frost-bite ; the tip of the nose is easily frost-bitten, and the nose remains red long after it has been frost-bitten. The hands and feet are affected with inflammation, painful eruptions, cracks. There is also a "frost-bitten feeling" in the toes. All these point to a lowered state of vitality. *Peculiar Sensations* are : As if she had a large goître which she could not see over. As if hair bristled. Uneasy, as if he had committed a crime. As if he would have apoplexy. As if scalp were drawn together. Pains as if between the skin and the flesh. As if head were moving up and down, with a similar floating of images of his fancy. As if he saw through a mist. As if he would fall over to other side. As if head were swaying back and forth. Nauseating weakness as after smoking too strong tobacco. As if eyes were drawn together by a cord. Stupefying headache as from coal gas. As if root of nose would be pressed into head. As if head would be drawn backward. As if air forced itself into frontal sinuses. As if head would burst. As if strained in occiput. As if scalp wrinkled up and kept tightening. As if insects were crawling from occiput to forehead. Feeling in eyes as if she had wept much. As if sand in eyes. As if upper lids paralysed. As if teeth would be pulled out with neuralgia. As if teeth long and loose. As if a web drawn across throat. As if a hard body were opposing pressure from pharynx into abdomen. As if food remained sticking in pharynx after dinner. As if stomach compressed or empty. As of a heavy weight in hypochondria. As if abdominal walls were retracted against spine. As if flatus pressing against coccyx. As from worms crawling in anus. As if testicles tightly compressed and drawn up. As if pudenda swollen. Cough with stitches in chest and feeling as if chest would burst. Chest : as if hollow and cold ; constricted ; cut to pieces. As if a foreign substance rising up throat. Emptiness behind sternum. As if a cap on heart. Pain in cervical muscles as if head had been in uncomfortable position. As if cold water were poured down her back. As if muscles of wrist too short. As if kidney would be twisted off. Wrist and foot as if sprained. As if soles swollen. As if tendons of right sole too short. As if ball of great toe frozen.—The headache and eye symptoms of *Zn.* are well marked, and "Headache with sympathetic amblyopia" may be regarded as a keynote: Kafka (*H. R.*, x. 153) relates the case of a "pale yet vigorous lady of forty" who for two years had had a headache recurring periodically every ten to fourteen days without warning. Simultaneously with the headache was *a weakness of vision*, she seemed looking through a fog, and could not distinguish even large objects. The pain, which lasted two or three days, now increasing, now diminishing, was a pressure on vertex and forehead from without inward. Face pale, appetite deficient, head muddled, mood cross and peevish. In forenoon the pain was bearable, in afternoon <, and still < evening, when reflex nausea, and even vomiting, occurred. The amblyopia went *pari passu* with the severity of the pain, and disappeared as the pain left off. Pupils rather contracted, eyes otherwise normal. *Zn.* 3 was given morning and evening. The pains diminished immediately and were gone in twenty-four hours. The remedy was taken in the evening daily for a week. There was no relapse. F. W. Payne (*N. A. J. H.*, xiv. 131, quoting *A. M.*) reports this case of cataract: Right eye partially affected, and left practically useless for vision, with bruised, sore, smarting, burning, itching, and stinging sensation; at intervals, suddenly, sensation as if pepper had been thrown into it, causing scalding lachrymation and spasm of the lids. These spells were < in evening. Burning dryness as if a stick under lid scratching eyeball. Flickering before left eye; blue and green rings; green halo round gas-jet at times. Slight irritation of conjunctiva and tendency of lids to adhere. < By warmth, on warm days, by artificial light. Patient nervous, tremulous, impatient, < by mental emotion. Choreic jerkings of individual muscles. *Zn.* 200, given occasionally, steadily improved the case. In six months right eye was quite clear, and the left steadily gaining. Eleven years later vision was practically perfect, though some small streaks could still be found in the left lens. Gerstel (*H.R.*, x. 97) calls attention to the action of *Zn.* in fevers with inflammation of the brain. In these cases the seat of inflammation was the meninges. He refers to a case of a child suffering from scarlatina who was in this condition: Entirely motionless; extremities icy cold, body cold, skin all over body bluish red, *except the parts about the eyes, forehead and chin, which were white.* *Zn.* was given, and the child gradually recovered. In a case of typhoid (16th day) in a man, in whom mental symptoms had set in: "Muddled feeling in the head, an incapacity to relate anything connectedly, and a sort of *half-smiling loquacity;*" and later: Staring look, almost hippocratic appearance, *pale as wax;* carphologia, subsultus tendinum, constant trembling of the hands—*Zn.* 2 saved the patient.—The symptoms of *Zn.* are: < By touch. Pressure <; (> conjunctivitis; toothache; left ovarian pain). Rubbing and scratching >. Jarring, riding <. Rest <. Sitting <. Lying <; (> vertigo). < By motion, active or passive: "Child screams out whenever it is moved." Walking; lifting; exertion <. Looking up = vision of falling luminous objects, and dizziness. < Evening and night. 11 a.m. to 12 sinking <. Rheumatism < from over-heating. Wails and moans during sweat. < By chill when heated. Warm room <. Warm water > conjunctivitis.

Open air < ; (> headache and drowsiness). Very sensitive to draught. < By cold touch (*i.e.*, when patient touches anything cold). Sea bathing = herpes in mouth. Approach of storm = chills. > While eating ; < after. Eating <. Drinking < (as soon as liquid reaches stomach he vomits). < From : Sugar ; wine ; milk. Emissions > (temporarily). Sensitive to others talking and to noise.

Relations.—*Antidoted by :* Hep., Ign., Camph. (Lobel., Teste). *Antidote to :* Baryt. c. *Incompatible :* Wine, Cham., Nux. *Followed well by :* Sep., Sul. (best—H. N. G.) ; Puls., Ign. *Follows well :* Ap., Bell. *Complementary :* In hydrocephalus, Calc. p. *Compare :* Erratic temperature in fevers, Puls. Colics, Pul., Lyc. Abdominal symptoms, Plb., Pod. Tremors, Arg. n. Spinal pains, Cob., Sep. Asthma accompanying great constriction of chest, Cad. s., K. chl., Cact. Boring fingers in nose, Cin., Ver., Ar. t. Scarlatina, Bell. (Zn. follows well when rash fails to come out and child screams whenever moved). Hydrocephalus, Calc. ph. Pain in back < sitting than walking, Sep., Cob., Arg. n. (Arg. n. has pain when rising). Goneness 11 a.m., Sul., Nat. c., Pho., Indm. Paralysis and brain softening, Pho., Pb. Spermatorrhœa, testes drawn up, Con. (Con. lacks the excessive irritability of Zn., and Zn. has temporary > from the emissions). Fag, nervous exhaustion, Pic. ac. Neuralgia, nervous exhaustion, Mg. c. Spinal irritation, Act. r. (Zn. has < sitting and < from wine). Sinking sensation, inability to throw out eruption, Hell. Crying out in sleep, wakes terrified ; puts hands to genitals, Stram. Suppressed or undeveloped eruption, Bry. Fidgety feet, Trn. Boring in left ovary ceasing with flow, Lach. Fear of ghosts, Aco., Ars., Bro., Carb. v., Cocc., Lyc., Pho., Pul., Ran. b., Sep., Sul. Pain in right chest, Phell. Pain in throat > when not swallowing, Ign. Too weak to develop exanthemata, Cup., Sul., Bac. Convulsions *with pale face*, no heat except in occiput, no rise of temperature (Bell. opp.). Automatic movements of hands and head or one hand and head, Apoc., Bry., Hell. Cannot bear back touched, Chi. s., Trn., Ther. Twitching or jerking of single muscles, Agar., Ign. Incipient brain disease from suppressed eruptions, Bac., Hell. Unconquerable sleepiness, Nux m., Op. Diarrhœa with stupor, Op. < From sea-bathing, Ars. Too speedy ejaculation in coitus, Titan. Burning in spine, Pho., Lyc. Headache at root of nose, Ign. Affections of palate, Mang.

Causation.—Grief. Anger. Fright. Night-watching. Operations. Frost-bite. Suppressions : eruptions ; otorrhœa ; menses ; lochia ; milk.

SYMPTOMS.

1. **Mind.**—Hypochondriacal humour.—Thoughts of death, as if the end were approaching.—Fear of robbers or of frightful spectres.—Stares as if frightened on waking, rolls head from side to side.—Fretful, peevish humour, morose, with dislike to conversation, esp. in evening.—Child cross towards evening, brain affected.—The patient is powerfully affected by conversation or by noise.—Irascibility and impatience.—Tendency to fits of passion, and great uneasiness when left alone.—Aversion to labour (and to **walk**).—Fickle-

ness (very variable mood), with sadness towards noon and joy (hilarity) in evening, and *vice versâ*.—Weakness of memory.—Forgetfulness (forgets what has been accomplished during the day).—Weak memory with stinging pains in head.—Unconquerable drowsiness after prolonged night-watching.—Absence of ideas.—Difficult conception.—Incoherent ideas.—Thoughtlessness and dulness of intellect.—Repeats all questions before answering them.

2. **Head.**—Continued confusion and cloudiness in head.—Vertigo deeply seated in brain, principally in occiput (cerebellum), causing patient to fall sidelong (to l.).—Vertigo : as if he would have apoplexy ; as if head moving up and down ; as if he would fall to r. when on a height ; with flushing heat ; on staying up late, as after smoking too strong tobacco.—Vertigo, as if the seat were undulating when sitting up in bed in morning.—Vertigo and delirious feeling : kept continually talking in his sleep (agg. from 3x trit.—R. T. C.).—Stupefying vertigo, with clouded sight (everything gets black before the eyes ; < in morning in warm room and after eating ; > in open air) ; and general weakness.—Frequent attacks of vertigo, preceded by sharp pressure at root of nose, and a sensation of drawing together of eyes, as if by a cord, followed immediately by excessive nausea, faintness, and trembling of hands.—Pain as from a tearing in whole brain.—Headache at night, or in evening after lying down.—Headache after drinking (even small quantities of) wine.—Fit of headache, with nausea and vomiting.—Sharp pressure on a small spot in forehead, evening.—Pressure at root of nose as if it would be pressed into head.—Pressive cephalalgia, principally in morning and in forehead, with confusion ; or else in temples and occiput.—Pain in sinciput, with dulness, extending into the eyes.—Compressive boring, or expansive pressure in head.—Drawing in occiput and forehead.—Shootings and tearing in the head, esp. in the sides, temples, forehead, and occiput, < after dinner.—Hemicrania ; < after dinner ; tearing and stinging.—Frequent screwing together pain in both sides of head in evening.—Chlorotic headaches, esp. in patients saturated with iron.—Cerebral and nervous exhaustion ; brain-fag ; anæmia.—Pain as from excoriation in head.—Pulsative pains in head.—Buzzing in head.—The headaches are > in open air and < in a room.—Itching and sensation of excoriation in the scalp, or pain as from ulceration.—Sensitiveness of vertex, as from soreness or ulceration, without regard to touch ; < in evening in bed and after eating ; > in open air.—Forehead cool, base of brain hot.—Sensation as if hair were standing on end.—The hair falls off from the vertex causing complete baldness, with sensation of soreness of the scalp.—Hydrocephalus.

3. **Eyes.**—Pain in the eyes in evening after lying down or drinking wine.—Pressure on eyes or sensation as if pressed or sunk into head.—Pressive and lancinating tearing in eyes.—Photophobia ; dread of sunlight with watery eyes.—Sensitive to light ; brain affected.—Burning and biting in eyes, esp. in r., as from dust ; photophobia and lachrymation ; < evenings.—Itching, smarting, and feeling of excoriation in eyes, eyelids, and internal canthi ; < evening and night ; also during menses.—(Pterygium.)—Burning and inflammation of eyes and lids.—Redness and inflammation of internal canthi, with suppuration.—Dryness of eyes.—Agglutination of lids at night, with pressing, sore feeling.—Intense burning in eyes after operations.—Falling down and paralysis of upper eyelids.—Pupils contracted.—Luminous flakes before eyes when looking into the air (at the sky).—On looking up felt

giddy and saw showers of gold descending (cured with hysterical retention of urine.—B. Simmons).—When looking up, a dark, diagonal line before l. eye, directed upwards and to the r., about six feet in length.—Diplopia, l. eye most affected; strabismus developed.—Amaurosis: during severe headache, passing away with headache.

4. **Ears.**—Earache, with tearing lancinations and external swelling, esp. in children.—Frequent, acute stitches in r. ear, near tympanum.—Earache of children, esp. boys.—Increased ear-wax, l. ear, thinner than usual.—Tickling in l. ear not > by rubbing.—Itching in r. ear, > by boring into it.—Flow of fetid pus from ears.—Noises: humming; whizzing; ringing; crash as from breaking glass on falling asleep.

5. **Nose.**—Pain as from excoriation in interior of nose.—Troublesome pressure at the root of nose, as if it were squeezed.—Cutting, crawling in evening, then sneezing.—Swelling of nose, internally and externally, sometimes semilateral, with anosmia.—Obstruction of nose.—Fluent coryza, with hoarseness and burning sensation in chest.—Redness of nose, remaining after freezing; tip of nose easily frosted.

6. **Face.**—Pale and earthy countenance.—Pale; alternating with redness.—Face: cadaverous; pinched; unnatural; earthy, as after long illness; cachectic, bluish-white; waxy, white or yellow; pewter-like.—Gloomy and wandering look; vacant; apathetic.—Tearing, pressing, stitches, and pain as of a fracture in the bones of the face.—Sudden pressing stitch from r. zygoma to upper margin of orbit, deep in bone, followed by great sensitiveness on the spot; evening.—Neuralgia of fifth pair of nerves, < from touch and in evening.—Spasmodic twitching of musculi risores, with constant inclination to laugh.—Cracks in lips and commissures, with internal ulceration.—Lips: swollen; dry.—Upper lip: violent muscular twitches in l. side; sore; ulcerating in middle; jerking tearing in r. side; fine stitches.—Lower lip: tensive, painful smarting: burning smarting on inner surface.—Sticking pain in jaw-joint, beneath and in front of l. ear, on moving jaw back and biting strongly, and on pressing finger on joint.—Thick, viscid, tasteless mucus on lips.—Itching eruption and redness on chin.

7. **Teeth.**—Toothache during mastication.—Tearing, lancinating, or drawing toothache, esp. in molars.—Pain in teeth, as from excoriation.—Frequent toothache, a drawing pain in roots of incisors.—Painful jerking in a tooth.—Looseness of teeth.—Teeth: feel sore; feel elongated.—Grits teeth.—Copious bleeding of teeth and gums (on slightest touch).—Gums white and swollen, with pain as from excoriation.—Ulcers in gums.

8. **Mouth.**—Small yellow ulcers in mouth, on internal surface of cheeks.—Tingling (crawling) of internal surface of cheeks, and copious secretion of saliva, having a metallic taste.—Sticking, biting on palate, close to and in the roots of incisors.—Vesicles on tongue.—Tongue: dry, doesn't want to talk; coated at root and edges (brain diseases); swollen l. side, hindering talking; covered with vesicles; white or yellowish white; white as from cheese, without taste; covered with white mucus; blistered, painful on eating.—Inflammation of palate.—Pain in palate and velum palati, esp. on yawning.—Herpes in mouth from sea-bathing.

9. **Throat.**—Drawing tearings in bottom of gullet, more frequently when not swallowing than during deglutition (or worse between acts of

swallowing than on empty swallowing).—Sensation of contraction and cramp in œsophagus, near pit of throat.—Dryness and roughness in palate and throat, with rawness, smarting, and scraping.—Pain as from excoriation in throat.—Copious accumulation of mucus in the throat, which frequently enters the mouth through the posterior nares.—Bluish herpes in throat after suppressed gonorrhœa.—Pain in throat as from an internal swelling.

10. **Appetite.**—Taste of blood in mouth.—Salt taste in mouth.—Taste: sweetish; metallic; like spoiled cheese; as after raw peas.—Violent thirst: from forenoon till evening; with heat in palms; in afternoon; in afternoon during menses; with hasty drinking; for beer in evening.—Diminution of appetite; loss of appetite.—Insatiable voracity.—Hunger: ravenous, esp. 11 a.m. or 12 noon, with weakness of legs and trembling; greediness and hasty swallowing.—Loss of appetite, with a perfectly clean tongue.—Dislike to meal (veal), sweet things, fish, cooked and hot food; to wine and brandy. —Pressure at stomach, with nausea, after eating bread.—Hypochondriacal humour, with aching under false ribs; choking, clawing in abdomen, and fulness, pressure, or burning in the stomach after a meal.—< From sugar (heartburn); wine; milk (loud eructations).

11. **Stomach.**—Rising, with pressive pain in chest.—Sour risings after a meal, esp. after drinking milk.—Pyrosis after taking things sweetened with sugar.—Hiccough, esp. after breakfast.—Nausea, with retching and vomiting of bitter mucus, renewed by slightest movement.—Nausea and headache from least drop of wine.—Vomiting: as soon as first spoonful of liquid reaches stomach; of pregnancy; easy, of watery bile, followed by great relief; acrid, causing burning on face and rawness in throat; almost continuous.—Vomiting of blood.—Stomachache.—Unpleasant sensation in cardia and along œsophagus.—Squeezing and pressure in scrobiculus.—Tearing and shootings in scrobiculus; from both sides towards each other.—Burning in stomach.—Burning sensation in epigastrium (extending to œsophagus).—Sudden oppression of stomach, has to unfasten dress.—Spasm in stomach and constriction of œsophagus; < during inspiration.

12. **Abdomen.**—Spasmodic pains in the hypochondria, alternating with oppression of chest (dyspnœa) after eating.—Sticking in r. hypochondrium. —Enlarged liver.—Violent pressure in hypochondria and sides of abdomen, < by movement and walking.—Squeezing, pressure, and shootings in the hepatic region.—Shootings in region of spleen.—Pressure, shootings, and pain as from excoriation in lumbar region.—Sticking in diaphragm.—Pains in abdomen in evening after lying down.—Violent pressure and tension in abdomen (and sides), with distension.—Pain after a light meal, with tympanites.—Pressure under short ribs, after eating, with depression of spirits.—Pain as from an internal induration in a spot beneath navel.—Sensation of pressure on internal surface of trunk, of a nervous character, without flatulency.—Spasmodic pain in umbilical region.—Squeezing in abdomen.—Gripings and pinchings in abdomen, with diarrhœa.—Griping after breakfast or cutting after dinner.—Tearings and shootings in abdomen.—Severe stabbing pains in abdomen.—Accumulation of much flatulence, with grumbling (loud rumbling, gurgling rolling) and borborygmi in abdomen, esp. after a meal.—Flatulent colic, esp. in evening.—Frequent expulsion of hot and putrid flatus.—Inguinal hernia.—Pressive aching in pubic region.—(Eroto-

mania ; patient always pressing on pubes.)—Cutting upward in l. iliac region, in paroxysms; in a pregnant woman.—Swelling of inguinal glands; buboes (l.).

13. **Stool and Anus.**—Constipation.—Hard, dry (crumbling), insufficient fæces, often evacuated with violent straining.—Constipation of the new-born.—Loose, soft evacuations of consistence of pap, or liquid, and often accompanied by a discharge of bright red (or pale) blood.—Diarrhœa with stupor.—Nervous diarrhœa from depression of nerve centres.—Involuntary evacuation.—Pain in abdomen during and after evacuation.—Tearings, shootings, burning, feeling as of excoriation, and violent itching in anus.—Burning in anus during stool.—Feeling in rectum as if flatus pressing against coccyx, by which it is retained.—Crawling tingling in anus, as from worms.

14. **Urinary Organs.**—Pressing, stinging, and soreness in the kidneys.—Pressure in region of l. kidney.—Stones (gravel) of kidneys and bladder.—Retention of urine when beginning to urinate.—Sitting with legs crossed, bending forward, and cannot pass water, or but very little, and feels as if his bladder would burst.—Can only pass urine (which she must do every hour) while sitting bent backwards.—Hysterical retention of urine (with vision of a golden shower on looking up.—B. Simmons).—Excessive desire to urinate, also at night.—Violent pressure of urine on the bladder.—Painful emission of urine.—Involuntary emission of urine, esp. when walking, coughing, or sneezing.—Frequent emission of a clear yellow urine, which afterwards deposits a white, flocky sediment.—The urine becomes turbid, like clay-water, after standing.—Sanguineous urine.—Burning sensation during and after emission of urine.—Acute drawing in forepart of urethra and in penis.—Incisive pains in orifice of urethra.—Discharge of blood from urethra after painful micturition.

15. **Male Sexual Organs.**—Testes retracted, swollen, painful.—Drawing in testes and along spermatic cord (one or the other testicle is drawn up).—Pain as from excoriation in scrotum.—Contraction of scrotum and shuddering in that part.—Orchitis ; from suppressed otorrhœa.—Strong sexual desire, with difficult or too speedy emission.—Permanent erections at night.—Emissions at night, without lascivious dreams.—Easily excited; the emission during an embrace is difficult or almost impossible.—Flow of prostatic fluid (without any cause).—Great falling off of hair of genital organs.—Hands constantly on the genitals.—The child grasps the genitals when coughing.

16. **Female Sexual Organs.**—Sensation of bearing down towards the genital organs.—Complaints coming on while the menses are absent, but feels perfectly well during the flow : suffers much pain, particularly in ovaries, will lie so as to press on the affected side, and dangling the limb will swing it about, patient can't keep still.—Menses flow more at night.—Nymphomania of lying-in women, with great sensitiveness of the genitals.—Hands constantly on the genitals.—Irresistible sexual desire at night; desire for onanism.—Menses too early.—Discharge of large clots during the menses.—Menstruation too late.—Catamenia premature ; suppressed.—Suppressed menstruation with painfulness of the breasts and genitals.—Catamenia retarded.—Spasmodic colic on appearance of catamenia.—During the catamenia : distension of the abdomen, cuttings, and pressure towards abdomen and loins, with great heaviness and lassitude in legs ; cough.—Leucorrhœa of thick mucus (bloody

mucus; excoriating after menses), sometimes preceded by pains in abdomen.—Leucorrhœa with much itching; pain in l. ovary, only > by menstrual flow.—Pruritus vulvæ; causes masturbation.—Itching of vulva during menses.—Varicose veins of external genitals, with fidgety feet.—Profuse falling off of hair of genitals.—Varices during pregnancy; stagnation of blood in l. leg.—Tendency to miscarry.—Puerperal convulsions with suppression of (chronic) eruption.—Suppressed lochia; nymphomania.—Pain as from excoriation in nipples.—Suppressed secretion of milk.

17. **Respiratory Organs.**—Roughness and dryness in throat and chest, esp. in morning and after dinner.—Hoarseness; with burning in trachea as if chest filled with mucus.—Frequent tickling in region of larynx.—Discharge of black blood when hawking.—Cough, with oppression.—Violent cough.—Cough, with stitches in the head.—Dry cough also at night, with violent stitches in chest and feeling as if it would burst.—Cough, with expectoration of viscid mucus, followed by a sensation of coldness and excoriation in chest as if it were raw.—Cough, with expectoration of blood, burning sensation, and pain as from excoriation of chest.—Debilitating, spasmodic cough from tickling in larynx, extending to middle of chest, with expectoration of yellow, purulent, blood-streaked, tenacious mucus, tasting disagreeably, sweetish-putrid, metallic; or of pure blood in morning or during day.—The cough is < after eating, during rest, sitting, standing, from milk, sweets, spirituous liquors, during menstruation.—Child grasps genitals when coughing.

18. **Chest.**—Difficult respiration and oppression, with pressive pain in the chest, esp. in evening.—Constrictive sensation around the chest, with pain in the chest, as if cut to pieces.—Dull stitches in r. side of chest.—Stitches in a spot in l. side of chest, with feeling as if corroded and bruised.—Tightness in evening, with pressure in middle of sternum; small, rapid pulse.—Spasmodic dyspnœa.—Shortness of breath, caused by flatulence after a meal.—Sensation of emptiness in the chest.—Chest loaded with mucus.—Pressure at chest.—Tensive pain in sternum.—L. intercostal neuralgia < by motion; fatigue; at times with palpitation.—Sticking beneath l. breast.—Tearings in chest.—Shootings in chest, esp. in region of heart.—Burning sensation in chest.—Pain beneath costal arches.

19. **Heart.**—Palpitation of heart, with or without anguish.—Irregular movements of heart.—Shocks in heart and intermittent palpitation, with suffocation.—Tension and stitches in the præcordial region, < by violent expiration.—Stitches at apex.—Sudden, spasmodic, bursting sensation about heart.—Feels as if a cap were over heart; spine affected.—Violent pulsations in blood-vessels during heat.—Rapid pulse.

20. **Neck and Back.**—Lancinating tearings, stiffness, and tension in nape.—Tearing in r. side of neck.—Nape of neck feels weary from writing or any exertion.—Spinal irritation with prostration; numbness of lower limbs.—Pains in loins, esp. when walking and seated.—Sensation of paralytic weakness in back and loins.—Rheumatic pains in back.—Itching tetters on back.—Tension and shootings in and between shoulder-blades.—Burning in scapulæ.—Pressive tension beneath the r. scapula.—Burning pressure upon spine above small of back.—Burning along whole spine, < when sitting.—Pains at last dorsal vertebra.—Violent, long-lasting ache about last lumbar vertebræ.—Stiffness and pain in upper dorsal muscles.—Pushing, aching, at times pinching

pains in coccyx ; lancinating in sacrum ; pressive tension and weakness in lumbar and sacral regions.

21. Limbs.—Tearing in limbs, < when over-heated or when taking exercise.—Drawing tearing in hollow bones, with pain so violent that the limbs can give no support.—Stiffness of joints, with sharp, lancinating pains above joints, always transverse, not lengthwise of the limb.—Coldness of extremities.—Drawing, tearing pains in all limbs.—Violent itching in all joints.—Spasmodic pain and cramp in the limbs.—Visible quivering and jerking in different parts of the muscles.—Tingling in the limbs.

22. Upper Limbs.—Rheumatic drawing and lancinating tearing in shoulders, arms, elbows, joints of hands and fingers.—Painful sensation of paralysis in arms.—Furunculi in arms.—Burning in l. forearm at night.—Paleness and paralysis of hands.—Weakness and trembling of the hands when writing.—Spasmodic tension in r. hand.—Lameness and deadness of hands ; they look bluish.—Herpetic, rough, and itching spots on hands.—Dry skin, with rhagades on hands.—Dry herpes on the hands and fingers ; they are rough and itch.—Chilblains itch and swell.—Cracks between the fingers.—Numbness of fingers when rising in morning.

23. Lower Limbs.—Rheumatic drawings and tearings in legs, knees, ankles and joints of the feet.—Varices in thighs and legs.—Legs œdematous.—Itching of thighs and hollow of knees.—Tensive pain in knees.—Nocturnal pains in knees.—Sensation as if the blood did not circulate in the legs.—Drawing and tensive stiffness in calves when walking.—Tingling in calves.—Burning pain in tibia.—Erysipelatous inflammation and swelling of tendo Achillis.—Intolerable boring pain in heel after drinking wine.—Stiffness of joint of the foot after being seated for some time.—Wrenching pain in joints of feet and toes.—Burning sensation in feet.—Inflammatory swelling of feet.—Weakness and trembling of feet.—Paralysis of feet : from spinal or chronic nervous disease, softening of brain or cerebral hæmorrhage ; from suppressed foot-sweat.—Feet sweaty and sore about toes ; fetid suppressed foot-sweat with much nervous excitement.—Coldness of the feet at night.—Nervous, fidgety movement of the feet ; after retiring and during sleep.—Tearing in margin of r. foot.—Painful chilblains on feet.—Itching, heat, redness, and swelling of toes as if they were frozen.—Pulsative lancinations in toes.—Sprained pain in bends of toe-joints.—Ulcerative, boring pains in heels ; < when walking than when sitting.—Profuse sweat on the feet.

24. Generalities.—[Affections in general appearing in the l. inguinal ring ; l. side of back ; upper jaw, and troubles of the teeth in lower jaw ; loins ; posterior surface of thigh ; tendo Achillis ; big toe ; joints of toes.—Patient can't keep still, must be in motion all the time.—Chilblains of the hand, much swollen, very painful.—In fevers or nervous complaints one keeps the feet in continual motion.—Variable mood ; clay-like sediment in the urine ; biting, pungent pain ; lancinating pains ; exanthema of long standing, esp. with a biting sensation.—< In the evening, sometimes lasting all night ; after swallowing food.—> While eating.—H. N. G.]—Pain as from excoriation.—Varices.—Pain, which sometimes seems to be between the skin and the flesh.—Formication on the skin.—The symptoms are aggravated to an extraordinary degree by *Chamomile, Nux,* and wine, substances which also excite them, particularly the nocturnal uneasiness and constipation.—The majority of the symptoms manifest themselves after dinner and towards evening.—Sensation of soreness in internal and external parts.—General insensibility of the body.—Sensation of coldness in bones.—Violent pulsation throughout body.—Violent trembling (twitching) of whole body, esp. after mental emotion.—Twitching of children.—Chorea.—Heaviness, lassitude, and excessive weakness, < when walking or on waking in morning.—Aversion to movement.

25. **Skin.**—Itching in bends of joints.—Itching, with violent lancinations, esp. in evening in bed, disappearing immediately on being touched.—Tingling between the skin and the flesh.—Chronic eruptions.—Eczema of back of r. hand with terrible irritation, little oozing and fissuration, < in cold weather and excited by rubbing (R. T. C.).—Tetters and herpetic ulcers.—Ganglia, chilblains, and liability of the external parts to become frozen.—Rhagades.—Small furunculi.—Varicose veins.

26. **Sleep.**—Sleep by day, and continued disposition to sleep, esp. in morning or after a meal; with inclination to yawn.—Unconquerable drowsiness.—Retarded sleep.—Disturbed sleep, with frequent waking.—Unrefreshing sleep (with unpleasant dreams).—Fantastic, frightful, agitated, or disgusting and terrific dreams, with talking and cries during sleep.—Excessive coldness of the feet at night.—Shocks in body during sleep and frequent starts.

27. **Fever.**—Febrile shuddering along back.—Constant shivering, with increased internal heat.—Chill begins generally after eating, and continues till late in evening and during the night.—Chilliness in open air and when touching a cold object.—Chilliness on approach of stormy weather.—Febrile shuddering, with flushes of heat; violent trembling of limbs, short and hot breath, and pulsation throughout the body.—Pulse small and rapid in the evening, slower in morning and during the day.—Pulse at times intermitting.—Violent pulsations in the veins during the heat.—Internal heat, with sensation of coldness in abdomen and on feet.—Tendency to perspire in the day.—Night-sweat.—Profuse perspiration during whole night, with inclination to uncover oneself.—Badly-smelling perspirations.—[" Brass-founders ague," which is supposed to be due to inhalation of Zinc fumes, begins with malaise and feeling of constriction across the chest, nausea occasionally, the symptoms occurring in after part of day are followed in evening at bed-time by shivering, sometimes by an indistinct hot stage, but always by profuse sweating; the worse the sweating, the less violent the attack; attacks always irregular. (R. T. C.).]

Zincum Aceticum.

Acetate of Zinc. $Zn(C_2H_3O_2)_2 3H_2O$. Solution.

Clinical.—Diarrhœa. Erysipelas. Gastritis. Night-watching, effects of. Toothache.

Characteristics.—*Zn. ac.* was proved by Hahnemann and others. The most *Peculiar Symptoms* were these: " Brain feels sore and as if sprinkled with salt." " Throat seems too tight and tongue too short."

There was toothache < by touch. Shaking chill during and after vomiting. Empty, hungry sensation. Pain and paralytic condition of arms. The symptoms were < in evening. < By motion. < Walking in open air. The only clinical uses of *Zn. ac.* I am acquainted with I learned from Burnett. He used Rademacher's solution of Zinc in Acetic Acid, and gave 5-drop doses three times a day in water to nurses and others who were compelled to work on an insufficient amount of sleep. I have verified the great utility of this. Another use to which Burnett put it was in erysipelas of old people. In the provers it produced a pustular eruption on forehead and knee; and the latter was attended with voluptuous itching.

Causation.—Night-watching.

SYMPTOMS.

1. **Mind.**—Anxious, quiet, does not speak a word; asked how she feels, says, "Let me alone, I shall soon be better."

2. **Head.**—Heaviness of head.—Throbbing headache, as if it would come out at forehead.—Frontal headache, as if brain sore and sprinkled with salt.—Dull, sticking, painful sensation in forehead.—Stitches: in forehead; needle-like in l. temple.

4. **Ears.**—L. ear swollen internally, painful on inserting finger and on external touch.

6. **Face.**—Face pale; look anxious.

8. **Mouth.**—Tearing pain in teeth, esp. when touched.—Blister on fore-part of gum, painful as if burnt.—Mouth feels burnt.—Bitter taste in mouth.

9. **Throat.**—Throat feels too tight and tongue too short.

11. **Stomach.**—Eructations: empty; ineffectual; sour, with shaking chill; tasting of food eaten three hours before.—Nausea followed by needle-like stitches in throat, then vomiting of bitter, sour mucus, whereby the sticking was <; afterwards chilliness of back.—Vomit with salivation.—Sensation of a small swelling in pit of stomach, painful to touch, previous to menses.—Pressure; and sticking in pit of stomach, < by motion, late in evening.—Empty, hungry sensation two hours after dinner.

12. **Abdomen.**—Violent griping in abdomen, obliged to lie down.

13. **Stool and Anus.**—Urging to stool a few times at night, followed by pasty stool.—Diarrhœa every hour during day.—Diarrhœa of black colour after dinner.

14. **Urinary Organs.**—Urethra: contraction of; biting in.—Frequent increased desire to urinate and irritation to urinate (like a burning).—Much watery urine.

18. **Chest.**—Much mucus comes from chest in afternoon, with a kind of nausea.

20. **Back.**—Back much affected, on stooping sudden shooting in it as if all strength had left him.

22. **Upper Limbs.**—Weakness in both arms.—Pain in l. arm, heavy, wrist hurts, no position easy at night (from injection into urethra).—Drawing, trembling, loss of power in r. arm.—Pressing, tearing, and stitches in muscles of r. arm during rest and motion.—Pressing pain in ball of r. hand.

23. **Lower Limbs.**—Pressive sticking in muscles of l. thigh while walking in open air.—Tensive pain in upper r. calf while walking in open air.

24. **Generalities.**—She wishes to walk, contrary to habit.—Frequent alternation between sitting and walking about.—Feels bad in afternoon.—(Effects of insufficient sleep.)

25. **Skin.**—Papular eruption filled with pus on forehead and neck; when opened it discharged pus and blood (from external application to urethra).—Red, papular eruption about both knees, which caused a tickling and voluptuous itching.—(Erysipelas of old people.)

26. **Sleep.**—Sleepy during day, frequent yawning.

27. **Fever.**—Shaking chill; during and after vomiting.—Several times a day feels hot, as though throat had been burnt with alcohol.—Burning heat in face, evening, and heat over whole face and redness of cheeks without sweat.—Night-sweat.

Zincum Bromatum.

Bromide of Zinc. Zincic bromide. $ZnBr_2$. Solution.

Clinical.—Chorea. Dentition. Hydrocephalus.

Characteristics.—Hale has used *Zn. br.* on its double indications for teething children who suffer intensely from pain in nerves of head and face, pains which throw the children into a state of stupor alternating with wakefulness. He uses the 3rd and 6th attenuations.

Zincum Cyanatum.

Cyanide of Zinc. Zincic Cyanide. $Zn(CN)_2$. Trituration. (Low attenuations should be freshly made.)

Clinical.—Chorea. Convulsions. Epilepsy. Hysteria. Meningitis. Paralysis agitans. Petit mal.

Characteristics.—*Zn. cy.* produces the nervous and mental symptoms of *Zn.* with great intensity, and it has been chosen in consequence as the salt for use in convulsions and paralytic conditions in which *Zn.* is indicated. The few symptoms of Kopp's proving show its suitability.

SYMPTOMS.

1. **Mind.**—Great excitement.—Bad temper.—Great sensitiveness.

2. **Head.**—Congestion to head.

6. **Face.**—Face suddenly changes colour.

13. **Stool and Anus.**—Constipation.

24. **Generalities.**—Great physical agitation.—General trembling from time to time.

Zincum Iodatum.

Iodide of Zinc. Zincic iodide. ZnI_2. Solution in syrup. Trituration.

Clinical.—Constipation. Cough. Phthisis.

Characteristics.—*Zn. i.* has been proved by American provers, and some well-defined symptoms were produced (*C. D. P.*). Among them were: Splinter-like pain in throat. Coldness in stomach and bowels with tendency to perspire. A cough from tickling in the throat, and the more he coughed the worse the tickling became. A peculiar tingling in right side of face to vertex, with tension in skin of the part. Undulating pain at border of right free ribs, extending to third rib on same side.

Relations.—*Compare:* Splinter pain in throat, Hep., Arg. n. The more he coughs the < it tickles, Ign.

SYMPTOMS.

1. **Mind.**—Brain seems clouded, hard to remember what he reads.

2. **Head.**—Vertigo and belching of wind, attended with coldness in lumbar region.

5. **Nose.**—At 8.30 a.m. constant tickling in nose, causing ineffectual desire to sneeze.

6. **Face.**—Peculiar tingling r. side of face, extending to vertex; skin of same region feels tense.

8. **Mouth.**—Taste in mouth like carbonate of soda.

9. **Throat.**—Splinter-like pain in throat at intervals.

11. **Stomach.**—Emptiness in pit of stomach accompanied all symptoms.—Coldness in stomach and bowels, with tendency to perspire.

12. **Abdomen.**—Cold sweat in umbilical and lumbar regions.—Lancinating pains in r. groin.

13. **Stool and Anus.**—Constipation; ineffectual efforts for stool; stool when passed scanty and insufficient.

17. **Respiratory Organs.**—Tickling in throat giving rise to a dry cough: the more he coughs the worse the tickling becomes.

18. **Chest.**—Painful undulation from free border of r. ribs up to 3rd r. rib.—Tingling in region of l. nipple.

20. **Back.**—Slight pain in l. lumbar region.—Coldness (and cold sweat) in lumbar region.—Aching in lumbar vertebræ.

21. **Limbs.**—Trembling feeling in lower limbs, later in arms.—Tired, aching sensation in legs and arms.

22. **Upper Limbs.**—Cold, clammy sweat of palms.

23. **Lower Limbs.**—Cramp-like pain in l. thigh.—Shifting, crampy pains in muscles of legs.—Creeping sensation in backs of legs and soles of feet.

25. **Skin.**—Skin very dry ; scattered over face are scaling patches, giving the appearance of whitish spots.

26. **Sleep.**—Very sleepy, with slight headache.—Slept very uneasily.

27. **Fever.**—Coldness : in stomach and bowels ; umbilical and lumbar regions.—Tendency to sweat.—Cold sweat on palms.

Zincum Muriaticum.

Chloride of Zinc. Zincic Chloride. $ZnCl_2$. Solutions in water or alcohol.

Clinical.—Bright's disease. *Constipation.* Convulsions. Cramps. Diphtheria. Dysentery. Emaciation. Hæmatemesis. Hiccough. *Hydrocephalus.* Smell, perverted. Taste perverted. Typhoid fever. Wounds.

Characteristics.—The bulk of the symptoms of *Zn. m.* are derived from poisoning cases. Chloride of Zinc is an active poison and a powerful disinfectant, and being readily accessible in the form of "Sir Wm. Burnett's Disinfectant Fluid," has occasioned many poisonings, both accidental and suicidal. Most of the symptoms are the usual effects of a corrosive poison, but some characteristic symptoms appear. One of them was the perversion of the senses of smell and taste : Things had a putrid smell and taste which were not putrid ; and fæces had no odour at all. Quinine had no bitter taste, and acids and alkalies had no acid or alkaline taste. Insipid things were most relished. Other symptoms were : "No natural appetite, but a morbid craving for something to allay the irritation at the stomach." "Vomiting of all food except boiled milk." "Occasional attacks of tetanic spasms of right forearm and hand." "Emaciation ; skin looked as if stretched tightly over bones of face and hands." "Bluish and blue-mottled skin." "Sleeps on right side with legs drawn up, grinds teeth." Spasmodic twitchings of face and hands, sprains and convulsions were prominent features. De Noë Walker used a dilution of *Zn. m.* as an application to fresh wounds, and found it very effectual in securing rapid healing.

SYMPTOMS.

1. **Mind.**—Excessive nervous derangement and prostration.—Picks bedclothes.—Anxiety, dulness.—Depressed.—Intellect clear by day, wanders at night.—Semi-comatose.

2. **Head.**—Vertigo : and fainting ; and rush of blood to head.—Headache, occipital and frontal.

3. **Eyes.**—Eyes sunken.—Pupils : widely dilated ; contracted.—Sight lost.

5. **Nose.**—Smell perverted : putrid and fæcal matter had no odour ; scents smelt like hemlock ; meats if the least bit burnt smelt intolerably putrid.

6. **Face.**—Face: distorted with agony and livid; pale and anxious; dusky; flushed; convulsed and twitching.—Swelling of lips, with thick, transparent mucus adhering.—Vesication of lips and tongue.

8. **Mouth.**—Toothache in carious teeth.—Gums: spongy; red and covered with white sordes.—Tongue: coated with white fur; thick yellow fur; intensely red; covered with brown sordes.—Frothing at mouth.—Peculiar fetor of breath.—Taste: astringent; metallic; perverted not less than the sense of smell, roast things intolerable, most foods, esp. *raw* oysters, tasted of burnt flour, quinine was not bitter, nor acids acid.

9. **Throat.**—Throat: inflamed; painful; burning.—Diphtheritic-like membrane on fauces.—Constriction of throat.—Burning along œsophagus.—Swallowing difficult.

11. **Stomach.**—No natural appetite, had a morbid craving to allay irritation of stomach.—Anorexia.—Constant thirst, but aversion to swallowing any fluids.—Nausea.—Vomiting: distressing; violent; of all food except boiled milk; of shreds of membrane; most offensive; of blood.—In stomach: clawing and burning pain.

12. **Abdomen.**—Severe pain in l. hypochondrium, < by food.—Abdomen shrunken, edge of liver sharply defined.—Intense abdominal pain and tenderness.

13. **Stool and Anus.**—Diarrhœa: violent, with vomiting and collapse.—Stools: thin, dark brown; fetid; coffee-ground; pitchy; olive-green; pale, clayey, dry, crumbling.—Constipation.

14. **Urinary Organs.**—Nephritis (*H. W.*, xxxii. 428).—Urine excessive, seven pints in five hours.

17. **Respiratory Organs.**—Voice: in whispers; lost.—Breathing: difficult; thoracic, rapid.

19. **Heart.**—Pain in præcordial region; pulse rapid, fluttering.

21. **Limbs.**—Tremor in limbs.

22. **Upper Limbs.**—Spasmodic pains at shoulders and back.—Tetanic spasms occasionally in r. forearm and hand.

23. **Lower Limbs.**—Legs drawn up on belly.—Severe cramps.

24. **Generalities.**—Emaciation extreme.—Nervous prostration, hyperæsthesia.—Spasmodic movements of muscles of face and arms.—Convulsions.—Faintness.—Collapse.

25. **Skin.**—Skin: dusky; ghastly bluish green; harsh and dry, with odour as in starvation; bluish mottled; dry; hot.—Skin of legs covered with thick scales.

26. **Sleep.**—Utter inability to sleep.—Slept restlessly, lying always on r. side with legs drawn up, and ground teeth during sleep.

27. **Fever.**—Surface cold, wet, and clammy.—Alternations of cold and heat.—Complained of cold though skin moderately warm to touch.—Forehead bathed in sweat, general surface warm.—Cold, clammy sweat.

Zincum Oxydatum.

Flowers of Zinc. Oxide of Zinc. Zincic oxide. ZnO. Trituration.

Clinical.—Coryza. Debility. Deltoid, pain in. Diaphragm, neuralgia in. Elbow, pain in. Hiccough. Hypochondriasis. Laughter, involuntary. Sleeplessness.

Characteristics.—An extensive proving of *Zn. o.* was made by Wernek, Buchner, and Michaelis. These symptoms have been included by Allen in the pathogenesis of *Zincum*, and some of them will be found in my Schema of *Zincum*. Jahr kept a separate record of *Zn. o.* I append his account. The contracting, shrivelling-up effect of Zinc was marked in these provings. Among the more *Peculiar Symptoms* were: Undulating movement in some muscles. Contraction of the risible muscles and constant impulse to laugh. Teeth blunted; incisors feel soft and glued together. Hiccough, > after regurgitation of bile. Liquid stools which > all symptoms. In these provings the *left* lung was very markedly affected. There was coryza < after a meal, with difficulty of respiration and nasal secretion. Stoppage of the nose was much complained of. Anorexia > after a meal. Farrington says *Zn. o.* is very like *Con.* in hypochondriasis and melancholy from masturbation, the difference being that *Zn. o.* is irritating as well as weakening and depressing.

SYMPTOMS.

1. **Mind.**—Anguish and agitation, as from a consciousness of having committed some crime.—Ill-humour, sometimes very great.—Unfitness for serious occupation.—Spasmodic laughter (sardonic).

2. **Head.**—Confusion in head: on awaking, with vertigo; with aching in forehead, in occiput, with heaviness; giddiness; violent, with transient heat.—Vertigo, sometimes with transient heat.—Headache: with slight vertigo; tension in forehead, sometimes with pressure; at night, lancinations and tearing pains in r. side of head, above temple.

4. **Ears.**—Pulsation and noise in ears, esp. in l., with increased secretion of liquid cerumen and hardness of hearing.

5. **Nose.**—Tickling in nose and impulse to sneeze.—Inability to breathe through nose (nose stopped), with anxiety and oppression; or else as during a violent coryza.—Coryza < after a meal, with difficulty of respiration and nasal secretion.

6. **Face.**—Paleness of complexion; convulsive drawing in facial muscles, sometimes with constant nausea; or else with contraction of the risible muscles, and constant impulse to laugh.—Dryness of lips.

7. **Teeth.**—Teeth as if blunted on closing them; the incisors appear to be soft and glued together.

8. **Mouth.**—Flow of an acrid and bitter water into mouth; frequent flow of saliva, with nausea; salivation increased.

9. **Throat.**—Pressure in throat; accumulation of mucus, with tickling in larynx.

10. Appetite.—Anorexia: total, with violent thirst; at breakfast, with loathing, > after a meal.—Disgust, which, however, may be overcome.—Ardent thirst.—Strong desire for cold water, which affords great relief.

11. Stomach.—Frequent risings: empty; bitter; after partaking of broth, with hiccough.—Regurgitations: of a yellow, bitter, bilious water after a meal.—Violent hiccough, ceasing after a regurgitation of bile.—Nausea: after supper, proceeding from the stomach, with acidulated taste in mouth and flow of acid water; with heat, followed by vertigo; with transient heat, spasmodic pulse, and general depression.—Nausea, with loathing.—Retching, with risings and want to evacuate.—Vomiting: often sudden and involuntary, in the case of children; of a mucous water after the nausea, succeeded by another fit of nausea, and then the headaches are dissipated; bilious vomiting, sometimes very violent, of a yellow colour and bitter; vomiting and diarrhœa.—Pressure in stomach: after supper, with risings; spasmodic, sometimes chiefly in pit of stomach, or else with tension and sensitiveness of the stomach; burning pain in region of stomach, sometimes with loathing.—Fulness of stomach, sometimes with sweat on hands and head, followed by easy vomiting of contents of stomach, which are rather acrid, and occasioning a burning of the parts touched; the throat also preserves a long time afterwards a sensation of roughness, which is succeeded by a keen appetite.—Lancinations in diaphragm.

12. Abdomen.—Colicky pains below navel, tearing pains from side to side until evening; dull pain in umbilical region; spasmodic drawing in abdomen, with dull pain.—Lancinations in hepatic region.—Pinchings in abdomen.—Inflation of abdomen.—Borborygmi in abdomen, sometimes with aching.—Boil above the genital parts, first red then dark-blue, with hard areola; later, discharge of a yellow foul pus, after which the areola remains for a long time, red and hard.

13. Stool.—Liquid stools: with tenesmus and pinchings in abdomen, and followed by a marked > of all symptoms.

17. Respiratory Organs.—Abundant accumulation of mucus in larynx, with dryness of throat and constant want to hawk, with viscid and mucous saliva.—Impeded respiration, esp. in the l. lung.

18. Chest.—Great oppression of chest.—Constriction of the entire thorax.—Spasmodic sensation in lungs and heart.—Spasmodic aching in chest and pit of stomach.—Lancinations in l. side of chest, sometimes with aching, or else with soreness of the l. nipple.—The l. lung is affected.—Externally ribs painful to touch.

19. Heart.—Frequent palpitation of heart, with anguish, sometimes chiefly in evening, and with spasmodic pulse; pulsations more rapid.—Sensation of pressure, weight, and spasmodic tension in the heart itself.

20. Back.—Sacral pains: at night on turning body in bed; on stooping, extending to lumbar vertebræ.—Sensation of paralysis, extending to hips.—Tearings and lancinations between shoulders; or else pains extending to loins and sacrum.—Throbbing below l. shoulder-blade.—Pressure on the shoulders on waking in morning, with confusion in head.

21. Limbs.—Drawing pain in the limbs, sometimes with sacral pains.—Tearing pains in limbs.—Tingling which passes along limbs.—Undulating movement in some muscles.—Trembling of limbs, sometimes with jerking of muscles of legs.—Lassitude in limbs.

22. Upper Limbs.—Arms: Pain as if broken, sometimes chiefly in deltoid muscle, or else in bend of elbow; heaviness and paralytic aching in the bend of the l. elbow.

23. Lower Limbs.—In lower extremities: permanent debility, pain as if broken, sometimes chiefly in the l. leg, or else in joints of hip and knee; pulsations in the l. buttock; tension in the l. leg, in the l. knee-joint, frequent tingling in l. foot; drawing pains in the bones; trembling of the feet.

24. Generalities.—Tension in muscles and painful sensation during movement; pain throughout body > during repose; pains in all limbs.—Depressed state of whole body, sometimes with lassitude.—Perceptible failing of the strength, sometimes with general internal uneasiness.—Conversation occasions fatigue.—Turgor vitalis sensibly diminished.

26. Sleep.—Very restless nights.—Agitated sleep, with concourse of dreams of all kinds; with dreams of fire, of falling, of false coin; with fanciful ideas, and towards morning general perspiration.

27. Fever.—Sensation of coldness: of the extremities; constant, with general uneasiness; followed by febrile movement throughout the body, with shuddering and drawing pains in back; with shivering of whole body.—Shivering which passes over the whole body.—Coldness of hands and feet.—Shuddering over the whole abdomen, with retching.—Pulse small and hard, sometimes to a very great degree; spasmodic, and sometimes small at the same time; wiry, accelerated, irregular, hard, and dull.—Perspiration, esp. towards morning, sometimes while sleeping.

Zincum Phosphoricum.

Phosphide of Zinc. Zincic Phosphide. Zn_3P_2. Trituration.

Clinical.—Brain-fag. Delirium tremens. Headache. Herpes zoster. Impotence. Kidneys, irritable. *Neuralgia*. Paralysis. Sleeplessness. Tremors, mercurial.

Characteristics.—Ashburton Thompson gave pills, each containing $\frac{2}{3}$ gr. of *Zn. ph.*, to two patients, and both experienced a severe frontal headache with frequent stabs of pain backward, deep in the head, to occiput. Hale has used it on a combination of the indications of the elements, and especially in brain-fag of business men. Hammond has cured with it nervousness, and vertigo > lying down. In some patients the 3rd potency has caused sexual excitement and sleeplessness after 3 a.m. According to him, *Zn. ph.* removes the mental depression and paralysis following cerebral congestion and apoplexy. J. E. Baldwin (*N. A. J. H.*, xiii. 266) reports this case: A lady in perfect health prepared a long report and read it to a large audience without undue excitement. Next day had some pressure in occiput to cervical spine, lasting four days. Feeling of fatigue with disinclination to any mental exertion. *Zn. ph.* 2x cured in a few doses. *Zn. ph.* 6x has cured irritable kidney with loss of memory in an old man.

SYMPTOMS.

2. Head.—(Vertigo > lying down.)—Severe frontal headache, accompanied by frequent stabs of pain, apparently darting from before backward to occiput, but intra-cranial, and not attended with altered sensation in scalp.—Bursting headache.

11. Stomach.—Vomiting.

14. Urinary Organs.—(Irritable kidneys with loss of brain-power even when calculus is present.)

15. Male Sexual Organs.—Erections with unusual voluptuousness and desire.—Emissions with voluptuous dreams and intense nervous thrill.

18. Chest.—Neuralgic pains and skin symptoms like those of zoster (Mohr, *M. A.*, xxi. 259).

26. Sleep.—Sleepless after 3 a.m.; "it wakes me at three, and I feel as if under the influence of pleasant and quick music" (from third trit.)

Zincum Picricum.

Picrate of Zinc. $Zn[C_6H_2(NO_2)_3O]_2$. Trituration.

Clinical.—Bright's disease; headaches of. Exhaustion. Facial paralysis. Headaches. Nymphomania. Paralysis agitans. Priapism. Satyriasis. Seminal emissions. Spinal weakness.

Characteristics.—Hale gives this indication of *Zn. pi.*: "Cerebro-spinal troubles of the erethistic character." Hugh Pitcairn (quoted *H. W.*, xix. 366) gives these indications: (1) Brain-fag. (2) Nervous exhaustion from over-worked brain or sexual excess. (3) Chronic occipital headaches, periodic. (4) Headache occurring in Bright's disease. (5) Threatened cerebral paralysis, especially in children. (6) Profound neurasthenia, when nervous exhaustion has passed beyond stage of erethism. (7) Seminal emissions. (8) Erotomania. He gives this case: Mr. M., 36, merchant. Above ordinary intelligence. Single; correct in his habits, but subject to seminal emissions since early manhood, occurring about 3 a.m. every third night, leaving him very weak and debilitated; < every change of weather, especially in hot weather and before and during thunderstorms. Never masturbated. Complains of loss of memory and energy; dull, heavy feeling in head; sticky, pasty mouth; dry throat, poor appetite. Belches torrents of tasteless flatus after eating, followed by relief and diarrhœa. At other times inclined to constipation. Languid, heavy feeling throughout body. Dull, aching pain in back. *Zn. pi.* 2nd trit. caused steady improvement, the emissions being reduced in frequency to one in six weeks. Halbert (*Clinique*; *H. W.*, xxxiv. 511) reports: (1) A case of recent facial paralysis from cold cured by *Zn. pi.* 3x, and (2) Paralysis agitans in lady, 45, very greatly improved by the same.

Relations.—*Compare*: Fag, Pic. ac., Fe. pic., and picrates generally.

Zincum Sulphuricum.

White Vitriol. Sulphate of Zinc. Zincic Sulphate. $ZnSO_4 7H_2O$.
Solution. Trituration.

Clinical.—*Convulsions.* Cornea, opacity of. Dysentery. Granular lids. *Headache.* Heartburn. Laughter, involuntary. Metrorrhagia. Œsophagus, stricture of. Prurigo. Tongue, paralysis of.

Characteristics.—A large number of poisonings with *Zn. s.* are on record, and these have furnished the symptoms of the Schema. The use of *Zn. s.* in solution as an eye lotion is founded on a specific relationship, and in homœopathic attenuations it has cured corneal opacities. Severe gastric and dysenteric symptoms were induced, and *Zn. s.* has cured many cases of dysentery. Farrington says it is chiefly in subacute cases that it is indicated, when the pains are confined to the *sides* of the abdomen, probably to the colon. *Peculiar Symptoms* are : Burning, acute pain in head. Immediately sensation as if a strong electric shock passed through head, he expected his brains would have burst through his skull. Abdomen contracted. She felt as if the blood could scarcely struggle through the veins. Titillation all over, with an irresistible desire to laugh. A " milk-like pallor of the surface looks like a characteristic." Gerstel (*H. R.*, x. 155) relates this case, treated by Arnold : A lady had suffered from headache from childhood. During childhood she was unable to study in consequence of it. Menses began in her sixteenth year, were weak and irregular, recurring only every six weeks. In her eighteenth year she had serious inflammation of the brain, with unconsciousness, and was treated by venesection and leeches. When Arnold saw her she was married and a mother, the state being as follows : Dull, pressive pain running right across forehead, as if head compressed in a vice. (Formerly it had been more throbbing and shooting.) Eyes inflamed. Forehead red and swollen. She was compelled to lie down, and had most frightful visions, saw her child with its head shattered, while she heard everything that passed around her. It required a strong effort to realise the emptiness of the visions. With them the headache reached its highest point, an abatement would follow, then sleep. The head during the attacks was cold and dry to touch. The acute stage lasted one day, but the whole attack fourteen days, during which time the pain would increase and decrease, and the patient was well satisfied if it was bearable. Pain < at times when menses should appear ; a few days before and after menses painful burning and sensation of weakness in spine. She did not look ill, and had a good colour. *Puls.* did her no good. *Bell.* 6 strengthened the periods and diminished the frequency and severity of her headaches considerably ; but she was *now seized with an irresistible drowsiness*, and troubled with a frequently recurring vomiting. *Zn. s.* 2nd trit. was given for sixteen days, one dose daily, then intermitted for eight days. The headaches now appeared before, during, and after the period in a *moderate* degree but in the intermediate time she was free from pain. *Zn. s.* was repeated in the same way three times, and then she was free from all pain. She wrote the doctor three months later, "You have radically cured me of a great bodily ailment, and what is more, you have saved my mind from a yet more dreadful one."

SYMPTOMS.

1. **Mind.**—Delirium.—Great nervous anxiety and depression.—Frightful visions during headache; saw her child with its head shattered (cured with the headache).

2. **Head.**—Dizziness.—Headache: violent, with thirst.—Burning, acute pain in head.—Immediately felt as if a painful electric shock had gone through his head; he expected his brains would have burst through his skull.

3. **Eyes.**—Bluish rings round eyes.—Eyes: heavy, dull; staring; fixed, with peculiar bright lustre; convulsed, with upper limbs.—Lachrymation.—Obstinate keratitis in r. eye goes away from a 3x lotion (R. T. C.).—Diffuse opacity of each cornea goes away on using a lotion round both orbits externally.—Pupils dilated.

4. **Ears.**—Roaring in ears.

6. **Face.**—Face: pale; sunken; with cold extremities and convulsed pulse; leaden tint, contracted features.

8. **Mouth.**—Tongue: moist, a little blanched; partially paralysed.—Tongue, mouth, and lips greatly swollen.—Gums swollen and red on outer edge.—Irritation of whole buccal membrane.—Very sour taste.

9. **Throat.**—Inflammation of throat, threatening suffocation.—Tenderness in throat.—Burning and constriction in fauces.—Œsophagus so contracted he fears choking.

11. **Stomach.**—Thirst: intolerable; and dry mouth.—Heartburn.—Vomiting; and purging; with cramps, severe pain, and burning in stomach, and extreme prostration.—Burning heat in stomach; with acute pain in epigastrium.

12. **Abdomen.**—Inflammation of abdomen, with retraction of umbilicus and terrible colic.—Sharp, continuous colic.—Pain: in abdomen and esp. in bladder region; in groin.

13. **Stool and Anus.**—Rectal tenesmus.—Constant desire for stool.—Purging and vomiting.—Bilious diarrhœa.—Stools infrequent.—After three months stools became bloody, with sticking and cutting pains in both sides of abdomen and along colon.—Obstinate dysentery, with emaciation; pale, bloody stools; painful tenesmus, and desire for food that failed to nourish (cured.—A. E. Small).

16. **Female Sexual Organs.**—Has been given for metrorrhagia (R. T. C).

17. **Respiratory Organs.**—Violent cough, with bloody and purulent expectoration.—Breathing: weak, slow; difficult.

18. **Chest.**—Pains in chest, with vomiting.—Violent burning pains beneath chest.—Sense of choking and constriction round chest.

19. **Heart.**—Palpitation on every motion.—Pulse: fluttering; indistinguishable; dicrotic; almost lost, as in cholera.

21. **Limbs.**—Trembling and cramps.

22. **Upper Limbs.**—Convulsive movements of upper limbs and eyeballs.

24. **Generalities.**—Anæmia.—Tremors.—Convulsions.—Prostration.—Heaviness.—Feeling as though her blood could scarcely struggle through her veins.—Titillation all over body, with irresistible inclination to laugh.

25. **Skin.**—Skin pale yellow.—Deadly pallor, skin milky white.—Blisters on neck discharge first bloody water, later thin, green, ill-smelling pus.—Frightful prurigo of chiidren affecting the back (cured with diluted lotion.—R. T. C.).

26. **Sleep.**—Sleepy and stupid, wanted to sleep and die in peace.

27. **Fever.**—Coldness.—Shivering: violently, and slight quivering of lips.—Skin and extremities cold and clammy.—Fever followed by profuse sweat.—Constant heat, preventing sleep.—Burning heat of extremities.—Profuse sweat.—Hands covered with cold, clammy sweat, but to herself they felt hot, and she tried to get hold of anything to cool them.

Zincum Valerianicum.

Valerianate of Zinc. Zincic Isovalerate. $Zn(C_5H_9O_2)_2$. Trituration.

Clinical.—Angina pectoris. Asthma. Brain-fag. Deltoids, pain in. Diarrhœa. Emaciation. Epilepsy. Hæmorrhoids. Hypochondriasis. Hystero-epilepsy. Priapism. Seminal emissions. Stiff-neck.

Characteristics.—*Zn. v.* is a favourite anti-hysteric medicine in old-school practice. There is one proving with substantial doses by C. B. Finney, which brought out a strong action on the genital sphere, the usual starting-point of hysteria. Finney had the brain-fag symptoms of *Zn.*, and gastro-intestinal disturbance. The abdominal pains waked him from sleep, and he had to rise at 6.30 to stool, which was partly fœcal and partly fluid. Later he was constipated and had tenesmus. Hale quotes C. Dradwick as saying that a considerable number of patients having piles, who were taking *Zn. v.* for other troubles, had their piles relieved by the remedy. Finney had distinct heart pains, and Hale mentions angina pectoris as having been cured by *Zn. v.* Other conditions named by him are: Prosopalgia, spinal neuralgia, sciatica, ovarian neuralgia, cerebro-spinal meningitis, and tubercular meningitis. *Zn. v.* is indicated in hysteria with fidgety feet; hypochondriasis; groundless fears. Hansen gives "epilepsy without aura." Finney had "Sensation as if a very heavy weight on chest"; and dull headache and stiffness of muscles of neck.

SYMPTOMS.

1. **Mind.**—Dulness of mind and headache with erections.—Great fulness of head, with difficult thinking.—Distressed mentally, mind all mixed up.

2. **Head.**—Slight pain in l. temple and l. mastoid process.—Fulness in head, esp. occiput.

3. **Eyes.**—Slight pain over r. eye, with dull headache.

5. **Nose.**—Hard sneezing.

8. **Mouth.**—Tongue coated white.

11. **Stomach.**—No appetite.—Belched up bitter fluid.—Woke with empty feeling in pit of stomach.

12. **Abdomen.**—Rose 6.30 a.m. with colicky pains.—Abdominal pains > by passing flatus.—Crampy pain in abdomen.—Drawing pain at umbilicus and sense of pressure in rectum when standing.—Pain in bowels while dressing and after breakfast.

13. **Stool and Anus.**—At 2 p.m. evacuation of fæcal matter, followed by watery flow, with pain in belly.—Pressure on rectum when standing.—At 6.30 had to get up to stool, which was small, brown, and mushy, discharged with much wind.—Ineffectual desire for stool.—Stool scanty, much tenesmus.

15. **Male Sexual Organs.**—Tendency to erections all day.—Strong erection 8.15 a.m.; with dulness of mind and headache.—Nocturnal emissions on several successive nights; after them weight and constriction in perinæum.

17. **Respiratory Organs.**—Spell of coughing, with sense of fulness in chest.

18. **Chest.**—Sensation as if very heavy weight lying on chest.

19. **Heart.**—Cramp-like pain in heart.

20. **Neck.**—Dull headache and stiffness of muscles of neck, lasting all evening.

22. **Upper Limbs.**—Pain in l. deltoid; later in r.

Zingiber.

Zingiber officinale. Ginger. *N. O.* Zingiberaceæ. Tincture of dried rhizome.

Clinical.—Albuminuria. Asthma. Breath, offensive. Deltoid rheumatism. Diarrhœa. Dropsy. Flatulence. Ozæna. Post-nasal catarrh. Seminal emissions. Spleen, pains in. Urine, suppressed.

Characteristics.—*Zng.* was proved by Franz and others, and their symptoms make a full pathogenesis. The genito-urinary and respiratory systems were strongly affected. Farrington says ginger is not a safe food to give in kidney affections, as it has caused Bright's disease. Prolonged retention of urine; or complete cessation of the function of the kidneys is an indication for *Zng.* In the provers it produced a cheerful, good-humoured state of mind; and when this occurs when the opposite might rather be expected, *Zng.* will probably be the remedy. For instance, in asthma, Farrington gives this indication: Asthma, of gastric origin; attacks come in the night, towards morning. Patient must sit up to breathe; but *despite the severity of the paroxysm, there is no anxiety.* The nasal mucous membrane is affected as markedly as that of the lungs. Ozæna and post-nasal catarrh are among the symptoms. Like most condiments, *Zng.* has a specific action on the digestive organs, causing flatulence and other symptoms of indigestion ; pressure in stomach as from a shot. *Zng.* has < from eating bread ; and especially from eating melons. It causes diarrhœa or constipation, and sets up some irritation of the rectum. *Peculiar Sensations* are : As if head too large. Confused and empty in head. As if contents of head pressed into forehead and root of nose on stooping. As if right eye were pressing out, with headache. As if a board pressing through head. As if head were pressed. As from a grain of sand in eye. As if there were an obstacle in throat to swallow over. As of a stone in stomach. Empty feeling in stomach. As if beaten in lower back. A shock-like moving downward as from a dropping fluid in left loin. Pain as from weakness in sacral region. Pain as from over-work in left deltoid. As from over-strung muscles in bend of knee. As if going to faint. The symptoms are : < By touch. < Lying. > Sitting ; standing. Motion <. Rising <. Laughing and talking < headache. < Evening and night. > Uncovering. < In cold air ; cold, damp air. < From bread : from melons.

Relations.—*Antidoted by :* Nux. *Compare :* Weight in stomach, Ab. n. Prepuce cold (Sul. glans cold). Wakes 3 a.m., Bels., Nux.

Causation.—Melons. Bread.

SYMPTOMS.

1. **Mind.**—Cheerful, good-humoured, a pleasing sensation in her system. —Asthma without anxiety.—Increased activity of brain.—Forgetful; weak memory.—Irritable and chilly in evening and during menses.—Nervous and fidgety.—Feet very uncomfortable, and did not know what to do.

2. **Head.**—Vertigo, limbs heavy.—Feels confused and empty in his head.—Head feels too large.—Frontal headache (drawing and pressive pains) over eyes and at root of nose ; also when he exerts himself.—Headache (pressure) < over l. eye ; aching (drawing) over eyebrows, followed by nausea; later over r. eye and pressing in l. occiput ; < in warm room, but continued in cold, damp air, in motion or sitting.—Pressive drawing headache as if r. eye pressing out.—Pain encircling head ; dull, heavy pain, like a board pressing through whole head, 11 a.m.—Heavy pressure in head from without inward, when walking in cold, damp air.—Hemicrania ; nervous headache.—Congestion of blood to head, esp. temples.—Itching on scalp, head, and cheeks.

3. **Eyes.**—Smarting and burning in eyes ; sensitive to light, with stinging pain in them ; feeling as of sand in eyes.—Pressure on eyes ; on l.—Weakness of sight ; dimness of cornea.

5. **Nose.**—Coryza, watery, sneezing, more in open air.—Insupportable itching, tingling in nostrils.—Dryness and obstruction in posterior nares, with discharge of thick mucus.—Ozæna.

6. **Face.**—Hot, red face.—Exhausted look, blue under eyes, before menses.—Dry lips and mouth.

7. **Teeth.**—Painful sensibility of teeth, with pressive, drawing pain in their roots.

8. **Mouth.**—Slimy, bad taste in mouth in morning.—Mouth smells foul to herself, as from disordered stomach.

9. **Throat.**—Dryness of throat and difficulty of swallowing, as from an obstruction, with dryness of posterior nares.—Increased mucous secretion ; no fever.

10. **Appetite.**—Much thirst ; mouth dry.—Headache and pressure in stomach after eating bread.—Complaints from eating melons.

11. **Stomach.**—Belching and diarrhœa.—Nausea ; vomiting of mucus in drunkards.—Acidity of stomach.—Weak digestion, stomach heavy, like a stone.

12. **Abdomen.**—Stitches in spleen.—Unbearable sore pain on a small place in r. side of abdomen.—Contractive pain passes through abdomen while standing ; soon after, desire for stool.—Sharp pain in l. iliac region.—Great flatulency ; in gouty persons.—Constipation.

13. **Stool and Anus.**—Diarrhœa : from drinking impure water ; of brown mucus ; < mornings ; < from deranged stomach ; from damp, cold weather.—Diarrhœa in morning, followed by nausea.—Belching with constipation.—Redness, inflammation, burning-itching at anus and higher up back.

14. **Urinary Organs.**—Increased secretion of urine.—Urine thick, turbid ; dark brown, of strong smell.—Retention of urine (after typhus).—Acute pain in orifice of urethra while urinating.—Dull aching in both kidneys, with frequent desire to urinate.—Dull aching, with sensation of heat in l. kidney ; < while sitting, with frequent desire to urinate.

15. **Male Sexual Organs.**—Itching on prepuce, which feels cold.—Painful erections.—Increased sexual desire ; nightly emissions.

16. **Female Sexual Organs.**—Menstruation too early and too profuse; irritable ; blood dark, clotted.

17. **Respiratory Organs.**—Burning, smarting sensation below larynx, followed by a cough, with rattling of phlegm, and sometimes with expectoration of thick mucus.—Asthma humidum.—Painful respiration ; < at night, must sit up in bed ; < two or three hours every morning ; asthma.—Dry, hacking cough, from tickling in larynx on l. side of throat ; from smarting or scratching ; with pain in lungs ; difficult breathing ; morning sputum, which is copious.

18. **Chest.**—Stitches in (through) chest ; pleuritic pains.

19. **Heart.**—Violent stinging-pressing pain in l. side of chest, in region of heart.

20. **Neck and Back.**—Stiffness of back of neck, with headache and nausea.—Backache, as from weakness ; < sitting and leaning against something ; lower part of back lame, as if beaten, or from walking or standing ; feels stiff.

21. **Limbs.**—Dull, heavy, lame feeling in limbs ; numbness.—Rheumatic, drawing pains.—Joints feel weak, stiff, lame.

22. **Upper Limbs.**—Rheumatic drawing in backs of hands.

23. **Lower Limbs.**—Painful swelling of feet.—Soreness of heels after standing a long time.

24. **Generalities.**—Foaming at mouth ; free urination ; spasms.—Faint, weak, wants to lie down.—Nervous, fidgety feeling at night.

26. **Sleep.**—Sleepy and exhausted ; coma.—Sleepless, wakes at 3 a.m. ; falls asleep again late in morning.

27. **Fever.**—Chilliness beginning in lower limbs, going upwards.—Chilly in evening.—Chilliness and sensibility in open air.—Hot and chilly at same time.

Zizia.

Zizia aurea. Thapsium aureum. Carum aureum. Meadow Parsnip. *N. O.* Umbelliferæ. Tincture of root.

Clinical.—Asthma. Brain, affections of. Catarrh. Chorea, in sleep. Convulsions. Dropsy. Epilepsy. Hypochondriasis. Hysteria. Influenza. Leucorrhœa. Menses, suppression of. Migraine. Ovary, intermittent neuralgia of. Pleurisy. Stye.

Characteristics.—The Meadow Parsnip is a common plant indigenous to the United States on the moist banks of streams and in open wet woods, where it flowers in June and July. Rafinesque speaks of it as vulnerary, antisyphilitic, and sudorific (Millspaugh). Marcy proved *Ziz.* on himself and some others, and symptoms of poisoning have been added. Exhilaration with increased physical strength was noted; but a slight amount of exercise caused fatigue. The spasms and convulsions of the Umbelliferæ were elicited. The generative organs in both sexes were excited. *Ziz.* is indicated in uterine affections characterised by increased nervous and vascular excitement. The menses are profuse, and followed by acrid leucorrhœa. Burning, smarting backache. Spasmodic movements of face and limbs. Mind first exhilarated, then depressed, finally indifferent. The restlessness of *Ziz.* runs into chorea; and the chorea has this distinguishing feature, that the movements continue or are even < during sleep. Connected with the uterine congestion there is migraine, the region of the right eye being most affected. There was rush of blood to the head. Marcy considered *Ziz.* especially suitable in brain affections; catarrhal, asthmatic, and pleuritic diseases; in ovarian neuralgia. Among *Peculiar Symptoms* are: Surface of body paler than natural; white, puffy appearance of whole body. Laughs and weeps alternately. One cheek red. Craves acids and stimulants. The symptoms are: < By touch. Pressure = pain in intercostal muscles; on stomach = nausea and faintness. < Lying; stooping; motion; coughing.

Relations.—*Antidoted by:* Puls. (migraine), Carb. an. (stye). *Compare:* One cheek red, Cham. Uterine congestion, backache, indifference, Sep. Chorea in sleep, Trn. As if in a dream, Amb., Anac., Calc., Can. i., Con., Cup., Med., Rhe., Val., Ver. Laughing alternately with weeping, Calc., Ign., Merc., Nux m., Puls., Stram.

SYMPTOMS.

1. **Mind.**—Exhilaration; like intoxication; followed by strong desire to sleep.—Depression following exhilaration.—Laughing and weeping alternately.—Depression followed by exhilaration.—Irritable, low-spirited, indif-

ferent.—Nervous irritability and depression, culminating in a paroxysm of self-dissatisfaction with weeping.—Indolence with contentment.—Behaviour quiet, with much apparent suffering and sadness.

2. **Head.**—Giddiness ; swimming ; light-headedness.—Rush of blood to head and face, with feeling of fulness.—Sensation of tightness round head.—Intensely painful, sharp headache over r. eye ; *Puls.* > first days, not later ; fully developed seventh day, must lie still in dark room ; < evening (the usual headache is < morning) ; associated with backache ; < by coughing.—Severe pain in r. temple, with nausea.—Pressure on top of brain.—Dull pain in occipital region, extending down neck muscles.

3. **Eyes.**—Redness of both eyes.—Pain affects r. eye most.—Shooting pains through orbits.—Sharp pain through r. orbit, < moving eyeballs, stooping, or stepping.—Eyelids agglutinated on rising by yellowish muco-purulent secretion.—Stye, r. lid.—Stye middle of upper lid, very painful, > *Carb. an.*—Eyes sensitive to light.

5. **Nose.**—Nasal catarrh, with sneezing and coughing from first inhalation.—Nasal discharge of thick mucus.—R. nostril congested, sore ; with injection of pharynx and conjunctiva.

6. **Face.**—Face : pale and puffy.—One cheek red, other pale.—Boring pains in cheek-bones.—Dull pains in jaws.—Painful tenderness in lower jawbone, an inch below root of ear.

8. **Mouth.**—Tongue : red and unusually sensitive to cold and warm drinks ; covered with whitish fur ; yellow fur on tongue and oppressed respiration ; broad, furred in middle, red at tip and sides.—Mouth dry.—Taste : bitter ; bilious.

9. **Throat.**—Mucus increased.—Slight redness of tonsils and palate, with soreness.—Inflamed pharynx.

11. **Stomach.**—Craving for acids and stimulants.—Appetite : diminished ; lost.—Thirst.—Nausea.—Vomiting : acid, bilious ; immoderately.—Stomach sensitive to touch ; pressure = nausea and faintness.

15. **Male Sexual Organs.**—Involuntary emission two nights in succession.—Excitement.—Lassitude and prostration after coitus, which had existed a long time, was completely removed in the proving.

16. **Female Sexual Organs.**—Increased vascular and nervous excitement.—Leucorrhœa : bland ; acrid ; acrid at first, later copious and bland.—Profuse menses one day, followed by acrid leucorrhœa.—Menses appeared in due time but ceased after twelve hours.—Sudden suppression of menses.

17. **Respiratory Organs.**—Roughness in upper part of larynx when inspiring or coughing.—Larynx raw from coughing.—Trachea sensitive to touch.—Dry cough, with shooting pains in chest.—Tight cough, from deep breath ; from dryness of larynx.—Short, dry cough, with severe stitching in r. side and sense of suffocation.—Breathing oppressed, cannot keep lying down.—Asthma.

18. **Chest.**—Severe pains in pleuræ.—Bruised feeling in muscles of chest.—Pressure = pain in intercostal muscles.—On and around xiphoid cartilage pain and tenderness to touch.—Dull, aching pain under r. scapula.—Severe shooting from front of thorax to scapula.—Sharp pains from sides and chest to both scapulæ.—Severe stitching pains accompanied by feverish symptoms.—Pleuritic stitches < by coughing or deep breath.

20. **Back.**—Pains in posterior margin of scapulæ, aching, smarting, stinging, with aching in small of back when at their worst.—Dull pains in loins, < by movement.—Smarting burning in small of back.

22. **Upper Limbs.**—Lameness in muscles of both arms, from shoulder to elbow.—Pricking sensation in r. arm, with steadily diminished sensibility of the part.

23. **Lower Limbs.**—Dragging sensation in both hips.—Unusually tired feeling in legs after slightest exertion.

24. **Generalities.**—Increased strength with inclination for exertion.—Aspect of grave and chronic illness.—Whole body white and puffy.—Œdema of face and ankles.—Convulsions, epilepsy.—Spasms, swooning convulsions, and fainting fits, ending in death in three hours.—Spasms of face and extremities.—Surface of body sensitive to touch.—Pains fixed, < by movement, noise, light, contact ; < evening.

25. **Skin.**—Itching pimples on forehead, wrists, and legs.

26. **Sleep.**—Drowsiness ; with sense of fatigue.—Sleep prevented by pains.—During sleep : spasmodic twitches ; talking ; unpleasant dreams.

27. **Fever.**—Chilliness and heat alternating with faintness, nausea, pain in r. temple, redness of eyeballs, dry and red tongue, and thirst for cold water.—Chilliness accompanied by spasmodic twitchings of muscles of face and upper limbs, followed by fever.—Fever, with headache, pain in back, thirst.—Fever with stitching pain in chest.—Some sense of heat and fulness in both cheeks.—Flushed cheeks, hot head, visible pulsations of carotid and temporal arteries, coldness of hands and feet, drowsiness and irritability.—Redness and heat of cheeks.—Hot flushes in face and head followed by perspiration.

END OF VOL. II.

A NEW APPENDIX

TO THE

DICTIONARY *of* PRACTICAL

MATERIA MEDICA

BY

JOHN HENRY CLARKE, M.D.

ISSUED AS A SEPARATE SUPPLEMENT TO THOSE DESIROUS OF ADDING TO THE VALUE OF THEIR PRESENT VOLUMES

CONTENTS

Calcarea Lactica.

Lactate of Lime. $Ca_6H_{10}O_6$, $5H_2O$. Trituration.

Clinical.—Chilblains. Headache. Migraine. Rhinitis. Sprue.

Characteristics.—With the introduction of colloidal preparations of the metals preparations of Calcium and its salts have come into much more general use in old-school practice of late, and valuable experiences have resulted which may be utilised by homœopaths, since they are all in agreement with the uses of the *Calcareas* of the Materia Medica. Remedies for sprue are not very numerous, and as *Calc. lact.* has been credited with cures of this troublesome complaint it should be kept in mind. It has been prescribed in the crude, but homœopaths may begin with eight-grain doses of the 3x trit. three or four times a day. Migraine is another sphere of its action. A Danish writer, C. I. Bȧastrup (quoted *Homœopathic World*, September 1923), described a type in which he found *Calc. lact.* "dramatically successful." It is accompanied by slight œdema affecting the eyelids, upper lip, or one hand. This is apt to run in families. The œdema is associated with no abnormal sensations. Baastrup suggests that the migraine may be due to an œdema of the meninges. He gives 1 gramme of *Calc. lact.* once or twice a day for three weeks. It not only removes the headache, " but also such troublesome symptoms as vasomotor rhinitis." That the action is homœopathic is proved by an experience recorded in *British Medical Journal*, December 22, 1923, and quoted *Homœopathic World*, July 1923. The writer was subject to a dull headache with sickness. Two years previously he took ten grains thrice daily of *Calc. lact.* " as a blood tonic." One day, " while conscientiously and methodically finishing my second bottle, I experienced a severe attack of migraine, starting with visual phenomena (zigzag lines and balls of light before the left eye), and finishing up with dizziness and a diabolical headache in r. temple." He had never had eye-symptoms with headache before, and a later repetition of the drug produced a similar effect.

Relations.—*Compare:* Kali bich. and Iris in migraine and Apis in œdema.

SYMPTOMS.

2. Head.—Migraine with œdema, visual disorders and dizziness.

3. Eyes.—Zigzags and balls of light before left eye, followed by dizziness and violent headache in r. temple.

5. Nose.—Vasomotor rhinitis.

6. Face.—Œdema of eyelids, upper lip and hand.

12. Abdomen.—Sprue.

Calcarea Lactica Natronata.

Lactate of Calcium and Sodium.

Clinical.—Alkaline blood. Asthma. Chilblains. Hæmorrhage. Hay fever. Urticaria.

Characteristics.—A colloid of metallic Calcium has been prepared by the Crooke's laboratory, and its use subcutaneously has met with success in checking hæmorrhages, notably of the lungs. The double lactate of Calcium and Sodium appears to possess these properties. It apparently acts on the blood, reducing its alkalinity, relieves chilblains, urticaria, asthma, and hay fever. It is given for all these conditions in old-school practice in tablets of the crude substance. Homœopaths may use it for similar conditions in the 3x and higher. I have done this with much success with *Calc. mur.* in chilblains.

Relations.—*Compare:* In asthma and hay fever, Cr. k. s.; in urticaria, Apis, Urt. ur., Ast. fl.; in chilblains, Calc. mur., Agar.

Carcinosinum.

Carcinomin. The nosode of Carcinoma.

Clinical.—Cancer Melancholia. Worms.

Characteristics.—This is one of the principal nosodes of cancer, and is one of Dr. Burnett's preparations. I use it more frequently than any other as a diathesic remedy. Burnett had a number of different cancer preparations, and followed his instinct largely in their use and selection. In addition to *Scirrhinum,* of which I have given an account in the *Dictionary,* he had a preparation which he named *Durum* (a Latinised form of *Scirrhinum,* as I take it). This he used in treating depraved inherited conditions in children, such as infantile self-abuse, with good effects, which I have confirmed. I have met with a suicidal tendency in several cancer patients, so that the cancer nosodes may be appropriate in many mental cases, especially where the heredity points that way.

Relations.—*Compare* Scirrhinum.

Chromium Kali Sulphuratum.

Chrome Alum. Potassic-Chromic Sulphate ($Cr_2K_2S_4O_{16}$, $24H_2O$).

Clinical.—Catarrh. Hay asthma. Hay fever.

Characteristics.—*Cr. k. s.* was introduced into homœopathic practice some years ago by Dr. Mersch, of Brussels, and in my experience it is by far the most valuable remedy for hay fever that we possess. I use it on Dr. Mersch's indications in the 6x trituration and downwards. Because it sometimes succeeds in the 3x, and even the 1x, when higher numbers fail. I generally give eight grains of the 5x to begin with, three or four times a day. There is no proving that I am acquainted with, but it can be used on general indications for coughs and catarrhs which its constituents will readily suggest.

Relationships.—*Compare:* Cep., Psor., Sabad., Naphthal., Sang. Ka. bi.

Coqueluchinum.

Pertussin. The nosode of Whooping-cough.

Clinical.—Cough, paroxysmal. Whooping-cough.

Characteristics.—In 1906 Messrs. Epps published a little book of mine dealing with this nosode, to which I then gave the name of *Pertussin.* But it appeared that a German firm of chemists had registered in England a patent medicine under that name, and threatened the publishers with an action unless the book was withdrawn! As the matter was not worth a law-suit, I adopted the French name for the nosode, and a second revised and enlarged edition was brought out by the Homœopathic Publishing Co. under the title *Whooping-cough Cured with Coqueluchin.* Since that date later experience has fully confirmed all that was then written, and many patients, old as well as young, have experienced the virtues of *Coqueluchin.* In all cases of whooping-cough suspected or defined I give the remedy in the 30th attenuation every four hours as a matter of routine, and as a rule it quickly assumes control of the case and does all that is necessary. In my experience it agrees well with all other whooping-cough remedies, and when their specific indications appear

I give them also in alternation, or else alone. *Coqueluchin* is an "unproved" remedy, except in the sense that every case of the disease is a "proving," but I have noted a few special symptoms removed by it, and I have arranged them in a subjoined "Schema." It is equally applicable to cases of cough of the same type, though not caused by the same infection, such as appear in some cases of influenza.

Relations.—*Compare:* Bell., Cocc. c., Coral. r., Dros., etc.

SYMPTOMS.

3. Eyes.—Coryza with hacking cough.

6. Face.—Intense flushing with cough.

8. Mouth.—Itching of the palate on lying down at night.

9. Throat.—Intense tickling in throat causing cough.

11. Stomach.—Vomiting or nausea at end of cough.

17. Respiratory Organs.—Dyspnœa with cough.—Sobbing or sighing at end of cough.—Strangling sensation with cough on waking.—Cough provoked by intense tickling in throat—fauces or trachea.—Hacking cough; with coryza.—Deep-sounding croupy cough.—Spasmodic choking cough.—Spasmodic cough with intense flushing of face.—Cough in frequently repeated paroxysms.

18. Chest.—Stinging pain in or on the chest with cough.

Epihysterinum.

Epiphysterin. A nosode.

Clinical.—Fibroma. Menorrhagia. Metrorrhagia.

Characteristics.—This is one of Dr. Burnett's nosodes, used by him in cases of hæmorrhage and obtained, as I conclude, from a case of hæmorrhage in a patient suffering from fibrous tumour, possibly with malignant elements. At any rate, I have found it of great value in controlling uterine hæmorrhage, whether connected with fibrous growth or not. I have used it in the 30th upwards, giving one or two doses weekly.

Relations.—*Compare:* The cancer nosodes; in fibrous tumours and uterine hæmorrhages, Thlaspi b. p., Fraxin., Hydrastis and its alkaloids.

Gunpowder.

Black Gunpowder. Carbon-Sulphur-Kali-Nitricum.

Clinical.—Abscesses. Acne. Bites. Blood-poisoning. Boils. Carbuncles. Cuts, poisoned. Ivy (Hedera) poisoning. Osteo-myelitis. Tonsillitis, septic. Vaccinosis. Worms.

Characteristics.—*Black Gunpowder* is a mixture and not a chemical compound. But for all that, it is a unit, and can be used as such in medicine. As it contains three potent remedies, two of them polychrests, there is little wonder at its medicinal powers. A fourth substance may have some share in its working, as a correspondent of *The Homœopathic World* writes that *Graphites* is used in its manufacture to give a coating to the grains. In its crude form it is an old-established remedy among the rank and file in the Army for gonorrhœa, syphilis, and blood disorders in general, especially boils. The London Police Force also know it as a boil remedy. "Get sixpennyworth of gunpowder from an oil store and take as much as would lie on a sixpence night and morning for four days, and then leave it off for the same time, and resume if necessary" is one prescription which has reached me for recurrent boils from the "Force." Canon Roland Upcher has related the experiences of Norfolk and Suffolk shepherds, who sprinkle gunpowder on their bread and cheese to cure and prevent infection when handling sheep affected with "rot." There is no proving of *Gunpowder*, but I made an experiment on myself with the 2x, as I have mentioned in my article on *Kali nitricum* in my *Dictionary of Materia Medica*. This resulted in a severe attack of herpes of right eyebrow and side of the nose, leaving permanent scars. I have used almost exclusively the 3x trituration, which I have prescribed in 4-, 6-, or 8-grain doses, three or four times a day, either in the form of powder or tablets. In August 1915 I put the recorded experiences into the form of a pamphlet, *Gunpowder as a War Remedy*, and since then many more experiences have seen the light, principally in the pages of *The Homœopathic World*. The indications for the remedy are broad and clear, so that no fine differentiating of symptoms is required. The list of diseases named under "Clinical" will be a sufficient guide, coupled with the broad indication "Blood-poisoning." *Gunp.* corresponds to suppuration in a great number of forms, many of them septic. I have not found it disagree with any other remedy, so that there need be no fear of alternating it with some other remedy if particularly indicated.

Canon Upcher has recently published cases of skin eruption mistaken for scabies by medical men, but actually produced by handling ivy, and quickly cured with *Gunp.* 3x. In some country districts a decoction of gunpowder is given to children for worms, lumbrici chiefly, and with much success.

Relations.—Canon Upcher finds that occasional doses of Hepar highly increase its effects. Calendula externally is also complementary. Thuja, Silica, Baryta carb. (septic tonsils) agree very well.

Causation.—Blood-poisoning.

Influenzinum.

The nosode of Influenza.

Clinical.—Catarrh. Colds. Influenza.

Characteristics.—The nosode of influenza has with many practitioners taken the place of *Baptisia* as the routine remedy in epidemics. It may be given in the 12th or 30th potency, either in the form of tincture, pilules, or discs; or ten globules may be dissolved in six ounces of water, and of this a dessertspoonful may be given for a dose. It may be repeated every two hours. This will be found sufficient to control a large proportion of the cases. The general directions I give to my patients are these: When "colds" appear in a family let all those who are unaffected take *Arsen.* 3 thrice daily, and let the patients take *Influ.* 30 every hour or two. This generally prevents the spread of the trouble and clears up the "colds," whether they are of the influenza type or not. Influenza has the property of developing old troubles, and thus it takes an infinite variety of forms in different persons, so that *Influ.* need not be expected to cure all cases unaided, or, indeed, to be appropriate to every case.

Relations.—I find Influ. compatible with Act. r., Ars., Bell.. Bry., Hep., Merc., and many others.

Morbillinum.

Morbillin. The nosode of Measles.

Clinical.—Catarrh. Coryza. Cough. Ear, affections of. Eye, affections of. Measles. Skin, affections of.

Characteristics.—The well-known symptoms which characterise an attack of measles may all be taken as guides for its homœopathic use. Its chief use hitherto has been as a prophylactic against infection, and to clear up after-effects of an attack. My own use of it has been confined to the 30th and higher, but there is no bar upon lower potencies, and those who prefer them may begin with the 6th. As a prophylactic given to those who are, or may be, exposed to infection,

I prescribe a dose of the 30th twice or thrice daily. For an attack of the disease I find nothing better than *Morbil.* 30, eight or ten globules in six ounces of water, a dessertspoonful every two hours. The effect of this is heightened by giving alternately *Bell.* 30 in the same way. These two medicines will be sufficient to carry through any uncomplicated case, and in my experience do even better than *Pulsatilla.* As the measles poison has a great affinity for the mucous passages, the eyes, the ears and the respiratory mucous membranes, *Morbil.* may be used in such cases like any other homœopathic remedy, when the symptoms correspond.

Relations.—*Complementary:* Bell. *Compare:* Puls., Hep., Merc., Sul.

Parotidinum.

The nosode of Mumps.

Clinical.—Glandular affections. Meningitis. Mumps. Orchitis. Salivation;

Characteristics.—*Parotidinum* has been used as a prophylactic against infection by mumps. In this instance it is generally given in the 6th or 30th two or three times a day to those exposed to infection. In the disease itself it may be given every four hours, either by itself or alternated with other indicated remedies. The well-known complications which sometimes occur with mumps, cerebral inflammation and orchitis suggest its possible use in these conditions.

Relations.—*Compare:* Merc.

Radium Bromatum.

Radium Bromide. Ra br_2, $2H_2O$. Trituration.

Clinical.—Acne. Arteritis. Albuminuria. Appendicitis. Arthritis. Atheroma. Bones, affections of. Callosities. Cancer. Carcinosis. Carucle of Urethra. Climacteric flushes. Corns. Dermatitis. Diarrhœa. Duodenal ulcer. Eczema. Epistaxis. Epithelioma. Erythema. Eyes, affections of. Gout. Hæmorrhage. Headache. Lumbago. Lupus. Nævus. Neuralgia. Neurasthenia. Nose: affections of; catarrh of; redness of. Ophthalmia. Phimosis. Prurigo. Pruritus Ani et Vulvæ. Psoriasis. Rheumatism. Rodent ulcer. Sclerotitis. Skin, affections of. Tic douloureux. Trachoma. Ulcers. Warts. X-ray Dermatitis.

Characteristics.—The discovery of *Radium* and its properties in 1898 by Pierre Curie and his wife set many persons thinking, and among them, naturally, those who are engaged in the healing of the sick. Curie himself made the first "proving." He put a tiny bit of *Radium* salt in an indiarubber capsule and fastened it to his arm, leaving it there for ten hours. When he took it off the skin was red, the place turned into a wound, which took four months to heal, leaving a white scar the size of a shilling surrounded by discoloured puckered skin. On another occasion he left it for half an hour. A wound appeared at the end of a fortnight and took another fortnight to heal. On a third occasion, left for eight minutes only, *two months later* the skin became red and a bit sore, but it soon passed off.—In 1904 I began to make a few provings with the 30th, and in 1908 I published them in *Radium as an Internal Remedy*, along with some observations by Dr. Molson, experienced by himself when making triturations, and by Dr. Stonham with the 30x. A full account of these will be found in my book. By far the most important proving is that by Dr. William H. Dieffenbach, of New York City, published in *The Journal of the American Institute of Homœopathy*, August 1911, and afterwards reprinted in pamphlet form the same year. Dieffenbach had the co-operation of Drs. R. S. Copeland, W. G. Crump, H. C. Sayre, and Guy B. Stearns in his proving, and this leaves little to be desired. It was carried out on both men and women on a much more heroic scale than mine, with 30x, 12x, and 6x, in repeated doses, but the 6x produced such severe symptoms that Dieffenbach warns against its use medicinally. Pure *Radium* is a white metal which "oxidises in water, burns paper, turns black on exposure to air, and has the property of adhering firmly to iron." This last quality is not without significance, and shows a close affinity with *Ferrum*. Its atomic weight is 225. It is found in the ore pitchblende, and Drs. E. Stillman Bailey and F. H. Blackmarr, of Chicago (*J.A.I.H.*, September 1911), have used triturations of this combined with *Thorium* for radio-treatments. Although Dieffenbach used much more crude preparations than I did, his results confirm most of mine, and also greatly extend them, the eyes, skin, joints, and alimentary tracts being particularly affected. Dieffenbach quotes Professor William His, of Berlin, who published an article on the "Use of Radium in Gout and Rheumatism." His used *Radium emanations* (inhalations of the gas), *Radium* injections into joints and muscles, and the drinking of *Radium* water. The provings show the homœopathicity of the drug to these conditions, although His used it empirically. Dieffenbach, who had been investigating *Radium* for ten years before he published his pamphlet, records that as a result of former X-ray and Radium-ray experiments one prover's hands had, when the proving commenced, eczematous eruptions, cracks, scaly excrescences, and wart-like outcroppings. After his proving with 6x these gradually disappeared. This is confirmed by a case reported to me by Mr. E. S. Pierrepont. A girl employed in the X-ray Department of the hospital with which he is connected developed dermatitis of the r. hand and fingers. An ointment was prescribed without benefit, and cracks appeared on the skin. Two doses of *Radium b.* 30 were given, on Mr. Pierrepont's suggestion, one in the morning and one in the evening. The following day the patient came out in a rash, which the matron mistook for measles, eyes watering, fingers very sore, and she felt very ill. By the following day the rash had disappeared and she felt well. The *fingers were now better*, and they got quite well, except that a sore feeling was left after washing.—A noticeable feature of both Dieffenbach's proving and mine was the disappearance of small nævi, which is significant, seeing that the rays are used for the destruction of nævi.—Among the most successful local uses of *Radium* may be mentioned cases of lupus, epithelioma, carcinoma of the cervix uteri, and urethral caruncle. That *Radium*, like X-rays, can cause as well as cure cancer is on record. I have quoted a case (*H.W.*, August 1923) in a practitioner who contracted squamous-celled carcinoma from a careless handling of Radium tubes. Cases of cure of skin cases with *Radium* in potencies are numerous. T. Simpson (*H.W.*, April 1923) records one such. A retired excise officer had an intractable eruption on the genitals, inner surface of thighs and legs, which had prevented him getting any *refreshing* sleep for three years. One tablet of *Rad. b.* 30 each morning was prescribed for a month. All conditions were vastly improved, and the patient got well without further medication. I have recorded another (*H.W.*, May 1924). A young unmarried woman, after the application of a Belladonna plaster to the back for lumbago, developed an œdematous rash involving the whole face and neck, extremely irritating, < at night, preventing sleep. At the back of the neck was a sore, oozing patch. After temporary relief from some remedies, there still remained an irritating oozing rash, sore eyes—first right, then left—lids swollen, oozing from corners, lips hard, swollen. One dose of *Rad. b.* 30 was given. The result was dramatic. The first night she was able to sleep with only once waking. Two days later the rash had nearly gone, and the eyes had ceased to water. In a few days all had vanished, and the patient could enjoy open air. In *H.R.* (April 1923) Dr. S. L. Guild-Leggett records the case of a girl aged 2½ years who had shifting rheumatism—l. foot to r. knee, then to l. knee, hands, and toes. She had also a peculiarity about her stools. They were slate-coloured, very offensive, urgent, and came *at noon* during a meal. On these symptoms of Dieffenbach's proving: "Defecation at noon; stool soft, dark, or offensive, slate-colour, clay-colour; pains in extremities, wakes 4 a.m., pains in all joints—knees, ankles, feet; could not walk, *had to lie down*," *Rad. b.* was given, and cured entirely. Other of my cured cases will be found in the Schema marked (°). I have also distinguished the symptoms from my proving with the letter (C) appended to each symptom. All the rest are from Dieffenbach. This enables a comparison to be made between the two.

Peculiar Sensations are: As if skull too small; as if foreign body (lash) in eye; as if something dropped into trachea. Knees feel as if the bones would protrude. Intolerance of tobacco was produced.

The *Conditions* of *Radium* are very marked in the general > by motion, < by warmth of the bed, and > in open air; > lying down; > after sleep; > by pressure. < at night. < by shaving, by washing. < by smoking. < 3 a.m., 4 a.m., 7 a.m., 11 a.m., noon, night.

Relationships.—Rad. bro. is *antidoted* by Rhus and Nux mos. (dry mouth); Rhus ven. acted promptly in my cases. Dieffenbach used both Rhus ven. and Rhus tox. with success, and the homœopathicity is evident enough. Rad. *is followed well* by Rhus; (in some cases I have given intermediate doses of Rhus v. 3x without interfering with the curative effects and avoiding unpleasant aggravations); by Kali iod., Sep., Calc.—Rad. b., *antidotes* Bell. (*H.W.*, May 1924). *Compare:* Cancer nosodes, Hydrast., Con., Cundur., Uran. (Rad. is found in pitchblende, which is an Uranium ore. Tellur. is also associated with Rad. in origin, and its symptoms are closely similar in many respects). Lyc. corresponds in r. to l. direction, flatulent symptoms, and sudden pains; in stomach symptoms, Cad. sul., Ornith., Arg. n., and Uran. n. are allied; in sclerotitis, Act. r.; alternate constipation and diarrhœa, Ant. c. Rad. b. has warming sensation down œsophagus, Manc. has the same sensation rising up œsophagus. Carb. an. has < by shaving.

Causation.—Effect of X-ray burns.

SYMPTOMS.

1. Mind.—Apprehensive.—Depression; hardly able to move about.—Fear of being alone; of the dark; wants to have someone near.—Irritable, cross, easily vexed.—Mind cloudy and unable to think clearly; stupid with dull frontal headache all day.—After taking a single dose felt in much better spirits (curative).

2. Head.—Vertigo with pains in occiput; > after sleep.—Vertigo after rising; tendency to fall to left; > noon and after eating; > lying down; > in open air; > after eating.—Dizziness with palpitation of the heart in afternoon.—Vertigo with tendency to fall to l.; > open air.—Lightness of head with nausea and sinking in epigastrium; pulsation outward; skull felt too small.—Numbness or compression of bones of head.—Fulness of head.—Head heavy; dull ache.—Dull frontal headache; lasts all day; head feels light; > pressure; with clouded mind, unable to think.—Terrific pain over r. eye, spreading back to occiput, continued next morning.—Intense sharp headache commencing over l. eye and spreading over the head; > heat, < cold and pressure.—Sharp pain over r. eye, extending to vertex, > in open air.—Head heavy all day; began occiput; sharp over r. eye; throbbing, pulsating, < motion, < lying down, < by warm air, > sitting down with head back, > cold air, > pressure over forehead and r. eye; unable to lie in bed until 5 a.m.—Sharp sticking pain r. side of head; also in l. temple; on going to bed.—Headache in occiput in morning; a tight feeling, < motion (C).—Dull occipital headache, > pressure and open air.—Dull headache, mostly occipital.

3. Eyes.—Eyes smart and look red (C).—Eyes have sticky feeling and are reddened; as if sand in them.—Sensation as if piece of cotton in eyes, > rubbing.—Both eyes sore, < l.—Swelling of tissues of l. orbit with slight itching.—Lids heavy, hard to keep them open.—Discharge from right eye runs down on nose and forms yellow crusts.—Margins of lids inflamed and burning.—Both eyes ache along margin of lids.—Burning, stinging in eyes.—Eyes sensitive to light.—Some secretion on lashes r. eye on waking (C).—R. eye began to feel sore with occasional sticking pains and increased secretion, < reading, < artificial light, > closing eye; sclerotic vessels injected running to cornea from both sides; occasional itching in lids, < upper (C).—Blenorrhagia of r. eye; injection of sclerotic, slight injection of lower part of cornea; pupil of r. eye dilates and contracts more sluggishly than l. (C).—Woke with r. eye very painful, with feeling of foreign body in it, > open air (C).—Sensation as if lash in l. eye, slight soreness of ball (C).—When reading for a while letters dance and get blurred.

4. Ears.—Tickling in ears, very severe at night.—Sharp sticking pain just over r. ear.—Earache, much pain in (r.) ear, stitching and throbbing (C).—Sound of rushing water (associated with rapid heart-action following vivid dreams).

5. Nose.—Much mucus without having taken cold (C).—Pricking and peppery sensation in l. nostril (C).—° Nævus-like spot on tip of nose (C).—° Catarrh with green discharge (C).—° Epistaxis (C).—° Burning sensation in nose (C).—Itching and dryness of both cavities.—Pricking and hard crusts.—Itching of nose.

6. Face.—Flushed face.—Slight patchy erythema diffused over forehead (C).—Succession of little pimples on forehead and chest, raised, red, exuding when punctured serum, blood, and a small amount of pus.—Small papule in centre of l. cheek, which dried off and recurred many times. Heavy crust formed over area when papule scratched. This also recurred many times.—Skin of face very irritable; this gradually got worse and lasted two months; the skin became thickened and broke in places, exuding clear moisture; > scratching, < by washing, which caused oozing; > bathing in very hot water; < shaving (only possible on alternate days); < night when warm in bed. (Finally cured by *Rhus ven.*) (C).—Small nævus on chin turns black and scales off and disappears (C).—Sudden and violent shocks of pain in lower branches of 5th cranial nerve, l., so intense and of such lightning-like suddenness as to call forth an exclamation (C).—Severe aching pain at angle r. lower jaw.—° Erythema of nose and face.—° Acne.—Twitching and burning sensation in lips.—Lower lip drawn and stiff, feels as if swelling.

7. Teeth.—Teeth painful, feel elongated.—Gumboil r. lower jaw back of molar teeth, swelling and soreness prevented talking.

8. Mouth.—Dry in the morning (C).—Parched, dry sensation in roof of mouth, > cold water but soon returns, > *Nux moschata*.—Mouth dry, breath seems hot.—Saliva runs into mouth.—Tongue very sore r. side, about middle (C).—Tongue white (C).—Tongue bluish white and thick, swollen sensation; speech difficult and heavy.—Taste: peculiar metallic; bitter-sour; of chalk with increased salivation; bitter and oily.—° Power of taste returns (C).

9. Throat.—Dry mouth and throat.—Warming sensation in œsophagus and stomach, lasted half an hour after the dose.—Throat sore with earache (C).—Wanted cold drinks to quench parched condition of throat.—Sore throat followed by tickling cough.—Stitching in throat on swallowing.—Sensation of lump and constriction.—Throat dry and raw, > swallowing and drinking cold water.—Throat dry and congested, < r. side; as if he had smoked too much.—Throat sore at bedtime, < r. side.—Feeling in throat as from eating pepper.

10. Appetite.—No appetite (C).—Loss of appetite, esp. for meat (C).—Loss of appetite with colic.—Aversion to meat; to bacon for breakfast (° *Rhus ven.*) (C).—Aversion to sweets.—Aversion to ice-creams, of which she is usually very fond.—Great hunger an hour before meals, soon satisfied.—Loss of appetite with colic.—Usual food not relished; sour things taste good.—Distaste for tobacco.

11. Stomach.—Intense emptiness (lasted an hour).—Emptiness one hour before meals.—Warm, empty feeling > after eating.—Nausea (C).—Nausea 5 p.m., desire to vomit but cannot.—Nausea and sinking sensation in pit of stomach < walking, lightness of head.—Nausea in abdomen, before meals, > by eating.—Food slow of digestion, though appetite good.—Colicky pains in stomach.—Much pain and distress in stomach, > by much belching of gas and eructations of wind.—Frequent belching.

12. Abdomen.—Distended feeling and indigestion after food, alternating with earache (C).—Inflammation of umbilicus (C).—Severe aching pains over pubes.—Slight colicky pains with passage of foul flatus.—Pain over McBurney's point.—Pain after dose > bending double and after defecation.—Violent cramps 11 p.m., > bending double.—Nausea in abdomen > by eating.—Awoke 4 a.m. with colic in abdomen and stitching in rectum, > by passage of dark, watery stool, other stools less dark followed later.—Cramping whilst eating > by stool.—Cutting pains in intestines after waking, with great sensitiveness to pressure.—Sharp sudden pains at McBurney's point, also at sigmoid flexure above crest of ilium; attacks recurred several times in the week, came quickly like shocks and passed off quickly.—Abdomen distressed evening.—Two red macules on r. and l. sides of abdomen slightly itching.—Lameness in both groins after sitting and first beginning to move.

13. Stool and Anus.—Stools paler than normal (C).—Stools relaxed, almost watery, tags of mucus (C).—Constipation (C).—Constipation, difficulty of evacuation even after the use of an enema.—Dry, hard, scanty stools.—Alternate constipation and looseness.—Soft yellow stool with much flatulence.—Severe sacral pains with much flatulence, > by stool.—Much flatulence; hot, following diarrhœa.—Gushing stool of bad odour.—Yellow, soft stools alternately with hard brown stools, foul flatus.—Burning stool.—Rectum feels dry.—Very large, dark brown stool, very offensive.—Constipated for four days, no desire except twice, when passed three little black marbles; at noon, small diarrhœic stool.—Constipation of years' standing removed in one prover.—After several watery stools rectum feels sore and as if prolapsed.—Yellow-brown or slate-coloured stools, bad odour.—No desire, had to force a stool, which was soft and clay-like.—° Eczema about anus (C).

14. Urinary Organs.—Urine becomes more profuse.—Urine slightly burning.—Has to wait some minutes before he can micturate.—Urine radio-active; clayey or brick-dust sediment.—Albuminuria (five provers, one of whom showed hyaline and granular casts).—Increased elimination of solids, particularly chlorides.

15. Male Sexual Organs.—Eruption of psoriasis on penis with circular or serpiginous edges (C).—° Eczema of penis and inner surface of prepuce (C).—Sexual desire diminished or absent for one month.—Three weeks after cessation of drug desire stronger than usual.—Desire increased. —Nocturnal emissions; once whilst sleeping in afternoon.—Two emissions in one night.—Slight pains in l. spermatic cord when walking.—Previous to taking the drug (12x) had slight phimosis, this was worse during the proving, head of penis itching and burning; after the proving phimosis was better.

16. Female Sexual Organs.—Period delayed; rather less painful than usual (C).—Aching over pubes when menses came on (an unusual occurrence); flow copious first two days, then stopped gradually.—Menses delayed three days.—During period, bearing-down pains in the back.—Flow during night very copious and dark red.—Leucorrhœa, white and scanty; curdy and cheesy.—° Urethral caruncle.

17. Respiratory Organs.—Feels as if she could not get air enough (C).—Tickling in larynx, < lying down.—Tickling in supra-sternal fossa very pronounced; could not stop coughing after once started.—Aversion to sweets (of which ordinarily very fond) during cough; after three nights controlled by *Rhus tox.*—Dry, spasmodic cough < smoking, < indoors, > eating, > out of doors.—Tickling in throat and hacking cough with frothy expectoration.—Tickling in trachea, as if something had dropped into it, causing a dry, hacking cough, > in open air.—Occasional dry paroxysms of coughing, with sensation as if dust had reached the larynx or bronchi; > by coughing.

18. Chest.—Chest feels tight as if she could not get air enough (C). —Eruption disappeared from chest in prover (C).—Pain in chest alternating with indigestion and stuffed-up feeling (C).—Sharp pain in l. chest, comes and goes.—Constriction of chest; in heart region.—Beating pain r. of sternum, < at end of respiration.

19. Heart.—Sharp pains in region of heart, > after walking.—Palpitation on waking from dreams with sound in ears of rushing water.—Constricting sensation about heart, with anxiety and desire for air, > in open air.—[Applied locally in massive doses, *Rad. bro.* has produced endarteritis, atheroma, and sclerosis of the vessels acted on.]—Examination of the blood of the provers showed a marked increase in polymorphonuclear neutrophiles—"the police" of the blood corpuscles which attack invading bacteria.—Lowered blood pressure (in all Dieffenbach's provers).

20. Neck and Back.—Sensation of swelling in back of neck (C).—Itching back of neck and upper part of both arms.—Dull throbbing; and sharp pains, r. side neck.—Catch (and lameness) in r. sterno-mastoid muscle.—Evening, stiffness muscles l. side neck.—Pain and lameness in cervical vertebræ.—On waking pain between 6 and 7 cervical vertebræ,

> motion.—Red spot l. side neck; this disappeared and later similar spot appeared r. side.—Pain under l. scapula, < on moving, < putting shoulder back, > after rising (C).—Sharp, sticking pain under l. scapula, extending through to front of body, caught breath as if could not raise diaphragm.—Dull backache lower lumbar region, > after exercise.—Aching lumbo-sacral region; > after hot bath.—Severe lumbo-sacral pain, appears to be in the bones; < going upstairs.—Sharp shooting pains (also electric shocks) in lumbar muscles, > by continued exercise.—Sudden severe pain l. lumbar region, > pressure.—Dull pain runs from sacrum up to shoulder, or to between shoulders, > by exercise.—Soreness of latissimi dorsi (esp. l.).—Sacral pains with flatus > by stool.—Swelling over sacrum, > lying on something hard.—Backache extending through abdomen to iliac crests.—Gnawing sensation in lumbo-sacral bones.

21. Limbs.—Pain in all limbs and whole body during the night.—Waked 4 a.m. with pains in all limbs, could not keep them quiet, > after warm bath.—Pains in all joints, esp. knees and ankles; had to lie down, feet gave out.

22. Upper Limbs.—Sharp pain r. shoulder-joint; < motion, > by heat; lame sensation r. arm, forearm, and hand, > exercise, > warmth; sharp stitch l. shoulder-joint.—Catch in l. shoulder-joint, > exercise.—Lameness l. shoulder-joint, under deltoid, > motion.—Cracking r. shoulder-joint on raising arm.—Very lame r. arm and sore muscles over r. breast.—Severe drawing in flexor muscles of l. arm.—R. elbow stiff and slightly lame after writing.—In morning twinging pain in l. elbow.—Hands cold (C).—Serpigenous ulcer on hand (C).—Blisters on dorsal aspect of first three fingers (l.) just above nails (C).—Small pustule on centre of dorsum of r. hand.—Itching on upper part of both arms and back of neck.—Bruised pain l. wrist.—Dull pains in whole r. hand, all fingers affected, esp. distal phalanges; > rubbing and continued exercise.—Sharp pains in finger-joints, > exercise.—Lameness in l. thumb-joint after holding a book.

23. Lower Limbs.—Dull pain in hip-joint, located in head of femur; also under l. patella.—Kink in r. hip-joint, > after walking some time.—Beating pain in r. hip while sitting at desk writing, > beginning to move.—Lameness in both groins after sitting; left groin aches, but thighs seemed lame on beginning to move.—Dull pain r. knee-joint, < motion, > after continued motion.—Pain in legs, beginning in knees and running down legs. > after exercise.—Very severe pains in knee-joints, very deep, > from cold and exercise.—Dull pains in both legs and back, running up to shoulders.—Dull, tired pains in popliteal spaces.—Soreness in calves and thighs.—Muscles in front r. leg lame.—Soreness and pain in both knees, feel as if bones would protrude.—When crossing legs they became asleep in a little while; a few days later legs heavy, difficulty in going upstairs.—Sharp, lightning-like pain, l. anterior tibial surface, as if in periosteum.—Muscles of antero-exterior part of r. leg lame, < from walking and rubbing.—Sharp, darting pains in l. calf, come and go suddenly.—Pain under l. patella, > when foot still, < walking and moving.—Bruised feeling in calves.—On rising from sitting, ankles and feet lame and stiff could hardly stand or walk.—Lameness and catch in r. ankle, descending stairs.—R. Achilles tendon sore on ascending stairs.—Sharp pain in l. great toe (also both), < motion, > continued motion.—Numbness of both great toes.—Pains in and round r. great toe.—Dull aching pain in l. great toe-joint, after dancing.—Burning pain in l. great toe as from acid.—Needle-pricking in the two middle toes (r.) with some burning.—Sharp sticking pain in arch of r. foot.—Corns of feet over sensitive.—A callosity or corn on inner border r. foot, which had been there for twenty years, disappeared completely (C).—A corn fell off r. foot (C).—Irritable patch appeared on r. foot in patient taking *Rad. bro.* 30 fourteen days after the dose (C).—Fetid foot-sweat relieved (C).

24. Generalities.—Looked ill all time of proving, lost 3¾ lb. in weight (C).—Felt as if going to be ill, could hardly crawl about (C).—Aching pains all over body; very restless, had to keep moving about.—Hardly able to move about; unable to work properly.—Tiredness; weakness; lassitude; exhausted, wants to take off clothes and rest.—Pains all over, > in open air and moving about.—Entire body feels as if afire; with sharpest kind of needle-pricks or electric shocks all over body; also itching all over.—Sudden, lightning-like "shock"-ing pains (C).—Electric shock through body during sleep.

25. Skin.—Psoriasis (of penis) (C).—° Serpigenous eczema (C).—Itching eruption on face, oozing, < shaving, lasting weeks, finally cured with *Rhus* (C).—Small nævi cured (C).—Skin of face dry (C).—Patchy erythema on forehead (C).—Pimples.—Papules.—Itching all over at night.—Red itching rash between scapulæ.—Eczematous dermatitis of hands caused by *Radium* and X-ray burns disappeared in the proving.—Red papules on side of mouth; chest; back; neck.—Eruption on chest disappears.—° Acne.—Burning sensation and itching all over.—Exposure to rays causes dermatitis, proceeding to ulceration and necrosis and epithelioma.—Corns.

26. Sleep.—Irresistible sleepiness and lethargy.—Tired and sleepy all day.—Sleeps well, wakes tired, with desire to stretch.—Restless from dreams, awakes in fright.—Restless all night, kept moving about in bed.—Dreams: of passing urine; fires; suicide; alarming; busy; active; with palpitation.—° Sleeps regularly without opiate (in cancer case) (C).

27. Fever.—Shivering bilious feeling (C).—Cold sensation all day; chilliness with chattering teeth till noon; > afternoon (during menses).—Internal chilliness, followed by heat without sweat, though usually perspires.—Internal chilliness with many movements of the bowels.—Felt hot all over, had to take off bed covers.—Entire body feels afire, with sharp needle-pricks and electric shocks.—Fetid foot-sweat relieved (C).

Scarlatininum.

The nosode of Scarlatina or Scarlet Fever.

Clinical.—Albuminuria. Nephritis. Scarlet fever. Skin affections. Throat, sore.

Characteristics.—*Scarlatinin* has been used, like other nosodes, for the prevention and for cure of the disease from which it takes origin. But its well-known affinity for the skin, throat and kidneys suggests its applicability for affections of those organs.

Relations.—Bell. is the nearest analogue and should be its *antidote*, and the various Mercuries come next. *Compare also:* Apis, Arsen., Rhus, Morbillin, Diphtherinum.

Simaruba.

Simaruba amara. Mountain damson. *N. O.* Simarubaceæ. Tincture of the dried root-bark.

Clinical.—Diarrhœa. Dysentery. Snake-bite. Worms.

Characteristics.—*Simaruba* is a native of the West Indies and tropical America. "Simaruba bark" is used as a bitter tonic and as a local remedy for dysentery and diarrhœa. The part used is the "bark," which is really the rind of the root, of which, domestically, a decoction is made. "In large doses," says *Treas. of Botany*, "it is said to act as an emetic, purgative and diaphoretic." *S. versicolor*, a Brazilian species, has similar properties. The fruits and bark are used as anthelmintics; an infusion of the latter is employed in cases of snake-bite. The plant is so bitter that insects will not attack it, on which account the powdered root has been used to kill vermin. *S. glauca*, a native of Cuba, furnishes a glutinous juice which is employed in certain cases of skin-disease." This very well sums up the place and properties of *Simaruba*. And it is well to remember that *Cedron*, which is "*Simaba Cedron*," belongs to the same order. My first practical acquaintance with *Simb.* as a homœopathic remedy was in the case of a much-travelling patient who suffered from a chronic tendency to looseness of the bowels. He had stools like yellow ochre, for which *Gamboge* had been very helpful. When in the South of France he consulted a homœopathic practitioner, whose name has escaped my memory, and he prescribed *Simaruba* with excellent effect. Since then I have used it in similar cases. H. H. Beamish (*H.W.*, April 1925) says that on the Zambesi for dysentery the *Simaruba bark* is boiled, and, by way of strengthening the astringent effect, *Alum* is added to the decoction. But *Simaruba* is the specific agent.

Relations.—*Compare :* (Botan.) Cedron, Ail., Chap. am., Quassia. *Compare also :* Vacc. myrt., Chi., Rheum, Gamb.

Vaccinium Myrtillus.

Whortleberry. Bilberry. *N. O.* Vacciniaceæ. Tincture of fresh berries.

Clinical.—Diarrhœa. Dysentery.

Characteristics.—My attention was first drawn to this remedy by Dr. A. H. Croucher in an article published in the *Homœopathic Review* many years ago, giving cases of inveterate diarrhœa cured by it. This experience I have repeatedly confirmed. I have always used it in the ϕ tincture, generally giving 5-drop doses every four hours. It is especially applicable to vaccinal, malarial, and dysenteric cases. Whortleberry is a close relative of Cranberry, and the natural order is allied to the Ericaceæ. It is a native of heathy and swampy mountainous regions.

Relations.—*Compare :* Simaruba, China, Rheum, Merc.

Printed in Great Britain by
UNWIN BROTHERS, LIMITED, LONDON AND WOKING

NOTES